W9-DBA-834

*Jim Powers*

# PUBLIC HEALTH
## ADMINISTRATION AND PRACTICE

SIXTH EDITION

# PUBLIC HEALTH

ADMINISTRATION AND PRACTICE

## JOHN J. HANLON
M.S., M.D., M.P.H.

Assistant Surgeon General, Public Health Service,
U. S. Department of Health, Education, and Welfare

*Formerly*

Director of Community Health Services, Philadelphia

Commissioner of Health, Detroit and Wayne County

Chairman, Department of Community Medicine,
Temple University School of Medicine, Wayne
State University School of Medicine

Professor of Public Health Administration and Practice,
University of Michigan School of Public Health, University
of North Carolina School of Public Health

WITH 45 ILLUSTRATIONS

THE C. V. MOSBY COMPANY

SAINT LOUIS   1974

SIXTH EDITION

**Copyright © 1974 by The C. V. Mosby Company**

All rights reserved. No part of this book may be reproduced
in any manner without written permission of the publisher.

Previous editions copyrighted 1950, 1955, 1960, 1964, 1969

Printed in the United States of America

**Library of Congress Cataloging in Publication Data**

Hanlon, John Joseph, 1912-
    Public Health: administration and practice.

    Previous editions published under title: Principles
of public health administration.
    Includes bibliographies.
    1.  Public health administration.  2.  Hygiene,
Public.  I.  Title.  [DNLM:  1.  Health administration.
WA525   H241p]
RA425.H29   1974        362.1        74-8669
ISBN 0-8016-2045-7

GW/CB/B    9    8    7    6    5    4    3

*To* FLORENCE,
FRANCES,
DON, and JON

# Preface

About 25 years ago, in a surge of dissatisfaction and as a personally imposed challenge, I decided to write the first edition of this book, which appeared in 1950. After several abortive attempts, I well remember completing the writing while waiting in an anteroom for the birth of my second son and some months later the drudgery of page proofing in the almost unreal environment of the Bolivian *altiplano* 2½ miles above sea level.

Since then, many professionally rewarding experiences have come my way: the direction of the United States health technical assistance programs throughout the world, the administration of the official health agencies of the two large and complex cities of Philadelphia and Detroit, the invariable stimulation from contact with students in numerous professional schools, attendance at countless professional meetings and conferences, and a wanderer's return a half-dozen years ago to an early love, the Public Health Service, to be swept up first in an ecologically based revitalization of environmental concerns and more recently in a systems approach to the long-ignored and neglected field of comprehensive emergency medical services. Each experience so far and especially the students and associates with whom I have been privileged to have had contact have all enriched my personal and professional life and my perspective. Hopefully this will be evident in this latest edition.

Concurrently, the nation and the world have changed significantly. In 1950 the United States population was 150 million. Now it is over 210 million, while the world's people have increased from 2.5 to almost 4 billion. During the same period the phenomenal human agglutination in urban and metropolitan centers has occurred everywhere. The number of American cities with more than 500,000 inhabitants has risen from only 18 in 1950 to 27 in 1973. During the same interval, our states have increased in number from 48 to 50, while membership in the United Nations has soared from 60 to 133.

Public health also has changed dramatically. When this book first appeared, there was no federal Department of Health, Education, and Welfare, and the original Social Security Act had only recently been enacted. Now the former has become an enormous organization with a budget in 1974, just for medical and health-related programs but not including Medicare and Medicaid, of well over $4.5 billion. For its part the Social Security Act has been significantly amended to provide not only greatly expanded retirement and related benefits but also to include medical care insurance benefits of far-reaching social consequences.

The perimeters of public health have undergone considerable expansion. Gone is the long-standing dichotomy of disease prevention and health promotion, in contrast to therapy and rehabilitation. Gone is the categorical approach. Disappearing is the distinction between official and voluntary action. Now the watch words are decentralization, comprehensive health planning, continuity of neighborhood health services, consumer involvement, allied health personnel, revenue sharing, and the like. Many agencies and organizations share the credit for bringing these changes about. These concepts as well as others have been manifest by a plethora of new social legislation, demonstrations, programs, and personnel. All this bodes well for the future of the health of people in America and throughout the world. Certainly there will be no lack of challenges for health workers of the future. The tools have been placed in our hands. Let us make the most of them.

He who attempts a book of this type is one of the most indebted of men. So many individuals contribute and assist directly and indirectly and in so many known and unknown ways that adequate, much less complete, recognition becomes impossible. How can one adequately evaluate the influence of past and present friends, associates, and teachers? How can one adequately express gratitude to the wonderfully patient and helpful secretaries who assist in so many important ways? All that can be done is humbly to acknowledge their great value and assistance. Special credit is due my wife not only for her many suggestions and critical judgments but especially for her many years of patient understanding and encouragement. To her and to all the others, a deep felt thanks.

JOHN J. HANLON

# Introduction

The policy that has developed in the United States and elsewhere is to place at the executive helm of organizations conducting public health programs individuals whose primary qualification is the possession of a medical education. There was a time in the formative days of the profession and in a less complex society when that single qualification perhaps sufficed. But neither public health thought nor society has been static. Remarkable and intimately inter-related changes and progress have occurred at a rapid pace containing far-reaching implications for those who would successfully strive for the protection and promotion of the public health. No longer is it adequate merely that the health officer be a good diagnostician and therapist. If his ability and inclination are restricted to these, his most fruitful and satisfactory work will be performed in the private practice of medicine.

Should an individual, on the other hand, have a deep-seated wish to participate in the promotion of the well-being of the public en masse through the work of the increasing numbers of public health agencies, he soon finds himself involved in fields and problems whose importance, even existence, he was hardly aware of during his basic education. An indication of this was given some years ago by Donald C. Stone while Assistant Director of the United States Bureau of the Budget in a discussion of the role of the government executive.

The specialized conditions surrounding governmental programs put extraordinary demands on their directors in terms of knowing how to weave the competing and disparate elements into a unified whole and producing an organization capable of accomplishing its mission. Public pressures, the need to adjust to the views of legislative bodies, the rigidities in procedures attendant upon management according to law and executive regulation are elements present in any public service enterprise. All of these are related to that central characteristic that distinguishes executive positions in the public service from those in private management—the fact that the government executive is the guardian of the public interest and is accountable to the electorate, directly or indirectly, for what he does. This is very different from the concern for the public which the private executive has in relation to the marketability of his product and the good name of his firm. *

In a more specific sense, the neophyte in community health administration, when first opening the door to the organization for which leadership is expected, finds himself face to face with a series of quite unexpected problems for which he usually has been unprepared. His record of clinical or academic prowess and acumen may be excellent, but he will find it of relatively little value. When he pulls the knob and enters, his first problem is always one of personnel management. In rapid succession he finds himself involved with problems implying an understanding of the principles of organization, government, and law. Before much of his first day has passed, he is certain to have participated in several situations that require personal relationships with the public, the press, the medical and other professions, and labor unions, to mention only a few. He then realizes that although a satisfactory bedside manner is one thing, an acceptable public manner is another. Sooner or later he awakens to the fact that the program and the personnel he is directing involve the expenditure of money. Where does it come from? How to go about obtaining it? The probability is that his acquaintance with the word *budget* was in connection

---

* From Stone, D. C.: Notes on the government executive: his role and his methods; new horizons in public administration, a symposium, University, Ala., 1945, University of Alabama Press, pp. 47-48.

with his personal financial struggles at the end of each month. Now demands are made on him to produce in some baffling manner what seems to him a complicated document to depict the financial working, past, present, and future, of the program or agency for which he is held accountable. And this last is likely to be a new and disturbing realization!

These are only a few of the unforeseen and unprepared-for problems and worries encountered by one who decides to devote his professional life to the field of public health administration. What is expected of him appears to be the impossible. Physician, engineer, lawyer, political scientist, economist, sociologist —must he be all of these and more? In the literal sense this, of course, would not be possible. It is not too much to expect, however, that he have at least an understanding of the fundamental principles involved in the various fields related to his office. Experience will teach much, but at least a modicum of information beforehand might be helpful. It is with this in mind and with the hope of stimulating an interest for further study that this book is presented.

# Contents

# PUBLIC HEALTH
ADMINISTRATION AND PRACTICE

# PART ONE

# Roots of
# public health

Before embarking on the main purpose of this book it is well to consider the origins and meaning of present-day public health. It has been interesting and enlightening to hear the replies of fellow workers and particularly those of students when they are asked why they have chosen or are planning to enter the public health profession. It must be admitted that the occasional vague and indefinite replies are discouraging. It is desirable, therefore, to admonish students to question seriously the advisability of becoming public health workers, as, of course, they should question the pursuit of any calling. The disadvantages as well as the advantages that are honestly believed to exist should be considered. Each of us has one life to live, and for practical if not selfish reasons we should each exercise jealous care of what we do with it. It is foolish indeed for an individual to cast away his one great experience in a field for which he is unsuited or unhappy or to work for a cause in which he does not sincerely believe. Every enterprise requires understanding and belief so that it will be satisfying and fruitful.

In the belief that an acquaintance with the history of society, its health problems, and its attempts to solve them might contribute to greater understanding and satisfaction, these introductory chapters are presented. Similarly an awareness of man's state of illness or health is important. These are a few of the phases of the subject that are presented in brief form hopefully to stimulate interest in more extensive reading, analysis, and thought.

*Health frees the individual to live up to his potential.*

JOHN W. GARDNER

# CHAPTER 1

# Philosophy and purpose
# of public health*

## PUBLIC HEALTH AS A PROFESSION

It is significant that many outstanding persons who otherwise might have gained greater material benefits have devoted their lives to the public health movement. One of their characteristics has been a special enthusiasm for their work. What makes such ardent proponents of those who have given sincere thought and effort to this field? Does it present some unique challenge? Perhaps here more than elsewhere man at last has the opportunity successfully to adapt the creatures and environments of nature to himself and his welfare rather than to submit helplessly to them.

But, one might ask, what can a sincere and honest person hope to accomplish in the face of superstition and ignorance of a large part of the public, political interference, inadequate funds, and sometimes personnel of poor quality? Is not impatience justified? One is reminded of a statement by the Irish parliamentarian Edmund Burke (1729-1797) in the face of repeated criticism: "Those who carry on great public schemes must be proof against the most fatiguing delays, the most mortifying disappointments, the most shocking insults, and what is worst of all, the presumptuous judgments of the ignorant." Sir Henry Cole once showed this statement to his close friend, the public health pioneer Edwin Chadwick, with the com-

ment that he should have it pinned to his sleeve as an epigraph.

Perhaps the essential point is that despite all handicaps, spectacular successes of far-reaching consequences have been achieved during a brief period of man's history. At the time of Cole's comment to Chadwick in the midnineteenth century the average age at death in large English cities was only 36 years for the gentry, 22 years for tradesmen, and 16 years for the laboring class! More than one half of the children of the working class and one fifth of the children of the gentry died before their fifth birthday. During the century and a half since, the average life expectancy at birth has been increased in the United States and several other countries to over 70 years, and deaths before the fifth birthday have decreased about 95%.

A justification for patience was suggested to the author by the late Milton J. Rosenau. His reasoning was that relatively few generations have existed throughout the recorded history of Western civilization. Only 3,500 years have passed since the time of Moses; and if the average length of one generation were considered to have been approximately 35 years, there have been only about 100 successive generations or direct steps back to the time of Moses. To pursue this reasoning further, when one considers that the majority of those generations might be ignored as having failed to contribute significantly to the knowl-

---

*For a discussion, see Hanlon, Rogers, and Rosen.[1]

**2**

edge and social advancement of man, there remains perhaps a scant dozen, most of them in the immediate past, to whom mankind owes a real debt.

The practice of medicine is commonly referred to as one of the oldest professions. Yet modern medicine can hardly be considered more than a century old. It is said that it was not until 1910 that the average patient in the United States had a fifty-fifty chance of being diagnosed correctly. Proper treatment was something else again. Indeed the present-day practice of medicine is quite different from that of only a decade ago. Still more recent in origin is the public health movement, which although presaged by occasional and sporadic earlier glimmerings, dates back only a brief half century. Health workers are naturally led to a consideration of the significance and purpose of this public concern for health. Far from being a thing apart, it is intimately related in its conception and development to a broad philosophic and social revolution with many facets that has as its driving force a growing appreciation of the innate dignity of man. It has been a critical part of a spectrum of social reforms that include public education, public welfare, rights of labor, humane care of the mentally ill, and penal management, to mention only a few.

## DEFINITION

There have been many attempts to define public health. When arranged chronologically, it is interesting to observe that the definitions present a word picture of the evolution and progress of the field. Early definitions were limited essentially to sanitary measures invoked against nuisances and health hazards with which the individual was powerless to cope and that, when present in one individual, could adversely affect others. Insanitation and later communicability were the criteria followed in deciding whether a problem fell within the concern and jurisdiction of public health. With the great bacteriologic and immunologic discoveries of the late nineteenth and early twentieth centuries and the subsequent development of techniques for their application, the concept of prevention of disease in the individual was added. Public health then came to be regarded as an integration of sanitary science and medical science.

As far back as 1847, Solomon Neumann in Berlin propounded that "medical science is intrinsically and essentially a social science, and as long as this is not recognized in practice we shall not be able to enjoy its benefits and shall have to be satisfied with an empty shell and a sham." Despite this, it is only recently that medicine and, indeed, public health have become widely recognized as applied social sciences. Many writers still find it necessary to emphasize this relationship.[2,3] The enigma of the delay in acceptance of this relationship has been particularly well analyzed by Rosen[4]:

In Great Britain, as in the United States, interest in the development of a concept of social medicine is a recent phenomenon. The social relations of health and disease had been recognized by physicians and laymen, but owing to a number of causes no concerted effort had been made to organize such knowledge on a coherent basis and thus make it available for practical application. In part this was due to the dominant role that laboratory sciences and techniques had come to play in medicine, in part to the concurrent rise and expansion of medical specialism, and in part to the limited view of public health that had been current in both countries. Furthermore, the bias created by these factors was reinforced by powerful social ideologies still rooted in the nineteenth century version of natural law.

During the past few decades, however, influences within medicine itself and in society as a whole have acted to overcome these factors. The development of such branches of medicine as endocrinology, nutrition and psychiatry tended to break down the compartmental thinking of the physician, and to bring back into mental focus the sick person, the patient. Moreover, within society as a whole, the ideology of the complacent individualism was wearing thin, and the consciousness of social problems, including those involving health, became exceedingly acute.

One of the most forceful advocates of this broader point of view was Winslow,[5] who crystalized his thought into what became the best known and most widely accepted definition of public health and of its relationship to other fields. For analytic purposes it is presented in the following manner:

Public Health is the Science and Art of (1) preventing disease, (2) prolonging life, and (3) promoting health and efficiency through organized community effort for

    (a) the sanitation of the environment,
    (b) the control of communicable infections,
    (c) the education of the individual in personal hygiene,
    (d) the organization of medical and nursing services for the early diagnosis and preventive treatment of disease, and

(e) the development of the social machinery to insure everyone a standard of living adequate for the maintenance of health,

so organizing these benefits as to enable every citizen to realize his birthright of health and longevity.

Winslow's definition certainly cannot be criticized for lack of comprehensiveness. It provides for inclusion of almost everything in the fields of social evolution and service. In addition, it provides a rather complete summary not only of public health and its administration but also of its historic development and present-day and probable future trends.

From a somewhat different viewpoint, I have considered the multifaceted relationships of health and public health in the following terms:

Health is a state of total effective physiologic and psychologic functioning; it has both a relative and an absolute meaning, varying through time and space, both in the individual and in the group; it is the result of the combination of many forces, intrinsic and extrinsic, inherited and contrived, individual and collective, private and public, medical, environmental, and social; and it is conditioned by culture, economy, law, and government.

Accordingly,

Public health is dedicated to the common attainment of the highest level of physical, mental and social well-being and longevity consistent with available knowledge and resources at a given time and place. It holds this goal as its contribution to the most effective total development and life of the individual and his society.

There are two other definitions to which attention should be directed. One is the official statement of the House of Delegates of the American Medical Association, formulated in 1948. This rather conservative statement defined public health as:

The art and science of maintaining, protecting and improving the health of the people through organized community efforts. It includes those arrangements whereby the community provides medical services for special groups of persons and is concerned with prevention or control of disease, with persons requiring hospitalization to protect the community and with the medically indigent.

From its inception the protection and promotion of public health has been one of several stated concerns of the American Medical Association. This definition of public health is of particular interest and significance in view of subsequent social and legislative trends.

Another definition is that which is included in the Constitution of the World Health Organization:

Health is a state of complete physical, mental and social well-being and not merely the absence of disease or infirmity.

In a sense this may be considered not so much a definition as a statement of aims and principles.

It is evident from the various definitions that there has occurred a gradual extension of the horizons of public health. In conformance with the advances of medical and scientific knowledge and keeping pace with social and political progress, public health work has expanded from its original concern with gross environmental insanitation to, in sequence of addition, sanitary engineering, preventive physical medical science, preventive mental medical science, the positive or promotive as well as social and behavioral aspects of personal and community medicine, and more recently, the promotion and assurance of comprehensive health services for all.

The inevitable and continuous extension of the boundaries of public health was clearly recognized some years ago by Mountin,[6] who stated:

The progressive nature of public health makes any restricted definition of the functions and responsibilities of health departments difficult. More than that—there is a real danger in attempting to narrow down a moving or growing thing. To tie public health to the concepts that answered our needs 50 years ago, or even a decade ago, can only hamstring our contribution to society in the future.

## THERAPEUTIC MEDICINE, PREVENTIVE MEDICINE, AND PUBLIC HEALTH

A question sometimes arises as to the distinctions between therapeutic medicine, preventive medicine, and public health. Until the present the private practice of medicine has been concerned essentially with diagnosis and therapy of damage already done—the realignment of a broken limb, the healing or removal of a diseased organ, or the readjustment of an unsettled mind. The nature of the problems involved necessitates a highly personalized and individualized approach. Preventive medicine goes a step further, but its primary goal still represents a negative ideal: prevention of disease in the individual. In this sense preventive medicine can be said to consist of the following three areas of activity[7]:

1. The prevention by biologic means of certain preventable diseases such as acute communicable and deficiency diseases
2. The prevention of some of the consequences of preventable or curable chronic diseases, such as syphilis, tuberculosis, cancer, and diabetes
3. The prevention or retardation of some of the consequences of nonpreventable and noncurable diseases, such as many cardiac ailments

Increasingly it has become obvious that as the number of possible applications of preventive care to the early diagnosis and treatment of incipient or established diseases are multiplied, preventive medicine becomes all but indistinguishable from good clinical medical practice. Among the results have been the increased teaching of community medicine, the development of comprehensive medicine, continuity of care, and a growing tendency by private physicians to incorporate preventive medicine in their practices.[8]

It is necessary to go still further, however, and encourage the development of constructive and promotive medicine in which the center of interest is still the individual but now as a social or community integer, a member of a family and social group. Health workers must not be content with the mere preservation of his health but must strive for the development of its maximum potentials. Referring again to Winslow's definition, it is of interest to note that the emphasis in public health has changed from the physical environment or sanitation to preventive medicine and, more recently, back to the individual and his environment but now in terms of the individual's relationship with his complex social and physical environment. This change has brought a more mature realization on the part of both organized medicine and public health workers that each is an adjunct to and a true partner of the other and that both in turn exist to serve society. Thus Murphy,[9] in attempting to answer whether health is a public or a private matter, indicated that "it is neither and it is both." In considering the many and complex health and medical problems that challenge public health workers, he argued that "their effective resolution will be hastened as we blend public and private effort on the basis of logic and need." Appropriately he concluded, "There may be times when we can afford the luxury of foolish, unproductive infighting, but this is not one of them." In a sense this was an echo of a statement a third of a century ago by Vaughan[10] who, while ex-

tolling the success of various public health programs, nevertheless cautioned:

Notwithstanding these reasonable and warranted activities, supported in the main by tax funds cheerfully and eagerly appropriated by our elected officials, public health will never rise higher than the level of health established for the individual. The health of the many is but a summation of personal health. A nation can never be healthier than its citizens, and it is upon the welfare of the latter that our effort must be concentrated.

It would be preferable, of course, if medical practitioners served in a total sense—as personal or family health counselor, therapist, and provider of all preventive and health promotive services. To be able to do so, however, would require some philosophic reorientation, some reorganization, more time, and a more extensive use of allied health personnel and automated and electronic technology. One method of great potential by which this might be accomplished is through the application of prospective medicine.[11-14] The widespread acceptance and use of this developing approach will probably depend on effective cooperative efforts of public health organizations, schools of medicine, and practitioners of medicine. Briefly the concept is based on the fact that whereas a given individual theoretically may be subject to a vast array of health risks that may lead to a large number of possible illnesses or injuries (i.e., causes of death), in actuality at any given point in life for a particular type of individual a few conditions, perhaps five or six, constitute most of the risk for the succeeding 5 to 10 years. This is a time span that the usual person is able to comprehend and more willing to plan for. For each given type of person, categorized by age, sex, race, and perhaps occupation and location, the probability of illness or death from each of the predominant conditions during the next 5 or 10 years is provided. These probabilities are then adjusted in terms of the specific patient's history, habits, and physical examination. Indicated laboratory and clinical tests may be performed to refine them more. It is then possible to tell the individual that although people of his age, race, sex, and occupation have, for example, 780 chances out of 1,000 of surviving the next decade, his chances are only 590 out of 1,000. It is also possible then to pinpoint the specific changes that might be made to raise his chances to those of the average person of his type. For example, a certain amount of weight reduction

Name.... *William Smith* ........Age .*45*.......Sex .*male*.......Race .*white*..........

| Rank | Cause of death | Average risk* | Pertinent observations | Present personal risk† | Prescription | Adjusted personal risk‡ |
|---|---|---|---|---|---|---|
| 1 | Arteriosclerotic heart disease and chronic endocarditis | 35.07 | 10 lbs overweight, 2 packs cigarettes/day; coronary thrombosis 35± | 350 | weight reduction, exercise and coagulant refused alcohol and tobacco | 70 |
| 2 | Malignant neoplasms, pulmonary | 4.86 | 2 packs cigarettes/day | 50 | stop smoking | 25 |
| 3 | Vascular lesions of central nervous system | 4.28 | see 1 | 14 | same as 1 | 5 |
| 4 | Cirrhosis of liver | 3.70 | heavy smoker, heavy drinker (8-12 oz/day) | 15 | reduce alcohol intake | 4 |
| 5 | Suicide | 3.13 | other release | 2 | | 2 |
| 6 | Accidents, vehicular | 3.13 | overweight, heavy drinker hypertensive | 9 | same as 1; seat belts, periodic vision tests | 3 |
| 7 | Chronic rheumatic heart disease | 2.20 | no history | 1 | | 1 |
| 8 | Pneumonia | 1.85 | no significant findings | 2 | | 2 |
| 9 | Malignant neoplasms, intestinal, rectal | 1.85 | " | 2 | | 2 |
| 10 | Other diseases of the heart | 1.50 | " | 1 | | 1 |
| 11 | Malignant neoplasms, stomach, esophagus | 1.50 | " | 1 | | 1 |
| 12 | Hypertensive heart disease | 1.50 | 160/110 overweight, history of coronary | 15 | hypotensive treatment regime | 7 |
| 13 | Lymphosarcoma | .93 | no significant findings | 1 | | 1 |
| 14 | Tuberculosis | .93 | | 1 | | 1 |
| 15 | Diabetes | | family history | 2 | periodic blood sugar tests | 1 |
| 16 | | | | | | |
| 17 | All other causes | 25.24 | | 25 | | |
| 18 | Total risk | 91.67 | | 490 | | 124 |

* Chance in 1,000 of the individual dying from this cause during next ten years
† Present personalized risk—average risk modified by personal history, physical, laboratory and social findings
‡ Adjusted personalized risk—present personalized risk as it might be modified by certain specific preventive measures

**Fig. 1-1.** Probability of death in next decade from specific causes.

would lower the chances of heart attack, a reduction in alcohol consumption would reduce the risk from accidents, and elimination of smoking would lower the chances of carcinoma of the larynx and lungs. An example of such a health hazard chart is shown in Fig. 1-1.

The various shifts in opportunity, attitude, and practice that have occurred over the years have led inevitably to a reevaluation of the meaning and purpose of health. Until recently, to the extent that it has been possible, many people, including many health workers, have pursued health as an ultimate goal in itself. Increasingly, however, it is realized that health has value only to the extent that it promotes efficiency and a satisfactory total living experience. After all, it is the quality of life that is meaningful, not merely the quantity. Health in and of itself is therefore of little if any use. Its true value lies in worthwhile activities made possible by virtue of it; nor should one fall into the trap of regarding complete and lasting health as attainable. Dubos[15] has used this point as the theme of his provocative book, *Mirage of Health*. In it he emphasizes that health and happiness, for so long regarded as absolute and permanent values supposedly achieved by some in the golden ages of the past and still universally sought after as man masters the arts of living through power and knowledge, now in our time appear to be illusions. To be otherwise is unnatural because, as he indicates, complete freedom from disease, from stress, from frustration, and from struggle is incompatible with the process of living and evolution. He muses:

Life is an adventure in a world where nothing is static, where unpredictable and ill-understood events constitute dangers that must be overcome, often blindly and at great cost; where man himself, like the sorcerer's apprentice, has set in motion forces that are potentially destructive and may someday escape his control. Every manifestation of existence is a response to stimuli and challenges, each of which constitutes a threat if not adequately dealt with. The very process of living is a continual interplay between the individual and his environment, often taking the form of a struggle resulting in injury or disease.

He adds wryly, "Complete and lasting freedom from disease is but a dream remembered from imaginings of a Garden of Eden designed for the welfare of man."

## HEALTH AND GOVERNMENT

Occasionally one encounters objection to the concept that the protection and promotion of the public's health is an appropriate responsibility and activity of government. It must be realized that social and political philosophy was not always such as to lead to acceptance of this idea. The Roman Empire was notable for its wise concern for the protection and enhancement of the health and well-being of its people. During most of history, however, the prevailing attitude has been to regard any such proposition as constituting unnecessary and dangerous pampering of the masses. Indeed, this was one of the basic points made by Malthus[16] that not only should the genetically and otherwise inferior be allowed to die according to nature's plan but that the conditions of the poor should not be improved lest they lose a sense of responsibility and moral restraint. Subsequently, lack of positive action was also justified on the basis of unwarranted and improper interference on the part of government in the private rights of the individual. Beck-Storrs[17] describes the dilemma well in her discussion of the beginning of public health legislation in England as recently as the late nineteenth century against a background of liberalism and individualism. She points to the conflict presented by the basic concept of public health and the prevailing idea of freedom of the individual:

It suddenly dawned upon Englishmen that the modern apostles of health challenged the tradition of local government. They thought that they were called upon to make a decision between two evils, namely, either to let disorder and disease continue as before, or to suffer the monster of a civilized state.

She points out that public health threatened the Englishman's "right to be dirty" if he were so inclined. The well-to-do and the legislators, in the face of widespread communicable disease, were willing to agree to certain changes to protect themselves, but they did not want to go too far. The recommendations of The Royal Sanitary Commission of 1869 required the services of inspectors—but how could their authority be limited? To control the spread of infectious diseases a system of compulsory notification would be necessary. Rules would have to be enforced for slum clearance. Minimum specifications for low-cost housing for workers were likely to force landlords and landowners to spend more money than they had intended. She writes:

Here for the first time in the modern period, arose the problem of state supported welfare measures which threatened to interfere with the economic activities of private citizens. And this happened at a time when economic liberalism was believed to be the principle reason for the prosperity of the 19th century.

To the extent possible the government of England attempted to present the desired changes in a positive context—rights rather than restrictions, protections rather than prohibitions. Thus the state was empowered to ensure that a man was no more likely to have his well poisoned through the neglect of his neighbor than he was to be robbed with impunity. Health inspectors were given the responsibility of surveillance over drainage and sewerage systems, water supplies, bathhouses and washhouses as well as health conditions in workshops, mines, and bakeshops. Under the existing circumstances the inspectors were natural targets of a public highly sensitive to its freedoms. Success depended on their training and tact and also on whether the instinctive resentment against such invasions of a person's private affairs could be overcome. The Royal Sanitary Commission, anticipating this reaction, therefore recommended "employment of only well-trained men, capable of administering on a national level the measures instituted by the proposed central authority." It may be worth observing parenthetically that this recommendation is as valid now and in America as it was in England at the time it was made.

In the developing United States, attitudes were if anything more individualistic. As Roemer[18] has pointed out, the Western world's negative attitude toward government has deep roots, especially in America, where the colonists revolted against a domineering British monarchy. One result was the explicit limitations placed on the central government in the Constitution and the absence of Constitutional reference to health, either as a personal right or a governmental responsibility. Roemer also emphasizes that the medical profession, having much earlier achieved independence from feudal landlords and religious authority in Europe, was doubly suspicious of governmental interference. As a result, as Shryock[19] has reasoned, medicine had little tangible impact on American society prior to 1875. Since then, however, medicine

and related fields, either by their presence or absence, have had an increasingly significant influence on the problems, nature, and even survival of society. This no government can afford to ignore.

Mustard[20] analyzed the situation in more colorful but effective terms:

Public health service at any given time and place represents, in a way, the confluence of two streams in human progress. First there is the fairly clear and clean, but somewhat cold, trickle that filters down through the very fine sands of science; and second, there is the somewhat muddy flow of varying temperature that gushes intermittently from the rich but unpatrolled sociopolitical pastures. Taking their rise as they do in such entirely different sources, it is not astonishing that these tributaries do not completely or smoothly mix on their conjunction; nor need one be discouraged because there are eddies and backwashes, flotsam and froth. It is a powerful stream and one that will continue to flow.

There is no longer any question concerning health as a human right and its protection as a governmental responsibility. Thus commenting on the National Hospital Act of 1940, Senator James E. Murray said, "It is the function of government to preserve the person as well as the property of man . . . and there can be no natural progress except through promoting the health and welfare of the citizens of the Nation." The same thought has been emphasized on an increasing number of occasions by each recent President of the United States and other leading governmental figures.[21]

In American society there are numerous reasons for governmental action in public health. Many public health activities can be carried out only by group or community action. This is particularly true in urban areas, which are so characteristic of the increasingly mechanized industrialized societies. Sanitary water systems and sewage disposal facilities are obvious examples; so too, however, is the organization of quality comprehensive health care. Many necessary health activities must have an authoritative and legal base such as is available only to government. Isolation and quarantine regulations and many aspects of environmental health work are obvious examples. Some other activities such as the collection and analysis of vital records can be carried out only through a well-organized, well-staffed, stable, and continuing governmental agency. The most important organizing force is government, which passes, enforces, and finances health legislation that in the final analysis determines the content and pattern of health services and protection for all of the people. It is the only mechanism that can do this in the total sense. However, as Kruse[22] indicates, "This concentration of political, economic, and social power, with its vast organization, is at the expense of the individual. . . . He surrenders liberty for opportunity and security."

## SCOPE OF PUBLIC HEALTH

During recent years, the perimeters of generally acceptable areas of public health concern have been moving outward at a rapid rate. Whereas not long ago many would limit public health matters to general sanitation and the control of infectious disease, today all aspects of Winslow's famous definition are not only included but even surpassed. With reference to man's environment, public health workers now think in the broadest possible terms—the total ecologic relationship between man and the environment of which he is a part. This forms the basis of recent comprehensive studies of environmental health, one of which is cited in the references.[23] Similarly, with reference to personal health services, health agencies are already deeply involved not only in problems of distribution and quality of health personnel and facilities, but also in the assurance of adequate comprehensive health care for all. This is evidenced by a spectacular increase in significant federal legislative actions and programs during recent years.[24,25]

In general terms it has been stated that public health is concerned with the following two broad areas: (1) environmental problem sheds and (2) health service marketing. More specifically, public health activities appear to fall into the following seven categories:

1. Activities that must be conducted on a community basis
   a. Supervision of community food, water, and milk supplies as well as medications, household products, toys, and recreational equipment
   b. Insect, rodent, and other vector control
   c. Environmental pollution control, including atmospheric, soil, and aquatic pollution control, prevention of radiation hazards, and noise abatement
2. Activities designed for prevention of illness, disability, or premature death from
   a. Communicable diseases, including parasitic infestations
   b. Dietary deficiencies or excesses

c. Behavioral disorders, including alcoholism, drug habituation, narcotic addiction, certain aspects of delinquency, and suicide
d. Mental illness, including mental retardation
e. Allergic manifestations and their community sources
f. Acute and chronic noncommunicable respiratory diseases
g. Neoplastic diseases
h. Cardiac and cerebrovascular diseases
i. Metabolic diseases
j. Certain hereditary or genetic conditions
k. Occupational diseases
l. Home, vehicular, and industrial accidents
m. Dental disorders, including dental caries and periodontal disease
n. Certain risks of maternity, growth, and development
3. Activities related to provision of comprehensive health care
   a. Promotion of development and equitable distribution of medical and allied health personnel and facilities
   b. Assistance in development and maintenance of the quality and quantity of community resources and facilities, including establishment and application of standards for and categorization of hospitals, nursing and convalescent homes, and day care centers
   c. Operation of screening programs for early detection of disease
   d. Promotion and sometimes operation of emergency medical service systems
   e. Promotion and sometimes operation of treatment centers, varying from disease-specialty clinics to comprehensive health centers
   f. Facilitation of and participation in pregraduate and continuing professional and paraprofessional education
4. Activities concerned with collection, preservation, and analysis of vital records
5. Public education in personal and community health
6. Comprehensive health planning and evaluation
7. Research—scientific, technical, and administrative

Obviously many public health agencies do not find it possible or necessary to engage in all of these activities. In each case it is desirable to determine local needs, wishes, resources, and capabilities and to adapt the program of the community to them. Various administrative and planning tools exist to aid in accomplishing this; one is the *Guide to a Community Health Study*,[26] developed by the American Public Health Association. This and several others are considered in Chapter 12.

In addition, it must be realized that public health agencies cannot and should not attempt to carry out the foregoing activities by themselves. To be successful and acceptable requires that most if not all of them be done in cooperative partnership with many other agencies, organizations, professions, and community groups. The encouragement of this was the purpose, in part, of the Comprehensive Health Planning and Public Health Service Amendments of 1966 (P.L. 89-749).[27] Increasingly this philosophy is spreading also to international health planning.[28]

## PUBLIC HEALTH AS OPPOSED TO NATURAL SELECTION

A worrysome objection to public health activities that is encountered not infrequently is that it promotes the survival and propagation of the biologically or genetically unfit at the expense of the fit and to the ultimate detriment of the human species.[16] Advocates of this viewpoint claim that public health activities interfere with or negate the forces of natural biologic selection, which in a coldly impersonal manner supposedly weeds out "the lame, the halt, and the blind" as well as protoplasm of poor genetic quality. Thus referring to public health as unnatural, Huxley[29] called it the very essence of the myth of progress. Bowes,[30] another British writer, concludes that whereas modern public health measures will continue to make life comfortable during the few remaining generations of Western civilization, a few "good old-fashioned epidemics" such as the Black Death might be desirable because they tend to wipe out many mental and physical weaklings who at present are coddled through life. Other examples among many that can be cited are those of a sociologist,[31] on the one hand, and a physician,[32] on the other, who point to the public health efforts that protect the unfit while more desirable human specimens are sent off to war. Goldstein[33] provides a critical analysis of these various arguments.

One may ask, however, how the "fit" (whoever they may be) can survive if disease is allowed to run rampant among the "unfit." It is true that uncontrolled disease tends to eliminate those who appear to be weak or inferior according to certain standards. Those who are chronically tired, hungry, and cold are indeed more likely to succumb. In most instances, however, uncontrolled disease strikes blindly, producing malaria, tuberculosis, and other diseases that attack with limited selectivity among allegedly superior individuals if they are unprotected as well as among so-called inferior individuals. Disease and death have often entered palaces and mansions through the back door. A normal infant, or for that matter a gifted infant, may be disastrously affected by the presence of disease. Generally speaking, the use of the terms *unfit, undesirable,* or *inferior* represents psychologic, socially produced blind spots based on subjective biases and judgments.

The risk involved in uncontrolled disease is strikingly illustrated by the entries on the church register at Stratford-on-Avon. At that shrine of civilization, enclosed in a glass case, is a church register opened at the page on which is entered the statement of birth of William Shakespeare. Several lines above may be seen the entry "juli 11, 1564, Oliverus Gume—hic incipit pestis." During the year 1564, that little village suffered 242 deaths from plague. This probably represented one third to one half of the population. During the upswing of the epidemic, there was born a helpless infant who easily could have been one of those affected but who, by chance alone, was spared, subsequently to give us some of the greatest cultural treasures of this civilization. If he had become infected and died, would that infant have been considered unfit or inferior?

The question arises therefore—who are the fit and the unfit? Observation indicates that the definition varies with time and place. Steinmetz was a congenital cripple; Toulouse Lautrec was afflicted with hereditary osteochondritis fragilitas; Mozart, Chopin, and many other great figures in the arts and sciences died at early ages from tuberculosis,[34]; and Schumann and numerous other notable persons died from typhoid fever. Would anyone dare label these and thousands like them unfit? Americans can least afford to point the finger. Most citizens of this great nation are descendants of persons who by one standard or another would have been considered undesirable or unfit. The reasons have varied—religious, ethnic, economic, social, political, and cultural—whatever reason has been most expedient to those in power at the moment. Testimony to this is given in the statement by Emma Lazarus that is enshrined in the Statue of Liberty:

Give me your tired, your poor,
Your huddled masses yearning to breathe free,
The wretched refuse of your teeming shore.
Send these the homeless, tempest-tossed to me.
I lift my lamp beside the golden door.

Although some individuals or even groups admittedly may suffer from physical or other handicaps, it is false reasoning to suppose that they are necessarily stigmatized for all time or useless for all purposes. No public health worker would deny that his profession makes it possible for many to live who otherwise would die. These beneficiaries and their progeny have lived, and although much yet needs to be done, they have prospered. Each new Olympic tournament sees the establishment of new records of physical prowess. The descendants of immigrants are taller and of greater physical stamina than were their forebears or are their counterparts in their countries of origin. This is not meant to deny the need to apply the increasing knowledge of genetics in personal and marital counseling, which will be considered subsequently. At this point, however, one cannot help ponder the potential magnitude of the benefits that would accrue to the human race from a truly vigorous application of present knowledge. Rosenau had this in mind when he wrote concerning preventive medicine and public health as follows:

It dreams of a time when there shall be enough for all, and every man shall bear his share of labor in accordance with his ability, and every man shall possess sufficient for the needs of his body and the demands of health. These things he shall have as a matter of justice and not of charity. It dreams of a time when there shall be no unnecessary suffering and no premature deaths; when the welfare of the people shall be our highest concern; when humanity and mercy shall replace greed and selfishness; and it dreams that all these things will be accomplished through the wisdom of man. It dreams of these things, not with the hope that we, individually, may participate in them, but with the joy that we may aid in their coming to those who shall live after us. When young men have vision the dreams of old men come true.

Some people may easily dismiss all this as impractical, starry-eyed idealism. But the achievement of the greatest success and satisfaction in a social field such as that represented by public health demands a full share of idealism. Perhaps this is the answer to the question raised early in this chapter, since it can be said fairly that public health officials through their efforts have rarely aimed at the improvement of personal fortunes or the creation of new positions in which they have a personal vested interest. Nevertheless, as a final word of caution, it must be realized that idealism and practicality are not necessarily immiscible as are oil and water. In fact their admixture is sorely needed now more than ever before in this incredibly rapidly evolving age. The prefacing statement by Lowell[35] in *Conflicts of Principle* is as timely and pertinent now and to the present public health purpose as when he wrote it half a century ago:

People often call some men idealists and others practical folks as if mankind were by natural inclination so divided into these two groups that an idealist cannot be practical or a man of affairs have a lofty purpose whereas in fact no man approaches perfection who does not combine both qualities in a high degree. Without either he is defective in spirit and unscientific in method; the idealist because he does not strive to make his theory accurate, that is consonant with the facts; the so-called practical man if he acts upon the impulse of the occasion without the guidance of an enduring principle of conduct. Hence both lack true wisdom, the idealist more culpably for he should be diligent in thought and seek all the light he can obtain. It is useful to repeat that many men have *light* enough to be visionary, but only he who *clearly sees* can *behold* a vision.

## REFERENCES

1. Hanlon, J. J., Rogers, F. B., and Rosen, G.: A bookshelf on the history and philosophy of public health, Amer. J. Public Health **50:**445, April 1960.
2. Boek, W. E., and Boek, J. K.: Society and health, New York, 1956, G. P. Putnam's Sons.
3. Terris, M.: Social medicine as an academic discipline, J. Med. Educ. **33:**565, Aug. 1958.
4. Rosen, G.: Approaches to a concept of social medicine, Milbank Mem. Fund Quart. **26:**7, Jan. 1948.
5. Winslow, C.-E. A.: The untilled field of public health, Mod. Med. **2:**183, March 1920.
6. Mountain, J. W.: The health department's dilemma, Public Health Rep. **67:**223, March 1952.
7. Smith, G., and Evans, L. J.: Preventive medicine, attempt at definition, Science **100:**39, July 21, 1944.
8. National Commission on Community Health Services: Comprehensive health care, Washington, 1967, Public Affairs Press.
9. Murphy, F. D.: Health—public or private? Amer. J. Public Health **46:**15, Jan. 1956.
10. Vaughan, H. F.: The way of public health, Trans. Coll. Physicians Phila. **9:**86, June 1941.
11. Sadusk, J. F., and Robbins, L. C.: Proposal for health-hazard appraisal in comprehensive health care, J.A.M.A. **203:**1108, March 25, 1968.
12. Campbell, R. W., and Stuart, B. A.: A teaching case in health hazard appraisal, Indianapolis, 1970, Department of Internal Medicine, Methodist Hospital of Indiana.
13. How to practice prospective medicine, India-

napolis, 1970, Department of Internal Medicine, Methodist Hospital of Indiana.

14. Probability tables of deaths in the next ten years from specific causes, Indianapolis, 1972, Methodist Hospital of Indiana.

15. Dubos, R. J.: Mirage of health, Garden City, N. Y., 1960, Doubleday & Co., Inc.

16. Malthus, T. R.: An essay on the principle of population as it affects the future improvement of society, London, 1798. Reprint, London, 1926, Royal Economic Society.

17. Beck-Storrs, A.: Public health and government control, Social Stud. **45:**211, Oct. 1954.

18. Roemer, M. I.: The influence of government on American medicine, Oslo, 1962, Gyldendal Norsk Forlag, p. 226.

19. Shryock, R. H.: The interplay of social and internal factors in the history of modern medicine, Sci. Month. **76:**221, April 1953.

20. Mustard, H. S.: Government in public health, New York, 1945, Commonwealth Fund.

21. Government and public health, Bull. N. Y. Acad. Med. **43:**4, April 1967.

22. Kruse, H. D.: The great bane, Bull. N. Y. Acad. Med. **42:**2, Feb. 1966.

23. Linton, R. M., and others: A strategy for a livable environment, Washington, D. C., 1967, Government Printing Office.

24. U. S. Senate, Committee on Government Operations: Federal role in health, Rept. 91-809, 91st Cong., 2nd sess., Washington, D. C., 1970, Government Printing Office.

25. U. S. Department of Health, Education, and Welfare: HEW catalog of assistance, DHEW pub. no. (OS)73-44, Washington, D. C., 1972, Government Printing Office.

26. American Public Health Association: Guide to a community health study, New York, 1961, The Association.

27. U. S. Department of Health, Education, and Welfare: Comprehensive health planning: Why is it needed? How does it work? Who makes it work? DHEW/HSM pub. no. 72-750, Washington, D. C., 1972, Government Printing Office.

28. Hilleboe, H. E., Barkhuus, A., and Tomas, W. C.: Approaches to national health planning, Geneva, 1972, World Health Organization.

29. Huxley, A.: Brave new world, Life **25:**63, Sept. 20, 1948.

30. Bowes, G. K.: Epidemic disease; past, present, and future, J. Roy. San. Inst. **66:**174, July 1946.

31. Gillette, J. M.: Perspective of public health in the United States, Sci. Month. **53:**235, Sept. 1941.

32. Johnson, A. S.: Medicine's responsibility in the propagation of poor protoplasm, New Eng. J. Med. **238:**715, May 27, 1948.

33. Goldstein, M. S.: Theory of survival of the unfit, J. Nat. Med. Ass. **47:**233, July 1955.

34. Moorman, L. J.: Tuberculosis and genius, Chicago, 1940, University of Chicago Press.

35. Lowell, A. L.: Conflicts of principle, Cambridge, Mass., 1932, Harvard University Press.

*Those who forget the past
are doomed to repeat it.*

GEORGE SANTAYANA

CHAPTER 2

# Background and development of public health *

## A LOOK AT THE PAST

Although the primary purpose of this book is to consider the various administrative factors involved in the practice of public health, it is also important to consider its genesis. This is done not merely to pay tribute to those who preceded today's public health workers but also for practical reasons. Osler[4] once claimed it to be a sign of a dry age when the great men of the past are held in light esteem. Furthermore, historic review might enable readers to grasp the social significance of the public health movement.

In the process a better understanding might thereby be achieved of where public health workers are and in which direction they should be going. It is important to glance backward occasionally to see whence and how the public health movement originated. Many circumstances and events of the past help to explain some present-day administrative problems and trends that otherwise might be puzzling. As mentioned earlier, as with all other constructive social movements, numerous difficulties have been encountered in the field of public health; superstition, public apathy, political interference, inadequate funds, and inadequate per-

*For two extensive and scholarly presentations of this subject, see *A History of Public Health* by Rosen[1] and *The History of American Epidemiology* by Top.[2] For more detailed references, see Hanlon, Rogers, and Rosen.[3]

sonnel are only a few. One sometimes hears shortsighted, impatient, and intolerant persons, even within the public health profession, condemn past and present public health practices in terms of these factors or because progress appears to be slow. Learning something of the backgrounds of different social structures and of the public health movement may provide better perspective and greater understanding of the relative importance of these factors and the reason why they still exert some influence. This is not meant to condone or encourage complacency or comfortable self-satisfaction but merely to point out that sound planning for the future is best accomplished by honest evaluation and understanding of the past and present.

## THE PRECHRISTIAN PERIOD

Little is known about the prehistoric origins of either personal or community hygiene. Some hints may be gleaned, however, from a study of the customs and tribal rules of contemporary groups that are low in the scale of civilization. With few exceptions primitive tribes have a certain amount of group and community hygienic sense usually derived from experience with survival. Rules against the fouling of family or tribal environments are almost universal. Many have taboos against the use of the upstream side of the camp site for excretory purposes. Burial of excreta is not uncommon. However, this practice is sometimes based on superstition rather than on sanitary intent.

**13**

Many groups have elaborate provisions for disposal of the dead. Almost all primitive people recognize the existence of disease and engage in forms of voodoo, quarantine, tribal dancing, and the use of smoke and noise to drive away the evil spirits of disease. Indeed, as recently as the end of the nineteenth century, the practice of burning pitch and firing cannons was used to combat yellow fever in some American communities.

Archeologic evidence and other records show that the Minoans, 3000 to 1500 B.C., and the Cretans, 3000 to 1000 B.C., had advanced to the point of constructing drainage systems, water closets, and water-flushing systems. Herodotus wrote that the Egyptians of about 1000 B.C. were the healthiest of all civilized nations. They had a considerable sense of personal cleanliness, possessed numerous pharmaceutical preparations, and constructed earth closets and public drainage pipes. The Hebrews extended Egyptian hygienic thought and behavior by stating in Leviticus, written about 1500 B.C., what is probably the world's first written hygienic code. It dealt with a wide variety of personal and community responsibilities, including cleanliness of the body, protection against the spread of contagious diseases, isolation of lepers, disinfection of dwellings after illness, sanitation of campsites, disposal of excreta and refuse, protection of water and food supplies, and the hygiene of maternity.

The Athenian civilization is of particular interest for two reasons. It was there that personal hygiene was developed to a degree never previously or subsequently approached. Much concern was given to personal cleanliness, exercise, and dietetics in addition to environmental sanitation. Another point of interest is that in contrast with present-day public health thought the weak, the ill, and the crippled were ignored and in some instances deliberately destroyed.

The Roman Empire is well known for its administrative and engineering achievements. At its zenith it had laws for the registration of citizens and slaves, for a periodic census, for the prevention of nuisances, for inspection and removal of dilapidated buildings, for the elimination of dangerous animals and foul smells, for the destruction of unsound goods, for the supervision of weights and measures, for the supervision of public bars, taverns, and houses of prostitution, and for the regulation of building construction. An uninterrupted supply of good and cheap grain to the population was assured. Numerous public sanitary services were provided. Many streets were paved; some even had gutters and were drained by a network of underground conduits. Provision was made for the cleaning and repair of streets and the removal of garbage and rubbish. Public baths were constructed and extensively used. An adequate and, for that time, a relatively safe public water supply was made available by the construction of magnificent aqueducts and tunnels. It is of interest to note that several of the aqueducts and subsurface drains (cloacae) constructed by the Romans are actually still in use, having been incorporated in the present-day water and sewerage systems of Rome.

## THE MIDDLE AGES

With the dawn of the Christian era there developed a reaction against anything reminiscent of the Roman Empire and its attendant paganism. The early Christian Church, which represented the consensus of the period, took the attitude that the Roman and Athenian lifestyles pampered the body at the expense of the soul. Accordingly, belittlement of worldly and physical matters and "mortification of the flesh" became the preferred patterns of behavior. This philosophy contributed to the prolonged intermission in the progress of civilization known as the Dark Ages, marked by superstition, mysticism, and the rigorous persecution of freethinkers.

So intense was the reaction that it even included a significant change in attitude toward sanitation and personal hygiene. It was considered immoral to view even one's own body; therefore people seldom bathed and wore notoriously dirty garments. This is said by some to have been partly responsible for the eventual widespread use of perfume in the latter part of this period. Diets in general were apparently poor and consisted of badly prepared or preserved foods. This contributed to the eventual great interest in the use of spices and in the search for trade routes to obtain them. Sanitation was ignored. Refuse and body wastes were allowed to accumulate in and around dwellings. Slops were customarily emptied out of windows, giving rise to the familiar outcry *gardez l'eau*. These and other unsalubrious customs lasted until relatively recent times, as evidenced by Hogarth's prints of life in eighteenth century England.

However, some important medical and hygienic developments did occur during this period. Generally speaking, they were forced on the people by the disastrous effects of an uncontrolled nature and as fruits of their self-made, ill-conceived habits and customs. Terrifying pandemics of disease occurred that were among the most commanding and intense experiences in the entire history of the human species. During the seventh century a new religion Islam appeared. Its philosophy spread and gathered many followers in Africa, the Near East, Asia, and to some extent the Balkans and the Iberian peninsula. As with Judaism, it placed much emphasis on cleanliness. However, after the death of Mohammed, it became a religious custom to make a pilgrimage in the company of a large number of people to Mecca, the place of the prophet's birth, about A.D. 570. During each great pilgrimage, among the many thousands who converged on the small city were some from far-off Asia, especially India, which was and still is the endemic center of cholera. Cholera naturally spread rapidly throughout the thousands of pilgrims, who disseminated it along their homeward routes of travel and throughout their respective homelands. Thus each great pilgrimage was almost invariably followed by a pandemic of cholera. Added to this were the hordes of Christian crusaders from all parts of Europe whose wanderings inevitably resulted in periodic seeding of the European continent with the vibrio of cholera as well as other agents of disease. The vibrio prospered in a gradually urbanizing Europe, whence centuries later it was transferred to America by the invading settlers. During the period from 1830 to about 1880, cholera repeatedly reentered America, spreading along the water routes and accompanying the prospectors to the gold fields of California. At one time or another most settlements were affected by cholera, often resulting in the death of one third to one half of the population.

During the early Dark Ages, leprosy spread probably from Egypt to Asia Minor and eventually throughout Europe, aided again by the Crusades and other great migrations. It apparently was a far more acute and disfiguring disease than is presently observed in the Western world, and because of the terror to which it gave rise, laws were passed to regulate the conduct and movement of those afflicted. In many places lepers were declared civilly dead and were banished from human communities. They were compelled to wear identifying clothes and to warn of their presence by means of a horn, bell, or clapper and by crying the word "unclean." This had a twofold result in that it was an effective isolation measure and also usually brought about a relatively rapid death from hunger and exposure as well as from lack of treatment and care. These measures, inhumane as they were, almost eradicated leprosy in Europe, but by no means in the world, by the sixteenth century and may be regarded as an early, although unplanned, victory in epidemiology.

## The Black Death

No sooner had leprosy passed its zenith and begun to decline than an even deadlier menace appeared in the form of bubonic plague. Its spread was largely the result of the development of trade contacts between Europe and the Near East and Asia. It has been said with considerable justification that nothing before or since came so close to exterminating the human species. To quote a few historic figures,[5] during the 1340s more than 13 million people are said to have died from the disease in China. India was almost depopulated; Tartary, Mesopotamia, Syria, and Armenia were literally covered by dead bodies. When the disease was raging in its greatest violence, Aleppo lost about 500 people and the larger city of Cairo, from 10,000 to 15,000 people daily. In Gaza 22,000 people and most of the animals were carried off within 6 weeks; Cyprus lost all of its inhabitants, and ships without crews were often seen in the Mediterranean, as afterward in the North Sea, drifting about aimlessly, spreading the plague wherever they were driven ashore. When Pope Clement VI asked for the number of the dead, some said that half of the population of the known world had died. The figure he was finally given was about 43 million. The total mortality from the Black Death is thought to have been over 60 million.

Europe, particularly during 1348, was devastated. Florence lost 60,000 people, Venice 100,000, Marseilles 16,000 in 1 month, Sien 70,000, Paris 50,000, St. Denys 14,000, Strasbourg 9,000, and Vienna 1,200 daily. In many places in France not more than 2 out of 20 people were left alive.

In Avignon, where 60,000 people died, the Pope found it necessary to consecrate the Rhone river so that bodies might be thrown into it without delay, the churchyard no longer being able to hold them. In Vienna, burial within churchyards or churches was prohibited; the dead were arranged in layers by thousands in six large pits outside the city, as had already been done in Cairo, Paris, and other cities. Crossing the channel, the Black Death destroyed one half of the population of medieval England, at least 100,000 in London alone.

Altogether it is estimated that Europe's tribute in the pandemic of the midfourteenth century was about 25 million. Furthermore, this one horrifying visitation was just beginning; plague continued to ebb and flow like a tide, periodically sweeping over the dirty, miserable European continent. For example, in the city of London in 1603 over one sixth of the population succumbed to the disease, in 1625 another sixth, and in 1665 about one fifth. During 1790, Marseilles and Toulon lost 91,000 people; in 1743, Messina lost 70,000; and in 1759, about 70,000 died on the island of Cyprus. It must be recognized that as great as are these figures, they are proportionately enormous in relation to the populations of those times.

Growing out of these terrifying experiences and despite the then current view of divine or cosmic causation of disease, certain groping attempts were made to forestall the apparent inevitability of epidemic disaster. In 1348 the great trading port of Venice banned entry of infected or suspected ships and travelers. In 1377 at Ragusa it was ruled that travelers from plague areas stop at designated places outside the port and remain there free of disease for 2 months before being allowed to enter. Historically this represents the first quarantine measure, although it involved a 2-month interval rather than the literal 40 days. This procedure is of particular interest in that it implied a vague realization of the existence of an incubation period for a communicable disease. Six years later, in 1383, Marseilles passed the first actual quarantine law and erected the first quarantine station. These are historic landmarks in public health administration and epidemiology, but unfortunately their effectiveness was impaired by the fact that although great attention was paid to humans, the role of the rat and the flea was not discerned.

**Other diseases**

Some mention, even if necessarily inadequate, should be made of the rapid dissemination of syphilis throughout Europe and the Near East after the discovery of America, whence it is commonly thought to have originated. Some measure of its incidence and seriousness is indicated by its vernacular name, "the great pox," which was used to distinguish it from smallpox, now considered serious enough. Incidentally, it is curious that little historic reference is made to many of the other diseases that are known to have existed with incidences far exceeding any now occurring, for example, diphtheria, the streptococcal infections, the dysenteries, typhoid, typhus, and others. The most probable reasons for the paucity of mention of these diseases are that, in the first place, people undoubtedly became accustomed to their inevitable endemicity and accepted them as part of the routine risk of life and, second, that they were so dramatically overshadowed by the tremendous impact of the great periodic pandemic killers as to merit relatively little mention in the historic writings of the times. In summary therefore the people of Europe emerged from the Middle Ages and, in fact, came all the way to recent times with little substantial comprehension of any principles of public health other than those of crude, inhumane, and inefficient isolation and quarantine.

## RENAISSANCE AND REASON

In a period marked by expanding trade and population movement and concentration, the risks presented by disease were necessarily magnified. The great pandemics of the Middle Ages therefore must have caused considerable social and political frustrations that could lead only to attitudes of fatalism and general disregard for the welfare of individuals. In this regard Hecker[5] commented as follows:

> The mind of nations is deeply affected by the destructive conflict of the powers of nature, and . . . great disasters lead to striking changes in general civilization. For all that exists in man, whether good or evil, is rendered conspicuous by the presences of great danger. His inmost feelings are aroused—the thought of self-preservation masters his spirit—self denial is put to severe proof, and wherever darkness and barbarism prevail, there the affrighted mortal flies to the idols of his superstition, and all laws, human and divine, are criminally molested.

The way of life of a people likewise has a significant effect on their state of health or illness. In this respect it is of interest to learn from a letter of Erasmus to the personal physician of Cardinal Wolsey the manner of life in the average English household of the sixteenth century:

> As to floors, they are usually made with clay, covered with rushes that grow in the fens and which are so seldom removed that the lower part remains sometimes for twenty years and has in it a collection of spittle, vomit, urine of dogs and humans, beer, scraps of fish and other filthiness not to be named.

Winslow,[6] in his precis of the modern public health movement, pointed out how long it has taken the human race to improve such conditions, presenting examples as disgusting as the preceding from England in 1842 and New York City in 1865. Indeed, even now in some parts of the world, including some urban and rural areas in the United States, circumstances such as these are occasionally encountered.

Gradually there developed in the minds of a few some doubt of the teleologic origin of disease as a punishment for sin. It might be noted in passing, however, that this stigma has only recently been removed from cancer and tuberculosis and that venereal infection is still considered by many as a punishment for immorality. By the end of the Middle Ages several diseases had been differentiated. Among them were leprosy, influenza, ophthalmia, trachoma, scabies, impetigo, erysipelas (St. Anthony's fire), anthrax, plague, consumption, syphilis (the great pox), smallpox, diphtheria and scarlet fever considered as one, and typhus and typhoid fever also considered together.

The people of Europe emerged from this stunted and rather barbaric period of history slowly and cautiously and began to open their eyes and think as free individuals. An increasing number of outstanding thinkers appeared, among whom were Montaigne, Paracelsus, Galileo, Spinoza, Bacon, Descartes, to mention only a few. Each in his own way hammered at the bars imprisoning the minds and bodies of men. Their combined efforts resulted in remarkable subsequent accomplishments, especially in the late eighteenth century and throughout the nineteenth century. The concepts of the dignity and the rights of man began to be emphasized more and more. The search for scientific truth was at last advocated for its own sake.

## THE EIGHTEENTH AND NINETEENTH CENTURIES

### The plight of children

Meanwhile, other changes were occurring. Among them were the development of national-

ism, imperialism, and industrialization, with their tragic and degrading concomitants. The false gods of power and profit were placed on ever higher pedestals, and individual liberties, labors, and lives were sacrificed on a scale probably unprecedented since the building of the pyramids. As an example, in one of the most shameful actions in history there came about in England a legally condoned practice of apprentice slavery, whereby pauper children were indentured to owners of mines and factories. The socially accepted pattern was for parishes to assume responsibility for orphans and pauper children. This responsibility was met at first by paying private "nurses" for taking the infants and younger children into their homes for a few years and putting them out to work as apprentices when they grew older. Partly because of the increasing numbers and partly as a remedy for frequent abuse of young children, parish workhouses began to be established in the late seventeenth and early eighteenth centuries as a substitute for parish nurses.

Theoretically the workhouses were also intended to provide some training for the children, but this was kept at a minimum and was largely concerned with inculcating the ideals of obedience, labor, industry, virtue, and religion. It was hoped that the workhouses would ". . . cure a very bad practice in parish officers, who to save expence, are apt to ruin children by putting them out as early as they can to any sorry master that will take them, without any concern for their education and welfare."[7]

In her authoritative review of life in England in the eighteenth century, George[7] gives a picture of these methods and ideals in practice by describing the London Workhouse in Bishopsgate Street in 1708:

> . . . thirty or forty children were put under the charge of one nurse in a ward, they lay two together in bunks arranged round the walls in two tiers, "boarded and set one above the other . . . a flock bed, a pair of sheets, two blankets and a rugg to each." Prayers and breakfast were from 6:30 to 7. At 7 the children were set to work, twenty under a mistress, "to spin wool and flax, knit stockings, to make new their linnen, cloathes, shooes, mark, etc." This work went on till 6 P.M. with an interval from 12 to 1 for "dinner and play." Twenty children were called away at a time for an hour a day to be taught reading, some also writing. Some children, we are told, "earn a halfpenny, some a penny, and some fourpence a day." At twelve, thirteen or fourteen, they were apprenticed, being given, at the master's choice, either a "good ordinary suit of cloaths or 20s, in money."

When children reached the age of apprenticeship, their lot became infinitely worse. A writer on the Poor Laws in 1738 said the following:

A most unhappy practice prevails in most places to apprentice poor children, no matter to what master. Provided he lives out of the parish, if the child serves the first forty days we are rid of him for ever. The master may be a tiger in cruelty, he may beat, abuse, strip naked, starve or do what he will to the poor innocent lad, few people take much notice, and the officers who put him out the least of anybody . . . . The greatest part of those who now take poor apprentices are the most indigent and dishonest, in a word, the very dregs of the poor of England, by whom it is the fate of many a poor child, not only to be half-starved and sometimes bred up in no trade, but to be forced to thieve and steal for his master, and so is brought up for the gallows into the bargain. . . .

Children apprenticed to chimney sweepers fared among the worst. In 1767 Hanway, a leading reformer of the period, described the miseries of their neglect and ill-treatment, of their being forced up chimneys at the risk of being burnt or suffocated, and of their being forced to beg and steal by their masters. "Chimney-sweepers," he says, "ought to breed their own children to the business, then perhaps they will wash, clothe and feed them. As it is they do neither, and these poor black urchins have no protectors and are treated worse than a humane person would treat a dog." In apprenticing children in large groups the provision was not uncommon to require that for every 30 normal children 1 idiot would have

to be taken. These unfortunates, forced to work from 15 to 18 hours a day, sometimes literally chained to their machines, fed a minimum of food scarcely fit for consumption, and housed under the most crowded and filthy conditions, usually were released from their sufferings and abuse by early death.

In 1842 Edwin Chadwick pointed out that more than one half of the children of the working classes died before their fifth birthday and that in cities such as Liverpool the average ages at death of the various social classes were 36 years for the gentry, 22 years for tradesmen, and 16 years for laborers![8] The breakdown for London, obtained by the Sanitary Commission for the Metropolis in 1843, is given in Table 2-1.

**Sanitary conditions**

During this period the condition of the streets of most European cities became deplorable, due in part to nightmen and scavengers emptying their carts in the streets instead of in the places assigned for the purpose. The accumulated filth of the eighteenth century house was in many cases simply thrown from the doors or windows.

Although eighteenth-century London was incredibly dirtier, more dilapidated and more closely-built than it afterwards became, was there no compensation in its greater compactness, the absence of straggling suburbs, the ease with which people could take country walks? This is at least doubtful. The roads round London were neither very attractive nor very safe. The land adjoining them was watered with drains and

**Table 2-1.** Deaths by social class, London, 1840*

| Class | Proportion of deaths from epidemics to total deaths of each class (%) | Proportion of deaths of children under 1 year to births in that year | Proportion of deaths of children under 10 years to total deaths of each class (%) | Mean age of death of all who died– men, women, and children | Mean age of all who died above age 21 years |
|---|---|---|---|---|---|
| Gentry, professional persons, and their families | 6.5 | 1 to 10 | 24.7 | 44 | 61 |
| Tradesmen, shop-keepers, and their families | 20.5 | 1 to 6 | 52.4 | 23 | 50 |
| Wage classes, artisans, laborers, and their families | 22.2 | 1 to 4 | 54.5 | 22 | 49 |

*Modified from Chadwick as quoted by Richardson, B. W.: The health of nations, a review of the works of Edwin Chadwick, London, 1887, Longmans, Green & Co., vol. II, p. 80.

thickly sprinkled with laystalls and refuse heaps. Hogs were kept in large numbers on the outskirts and fed on the garbage of the town. A chain of smoking brick-kilns surrounded a great part of London and in the brick-fields vagrants lived and slept, cooking their food at the kilns. It is true that there was an improvement as the century went on. In 1706 it was said of the highways, tho they are mended every summer, yet everybody knows that for a mile or two about this City, the same and the ditches hard by are commonly so full of nastiness and stinking dirt, that oftentimes many persons who have occasion to go in or come out of town, are forced to stop their noses to avoid the ill-smell occasioned by it.[7]

These conditions under which so many hundreds of thousands of people lived and worked had dire results indeed from a hygienic standpoint. Smallpox, cholera, typhoid, tuberculosis, and many other diseases reached exceedingly high endemic levels, and the contamination of sources of water became so extensive as to prompt that famous statement in Parliament on the condition of the empire in 1859: "India is in revolt and the Thames stinks." Southwood Smith pointed out at the time that the annual slaughter in England and Wales from typhus and typhoid fevers was double the number of lives lost by the allied armies in the battle of Waterloo.

The circumstances described were by no means confined to England—they concerned the inheritors of the age of reason in many lands. Increasingly liberal views of the nature and role of man were expressed and broadcasted, especially by philosophers and writers such as Smith, Hume, Bentham, and Mill in England; Montesquieu, Voltaire, Diderot, and Rousseau in France, and Jefferson, Franklin, Dickinson, and Samuel Adams in the American colonies. In a very real sense the broader concerns of these men and others like them constructed the political and social platform on which it was possible to promote and develop sanitary reforms and other measures for the protection of the public health.

## ENGLISH SANITARY REFORMS

Concern with the economic consequences of existing social and sanitary conditions began to appear, providing leaders in sanitary reform with forceful arguments. Thus Chadwick[8] reported the following:

This depressing effect of adverse sanitary circumstances on the labouring strength of the population, and on its duration, is to be viewed with the greatest concern, as it is a depressing effect on that which most distinguishes the British people, and which it were truism to say constitutes the chief strength of the nation—the bodily strength of the individuals of the labouring class. The greater portion of the wealth of the nation is derived from the labour obtained by the application of this strength, and it is only those who have had practically the means of comparing it with that of the population of other countries who are aware how far the labouring population of this country is naturally distinguished above others. . . . The more closely the subject of the evils affecting the sanitary condition of the labouring population is investigated, the more widely do their effects appear to be ramified. The pecuniary cost of noxious agencies is measured by data within the province of the actuary, by the charges attendant on the reduced duration of life, and the reduction of the periods of working ability or production by sickness. The cost would include also much of the public charge of attendant vice and crime, which come within the province of the police, as well as the destitution which comes within the province of the administrators of relief. Of the pecuniary effects, including the cost of maintenance during the preventible sickness, any estimate approximating to exactness could only be obtained by very great labour, which does not appear to be necessary.

Public health went unrecognized in a legal sense in England until 1837, when the first sanitary legislation was enacted. It established a National Vaccination Board and appropriated 2,000 pounds for its support. As a result, a few vaccination stations were set up in the city of London. This modest beginning was followed shortly in 1842 by Edwin Chadwick's momentous *Report on an Inquiry into the Sanitary Condition of the Labouring Population of Great Britain,* one of the results of which was the establishment in 1848 of a General Board of Health for England. Significantly, the same year saw the appointment as first medical officer of health for London of John Simon, who 7 years later was to assume that office for the nation as a whole. Improvements rapidly followed one another. These advances in sanitation and hygiene did not go forward alone. Legislation was passed concerning factory management, child welfare, care of the aged, the mentally ill, and the infirm, education, and many other phases of social reform.

It was not long before the horrors of previous conditions were forgotten, and the standards of order, decency, and sanitation began to be taken for granted.

. . . pride was based on real achievements, which had an undoubted effect on the health of the town, and in which London was a pioneer among large cities.

The foot-pavements, the lamps, the water-supply, the fire-plugs, the new sewers, defective enough by later standards, were admired by all. . . . Beneath the pavements are vast subterraneous sewers arched over to convey away the waste water which in other cities is so noisome above ground, and at a less depth are buried wooden pipes that supply every house plentifully with water, conducted by leaden pipes into kitchens or cellars, three times a week for the trifling expense of three shillings per quarter. . . . The intelligent foreigner cannot fail to take notice of these useful particulars which are almost peculiar to London.[8]

The seeds of sanitary and social reform spread rapidly to other large urban centers of England. However, participation in these benefits by the smaller towns and rural areas was understandably slower. As early as 1830, Chadwick had recommended the employment of a large number of local sanitary officers, including medical personnel, for the adequate coverage of the nation. As might be expected, his proposals originally met with considerable opposition, some of which continued even when he subsequently was able to demonstrate the economic soundness of the costs incurred.

### ENGLISH INFLUENCE ON AMERICA

Conditions and developments in Great Britain may seem to have been unduly stressed. In view of the purpose of this book, however, any discussion of backgrounds must necessarily emphasize those extraterritorial developments that have exerted the greatest influence on North America. It is true that many advances had been made elsewhere, notably in the Low Countries, in Germany, and on the Scandinavian peninsula. By midnineteenth century France had long since embarked on significant studies and activities relating to public health and sanitation, and many scientific papers were being published. The establishment of the *Annales d'Hygiene Publique* gives testimony to this. The work of the Belgian, Quételet, was already widely known, and Pettenkofer in Munich and Virchow in Berlin already had far-reaching influences.

Nevertheless, the early intimate ties, social, economic, and otherwise, between the North American continent and Great Britain made events in the latter of particular significance to the former. The relationship was aptly described in 1876 by Bowditch,[9] first president of the Massachusetts State Board of Health:

But by far the greatest influence has been exerted upon us in America by England, who, by her un-bounded pecuniary sacrifices and steady improvement in her legislation, and her able writers, has far outstripped any country in the world in the direction of State Preventive Medicine. . . . The consummate skill in the discovery, removal, and prevention of whatever may be prejudicial to the public health, shown under the admirable direction of Mr. Simon, late Medical Officer of England's Privy Council, by his corps of trained inspectors is wholly unequalled at the present day, and unprecedented, I suspect, in all past time in any country on the globe.

Although scientific researchers may have progressed further in some other countries, the application of the new knowledge, especially in terms of administrative organization and procedure, occurred more rapidly and more successfully in England than elsewhere. Since the administrative organization depends to a considerable degree on legal procedure, it is noteworthy that America, from the beginning, followed the pattern set by English law. Thus when the time came for American communities to pass sanitation ordinances, they did so in the tradition of the English common law.

### COLONIAL AMERICA

Transferring attention to the developing North American continent, certain public health problems were soon recognized by the colonists. They had good reason for being conscious of the threat of disease. Many of the early settlements had been completely obliterated by epidemic diseases, particularly smallpox. Among these were the colonies at Jamestown and undoubtedly the colony at Roanoke Island. On the other hand, it was ironically probably due to disease that colonial powers were able to establish footholds in the Western Hemisphere. The settlers of the Massachusetts Bay Colony, for example, came to a territory in which the natives were by no means peaceful. Yet by the time the Pilgrims landed at Plymouth the hostile natives of the surrounding countryside had been all but eliminated, apparently by smallpox introduced by the Cabot and Gosnold expeditions. Smallpox also appears to have played some role in the weakening and eventual conquest of the Aztec Empire. In this instance it is known to have been introduced by a servant of Narvaez who joined Cortez in 1520.[10] It has been estimated that during the early periods of colonization of Central and North America, the Indian population was decimated by diseases introduced by the invaders, whether peaceful or otherwise.[11]

The registration of vital statistics is generally considered to be one of the essential cornerstones of sound, efficient public health awareness and practice. It is not without interest that the recording of these data was an early concern of the New England colonists. As early as 1639, an act was passed by the Massachusetts colony ordering that each birth and death be recorded; subsequent acts outlined the necessary administrative responsibilities and procedures. Not only was the information made available locally but copies had to be made by the town clerks and transmitted to the clerks of the county courts. The law also provided for fees and penalties. Similar laws were enacted at about the same time by the Plymouth colony.[12]

Most of the early activities of a public health nature in America were concerned with gross insanitation and attempts to prevent the entrance of exotic diseases. For example, as early as 1647 the Massachusetts Bay Colony passed a regulation to prevent pollution of Boston Harbor. Between 1692 and 1708 Boston, Salem, and Charleston passed acts dealing with nuisances and trades offensive or dangerous to the public health. In 1701 Massachusetts passed laws for the isolation of smallpox patients and for ship quarantine, to be used whenever necessary. The difficulty with these and other early measures was that no continuing organization or even committee existed to assure ready recognition of undesirable situations or noncompliance with the requirements of the legislation enacted.

In the century during which the American colonies developed, drew together, and eventually formed a federation of states, little progress of a public health nature was made. After the American Revolution the threat of various diseases, particularly yellow fever, which caused the abandonment of the national capital in Philadelphia, led to widespread interest in the development of legislation for the establishment of permanent boards of health. Permissive legislation of this type was passed in 1797 by the states of New York and Massachusetts, followed in 1805 by Connecticut. There is some controversy over the establishment of the first permanent local board of health. Boston is commonly said to have organized the first in 1799, with Paul Revere as its chairman. However, this has been contested by the cities of Petersburg, Va. (1780), Philadelphia (1794), New York (1796), and Baltimore (1793). The latter claim has been supported more or less by the American Public Health Association.[13]

By the end of the eighteenth century New York City, with a population of 75,000, had formed a public health committee concerned with the "quality of the water supplies, construction of common sewers, drainage of marshes, interment of the dead, planting of trees and healthy vegetables, habitation of damp cellars, and the construction of a masonry wall along the water front." In July 1798 the new American Congress created a Marine Hospital Service to provide for the care of sick and disabled merchant seaman. This service was later to become of interest and significance for three reasons: (1) it was the origin of what eventually became the United States Public Health Service; (2) it was to furnish the organization for effecting national quarantine; and (3) it represents one of the earliest examples of prepaid medical insurance. For 20 cents a month each merchant seaman was provided with medical and hospital care. As early as 1800, the first marine hospital was constructed in Norfolk, Va.

## THE NINETEENTH CENTURY IN AMERICA

Between 1800 and 1850 the United States underwent great expansion, but public health activities remained stationary. What did not remain stationary, however, was the development of threats to public health and welfare and the resulting incidence of disease. Many epidemics, especially of smallpox, yellow fever, cholera, typhoid, and typhus, repeatedly entered and swept over the land. Tuberculosis and malaria reached high levels of endemicity. In Massachusetts in 1850, for example, the tuberculosis death rate was over 300 per 100,000 population, the infant mortality was about 200 per 1,000 live births, and smallpox, scarlet fever, and typhoid were leading causes of deaths. As a result, by 1850 the average life expectancy in Boston and most of the other older cities in America was less than that in London, which at that time was itself the object of wide criticism for its sickening scenes of misery and depravity. The American social scene was the subject of scathing comments by visitors from abroad who were impressed with the crudity and "barbarism" of life in the United States and the generally unkempt appearance of its communities. As so often has happened, improvements in sanitation and public health were delayed by lack of progress in other fields. Newsholme,[14] the noted British hygienist, described this period of American social history in the following manner:

The rapid growth of cities tended to out run the forces of law and order and to smother under the weight of numbers any attempts at civic reform. Before public health measures could be adopted or enforced, other more pressing problems had to be solved. An effective police force, the first requisite of community life, did not make its appearance in the Atlantic seaboard cities until 1853, and satisfactory fire prevention came even later. Protection against the dirt and filth of human aggregation, which threatened the life of every man, woman, and child, had to wait upon the adequate enforcement of law and order.

The inadequacies of the times were reflected in the low quality of medical care available to the people. Professional teaching facilities were few and inadequate. Many "physicians" were self-designated and itinerant. The prestige of the medical profession was at its lowest ebb, and its ranks were disorganized and split by the development of numerous healing philosophies and cults. One writer[15] summarized the situation: "The doctors were victims of their own want of knowledge, of the absence of adequate medical standards and of a chaotic educational system." Healing agents used included not only empiric remedies left over from medieval Europe but, in addition, many newly discovered "remedies" often borrowed from the American aborigines. This state of therapeutic affairs led Holmes[16] to remark that "if the whole materia medica as now used, could be sunk to the bottom of the sea, it would be all the better for mankind—and all the worse for the fishes."

## CITY HEALTH DEPARTMENTS

The first half of the nineteenth century saw a gradual trend toward the more or less full-time employment of persons to serve as the functional agents of local boards of health, which now were increasing in number. This represented the first step in the formation of full-time local health departments. Some of the earlier of these organizations were established in Baltimore (1798), Charleston, S. C. (1815), Philadelphia (1818), Providence (1832), Cambridge (1846), New York City (1866), Chicago (1867), Louisville (1870), Indianapolis (1872), and Boston (1873). The last is of interest in illustrating the lag, in this instance three quarters of a century, that occurred between

the formation of many local boards of health and the establishment of functional health departments. As might be expected, the activities of these health departments were determined by the current epidemiologic theories that placed particular emphasis on the elimination of sanitary nuisances. For example, at the midpoint of the nineteenth century the population of New York City had reached 300,000. Its board of health was concerned only with crowded living conditions, dirty streets, and the regulation of public baths, slaughterhouses, and pigsties.

## THE SHATTUCK REPORT [17]

In terms of American public health history the midnineteenth century is most notable for the extraordinary *Report of the Sanitary Commission of Massachusetts*. Its author, Lemuel Shattuck (1793-1859), a most unusual man, led the diversified life of teacher, historian, book dealer, sociologist, statistician, and finally legislator in the state assembly. Although in a medical sense a layman, he had a keen interest in sanitary reform, originating apparently with his work when gathering and tabulating the vital statistics of Boston. Because of his persistent complaints regarding the current lack of sanitary progress, he was appointed chairman of a legislative committee for the study of health and sanitary problems in the commonwealth. From this committee and essentially from Shattuck's pen issued the aforementioned report. With remarkable insight and foresight the report included a detailed consideration not only of the present and future public health needs of Massachusetts but also of its component parts and of the nation as a whole. This most remarkable of all American public health documents, if published today, in many respects would still be ahead of its time.

The content of the Sanitary Commission report may be appreciated in its true light when it is realized that at the time it was written there existed no national or state public health programs, and such local health agencies as by that time had been organized were still in an embryonic stage of development. Medical practice in general was then far from scientific; facilities for medical training were few and in a most confused state; and provisions for nurses' training was entirely lacking. Almost another half century was to pass before the spectacular era of Pasteur, Koch, and the other contributors to the golden age of bacteriology would begin.

Among the many recommendations made by Shattuck a century and a quarter ago were those for the establishment of state and local boards of health, a system of sanitary police or inspectors, the collection and analysis of vital statistics, a routine system for exchanging data and information, sanitation programs for towns and buildings, studies on the health of school children, studies of tuberculosis, the control of alcoholism, the supervision of mental disease, the sanitary supervision and study of problems of immigrants, the erection of model tenements, public bathhouses, and washhouses, the control of smoke nuisances, the control of food adulteration, the exposure of nostrums, the preaching of health from pulpits, the establishment of nurses' training schools, the teaching of sanitary science in medical schools, and the inclusion of preventive medicine in clinical practice, with routine physical examinations and family records of illness.

Unfortunately, although this document laid down the principal ideas and modes of action that would ultimately form the basis of much of today's public health practice, its importance was not appreciated at the time it was submitted, and it was destined to lie dormant for nearly a quarter of a century. One of the earliest appraisals of it was given in 1876 by Bowditch,[9] first president of the State Board of Health of Massachusetts, in an address before the International Medical Congress at Philadelphia:

The report fell flat from the printer's hand. It remained almost unnoticed by the community or by the profession for many years, and its recommendations were ignored. Finally, in 1869, a State Board of Health of laymen and physicians, exactly as Mr. Shattuck recommended, was established by Massachusetts. Dr. Derby, its first secretary, looked to this admirable document as his inspiration and support. In giving this high honor to Mr. Shattuck, I do not wish to forget or to undervalue the many and persistent efforts made by a few physicians, among whom stands pre-eminent Dr. Edward Jarvis, and occasionally by the Massachusetts Medical Society, in urging the State authorities to inaugurate and to sustain the ideas avowed by Mr. Shattuck. But there is no doubt that he, as a layman, quietly working, did more towards bringing Massachusetts to correct views on this subject than all other agencies whatsoever. Of Mr. Edwin Chadwick, I need say nothing. You all know him. Fortunately for himself, he has lived to see rich fruits from his labors. That was not granted to Mr. Shattuck.

The comparison of Shattuck, the American, and Chadwick, the Englishman, is of more than passing interest. Some lessons may be learned by comparing the effects of the work of the two men. Shattuck's report consisted essentially of straightforward, unembellished, unillustrated statements of fact, followed by specific and detailed recommendations. This is in contrast with Chadwick's *Report on an Inquiry into the Sanitary Condition of the Labouring Population of Great Britain,* which included many vivid descriptions of the appalling conditions in existence. The latter caused an immediate emotional response on the part of all who read or heard of the report. One wonders if Shattuck's report might have had a more immediate effect had it provided the reader with mental images of existing conditions for contrast with further mental images of desirable conditions attainable. Another point of contrast is that although Chadwick's report brought about a prompt reaction resulting in the establishment of a General Board of Health in 1848, the response was not long lasting. Chadwick's overenthusiasm and impatience demanded immediate action, for which the British people were not yet ready.[18] Certain aspects of this were discussed in Chapter 1. Considerable antagonism and resistance were generated in many quarters, resulting in the early demise of the General Board of Health after only 4 years of existence. This reversal caused an unfortunate delay in the ultimate development of a sound national health program in Great Britain. The reports of Chadwick and Shattuck, therefore, remarkable as they were, provide examples of administrative failure, one because of underpromotion and the other because of overpromotion.

## THE FIRST STATE HEALTH DEPARTMENT

The repeated outbreaks of yellow fever and other epidemic diseases caused the state of Louisiana in 1855 to set up a board or commission to deal with quarantine matters in the port of New Orleans. This has led some to claim priority for Louisiana in the establishment of a state board of health. However, in terms of the more usual concept of the general functions of a state board of health, it is generally considered that Massachusetts, despite its lack of response to Shattuck's recommendations, merits recognition for establishing the first true state board of health in 1869. The act creating it directed:

The board shall take cognizance of the interests of health and life among the citizens of this Commonwealth. They shall make sanitary investigations and inquires in respect to the people, the causes of disease, and especially of epidemics, and the sources of mortality and the effects of localities, employments, conditions and circumstances on the public health; and they shall gather such information in respect to these matters as they may deem proper, for diffusion among the people.*

In determining policy at early meetings, the board, under the leadership of Bowditch, decided to concern itself with public and professional education in matters of hygiene, various aspects of housing, investigations of various well-known diseases and measures for their partial or entire prevention, prevailing methods of slaughtering, sale of poisons, and conditions of the poor. It was decided also to send a circular letter to local boards of health to inquire about their powers and duties and to collect for publication the number and prevailing causes of deaths in the most populous cities and towns in the state. The board requested that each community designate a physician to act as correspondent. Patterson and Baker,[19] in discussing the early history of this board, made the pertinent observation that "one by-product of this correspondence was the beginning of a productive cooperation between the state and local authorities." One reads with annoyance of the merger in 1878 of the Massachusetts Department of Health with the Department of Lunacy and Charity because of political pressure and a desire for "economy." As a result, matters dealing with the public health were effectively submerged by the weight of the other two interests. Eventually the light was seen, and a sound program was made possible by reestablishment of the health agency as an entity.

It is interesting to note the establishment of the second state health department the next year, on the opposite side of the continent in California. By the end of the nineteenth century 38 other states had followed suit, to be joined during the early decades of the twentieth century by the remainder.

## THE QUARANTINE CONVENTIONS AND THE AMERICAN PUBLIC HEALTH ASSOCIATION

Other events of great public health potential were occurring in the midnineteenth century. Those concerned with the public health felt the need to maintain closer contact to solve

*Act of 1869, General Court of Massachusetts.

problems of mutual concern. Due especially to Wilson Jewell, the health officer of Philadelphia who had recently attended the Conference Sanitaire in Paris in 1851-1852, a series of National Quarantine Conventions was called.[20] The first, a 3-day meeting, was held in Philadelphia in 1857. It organized itself formally, and the 54 members in attendance discussed many subjects of common interest, including prevention of the introduction of epidemic diseases such as typhus, cholera, and yellow fever, port quarantine, the importance of stagnant and putrid bilge water, putrescible matters, filthy bedding, baggage and clothing of immigrant passengers, and air that has been confined. It recommended that immigrants not previously protected against smallpox be vaccinated. The second convention, held in Baltimore in 1858, was noteworthy for proposals for a uniform system of quarantine laws and the organization of a Committee on Internal Hygiene or the Sanitary Arrangement of Cities. In these days when much is made of "multidisciplinary and consumer representation," it is interesting that 42 of the 86 persons attending the second convention were not physicians. Two more conventions were held, New York in 1859 and Boston in 1860, before the outbreak of the American Civil War precluded further meetings.

The seed planted by the quarantine conventions by no means died. On April 18, 1872, after the termination of the war, 10 men, including Elisha Harris and Stephen Smith, met informally in New York City to reactivate interest in national meetings for the consideration of public health matters. Meeting again at Long Beach, N. J., in September with several additional representatives, they chose a name, adopted a constitution, and elected Dr. Stephen Smith first president of the American Public Health Association. In a later discussion of the early days Smith[21] said, "The American Public Health Association had its origin in that natural desire which thinkers and workers in the same fields, whether of business or philanthropy, or the administration of civil trusts, have for mutual council, advice and cooperation."

Since the National Quarantine Conventions were necessarily concerned primarily with quarantine matters, the formation of the American Public Health Association represented a considerable advance in that the scope of interest was greatly broadened. This was reflected in its earliest meetings, wherein were presented papers on many aspects of sanitation, on the transmission and prevention of diseases, on longevity, on hospital hygiene, and on other diverse subjects. In addition, discussions on quarantine were held. Through the 100 years of its existence, the association has served its members and the public well, providing a common fount of knowledge, information, and encouragement and a means of presenting a united front for the improvement of the health of America.

## THE NATIONAL BOARD OF HEALTH

One of the earliest concerns of both the quarantine conventions and the American Public Health Association was with the need for a national board of health. Smillie[22] described the circumstances that led to the ultimate formation of such a national board, its controversial 4 years' existence, and its painful, premature death from deliberate financial starvation. Meetings were held in Washington in 1875 attended by representatives of many state and city health departments for the purpose of considering plans for the formation of a federal health organization. The meeting degenerated into a jurisdictional dispute involving the army, the navy, and the Marine Hospital Service, the three existing federal agencies that already provided certain services in this field. In 1878 a devastating epidemic of yellow fever swept over much of the country. Since the disease was known to have entered through the port of New Orleans, the Louisiana authorities were charged with laxity. Public sentiment was aroused; as a result, not only the army and the Marine Hospital Service but also the American Public Health Association sponsored legislation for the establishment of a national health department. It was the bill proposed by the American Public Health Association that was finally passed by Congress in 1879. This bill transferred from the Marine Hospital Service all health duties and powers, including maritime quarantine. The act created a board of presidential appointees consisting of seven physicians and representatives from the army, the navy, the Marine Hospital Service, and the Department of Justice. About 2½ months later another act was passed that gave the board extensive quarantine powers and authorized an appropriation of $500,000 for its work. This second act included an unfortunate clause that limited the powers to 4 years, necessitating a reenactment of the bill in order for the work to continue.

The membership of the first board was notable, including J. L. Cabell, J. S. Billings, J. T. Turner, P. H. Bailhoche, S. M. Bemiss, H. I. Bowditch, R. W. Mitchell, Stephen Smith, S. F. Phillips, and T. S. Verdi. The 4 years of life of the National Board of Health were marked by an ambitious and efficient program of studies and services marred by the persistent and vociferous opposition of Joseph Jones, secretary of the Louisiana Board of Health, who objected to the presence of "Federal agents and spies" and seized every opportunity to belittle and misrepresent the activities of the National Board of Health. Intent as he was on destroying the new organization, he was saved the trouble by John Hamilton, the Surgeon General of the Marine Hospital Service. Hamilton, although professionally inept, possessed considerable political astuteness. Realizing that the National Board of Health would pass out of existence unless the law of 1879 was reenacted in 1883 and that in such an event its powers and functions would revert to the Marine Hospital Service, he worked quietly and effectively to prevent reenactment. Charging misuse of funds, extravagance, and incompetence, he succeeded in bringing the National Board of Health to an untimely death.

One of the members of the board, Stephen Smith, from the first had favored conferring all national public health duties and powers on the National Board of Health but incorporating in it the officers, staff, and activities of the Marine Hospital Service and any other agencies concerned with public health matters. Smillie[22] analyzed the situation in the following terms:

He foresaw that Congress would lose interest in the National Board of Health, but would continue to support a service agency that had full-time career officers and was incorporated as an integral part of national government machinery.

In retrospect we realize that Stephen Smith was right. The unwieldy board of experts, each living in a different community and attempting to carry out administrative duties, with no cohesion, no real unity of opinion and no central authority, was an impossible administrative machine. A centrally guided service, such as actually developed, had unity and purpose, but unfortunately lacked intelligent leadership. The public health policies for a great nation for many years were determined solely by the opinions—sometimes the whims and personal prejudices—of a single individual. It would have been a much better plan if Dr. Stephen Smith's half formulated plan of 1883 could have been carried out, thus salvaging the really important features of the National Board of Health and incorporating in it a service agency with a full-time personnel, an esprit de corps, and a strong central administrative machine. The members of the Board of Health selected by the President of the United States because they were public health experts, should have been continued as a Board of Health and should have served as a permanent policy-forming body, advising and aiding their administrative officer. The Marine Hospital Service was the most logical existing national agency with which to vest this national public health function. The Surgeon General should have been made the executive officer of the board, and all actual administrative responsibility should have been centered in him. It was a great opportunity to have organized a close-knit, effective National Health Service, but there was no single man who had the vision or the power to solve this simple problem.

This provides much food for thought and guidance at the present time, when ironically active attempts are underway to establish a separate National Department of Health and at the same time to scuttle the time-proved effective Public Health Service.

## THE PUBLIC HEALTH SERVICE

To consider the history and development of the Public Health Service, the most important federal health agency, it is necessary to retrace our steps to the year 1798. The United States of America had just come into existence. Although still largely undeveloped, it was already vigorous and enterprising, one manifestation of which was its expanding maritime trade. Sailing ships for world commerce were coming down the ways at an ever-increasing rate, and the maritime service was becoming one of the nation's most important resources.

The farmer of Virginia and the tradesman of Boston had roots that were firmly established in their respective communities, which they supported through taxes. The merchant seaman on the other hand, led a precarious existence somewhat resembling that of the itinerant or vagabond. Often he had neither a permanent abode nor a permanent route. His ship was the closest approach to a home, and his ship might be in New York harbor one week, in Charleston the next, and in Liverpool within a month. Despite this, he too was an American citizen and deserved whatever security and assistance his nation could find possible to provide its citizens. For a period, however, things did not work out that way. Like anyone the sailor was subject to injury or illness. In fact, because of the unusual hazards of his occupation, he was subject to greater than average risk. Furthermore, he was underpaid, and whatever he received at the end of a journey was more often than not quickly removed from him in the taverns and brothels that thrived in the vicinity of the wharves. As a result, he usually found it difficult or impossible to pay for whatever medical or hospital care he needed. Because he paid no local or state taxes and generally was not a member in good standing of whatever port city he happened to be in when ill, responsibility for him was usually avoided by the local authorities.

The young American Congress, becoming conscious of this undesirable state of affairs, passed the Marine Hospital Service Act in June 1798, which authorized the President to appoint physicians in each port to furnish medical and hospital care for sick and disabled seamen. Twenty cents a month was deducted from the pay of each man, the money being collected from the paymasters by the customs officers of the Treasury Department. Since the money was placed in the custody of the Treasury Department, there came about the anomalous situation whereby until 1935 most federal public health services were carried out under the egis of the Treasury Department. The small sum of 20 cents a month, subsequently increased to 40 cents a month, is of particular interest in that it actually represented a sickness insurance payment and provided the precedent for the first prepaid comprehensive medical and hospital insurance plan in the world, under the administrative supervision of what eventually became a public health agency. In 1884 the tax of 40 cents a month was discontinued and replaced by a tonnage tax. The tonnage tax is still collected but now goes into the general Treasury, from which the hospitals are supported through appropriations to the Public Health Service.

At first the physicians who served the plan were also engaged in the private practice of medicine, but before long the need became so great that physicians were employed full time. Originally, sailors who needed hospital care were placed in whatever public or private hospitals existed at the ports. However, as in the case of the physicians, the demand for hospital services soon became so great that within 2 years (1800) the first marine hospital was constructed at Norfolk, Va. This was followed by similar hospitals throughout the country, at first at certain seaports and later at a number of places along inland waterways. With improvement and extension of other sources of hospitalization, the need for Public Health Service hospitals has decreased. At present there are eight: Staten Island, Baltimore, New Orleans, Seattle, San Francisco, Norfolk, Boston, and Galveston. Outpatient facilities are operated in 38 cities. The Public Health Service also maintains contract arrangements in many communities, where the use of nonservice facilities is economically more feasible. In addition, a large number of hospitals, community health centers, and other health facilities are operated exclusively for American Indians and Eskimos by the Indian Health Service. A clinical treatment and clinical research center for drug addicts and certain mental patients is operated at Lexington, Ky., by the National Institute of Mental Health. In addition, the Public Health Service operates The National Leprosarium at Carville, La.

Through time, eligibility for admittance to Public Health Service Hospitals has been broadened, and now United States merchant seamen constitute fewer than 50% of all patients. Eligibility now includes the following:

1. Seamen employed on vessels of the United States, registered, enrolled, and licensed under the maritime laws thereof, other than canal boats engaged in coastal trade
2. Enrollees in the United States Maritime Service on active duty and members of the Merchant Marine Cadet Corps
3. Cadets at state maritime academies or on state training ships
4. Federal Civil Service employees injured or taken ill in line of duty and falling within purview of regulations governing the administration of Federal Employee's Compensation Act
5. Officers and enlisted men of the United States Coast Guard, active or retired, and their dependents
6. Officers of United States Public Health Service, active or retired, and their dependents
7. Ships' officers and crew members of vessels of the United States Environmental Science Services Administration (formerly, Coast and Geodetic Survey), active and retired, and their dependents
8. Officers and enlisted men of the United States army, navy, marine corps, and air force, active or retired, and their dependents
9. Any person requiring immunization for yellow fever

Foreign seamen and nonbeneficiary emergency cases are charged for outpatient and/or inpatient medical care according to rates established by the Office of Management and Budget.

At present, steps are underway to phase out direct operation of hospitals and other clinical facilities by the Public Health Service. This move has been accelerated by the large number of persons provided for by various public and private medical and hospital insurance plans.

It is interesting that a medical director or supervising surgeon for the Public Health Service was not appointed until 1870. Compensation at the time amounted to a salary of $2,000, plus travel expenses. This position was later to become that of Surgeon General.

The growing concern of the federal and state governments with the need for preventing the introduction of epidemic diseases led to the passage in 1878 of the first port quarantine act. Entry into the country was limited to its ports, and as a consequence it was readily realized that the ports were the nation's first line of defense against epidemic diseases. Since the incidence of these diseases was invariably greater at ports, the physicians of the Marine Hospital Service had more opportunity to see and become acquainted with them. In addition, since epidemics usually began at the ports and frequently got out of hand, the states had developed the custom of asking or authorizing the federally employed Marine Hospital Service physicians to aid in the control of local situations. It was logical therefore that the responsibility for carrying out the new port quarantine activities should have been placed in the Marine Hospital Service. In recent years this has been extended to include international airports.

The law of 1878 embodied another important feature in authorizing the investigation of the origin and causes of epidemic diseases, especially yellow fever and cholera, and the best methods of preventing their introduction and spread. With little delay attempts were begun to prevent the entry of communicable disease by means of control measures applied at the ports of origin to those who might potentially be carriers of disease. Marine Hospital Service physicians were attached to the offices of the U. S. consular service in major foreign ports, and a system of reporting communicable disease through the consular service was put into effect. In 1890 domestic quarantine was added to provide interstate control of communicable disease. This was an immediate outgrowth of another particularly devastating epidemic of yellow fever that entered at New Orleans and spread throughout the Mississippi Valley. Between the time of the Louisiana Purchase in 1803 and the beginning of the twentieth century, New Orleans experienced no fewer than 37 severe epidemics of yellow fever in addition to constantly recurring outbreaks of cholera, plague, and smallpox.

In 1890 Congress gave the Marine Hospital Service authority to inspect all immigrants. This was intended first to bar lunatics and others unable to care for themselves, but the following year "persons suffering from loathsome and contagious diseases" were added. In that year Congress also provided quasi-military status for the personnel of the Marine Hospital Service so that the men were given commissions and uniforms. The Hygienic Laboratory was established in 1901. Fortunately, from the start it was developed with such skill, imagination, and foresight that it soon became one of the world's leading centers of public health and medical research. Originally organized in three divisions of chemistry, zoology, and pharmacology, its functions were expanded in 1912 by an act authorizing the laboratory to "study and investigate the diseases of man and conditions influencing the origin and spread thereof including sanitation and sewage, and the pollution directly or indirectly of navigable streams and lakes of the United States and may from time to time issue information in the form of publications for the use of the public." Under consistently able direction the Hygienic Laboratory, which was later to become the National Institutes of Health, attracted and developed a steady stream of outstanding investigators, including Carter, Sternberg, Rosenau, Goldberger, Frost, Leake, Armstrong, Stiles, Lumsden, Francis, Spencer, Maxcy, and Dyer, to name only a few. The contributions of these men and their co-workers caused William H. Welch to state publicly that there was no research institute in the world that was making such distinguished contributions to basic research in biology, medicine, and public health. In recent years several members of its staff have been recipients of much coveted Nobel, Lasker, and similar awards. The subsequent development of the National Institutes of Health will be discussed later.

In 1902, recognizing that the Marine Hospital Service had come of age, Congress renamed it the Public Health and Marine Hospital Service and gave it a definite form of organization under the direction of a Surgeon General. The re-organization act was of further significance in that for the first time the Surgeon General was authorized and directed to call an annual conference of all state and territorial health officers. In 1912 the service experienced another change in title, this time to the United States Public Health Service.

From this point on the Public Health Service grew rapidly under the impetus of an increasingly complex society, two great wars, and an economic depression. In 1917 the National Leprosarium at Carville, La., was established. In the same year the service became responsible for the physical and mental examination of all arriving aliens. The year 1917 was also noteworthy for a congressional appropriation of $25,000 to the Public Health Service for studies and demonstrations in rural health work in cooperation with states. This modest appropriation represented the beginning of a new administrative approach in federal-state public health relationships. In 1918, because of problems brought to public awareness by the entry of the United States into World War I, a Division of Venereal Diseases was created, with power to cooperate with state departments of health for the control and prevention of these diseases. In 1929 a Narcotics Division, later expanded to the Division of Mental Hygiene, was created with hospital facilities at Lexington, Ky., and Fort Worth, Texas, for the confinement and treatment of narcotic addicts.

The passage of the Federal Social Security Act in 1935 set in motion many developments of far-reaching consequence. Title VI of the act, which relates to the Public Health Service, was written "for the purpose of assisting states, counties, health districts, and other political subdivisions of the states in establishing and maintaining adequate public health service, including the training of personnel for state and local health work. . . ." Associated with the act was an appropriation that made possible grants-in-aid to the states and territories according to budgets submitted to the Surgeon General and approved by him. This brought with it a most difficult administrative problem for the Public Health Service, which has constantly attempted to determine an equitable basis on which to distribute grant-in-aid funds. Although subject to frequent adaptation, an attempt has been made to allocate these funds on the basis of four factors: (1) population, (2) public health problems, (3) economic need, and (4) training of public health personnel. The method of allocation has carried with it an educational value for state legislators, since considerable proportions of the grants-in-aid must be matched by state and local appropriations. Results were rapidly forthcoming. More than a year after the funds were first made available not only was there a great increase in the number of new local health departments but in addition 19 states that did not already have such service set up central facilities for the promotion and supervision of local health administration; 33 state health departments strengthened their public health engineering forces; 11 states added new units for the investigation and promotion of industrial hygiene; preventable disease control groups were materially strengthened in 24 states; laboratory facilities were augmented in 27 states; 19 states made needed improvements in the personnel and equipment for vital statistics; public health nursing was strengthened either directly or indirectly in almost all states; 11 states provided special measures for syphilis control; and 13 states provided measures for the control of tuberculosis.[23] In 1938 a second Federal Venereal Disease Control Act was passed, designed to promote the investigation and control of venereal diseases and to provide funds for assistance to state and local health agencies in establishing and maintaining adequate measures to that end.

In 1939, as part of President Roosevelt's program for the reorganization and consolidation of federal services, a Federal Security Agency was created for the purpose of bringing together a large part of the health, welfare, and educational services of the federal government. After 141 years, only 9 years less than the life of the nation itself, the Public Health Service left the now anachronistic administrative jurisdiction of the Treasury Department. At that time the service had the following 8 divisions, each under an assistant surgeon general:

Division of Scientific Research (including the National Institute of Health and the National Cancer Institute)
Division of Domestic Quarantine (including State Relations)
Division of Foreign and Insular Quarantine
Division of Sanitary Reports and Statistics
Division of Marine Hospitals and Relief
Division of Mental Hygiene
Division of Venereal Disease Control
Division of Personnel and Accounts

Since that time, to achieve greater organi-

zational response and efficiency and to bring the benefits of research and federal health legislation more quickly and effectively to the people of the nation, the Public Health Service has undergone several reorganizations in 1944, 1954, 1963, 1968, and 1973.[24,25] As a result of the last, the Public Health Service consists of six components: (1) the Center for Disease Control, (2) the Food and Drug Administration, (3) the Health Resources Administration, (4) the Health Services Administration, (5) the National Institutes of Health, and (6) the Alcoholism, Drug Abuse and Mental Health Administration (Fig. 11-4).

Meanwhile, many other developments of consequence occurred. In 1946 the Congress passed the Hospital Services and Construction (Hill-Burton) Act, which placed on the Public Health Service administrative responsibility for a nationwide program of hospital and health center construction. Each year since 1947 the Congress has appropriated substantial amounts of monies for this purpose. The federal contributions had to be matched by one third to two thirds state and local funds. Through time, increased emphasis was placed on loans at favorable rates rather than outright grants. In 1954 the Congress enlarged the program to permit federal assistance in the construction of other types of health facilities as well as hospitals and health centers. Included were general hospitals, mental hospitals, tuberculosis hospitals, chronic disease hospitals, public health centers, diagnostic and treatment centers, rehabilitation facilities, nursing homes, state health laboratories, and nurses' training facilities. The construction challenge is now considered met, and a shift is underway toward a program of loans for improvement and modernization.

The research activities of the Public Health Service date back about three quarters of a century to a one-room Laboratory of Hygiene in the Marine Hospital on Staten Island that was devoted to bacteriologic studies of returning seamen. This grew slowly to become the National Hygienic Laboratory, later renamed the National Institute of Health in Bethesda, Md., about 10 miles from Washington. From these humble beginnings has grown the greatest medical research center in the world. In 1937 the Congress indicated its concern over a rapidly growing health problem by passing the National Cancer Act, which provided for the establishment of a National Cancer Institute for research into the cause, diagnosis, and treatment of cancer, for assistance to public and private agencies involved with the problem, and for the promotion of the most effective methods of prevention and treatment of the disease. In 1946 the National Mental Health Act was passed. This measure authorized $7.5 million for the construction and equipment of hospital and laboratory facilities to be operated by the Public Health Service as a stimulating center for research and training in the field of mental health; $10 million for grants to states; and an additional $1 million for demonstrations and personnel to assist the states.

In 1948 the National Heart Institute (subsequently the Heart and Lung Institute) was authorized by Congress, and three other institutes—the Microbiological Institute, the Experimental Biology and Medicine Institute (these two joined in 1955 to form the National Institute of Allergy and Infectious Diseases), and the National Institute of Dental Research—were established by regrouping existing units. The National Institute of Health thus became the National *Institutes* of Health.

In 1949 the activities of the Mental Hygiene Division were transferred from the Bureau of Medical Services to the National Institutes of Health to form the National Institute of Mental Health. As a result of various program additions and organizational changes, it is now a separate entity, the Alcoholism, Drug Abuse and Mental Health Administration. In 1950 the National Institute of Neurological Diseases and Blindness was founded, and in 1959 the National Institute of Arthritis and Metabolic Diseases came into being. In 1962 legislation raised the Division of General Medical Sciences to institute status and also established an Institute of Child Health and Human Development. In 1966 a Division of Environmental Health Sciences was established in the Public Health Service; 3 years later it was given institute status and moved to the "Research Triangle" in North Carolina—a complex of public, private, and academic research and development organizations.

As time passed, an increasing amount of the National Institutes of Health's function came to be fulfilled by grants to universities and other extramural research centers. By now about 60% of its budget goes to finance research in such centers throughout the United States and abroad. By 1972 the institutes provided about 12,000 health research grants and contracts and about 9,500 health research, education, and training awards.

Because of the evergrowing grant programs, the National Institutes of Health found it necessary to establish certain organizations to handle them. In 1947 it formed a Division of Research Grants, in 1955 a Division of Research Services, and in 1962 a Division of Research Facilities and Resources. With the burgeoning of the pharmaceutical industry and market, it also became necessary to establish in 1955 a Division of Biological Standards.

To accelerate research and its confirmation and final application the Public Health Service in 1952 completed and opened the National Clinical Center on the grounds of the National Institutes of Health in Bethesda, Md. This is a research hospital of 516 beds, with twice as much space for laboratories (about 1,000 of them) as for patient care. Each institute of the National Institutes of Health has space for patients and laboratories in close proximity. Patients are admitted only when they meet the requirements of a particular study being conducted by one or more institutes. A patient chosen by a particular institute, for example, may be one of a group of patients having the same type of condition at the same stage and site. Often factors such as the patient's sex, age, and weight must also be taken into consideration. Patients may be accepted from any part of the country.

The planning and conduct of research in the National Clinical Center is the responsibility of each institute. When a problem is selected, the methods of approach are determined by a research team, which may include scientists from more than one institute and from other research organizations. Special provisions are made so that outstanding laboratory scientists and research physicians from other institutions in the United States or abroad may work in the clinical center for periods ranging from a few months to a year or more on problems of their own choosing. As a result, investigations involve numerous scientific fields and widely varying viewpoints, bringing laboratory and clinical workers into close daily association in a search for answers to both basic scientific and practical problems.

The staff of the National Clinical Center immediately responsible for the care of a patient maintains intimate working relationships with the physicians and institutions who send patients to the center. This professional liaison is so close that for all practical purposes the referring physician is a member of the research team, and the clinical center becomes a major addition to the resources available to the physician for the study and benefit of his patient. Through the years Congress has shown an intense and growing interest in health research. Appropriations have consistently increased to a present budget for the National Institutes of Health that approaches $2 billion.[27] It is also noteworthy that in 1965 the Congress authorized an additional $280 million for the construction of other health research laboratories throughout the nation during the following 3 years.

To return for a moment to 1956, another significant event was the transfer of the Army Medical Library to the Public Health Service, which has since established it as an expanded National Library of Medicine in an excellent structure on the grounds of the National Institutes of Health. In 1968 the library became a constituent of the institutes complex. An innovative activity at the library has been the development and implementation of the computer-based MEDLARS (Medical Literature Analysis and Retrieval System), which is a computerized bibliographic service to assist users in the library itself or in selected medical centers in the nation in obtaining prompt abstracts of material pertinent to their area of interest. It has become necessary because of the inability of conventional methods to keep current with the tremendous growth of medical literature. This development probably leads the way for the National Library of Medicine to become, among other things, a center for research in biomedical communications. It is intended to extend this service to centers in other nations by way of communications satellites. In this regard a Division of Computer Research and Technology has been developed as a component of the National Institutes of Health.

Mention should be made of several other important post-World War II additions to the resources of the Public Health Service. One was the development of the National Office of Vital Statistics, later renamed the National Center for Health Statistics. This valuable staff unit provides a vast amount of detailed data concerning health, illness, injuries, and death. Of great significance was the establishment during World War II of the Communicable Disease Center in Atlanta, Ga. This renowned institution, now known as the National Center for Disease Control, has grown to become not only one of the world's great epidemiologic centers but also an outstanding training center for various types of health personnel and a leading center for health communications and educational methods. Another important postwar development was the establishment in 1954 of the Robert A. Taft Sanitary Engineering Center in Cincinnati as a center for research and training in various aspects of environmental health. In 1966 this institution and the responsibility for water pollution control were transferred to a new Federal Water Pollution Administration in the Department of Interior and subsequently in 1971, in company with most of the other environmental programs of the Public Health Service, to a new Environmental Protection Agency. In 1971 a National Center for Toxicological Research was established at Pine Bluff, Ark., under the direction of the Food and Drug Administration, which by this time had become part of the Public Health Service. About the same time a National Institute on Alcohol Abuse and Alcoholism was also established.

Mention has been made of the growing interest of Congress in health affairs. This has by no means been limited to research. In fact the past several Congresses have raised repeated questions about the application of the growing fund of knowledge in the health and medical field—how to close the gap between the acquisition of knowledge and its application for the welfare of the people. The Eighty-ninth Congress was especially notable in this regard. It had the distinction of being known as the most "health minded" Congress in the history of the United States.[26] An astounding number of legislative acts were passed that, combined with the highly significant acts passed by subsequent Congresses, if wisely used, will completely recast the nature, structure, and effectiveness of public health, medical care, and social security in the United States.

Significant health legislation enacted by Congress between 1965 and 1973 includes the following:

The Drug Abuse Control Amendments (P.L. 89-74)
The Federal Cigarette Labeling and Advertising Act (P.L. 89-92)
The Mental Retardation Facilities and Community Mental Health Centers Construction Act Amendments (P.L. 89-105)
The Community Health Services Extension Amendments (P.L. 89-109)

The Health Research Facilities Amendments (P.L. 89-115)

The Public Works and Economic Development Act (P.L. 89-136)

The Water Quality Act (P.L. 89-234)

The Heart Disease, Cancer, and Stroke Amendments (Regional Medical Programs) (P.L. 89-239)

The Clean Air Act Amendments and the Solid Waste Disposal Act (P.L. 89-272)

The Health Professions Educational Assistance Amendments (P.L. 89-290)

The Medical Library Assistance Act (P.L. 89-291)

The Appalachian Regional Development Act (P.L. 89-4)

The Older Americans Act (P.L. 89-73)

The Social Security Amendments (Medicare, Medicaid, Comprehensive Child Health Care) (P.L. 89-97)

The Vocational Rehabilitation Amendments (P.L. 89-333)

The Housing and Urban Development Act (P.L. 89-117)

The Extended Comprehensive Health Planning and Public Health Services Amendments (P.L. 89-749)

The Allied Health Professions Personnel Training Act (P.L. 89-751)

The Demonstration Cities and Metropolitan Development Act (P.L. 89-754)

The Air Quality Act (P.L. 90-148)

The Vocational Rehabilitation Amendments (P.L. 90-99 and P.L. 90-391)

The Clinical Laboratories Improvement Act (P.L. 90-174)

The Social Security Amendment (P.L. 90-248)

The Health Manpower Act (P.L. 90-490)

The Older Americans Act (extension) (P.L. 91-69)

The Child Protection Act (P.L. 91-113)

The Federal Coal Mine Health and Safety Act (P.L. 91-173)

The Occupational Health and Safety Act (P.L. 91-596)

The Migrant Health Amendments (P.L. 91-209)

The Community Mental Health Centers Amendments (P.L. 91-211)

The Comprehensive Drug Abuse Prevention and Control Act (P.L. 91-513)

The Developmental Disabilities Services and Facilities Construction Amendments (P.L. 91-517)

The Drug Abuse Education Act (P.L. 91-527)

The Family Planning Service Amendments (P.L. 91-572)

The National Environmental Policy Act (P.L. 91-190)

The Environmental Quality Improvement Act (P.L. 91-224)

The Environmental Education Act (P.L. 91-516)

The Environmental Protection Agency Personnel Act (P.L. 91-604)

The Comprehensive Alcoholism Prevention Treatment and Rehabilitation Act (P.L. 91-616)

The Lead-Based Paint Poisoning Prevention Act (P.L. 91-695, Sec. 401)

The Social Security Amendments Act (P.L. 92-5)

The Comprehensive Health Manpower Training Act (P.L. 92-158)

The Nurse Training Act (P.L. 92-158)

The National Cancer Act (P.L. 92-218)

The Communicable Disease Act (P.L. 92-449)

The Consumer Product Safety Act (P.L. 92-573)

The National Sickle Cell Anemia Protection Act (P.L. 92-294)

The Drug Abuse Office and Treatment Act (P.L. 92-255)

The Heart, Lung and Blood Act (P.L. 92-423)

The Cooley's Anemia Act (P.L. 92-414)

The Uniformed Services University of the Health Services Act (P.L. 92-426)

The General Revenue Sharing Act (P.L. 92-512)

The Social Security Amendments Act (P.L. 92-603)

The Emergency Medical Services Act (P.L. 93-154)

The Loans for Nursing Homes and Intensive Care Facilities Act (P.L. 93-204)

The Health Maintenance Organization Act (P.L. 93-222)

The Social Security Amendments Act (includes the Professional Standards Review Organization provision) (P.L. 93-233)

The Sudden Infant Death Syndrome Act (P.L. 93-270)

The Child Abuse Prevention and Treatment Act (P.L. 93-247)

The preceding partial list[28] of recent federal health legislation represents a formidable health legislative record indeed! Its significance was well indicated by Forgotson[29]:

The deep and long-term significance of the 1965 federal health legislation . . . lies in the changing role of government in the direction of widening the responsibility of the public sector (as exemplified by the Medicare amendments) and in developing new patterns of medical service and continuing education (as exemplified by the Regional Medical Programs). The introduction of systems engineering and operations analysis into the total health endeavor will permit the development of sound priorities, effective controls, and improved administration. Comprehensive legislation covering every facet of resources and services makes 1965 the turning point in health legislation.

The cumulative effect of all the foregoing developments has been a remarkable growth in the size and usefulness of the health component of the Department of Health, Education, and Welfare. This growth may be illustrated in terms of expenditures. In 1900 the budget of the Marine Hospital Service was about $1.4 million; by 1950 it was almost $120 million; by 1960 it had reached about $300 million. By 1972 total federal expenditures for health totaled about $24 billion, of which about $4.5 billion was budgeted for the Public Health Service.

Through the years since 1798, great responsibilities have been placed on the Public Health Service. It is fortunately appropriate to state that throughout its long history the service has met its responsibilities and opportunities as a governmental agency remarkably well, as is readily evident from its admirable record. It is probable that no one in the nation passes a day without being affected by its efforts in some way. Currently the service is undergoing much study and change in company with the entire federal structure. Whatever the outcome in form or name those dedicated to its goals will continue to fulfill their responsibilities.

## THE CHILDREN'S BUREAU

The conception, establishment, and development of this specialized agency, The Children's Bureau, is worthy of considerable study by students of public administration. Although appearing on the surface to be concerned with matters of a noncontroversial nature, the bureau from its inception was a principal in many disputes and the target of several administrative and ideologic struggles.

The idea of a separate Children's Bureau was first suggested to President Theodore Roosevelt in New York City.[30] As pointed out later by Lathrop,[31] who served as the first chief of the bureau from 1912 to 1921, it was no coincidence that "this bureau was first urged by women who have lived long in settlements and who by that experience have learned to know as well as any person in this country certain aspects of dumb misery which they desired through some governmental agency to make articulate and intelligible."

The support of numerous protagonists was obtained with little delay, among them the National Consumers League, the National Child Labor Committee, and many national women's organizations and church groups. Arguing for a center of research and information concerning the welfare of mothers and children, they maintained an active lobby and pressure group in Washington until their goal was ultimately obtained. One of their most effective arguments was that the federal government had already set a precedent by establishing centers of research and information in other fields relating to national resources and that it might well become similarly concerned with its most important resource, the mothers and children of the nation. Between 1906 and 1912 many bills concerned with the establishment of a Children's Bureau were introduced and extensive hearings held on each. Both President Theodore Roosevelt and, later, President Taft gave support to the movement, which incurred little opposition. Eventually Congress was spurred to final action and passed a measure sponsored by Senator Borah on April 9, 1912.

One of the reasons for delay was controversy over the placement of the bureau in the federal governmental structure. The three possibilities suggested were the Bureau of Labor and the Bureau of the Census, both in the Department of Commerce and Labor, and the Bureau of Education, in the Department of the Interior. It should be noted that the United States Public Health Service, then a part of the Treasury Department, was not considered. This may have been because of the submergence of the health aspects by the broader social service aspects of the proposed bureau. The failure on the part of the Public Health Service to concern itself with the problem at the time was to lay the groundwork for subsequent controversies over administrative jurisdiction and organization.

The Act of 1912, which established the Children's Bureau,[32] placed it as an agency in the Department of Commerce and Labor. When this department was divided the following year, the bureau was retained by the Department of Labor. The act directed that the "said Bureau shall investigate and report . . . upon all matters pertaining to the welfare of children and child life, among all classes of people, and shall especially investigate the questions of infant mortality, the birth rate, orphanages, juvenile courts, desertions, dangerous occupations, accidents, and diseases of children, employment, legislation affecting children in the several states and territories." Although originally given authority merely to *investigate* and *report*, the Children's Bureau trained a highly technical staff of experts who rapidly gained in experience. The bureau thus became the natural agency to be entrusted with new programs dealing with problems of maternal and child welfare. During the early years of its existence, the bureau, in accordance with Congressional direction, followed a path of extensive and fruitful scientific research and dissemination of information. Many studies were made of the effect of income, housing, employment, and other factors on the infant and maternal mortality rates. These studies led to the White House Conferences on child health, the first of which was held in 1919. Evidence gathered in some of the investigations was used by the National Child Labor Committee in obtaining the passage of the Federal Child-Labor Law in 1915. This law, with the Children's Bureau designated as the administering agency, was effective from 1917 to 1918, when it was declared unconstitutional by the Supreme Court.

Study of maternal and infant care problems of rural areas led to the introduction of proposed national legislation to encourage the establishment of maternal and child welfare programs by means of grants-in-aid to the states. The Children's Bureau, designated in the bills as the administering and supervising agency, quickly found itself the subject of attacks from several quarters. It was argued that the adoption of the Sheppard-Towner Bill would provide an entering wedge for socialized medicine, that it would centralize power in the hands of federal bureaucrats, and that personal, family, and states' rights would be violated. The American Medical Association, the Anti-Suffragists, the Sentinels of the Republic, and several other organizations arrayed themselves in opposition.

During the hearings a controversy that had begun to smolder between the Public Health Service and the Children's Bureau broke through. Some of the opponents of the bill were willing to compromise by favoring administration by the Public Health Service. The decision depended on whether the chief concern of the bill was with health or with general child welfare. Congress, deciding on the broader viewpoint, retained the Children's Bureau as the administering agency when final approval was given in 1921. One authority[33] has pointed out that unquestionably the bureau was able to maintain its position "by right of discovery and occupation and that the Public Health Service had been derelict in not promoting this type of work with sufficient vigor to maintain its belated claim to jurisdiction." It has been observed[34] that this conclusion merits reading and rereading by public health officers today. When the suggestion of a governmental health plan arises, one of the first concerns is with the agency of ad-ministration and that control by right of occupation has occurred more often than not in government.

The Sheppard-Towner Act established a pattern for maternal and child health programs throughout the country. It provided for federal assistance to states in the form of grants-in-aid for use in attacking problems of maternal and infant welfare and mortality. The states were given authority to initiate and to administer their own plans subject to approval by a Federal Board of Maternity and Infant Hygiene, consisting of the Chief of the Children's Bureau, the Surgeon General of the Public Health Service, and the Commissioner of Education. Prior to the passage of the act, 32 states had established divisions or bureaus of child hygiene. During the following 2 years an additional 15 states developed programs of this nature. Although it is difficult to conclusively prove a causative relationship, the Children's Bureau is generally given major credit for the increased interest and action.

The original act provided for a 5-year program. In 1926 a bill was introduced for the extension of the act to 7 years. This provided opponents with another opportunity for attack. The 2-year extension, although granted, signaled the end of the program, further efforts to continue it being fruitless. The importance of the federal aid was well illustrated by the fact that after expiration of the program 35 states decreased appropriations, 9 states eliminated appropriations, and only 5 states reported increases for the maternal and child health program.

With the adoption of the Social Security Act in 1935 the Children's Bureau not only regained its lost functions but added to them. Under Title V of the Social Security Act the Children's Bureau was given responsibility for the administration of programs dealing with maternal and child health, crippled children, and child welfare services. To implement these ends the bureau was allotted an annual budget of $8.17 million for grants-in-aid exclusive of administrative costs. In 1939 this sum was increased to $11 million and in 1946 to $22 million. Within 10 months after the grants-in-aid became available all of the 48 states, the District of Columbia, Alaska, and Hawaii submitted requests and plans for approval. In this way state maternal and child health programs received a much needed transfusion.

Through time there has been ample evidence of the success of the pioneering and stimulating efforts of the Children's Bureau. Thus in 1940 federal contributions accounted for 48% of the total sum spent for maternal and child health activities; since then, state and local governments have assumed increasing proportions of the costs.

With the entrance of the United States into World War II and the subsequent draft of a large proportion of the male population, many wives, expectant mothers, and infants found themselves in somewhat precarious economic positions, reflected in their inability to pay for private obstetric and medical care. Congress, becoming aware of the problem in 1943, decided to take action and established the Emergency Maternity and Infant Care Program, which functioned throughout the war years.[34] It considered the Children's Bureau to be the logical federal agency for the administration and supervision of the program of aid on which it decided. Once again the factor of prior interest and occupation decided the issue of administrative jurisdiction. The Children's Bureau had attempted, to the best of its ability and using some of its grants-in-aid funds, to do what it could to alleviate the situation. Congress decided to take action by means of supplementing the grants-in-aid funds of the bureau. As a result, a series of appropriation acts were passed involving a total of more than $130 million. The use of these sums made possible the provision of much needed obstetric care for about 1.2 million expectant mothers and pediatric care for about 200,000 infants. An incidental but significant result was that the staffs of the Children's Bureau and of many state health departments obtained an invaluable experience in medical care administration.

The Children's Bureau continued to expand its leadership in many fields, including audiology, perinatal mortality, prematurity, rheumatic fever, epilepsy, cerebral palsy, mental retardation, juvenile delinquency, nutrition of growth and development, problems of children of migratory workers, and children's dentistry.[35] It shared in the momentous legislative advances of the mid-1960s. Because of increased awareness and concern about the relatively high rate of perinatal mortality as well as premature births, handicapping conditions, and mental retardation, Congress passed the Maternal and Child Health and Mental Retardation Planning Amendments of 1963. This law authorized project grants to meet up to 75% of the costs of projects to provide comprehensive maternity

care for high risk mothers in low income families and care for their children. Two years later in 1965, when Section 532 of Title V, Part 4, of the Social Security Act was amended, provision was made for the development of high quality comprehensive health services for children and youth.

The combined objective of these two pieces of legislation was the reduction of maternal, infant, and child morbidity and mortality by assisting communities to organize and use their services and resources to maximum efficiency. For improved maternal and infant care, funds were used for the establishment of prenatal and postpartum clinics, hospitalization, medical salaries or fees, salaries of public health nurses, health education, and various other services. The Social Security Amendments of 1965 made possible some major departures from traditional public health services. Comprehensiveness and continuity of care are stressed. There is no separation of preventive and promotive health services from treatment and rehabilitation, nor are services limited to particular illness categories. All health problems of the children involved are taken care of by the program, either by direct services or by referral to appropriate resources in the area concerned. Medical, dental, and emotional health problems are all included, and since particular emphasis is placed on children of families often unaccustomed to seeking care, outreach casefinding is provided. These two programs are especially needed in areas where there are many people of low incomes and where there are likely to be few practitioners of medicine and dentistry, a situation common to city slums. These efforts are bringing convenient, well-organized, high-quality, comprehensive health services to those who need them the most and have obtained them the least. In the process, public health agencies of many cities have developed some new, interesting, and effective working relationships with medical schools and other organizations in their jurisdictions. Furthermore, wherever programs exist through the aegis of the Economic Opportunity Act to assist the socioeconomically disadvantaged, the maternal and child health programs have been intimately coordinated with them.

From the standpoint of organization early in 1963, soon after its fiftieth anniversary, the Children's Bureau became part of a new Welfare Administration in the Department of Health, Education, and Welfare. Subsequently, in

August 1967 it became part of another new major unit in the department. This unit, named the Social and Rehabilitation Service, also included the functions of the former Welfare Administration, the Vocational Rehabilitation Administration, the Administration on Aging, and the Mental Retardation Division of the Public Health Service. This new agency was designed to join under single leadership both the income-support programs for those in need and the social service and rehabilitation programs that many individuals and families require.

Eventually, in 1973, the health functions of the Children's Bureau were split off to form the Maternal and Child Health program of the present Bureau of Community Health Services of the Health Services Administration.

## THE DEPARTMENT OF HEALTH, EDUCATION, AND WELFARE

In 1946 the Federal Security Agency underwent further accretion, and the various federal health services were further consolidated by the transfers of the Children's Bureau from the Department of Labor and of the Food and Drug Administration from the Department of Agriculture. At about the same time the National Office of Vital Statistics was transferred from the Bureau of the Census of the Department of Commerce to the Public Health Service. In this way the activities of the agencies concerned with various aspects of health and sanitation were brought into closer working relationship. Then in 1953 the first move taken by President Eisenhower to reorganize the Executive Branch of the Government was to propose that the Federal Security Agency be granted Cabinet status. The proposal became fact on April 11 1953, when Congress established a Department of Health, Education, and Welfare. On the same day the first Secretary of the newly created Executive Department of Health, Education, and Welfare was sworn into office.

The purpose of this plan was to bring together and improve the administration of the important health, education, and social security functions then being carried on by the federal government. Up to the present this plan has succeeded only partially; the functions, relations, and organization of the basic components have not yet meshed substantially toward a clearly defined and understood purpose or mission. This has led some to refer to the department as an enormous social welfare "holding company," a "bureaucratic maze" for which no effective guide exists or perhaps is even possible.

The Department of Health, Education, and Welfare therefore is not truly an administrative or functional unity. It consists of units of differing organization, expertise, and interests. Most units have strong traditions and histories that antedate the department considerably. Many have separate, strong, and effective congressional ties and public or professional constituencies and do not hesitate to use them unilaterally. Yet the need is increasingly clear to bring about a more effective operational relationship among those working in the fields of health services, education, welfare, and social security. The awareness of this, and the chronic administrative frustration which derives from it, is evidenced by the fact that in the past decade the department has been subjected to eight substantial organizational changes.[24,25,28] The probability of an even more extensive reorganization in the near future is excellent. The organization in effect at the beginning of 1974 is shown in Fig. 15-4.

## VOLUNTARY HEALTH AGENCIES

While the official, governmental, or public health agencies were still in the process of development, a complementary and supplementary force appeared in the form of voluntary or nonofficial health agencies. This is considered in detail in Chapter 16. Beginning with the establishment of a local antituberculosis society in Philadelphia in 1892, the voluntary health movement soon developed considerable force and magnitude. Spurred by public interest, by private philanthropy, and sometimes by impatience or dissatisfaction with governmental programs, over 20,000 such agencies have been established during the ensuing half century. They draw voluntary support from literally millions of persons and serve millions of others.

Not infrequently the development of these agencies has been related to certain strong and appealing personalities such as Beers, Trudeau, Wald, and Franklin Roosevelt. One interesting aspect of their development is that although some agencies such as the antituberculosis associations began locally and spread upward to state and national levels, others such as the National Foundation (for Infantile Paralysis) began on the national level and spread downward. Still others, notably the mental hygiene associations, began on the state level and spread both upward and downward.

One phase of the voluntary health movement, visiting nursing, deserves particular mention. William Welch once singled out public health nursing as perhaps America's greatest contribution to the public health movement. It had its origin in 1877 in the Women's Branch of the New York City Mission and was organized for the purpose of teaching hygiene in the homes of the underprivileged. In 1902 Lillian Wald organized the first school nursing program in New York City, setting up a pattern that was rapidly followed throughout the nation. Largely from these modest beginnings developed the adoption of public health nursing as a most important part of any public health program. Among the important recent developments, as discussed in Chapter 36, is the move toward merger of official and voluntary visiting nursing programs and the development of and experimentation with new types of auxiliary personnel, such as Home Health Aids.

## COUNTY HEALTH DEPARTMENTS

In 1910-1911 one of a series of severe typhoid fever epidemics occurred in Yakima County, Wash. Because it was uncontrolled by local authorities, L. L. Lumsden of the United States Public Health Service was loaned to bring it under control. Lumsden not only solved the particular epidemiologic problem but suggested ways of preventing its recurrence. One strong recommendation was the establishment of a full-time resident staff to deal with all public health matters. Meanwhile the Rockefeller Sanitary Commission, which had been active in hookworm control in the southeastern United States and Central and South America, concluded that no single disease or sanitary or public health problem could be successfully attacked without concurrent efforts aimed at all phases of public health. As a result, they also strongly recommended the establishment of local full-time resident public health staffs. Thus there occurred the coincidence of the same idea at almost the same moment at two different places for two different but related reasons, resulting in the establishment of the first full-time county health departments in Guilford County, N. C., June 1911 and Yakima County, Wash., July 1911.* The basic soundness of the principle is indicated by the subsequent growth

of local health units, which now serve most of the population of the nation. With the increased trend toward core city-suburbia complexes as well as metropolitanization, a growing movement is underway toward merger of city and county health departments. This trend, although fraught with difficulties of a political and fiscal nature as a result of an outdated intergovernmental system, to the extent that it succeeds can only bring about greater efficiency and improved public service. In discussing county health organization the Association of County Health Officers should be mentioned, which is associated with the National Association of Counties, an organization of ever-growing significance and national influence.

## DEVELOPMENT OF PROFESSIONAL TRAINING

The appointment of health officers for many towns and districts in midnineteenth century England led to the establishment of a course of lectures on public health at St. Thomas' Hospital in London. This was the first training of its kind in England and resulted in the development of several excellent curricula and schools devoted specifically to the subject. Despite the many parallel interests and activities, no similar facilities existed in the United States until 1910. Since insanitation was of predominant interest at the time, it was logical that the first teaching of public health was particularly in relation to engineering. The first specific public degree was awarded in 1910 at the University of Michigan; in 1912 a program of study was organized at the Massachusetts Institute of Technology by William T. Sedgwick, whose strong personality sent forth over many years a large number of outstanding disciples in the new profession. After a few years, realizing that the environmental phases represented only a part of the total public health picture, there was formed a joint Massachusetts Institute of Technology–Harvard School of Public Health, which later divided when Harvard University established its separate School of Public Health. Meanwhile the first institution designated as a School of Public Health (now defunct) was organized at the University of Pennsylvania.

In relation to these early steps toward professionalization of public health the name of Milton Rosenau is again encountered. Having left the National Hygienic Laboratory (later the National Institutes of Health), he served as

---

*Some difference of opinion exists with regard to priority, many contending that Jefferson County, Ky., was the first in 1908.

codirector of the joint M.I.T.–Harvard school and also became the first chairman of the division of preventive medicine in the Harvard University School of Medicine. It was about this time (1913) that Rosenau brought out the first edition of his world-famous volume, *Preventive Medicine and Hygiene*. One public health authority, Wilson G. Smillie, commented that this one book did as much to advance public health as any other single factor. It is notable that Rosenau, on retirement from Harvard University in 1936, went on to establish and direct another school of public health at the University of North Carolina before his death in 1946.

Recent years have seen much progress in professional education and training in public health. The Committee on Professional Education of the American Public Health Association played a significant role in stimulation of thought and discussion, crystalization of ideas, and development and implementation of programs for the improvement of the quality of public health personnel. This is exemplified in its current activities, which include the accreditation of schools of public health, the development of statements on educational qualifications of personnel in the various public health disciplines, the development of field-training methods and standards, the promotion of a professional examination service, the development of recruitment programs, and the study of public health salaries. Mention should also be made of the great professional development value of the scientific sessions at its annual meetings.

As more demand developed for public health services, many schools and universities began to offer a wide variety of degrees in public health, often on a questionable basis. In 1941 the leading schools formed an Association of Schools of Public Health. This stimulated a study by the Committee on Professional Education of the American Public Health Association that led to the development and application by the committee in 1946 of a system of accreditation for the granting of recognized degrees in public health. At the present time (1974) 18 schools are so accredited—University of California at Berkeley, University of California at Los Angeles, Columbia University, Harvard University, University of Hawaii, Johns Hopkins University, University of Illinois, Loma Linda (Cal.) University, University of Michigan, University of Minnesota, University of North Carolina, University of

Oklahoma, University of Pittsburgh, University of Puerto Rico, University of Texas at Houston, Tulane University, University of Washington, and Yale University. The American Public Health Association maintains contact with other centers of public health education elsewhere in the world, especially those in Latin America, Great Britain, France, and the American University at Beirut in Lebanon. Recognizing that the accredited schools in the United States serve regional, national, and indeed, international needs, several bills calling for the provision of federal subsidization were introduced into Congress. The first result occurred in 1958 when $1 million was appropriated for strengthening the accredited schools by providing grants for construction and improvement of teaching facilities. The present law also provides funds for scholarships and loans to students who otherwise would be unable to pursue professional education.

In early 1949, recognizing that the full-time practice of preventive medicine and public health had long since become a specialty in the medical profession, the American Board of Preventive Medicine and Public Health was organized under the joint sponsorship of the American Medical Association, the American Public Health Association, the Association of Schools of Public Health, The Canadian Public Health Association, and the Southern Medical Association. Rigid standards and requirements with regard to training and experience were developed, and an examination system was established, on the satisfactory completion of which candidates become certified as specialists in this field of medical practice. Soon after, in 1950, steps were taken for the development of approved field residency programs in acceptable public health organizations. Supervision and accreditation of these are under the joint aegis of the American Board of Preventive Medicine and Public Health and the Council on Medical Education and Hospitals of the American Medical Association.

Since these latter developments apply only to physicians, several other professional disciplines involved in public health work have developed or are developing similar accreditation procedures.

An important impetus was provided by the passage in 1963 of the Health Professions Education Assistance Act. It formally recognized the necessity of the federal government to participate significantly in the development of an adequate health manpower resource. A Bureau of Health Manpower was established in the Public Health Service and is now organizationally located in the Health Resources Administration.

As a result of these many activities the past 15 years have seen extensive improvements in all aspects of training, education, experience, and status of those who are devoting the energies of their professional lives to the improvement of the health of the public. Some aspects of these training and accreditation subjects are discussed further in Chapter 11.

## SUMMARY

There appear to have been three great turning points in public health history in the United States, and it is interesting that they have been about 50 years, or two generations, apart: the 1860s, when the Shattuck Report began to exert an influence; the 1910s, when the groundwork was laid for so much of public health development since; and the 1960s, when public health really began to broaden its horizons and abandon the barrier between it and medical care and when Congress decided to make undreamed-of resources available for undreamed-of accomplishments. It would appear that public health has now come of age.

## REFERENCES

1. Rosen, G.: A history of public health, New York, 1958, MD Publications, Inc.
2. Top, F. H.: The history of American epidemiology, St. Louis, 1952, The C. V. Mosby Co.
3. Hanlon, J., Rogers, F., and Rosen, G.: A bookshelf on the history and philosophy of public health, Amer. J. Public Health **50:**445, April 1960.
4. Osler, W.: The functions of a state faculty, Maryland Med. J. **37:**73, May 1897.
5. Hecker, I. F.: The epidemics of the Middle Ages, Philadelphia, 1837, Haswell, Barrington & Haswell.
6. Winslow, C.-E. A.: The evolution and significance of the modern public health campaign, New Haven, 1923, Yale University Press.
7. George, M. D.: London life in the XVIIIth century, New York, 1925, Alfred A. Knopf.
8. Richardson, B. W.: The health of nations, a review of the works of Edwin Chadwick, London, 1887, Longmans, Green & Co., vol. II.
9. Bowditch, H. I.: Address on hygiene and preventive medicine, Transactions of the International Medical Congress, Philadelphia, 1876.
10. Prescott, W. H.: History of the conquest of Mexico, New York, 1936, Random House, Inc.
11. Woodward, S. B.: The story of smallpox in Massachusetts, New Eng. J. Med. **206:**1181, June 9, 1932.
12. Chadwick, H. D.: The diseases of the inhabitants of the commonwealth, New Eng. J. Med. **216:**8, June 10, 1937.
13. Editorial: Has Baltimore the oldest health department? Amer. J. Public Health **35:**49, Jan. 1945.
14. Newsholme, A., Sir: The ministry of health, London, 1925, G. P. Putnam's Sons, Ltd.
15. Kramer, H. D.: The beginnings of the public health movement in the United States, Bull. Hist. Med. **21:**369, 1947.
16. Holmes, O. W.: Writings, IX, medical essays, Boston, 1891, Houghton, Mifflin Co.
17. Shattuck, L., et al.: Report of the Sanitary Commission of Massachusetts: 1850 (Dutton & Wentworth, State Printers, Boston, 1850), Cambridge, 1948, Harvard University Press.
18. Beck-Storrs, A.: Public health and government control, Social Stud. **45:**211, Oct. 1954.
19. Patterson, R. S., and Baker, M. C.: Seventy-five years of public health in Massachusetts, Amer. J. Public Health **34:**1271, Dec. 1944.
20. Cavins, H. M.: The National Quarantine and Sanitary Conventions of 1857 to 1860 and the beginnings of the American Public Health Association, Bull. Hist. Med. **13:**404, April 1943.
21. Smith, S.: Historical sketch of the American Public Health Association, Public Health **5:**7, 1889.
22. Smillie, W. G.: The National Board of Health, 1879-1883, Amer. J. Public Health **33:**925, Aug. 1943.
23. Annual Report of the Surgeon General of the Public Health Service, Washington, D. C., 1936, Government Printing Office.
24. U. S. House of Representatives, Special Subcommittee on Investigation of the Department of Health, Education, and Welfare of the Commission on Interstate and Foreign Commerce, 89th Cong., 2nd sess., Oct. 13, 1966, Rep. 2266.
25. Sims, L. B.: Organizational history of HSMHA, Health Services Rep. **88:**117, Feb. 1973.
26. Rusk, H.: Congress and medicine, The New York Times, Nov. 20, 1965.
27. Basic data relating to the National Institutes of Health, Washington, D. C., 1972, Government Printing Office.
28. U. S. Department of Health, Education, and Welfare: A common thread of service—an historical guide to HEW, DHEW pub. no. 73-45, Washington, D. C., 1973, Government Printing Office.
29. Forgotson, E.: 1965, The turning point in public health law—1966 reflections, Amer. J. Public Health **57:**934, June 1967.
30. The Children's Bureau, yesterday, today and tomorrow, Washington, D. C., 1937, Government Printing Office.
31. Lathrop, J. C.: Children's Bureau, Amer. J. Sociol. **18:**318, Nov. 1912.
32. 37 Stat., 79, 737, 1912.
33. Key, V.O.: The administration of federal grants

to states, Chicago, 1937, Public Administration Service.

34. Sinai, N., and Anderson, O. W.: E.M.I.C., a study of administrative experience, 1948, University of Michigan.

35. Eliot, M. M.: The Children's Bureau, fifty years of public responsibility for action in behalf of children, Amer. J. Public Health **52:**576, April 1962.

*The twentieth century will be remembered chiefly,
not as an age of political conflicts and astonishing
technical inventions, but as an age in which human
society dared to think of the health of the whole
human race as a practical objective.*

ARNOLD TOYNBEE

# CHAPTER 3

# World health

## HEALTH: A GLOBAL ISSUE

The ultimate measure of a nation is found in the numbers and quality of its people. Everything else, including agricultural, mineral, industrial and economic potential, is of value only to the extent and manner in which it may be related to people. The quantitative measure of a people is the population, especially the number of persons who are able to produce goods or children. This, of course, had best be closely balanced with resources, present and future, of the nation and the world of which it is a part. The qualitative measure of a people is largely determined by the degree of illness or health and the rates by which it dies or survives. Four factors influence the growth or decline of a nation's population: the numbers of births, deaths, immigrants, and emigrants. At the moment this book is not concerned with the last two. The first two, numbers of births and deaths, are of major social, economic, political, public health, and medical importance to every nation. Beyond this their relationship to similar factors in other countries, especially those nearby, is also important. It is fundamental therefore to any consideration of international problems or relationships that an adequate fund of accurate statistical data be readily available, relating to the number of persons in each nation as well as the rates and manner in which they are born, live, and die. Unfortunately this is not the case. The student of international health problems is confronted at the outset by gross inadequacies in this respect and is forced to think, plan, and function to a considerable degree on the basis of impressions, estimates, and generalizations.

It is not the purpose here to evaluate the completeness, accuracy, or comprehensiveness of various national or international vital statistics. However, it should be recognized that understandably the most complex, industrialized, and highly developed countries have the most exact and adequate vital data, whereas the least developed and youngest nations, and unfortunately many of those with the most outstanding health problems, tend to have the least satisfactory information about their people. One might generalize that population enumeration and birth and death registration are relatively good in the countries of northern and western Europe, parts of central and southern Europe, the British Isles, North America, Australia, New Zealand, and Japan. Conversely, they are less accurate, to varying degrees of course, in most countries of Central and South America, parts of eastern and southern Europe, and most of Africa, the Middle East, and Asia.

## GENERAL OBSERVATIONS

Despite these limitations, there is sufficient information to indicate considerable variation among countries with regard to the fertility, health, and longevity of their populations. For detailed information the reader is referred to the various statistical and epidemiologic reports of the World Health Organization.[1] In evaluating these variations, it is important to realize that many biologic, environmental, and social factors are involved. Thus climate, the nature of the soil, food consumption and habits, physical inheritance, folk customs, superstitions, and habits of work or exercise may affect the

**41**

fertility, health, and mortality experiences of populations. Beyond these there are, of course, the influences of public health personnel, facilities, medical and nursing services, housing standards, and occupational conditions.[2] In the broadest sense economics, education, and national political policy are probably the most important factors.

The key factor in determining the size of a population is the extent to which it can reproduce and maintain or increase itself. Various methods have been devised to measure this, the commonest of which is the birthrate. In general, an inverse relationship appears to exist between the birthrate and the degree of development or complexity of a nation. Thus the greater the degree of industrial and scientific progress, urbanization, and elevation of the standard of living the more the birthrate tends to be depressed. There are, of course, several exceptions to this generalization. Nevertheless, birthrates have declined rather consistently in the European countries, the British Isles, North America, and Japan. By contrast, birthrates have tended to fall more slowly or to increase in the countries of Asia, Africa, and Central and South America.

The birthrate in itself is neither a true measure of human fertility nor indicative of the extent to which the number of births is sufficient to maintain or to increase the population of a nation. Because of this, additional indices such as the rate of natural increase and fertility rates have been devised. The rate of natural increase is simply the annual excess of births over deaths per 1,000 population. In general this rate is highest in the countries of Africa, the Middle East, Asia, southeastern Europe, and parts of Central and South America and is lowest in northern and western Europe and North America. Even this rate of numerical excess of births over deaths, however, is not a conclusive indication of the ability of a country's population to reproduce itself. A particular country at a given time may have an extremely large excess of births over deaths, yet its birthrate, especially when determined in relation to the number of persons of childbearing age, may not be high enough to maintain the present population eventually. This can occur when a country has a temporarily high porportion of young adults as a result of immigration or as a result of a mass delayed reproductive action such as occurs during a period of warfare followed by the return home of large numbers of young men. As a result of such circumstances, the birthrate temporarily may be much higher than the death rate, but the gross number of births may not be large enough to maintain such a favorable age distribution permanently. There results eventually a population with a relatively high proportion of older persons and a concomitant fall of the birthrate, even below the level of the death rate.

As a result of these influences, it is fair to expect not only continued variations in population numbers, rates of increase, and density but also significant accentuation of the differences in these factors among the nations and regions of the world (Table 3-1). North America, the United Kingdom, Japan, the USSR, and western Europe will probably experience stabilized or even decreasing populations, unless net reproductive rates increase, mortality rates decrease even more than they have, or major immigrations occur. Most of Asia, Africa, the Middle East, and Central and South America, on the other hand, appear destined to experience great, dangerous, and unsupportable increases in population if present fertility rates continue. In addition, barring the influence of other factors, these increases will be greatly magnified as mortality rates decline. There are many factors that might change or even reverse these trends. Important among them are improved education and standard of living combined with prompt and energetic sustained family planning programs.

The crude death rate is one of the commonest and most convenient indices of the state of health of a community or nation. In viewing the world scene, despite inadequate information, it is readily observed that in general the highest death rates occur in the countries of Africa, the Middle East, Asia, and parts of Central and South America as well as in a few southern and eastern European nations. Significantly lower death rates are experienced by western Europe, the USSR, the British Isles, Australia, New Zealand, North America, Japan, and a few countries in South America. It is immediately apparent that the difference observed in the case of birthrates between more highly developed industrialized countries and less developed and primarily agricultural countries exists also in the case of death rates but in a reciprocal sense. Progress in combating preventable disease and reducing mortality has been closely related to the widespread application of advances in medical, physical, and chemical sci-

**Table 3-1.** Vital statistics of the world, 1969*

| | Region | | | | | | | |
| Index | Latin America | Africa | Asia | Oceania | North America | USSR | Europe | World |
|---|---|---|---|---|---|---|---|---|
| Population estimates Mid-1969 (millions) | 276 | 344 | 1,990 | 19 | 225 | 241 | 456 | 3,551 |
| Birthrate per 1,000 population | 39 | 46 | 38 | 24 | 18 | 18 | 18 | 34 |
| Death rate per 1,000 population | 10 | 22 | 18 | 11 | 9 | 8 | 10 | 15 |
| Current rate of population growth | 2.9 | 2.4 | 2.0 | 1.8 | 1.1 | 1.0 | 0.8 | 1.9 |
| Number of years to double population | 24 | 28 | 35 | 41 | 63 | 70 | 88 | 37 |
| Infant mortality rate (deaths under 1 year per 1,000 live births) | 65† | 137† | 80† | 18 | 22 | 26 | 30† | |
| Population under 15 years (%) | 43 | 43 | 40 | 30 | 30 | 32 | 25 | 37 |
| Population projections to 1980 (millions) | 376 | 456 | 2,472 | 23 | 264 | 278 | 499 | 4,368 |
| Per capita gross national product (US$) | 385 | 140 | 184 | 1,857 | 3,399 | 890 | 1,230 | 589 |

* Modified from World Population Data Sheet, Washington, D. C., 1969, Population Reference Bureau.
† Very crude estimates.

ences. This has occurred to the greatest extent in the western European countries and in North America, the most highly industrialized and urbanized areas in the world. To the extent to which this has been accomplished in the lesser developed countries it has been due largely to assistance from outside—from some of the more developed nations and from international agencies and foundations, which in turn are supported largely by the more developed nations. One may generalize therefore that death rates are lower in the more highly developed countries and higher in the more underdeveloped countries. Similarly, death rates tend to be lower in the more urbanized and industrial countries and higher in the more rural and predominantly agricultural countries.

Although this relationship appears to apply to many specific death rates, it is by no means universally true. Certainly the relationship applies to the infant death rate and the maternal mortality rate, as it also applies to the specific rates of death from almost all of the communicable diseases that can be controlled by public health, sanitation, and immunization methods. One outstanding group of exceptions, however, does exist. Death rates for the degenerative diseases of middle and later life, such as cancer, hypertension, and the like, are generally much higher in the economically more advantaged and industrially and scientifically advanced countries of western Europe, the USSR, the British Isles, North America, Australia, New Zealand, and Japan. This apparent difference is undoubtedly due to the higher proportion of persons who reach later life as a result of public health measures and also to more accurate cause-of-death reporting in the more advanced countries.

In addition to birthrates and death rates, but as a function of the latter, average expectation of life should be considered briefly. The average life expectancy varies considerably among the different nations of the world, from a low of perhaps about 30 to 35 years to a high of about 70 years. As would be expected from the preceding consideration of death rates, the average life expectancy is much greater in Western Europe, the USSR, the British Isles, North America, Australia, New Zealand, and Japan than it is in most of the rest of the world. The differences among countries in this respect are significant at all age levels but appear to diminish consistently as one approaches the older ages. The logical conclusion, upheld by a consideration of age-specific death rates, is that the greatest risks to life in the underdeveloped and less advantaged countries are experienced by infants and young children and that once they reach a certain age, they have a reasonable chance in most places of attaining an advanced age.

One other interesting aspect of the variation in death rates and life expectancies relates to the differences that are observed among the races. That such differences generally exist is not subject to question. It is not known, however, whether the differences are related to inherent racial characteristics or to social and economic environment. In general, one is inclined to think that the difference is circumstantial rather than inherent. This appears to be borne out by the fact that the black in Europe and North America, although he still has a somewhat lower life expectancy and higher death rate than his white compatriot, nevertheless is in a decidedly more advantageous situation than the members of his race who are still living in Africa. Furthermore, the discrepancy between the rates for whites and blacks in the Western Hemisphere has consistently become less. That the problem is not simple, however, is indicated by the situation in Hawaii, where the life expectancy of native Hawaiians is significantly less than that for other races at every specified age except under 1 year. In fact, Caucasian-Hawaiians also have a shorter life expectancy than whites, Japanese, and Chinese who live on the islands. The explanation for this and similar phenomena remains to be determined.

## EXTENT OF WORLD HEALTH PROBLEMS

When one attempts to reduce world health problems to the lowest common denominators, the conclusion is inevitable that a sound knowledge and consideration of two important but related fields are prerequisites. These are the sciences of biology and climatology in their broadest senses. Man is a biologic being whose behavior, cultural development, physical devel-

**Table 3-2.** Morbidity and mortality from communicable diseases (world, 1963)*

| Disease | Deaths | Incidence | Prevalence |
|---|---|---|---|
| 1. Pneumonia and bronchitis | 6,786,000 | 125 to 350,000,000 | NA |
| 2. Gastritis, duodenitis, enteritis, colitis (excluding diarrhea of newborn) | 3,094,000 | 750,000,000 | NA |
| 3. Tuberculosis of respiratory system | 2,840,000 | 13,000,000 | 40,000,000 |
| 4. Infections of newborn | 1,131,000 | Unknown | NA |
| 5. Measles | 508,000 | 90,000,000 | NA |
| 6. Malaria | 326,000 | 25,000,000 | 200,000,000 |
| 7. Influenza | 313,000 | Unknown | Unknown |
| 8. Dysentery, all forms | 202,000 | 50,000,000 | NA |
| 9. Smallpox | 172,000 | 430,000 | NA |
| 10. Leprosy | † | 200,000 | 10,800,000 |
| 11. Diphtheria | 127,000 | 1,270,000 | NA |
| 12. Whooping cough | 112,000 | 70,000,000 | NA |
| 13. Typhoid | 98,000 | 2,000,000 | NA |
| 14. Syphilis and its sequelae | 68,000 | Unknown | Unknown |
| 15. Acute poliomyelitis | 35,000 | Unknown | NA |
| 16. Meningococcal infections | 31,000 | 150,000 | NA |
| 17. Cholera | 12,000 | 24,000 | NA |
| 18. Typhus | 7,000 | Unknown | NA |
| 19. Scarlet fever and streptococcal sore throat | 6,000 | Unknown | NA |
| 20. Plague | 500 | 860 | NA |
| 21. All other diseases classified as infectious and parasitic | 1,350,000 | NA | NA |
| 22. Yaws | † | Unknown | 10 to 15,000,000 |
| 23. Ankylostomiasis | † | Unknown | 716,000,000 |
| 24. Schistosomiasis | † | Unknown | 204,000,000 |
| 25. Taenia saginata (beef tapeworm) | † | Unknown | 61,000,000 |
| 26. Taenia solium (pork tapeworm) | † | Unknown | 4,000,000 |

*Modified from LeRiche, W. H.: World incidence and prevalence of the major communicable diseases. In Wolstenholm, G., and O'Connor, M., editors: Health of mankind, London, 1967, J. & A. Churchill, Ltd.
†Included in item 21.
NA = not applicable.

opment, feeding habits, clothing, housing, and at least to some degree, methods of political organization are determined largely by biologic factors, particularly his reaction to his environment. By like token most of the preventable illnesses to which man is subject involve other biologic beings: bacteria, viruses, protozoa, helminths, insects, and the like. Intimately influencing the extent of favorable development of man on the one hand and those factors that may act to his detriment on the other is the climate of the environment in which man and these agents are cast. A few examples may illustrate these points. Since man is a satisfactory host for the plasmodium of malaria and since he shares this unfortunate role with the mosquito, it is obvious that, in the absence of scientific interference, human beings affected by malaria are most frequently found in areas where the climate is most conducive to the propagation of the mosquito. Such conditions are found especially in the warm and moist tropical and subtropical zones of the world. In contrast, it is to be expected that the serious pulmonary infections are found most often in the less temperate climates that have wider and more frequent variations in temperature. These climatic conditions are conducive to frequent upper respiratory illnesses, which so often are the precursors of more serious diseases of the pulmonary system. Between these two situations one might point to typhus fever, which requires environmental and climatic conditions that are not so cold as to discourage the propagation of the louse vector yet are cold enough to cause the human host to wear considerable clothing, sometimes in a continuous and unwashed manner. If conditions are such as to combine a cold climate with continued inadequacy of water, thereby precluding bathing and the washing of clothing, so much the better for lice and some other "body-contact" insects that may cause disease.

In view of the foregoing one would rightly expect to find that the greatest amount of preventable disease at the present time is in the warmer areas of the earth. If the factors of biology and climatology are correlated with the degree of economic development and applied scientific knowledge (and, indeed, the latter would appear to be a function of the former), one observes a broad zone on the world globe, with necessarily indefinite borders and certain variations, which in general overlaps the equator about 20 to 25 degrees in both directions. This band or zone includes the areas in which the bulk of preventable infectious diseases and premature deaths now occur.

To most of those who reside permanently outside this zone the extent of preventable disease seems incomprehensible. Nevertheless, as Russell[4] has said, "Nothing on earth is more international than disease." Table 3-2[5] presents an inadequate, statistically unfeeling impression of the magnitude of the burden. The obvious shortcoming is the different feeling experienced from seeing one suffering fellow human to that experienced from glancing over some columns of numbers. A few descriptive paragraphs may help to fill the gap.

Consider first malaria, which is still the leading cause of death in the world. In India the Ministry of Health[6] stated the following:

No less than 75 million persons suffer from it every year, and during epidemic years the incidence may reach up to twice as much or even more. It has been calculated that approximately half of the 5.5 million annual deaths in India are accounted for by fevers. Nearly one seventh of these fever deaths are directly attributable to malaria. Apart from this high annual mortality, malaria is also responsible for untold sickness and suffering. Untreated or partially treated malaria leads to general debility and anaemia, and reduces the resistance of the individual to other diseases. This results in an unduly high rate of morbidity. Thus, by sapping the vitality of whole groups of population, malaria has been largely responsible for impeding the development of the country's agricultural and other natural resources. The economic loss to the nation is therefore incalculable.

In Liberia 90% of the children under 5 years of age have positive blood smears and 70% of the adults are continuously infected. Malaria is a constant scourge of a large part of the lowlands of South and Central America, large parts of Africa, and almost all of South and Southeast Asia. LeRiche[5] estimates a worldwide burden of 326,000 deaths, an annual incidence of about 25 million new cases, and a prevalence of about 200 million is commonly considered. The latter represents about 1 out of every 20 people in the world.

Schistosomiasis affects the populations of large parts of Africa, northeastern South America, Japan, and southeastern China. In the Middle East, it has been estimated that from 20 to 30 million people, or 90% of the rural population, suffer from this debilitating disease, which generally reduces the productivity of the population by at least one third.[7] In Egypt about three fourths of the population is affected. Some years ago Wright[8] estimated its cost to Egypt to be about 20 million pounds per year. Lower Egypt is affected more than Upper Egypt. In 1951 22% of army recruits from Lower Egypt were rejected because of physical defects, as compared with only 3% from Upper Egypt.

Helminthic or worm infestation represents one of the greatest drains on human energy and health. Some careful estimates have been made of their extent, and the resulting figures are staggering. To give a few examples: hookworm, the aptly termed assassin worm, one of the worst scourges to suck the lifeblood and strength of a population, affects about 460 million persons throughout the world, over 200 million in India alone. For the roundworm, *Ascaris*, an interesting and dramatic picture painted by Stoll[9] indicated that the total case load approached 650 million persons. China's load alone was estimated to be about 335 million cases, with about 6 billion adult ascarides. This number of worms would equal the combined weight of almost 500,000 adult men, and they consumed enough food annually from the bellies of the Chinese to feed the entire populations of Guatemala and Costa Rica at that time. Stoll further calculated that these many worms produced about 18,000 tons of microscopic eggs, which were broadcast continuously over the landscape.

Stoll also estimated that although the world's population was then about 2.2 billion people, including multiple infestations there were probably just over 2.2 billion cases of helminthic infestation. The largest amounts of infestations were in the so-called underdeveloped areas of the world. He described their significance dramatically by saying, "Helminthiases do not have the journalistic value of great pandemics like flu or plague . . . but to make up for their lack of drama, they are unremittingly corrosive."

In India more than 2 million persons are blind, mostly from trachoma, gonorrhea, and syphilis. Many millions more are affected by trachoma to a degree less than total blindness. A recent survey[10] based on a random sample in Egypt showed a blindness prevalence rate of about 3%. In many places in Africa one encounters what are referred to as "villages of the blind." An idea of the economic burden involved may be obtained from figures from a much smaller country. Tunisia with only 4.8 million inhabitants loses an estimated 30 million workdays a year because of trachoma. Leprosy claims a world total of from 5 to 7 million people. It is estimated that 1 million

persons in India and 2 to 4 million persons in China suffer from this disease. In Africa there are probably about 1.5 million affected persons. Some estimates for Latin America include Brazil, 40,000; Bolivia, 12,000 to 15,000; Paraguay, 10,000 to 12,000; Argentina, 12,000; Mexico and Colombia, 9,000 each; and Peru, Venezuela, and Cuba, about 3,000 each. Yaws is one of the most important economic disease handicaps. Throughout the world it is estimated that there are 10 to 15 million cases,[5] approximately half of them in the Republic of Indonesia.

With regard to tuberculosis, which may be rightfully considered a disease of poor economy, there are probably about 40 million cases and almost 3 million deaths each year throughout the world. Studies have indicated the existence of about 1.3 million cases and 35,000 deaths each year from this disease in the Philippines; India has an estimated 2.5 million cases and about 500,000 deaths annually. Recognizing the fact that in most of the world there is no, or at best only poor, reporting and statistics, several interesting attempts have been made to analyze the world prevalence of tuberculosis. One such study, although somewhat out of date, is particularly illustrative. It divides the countries of the world into the following four groups:

| Group | Cases per 100,000 population |
|---|---|
| I | Under 49 |
| II | 50 to 99 |
| III | 100 to 149 |
| IV | Over 150 |

At the time of the analysis in 1946 the rates ranged from a low of 34 for Denmark to 550 for Greenland. Only four countries, Denmark, Australia, Netherlands, and the United States, were in group I. Thirty-two countries were in group II, 26 were in group III, and 34 were in group IV. Even this does not tell the whole story. The picture became more shocking when populations affected rather than numbers of countries were considered. When this was done, the following results appeared:

| Group | TB death rates | Number of countries | Percent of world population |
|---|---|---|---|
| I | Very low | 4 | 8 |
| II | Low | 32 | 14 |
| III | Medium | 26 | 8 |
| IV | High | 34 | 70 |

This, it should be realized, was correlated on the basis of considering death rates of from 100 to 149 per 100,000 as medium!

The number of cases and deaths resulting from typhoid and paratyphoid fevers, the diarrheas and dysenteries, and other related illnesses acquired through the gastrointestinal tract is unknown. That their incidence is tremendous is common knowledge. Some years ago the Director General of the World Health Organization said, "One-fifth of all deaths throughout the world are due to faulty environmental conditions." He pointed out that "probably three-fourths of the world's populations drink unsafe water, dispose of human excreta recklessly, prepare milk and food dangerously, are constantly exposed to insect and rodent enemies, and live in primitive condition of insanitation." By virtue of the circumstances which tend to bring about such undesirable environment it is again obvious that these diseases are most widespread in the predominantly rural agricultural nations of the world.

LeRiche[5] has compiled world estimates as follows:

| Diseases | Annual cases | Cases per death |
|---|---|---|
| Typhoid | 2,000,000 | 20 |
| Cholera | 24,000 | 2 |
| Dysentery | 50,000,000 | 250 |
| Gastritis, enteritis, colitis, except in newborn | 750,000,000 | 250 |

Filarial infestations are another widespread cause of physical incapacitation and economic loss. *Wuchereria bancrofti* is found in most tropical countries, particularly in the Republic of Indonesia, northern Australia, parts of South Asia, Japan, Africa, the West Indies, the northern coast of South America, and the eastern coast of Brazil. In addition, *Wuchereria malayi* occurs frequently in the Malay peninsula, Sumatra, Borneo, New Guinea, India, Indochina, Sri Lanka, and southern China. Onchocerciasis is the best known filarial disease of the Western Hemisphere, occurring in Mexico, Guatemala, and Venezuela. It is also found on the west coast of Africa from Sierra Leone to the Congo Basin, then eastward across Africa through the Congo and the Sudan to Uganda, Malawi, and Kenya. The number of persons affected by filariasis is difficult to determine but is known to be large. Some idea of the magnitude is indicated by the incidence of infestation by one other filarial worm, *Dracunculus medi-*

*nensis*, or the guinea worm; approximately 50 million people act as hosts to it.

Another geographically widespread disease is leishmaniasis. Although its victims are unnumbered, it is known to occur in various forms across southern and southeastern Asia, the Middle East, northern and central Africa, and in a number of South and Central American countries. A somewhat related disease, trypanosomiasis, is of particular significance, since along with malaria it bars effective use of the tremendous area of central Africa, which many consider to contain some of the best agricultural and grazing land in the world, equal to or surpassing in quality that of Argentina or the central United States. The total area involved is about 4.5 million square miles, 50% again as large as the continental United States. The potential importance of the effective use of this tremendous area to the future world food supply is obvious.

The venereal diseases are truly worldwide in occurrence, but again their true extent is unknown. Guthe and Hume[11] have pointed out that if the discovered incidence of syphilis in Denmark and Finland in 1946 (i.e., 100 to 200 new cases of syphilis per 100,000 persons per year) were applied to the then world population of 2 billion, the result would be from 2 to 4 million newly acquired cases of syphilis annually. There is, of course, good reason to consider this incidence rate as low for the world as a whole. Beyond this if the conservative ratio of 1 case of syphilis to 3 cases of gonorrhea is applied, the result is an estimated minimum of 6 to 12 million new cases of gonorrhea per year. In terms of prevalence if the probably low rate of 2% is applied, an estimated total of 40 million cases of syphilis results. Granted that since this study was made, dramatic declines in the incidence of the venereal diseases occurred in many countries because of widespread use of antibiotics, the subsequent development of drug-resistant strains combined with changes in sexual mores appears to have set mankind back to a worldwide endemic, if not epidemic, state.

## HEALTH MANPOWER

One of the most serious problems is the shortage of health manpower of all types throughout most of the world. Indeed, the insufficiency not only of physicians but also of nurses, trained midwives, environmental health workers, and all other types of health personnel has been referred to by the Director General of the World Health Organization as the main reason why health levels throughout the world are not improving. The supply of physicians provides a good example, not only of the general inadequacies in numbers but also of the greatly skewed maldistribution. In 1973 the physician-to-population ratio in Israel is 1 to 400, the most favorable in the world. For the USSR it is 1 to 455; for New Zealand, 1 to 680; for the United States, 1 to 720; and for Canada, 1 to 890 inhabitants. By contrast Niger has 1 to 63,000; Indonesia, 1 to 41,000 and The Sudan and Vietnam, 1 to 29,000 inhabitants each. World regional figures reflect these variations. For Europe the ratio is 1 to 1,000, but of the 22 nations reporting, 10 nations average 1 physician per 500 to 750 inhabitants. For the western Pacific the ratio is 1 to 2,500, varying from Australia's 1 to 680 to Laos' 1 to 39,000 inhabitants. For Latin America the ratio is 1 to 3,500, varying from Cuba's 1 to 1,220 to Belize's 1 to 5,700 inhabitants. In the eastern Mediterranean region the ratio is 1 to 4,500 inhabitants. Of the 11 nations reporting, many have significant shortages, yet the area includes Kuwait with 1 to 800 and Egypt with 1 to 2,500 inhabitants. The Southeast Asia region, which includes Sri Lanka, India, Thailand, Burma, and Indonesia, averages 1 to 5,000, despite a highly unfavorable ratio of 1 to 41,000 inhabitants for Indonesia, which has a large population. In Africa south of the Sahara, with all but two countries reporting, the ratio is 1 to 18,000 inhabitants. In addition to the many quantitative inadequacies, differences in extent and quality of education of physicians must also be kept in mind. On the brighter side, mention should be made that training in public health has been increasing significantly both in quantity and scope. There are now (in 1973) 121 schools of public health in 44 countries, an increase of 34 schools in 6 years. Furthermore, postgraduate education in such schools is broadening to include not only the biomedical but also the behavioral and managerial aspects of public health and its administration.

## ECONOMIC, SOCIAL, AND POLITICAL RELATIONSHIPS OF WORLD HEALTH PROBLEMS

From what has been presented it may be obvious that the major portion of the vast mass of preventable disease in the world is concentrated in what is commonly referred to as *developing* areas or countries. It should be recognized that the term is unsatisfactory and that citizens of countries so described often object to it. Perhaps such understandable objection based on commendable national pride may be somewhat assuaged by pointing out that the term implies that there is something worth developing—a situation not without its desirable aspect. It would seem equally obvious that one cannot speak, think, or act about the health problems of these countries or areas within an isolated substantive framework. Large proportions of the human beings who live in these areas, and they constitute a majority of the population of the earth, eke out a miserable existence under circumstances that are undesirable from many different standpoints, of which ill health is only one. Their housing is inadequate, their economy unbalanced, their food supply precarious, their methods of performing daily tasks primitive, their educational horizons limited, and their daily work relatively inefficient and unproductive.

What is cause and what is effect? Widespread preventable disease unquestionably serves as a barrier to progress in any direction, be it economic, social, or political. A population that is chronically ill understandably has a decreased productivity. Thus in planning a program in the mid-1950s to provide safe water in rural Venezuela, it was found that about 2 million man-days of work were lost annually because of typhoid, paratyphoid, the dysenteries, and enteritis. This was estimated to represent a total productive loss of 2,321,000 bolivars. It was further estimated that the cost of medical treatment and care of persons stricken with these preventable diseases amounted to 1,643,000 bolivars a year, approximately $5.5 million. The loss of manpower in Rhodesia due to malaria has been reported to be from 5% to 10% of the total labor force, with the greatest incidence of the disease occurring at the peak period of agricultural production. Similarly in Indonesia a program for the mass treatment of yaws returned large numbers of previously incapacitated persons to work and increased the national production significantly.

It has been estimated by Russell[4] that any nation importing products of a highly malarious country pays the equivalent of a 5% malaria tax. For what the United States imports from such areas this would amount to a hidden cost of at least several hundred million dollars per year. Widespread disease also serves as an effective barrier to the development of agricultural lands and natural resources. The effective settlement of such areas as Sumatra, Borneo, central Africa, large areas of South America, and until recently, the Terai of India, Pakistan, Nepal, and large parts of Sardinia, to mention only a few examples, has been prevented by disease, primarily malaria and other insect-borne diseases. The accomplishments in the last two locations give some indication of the potential elsewhere. The control of malaria in Sardinia during the 1950s paved the way for the resettlement of about 1 million Italians from the overcrowded mainland. Similar measures in the Terai have made it possible to open this great fertile area so badly needed to feed the people of India. In terms of the world as a whole, the malaria eradication program begun by The World Health Organization in 1955 has accomplished much. Of an estimated 1,580 million people who in 1965 lived in previously malarious areas, 1,215 million now live in areas where the disease has been or is in the process of being eradicated. Even greater success has been achieved in the fight against smallpox, which will soon probably disappear as a threat to mankind.

For the individual, educational and intellectual development is difficult, if at all possible, when the body is chronically drained of its energy by illness and parasites. This was illustrated in the Philippines, where it was found that malaria control reduced school absenteeism from about 50% daily to 3%. At the same time industrial absenteeism was reduced from 35% to under 4%. Uncontrolled disease in the environment and the continuance of conditions that breed unproductivity and illiteracy also effectively discourage investment from within or without as well as industrial development. Finally, a low economy and standard of living attributable directly or indirectly to widespread ill health are a constant encouragement to political instability. Under such circumstances, people have many reasons for discontent and have little to lose in resorting to violence.

This situation, of course, is a vicious circle. Disease breeds poverty, and poverty in turn breeds more disease. A similar relationship exists between disease and illiteracy, political instability, and many other factors. It is difficult or impossible to state which factor is primary, which is cause, and which is effect. Once the cycle is established, however, it is clear that each factor contributes to the continuance of all other undesirable factors. This has been referred to as cumulative causation. The relationships are illustrated in Table 3-3, which presents data for countries of the world, distributed by regions—more developed regions and less developed regions. Although based on data collected about 1950 and although many changes and improvements have occurred, the relative picture remains essentially unchanged. For the sake of depicting broad geographic areas of relative development and for the sake of convenient general statistical handling, certain individual countries that are obvious exceptions to the region in which they are located are nevertheless included in that region. The more developed regions include North America, western Europe, the British Isles, southern Europe, Australia, New Zealand, and Japan. The less developed regions include Latin America, southeastern Europe, the Near East, Africa, and South and Southeast Asia. It will be observed, first of all, that twice as many people live in the less developed regions than in those that are more developed. Beyond this it will be noted that in the case of every index (and they measure health, agricultural development, industrial development, education, trade, and food consumption), the less developed regions are significantly disadvantaged as compared with the more developed regions.

The solution to the problem is not easy. Certainly it cannot be accomplished by an attack on health problems alone. In fact, such an approach would carry with it certain real dangers, if indeed it really were to succeed at all. Advancement must be made in many fields simultaneously. In this regard the statement of Myrdal[12] at the Fifth World Health Assembly is worthy of note in summarizing the complexity of the situation and outlining a guide for effective, lasting action:

> The task of social engineering is to proportion and direct the induced changes in the whole social field so as to maximize the beneficial effects of a given initial financial sacrifice. One important corollary to the theory of cumulative causation is that a rational policy should never work by inducing change in only one factor; least of all should such a change of only one factor be attempted suddenly and with great force. This would in most cases prove to be a wasteful expenditure of efforts which could reach much further by being spread strategically over the various

**Table 3-3.** Comparison of economic, health, and educational conditions in more developed and less developed regions of the world

| Condition | More developed regions | Less developed regions |
|---|---|---|
| Population in millions, 1950 | 534.0 | 1,061.0 |
| National income ($ per capita), 1949 | 690.0 | 70.0 |
| Nonhuman energy (metric tons of coal per capita or equivalent), 1950 | 3.8 | 0.2 |
| Males in nonagricultural employment (%) | 73.0 | 33.0 |
| Births per 1,000 population, 1950 | 21.7 | 43.5 |
| Deaths per 1,000 population, 1950 | 10.5 | 25.9 |
| Infant mortality per 1,000 births, 1950 | 45.0 | 183.0 |
| Expectation of life (years) | 63.0 | 34.0 |
| Crop yields (bushels per acre) | | |
|   Wheat, 1949 to 1951 | 26.0 | 13.0 |
|   Rice, 1949 to 1950 and 1951 to 1952 | 69.0 | 30.0 |
| Calories person per day | 2,800.0 | 2,000.0 |
| Animal protein per day (oz.) | 1.4 | 0.4 |
| Persons per physician, 1945 to 1950 | 1,000.0 | 14,000.0 |
| Daily newspapers per 100 persons, 1948 to 1951 | 31.0 | 2.0 |
| Radio sets per 100 persons, 1948 to 1951 | 28.0 | 1.0 |
| Illiterates per 100 persons | | |
|   Males | 5.0 | 64.0 |
|   Females | 7.0 | 83.0 |
| Elementary school teachers per 1,000 persons | 3.6 | 1.3 |
| Motor vehicles per 100 persons, 1950 | 12.0 | 0.4 |
| External trade ($ per capita), 1949 | 140.0 | 32.0 |
| Consumption of textiles (pounds per capita), 1948 | 21.0 | 5.0 |

factors in the social system and over a period of time. What we are facing is a whole set of interrelated adverse living conditions for a population. An effort to reach permanent improvement of health standards aimed to have a maximum beneficial effect on the well-being of the people will, in other words, have to be integrated in a broad economic and social reform policy. Such a policy will have to be founded upon studies of how in the concrete situation of a particular country the different factors in the plane of living are interrelated and how we can move them all upwards in such a fashion that the changes will support each other to the highest possible degree.

## HEALTH PROGRAMMING FOR DEVELOPING AREAS

Areas of the world in which socioeconomic development has been delayed are always confronted by several frustrating dilemmas. One of the most obvious that appears, especially if and when assistance becomes available, is what to do first. It is understandable that in such circumstances many individuals and groups, who have had to wait so long for the opportunity to move forward, clamor for many different, divergent, uncoordinated and sometimes im-

practical things. I remember a nation with a mammoth backlog of preventable illness and widespread malnutrition that, when offered public health technical assistance, vigorously requested an electron microscope and the services of a cardiorespiratory physiologist. Another country with similar problems held for a 1,000-bed general hospital, a 500-bed pediatric hospital, and a 500-bed tuberculosis hospital, despite the fact that there were not enough trained personnel in the entire region, much less in the particular nation to staff such institutions.

Such tendencies force the necessity of determining some kind of reasonably effective and satisfactory guidelines or "groundrules" for the hoped-for best application of health technical assistance. In doing so it is critical that one bear constantly in mind the total needs, problems, resources, and aspirations of the nation or area under consideration.[13]

Decisions relating to program choices should be based on two fundamental considerations or criteria:

1. The extent to which they strengthen the

economies of nations by health benefits that release effective human energy, improve citizen morale, improve environment for local and foreign investment, and open new land and project areas

2. The extent to which they contribute to desirable political objectives by aiding the stability of governments, by reaching large populations with highly welcomed personal service programs, and by demonstrating deep human interest in man and his dignity

Within this framework the suggested areas of program activity and assistance for developing countries appear to fall into three broad priority areas as follows:

1. Of highest priority are activities or programs that are always and unquestionably justified whenever the related problems exist. Malaria control is perhaps the example par excellence. It is always politically and culturally acceptable; the necessary technical and scientific knowledge and tools are at hand; their use is administratively feasible; results are rapid, recognizable, and appreciated; large numbers of people are affected at an extremely low cost per person, a cost so low that the host country can almost always take over the maintenance job; and, finally, the total economy of the family, community, and nation is favorably affected by the activity.

2. Of secondary importance are activities or programs that would not be favored in the absence of special precise explanation and justification because of reservations with regard to one or several evaluation criteria. Thus although antitrachoma programs may be favored on the bases of economic value and public and political acceptability, there may be some question about the technical feasibility of such programs in relation to certain organizational and administrative difficulties.

3. In the lowest category are activities or programs that are definitely not justified and that should not be encouraged or assisted except under unusual circumstances. In rare instances certain peculiar nonhealth considerations might result in a decision to engage in one of these activities. In this category would fall programs in relation to many of the noncommunicable chronic diseases, for example, or expensive equipment or training that would benefit only a limited number of people. Examples of public health activities that might fall into each of these categories are presented for consideration with the recognition that each place and circumstance is unique unto itself and that in the final analysis, final decisions should be made by those who will have to live with their success or failure.

**First priority (acceptable without justification)**

1. Programs to promote the widespread understanding, acceptance, and use of family planning, including the training of personnel

2. Mass campaigns against malaria and yaws where they are major problems and against selected gross nutritional deficiencies, such as kwashiorkor, beriberi, xerophthalmia, and goiter, where they may be readily attacked

3. Development of small, protected community water supplies

4. Demonstrations by health centers of services on a community-wide basis, including sanitation, communicable disease control, health records and statistics, home visiting, maternal and child health, nutrition, health education, laboratory, and general clinical services where required to gain acceptance of the community (Demonstration health centers should be used for subprofessional training and field experience for professional personnel and should be limited in scope and number to the national capacity to absorb and operate them.)

5. Advice and assistance in strengthening and lending stability to the organization and operation of the public health administration of the host government

6. Inclusion of training and health service projects in proposed or existing community or village development programs

7. Advice and assistance in planning, designing, and supervision of construction of hospitals, health centers, laboratories, and other health facilities

8. Development and support of basic training of nurses to demonstrate the proper status of nursing as a profession and to provide leadership for indigenous training

9. Training of various allied health personnel for specific health needs in preventive medicine, nursing, sanitation, limited medical services; such training to develop personnel for a planned program that must include professional supervision

and periodic refresher training (Where practicable, opportunity should be given for advancement of outstanding individuals to higher levels.)

10. Fellowships in public health, preferably project related, to physicians, engineers, sanitarians, nurses, health educators, laboratory technologists, public health statisticians, and health administrators (In all but exceptional cases, training should be provided in the host country or region if possible.)

11. Programs for training key medical and nursing school teachers in major clinical and preclinical specialties (Training should be provided in the host country or region if possible.)

12. Construction of demonstration health centers and nursing schools when necessary to the success of these programs by ensuring physically adequate, effective planned facilities

**Second priority (require special justification)**

1. Mass campaigns against other diseases where of major importance, for example, trachoma, louse-borne typhus, and leprosy

2. Consultation on urban water or sewerage systems

3. X-ray, audiovisual, or other major equipment for hospitals or health centers

4. Excreta disposal projects other than as an integral part of a community general sanitation program

5. Refuse disposal, fly control, and food protection projects

6. Assignment of extranational personnel to national institutions, except on a short-term consultation basis (3 months or less)

7. Occupational health services

8. Projects for tuberculosis immunization (BCG), case finding and ambulatory treatment where the problem warrants and facilities permit

**Third priority (only under most unusual circumstances)**

1. Mobile clinics requiring specialized motor equipment or mobile clinics for general medical care that require special staff and maintenance

2. Construction or financing of construction of hospitals, water and sewerage systems, or other major structures

3. Operation of hospitals by nonnational personnel or at nonnational expense

4. Training of private practicing physicians in clinical specialties

5. Dental health projects requiring individualized service

6. Mental hygiene projects requiring individualized service

7. Establishment, equipping, or operation of blood banks

8. Medical rehabilitation projects

9. Mass treatment for intestinal parasites

10. Geriatrics projects

• • •

It is fully recognized that any such priority grouping would not be subscribed to in every detail by all health professionals in all situations at all times. Application of such a list must be related to individual country conditions and the stage of development of its resources and health administration. Each nation and agency is urged to engage in a health problem and resource evaluation and program development based on considerations such as the foregoing and preferably in company with those from whom assistance might be sought and obtained. Despite its limitations, it is believed that thoughtful application of this procedure would result in more consistent policy and greater effectiveness in attainment of the objectives of technical assistance programs in public health and socioeconomic development.

## INTERNATIONAL HEALTH ORGANIZATION

A consideration of the field of international health may be approached from several directions: first, from the standpoint of the specific preventable diseases and health problems that exist under various local, national, or regional circumstances; second, from the standpoint of the various organizations that are or have been active in the field; and third, from the standpoint of the relationship to present or potential public health organizations or structures in the various political units of the world. In the final analysis it is this latter that is the most important. It must always be borne in mind that effective, fruitful, lasting action can occur only on the local level where the people, their problems, their communities, and their governmental structures are found. Therefore international health work cannot be thought of as a field unto itself. It has meaning only in its relation to the many national and local components of the total world health picture. It is with this reservation that certain aspects of the development and present status of international health activities are presented.

## World Health Organization

Movement toward international cooperation in health goes back several generations, based initially and until recently on concerns about epidemic disease.[14] The first real crystallization was the First International Sanitary Conference in Paris in 1851. It is significant that each of the 12 participating countries was represented by a physician and a diplomat. This was followed by a series of similar conferences, and in 1903 plans began to be formulated for the establishment of a permanent international health agency. This became a reality in 1907, when 12 nations signed an agreement for the creation of the Office International d'Hygiène Publique.[15] Meanwhile, for the same reason, (i.e., concerns about epidemic disease) representatives of 21 American Republics met at their first International Sanitary Convention in Mexico City early in 1902. On December 2, 1902, the International Sanitary Bureau was established. This organization has functioned continuously with several name changes, and as the present Pan American Health Organization, is the oldest international health organization. It also functions as the western hemispheric regional office of the World Health Organization.[16]

To return to the world scene, after World War I was ended the League of Nations was established. It formed as one component in 1921 a Health Organization. Because of obvious conflict and duplication as well as the desirability of broad international connections the Office International d'Hygiène Publique merged with the Health Organization of the league, which continued to function as did the Pan-American Sanitary Bureau, through the period of World War II.

In 1944, while the war was still in progress and Paris occupied by the Nazis, an international conference was held in Montreal to discuss the fate of the Health Organization of the League of Nations. Stemming from this and culminating at a further conference in New York in 1946,[17] a constitution for a World Health Organization was signed by 61 nations on April 7, 1948, and the organization came into official existence. The duties and powers of the Health Organization of the League of Nations and the health functions of the temporary United Nations Relief and Rehabilitation Administration were transferred to the new agency. Sub-

sequently the Pan-American Sanitary Bureau (now the Pan American Health Organization), although retaining a separate identity, became the World Health Organization's regional office for the Americas.

On June 24, 1948, the first World Health Assembly convened in Geneva with delegates from 52 member states plus observers from 11 non-member states, and 10 international governmental organizations.[18] By January 1974 the World Health Organization had a membership of 138 nations, which makes it the largest of the specialized agencies of the United Nations. The United States has been an active member since its formation in 1948 under authorization of P.L. 80-643.

The constitution of the World Health Organization, particularly in view of its definition of health as "a state of complete physical, mental, and social well-being and not merely the absence of disease or infirmity," has been aptly referred to as the Magna Charta of health because of its affirmation that health is "one of the fundamental rights of every human being, without distinction of race, religion, political belief, economic or social condition" and because of its recognition that "the health of all peoples is fundamental to the attainment of peace and security."[19]

With regard to its structure and management,[20] the headquarters of the World Health Organization is in Geneva, Switzerland. Regional offices are located at Brazzaville, for Africa; Washington, D. C., for the Americas (Pan American Health Organization); New Delhi, for Southeast Asia; Copenhagen, for Europe; Alexandria, for the eastern Mediterranean; and Manila, for the western Pacific. It is financed by prorated and special contributions from active member nations and from the United Nations Technical Assistance Board. For 1974 its regular budget was approximately $109 million. An annual World Health Assembly, usually held in Geneva in May, determines international health policy and program and serves as the agency's legislative body. Each member nation is allowed three delegates but only one vote at the Assemblies. An executive board has the responsibility of putting into effect the decisions and policies of the Assembly and deals with emergency situations in the name of the Assembly. Normally this technical nonpolitical group of 24 health experts, who are elected at the Assembly, meets twice a year. A secretariat, headed by a director-general, includes a technical and an administrative staff located at the Geneva headquarters and in the regional offices. It is responsible for the day-to-day work of the organization. The World Health Organization avoids one of the basic errors of the health office of the former League of Nations, that of overcentralization, in that it provides for regional committees comprising representatives of the member states in each region. These regional committees formulate regional policies and supervise the activities of the regional offices. In addition, panels and committees on various pertinent subjects involve more than 12,000 experts in various fields to advise the World Health Organization on its activities and keep it up to date on current scientific research.

The functions of the World Health Organization have been summarized as follows[21]:

1. It is the one directing and coordinating authority on international health work. It is not a supranational ministry of health but rather a worldwide cooperative through which the nations help each other to help themselves in raising health standards.

2. It provides to member countries various central technical services, that is, epidemiology, statistics, standardization of drugs and procedures, a wide range of technical publications, etc.

3. Its most important function is to help countries to strengthen and improve their own health service. On request it provides advisory and consulting services through public health experts, demonstration teams for disease control, visiting specialists, etc.

The World Health Assembly has given top priority to the following six major problems: malaria, maternal and child health, control of tuberculosis, control of venereal diseases, environmental sanitation, and nutrition. Special attention is also given to programs for the control of parasitic and virus diseases, activities in the field of mental health, and family planning. Technical assistance in the field of public health administration, originally placed in the second priority group, has been receiving ever-increasing attention. The relevance of these decisions was confirmed by a survey,[22] which asked member states to list their health problems in order of priority. A total of 46 major health problems were submitted, with the following in highest priority: (1) environmental deficiencies, (2) malaria, (3) tuberculosis, (4) malnutrition, (5) helminthiases, (6) communicable diseases (other than malaria, tuberculosis, and venereal dis-

eases), (7) chronic degenerative diseases and accidents, (8) administrative and organizational deficiencies (including personnel deficiencies), (9) venereal diseases, and (10) mental illness.

There are two important distinctions between the health office of the League of Nations and the World Health Organization, which replaced it. First, the functions and activities of the latter are extremely broad. For the first time in international affairs emphasis is placed not on quarantine, checking epidemics, and other defensive measures but on positive aggressive action toward health in its broadest sense. Second, whereas the former organization was an integral part of a political body, the World Health Organization, although related to the United Nations, is nevertheless a separate independent agency with its own constitution, membership, and sources of funds. As yet it is too early to determine with assurance what the future holds for this organization. Much depends on the ability of the nations of the world to live with one another in peace and cooperation. It has been commonly said that despite its political affiliation, the old health office was the most successful part of the League of Nations. In view of this fact one might hope that the World Health Organization has an even greater chance of success, effectiveness, and permanency. On the basis of its first 25 years, this expectation seems well founded.[23]

## Pan American Health Organization

The turn of the century saw the establishment in 1902 at the Second Inter-American Pan-American Conference in Mexico City of the Pan-American Sanitary Bureau, more recently renamed the Pan American Health Organization.[24] Its headquarters is in Washington, D. C. As has been mentioned, this was the first permanent international health agency and the longest lived up to the present. It was organized to be governed by an elected directing council and a director-general. It is supported by annual financial quotas contributed by each of the American Republics, augmented from other sources. For 1974 it has a budget of $45 million, of which about two thirds comes from assessments of member nations, about $15 million from The World Health Organization and other United Nations sources, and the remainder from miscellaneous inter-American, national, and private contributions. Under the provisions of the Pan-American Sanitary Code, which was ratified by all 21 of the American Republics in 1924, it became the center of coordination of international action and information in the field of public health in the Western Hemisphere. It holds an annual conference of high quality, which is attended by delegates from all member nations. Through its development it has been given the responsibility and authority to receive and disseminate epidemiologic information, to furnish technical assistance on request to member countries, to finance fellowships, and to promote cooperation in medical research. It has done much to promote professional education in Latin America.[25] It also serves as the regional office and agent in the Americas of the World Health Organization.

## United Nations Children's Fund

The United Nations Children's Fund is an agency whose history and activities have been intimately related to those of the World Health Organization. At the demise of the United Nations Relief and Rehabilitation Administration in 1946 certain of its funds were transferred to a newly formed agency organized to assist especially the children of war-torn countries. The program gradually expanded to include other activities and other areas, particularly under-developed countries.

It has spent large sums of money, especially on food and supplies, for the promotion of child and maternal health and welfare activities throughout the world. Beyond this, however, and usually through partnership with the World Health Organization it has been carrying out large and significant programs of BCG vaccination, yaws control, and malaria control demonstrations. The promotion of family planning in developing countries has been one of its major activities in recent years. Organized originally as a temporary emergency agency, it has filled such a need and attracted such support that in 1953 it was given permanent status, and its name was changed to the United Nation's Children's Fund. One of its most interesting and valuable enterprises has been the International Children's Center, established in the late 1940s.[26] The center brings together and coordinates the efforts of many disciplines: pediatricians, social workers, psychologists, educators, and health and social administrators. It is concerned with all three aspects of child development: physical, mental, and social. Its activities are fourfold: international teaching of child welfare problems and methods, medical-social research work, international documentation and publications, and international cooperation in matters of child welfare.

## Bilateral health assistance

So far consideration has been given to the development of what have been commonly referred to as the multilateral organizations in public health, that is, organizations whose financing, staffing, policy making, and operations are entered into and shared by more than 2 and usually many nations. In addition, there exists another type of international health cooperation that is carried out by what are referred to as bilateral agreements and organizations. This comes about when 2 nations for reasons of mutual interest agree to work together on certain matters dealing with public health.

The United States Government became significantly involved in bilateral international public health activities as a result of World War II. In January 1942 the Foreign Ministers of the American Republics, concerned over the turn of world events, considered areas wherein cooperation among the republics of the Western Hemisphere was necessary for the common good and survival. Health needs were placed high on the list. They recommended that through bilateral and other agreements the necessary steps be taken to solve the environmental sanitation and health problems of the Americas and that to this end, according to capacity, each country contribute raw material, services, and funds. The United States was asked to accept the responsibility of leadership, and an Office of the Coordinator of Inter-American Affairs was established. Originally it was attached to the Office of the President of the United States but later assumed a governmental corporate structure with the name Institute of Inter-American Affairs. It was given the responsibility of initiating and conducting bilateral technical assistance programs in health, agriculture, education, and other fields.

Promptly, in intimate relation with each of the other republics involved, cooperative health programs were established with 18 nations of Central and South America. The activities of each were financed by contributions from both the United States and the other governments concerned, and the programs were determined jointly by an official of the host government, usually the Minister or Director-General of Health, and the chief of the group of professionals assigned by the United States to the host country.

From the beginning the program had four areas of emphasis: (1) the development of local health services through health centers; (2) the sanitation of the environment, with particular emphasis on water supply, sewage disposal, and insect control; (3) the training and full-time employment of professional public health workers; and (4) the education of the public in health matters. It stressed complete community health development under full-time trained direction with active community participation.

With the end of World War II and stimulated by the tremendous needs for rehabilitation throughout the world, by requests for assistance from newly formed nations, and by the proved value of the approach of the Institute of Inter-American Affairs, the United States organized a succession of agencies, each to serve certain problem or areal needs. Predominant among these were the Mutual Security Administration and the Foreign Operations Administration. In July 1955 these and the Institute of Inter-American Affairs were joined to form the International Cooperation Administration. In 1961 it was further reorganized to become the Agency for International Development (AID) within the United States Department of State.

The Agency for International Development cooperates with other nations by providing military, economic, and technical assistance. A significant component of the last is assistance in public health matters. At the present time the public health personnel of AID is actively engaged in numerous types of health programs in various countries throughout the world in cooperation with the various assistance programs of the World Health Organization and other United Nations–related agencies, other nations, and private foundations. Many public health and related workers from the United States, representing a wide spectrum of professional disciplines are involved in its programs. One of the most significant contributions of AID and of its predecessors has been in the field of training. Fellowships for advanced training in the United States and elsewhere have been granted to several thousand professional health workers of other countries, and many thousands more have been given in-service training in connection with ongoing cooperative health programs.

During the 5 years 1961 through 1965, AID expenditures for health purposes (not including loans for water supply and waste disposal) totaled $515.76 million. In fiscal year 1972, beside large amounts for population control, AID's health-related budget included $20 million for 18 malaria eradication programs serving over 600 million people, about $15 million for major nutrition programs in 30 countries, and over $25 million on environmental and water supply programs. Cholera control was an important part of the latter. It is current national policy to carry out increasingly large parts of AID's function through the various multinational organizations.[27]

In addition to the United States several other nations provide technical and material assistance in health and other fields on a bilateral basis. Among these are Sweden, the United Kingdom, the Federal Republic of Germany, France, the USSR, and China.

## Peace Corps

Mention should also be made of the Peace Corps, established in 1961 as an agency within the United States Department of State. It has sent many thousands of volunteers, mostly young men and women but also some older well-experienced experts, to work on request in socially and economically underprivileged areas of the world. In many instances they augment significantly the technical assistance provided by AID and other technical assistance agencies.

## Nongovernmental agencies

No summary of international health cooperation would be complete without emphasizing, although briefly, the great contribution that has been made by nongovernmental agencies. As far as "shirt-sleeve" technical assistance is concerned, undoubtedly the earliest endeavors were those of the various church missions and medical missionaries. In addition, there have been certain philanthropic foundations with interest in international health based on the highest altruistic motives. Outstanding among these organizations have been the Unitarian Service Committee, the American Friends Service Committee, the various Catholic Mission groups, the American Bureau for Medical Aid to China, the Foreign Mission Agencies of the Baptist and Methodist churches, the Near East Relief Agency, and many others. Representatives of all these have performed yeoman service, working hand in hand with the people of villages and farms in many lands on a basis of true friendship and equality.

Among the foundations, the Rockefeller Foundation is the best known in the field of international assistance in health. It has operated in almost all countries of the world in the six decades of its existence. Its contributions and successes are many and great and include such activities as the control of malaria and yellow fever, the development of recognized centers of learning in medicine and public health, the provision of postgraduate fellowships to many individuals, and the demonstration of sound methods of organization and operation of health programs.[28] More recently it has been joined by several other foundations, notably the Kellogg Foundation, which is especially interested at the present time in further improving professional education in the Latin American countries.

## Conclusion

To some it may appear as if the programs of international health are too many, too varied, too dispersed, and too confusing. Although this may be true to some degree, it has been by no means unexpected or undesirable. The field of international cooperation for social and economic development is still rather new. Indeed, there are still many individuals in the world who do not comprehend the mutual cause-effect and supportive relationships that exist between the efforts to improve health and the achievement of socioeconomic development. This in itself represents one of the greatest challenges to health workers on both the domestic and the international levels.[29] It has been necessary and logical to approach international health with a combination of caution and courage and often on the basis of trial and error, rather than to attempt at some premature date to establish a fixed pattern that might have stifled future growth and thought. The last few years have seen the beginning of a process of pulling the pieces together both in the multilateral and in the bilateral areas, and it is to be expected that the future will see an ever more logical and fruitful organizational approach to the tremendous problems that still exist in public health throughout the world. The names of some organizations may have changed frequently. If so, it should be borne in mind that only results count and that titles are incidental.

Finally, it must be realized that there will always be an important place for all three types of international health work, that is, the multilateral, the bilateral, and the nongovernmental. Each in its way provides support to the others. Sound, effective, and cooperative correlation of all of their activities may result in the ultimate achievement of the universally desired goal of world health and through it indirectly in world peace.[30]

## REFERENCES

1. World Health Organization: World Health statistics report and world health statistics (annual), Geneva, The Organization.
2. Brockington, F.: World health, London, 1958, Whitefriars Press.
3. World population data sheet, Washington, D. C., 1969, Population Reference Bureau.
4. Russell, P.: A lively corpse, Trop. Med. News **5:**25, June 1948.
5. LeRiche, W. H.: World incidence and prevalence of the major communicable diseases. In Wolstenholm, G., and O'Connor, M., editors: Health of mankind, London, 1967, J. & A. Churchill, Ltd.
6. Summary proceedings of the First Meeting of the Central Council of Health, Jan. 29-31, Hyderabad, 1953, Government of India, Ministry of Health.
7. United Nations, Document E/1327/Add. 1.
8. Wright, W. H.: Medical parasitology in a changing world, J. Parasit. **37:**2, Feb. 1951.
9. Stoll, N. R.: This wormy world, J. Parasit. **33:**1, Feb. 1947.
10. Said, M., Goldstein, H., Korra, A., and El-Kashlan, K.: Blindness prevalence rates in Egypt, Health Services Rep. **88:**89, Jan. 1973.
11. Guthe, T., and Hume, J. C.: International aspects of the venereal disease problem, New York, 1948, American Social Hygiene Association.
12. Myrdal, G.: Economic aspects of health, WHO Chron. **6:**207, Aug. 1952.
13. Hanlon, J. J.: The design of public health programs for underdeveloped countries, Public Health Rep. **69:**1028, Nov. 1954.
14. Goodman, N. M.: International health organizations and their work, New York, 1952, Blakiston Division, McGraw-Hill Book Co.
15. The evolution of international cooperation in public health, WHO Chron. **12:**263, July-Aug. 1958.
16. Pan American Health Organization: sixty-five years of interamerican health, PAHO Info. Series no. 7, Washington, D. C., 1967, The Organization.
17. U. S. Department of State: International Health Conference, New York, June 19 to July 22, 1946, Pub. no. 2703, Washington, D. C., 1947, Government Printing Office.
18. Doull, J. A.: The first world health assembly, Public Health Rep. **63:**1379, Oct. 22, 1948.
19. World Health Organization: Basic documents, ed. 22, Geneva, 1971, The Organization.
20. The structure and working methods of the World Health Organization, WHO Chron. **12:**269, July-Aug. 1958.
21. Division of Information, World Health Organization: The world health organization, Geneva, 1967, The Organization.
22. The world health situation: major problems, WHO Chron. **22:**11, Jan. 1968.

23. The second ten years of WHO, WHO Chron. **22:**265, July 1968.

24. Pan American Health Organization: The Pan American Health Organization: what it is, what it does, how it works, Washington, D. C., 1972, The Organization.

25. Pan American Health Organization: Facts on health progress, Scientific pub. no. 166, Washington, D. C., 1968, The Organization.

26. Berthet, E.: Activities of the international children's center, Amer. J. Public Health **48:**458, April 1958.

27. AID health programs to be internationalized, U. S. Medicine, p. 22, Jan. 1, 1972.

28. Shaplen, R.: Toward the well-being of mankind, Garden City, N. Y., 1964, Doubleday & Co., Inc.

29. World Health Organization: Interrelationships between health programmes and socio-economic development, Public Health Paper no. 49, Geneva, 1973, The Organization.

30. Morison, R. S.: Medical overseasmanship—obligations, opportunities, operations, J. Med. Educ. **36:**207, March 1961.

*Every wise gardener knows better than to crowd his luck by crowding his plants too closely. Even the most aggressive organisms, such as weeds, rodents, and noxious insects, do not increase and spread indefinitely.*

PAUL B. SEARS

CHAPTER 4

# Population and public health

## STORM WARNINGS

Without question the single most significant phenomenon in man's history is his tremendous and rapid increase in numbers during the past few generations. The potential consequences of this biologic surge are so great and far reaching in terms of local and world politics, economics, morals, and even ultimate existence as to justify concern and possibly pessimism. Increasingly, public health workers are criticized for compounding the problems of the world by causing widespread overpopulation through their dramatic saving and extension of lives. Public health workers, sociologists, political scientists, and others have long been aware of a relationship between public health activities and increases in the populations of nations and of the world.[1] Awareness has been sharpened by recent world events, especially the sustained postwar rise in birthrates in many areas and the growth and success of international technical assistance programs in health and sanitation. This awareness has reached the point of acute concern, which increasingly is voiced in part by questioning, indeed even condemnation, of the activities of the "dangerous doctor," the "heedless hygienist," and the "cynical sanitarian."[2-8] On the other hand, there are those[9-11] who are optimistic concerning the ability of this planet to sustain us. In view of these divergent opinions it is pertinent to consider some of the facts, problems, and interrelationships of this important question.

## THE BIOLOGIC SURGE

On the basis of recent anthropologic research by Leakey and others[12] it would appear that man has existed as a distinct species for possibly 2 million years. One may assume that throughout this long period, and in fact during any part of it, man multiplied to the extent that his way of life and environment allowed. The best available evidence indicates that during most of man's existence, increase was gradual and often precarious. It is estimated that by 6000 B.C. the total world population was probably only about 5 million, an amount that is now added to the present world population every month. At the time of Christ it had reached about 250 million. Over 16 centuries were to pass before it doubled to about 500 million in 1650. Then an acceleration began; the population doubled during the next two and a half centuries, then doubled again in less than another century. It took all of man's long history to reach the current figure of about 3.8 billion people, but it will require only about 35 more years to double that figure to an anticipated 7 billion. If the current rate of increase—2.1% compounded annually—continues, by the year 2050 the world's population will reach an almost incomprehensible 20 billion, and this is only about 75 years in the future! Usually accepted estimates are that the earth can support a maximum of 15 billion people if all land cultivation is brought up to that of the Netherlands. It should be

**Table 4-1.** Rate of population increase by region, 1970*

| Region | Population (millions) | Annual increase (%) | Doubles (in years) |
|---|---|---|---|
| Europe | 455 | 0.9 | 70 |
| North America | 224 | 1.2 | 60 |
| USSR | 238 | 1.3 | 55 |
| Asia | 1,946 | 2.0 | 35 |
| Oceania | 19 | 2.1 | 32 |
| Africa | 336 | 2.4 | 28 |
| Latin America | 266 | 2.9 | 24 |
| World | 3,483 | 1.9 | 38 |

*Modified from Logan, W. P. D.: The world population situation, J. Roy. Soc. Health **4:**200, April 1971.

pointed out, however, that calculations such as this are subjects of disagreement.

Overall the world's population is currently increasing at the rate of over 200,000 per day, or about 75 million per year. This is equivalent to adding a city the size of Des Moines, Yonkers, or St. Petersburg each day or the total combined populations of the United Kingdom and the Scandanavian countries each year. The annual increase is also equivalent to about one tenth the population of China. Indeed, the increase of the past decade is equal to the population of all Europe, exclusive of the USSR. The rate of increase is not the same, however, in all parts of the world. In the well-developed nations it varies from only 0.5 to 1.7% per year. This is in contrast with rates of 2% to 3.5% per year in the lesser developed nations (Table 4-1).

## DYNAMICS OF POPULATION GROWTH

When population growth data are studied, it becomes apparent that many forces in addition to public health are involved.[14] Thus the onset of the upswing in world population actually antedates the modern public health movement. As indicated previously, a significant quickening in the rate of population increase began about 1650. It is difficult to determine the relative importance of the various factors that must have been involved in the reduction of mortality and in the resultant increase in population. However, the increases during the first part of this period could not have been due to public health measures because few if any existed. Rather, the determining factors appear to have been changing social organization, a rising standard of living, gradually improved nutrition and work conditions, and the appearance of certain social reforms.

In Europe a significant excess of births over deaths was already well established by the eighteenth century. This produced a steady population increase despite fluctuations due to frequent epidemics and occasional famine. Then in the midnineteenth century a great decrease in mortality began, with a consequent upsurge in the rate of population increase. A peak was reached in the early twentieth century, despite much emigration. This upsurge may be attributed to the development of improved transportation, which facilitated a wider distribution of goods and people; to the technologic progress of the Industrial Revolution, which provided more goods and improved living conditions for greater numbers of people; and more recently, to the acquisition and wide application of new knowledge concerning the cause and prevention of disease. Subsequently, despite continued decline in death rates, population growth in Europe decelerated as a result of a rapid fall in birthrates.

Population growth in the United States differed from that of Europe in three respects. First, during the early nineteenth century the rate of natural increase was much higher than in Europe, probably because of the young average age of those who came to America. Second, throughout the rest of the century the rate of natural increase declined due to rapidly dropping birthrates. Thus in the United States, births per 1,000 women 15 to 44 years of age dropped from 276 at the beginning of the nineteenth century to 208 at the midpoint and to 130 at the end. Finally, despite this considerable slowing in natural increase, the flood of immigrants prevented a drop in the rate of total population growth.

The relationship between population changes and economic and social conditions was reviewed in *The Determinants and Consequences of Population Trends,*[15] issued in 1953 by the Population Division of the United Nations Department of Social Affairs. This extensive review indicated not only that many basic aspects of the problem had been scarcely considered but also that there was much disagreement about interpretation of much of what had been studied. One thing appears obvious: In relation to population change no single factor, for example, public health activity, can be considered alone as if it existed in a social and historic vacuum. Indeed, a highly complex series of interrelationships is involved in the dynamics of population growth, stability, or retrogression. A partial list of factors to consider includes areal limitations; climate; present size, spatial distribution, and age structure of the population; present and potential resources for food; availability and use of efficient agricultural implements, machinery, and techniques; availability and quality of housing; policies and practices with regard to public health and education; existence, availability, and utilization of natural resources and sources of energy; methods of verbal and physical communication, with special emphasis on farm-to-market roads; trends toward urbanization and industrialization; tax and financial structure, especially the availability of short-term and long-term loans at reasonable rates of interest; policies relating to the composition, full employment, and adequate compensation of the labor force; and a multitude of cultural factors.

Space does not permit adequate consideration of these factors. A few examples, however, illustrate the manner and extent to which some of them may affect a population. It is well known that the addition of new sources or types of nutrient will result in increased bacterial growth or increased size of a herd. It is not surprising that this applies also to human beings. Thus in the eighteenth century the sweet potato was introduced into China as an inexpensive, easily grown and stored, and rich source of carbohydrate in place of or to supplement grain. As far as is known, no other significant factor was changed. Certainly no public health or sanitary activities were introduced. Within 50 years the population increased from an estimated 60 million to 160 million. It is also interesting to note that the inception of the population spurt in Europe dates from about the time of the introduction of the white potato from the Andean region of South America.

The larger the area effectively available to a species the more the species tends to move and also increase. Thus an inoculum multiplies and spreads throughout a container of nutrient broth. This has also been the experience of man, most noticeably when new lands were discovered or developed. It was obviously more than chance that the beginning population upswing in the world coincided with the great period of discovery, colonization, and exploitation, and with more widely available and more rapid means of transportation.

In the final analysis life depends on energy. The determinant school of sociology has analyzed the history of man from this viewpoint and noted that each time a new source of power or energy has been discovered, a period of unrest and strife has occurred, resulting in a smaller number of units of people—clans, tribes, nations, or alliances. Then an increase in production and a great upsurge in population has followed.[16]

However, as Sears[17] has observed, "No form of life can continue to multiply indefinitely without eventually coming to terms with the limitations of its environment. . . . Every wise gardener knows better than to crowd his luck by crowding his plants too closely. Even the most aggressive organisms, such as weeds, rodents, and noxious insects, do not increase and spread indefinitely."

Without doubt public health measures have contributed to population increase during the past century. They have done so in four ways: (1) by improving the chances of fruitful conception, (2) by greatly increasing the chances of survival among infants and young children, (3) by preventing the premature deaths of many young adults who comprise the most fertile component of a population and the group with the longest period of future fecundity, and (4) by greatly reducing the number of marriages dissolved by the death of one partner. This too has allowed a longer period of effective conjugal life.

Among the social and economic factors related to the dynamics of population, consideration must be given to the extent of urbanization and industrialization. These are two of the most notable phenomena of our time and are closely related. They have an interesting two-phased effect on population growth—initial encouragement, followed by secondary retardation. The sequence is complex but basically appears to be about as follows. Industry, concentrated in centers of population and offering a means to obtain cash income, tends to attract especially the more mobile, vigorous, and adventurous young adults. At first they tend to follow the old established, essentially rural customs of their kind—marry young and aspire to large families. Sexual union among them is more fruitful because of their youth and because of the long average remaining period of fecundity. To this extent, industrialization and urbanization result in a substantial initial increase in the rate of population growth.

However, with improved education, growing sophistication, stabilization of the labor force, the wish for an improved standard of living, social rivalries, and competition for time, energy, and income there develops an emphasis on rationality and independence from tradition, with a breaking away from the traditional conservative cultural ties. Marriages are delayed, and families are kept small for the sake of more education, increased income, or improved social position. Children come to be considered less an economic asset and more an economic burden. Family life becomes less cohesive because individuals have many contacts outside the home. Since life becomes increasingly complex, sexual intercourse becomes less frequent or more vicarious and chances of fertilization decrease. Added to this is the more ready availability of methods of contraception and the knowledge to obtain and use them. Hence industrialization and urbanization result eventually in a decreased rate of reproduction and population growth. This has been found to hold true in Eastern as well as in Western civilizations.[18]

Reference has been made to the lesser developed areas of the world. Understandably there is concern over the rapidly declining death rates occurring in these areas in the face of high birthrates. Certain considerations should be borne in mind, however. In such circumstances there are several reasons for rapid mortality decreases at this time. These areas are suddenly benefiting from technical knowledge that required long periods of investigation and experimentation by the presently advanced areas. The practical and immediate application of this lifesaving knowledge in the lesser developed areas is now possible at low per capita cost because of the development of relatively simple and inexpensive techniques and the provision of international cooperation and assistance. It is unfortunate that during the early and critical phase of these assistance programs, technical knowledge and the inclina-

tion and political courage to plan for and maintain a proper balance between lifesaving measures and birthrates were lacking. Belatedly, family planning activities are encouraged and included in technical assistance programs to developing countries. One hopes that the ecologic balance has not been already so upset as to make these efforts too little and too late.

Another important reason for rapid decline in mortality is the great striving for independence and national identity throughout the world. In the lesser developed nations great emphasis is understandably placed on catching up as quickly as possible in education, in health, and in technical, industrial, and economic progress. Because so much is needed, achievements have been rapid and dramatic. It would be unrealistic, however, to expect improvements in health or other fields to continue indefinitely at the present rate. In the field of health, preventable communicable diseases have accounted for a large part of the illness and death, and it is in this area that almost all the gains have occurred. Other gains will take longer and will be more difficult to achieve. This is borne out by the slowing in the rate of mortality decline in some countries such as Sri Lanka, British Guiana, Japan, and others.[19]

After studying many aspects of this question, Woytinsky and Woytinsky[20] concluded:

> The growth of world population in the past three hundred years obviously does not express the secular trend and cannot be projected indefinitely into the future. Rather, it has been a unique, unprecedented and unrepeatable phenomenon of limited duration. It had a beginning in the not too distant past, and it will have an end, perhaps, in the not too remote future. The slowing down and levelling off of growth in world population seems unavoidable. The question is only when will growth stop and at what level.

The possibility of a reversal must always be kept in mind. Overwhelming uncontrolled population increase itself would eventually produce a stifling effect. Furthermore, despite the great improvements that have occurred in the mortality picture, if concurrent progress in fields other than health does not occur, a slump in the curve of health progress may be anticipated. Thus Stolnitz,[21] who refers to social and economic factors more as permissive than precipitating, states, "It is obvious that the impact of medical skills on today's underdeveloped areas can be enormous. Whether the permissive elements will also be adequate is perhaps the foremost problem confronting half the world's population." Already a Zero Population Growth movement is underway,[22],[23] and its goal appears to be approaching achievement in several nations, including the United States.[24]

It should not be overlooked that some of the same social and economic factors that affect mortality also affect fertility. Their relationship to mortality is not necessarily the same as their relationship to other factors that contribute to population change. Thus factors that contribute to mortality decline may not necessarily raise the rate of population growth, since they may also contribute to a decline in the birthrate. In this regard public health activities can contribute to improved school attendance and cerebration, to industrial development and urbanization, to higher general income levels and improvement in the standard of living, and to an understanding of man's physiologic and reproductive functioning as well as a better appreciation of his place in society. Beyond this it is reasonable to expect that some of the same forces that have been speeding the decline in mortality will also effect the speeding of a lowered birthrate, hence the deceleration of population growth. In other words, it is possible that the so-called dangerous time lag between lowered mortality and lowered fertility may be telescoped.

Of necessity, much has been left unsaid. No mention has been made of the potentials of more efficient land use, development of new agricultural techniques, improvement of plant and animal strains, application of nuclear energy to power development, irrigation, water distillation, food preservation, more adequate utilization of solar energy, reduction of food wastage by insects and vermin, chemical soil treatment, and hydroponics; and there has been no mention of the release of land for food use as a result of inexpensive artificial fibers and plastics, the food value of algae, the possibilities of sea farming and sea breeding, the possibility of more artificially manufactured foods, and the need for less energy as a result of increasing mechanization of farms and industry. The technologic possibilities of the future seem vast indeed and give some cause for reasonable optimism and hope.

## POPULATION AND ECONOMIC PROGRESS

One of the most fundamental facets of a culture or society is the productivity of the individual and his group—the degree of success to which he can feed, clothe, and house himself and those dependent on him. In the simplest sense this constitutes the economy of the individual or the group. The concept of both society and its economy implies people, and the plurality of the word *people* implies relationships, one type of which is interdependence and mutual support. But there is always the potential reverse relationship of competition and mutual destruction. Either relationship appears to be the result of the degree of balance or imbalance between the two dependent variables mentioned— the nature of a population, on the one hand, and of its economy, on the other. A population necessarily depends on its economy, whereas economic development in turn requires a population and is pursued to serve that population's purposes. Theoretically at least the greater the population total, the more will be its productivity. On the other hand, the greater the population, the more it must produce. Furthermore, the more a population grows, the broader and deeper must be its economic base. The breadth and depth of the economic base are dependent in turn on the resources that nature has made immediately and potentially available. These have tangible limits, and the avoidance of their depletion depends on careful husbandry and conservation to allow for whatever natural regeneration and replenishment may be possible.

To this point the word *population* has been used in a loose and general sense. It is important to consider certain of its components. Each population contains a proportion of socially dependent nonproducers—the young, the elderly, the infirm, and the unemployed. It must be recognized also that these groups are constant consumers. Indeed, at least two of the groups, the young and the infirm, in many societies such as that in the United States tend to consume proportionately more of the products and services of society than does the rest. Obviously therefore the more dependents there are in a society the larger must be the corps of producers. Any circumstance that alters the number and proportion of the various types of dependents and producers affect the economy. Similarly any change in the extent or nature of the economy tends to affect the number and proportion of dependent nonproducers. The most obvious effect is an increase in unemployed persons. Usually close on the heels of unemployment, however, comes a decrease in the number of conceptions and births. Excellent recent examples of this sequence are provided by the economic recession and a major steel strike that occurred in the United States in the late 1950s.[25] If a lowered economy should persist, financial inability to obtain adequate nutrition and preventive and therapeutic medical care as well as other necessities and amenities results inevitably in an increase in the number and proportion of individuals who become acutely and chronically ill. Finally, because of the interplay between these last two effects, there eventually occurs at least a temporary increase in the proportion of dependent adults and elderly persons.

Much of the problem with which mankind is confronted results from the different rates and timings of these and other changes. To consider this in another dimension, certain highly and rapidly effective disease preventive measures have made it possible within a relatively brief period of history for large numbers of otherwise doomed infants and children not only to survive but also eventually to become parents. Not so prompt has been the effect on the number and proportion of persons of advanced age. Not so prompt also have been changes in cultural attitudes with respect to family size, the role of children in society, attitudes toward fertility, and the control of conception to compensate in time for the population changes noted. As Sears[17] has pointed out, this delay, uncertainty, and confusion are understandable in view of the overwhelming force of the reproductive urge, "whose consequences are far less immediate and far more complex than those that may result from mixing a solution or throwing a switch." The individual beset by this natural urge is equally beset by inertia, custom, tradition, and the voices of his time, which "despite their common belief in the dignity and worth of human life, do not always see eye to eye."

Chisholm,[26] the first Director-General of the World Health Organization, expressed a similar opinion in relation to underdeveloped areas. He considered it impossible under current circumstances for foreign development assistance to be increased sufficiently to make possible the necessary rapid economic development in the face of high birth and survival rates. He stated the following:

There are limits to the amounts of capital that can be absorbed usefully in an underdeveloped country at a given time. There are limits to the speed with which the people can be educated or trained. There are limits to the rate at which public administration can be improved, and to the rate at which public service can be expanded. And clearly, all these limits are narrowed by rapid population growth.

Many insist, however, that public health workers should be seriously concerned and pessimistic about the distribution of the world's food products and especially about the possibility of improving to any significant degree the standard of living of the average inhabitant of the earth during the remainder of this century.[27] Chisholm[26] illustrates this by pointing out that whereas a per capita income of $100 annually in a situation with a 1% population growth per year would increase to $135 annually over a 10-year period, it would increase to $106 annually in the face of a 3.5% population growth per year. As he indicates, there are already several places in the world that have approached or reached the latter high rate of population increase.

It has become commonplace to compare the economically advanced countries with those that are economically retarded. Fifty-four percent of the world's inhabitants exist in 12 countries with 9% of the world's income, whereas the 7% who live in the United States and Canada produce and consume 43% of the world's income. Similarly one can compile a long list of variables that measure different aspects of social and economic development as well as political stability and sophistication and find, as one would expect, a remarkable consistency of relationship. Then one can examine the densities of population and their respective rates of increase and income. Here the relationships are less clear cut and evident. The populations of Japan and the Netherlands are as dense as those of Egypt and Sri Lanka; those of Great Britain and the eastern United States are as dense as the populations of the Balkans and Indonesia. To pursue this further into another dimension one might compare the natural resources of the eastern United States with those of Indonesia and still be left with some unanswered questions.

It would appear therefore that no simple direct relationship exists between socioeconomic status and population. One is forced to conclude that the relationship is affected by or dependent on a third set of variables, and evidence appears to be mounting to point to

**Table 4-2.** Vital balance in three world areas by degree of industrialization*

| Nature of group | World population (%) | Death rate | Birthrate |
|---|---|---|---|
| *Industrialized* <br> Relatively balanced and stationary populations with relatively low birth and death rates and incipient population decline (USA, United Kingdom, Scandinavia, France) | 20 | 10 | 15 |
| *Transitional* <br> Somewhat imbalanced and expanding populations with significant control of deaths and beginning control of births (eastern and southeastern Europe, USSR, Japan, Brazil, Argentina) | 20 | 15 to 20 | 25 |
| *Preindustrial* <br> Relatively balanced populations with high birth and death rates but with high population expansion potential (Asia except USSR and Japan, Africa except South Africa) | 60 | 30+ | 35+ |

*Modified from Gordon, J. E., Wyon, J. E., and Ingalls, T. H.: Public health as a demographic influence, Amer. J. Med. Sci. **227:**326, March 1954.

the importance of the degree to which the combination of mobility, urbanization, mechanization, and industrialization has become a fundamental part of the way of life. This even appears to hold true in areas devoted essentially to mineral extraction and agriculture. Thus the populations of those areas that pursue such ends in a large-scale, mechanized, or industrialized manner fare better, at least temporarily, than do those that retain the more simple, primitive, and individualized way of life. This was illustrated some years ago by Gordon and co-workers[28] in a comparison of three groups of nations (Table 4-2). It indicated that the greater the degree of industrialization, hence presumably urbanization, mechanization, and mobility, the greater will be the degree of balance between birthrates and death rates. It should be noted that in the interval since the study, several nations, notably the USSR and Japan, have changed categories.

The fact that there is a worldwide trend toward urbanization and industrial development, as well as toward more efficient agriculture, would seem to provide some basis for optimism. These twin changes not only result in more food and goods for more people at less unit cost, and indirectly force facilities for greater mobility, but also tend to increase the ratio of those who recognize a smaller family as an advantage. This is related to a departure from outdated traditional beliefs, practices, and customs regarding family size, the purpose of the individual, interpersonal relationships in general, and the roles of children and women

in society. Meanwhile it is worth emphasizing the conviction that some social scientists have done a disservice to the concept of economic development and to the recipients of its benefits by totally decrying its effect on existing mores and social organization as if they should be regarded as completely inviolate. To the contrary, one should frankly recognize that it is often critically necessary to change family and group attitudes and practices to reduce birthrates as well as illness and death rates and to improve individual, group, and national living standards. To do otherwise is most unrealistic. Indeed, that in essence is what health education is all about. Some, for example, have advocated almost total emphasis on agricultural programs to the exclusion of efforts in other areas of economic development. This would be disadvantageous in the long run because the life of the typical farmer is highly traditional, and merely to make it tolerable would remove the necessity or incentive for him to alter or adapt his attitudes and behavior toward many things, especially his family's size and purpose.

To carry this line of reasoning into the area of health programs in relation to economic development and population control it might be considered best under certain circumstances, such as during a transitional period, to emphasize activities in certain selective fields or areas such as the following:

1. Activities that tend to emphasize urban industrial areas more than rural agricultural areas
2. Activities that tend to favor presently

productive components of the population more than dependants

3. Activities that tend to aid potential producers more than postproducers
4. Maternal and child health activities that convince women of the advantages of having fewer but healthier children
5. Activities that tend to improve the social and political position of women
6. Activities that tend to develop new sources of security for the individual in place of traditional social institutions that tend to encourage large families

In considering the foregoing, however, it must be realized that the circumstances that led to industrial and economic development in the West were different in certain important respects from those confronting much of the remainder of the world, including Asia, Africa, and much of Latin America.[29] In the West, as already indicated, urbanization and the introduction of successful attacks on the resulting rising mortality have accompanied industrialization. In fact, for a significant period economic and industrial development in western Europe and the United States has depended on a lowered mortality in company with a sustained high birthrate and immigration rate for its continuance. During that period, industry could be considered to have consumed human life at a rate faster than it could be produced locally. By contrast the present situation elsewhere in the world is quite different. By virtue of the sudden application of certain products and techniques of the industrial culture, mortality rates are declining rapidly in the face of sustained or increased birthrates. As a result, populations are soaring. The significant point is that these changes are precedents rather than necessary concomitants of the hoped-for economic, social, and industrial development. Many authors have commented on the dangerous time lag between lowered death rates and lowered birthrates. Another dangerous time lag to which perhaps not enough attention has been given is summarized by Van den Haag[30] in the following way:

> The endogenous industrialization of the West was prepared for by a cumulative historical development starting at least in the Renaissance, and including the rise of individualism, rationalism, empiricism and science, the fall of feudalism, and numerous other changes which led to the attitudes associated with successful industrialization. The sudden introduction of an alien economic system without

historical preparation is a far more difficult and dangerous operation. It is unavoidable by now, but we must be prepared for undesirable side effects.

The phenomenon is further compounded by the agglutination of large numbers of persons in urban centers, not because growing industries can absorb them but because of the magnetism of the hoped-for amenities of a culture that is not yet there to enjoy.

The foregoing general comments are only a few of the many complex aspects of the relationship of population to socioeconomic development. Although concern over these problems is rapidly increasing, it is by no means new. The lack of reference to Malthus may have been noted. Instead, attention is called to a statement made two generations ago in 1908 by Carver[31]:

> Fundamentally there are only two practical problems imposed upon us. The one is industrial and the other moral; the one has to do with the improvement of the relations between man and nature, and the other with the improvement of the relations between man and man. But these two primary problems are so inextricably intermingled, and they deal with such infinitely ranging factors, that the secondary and tertiary problems are more than we can count.
>
> But whence arises that phase of the conflict with nature out of which grows the conflict between man and man? Is man in any way responsible for it, or is it due wholly to the harshness or the niggardliness of nature? The fruitfulness of nature varies, of course, in different environments. But in any environment there are two conditions, for both of which man is in a measure responsible, and either of which will result in economic scarcity. One is the indefinite expansion of human wants, and the other is the multiplication of his numbers.

The difficulty therefore is that all the intimate, interlinked phenomena discussed so far do not proceed apace, and some of them eventually end up counterproductive. It sounds satisfying to speak of the potentials of increased production of food and goods by the application of new methods and technology so that the needs and wishes of more people can be met. But this assumes that there is no limit or end point to development and production on a finite planet. Such a view is obviously illogical and folly. It also ignores the fact that although production of food and manufactured goods is shifting from first into second gear, the production of more people or consumers has been and still is racing ahead in ultrahigh gear. The concerns and warning of Reverend Carter two generations ago have been updated, documented, and dramatically voiced by the so-called "Club of Rome,"[32] a loosely organized group of leaders in a variety of disciplines, professions, and occupations. Beginning in 1968, the group arranged for extensive and continuing amounts of data to be sent to a research group at the Massachusetts Institute of Technology. The data relate to the following six factors: (1) the rate of population increase, (2) the rate of food production, (3) the rate of urbanization, (4) the rate of industrialization, (5) the rate of natural resource consumption, and (6) the rate of environmental pollution. Briefly, no matter what combinations have been put into the computer model so far, none except one appears to offer a real hope for the continuation of the human species. The exception is an immediate and significant cutback on all six factors together. To make an exception of or to underemphasize even one of them will still result in failure and ultimate disaster. On the basis of past and present human behavior it is unrealistic to expect the kind of total worldwide coordinated effort indicated.

The human species, especially those responsible for education, industry, politics, theology, medicine, and public health, who play such determinant roles in the life and future of society, have now reached a point when a critical and prompt decision must be made, a decision that no degree of euphoria or optimism can allow to be delayed any longer. Something has to give. Mankind must either face reality and take rapid and forthright steps toward the deceleration of the increase in man's numbers and of the misuse of man's self-limited environment or accept the inevitable take-over by nature, manifested by widespread political unrest, pestilence, and famine. Thus all man's hard-won gains would be lost.

What may be concluded so far? First, public health effort has saved lives but thereby has contributed to population increase; second, public health is only one of many factors involved in both social improvement and population increase; third, public health measures tend to be more rapidly successful than do activities in other fields; fourth, interrelationships among all the fields involved are still little understood in terms of cause and effect; fifth, assistance to underdeveloped communities or areas should be multidisciplinary and never limited exclusively to public health or any other single field of endeavor and should always be associated with family planning programs; sixth, in conducting public health programs anywhere, rather than attempt the impossible of bringing about public health changes entirely within existing cultural patterns, as if they were static, public health workers should encourage changes that are consistent with the realities of desirable dynamic, social, and public health improvement; seventh, there are valid reasons to believe that time may be running out more rapidly than previously realized and that prompt and coordinated worldwide efforts in several problem areas are critically indicated.

## FAMILY PLANNING PROGRAMS

In view of the foregoing it is obvious that efforts toward agriculture or industrial development or individual family or community self-sufficiency must be accompanied by population or fertility control. Furthermore, data exist to indicate that the incidence of infant mortality, maternal mortality, prematurity, mental retardation, congenital malformations, and brain damage is significantly higher than average among fourth and subsequent births, among births to older women, and among first births to girls in their early teens. These undesirable phenomena are more likely to occur when pregnancies follow each other rapidly in economically underprivileged women whose health is below normal as a result of poor living conditions, undernutrition, and inadequate medical care. It has been estimated that about 2,200 infants' deaths would be prevented annually among each 500,000 low income patients if they were provided with voluntary family planning services.[33] With reference to maternal risks, it has long been known that puerperal death rates increase significantly with increased age and multiparity of the woman. In addition, a study by the World Health Organization has noted that 10% of maternal deaths are caused by abortions, many of which are induced because of large families.[34] The removal of the mother by premature death or by invalidism especially in such instances is a family catastrophe. Practical availability of family planning services would go far to eliminate these needless causes of suffering and death. Parents with large families necessarily tend to be inextricably caught in the dependency vortex, and children born into it escape only with great difficulty. All aspects of living tend to be inadequately attainable—housing, food, recreation, education, and health. Such families also tend to be more frequently broken.

For these and many other reasons, fertility control or family planning has been promoted for many years in the United States as well as in various other parts of the world. Until recently, however, the promotion has been largely by some private physicians and several private or voluntary organizations. Without question the greatest credit must go to the Planned Parenthood Federation of America, founded by the courageous and dauntless Margaret Sanger, who persisted over many difficult years for the fulfillment of an idea she considered humane, honorable, and important. Progress was discouragingly slow due to a variety of cultural blocks, political opposition, and technologic inadequacies. Gradually professional organizations also took a positive position. At present the list includes the American Public Health Association, the American Public Welfare Association, the American Medical Association, the National Academy of Science, and the United Nations and its various specialized agencies such as WHO, UNESCO, and UNICEF. These actions have coincided with several significant scientific and technologic advances, particularly the development of relatively inexpensive, easily used, and increasingly effective methods of contraception. At the same time and for a complex set of reasons a remarkable change in public attitude toward the subject has occurred. Greatly improved and extended public education, the rigors of economic depression and wars, affluence, the emancipation of women, the development of mass communications—these and many other factors have led to a considerable liberalization of public, religious, and political attitude. Of great impact in the United States have been the forthright statements of recent Presidents, beginning with the late John F. Kennedy. Another significant milestone was the invalidation by the Supreme Court of the United States on June 7, 1965, of the 1879 Connecticut antibirth control law. The Court ruled that such legislation violated the constitutional right of married couples to privacy. One member of the court, however, pointed out that the interpretation was a two-way street and must be regarded also to protect welfare clients against coercive promotional techniques.

Federal, state, and local health, welfare, and similar agencies have adopted enlightened policies at an increasing rate. The first state-supported family planning services in local health departments were established in 1937 in North Carolina. Six other southern states followed (Alabama, Florida, Georgia, Mississippi, South Carolina, and Virginia). Services were incorporated into maternal health clinics and home nursing programs and served primarily rural rather than urban areas. Mention should also be made of the development and operation during the 1930s of a large number of birth control clinics in Puerto Rico, using funds from the Children's Bureau. It is interesting that although the federal government still does not have a firm overall policy on family planning, many of its present component agencies are actively involved in a wide variety of services, research, and training programs in this field.[35] By now the majority of the states and many cities are included. Unfortunately policies vary considerably, as does the effectiveness with which they are carried out.[36] With reference to this, a study of 56 metropolitan counties with the largest number of infant deaths, accounting for 26% of the national need, has indicated that only about one fourth of the women who needed subsidized family planning services were actually obtaining them from some source. Only about one half of the services obtained were provided by health departments. By the mid-1960s schools of public health had begun to present special seminars and curricula designed for the training of various types of professionals to work in family planning programs.[37]

In July 1969 an important step was taken by President Nixon in the creation of a Commission on Population Growth and the American Future to study the various ramifications of the problem and to make recommendations relating to national research and action policy.[38]

**Methodology**

Although it is not the intent of this book to be a technical manual in any sense, the nature and importance of the subject at hand are such as to justify a few words about methods of contraception. The origins of attempts to prevent conception are lost in primitive history. Some indications of the wide variety of materials used may be obtained from a study by deLaszlo and Henshaw.[39] The Ebers Papyrus, 1550 B.C., includes an interesting recipe for a medicated tampon to control fertility. The compound consisted of a mixture of acacia and honey, which was to be inserted into the vagina as a suppository. Interestingly, on fermentation acacia breaks down into lactic acid, a rather effective spermicidal agent.[40]

At the present time there exists a wide variety of behavioral, physiologic, chemical, and physical methods of contraception. They vary widely as to effectiveness, acceptability, cost, and other factors. The use of many of them requires or indicates the assistance, advice, or supervision of a physician or other properly trained person. To a considerable extent the ultimate choice depends on individual preference.[41] The amount of research that is being carried out in this field is such as to anticipate further radical discoveries, hence changes in methodology, at any time.

Among the areas of active investigation are once-a-month oral contraceptives that combine a long-acting estrogen and a progestogen, a progestogen-impregnated Silastic vaginal ring implanted for a month at a time, a year-long capsule of progesterone for subcutaneous implantation, a long-lasting injectable preparation of medroxyprogesterone acetate, a postcoital, or "after-the-fact," pill based on a prostaglandin derivative, and the synthesis and possible use of the luteinizing hormone–releasing factor (LH-RH, or LRF) of the pituitary gland.[42,43] All the foregoing are for use by women as of course are the various intrauterine devices. For use by men, in addition to vasectomies, which are being done increasingly in the United States and several other countries,[44] there have been unsuccessful attempts to develop a contraceptive pill based on pituitary gonadotropin suppressants, to inhibit sperm production by the administration of large doses of androgens, which unfortunately increases the risk of heart attacks, and the oral use of a number of nonsteroid sperm-suppressive compounds that, unfortunately, were either toxic or could cause genetic damage. Attempts to immunize men with testicular antigens and protein hormones have so far met with limited success, but research in this direction is very active.[42,45]

Special mention should be made of abortion as a method of conception control or family planning. Reference was made previously to the severe physical and psychologic risks of self-induced, unsanitary, or unskilled abortion. Despite the considerable emotional, religious, and political conflicts that the subject has engendered, an increasing number of public and professional organizations as well as political jurisdictions have approved and endorsed the use of proper medically-induced abortion for a variety of reasons and justifications, including family planning. Recent reports in the United States indicate about 270 legal abortions per 1,000 live births, and in some other countries such as Japan the rate is much higher. The beneficial effects on maternal mortality rates have been notable. In Great Britain, out of 160,000 legal abortions performed in 1972, there were only 10 deaths, which gave a maternal abortion death rate of 6 per 100,000 compared with a former rate of 12 per 100,000. For simple abortions performed at less than 13 weeks gestation, the rate was only 3 per 100,000.[46] During the first year of legal abortion in South Australia, deaths attributable to abortion dropped to zero, and the total number of women dying in childbirth fell sharply.[47] In mid-1970, New York State liberalized its laws concerning abortion. During the three years July 1970 to June 1973, almost 600,000 legal abortions were performed in New York City. Only 20 of the women involved died, giving a rate of only 2 per 100,000 legal abortions. The comparison with the national maternal mortality rate of 24 per 100,000 live births in 1972 needs no comment. Beyond this was a beneficial effect on maternal mortality as a whole. During the three years preceding liberalization, the maternal mortality in New York City was 51 per 100,000 live births. During the first three years of liberalization it dropped to 38 per 100,000 live births.[46] Although most agree that abortion is a "second-best" approach to family planning as compared with successful contraception, the evidence of the beneficial effects of properly performed abortion in place of self-induced, unsanitary, and unskilled abortion is incontrovertible.

### REFERENCES

1. Hanlon, J. J.: The public health worker and the population question, Amer. J. Public Health **46:**1397, Nov. 1956.
2. Vogt, W.: Road to survival, New York, 1948, William Sloane Associates.
3. Osborn, F.: The limits of the earth, Boston, 1953, Little, Brown & Co.
4. Cook, R. C. In Russell, P. F.: Public health practice and population pressure in the tropics, Amer. J. Trop. Med. **1:**177, March 1952.
5. Cook, R. C.: Human fertility: the modern dilemma, New York, 1951, William Sloane Associates.
6. Rolph, C. H.: The human sum, New York, 1957, The Macmillan Co.
7. Brown, H.: The challenge of man's future, New York, 1954, The Viking Press, Inc.

8. Hill, A. V.: Nature **170**:388, 1952.
9. Boyd-Orr, J.: Proceeding International Congress of Population, Cheltenham, England, 1948.
10. deCastro, J.: The geography of hunger, Boston, 1952, Little, Brown & Co.
11. Coale, A. J.: The economic effects of fertility control in underdeveloped areas. In Hauser, P. M., editor: The population dilemma, Englewood Cliffs, N. J., 1963, Prentice-Hall, Inc.
12. Man's origin: mystery deepens, M.D. **9**:99, July 1965.
13. Logan, W. P. D.: The world population situation, J. Roy. Soc. Health **4**:200, April 1971.
14. Stanford, Q. H.: The world's population: problems of growth, New York, 1972, Oxford University Press, Inc.
15. Population Division of the United Nations Department of Social Affairs: The determinants and consequences of population trends, New York, 1953, United Nations.
16. White, L.: Man's control over civilization, Sci. Month. **66**:235, March 1948.
17. Sears, P. B.: Pressures of population, an ecologist's point of view, What's New **212**:12, 1959.
18. Tauber, I. B.: Population and labor force in the industrialization of Japan, 1850-1950; economic growth in Brazil, India, and Japan, Princeton, 1955, Princeton University Press.
19. Bourgeois-Pichat, J., and Pan, C.: Trends and determinants of mortality in underdeveloped areas, New York, 1956, Milbank Memorial Fund.
20. Woytinsky, W. S., and Woytinsky, E. S.: World population and production; trends and outlook, New York, 1953, The Twentieth Century Fund.
21. Stolnitz, J.: Comparison between some recent mortality trends in underdeveloped areas and historical trends in the West. In Bourgeois-Pichat, J., and Pan, C., editors: Trends and differentials of mortality in underdeveloped areas, New York, 1956, Milbank Memorial Fund.
22. Ehrlich, P. R.: The population bomb, New York, 1968, Balantine Books, Inc.
23. Notestein, F. W.: Zero population growth: what is it, Family Planning Perspectives **2**:20, June 1970.
24. Item, Amer. Med. News Jan. 17, 1972.
25. Westoff, C. F., Potter, R. G., and Sagi, P. C.: Some selected findings of the Princeton fertility study, 1963, Demography **1**:1, 1964.
26. Chisholm, B. In Jones, J. M., editor: Does overpopulation mean poverty? Washington, D.C., 1962, Center for International Economic Growth.
27. Hauser, P. M.: Demographic dimensions of world politics, Science **131**:3414, June 3, 1960.
28. Gordon, J. E., Wyon, J. E., and Ingalls, T. H.: Public health as a demographic influence, Amer. J. Med. Sci. **227**:326, March 1954.
29. Coale, A. J., and Hoover, E. M.: Population growth and economic development in low-income countries, Princeton, 1958, Princeton University Press.
30. Van den Haag, E.: Population and economic development, What's New **214**:4, 1959.
31. Carver, T. N.: The economic basis of the problem of evil, Harvard Theol. Rev. **1**:1, Jan. 1908.
32. Meadows, D.: The limits to growth, New York, 1972, Universe Books, Inc.
33. Family planning and infant mortality; an analysis of priorities (mimeographed report), New York, 1967, Planned Parenthood-World Population, p. 8 ff.
34. Beck, M. B., Newman, S. H., and Lewit, S.: Abortion: a national public and mental health problem, Amer. J. Public Health **59**:2131, Dec. 1969.
35. Report on family planning: activities of the U. S. Department of Health, Education, and Welfare in family planning, fertility, sterility, and population dynamics, Washington, D. C., 1966, Government Printing Office.
36. Eliot, J. W.: The development of family planning services by state and local health departments in the United States, supplement on family planning, Amer. J. Public Health **56**:6, Jan. 1966.
37. Corsa, L.: Introduction, supplement on family planning, Amer. J. Public Health **56**:3, Jan. 1966.
38. An act to establish a commission on population growth and the American future, Public Law 91-213, 91st Cong., S. 2701, March 16, 1970.
39. deLaszlo, H., and Henshaw, P. S.: Plant materials used by primitive peoples to affect fertility, Science **119**:626, May 7, 1954.
40. The first prescription for control of fertility, M.D. **9**:58, July 1963.
41. Calderone, M. S.: Manual of contraceptive practice, Baltimore, 1964, The Williams & Wilkins Co.
42. Duncan, G. W.: Fertility control: contributions for the future. In Progress in drug research, Washington, D. C., 1969, Pharmaceutical Manufacturers Association.
43. Arehart-Treichel, J.: Birth control in The Brave New World, Science News **103**:93, Feb. 10, 1973.
44. Vasectomy patients multiply, Amer. Med. News, April 24, 1972.
45. Contraceptives for men, M.D. **16**:88, Oct. 1972.
46. Barnett, M.: Legalized abortion credited with some health advances, Hosp. Tribune, p. 5, Feb. 11, 1974.
47. Hosp. Tribune, p. 2, March 26, 1973.

# PART TWO

# Socioeconomics of public health

The manner in which those engaged in public health view themselves and the field of activity in which they are engaged has undergone an interesting evolution through the years. Originally they regarded their work as part of medicine. As specialized knowledge and techniques were developed and applied, it came to be considered as a separate science—sanitary science. With the involvement of increasing numbers of individuals other than physicians, public health became known as a distinct discipline, then a profession in itself. More recently, as the effects or end results of public health programs on other aspects of life and society manifest themselves, those in the field have begun to recognize themselves for what they truly are—agents of social change. This places the public health worker squarely in the arena of applied sociology, sharing kinship with a broad array of other social scientists. It is some of the more pertinent of these fields with which the following section is concerned.

> *You see clearly that something more
> than a microbe is needed to make us ill,
> since we so often find the organism and
> so rarely the disease.*
>
> LOUIS PASTEUR

CHAPTER 5

# Social science and public health

## HUMANITY REQUIRES CHANGE

Although the term *public health* has been used for several generations, the significance of the *two* words seems often to be overlooked. Implied are both a product—health—and a recipient—the public. Obviously the most complete knowledge and understanding of one is pointless without corresponding knowledge and understanding of the other. Leavell[1] had this in mind when he wrote:

Two major types of changes with which public health must deal are going on in the modern world: "public" changes and "health" changes. Our professional training helps us most with the health changes. Our knowledge of biology, chemistry, and physics and their medical sub-specialties helps us find and use the proper immunizing agents to prevent disease, the right kinds of food to eat, the best sprays to kill mosquitoes, and so on. We can usually adjust rather readily to rapid changes demanded as a result of research which provides better tools with which to combat health problems.

The public changes that are so important in public health work are in many respects more difficult for us to appreciate. Most of us have limited backgrounds in the basic social sciences—sociology, anthropology, psychology, economics, and political science—that might help us understand better the people with whom we must work. Yet public changes are often of even greater importance than health changes.

. . . we need a great deal more research to be able to translate the findings of biological investigation into social application. When we meet a health problem, we must recognize that two kinds of diagnosis and treatment are necessary. We must understand and deal with the health problem. We must also understand and treat the social or public part of the situation. Our pharmacopeia in both fields must be strong. It is no longer sufficient to prescribe drugs and neglect the social factors in a given case.

## THE MEANING OF HEALTH TO SOCIETY

Typically each of us views his particular interests and activities as of paramount significance. Because of this, there is some danger that public health workers may consider public health goals as ends in themselves and the activities required for their achievement as necessarily of primary interest to society. If they do, disappointment and disillusionment are inevitable. This is particularly true if, as is sometimes the case, goals have been arbitrarily determined and activities planned and carried out by "experts" who themselves are necessarily biased, without concern for the needs, ideas, and wishes of the group to be served. The group or public may look on the goals and activities differently. Furthermore, for reasons of group pride, cohesion, or self-assertion, the group may be forced into the psychologic position of objection or resistance.

Actually, although health is a common need and the effort to attain it represents a common drive, it is of secondary rather than primary importance. Even primitive man is concerned with the achievement of a total or integrated way of life. Because of the complexity of its ingredients, this is not easy to define. Some distinctions are possible, however, especially through study of certain situations such as

**72**

primitive societies and societies under stress. In such circumstances it soon becomes clear that although man and his societies are subject to many needs, urges, or drives, only a few of them are primary or basic, that is, the need for food, for shelter, and for sexual expression or propagation. As for many other goals, of which health is only one, most individuals and society in general are interested only to the extent that they make possible the achievement of related goals, especially those that are primary in nature. Actually, comfort, the absence of pain, and well-being are relative terms. Thus in societies where the majority acquire malaria or trachoma, these conditions tend to be regarded as part of the normal pattern of life and are adapted to as well as possible. Under such circumstances ill health tends to be considered as the presence of any condition that is unusual or beyond these. This is put in another dimension by Dreitzel,[2] who indicates that since there is no objective definition of illness, one must ask in whose interest and for what purpose "illness" is defined by different social classes and ethnic and religious groups. Generally illness tends to be defined by patients as any impairment of their physical well-being that conforms with what society tends to accept as "being sick." Merely to feel unwell does not suffice if the individual is not seriously disabled for work or social interaction. "Only then," Dreitzel concludes, "does unwell become socially accepted and the role of the patient is granted, entitling the afflicted to attention, care and protection."

It might be said that man will strive for food, shelter, and sexual expression in the absence of complete health, but he will not strive for complete health in the absence of the others. A few examples may help to place the desire for health in its proper perspective. A man and woman stranded on an island will ordinarily seek to assure themselves of food, shelter, and sexual satisfaction before giving attention to other needs. In most instances they will seek to satisfy these three needs or urges in the order given because of the differing critical intervals involved. Furthermore, they will do so in the face of actual or potential threats to their health or safety. Thus if the only source of food or of materials for shelter is in or near an insalubrious spot, they will still seek them out. Later, perhaps, they may seek out a more desirable alternative. With regard to sexual expression and health, undoubtedly syphilis could be completely eradicated by abstinence from sexual inter-

course by everyone. The chances of this procedure being followed are obviously nil because when faced with a choice between the two, the risk of infection will be readily accepted by the majority. The example is more than theoretic, since the suggestion has been made on more than one occasion to individuals or special groups to no avail.

Another example of health being relegated to a secondary position was encountered in relation to technical assistance activities in malaria control in North Africa. In certain areas the date is the basic element in the food supply and economy. Despite the recognized relief from malaria, the activities eventually were opposed in some communities because the insecticide DDT killed not only the malaria-transmitting *Anopheles* but also the species of fly that normally carried the pollen from the male to the female date palm. To assure both desirable ends, modifications in control techniques had to be developed.

Sometimes public health or medical deterrents to death may be regarded as undesirable. This may come as a shock to those accustomed to regarding health and the preservation of life as universally desired goals. When conditions for life and survival are difficult and especially when disease and premature death are common, the social attitude toward death may differ from one's own. In some cultures, death of infants or the aged is not necessarily a grievous event. The infant does not yet have a fully developed personality and may be regarded as an added economic burden to the family. The child's timely removal may mean more food and other things for the rest of the family and less suffering and misery for itself in the long run. This is sometimes evidenced in funeral ceremonies in less developed societies with high death rates. The difference between the funeral of a productive adult and that of a very young child or of an elderly person is striking. In the former there usually is genuine regret shown by the mourners. The adult has been around long enough for people to know him as a personality. Beyond this his death is recognized as the economic loss of a producer for his family and the group. In funerals of elderly persons there is again genuine regret, but not as much as in the former case. True, the elderly individual's personality is well known and familiar in the local scene. However, he has served his economic purpose in life, as he has also served his social purpose by producing offspring and by transmitting through his life the mores of the group. He now has become an economic or even a social burden that has to be supported. Furthermore, he is now entitled to his well-earned release to the rewards and security of the hereafter. In the case of infants and young children the difference may be even greater. Often there appears to be surprisingly little mourning. The physical appearance of the funeral procession, if anything, may appear bright and, among some peoples, even rather joyous. Songs may be sung, bands may play, and when the small body is finally removed, there may be a somewhat enthusiastic social event, with dining, drinking, dancing, and indulgence in all other pleasures of the flesh. Even in more sophisticated societies, gradations of these differences in attitudes may be observed. Suffice to point to the oft-expressed ameliorating comment that a deceased child was "pure of heart" hence much more likely to achieve everlasting happiness.

Finally, attention is directed to certain societies in which to be ill and suffering is to be considered saintly or god-like. Then there are groups or cultures in which to become ill and die during a religious pilgrimage is regarded as a good omen for the Hereafter.

The foregoing is not intended to belittle or discourage efforts toward the improvement of public health; rather, the purpose is to point out that health is a relative concept, that its definition and value vary from one place to another, and, even in a given society through time, that it is only one facet of the total interest and welfare of the individual and his society and as such, is in constant competition with all other factors of greater or lesser importance to that individual and that society. It is important to realize this because as Koos[3] has pointed out: "What we can expect a community to provide, and its members to accept, in the way of health activities must therefore be viewed in a framework which is peculiar to that community. This in no way prevents the establishing of uniform goals or standards for health, but it does mean that community efforts directed toward better health are necessarily custom-built."

## SOCIAL ANALYSIS AND COMMUNITY ORGANIZATION FOR HEALTH

Each of us is many things. First, we are individuals, a composite or compromise of various strengths and weaknesses, interests and prejudices, abilities and failings. But as some philosophers have claimed, perhaps there is no such thing as a true individual; each of us is the product and a part of a series of environments beginning with the womb. Beyond being individuals we are members of families and beyond that, members of varying numbers and types of social groups with shared and common needs and interests—complexes of interrelated families, the guild, the village, the clan, eventually agglutinating to form various types of cultural and national entities.

Human beings everywhere are members of groups. To varying degrees they are dependent on one another for sustenance, education, inspiration, economic welfare, entertainment, and many other needs. The individual needs the group, but not necessarily only a particular group, or always the same group, or the same group for all needs. The same conditions also apply to the group's need for the individual. Although the bonds that link the individual to the group must be strong if they are to be of value, they are not necessarily fixed. They may be and in fact often are broken or transferred. Accordingly individuals are seldom found to be members of only one group. Different groups are needed for different purposes. Although this is less apparent in primitive societies, even there individuals have multi-group attachments—to the family, to a larger kinship group, to a totem group, and to a maturation cult or secret society as well as to the tribe. In more highly developed societies the plurality of group membership is more evident. In addition to the family there is the school, the church, the social club, the athletic club, the business and professional associations, and many others.

The question inevitably arises whether all of these many groups are necessary and important or whether, for health promotional purposes or for other reasons, it is possible successfully to approach and influence all individuals through one group. Stated otherwise, is it possible to focus all of man's interests toward one group? Is it possible to have one group that would satisfy all needs? Clearly the answer is found in reality. Innumerable groups exist because people develop them to meet their various and varying needs. An individual requires a social complex of many differing groups to obtain sufficient significant or fruitful relationships that will satisfy the various facets of his personality and interests. Repeated attempts have been and continue to be made to relate the complete allegiance and interest of people to one single supergroup, for example, the state. So far, in the long run such attempts have failed, and it would appear that all future attempts will experience the same fate. Life devoted exclusively to one group is necessarily extremely narrow and self-limiting. "The man who can live without society," said Aristotle, "is either a beast or a god. But the man who can live exclusively for the state, if indeed such a being exists, is either a tyrant or a slave."

Granted that it is the nature of man to identify with various groups, how does this affect his behavior and his receptivity? Important in this regard is that man's behavior as an individual is usually different from his behavior as a member of a group or of society, and that his social or group behavior varies from group to group. Furthermore, when a point of common concern or mutual interest exists and can be adequately identified, widely differing groups may join forces and with regard to that particular interest jointly behave differently from the way each group behaves alone. This does not mean that any one group forfeits its identity. As Skinner[4] points out, "Social behavior arises because one organism is important to another as part of its environment. A first step, therefore, is an analysis of the social environment and of any special features it may possess."

Since the intention here is social analysis for the purpose of community or social organization for public health improvement, it is important to distinguish and identify groups which may be of significance toward that end. There are three general categories of identifiable groups, the existence of which the specialist in community organization should be constantly aware. They are important because community organization for health cannot be carried on apart from the social worlds in which people for whom it is designed live, or can community organization ignore the strength of the factors that create distinctive values regarding health and that place these values high or low in the whole hierarchy of values that are an essential part of life.

The first of these groups provides for ethnic identification. This is represented by religious, racial, or nationality groups, each with its own prescriptions, prohibitions, and ideals, any one of which may be of significance in relation to health and sickness.

A second category is related to ethos identi-fication, that is, bonds which identify individuals as belonging to the same ethical, economic, or social group. Often this is coincident with a neighborhood. The economic, educational, or moral nature of the group may determine the extent or manner of participation in activities designed for the improvement of the public health.

Finally, there is the family, which usually represents the most powerful example of social cohesion. To ignore the predominant influence of the family in the development or conduct of a public health program usually guarantees failure. The pertinence of Koos'[3] remarks in this regard justifies their repetition here:

We may well question the logic of industry- or school-centered programs that ignore the importance of the family as a "conditioner of attitudes," and which may send the individual back into his family to face conflicting ideologies about health and its value. This is not a plea to abandon school- or industry-centered programs; it is to point out that such programs can work effectively only if they send the individual back to his family prepared to adjust differences that may have been engendered; to make him, in effect, a health organizer in his own small family world. If the individual is no so prepared . . . the cost in tensions and frustrations can outweigh any small good the program may have accomplished.

## SOCIETY AND CULTURE

In the foregoing discussion, reference has been made to several closely related fields. It is important to distinguish between society, the subject matter of sociology, and culture, the subject matter of social or cultural anthropology. A society is any community of individuals drawn together by a common bond of nearness and interaction, that is, a group of people who act together in general for the achievement of certain common goals. A society has both quantitative and qualitative characteristics. Thus it is possible to count and measure the number of individuals who constitute a society. One of the qualitative characteristics is its culture or the manner in which the group as a unit tends to think, feel, believe, and react to stimuli;—in other words, its basis for behavior. As Kluckhohn[5] described it, "a culture refers to the distinctive ways of life of such a group of people . . . a culture constitutes a storehouse of the pooled learning of the group." Every society has its own distinctive culture, and since there are innumerable societies in each community, in each country, and on each continent of the world, there are therefore innumerable cultures, each differing to a greater or lesser degree from all of the others. The study of these cultures, their components, and their relationships with each other is the subject matter of cultural anthropology, the purpose of which is to aid man in understanding himself. Kluckhohn graphically states, "Anthropology holds up a great mirror to man, and lets him look at himself in his infinite variety."

Throughout the entire course of history every member of the human race was born into some sort of culture. Some cultures were primitive, simple, and crude, whereas others were complex and highly developed. Some dwindled and died, whereas others flourished and grew. All of them, however, regardless of their degree of complexity or simplicity, developed techniques, religious beliefs, social systems, and art forms. Every child born into his particular group culture is certain to be influenced more by it than by anything else in his entire life. "As a matter of fact," says White,[6] "his culture will determine how he will think, feel and act. It will determine what language he will speak, what clothes if any he will wear, what gods he will believe in, and how he will marry, select and prepare his foods, treat the sick, and dispose of the dead. What else could one do but react to the culture that surrounds him from birth to death?"

This behavioral determining effect of culture on the individual and the importance of understanding it is further stressed by Benedict[7]:

... The life history of the individual is first and foremost an accommodation to the patterns and standards traditionally handed down in his community. From the moment of his birth the customs into which he is born shape his experience and behaviour. By the time he can talk, he is the little creature of his culture, and by the time he is grown and able to take part in its activities, its habits are his habits, its beliefs his beliefs, its impossibilities his impossibilities. Every child that is born into his group will share them with him, and no child born into one on the opposite side of the globe can ever achieve the thousandth part. There is no social problem it is more incumbent upon us to understand than this of the role of custom. Until we are intelligent as to its laws and varieties, the main complicating facts of human life must remain unintelligible.

Beyond this she says:

The study of different cultures has another important bearing upon present-day thought and behaviour. Modern existence has thrown many civilizations into close contact, and at the moment, the overwhelming response to this situation is nationalism and racial snobbery. There has never been a time when civilization stood more in need of individuals who are genuinely culture-conscious, who can see objectively the socially conditioned behaviour of other peoples, without fear and recrimination.

The importance of culture and the contribution that an awareness of cultural anthropology may make to public health programs have become somewhat more evident to those who have worked in countries other than their own and in the field of international health. They have come to realize, with Carothers,[8] that "the visitor to foreign lands is always most impressed by the general peculiarities of peoples, whereas in his homeland . . . he notices only the individual divergencies." This is a most significant choice of words! It is important to call attention, however, to the oft-overlooked fact that it is unnecessary to visit foreign or exotic lands to encounter different cultures. It is fundamental that the domestic health worker realize that he too has been born into and grown up in a particular culture, received his training in possibly still another culture, and in the conduct of his work must deal with additional different cultures in his own community.

It is well to realize that as Oliver Wendell Holmes so aptly remarked, "The people in every town feel that the axis of the earth passes through its main street." That is why so many tribal and national names, when traced to their origins, are found to mean "the human beings," "the real or principal people," and similar accolades. Thus as Gittler[9] has discovered, "The Greenland Eskimo believes that Europeans have been sent to Greenland to learn virtue and good manners from him. Their highest form of praise of an outsider is that he is or soon will be as good as a Greenlander." This is also why the English language contains such phrases as "beyond the pale" or "the other side of the tracks." It is unnecessary to go to the ends of the earth to find other cultures; we can find them, must understand them, and must live and work with them in our own communities.

In this connection, sound action in a field like public health presupposes sound evaluation of circumstances and situations, and it is important to recognize that the evaluations of public health workers are determined by their own cultural background. In discussing the relationship between science and culture, Bernard[10] says, "We have come to use the term 'definition of the situation' to describe the process which people go through in perceiving, evaluating, and interpreting what goes on about them. Even within a given culture, among people using the same language, the student and the teacher, the husband and the wife, the parent and the child, the employer and the employee, define an identical situation quite differently. They all see, hear, and perceive different things, and what they see, hear, and perceive, has different meanings for each." According to Benedict,[7] "The truth of the matter is that the possible human institutions and motives are legion, on every plane of cultural simplicity or complexity, and that wisdom consists in a greatly increased tolerance toward their divergencies. No man can thoroughly participate in any culture unless he has been brought up and has lived according to its forms, but he can grant to other cultures the same significance to their participants which he recognizes in his own."

What is the purpose of culture? All cultural traits, habits, prejudices, and the like are based essentially on a mixture of conscious and subconscious urges for individual and group survival and perpetuation. As Kluckhohn[5] indicates: "Any cultural practice must be functional, or it will disappear before long; that is, it must somehow contribute to the survival of the society or to the adjustment of the individual." Every society has developed institutions and methods of behavior to safeguard and perpetuate the practices and beliefs that its members consider the most important and valuable. In every society, social arrangements or organizations have been developed over long periods of time on the basis of proved group experience to meet life's basic needs. Programs such as public health necessarily involve the introduction of new and strange practices and changes in these arrangements into the culture of the society. If such programs are to be constructive rather than disruptive forces, the social structure and the traditional cultural way of life of the community must be taken into account and utilized.

Not only are the accepted value systems of a culture deeply ingrained but disadvantaged people adhere particularly strongly to their attitudes and beliefs. This is to be expected, since people who for a long time have been accustomed to crowded living conditions, low economic status, discrimination, and philosophic systems that serve to make life under these conditions bearable look on change or suggested change with misgivings and suspicion. Their greatest fear is that things might get worse, and to them, on the basis of their experience, change often implies that very possibility. One is reminded of Plautus' maxim "Keep what you have; the known evil is best."

Advantageous incentives to change and demonstrations of the value of new ideas, techniques, or actions are necessary to overcome the natural reluctance of people to change their ways and their fear of the possible risks involved in following new practices. They need to have proved to them in one way or another that the suggestions will make possible genuine and lasting improvements in their standard of living. Furthermore, they need to be assisted in their attempts to implement the suggestions made and to integrate them with the rest of their cultural pattern. A public health program must demonstrate to people that the continued improvement in their welfare and level of living is its true purpose. It is insufficient merely to enunciate general principles or objectives of health as if they were the end and to think of the people involved merely as a means to that end. Instead, people must be able to see clearly and unequivocally that the public health activity or program is one that attacks the problem not merely in terms of improved community health in the abstract but in terms of all the needs of people with much the same aspirations the world over for their families and for their neighbors.

It is true therefore as Paul[11] says:

The cultural system does limit the range of individual behavior and in this sense customs exert a restraining influence. Culture defines the values men hold, the goals they seek, the means they use. By thus organizing their outlook, culture is also a guide to action, a positive force that channels motivation and imparts meaning to existence. We are too inclined to perceive the negative and overlook the positive when we behold the customs of others. . . . Now a health program strikes at the uncertainties of death and disease, and it may seem ironical that the dissemination of improved medical practices should be impeded precisely by those superstitions that owe their vitality to the hazards of life deriving from inadequacies of medical knowledge. But faith is strong where risks are great, and people act slowly when it comes to shifting their faith from a familiar system of security to an unfamiliar one, however efficacious the new system may prove to be in the long run. It should not be overlooked that faith gives psychological security, whether faith is placed in magic, religion or science.

One aspect of culture that is easily overlooked is that it is much more than a collection of customs; it is a *system* of customs, each one more or less related to the others in a meaningful fashion. A culture has structure as well as content; it is not just like a haphazard pile of bricks. This gives a clue to the reason for the tenacity with which societies hold on to their customs. Each one is like a gear in a transmission system, important and necessary for the total function and directly or indirectly related to all of the other gears. As it is impossible to remove a gear from a transmission system and still have the system function without an adequate substitute, so it is impossible to remove a custom from a culture without providing for an equally satisfactory or better substitute custom. To carry the analogy further, the end result of a transmission system is the product of its component gears, not merely their sum. Similarly a total culture is the product of its component parts or customs—not merely the sum—and if any one basic part is destroyed or reaches zero, the entire culture collapses. Eisenhower had this in mind when, speaking at Supreme Headquarters Allied Powers Europe, he said: "The strength that a nation, or a group of nations, can develop is the product obtained by multiplying its spiritual or moral strength, by its economic strength, by its military strength. . . . There can be no army unless there is a productive strength with a productive power to support it. There can be neither a strong economy nor an army if the people are spiritless, if they don't prize what they are defending."

Benedict[7] narrates a significant and touching anecdote in this regard. She tells of her conversations with a chief of the Californian Digger Indians who had been "civilized" and integrated to a greater or lesser degree with Western civilization. He told her of life in earlier times, of the ceremonies, the agriculture, the tribal economy, and of how each of these and other customs were so meaningful to the tribe: "In those days," he said, "his people had eaten 'the health of the desert' and knew nothing of the insides of tin cans and the things for sale at butchershops." It was such innovations that had degraded his people in the latter days. Then he added one day: "In the beginning God gave to every people a cup, a cup of clay, and from this cup they drank their life. They all dipped in the water, but their cups were different. Our cup is broken now. It has passed away."

In discussing the social disorganization that developed in the little Guatemalan town of Tiquisate, site of an experiment in agricultural productive efficiency, Hoyt[12] warns:

The potential economic effects of increasing production cannot be abstracted from the actual psychosocial effects; and it is possible, if we are not careful, that the disorganization accompanying the latter may be greater than the constructive services of the former.

She continues:

If Tiquisate is an outstanding example of productive efficiency, it is also an outstanding example of social disorganization, even to the extent that the latter threatens the former. This is evidenced by a great deal of drunkenness and prostitution—which the people themselves deplore—by lax family relations, and by strong social antagonisms. . . . Although new values appeared, they did not take the place of the old; neither did they furnish a framework within which the psychic aspects of the people's old life could find their place and get the necessary response.

Some years ago I encountered a somewhat similar phenomenon on the lovely island of Bali. The government of the then new nation Indonesia, of which Bali is a part, wanting to take its rightful place in the modern society of nations, apparently deplored any custom that might cause other nations to consider it backward or primitive. It therefore passed a law that required the women of Bali to cover their breasts. According to observers who had lived there for some time, there soon came about a noticeable change in the attitude of Balinese males toward female breasts and toward women, and it is significant that within a brief time after that law was passed prostitution appeared on the island. That a causal relationship actually exists in this case, of course, is not possible to determine. The circumstances and timing, however, give some reason to wonder.

In summary to this point, therefore, all human beings are members of societies, each with its own culture consisting of a complex mosaic of interrelated customs. These customs have developed through the ages as a result of group experience in the struggle for survival and for a reasonably satisfactory life. Accordingly, people relinquish customs reluctantly, and it is well that they do because each custom has stood the test of time, and it or a truly adequate substitute is fundamental to the continued existence of the society. The great contribution of cultural anthropology to the conduct of programs in a field such as public health is constantly to identify and point out the importance of cultural patterns of the groups or societies that constitute a community or a nation. Social evolution inevitably disturbs cultural patterns, but that is one price of progress. However, cultural patterns need not and should not be disturbed more deeply or more rapidly than the people involved are able to tolerate and adapt to. This principle should underlie all of the actions of the public health worker.

## EFFECT OF CULTURAL PATTERNS ON HEALTH

With the previous considerations in mind it is obvious that many if not all cultural patterns bear some relationships to the degree of health of a people and the extent to which they will accommodate themselves or be receptive to efforts that might be made to improve their state of health. It does not seem necessary to discuss here the positive or scientifically desirable contributions of certain cultural patterns to health or the even more obvious contributions of sound public health measures in general to cultural development. Instead some examples will be given of cultural patterns that may have a disadvantageous effect on the health of a people.

There are many reasons for ill health, only a few of which will be discussed. One easily recognized reason is ignorance or lack of knowledge about the factors involved in the causation of illness and death. During a period when the infant mortality for the city of Detroit was significantly declining, several districts were not sharing in the improvement. Analysis indicated that they were populated predominantly by individuals from a particular European nationality. Study of their cultural attitudes indicated a considerable family attachment to the infant as well as a typically neat and clean household environment. However, further inquiry brought out that traditionally infants were taken off the breast at an extremely early age and fed essentially adult foods, often directly from the family table. Concurrent analyses of the causes of infant mortality in these areas indicated a high incidence of death due to severe digestive disturbances and intestinal infections. It was necessary over a period of several years to bring to bear the efforts of a reoriented and rather specialized public health nursing program, assisted by appropriate nutritional and pediatric consultation. In addition to this instance there are groups in which it is the custom for mothers to prechew solid foods for their babies and young children, not realizing the bacteriologic risk in their attempt to carry out what seems to them a logical procedure.

Frequently, economic factors are cultural reasons for ill health. Until recently in the United States, and even now in several other countries, certain methods of earning a living have resulted in high incidences of tuberculosis and other diseases. This has been particularly true of certain industrial and manufacturing activities and in areas where trading, with its increased contacts, forms the economic basis of a group. Difficult as it may be for some to believe, there are many societies in which excrement, both human and animal, represents one of the most valuable commodities because of its use either as a fertilizer or as fuel. The extent of the use of human feces for fertilizer and the inherent health risks involved are well known and need not be dwelt on.

With regard to the use of excrement as fuel, the following example may be pertinent. Some years ago an attempt was made to improve health conditions in several villages in Egypt by installing latrines, constructing wells, and killing flies with insecticides.[13,14] The project was regarded as less than successful, not just because the fly population repeatedly developed resistance to the insecticides used, but particularly because of various cultural features of the situation that could not be changed within the scope of the project. One factor was that the dung of the *gamous* or cow was exceedingly valuable as the only form of fuel for heating and cooking. Accordingly, all members of each household were constantly on the lookout for dung and would collect it, pat it into cakes, and store it within the confines of the household where it would be safe from thieves. There it constituted a continuous and effective breeding matrix for flies. An additional factor was that each house served as the shelter for both the family and its livestock. A significant and permanent improvement in the health of the people of these villages, of which there are many thousands, must depend on effective separation of the family and their livestock, especially the *gamous*. But aside from extremely difficult problems of finding adequate space and building materials for stables in a land where every inch of arable soil is at a premium and trees are rare, considerable social problems arose from such a contemplated change. One of these was the safety and security of the animals. In addition, however, it was learned by careful interviews that many women in the villages found the *gamous* their only source of companionship within the home during the day while the men and boys worked in the fields. Many therefore resisted attempts to end this sociable relationship. It was concluded that an attack on health conditions in the villages merely by methods of sanitary engineering and fly control was not enough. The abominable conditions could not be materially improved without an attack on a broad front involving economic, educational, and social measures as well as those that had been carried out.

Bogue and Habashy[15] have also described the attitude of the Egyptian villager toward his animals and its effect on attempts to improve health conditions by quoting a villager involved:

The fellah has his own habits and traditions which have come down with his long heritage. Many of these habits are good but many contribute to bad health because of lack of experience or ignorance of their effect. The poorest farmers keep their cattle and other animals in the same house they live in themselves. . . . In attempting to get at the basis of such a peculiar habit in this modern time, many approaches were made by the social workers. One old man explained it to a health educator simply that: "We like our animals and want them where we can see them at night. . . . They are our wealth. They are our most prized possessions on which we depend for our very food and livelihood." Such a realistic answer causes social maneuverers to stop and think before making a casual suggestion to move them to a shed.

Although these examples may seem somewhat bizarre, recognition should be given to the presence in innumerable homes in our own societies of all sorts of animal pets, some of which are none too clean, others transmitters of specific diseases such as psittacosis, and to many of which humans may become allergic. Despite all of this, they are maintained on a sentimental or a companionship basis similar to the Egyptian village woman and her *gamous*.

An example of misguided effort and of the effect of economic limitation deals with the attempts by some outsiders to change what they regarded as unhygienic traditional menstrual habits of the Chamorro women, as observed by David M. Schneider in the course of a cultural study on the island of Yap. The attempts to make them give up their practical, time-proved although strange custom were successful, and they were persuaded to use sanitary napkins. However, these are not made locally,

the supply is limited, and the native economy provides little cash for the purchase of manufactured goods. As a result, each individual pad was worn throughout the entire menstrual period, during which time the Chamorro women, following the example of their American sisters, continue to be active in their society where previously they were separated from it. This is cited by Paul[16] as an example of an unforeseen, undesirable consequence of a supposedly progressive social action. I am reminded of a rather impressive phenomenon of this nature observed in several communities in Java. Apparently at some time previously a highly effective promotional program on the merits of brushing teeth had been carried out. Imported toothpaste, however, was well beyond the economic capacity of many of the people. Nevertheless, it was very common to see individuals with toothbrushes in their pockets stopping to brush their teeth at the edges of the many canals that ran through the streets. Since these were actually open sewers used for bathing, laundering—and for brushing teeth—one could not help wondering if the dental hygienic gains might not better be forfeited in the interests of other health considerations.

Conflict of desirable health practices with other cultural values that are considered more important forms another basis for the development or perpetuation of health problems. Few things are as important to people as their religious beliefs. As a result, if it is a custom not to eat a certain type of food such as animal protein, individuals will tend to avoid them even if an adequate nonanimal substitute is unavailable. Similarly, although it is well known that certain of the great traditional pilgrimages mean sickness and death for many people, nothing can deter them from the tremendous cultural drive to participate in the event. Modesty or moral values are factors of considerable import to most people. There have been periods in history and there are still societies where to see the naked body, even one's own or that of one's child, is considered immodest and immoral. In such instances personal cleanliness and hygiene may be inadequate. The type of clothing customarily worn is part of the culture of a people and often has been developed in conformance with the environment. Sometimes, however, clothing acts as a deterrent to health and a spreader of disease. The barracan, worn by many people in North Africa, is a highly practical garment from the standpoint of protection from the environment. However, in some places with scarce water and soap and a common use of the long loose sleeves to wipe one's eyes, nose, and mouth and those of one's children, it becomes a factor in the spread of disease, particularly trachoma, which is so prevalent in that area.

Hyde[17] gives an example of a cultural value, this time the wish for fertility, that supersedes not only health but even convenience (see also Bogue and Habashy[15]):

I recall being told in Egypt of a wealthy landowner who had dug good wells, out of which his fellaheens could obtain clear and pure drinking water. After some three days' use of this safe water, the fellaheens returned to drinking the polluted water of the Nile. On inquiring into their reasons, the landowner was told that the people preferred the Nile water, that it was obviously better because the Nile made the fields fertile and would therefore make the people fertile.

One might speculate on the possible value of an explanation of the relationship between the river water and the ground water through subterranean diffusion as well as evaporation and precipitation. In addition, it might have been possible to point to families of desirable size who used water from a well rather than from the river.

## EFFECT OF CULTURAL PATTERNS ON PUBLIC HEALTH ACTIVITIES AND PROGRAMS

From the examples given, it is evident that public health programs are frequently hampered by failure to inquire into or understand customs that the members of a group consider important. It is a rare public health worker who can truthfully claim unqualified success of every program or activity he has undertaken. Each has had the experience of meticulously planning a program, bringing to bear all technical knowledge available, only to be thwarted or disillusioned by an apathetic or resistant public. Often the reason is human behavior or motivation.

There are many barriers to public health success. One of the most common is inadequate communication. Public health workers frequently think that since they understand what they are thinking and saying, everyone else does. Whorf[18] analyzes this as follows: "Western culture has made, through language, a provisional analysis of reality and, without correctives, holds resolutely to that analysis as final.

The only correctives lie in all those other tongues which by eons of independent evolution have arrived at different but equally logical, provisional analyses . . . An important field for the working out of new order systems . . . lies in more penetrating investigation than has yet been made of languages remote in type from our own."

Even within one's own communities or between age groups, language differences may serve as a communication barrier. Particularly in larger communities there are sizable groups whose ability to speak and understand the official national language is limited. More than one patient has received inappropriate diagnosis or treatment in a hospital, clinic, or health center because he and his examiner could not communicate. An irony of such situations is that the more educated of the two is the least likely to admit to his handicap or failing. Even where the same language is ostensibly spoken, there may easily be differences in interpretations of what is said. There are also such factors as regionalism and provincialism; many words and phrases in a language may have different meanings in different sections of a country, not to mention the varying accents that those who speak them may use. Note, for example, the use of the word *country* in the preceding sentence. It is intended to imply *nation,* but in some places it connotes *rurality.*

An interesting and valuable lesson on communication as a barrier was encountered in connection with a health education program in Bolivia. Few of the rural people could read so that the use of educational films along with other techniques was indicated. At first, for lack of others, films on health that had been produced for use in the United States were shown. As would be expected, they meant little if anything to those who saw them. The people, their clothes, houses, foods, behavior, in fact everything in the pictures was strange and foreign to the viewers. The medical and hospital environments presented conditions much too advanced to be of any practical use or applicability to the local situations. Then several health agencies in the United States had cartoon-type health education films made. These were better in that the characters shown had a more or less universal appeal. However, they were first used with English sound tracks, followed sometimes, it is true, by verbal explanations in the native language. But the crucial moment of maximum impact had passed, and their chief function had still been that of entertainment. After this the films were made with Spanish sound tracks, since that was the official language of the country. Now they became useful as health education films in some areas, notably in a few of the larger cities. However, they were still incomprehensible to the majority of the people who needed them the most because they were Indians, many of whom did not understand Spanish. Therefore we undertook to translate and dub in the sound tracks in the two commonest native languages of the Andes. Now the films really meant something to the people, and they began to respond. Incidentally, they were said to have been the first films with speech in the Quechua language of the Incas and the much more ancient language of the Aymara.

A different type of communication barrier results when the communicator is held in awe by the other person, who is ill at ease and nervous. Foster[19] relates that in the Cerro Baron Health Center in Valparaiso, Chile, 13 women were asked as they emerged from the physician's room to repeat his instructions. The remarks of 10 women indicated that they had failed to profit from the visit. This prompted similar investigations in other countries with similar results. Failure to comprehend the physician's instructions was attributed to several factors. Often a women patient would be nervous and uneasy in the presence of a man, particularly since she usually was in a lower social class than he. She would therefore be unable to concentrate on what was being said. The problem was partially resolved by having the physician write the instructions on the patient's record card, after which a more *sympatico* nurse would explain the instructions in greater detail and more in terms that the patient would understand.

Differences in behavioral patterns may negate carefully planned and well-intentioned public health endeavors. More than one American public health worker has had to learn that the manner in which people relieve themselves may vary. Many American-type privies have gone unused for failure to realize that some people by tradition are "sitters," whereas others are "squatters." Actually, as Leavell[1] points out, it is unimportant for its public health purpose whether the privy has a seat or whether the squatting method is used in defecation. Even where they are adopted and used, surprising cultural handicaps may appear. I recall seeing privies designed by Westerners for rural Burmese, using local materials. The use of convenient, inexpensive local materials was praiseworthy. However, the fact that in rural Burma, as in many other places, paper is a luxury was overlooked. But of even more consequence was the failure to learn that by custom, pieces of bamboo were used for the same purpose as paper in the Western toilet. As a result, before long the privy superstructure tended to have a rather moth-eaten appearance, and the privy hole became clogged with pieces of bamboo. I also recall a provocative conversation, through an interpreter, with a rural Thai. He said, in effect, "You Americans are strange. Before you came here, if I felt like relieving myself, I found a quiet spot in the open with gentle breezes and often a pleasant vista. Then you came along and convinced me that this material that comes from me is dangerous. In other words, I and others should stay as far away from it as possible. Then the next thing you told me was that I should dig a hole, and not only I, but many other people should concentrate this dangerous material in that hole. So now I have even closer contact not only with my own but everyone else's, and in a dark, smelly place with no view at that." Which of us was the more logical?

People will seek to attain and maintain health provided there are no conflicting cultural forces. Even in sophisticated societies people may react in what they know are illogical or ill-advised ways because of deep-seated folkways or cultural traits of which they are sometimes not even aware, much less understand. Here, too, behavioral science may be of great assistance to the public health worker, either through analysis of a situation at hand or by explanation of the same or similar problems in purer cultures, that is, in more simple or primitive societies. For example, why do some people resist hospitalization? It may be that their group customarily looks on a hospital as a place to go to die. Beyond that, behavioral scientists have found that an extremely common if not universal cultural trait is a strong feeling of identification with the land or, in a nonrural situation, at least with the home. Remote in the history of the human species, but in many places even yet, is the feeling that when one dies it should be at home, that the spirit will reside in the place where one dies, and that the spirit's place is with the family. To some people death away from home means that the spirit must wander homeless and will be in an unfavorable position from which to intercede with the gods on behalf of the family who remains behind.

Another common reason for resistance to hospitalization is reaction against its tendencies to break down the cultural sense of responsibility for a family member in distress. In addition to pride, this may be based on the concept that the individual is continuous with his family unit. Still another reason may be an unwillingness to admit that one is sick, weak, or inadequate. This is closely related to another cultural reason for resistance to surgery, that is, shame or a feeling of incompleteness. This is emphasized particularly if by custom much importance is placed on the part removed, notably a breast, the uterus, or the testes. Again one does not have to leave the domestic scene to observe this. Closely related to the concept of continuity of the individual with the land is the fear that the excised part or, in the case of obstetrics, the placenta or the dead fetus will not be destroyed or will be separated in space from the environment of the rest of the body or from the family. In more primitive societies, of course, the thought enters into the picture that the excised part, if not destroyed, may be used against oneself as a fetish.

In obstetrics and gynecology innumerable taboos or cultural barriers are encountered. One reason is hinted at in a study of Yap culture by Schneider.[20] Yap women believe their genitals to be the source of power over their husbands. Since sex organs enable one to secure and keep a husband and to raise a family, they constitute one's personal "trade secrets," which must not be revealed to women rivals. Yap women never allow other women to see their genitals; therefore attempts to use native female attendants in delivery rooms met with resistance. The substitution of nonindigenous female attendants proved somewhat more acceptable. Although women, they are alien to the native system of power and sex competition. A husband may see his wife's secrets, but she knows that no self-respecting Yap husband would allow any man, including an obstetrician, to see and manipulate his wife's secret parts. The wife herself does not believe that exposure before any man is as undesirable as exposure before another woman, but she is constrained by the knowledge that she would be violating her husband's personal rights if she allowed the former. A solution was found by the compromise of using nonnative female attendants and post-ponement of the mechanics of antisepsis and delivery by the physician until after anesthetization.

This leads logically to consideration of difficulties met with regard to nursing in many parts of the world. In many cultures the position of women is still subservient, and in some cultures, women are not even allowed to be seen or move about freely. Under such circumstances it is difficult to develop much-needed nursing training programs. In some other cultures a woman who would touch, cleanse, or come in contact with the discharges or internal parts of other people is customarily held in extremely low regard. In such circumstances it is difficult to elevate nursing to the status of a useful, esteemed profession, since among other things only the poorest, least educated, and least dependable women are free to engage in the activities necessary. As one other example of a cultural reason for resistance to nursing care, the fear exists in some societies that to be touched by or given food by a female nurse might, should she be menstruating, bring impotence, illness, or death.

Spectacular curative measures are more readily accepted than are preventive measures that in the long run might be more beneficial. This is true in the United States and Western Europe as well as elsewhere. In most parts of the world therefore it is impractical to disassociate promotive and preventive measures from those that are curative. Erasmus[21] points to the difference in reception and support of the campaigns against yaws carried on by the Institute of Inter-American Affairs in collaboration with the governments of Colombia and Ecuador in contrast with measures to prevent intestinal infections. The results of the treatment of yaws with antibiotics were rapid and dramatic, and even the native healers readily admitted that the modern medicine was much more effective than their own herbal and magical treatments. By contrast, many looked on the symptoms of intestinal infections in a young child as a manifestation of the "evil eye," outside the realm of scientific medicine. Since the conditions under which they lived and their failure to understand the rationale of the suggested measures made obvious rapid improvement impossible, the measures were not successfully adopted.

Summarizing his findings, Erasmus[21] concludes:

. . . Needs created by the process of specialization

and the desire for increased production and profit actually seem the easiest for technicians from another culture or subculture to meet. The solution is often largely technical, fewer cultural barriers to a common understanding are presented, and the perception and feeling of needs are more easily shared by the innovators and the people.

However, when change is being attempted in a field not directly related to increased production in a cash economy, in other words not directly in terms of profits, the difficulties increase. In the field of public health, for example, the innovator may consider it highly desirable to introduce basic disease prevention measures into an underdeveloped area. But the folk still subscribed to an age-old system of beliefs about the cause, prevention, and treatment of disease, a system so different that the preventive measures of the innovator were meaningless. Lacking an understanding of the modern concepts of the etiology of disease and consequently the reasons for modern methods of prevention, they may feel no need to adopt the prescribed changes. Thus, despite the fact that they feel a general need for assistance in combating the ailments common among them, they may fail to perceive the need for the specific measures proposed and may actively resist them.

Public health workers, particularly the medical component, should always realize that often they are in competition with ancient folklore, superstitions, and erroneous but well-accepted ideas, even in modern societies. The practice of the healing arts is the oldest specialized activity known and one of the few, along with the priesthood (with which it is closely allied), that appears to be a universal characteristic of all cultures. Despite this, the phrase "world's oldest profession" is commonly applied to a rather different activity. Yet as Murdock[22] points out:

> Prostitution, historically, is a relatively recent phenomenon. I have personally read accounts of many hundreds of primitive societies, and in not a single one of them is genuine prostitution reported. Many of them exhibit forms of such behavior that we would regard as exceedingly lax, but such laxity does not take the specific form of prostitution except in the so-called "higher" civilizations. . . . Specialized occupations are exceedingly few in the simpler societies, and with a single exception, none occurs more than sporadically. This exception is the medical profession. Specialized practitioners of the healing art are found, to the best of my knowledge, in every known society, however primitive. The "medicine man," in one form or another, is universal and hence must be regarded as the oldest professional specialist.

If this is true, medical and public health programs would appear to have an advantage over other types of social programs, provided they are designed to make possible ease of adequate transference from the old way to the new. The need to recognize the existence and acceptance of the old ways must be emphasized. If medical and public health measures have an advantage over the other social measures, it is also true that the medicine man, the *curandero,* and the medical superstitions and folkways have an advantage over the new and strange ideas of modern medicine and public health.

In all instances, from primitive societies in the most underdeveloped areas to groups in sophisticated Western communities, there would appear to exist an interesting dichotomous attitude toward illnesses and what might be done about them. The continued extensive use of patent medicines, the enormous amount of self-medication, and the extent to which various types of charlatans, faith healers, and pseudophysicians are consulted by sophisticated societies provide testimony to this. Documentation is provided by a study[23] sponsored by the Department of Health, Education, and Welfare at the suggestion of the Senate Committee on Aging. It was based on interviews of individuals in a national probability sample. The study showed that millions of consumers base important health decisions on the idea that in the light of individual difference there is a chance that almost any treatment may be beneficial. Faith in this approach is reinforced by psychosomatic effects and unaided recovery.

Forty-two percent of the persons interviewed would not be convinced by almost unanimous expert opinion that a hypothetic "cancer cure" was worthless. Only 45% thought such a medicine should be banned by law. Three fourths of the public believe that extra vitamins provide more pep and energy, the most common of the misconceptions investigated in the survey. Although their disorders had never been diagnosed by a physician, 12% of those interviewed reported that they had arthritis or rheumatism, asthma, allergies, hemorrhoids, heart trouble, high blood pressure, or diabetes. Twelve percent of the sample also indicated that they would self-medicate—without seeing a doctor—for longer than 2 weeks for such ailments as sore throats, coughs, sleeplessness, or upset stomach. Twenty-six percent had used nutritional supplements, expecting specific observable benefits, without a physician's advice. About 2% of the persons indicated that they did something every day or nearly every day to help with bowel movement and that they were not following a physician's advice. More than a third believed in various erroneous concepts of weight control, the most common being that sweating is a means of substantially losing weight. Other sworn-by nostrums are nonprescription appetite depressants, massage, and keeping up with the latest published diets. One of the most interesting findings was that older people are generally less likely than young people to make irrational decisions on health problems and are more skeptical about efficacy claims for drugstore remedies.

It may be of value to explore the background of these tendencies in less complex circumstances. In connection with a 10-year evaluation of the cooperative health programs of the Institute of Inter-American Affairs, Foster[19] studied the distinction between folk illnesses and those recognized by medical science. He found that certain types of disease are recognized as not responsive to treatment methods of *curan-deros* but curable or preventable by the scientific physician. On the other hand, there are other illnesses that are considered best treated by home remedies or with the aid of *curanderos*, that is, illnesses which are believed not understood by scientific physicians and the very existence of which they may deny. These illnesses, which may be referred to as "folk diseases," are particularly those considered to be of magical or psychic origin. "If an illness is diagnosed, for example, as 'evil eye,' obviously it is poor judgment to take the patient for treatment to a person who denies the existence of the disease." (Table 5-1.)

Sometimes the illness is actually admitted and recognized by a scientific physician. Even then, if individuals of the culture involved, on the basis of past experience and social custom, regard the condition a result of magical or psychologic etiology, they will tend to rule out the potential usefulness of the scientific physician —and it must be remembered that it is the

**Table 5-1.** Percentage of 48 schoolchildren in Quito, Ecuador, who would consult a physician or a *curandero* for specified illnesses*

| Illness | Would consult a curandero or treat with home remedies (%) | Would consult a physician (%) |
|---|---|---|
| Fright† | 98 | 2 |
| Air† | 93 | 7 |
| Witchcraft† | 86 | 14 |
| Colic | 79 | 21 |
| Evil eye† | 75 | 25 |
| Stomatitis | 72 | 28 |
| *Pasmo*† | 66 | 34 |
| Open infections | 66 | 34 |
| Urinary complaints | 64 | 36 |
| Skin disorders | 61 | 39 |
| Diarrhea and vomiting | 58 | 42 |
| Emaciation | 49 | 51 |
| Smallpox | 31 | 69 |
| Dysentery with blood | 25 | 75 |
| Pneumonia | 25 | 75 |
| Whooping cough | 20 | 80 |
| Liver complaints | 16 | 84 |
| Paralysis | 9 | 91 |
| Typhoid | 7 | 93 |
| Bronchitis | 6 | 94 |
| Malaria | 5 | 95 |
| Tuberculosis | 4 | 96 |

*Modified from Foster, G. M.: Use of anthropological methods and data in planning and operation, Public Health Rep. **68:**853, Sept. 1953.
†Diseases with magical or psychologic etiologies.

patient who makes the decision as to whom to ask for assistance. Attempts have been made to measure the practical effect of the distinction between "folk diseases" and "doctors' diseases." In Ecuador, for example, a list of the commonest complaints was given to 48 schoolchildren of both sexes, ages 11 and 12 years. On the assumption that their opinions would correspond reasonably well with those heard from parents and other adults, the children were asked to indicate which illnesses required a physician and which they would treat with home remedies or take to a *curandero*. The results are shown in Table 5-1. It is clear that even some distinctly physical ailments as well as certain psychologic conditions may tend to be cared for by other than a scientifically trained physician.

Similar surveys have been made in Chile, Colombia, and elsewhere with similar results. If conditions were customarily thought caused by the evil eye, bad air, fright, shock, or other magical or psychic causes of which most people believed modern physicians were ignorant, they were almost universally treated at home with folk remedies or by a *curandero*. This, of course, often prejudiced their chances of ultimate recovery, since often the symptoms were misleading and related to serious illnesses. On the other hand, certain clear-cut conditions such as anemia, appendicitis, hernia, meningitis, pneumonia, smallpox, typhoid, and the like generally, but not invariably, were considered to be within the province of a scientific physician.

Interestingly, a more recent study conducted by Banks and Keller[24] in metropolitan Columbus, Ohio, elicited a surprisingly similar picture. A representative sample of households was presented with a list of 29 symptoms and asked to rate them in terms of the following:

1. I would handle it myself because it is not very serious.
2. If it got worse or kept on I would go to a doctor.
3. I would see a doctor and have him check it out.
4. I would go to Emergency.

In general, symptoms such as bleeding, palpable lumps, frequent vomiting, urinary difficulties, or chest pain tended to be placed in the third or fourth category, whereas sore throat, overweight, poor appetite, frequent headaches or colds, nervousness, joint pains or stiffness, or dizziness were usually placed in the first or second category.

Despite this, it is tempting for those who have experienced only modern scientific thought glibly and arbitrarily to belittle, toss aside, or ignore the practitioners of folk medicine as if they were completely unworthy of consideration. The illogic of this was expressed by Elkins[25]:

Aboriginal medicine men are far from being rogues, charlatans or ignoramuses. They are men of high degrees . . . men who have undergone tests and have taken degrees in the secrets of life much beyond that which ordinary men have a chance to learn. This training involves steps which imply a discipline, mental effort, courage and perseverance. In addition, they are men of respected, and often of outstanding personality. Thus, they are of immense social significance, with the health of the group depending largely on faith in their powers. Furthermore, the various psychic powers attributed to them must not be readily dismissed as mere "make-believe," for many of them have specialized in the workings of the human mind and in the influence of mind on mind and mind on body. And, what is more, they are deeply convinced of their powers, so much so, that as long as they observe the customary discipline of their "order," their professional status and practice continues to be a source of faith and healing power to both themselves and their fellows.

Referring again to the Latin American scene, Foster's[19] analysis of the relationship between the scientific physician and the *curandero* is of particular pertinence and may be applied to our domestic scene with adequate provision for differences in degree and type of social camouflage.

The conflict between folk medicine and scientific medicine is summed up in the persons of the physician and *curandero*. Each represents the highest achievement in his field. The attitudes of the people of Latin America towards each, therefore, are pertinent to this study. Unfortunately, the physician frequently comes off second best. This is due in part to the inherent nature of the situation, and in part to native suspicion of individuals in other social classes, particularly those above them.

The *curandero* operates under conditions that are relatively more favorable than those of the physician, from the point of view of impressing the patient with concrete results and apparent success. He treats folk illnesses, the symptoms of which often are so ill-defined that he cannot help but succeed in alleviating them. If the vague physiological symptoms identified with the illness persist or reappear after the cure, the *curandero* can always say that the case has become complicated and requires another series of cures or a different cure, or that a new and different illness has attacked the patient. Also, most *curanderos* do not claim to cure all illnesses, and in many cases can even recommend that a patient consult a physician. These factors establish the *curanderos* in the minds of the folk as fair, open-minded individuals willing to admit their limitations. Finally, the *curandero's* diagnostic techniques do not require elaborate and eshaustive questioning of the patient as to symptoms, case history, and the like. He has certain magical or automatic devices which he applies to specific situations, and the answers follow almost like clockwork. Moreover, there are many cases reported by field observers in which a physician failed to cure an individual and a *curandero* had apparently genuine success.

The physician enjoys few of these advantages. His diagnosis is seldom cut and dried, he cannot guarantee quick results, and he seldom enjoys the faith and confidence accorded the *curandero* because he is from a social class instinctively distrusted by the majority of his patients. Moreover, the physician seldom admits that a *curandero* can cure things which he is incapable of treating, and this is interpreted as meaning that he conceitedly and selfishly believes himself to be the sole repository of medical knowledge—a point of view which the villager is loath to accept.

Criticisms of physicians and their professional methods are rife among the patients of the lower class, and such criticisms are usually based on a complete lack of comprehension of medicine, its methods, and its limitations. Several patients pointed out that physicians asked them questions about their symptoms, which showed that the physicians were not as smart as they thought they were. A good *curandero* doesn't have to ask questions, so why should a man who pretends to know a great deal more have to do so? Another patient scornfully pointed out that a President of Colombia died "even though he had 50 physicians at his bedside." The implication was that if 50 physicians could not keep a man from dying, a single doctor in a short interview was almost worse than worthless.

A final handicap of the physician is the general tendency of the people to exhaust home remedies and the arts of the *curandero* before appealing to the physician. The physician, therefore, gets many cases too late to effect a cure and many others which are simply incurable. Hence, the failures of folk medicine as well as those of his own profession are heaped upon his shoulders.

The consequences of the foregoing are sharpened by Dreitzel,[2] who after briefly describing the development of medicine from primitive superstition through the enlightenment to the successes of modern science, nevertheless makes the observation that at least 50% of patients suffer from "functional disturbances." He concludes therefore:

Necessary as it is in combination with what one might call an ecological view, the scientist's per-spective in medicine has become a serious impediment to a deeper understanding of the nature of health and illness in modern society *if* exclusively applied to diagnosis and treatment. And this still holds true for the overwhelming majority of medical practitioners in America in spite of the mental health movement, and in spite of much research effort in the sociology of medicine.

In fairness it must be admitted that there are many points of value in folk medicine. In a sense one might consider modern scientific medicine as a natural outgrowth, extension, or elaboration of folk medicine, thereby representing scientific folk medicine. The number of effective drugs that have originated in folk medicine is rather impressive: quinine, rauwolfia, mescaline, chaulmoogra, opium, coca, curare, and many laxatives, to mention only a few. As to physical techniques, one might mention massage, baths, sweating treatments, surgery, and even inoculation. In the field of mental health and psychotherapy a great deal can be learned from the practitioner of simple folk medicine.

It is interesting that although knowledge of the causative agents was lacking, certain illnesses traditionally have been considered communicable, and it was believed that those who suffered from them should be kept apart from the other members of society. Beyond this it is commonly believed that individuals subject to certain debilitating illnesses are in a weakened condition and that visitors may unintentionally harm them by strong "humors" which they may carry. Therefore, aside from possible communicability, isolation has been carried out for the patient's own good. It is worthy of note that the attitude of public health workers toward the value of isolation has shifted substantially to this point of view. Where concern exists with regard to the evil effects of *aire,* strong humors, or similar folk influences, it may be possible to take advantage of this, since whatever the reasoning, an essentially hygienic practice is followed—one that can with value be made use of by physicians and nurses in the treatment and prevention of spread of communicable diseases. Physicians need not express an opinion on the potential dangers of *aire.* They can simply say that visitors are undesirable for the patient's sake, and the family will probably follow the recommendation, even though physicians are thinking in terms of contagion and the family in terms of magic.

In most instances it is probably ill advised to ignore the patient's ideas about his illness and the relationship of established folkways to it. Foster[26] warns, "The common tendency on the part of doctors and nurses to ignore, if not to ridicule, folk concepts of illness, probably reduces their effectiveness. . . . " He illustrates this with several instances in which modern physicians and especially nurses wisely listen to patients' complaints and to their ideas of magical and metaphysical relationships thereto, then follow up by relating their suggestions for modern scientific treatment to those familiar, accepted ideas. This accomplishes several things. It raises the physician and nurse in the patient's estimation, since not only did they not belittle the patient's valued ideas and folk traditions, but they actually exhibited some interest and understanding of them. From this starting point there develops a rapport and a greater understanding and receptivity by the patient of scientific medicine and its practitioners. This is one of the most important ways that erroneous folk practices may eventually be dropped and more effective and suitable scientific practices substituted.

Sometimes professional individuals tend to make a fetish of terminology. After all, words and titles are of little consequence. It is the fundamental concept and effective action that are important. I once had the experience of serving as health officer of a county in a southeastern state, the county seat of which was the international headquarters of a fundamentalist religious group. This religious group not only refused to recognize the germ causation of some diseases but also refused to admit the existence of illness of any kind. If there was something the matter with an individual, he was not sick—rather, God was displeased with him or with something in his environment, and when God became happy again, the individual would recover. Meanwhile, of course, he might die from an otherwise preventable condition. These ideas were deeply ingrained in the religious beliefs of these people. It was obviously futile to try to convince them otherwise. In terms of their religious tenets, in which they had absolute faith, they were certain they were right, and after all, they were entitled to whatever religious beliefs they wished. Nevertheless, this posed a serious problem with regard to not only their welfare but also the welfare of everyone with whom they had contact.

Actually it worked out reasonably well. I went out of my way to become a good friend of the elderly bishop who was head of the church. He

was a good and sincere man. He believed that he and his people were doing the right thing. Who was I to say no? One day I said to him, "Bishop, you and I may disagree on a philosophic basis about certain things. We do however have one important common interest—we are both honestly interested in the well-being of your people and of all people. Furthermore, we also have an important point of agreement. We each recognize that at certain times something undesirable happens to people. Let us not argue about what causes that something to happen. After all, the cause is incidental to the effect. If you want to say that it is displeasure on the part of God, that is all right with me. On the other hand, if I happen to think that it is a bacterium, it can do no harm for me to think so. But let us, you and I, work together in doing something about the result." After that I had no more difficulty. If I wished to impose isolation on a person with a communicable disease, it was on the basis of preventing contact of the general public with influences that had displeased God. If I wanted to use immunizing agents, it was on the basis of injecting God-inspired material to help keep away unknown, displeasing factors that might harm people. If I wished to prescribe drugs and medicines, it was on the basis of giving materials to assist in driving out or removing from the body the things that had displeased the Lord. This approach succeeded so well that eventually I was consulted on various church matters.

How does the foregoing tie together? One may gain a clue if one accepts the idea that the goal as health workers must be to make good personal and community health practices an accepted part of the way of life and culture of people. This cannot occur spontaneously, and it cannot be done merely by destroying what to the health worker may seem to be erroneous customs. It requires careful planning and often much patience. Workers in public health must recognize the inadequacy of doing things to or even for people. The best way is to do things with people, and to do so the public health worker must understand as thoroughly as possible the cultural factors that make them believe and act the way they do and tailor his suggestions and programs as much as is practical to the accepted general cultural pattern of the group. The public health worker should constantly relate his efforts to something familiar, something most people already know, do, and accept. In addition, he must recognize that his own communities, sophisticated as they may appear to be on the surface, consist of numerous societies and numerous cultures. He must recognize that so-called sophistication may merely substitute city ways for folkways and that many of his customs are fundamentally the same as those found elsewhere, having merely been transferred, transformed, or adapted to a new environment or set of social conditions.

## EFFECT OF PUBLIC HEALTH ACTIVITIES ON CULTURAL PATTERNS

Discussion to this point has centered on the effect of cultural patterns on health and on public health activities. Brief consideration of the reverse relationship would seem in order. If public health programs successfully improve the physical and mental health of a people, invariably there follow complex, far-reaching effects on most other phases of the culture of the people. Thus if workers become healthier and more alert mentally, their ingenuity and inventiveness tend to increase. To the extent that they may produce more and better mechanical aids to their labors they then find it not only possible to produce more but they do it more easily and in less time. This makes possible a shorter average workday. With more leisure, people tend to engage more in the pursuit of various cultural activities, that is, recreation, study, reading, and the fine arts, and because of an increased standard of living, they have more money for such activities.

A measurable effect of public health activities is a decrease in the number of deaths and an increase in the average life expectancy. Thus in the United States since the beginning of the twentieth century, infant death rates have been lowered from about 200 per 1,000 live births to about 18 per 1,000 at the present time (1973). This means that instead of every fifth baby dying, only every fifty-fifth baby now dies. During the same period, the average life expectancy at birth has been raised from about 49 years to over 70 years of age. The social consequences of such a rapid effect of public health activities are many and far reaching. There are more mouths for families and the nation to feed, greater housing needs, more schools to be built, more school buses to be supplied, and more recreation facilities and other civic and social activities needed. Similarly, many more facilities are needed for the larger number of older citizens. On the other hand, it also means that less

money is needed for the care of preventable illnesses, much less family worry and sadness, a changed attitude toward illness and death, and healthier children who in a short time become more alert, better informed, and capable citizens and workers. One might generalize by saying that in many or all such situations rapidly improved health conditions tend to result first in increased social pressures and problems, followed by greatly multiplied social benefits.

The development of healthier people therefore sets off a chain of events, which result in general in the improvement of national culture and in an improved standard of living for everyone. More people become available to work in offices, businesses, farm lands, and factories, and because on the average they are healthier than their parents and grandparents, they can produce more. This means an increase in the individual share of the material things of life. At the same time, attitudes toward marriage and family life are strongly affected by the results of public health measures. To approach this negatively, if death rates are high in general and if maternal mortality rates are high in particular, family structure must be adapted accordingly. The husband and children must accept the possibility of having several wives and mothers. For the woman, childbirth is surrounded by fear and superstitions. Because of the frequency of deaths of the mothers, the position of the older surviving female relatives is more important in the total family picture than in the present typical American situation. Also, because of high infant and child mortality, husbands, public opinion, and nature conspire to keep the woman pregnant much of the time. One might say further that the generally pregnant wife results in the most significant accentuation of the double standard. The male tends toward more promiscuous relationships, which tend to be accepted more readily by society. This in turn incidentally invites a greater prevalence of venereal diseases.

Interestingly some of the same manifestations of cultural change have occurred among many young people of both sexes as a result of recent technologic and scientific advances in combination with increased affluence, mobility, and population concentration to all of which improved public health has contributed. In many places some consequences include significant changes in attitude toward family, religions, schools, property, interpersonal relations, morals, and other social institutions.

Lowered infant mortality and maternal mortality rates, on the other hand, tend eventually to bring about a pattern of smaller families that, in some respects at least, have stronger immediate family bonds. In current American society this has had a considerable effect on the size of houses and even their architecture and on the use that is made of the home. A social complication has resulted, however, from the concurrent lengthening of life and an increasing number of elderly individuals. This in relation to a change in social attitude or interpretation of family constituency and responsibility and to the change that has occurred in the size and design of the modern small home, has left many, especially grandparents and other elderly persons, with little or no home base. The development of such an unfortunate type of social problem results inevitably in a social reaction. This is evident in the increasing literature and social legislation dealing with the older or senior citizens' needs for medical care, housing, and other necessities.

Successful public health programs may bring about a great change in attitude toward previously deep-seated "health" customs. The wearing of charms of all types is a common practice in this and many other countries. Usually they are not readily relinquished. Because of the success of the antiyaws program of the Institute of Inter-American Affairs during the 1950s, it became necessary to place boxes at the treatment and health centers as receptacles for the charms and fetishes that some of the now convinced patients discarded in large numbers.

A final example of an effect which public health activities may have on a society illustrates that results not only may be unexpected but even undesirable. An effective venereal disease control program, like any other special health program, should take into consideration the social and behavioral problems and attitudes of the people and the social and cultural consequences of the activity. The many ramifications of such a program were emphasized dramatically in a joint international attempt to eradicate venereal diseases during World War II. Many United States military training camps were located close to communities in another nation. Large numbers of young soldiers when off duty had no place else to go for recreation except to those communities. Because of this, prostitution flourished, and large numbers of soldiers were infected with venereal diseases.

United States public health officials met with their counterparts in the other nation to solve the problem. From a strictly scientific and public health standpoint their jointly devised solution was sound. In line with recently developed antibiotic therapy and prophylaxis the basis of their approach was to require all prostitutes to receive large injections of residual penicillin each week, whether or not they appeared to be infected. Failure to be able to present evidence of the weekly injection meant a loss of permit to work in the registered houses of prostitution.

However, certain potential side effects had been overlooked. The first result was a dramatic drop in the incidence of new infection among the United States soldiers, the local population, and the prostitutes. Next, apparently as word of the situation got around, it was realized that these were desirable places in which to practice prostitution and relatively safe places to visit for such purposes. Understandably officials of the other nation complained that the program was actually promoting and increasing their prostitution problem. Finally a totally unexpected result began to appear. Many of the prostitutes had chronic gonorrheal inflammations that had prevented their becoming pregnant. Now, with the repeated routine injections of penicillin, many of these chronic inflammations cleared up, and some of the prostitutes became pregnant by unknown fathers. The international relations and social welfare aspects of this problem were considerable.

One should always be conscious of the delicate balance in which society operates. This applies particularly to activities in a field like public health that may have prompt and far-reaching influences. Whereas it is axiomatic that progress in one cultural direction inevitably results in progress in other aspects of a culture, it is equally true that the artificial stimulation of great sudden advancements in one phase of a culture alone may bring about at least a temporary social difficulty, if not even chaos. Thus workers in public health may actually be wielding a two-edged sword if they suddenly, rapidly, and exclusively apply all of the present public health knowledge to a situation. If this is done without consideration of family planning and the basic social needs of the additional people, there is real danger of causing irreparable distortion and harm to a culture or a society. There may develop increased food problems, social and economic imbalance and political unrest, to mention only a few potential results. Public health workers need not be pessimistic about this, however. The important thing is to realize the potentialities and implications and to emphasize the absolute necessity for public health workers always to work in conjunction with agriculturists, educators, political scientists, social service workers, behavioral scientists, and many others.

## CONTRIBUTIONS OF SOCIAL SCIENTISTS TO PUBLIC HEALTH

In *The Epic of America* James Truslow Adams claimed that America's greatest contribution to the total human culture was the "vision of a society in which the lot of the common man will be made easier and his life enriched and ennobled." Most certainly a well-chosen and successfully pursued public health program is one of the significant handmaidens to this goal of social order. But as Kluckhohn[5] warns:

Order is bought too dearly if it is bought at the price of the tyranny of any single set of inflexible principles, however noble these may appear to be from the perspective of any single culture. Individuals are biologically different, and there are various types of temperament which reappear at different times and places in the world's history. So long as the satisfaction of temperamental needs is not needlessly thwarting to the life activities of others, so long as the diversities are not socially destructive, individuals must not only be permitted but indeed encouraged to fulfill themselves in diverse ways. The necessity for diversity is founded upon the facts of biological differences, differences in situation, varying backgrounds in individual and cultural history.

Part of the function of the social scientist is to study these differences and to provide expert advice and consultation when programs or changes are contemplated. They can also provide warnings when those working in public health appear to be in danger of serious error because of misunderstanding the motivations of individuals and groups. Finally, if public health workers do find themselves in inexplicable difficulty, the social scientist, by virtue of his somewhat different way of looking at things, may be able to find out why and to point to a way out of the dilemma. For example, as Paul[11] describes, the health educator may approach an assignment with the preconception that it is merely to convey information to people who are uninformed. If this is the case, success will be doubtful or limited and the health educator may conclude that the slow acceptance of ideas is attributable to intellectual deficiency or willful stubborn resistance. In most instances the health educator's function is really to help people reorganize their existing conceptual system. As Paul states, "Knowledge of the local belief system enables the imaginative educator to present his data in such order and in such a way as to be most readily grasped by the recipients. It also enables him to anticipate the directions that 'misunderstanding' will take."

Meltzer[27] has provided an excellent example of the manner in which the foregoing approach to activity or program analysis may be of value. The study relates to topical fluoride demonstration programs in six communities; three were successful and three were failures. The purpose was to determine if possible the reasons for the failures as well as for the successes. By way of introduction she complains:

We in public health work have an unfortunate habit of talking and writing only about our successes, ignoring our failures, and seldom examining the principles we were trying to use when we failed. It does little good to study the methods that led to program success in one community, if we forget that the identical methods have failed miserably in other similar communities. When that happens, it is a case of using methods based on untested assumptions, rather than on sound principles.

In the analysis of the dental programs, as expected, no single reason for success or failure was found, since each of the six communities was a circumstance into itself with its unique cultural pattern. The failures were ultimately attributed to a variety of reasons, including inadequate communication between the public health workers and the public, the impression that the program was a self-contained short-term experiment, that it needlessly disrupted the school routine without real purpose, and that some significant groups in the community were not brought into the planning. The example illustrates that action teams such as groups of public health workers often define a problem and the anticipated reaction of a community in their own way and according to their own standards. They are often blind to the fact that these are rooted in the subculture of their own professional and social class. As Paul[11] emphasizes, this need to understand and overcome cultural differences "applies not only in the case of a health mission operating in a foreign country, but also in the case of a team working in a community within its own country. The difference in the two cases is one of degree."

The relevancy of the subject to public health

was formally recognized by the American Public Health Association in a resolution unanimously adopted at its Eighty-first Annual Meeting in New York on November 11, 1953:

WHEREAS, the field of health education is concerned basically with human behavior, its nature and how it may be altered for the improvement and promotion of individual and community health, and

WHEREAS, the social sciences contribute to knowledge of human nature and behavior, therefore be it

RESOLVED, that the American Public Health Association encourage collaboration between public health workers and social scientists to better promote the utilization of social science findings toward the solution of public health problems.

In discussing how social science may be helpful to the field of public health, Foster[26] has presented a list of factors to be considered, which, he warns, is intended to be merely suggestive and illustrative and not a definitive catalog. The list is sufficiently thought provoking, however, to merit repetition here:

Although it is desirable to know as much about a culture as possible, there are obviously strict limitations as to what can be known. Social scientists have barely made a beginning in the formidable task of describing the elements of the cultures of the world and interpreting their significance. It must be assumed that for any given program there are certain categories of information about the culture in which the work is to be carried out which are of primary importance, and others that are of lesser importance. A "trial run" in compiling a list of primary classes of data for public health programs gives the following picture.

*Folk medicine and native curing practices.* The importance of this has been discussed at some length above and need not be commented on further at this point.

*Economics, particularly incomes and costs of living.* Since in the final analysis the success of public health programs rests upon major changes in the habits of people with respect to diet, housing, clothing, agriculture, and the like, knowledge of the economic potential of an area is paramount.

*Social organization of families.* A bride often lives in her husband's home, under the domination of her mother-in-law. There are cases in which pregnant women failed to follow, or had difficulty in following, health center recommendations because these conflicted with what the mother-in-law thought was best.

Men and women who live together are frequently not legally married. Under such circumstances, a man is less likely to recognize obligations to his companion and their children, and it is therefore more difficult to persuade him to come to the health center for venereal or other treatment. Recognition of these and similar problems makes the responses of patients more intelligible.

*Education and literacy and comprehension.* Ability to comprehend the real nature of health and disease, to profit by health education, and to understand and follow the physician's instructions depends on the education and literacy of the people.

*Political organization.* Local conditions under which physicians and other staff members are appointed, the local attitude toward nepotism, bureaucratic rules which govern operations, and the like, are factors which will affect public health programs. In one country, for example, a large health center, not yet placed in operation, was seriously threatened by the conflicting interests of the state governor, the local nurses' union, and other bureaucratic factors.

*Religion.* A basic analysis of religious tenets is not essential, but some parts of the religious philosophy of the people should be known. Are there any beliefs which hinder or directly conflict with proposed programs? Is death, for example, at any age considered a welcome relief from a world of suffering? Are there food taboos based on religious sanction which should be taken into consideration in planning diets?

*Basic value system.* What are the goals, aspirations, fundamental values, and major cultural premises, consciously or unconsciously accepted, which give validity to the lives of the people in question? What is the practical significance, for example, of a fatalistic approach to life and death? What part does prestige play in determining customary behavior patterns of the people? Is male vanity and ego a factor to consider? What are the ideas of bodily modesty? What are the types of stimuli and appeal to which people respond most readily?

*Other types of data.* Planners and administrators of public health programs should also have at hand such information as credit facilities and money usages, labor division within the family, time utilization, working and eating schedules, cooking and dietary practices, and the importance of alcoholism.

Categories of culture in which precise knowledge would appear to be of lesser importance include agriculture, fishing, and other primary productive occupations, industrial techniques (except as working conditions may affect health), trade and commerce, religious fiestas and church observances, wedding ceremonies, burial customs, and music and folk tales.

In bringing to a close the brief consideration of social science in relation to public health it is appropriate to call attention to one final value that it has for public health workers. It has been stated by Murdock[22] as follows: "One of the greatest potential contributions of anthropology is to make those who are professionally concerned with health problems aware of the broad sweep of culture history and of their position in it."

## REFERENCES

1. Leavell, H. R.: New occasions teach new duties, Public Health Rep. **68:**687, July 1953.
2. Dreitzel, H. P.: The social organization of health, New York, 1971, The Macmillan Co.
3. Koos, E. L.: New concepts in community organization for health, Amer. J. Public Health **43:**466, April 1953.
4. Skinner, B. F.: Science and human behavior, New York, 1953, The Macmillan Co.
5. Kluckhohn, C.: Mirror for man: the relation of anthropology to modern life, New York, 1949, Whittlesey House.
6. White, L. A.: Man's control over civilization, an anthropocentric illusion, Sci. Month. **66:**238, March 1948.
7. Benedict, R.: Patterns of culture, New York, 1934, The New American Library of World Literature, Inc.
8. Carothers, J. C.: The African mind in health and disease, WHO Monogr. Series, no. 17, 1953.
9. Gittler, J. B.: Man and his prejudices, Sci. Month. **69:**44, July 1949.
10. Bernard, J.: Can science transcend culture? Sci. Month. **71:**270, Oct. 1950.
11. Paul, B. D.: Respect for cultural differences, Community Development Bull., University of London Institute of Education **4:**42, June 1953.
12. Hoyt, E. E.: Tiquisate: a call for a science of human affairs, Sci. Month. **72:**114, Feb. 1951.
13. Miller, W. S.: Some observations on enteric infection in a delta village, J. Egypt. Public Health Ass. **25:**45, 1950.
14. Wier, J. M., et al.: An evaluation of health and sanitation in Egyptian villages, J. Egypt. Public Health Ass. **27:**55, 1952.
15. Bogue, R., and Habashy, A.: Health education pilot project in three villages in Egypt, 1955, Unnumbered Publication of World Health Organization Regional Office, Alexandria.
16. Paul, B. D.: American medicine on the island of Yap, Harvard School of Public Health, 1951 (published paper).
17. Hyde, H. V.: Education and world health, Progressive Educ. March 1949.
18. Whorf, B. L.: Languages and logic, Techn. Rev. **43:**250, April 1941.
19. Foster, G. M.: Use of anthropological methods and data in planning and operation, Public Health Rep. **68:**853, Sept. 1953.
20. Schneider, D. M.: In Paul, B. D.: Health, culture, and community, New York, 1955, Russell Sage Foundation.
21. Erasmus, C. J.: An anthropologist views technical assistance, Sci. Month. **78:**148, March 1954.
22. Murdock, G. P.: Anthropology and its contribution to public health, Amer. J. Public Health **42:**8, April 1952.
23. National Analysts, Inc.: A study of health practices and opinions, Springfield, Va., 1972, National Technical Information Service.
24. Banks, F. R., and Keller, M. D.: Symptom experience and health action, Med. Care **9:**498, Nov.-Dec. 1971.
25. Elkins, A.: Aboriginal men of high degree, Sydney, 1944, Australasian Publishing Co., Ltd.
26. Foster, G. M.: A cross-cultural anthropological analysis of a technical aid program, Washington, D. C., 1951, Smithsonian Institution.
27. Meltzer, N. S.: A psychological approach to developing principles of community organization, Amer. J. Public Health **43:**198, Feb. 1953.

*It is bad enough that a man should be ignorant, for this cuts him off from the commerce of men's minds. It is perhaps worse that a man should be poor, for this condemns him to a life of stint and scheming, in which there is no time for dreams and no respite for weariness. But what surely is worst is that a man should be unwell, for this prevents his doing anything much about either his poverty or his ignorance.*

G. H. T. KIMBLE

CHAPTER 6

# Social pathology and public health

## THE BEHAVIORAL FACTOR

Now that public health has been viewed in relation to cultural behavior and the development of society it is important to consider some of the social factors that play significant causal, effectual, or augmenting roles with regard to the state of health or illness of the group or society. Simmons and Wolff[1] neatly state that "culture sets the stage, ascribes the parts, and defines the terms whereby society's drama is enacted." On the other hand, society is the instrument, the mechanism, the organization that provides the environment for a culture to develop, grow, and manifest itself. This is an area to which insufficient attention has been given not only by health workers but also by those in other disciplines who think, plan, and strive for the protection and promotion of the total well-being of society.

Paradoxically, as far as public health is concerned, the appearance of the great era of bacteriology actually resulted in delaying broad effective progress. The discovery that highly specific living organisms are related to plague, anthrax, and many other disease conditions, and that these clinical syndromes could not occur in the absence of their respective causative organisms, brought about a great flush of enthusiasm and hope. An unfortunate result, however, was the development of an attitude by some that effective bacterial exposure was the alpha and omega of disease causation. Indeed, this had much to do with the broad acceptance and support of certain sanitary measures in the late nineteenth and early twentieth centuries, since it became recognized that bacteria could invade the town house and the palace through the servants' quarters and that *Corynebacterium diphtheriae* could strike the children of the wealthy and privileged as well as the children of the poor.

As long as etiology was still indeterminate or uncertain, men tended of necessity to cast about widely in their search for causal relationships. Once a scientific or, better yet, a laboratory answer was forthcoming, there was a tendency to close the issue with a Q.E.D. This comparative attitude was well put by Stern[2] in a discussion of living conditions and health:

In contrast with the narrower focus of public health work after the modern science of bacteriology had developed, the objective of the pioneers of public health included demands for better housing conditions, nutritious food, unpolluted water, cleaner streets and improved working conditions. These men anticipated the fundamental truth of modern preventive medicine, that the health of the individual is intimately and indivisibly tied up with the social as well as the physical environment in which he resides.

Attention is directed to Chapter 2 on background and development to note that it was not coincidental that the midnineteenth century reports and recommendations of men like

Southwood Smith, Chadwick, and Shattuck were so extensive and far reaching. Similarly, it was not coincidental that they "fell flat from the printers' hands," and were underrated or set aside, appearing when they did on the eve of the era of dramatic bacteriologic discoveries. They simply had to wait until the more palatable and more easily dealt with vogue had run its course. It is equally interesting to note that those diseases for which etiologic agents were difficult to determine or that were matters of political, economic, and scientific controversy continued to be related almost fatalistically to social and environmental factors, which conveniently were regarded as too difficult to solve. This was true, for example, of tuberculosis, pneumonia, influenza, and malnutrition. One might state as an axiom that the easier it was to determine a specific relationship between a microorganism and a disease the more social, economic, and environmental factors were ignored.

In recent years it has been increasingly realized that man in his entirety is a combination of physical, psychologic, social, and cultural factors. If the recognition and acceptance of this is to be at all meaningful, practitioners of public health and medicine must cease to evaluate and treat man by the first of these factors alone. Sir Farquhar Buzzard,[3] Regius Professor of Medicine at Oxford, has stressed that the aim of workers in public health should be as follows:

... to expose the sources and bases whence arise ill health and disability, by investigating the influence of social, genetic, environmental, and domestic factors on the incidence of human disease ... [taking into consideration] ... such varying agents as heredity, nutrition, climate, and occupation ... [as well as] ... the part played by the individual and mass psychology.

A similar conclusion was reached by Ryle,[4] who after 30 years as a student and teacher of clinical medicine accepted the chairmanship of the first Department of Social Medicine (Oxford, 1942). He contemplated that during those 30 years he saw disease studied ever more thoroughly and mechanically, but not more thoughtfully, as if through the high power of the microscope. He commented:

Man, as a person and a member of a family and of much larger social groups, with his health and sickness intimately bound up with the conditions of his life and work—in the home, the mine, the factory, the shop, at sea, or on the land—and with his economic opportunity, has been inadequately considered in this period by the clinical teacher and hospital research worker. [And may I add—by a large number of health workers!]

In his prefacing statement Ryle avers:

We no longer believe that medical truths are only or chiefly to be discovered under the microscope, by means of the test tube, and the animal experiment, or by clinical examination and increasingly elaborate pathological studies at the bedside. Psychological and sociological studies have as important a part to play. Even so, it is not yet appreciated how intimately disease and social circumstance are interrelated. The whole natural history of disease in human communities, as well as in individuals, is ripe for a fuller and more exhaustive study.

The terms *social medicine* and *social pathology* have been used. They are much better known and understood in Europe than in America as a result of the work and writings of Pettenkofer, Neumann, Grotjahn of Germany, Sand of Belgium, and Southwood Smith, Chadwick, Simon, Buzzard, and Ryle of Great Britain. Nevertheless, the relationships between factors in the social environment and disease have long been a matter of concern in the United States, although it is only relatively recently that they have been considered as *social medicine*. Unfortunately, in the United States the term has often been confused with socialized medicine, and its content has been similarly confused with concerns about the organization and economics of the provision of medical care. Some have tried to solve this dilemma partially and indirectly by use of the term *comprehensive medicine*. In its present form this tends to limit itself to the relationship between an individual's physical illness and his psychosociologic stresses. This has been applied essentially toward the end of diagnosis, treatment, and prevention of recurrence of the particular malady.[5,6] The foregoing to the contrary, the United States had had its share of individuals who have contributed notably to the philosophy of social medicine and social pathology, albeit not always by their European designations. Among those who may be mentioned are Shattuck, Smith, Sydenstricker, Mountin, and Winslow. More recent contributions of significance have come from Galdston, Dunham, Rosen, and Wolff.[*]

---

[*] For historical review the reader is referred to *The Concept of Social Medicine as Presented by Physicians and Other Writers in Germany, 1779-1932* by Kroeger,[7] *Social Pathology and the New Era in Medicine* by Ryle,[8] *The Meaning of Social Medicine* by Galdston,[9] and *Approaches to a Concept of Social Medicine* by Rosen.[10]

The need to recognize the reality of the fields of social medicine and social pathology becomes more imperative in view of the twin revolutions now being witnessed in medicine and society. As an example, attention is directed to the dramatic changes in the types and extents of illnesses and deaths and in the resources with which to combat them. Thus the rate of major medical discovery has accelerated from one per century before 1900, to one per decade between 1900 and 1940, and to one or more per year since 1940. About 90% of the pharmaceuticals used today did not exist until recently. The nature and extent of the social revolution is discussed in Chapter 41. Suffice to point out here the tremendous increase in the population, its significant aging, the dramatic extent of urbanization and mechanization, and the great increase and equalization of the standard of living.

## DEFINITION

There have been numerous attempts to define social medicine and social pathology. One of the earliest and still one of the best definitions is that of Grotjahn,[11] who approached the problem of definition by enunciating several principles that, as he saw it, were necessary considerations in the proper study of a disease. These principles may be summarized as follows:

1. The social significance of a disease is determined primarily by its frequency. This emphasizes the importance of accurate medical statistics.

2. The most common form of a disease, its sociopathologic prototype, is also of social significance—more significant than its unusual or complicated rarer forms.

3. The etiology of every disease includes both biologic and social factors. The latter may affect a disease in several ways—they may be causative, predisposing, or they may influence the transmission or the course of illness.

4. The prevalence and outcome of disease may be influenced by attention to social and economic factors as they relate to the individual and the group.

5. It is important to determine the influence of successful treatment of a disease on the subsequent prevalence and on other social factors.

6. Diseases may themselves affect social conditions for the individual or for the group through recovery, predisposition to other illnesses, chronic infirmity, degeneration, or death.

The *British Journal of Social Medicine* attempted to clarify the issue editorially in January 1947 by the following statement[12]:

Social medicine is that branch of science which is concerned with: (a) biological needs, inter-actions, disabilities, and potentialities of human beings living in social aggregates; (b) numerical, structural and functional changes of human populations in their biological and medical aspects. . . . Social medicine takes within its province the study of all environmental agencies, living and non-living, relevant to health and efficiency, also fertility and population genetics, norms and ranges of variation with respect to individual differences and finally, investigation directed to the assessment of a regimen of positive health.

The importance of statistics of mass phenomena and relationships has again been stressed by Wolff[13] in his definition of social pathology:

The relation between disease and social conditions is the content of social pathology; its method is necessarily a sociological description of this relationship which, for simplicity's sake is mostly based on a statistical analysis of the quantitative findings.

In the discussion so far the terms *social medicine* and *social pathology* have been used almost interchangeably. Although similar and related, they are different. The following definitions are suggested therefore in an attempt to synthesize and simplify the several statements to which reference has been made and to indicate the relationship and the difference between the two terms:

1. *Social pathology* is a state of community imbalance evidenced by significant prevalence of disease and its related social disorders.

2. *Social medicine* is the study of the manner in which disease may result from, cause, or accentuate social problems and of the ways in which medical and public health efforts may contribute to their solution.

## MAN AND ENVIRONMENT

Even the most cursory consideration results in the empiric conclusion that there is a direct relationship between undesirable living circumstances and various types of problems. This is especially true and evident in urban situations where sheer numbers and crowding accentuate all such problems. The numerous social difficulties of cities are commonly observed to be concentrated particularly in the slum or substandard sections. Here houses tend to be small and crowded together, with a maximum amount of the area devoted to profitable subsistence living space. Little or no consideration is given to recreational needs. Often, and through no accident, industry is located nearby—close to a supply of labor eager for employment. The crowding of buildings, the generally narrow streets, the absence of open recreational areas, and the smoke of factories limit considerably the amount of sunshine and fresh air. Cleanliness and sanitation are difficult to maintain. Death or injury is invited by the narrow traffic-laden streets, the rickety abandoned structures, and the poorly planned flammable dwellings. Both education and nutrition also tend to be substandard and combine with insanitation and overcrowding to maintain a high incidence of illness. Lack of privacy encourages immorality and is conducive to a lowering of self-respect. These and other psychologic maladjustments in the developing child and adolescent breed attitudes of hopelessness, constant frustration, cynicism, resentment, and explosive pent-up hostility. Responsibility and initiative appear pointless, and what seem to be the only roads to self-expression and escape are socially undesirable. Undesirable positive reactions of rebellion such as destructiveness or crime or negative reactions of defeat such as addictions or prostitution tend to occur. It is perhaps not coincidental that the word for town dweller (*pagani*) has the etymologic root that it does. (See Chapter 27 on violence and delinquency for further discussion.)

These relationships have been repeatedly and conclusively shown to exist. Much of the writings of Southwood Smith and Chadwick discussed this subject. Earlier, in 1828, Villermé, one of the originators of social statistics, presented to the French Academy of Medicine a memoir comparing the death rates of the rich and the poor. Studies during the early 1930s in the United States showed about 20% of the land area of several metropolitan areas to be of a substandard, blighted, or slum quality. These areas, aside from factories, included the living quarters of a third of the populations of those cities. However, they accounted for 35% of the fires, 50% of the disease in general, 65% of the tuberculosis cases, 55% of the juvenile delinquents, and 50% of the arrests. Although they contributed only 6% of the tax revenue of the cities, they required 45% of the cities' expenditures.[14]

In the study of a specific community,

**Table 6-1.** Slum section of Cleveland, Ohio, 1934, compared with entire city

| Slum section | Percent of total in Cleveland |
|---|---|
| Population | 2.5 |
| Homicides | 21.0 |
| Prostitution | 26.0 |
| Tuberculosis deaths | 12.0 |
| Illegitimate births | 10.0 |
| Police protection expenditure | 4.5 |
| Fire protection expenditure | 14.5 |
| Health department expenditure | 8.1 |

Cleveland, Ohio, in 1934, the relationships shown in Table 6-1 were found to exist in connection with a slum section. As in other studies, whereas the area contributed only $225,000 per year in taxes, it required eight times that amount or $1.97 million per year to sustain it.

That this was not related to the times is evidenced by a recent study by the Sacramento City Planning Commission of the city's substandard housing area where most of the unemployed live. Although it contained only 20% of the population, it accounted for 42% of adult crime, 36% of juvenile delinquency, 26% of fires, and 76% of cases of tuberculosis. It required 25% of the city's fire protection, 41% of police protection, and 50% of the city's health services. On the other hand, it contributed only 12% of the city's taxes.[15] It has been estimated that the average person taken off welfare rolls and placed in a steady job will contribute $10,000 to the gross national product, pay $300 in state and local taxes, increase purchasing power for goods and services by $3,400, relieve the government of welfare or support payments of $1,308 a year, and cut unemployment costs and the need for other community services.[16]

With specific reference to the relationship of general environment to disease and death, a considerable body of data has now accumulated. For example, a study in Liverpool showed that crude death rates, infant mortality, and tuberculosis death rates were twice as high in the slum areas as in the city as a whole, with rates in tenements in between (Table 6-2).

At about the same time the National Health Survey in the United States brought to light many correlations between environment and health. Thus for urban white persons the relationships of crowding to amount of illness were

**Table 6-2.** Deaths by social area, Liverpool, England, 1923-1929

| City of Liverpool | Crude death rate | Tuberculosis death rate | Infant mortality |
|---|---|---|---|
| Entire city | 13.9 | 123 | 98 |
| Corporate tenement area | 18.2 | 164 | 131 |
| Slum area | 28.4 | 299 | 171 |

**Table 6-3.** Illness and crowding, United States, 1934

| Group | Degree of crowding (persons per room) | Percent of persons with illness 1 week or longer |
|---|---|---|
| A | 1 or less | 14.8 |
| B | 1 to 1½ | 15.7 |
| C | More than 1½ | 17.8 |

found to be highly significant (Table 6-3). The incidence of tuberculosis was found to be almost twice as high in group C as in group A, pneumonia was about one and a half times as frequent, and diphtheria occurred almost three times as often.

In a search for "the causes behind the causes of death" in the city of Cincinnati during 1949 to 1951, it was found that although significant declines in illness and death had taken place throughout the community during the previous quarter century, death rates still varied considerably from section to section. This was emphasized by the Basin area, the oldest section, which comprised about one seventeenth of the city's area but contained one fourth of the population. Most of the dwellings were substandard. In the Basin area infant mortality was twice as high, home accident fatalities were three times as high, the pneumonia death rate was eight times as high, and the tuberculosis death rate was thirty times as high as the corresponding rates for the remainder of the city. Interestingly there were no appreciable differences in the rates inside and outside the Basin for the non-communicable diseases of the older ages.[17]

Actually this is an increasingly complex question in a rapidly changing society. Thus Stockwell[18] in his comparative studies of Hartford, Conn., and Providence, R. I., found that the extent of association was not the same for all components of socioeconomic status, or did all aspects of mortality show similar associations

with the same components of socioeconomic status. He suggests that "the failure to realize this may lie behind much of the disagreement pertaining to the nature and extent of the relationship between socioeconomic status and mortality in the United States today." Whereas studies in the past indicated marked inverse relationship between socioeconomic status and all aspects of mortality, present evidence is much less conclusive. An additional precaution is brought out by Chilman,[19] who points out that although most studies of this nature relate to cities, actually socioeconomic disadvantage is more consequential in rural circumstances.

Admittedly it is difficult to determine direct cause-and-effect relationships between poor housing and ill health. Nevertheless, the consistency of their occurrence together cannot be ignored. As Pond[20] has reasoned:

A cautious and critical analysis of available data relating to the effects of housing on health leads to but one conclusion: one cannot state that substandard housing alone begets ill health. However, no reasonable student of the subject has yet stated that bad housing is compatible with good health. In the absence of irrefutable proof that housing has no ill effect on health, it may reasonably be hypothesized that good housing promotes the attainment of good health.

The quality of housing is, of course, only one reflection of socioeconomic status, and there are several other indicators of the latter that may be and have been used for comparative purposes. Thus Lawrence[21] followed a significant number of persons and families over a period of 20 years. He divided them into five socioeconomic groups and determined the prevalance of chronic illness as shown in Table 6-4.

A similar relationship has been found to hold true with regard to maternal and infant mortality. For example, Yerby[22] points to the significant differences between the mortality of black and Puerto Rican infants and mothers in the slum areas of New York City and the rates of the white population in that city (Table 6-5).

Even more striking are the results of a study in Aberdeen, Scotland, by Baird.[23] His method of distinction was to compare women who could afford delivery in private nursing homes with those who could not and were therefore delivered as charity patients in the Aberdeen Maternity Hospital. He found the results shown in Table 6-6.

Especially interesting is Baird's comparison

**Table 6-4.** Prevalence of chronic illness in families by socioeconomic status*

| Socioeconomic status | Adjusted † percent ill | |
|---|---|---|
| | 1923 | 1943 |
| Well-to-do | 27.7 | 29.3 |
| Comfortable | 47.3 | 39.8 |
| Moderate | 55.0 | 41.1 |
| Poor | 57.7 | 50.6 |
| Very poor | 61.3 | 44.0 |

*Modified from Lawrence, P. S.: Chronic illness and socio-economic status, Public Health Rep. **63:**1507, Nov. 19, 1948.
†Rates adjusted for age and family size.

**Table 6-5.** Infant and maternal mortality by race, New York City, 1963*

| Ethnic group | Infant mortality | Neonatal mortality | Puerperal mortality |
|---|---|---|---|
| Nonwhite | 39.2 | 28.1 | 11.8 |
| Puerto Rican | 28.2 | 20.7 | 10.2 |
| White | 19.9 | 15.0 | 4.1 |

*From Yerby, A. S.: The problems of medical care for the indigent populations, Amer. J. Public Health **55:**1212, Aug. 1965.

**Table 6-6.** Infant deaths by place of delivery, Aberdeen, Scotland, 1950

| Place delivered | Stillbirth rate | Neonatal death rate | Combined death rate |
|---|---|---|---|
| Charity hospital | 2.23 | 1.78 | 4.01 |
| Private nursing home | 0.99 | 0.50 | 1.49 |

of the characteristics of the two groups of mothers. He points out that all the women received the same standard of prenatal and postnatal care so that the differences in results were because of differences in health, physique, and intelligence. His epitomization is summarized in Table 6-7.

If one looks for them, relationships with factors in the social environment may be found with regard to almost all diseases. Their significance varies both to the particular group of individuals and their social environment and to the particular disease. In the case of diseases such as tuberculosis, silicosis, or gastric ulcer the relationship may be readily evident, whereas in others it may be somewhat obscure. The number of social factors potentially related to disease is undoubtedly legion. Furthermore, they are of several different types and affect health in a number of different ways—some directly, some indirectly. Certain factors such as tendencies to develop certain mental conditions, physical malformations, or blood dyscrasias are inherent in the members of the group; others such as exposure to siliceous dust or to fumes are related to occupation. Factors such as overcrowding or proximity to brothels are dangerous because they are conducive to exposure. Still others such as certain dietary habits or infant feeding customs are related to cultural factors.

In their stimulating discussion of social science in medicine, Simmons and Wolff[1] present the interplay of several aspects of man and his social and physical environment in an unusually descriptive manner well worth repeating:

. . . as an organism man is borne along by his physical environment, but he is also buffeted about

**Table 6-7.** Comparison by income group of women at delivery, Aberdeen, Scotland, 1950

| Characteristic | Low-income group | High-income group |
|---|---|---|
| Stature | Small | Tall |
| Physical grading | Poor | Good |
| Pelvis | Flat | Round or long |
| Functional grading | Poor | Good |
| Hygiene | Poor | Good |
| Knowledge | Limited | Adequate |
| Prenuptial conception | Frequent | Seldom |
| Housing | Poor | Good |
| Premature labor | Frequent | Infrequent |
| Fetal deaths | High | Low |
| Repeated pregnancies | Frequent; unplanned even when contraindicated | Limited; planned |
| Premature aging | Common | Seldom |

by some of its elements. As a member of society, he is supported and reinforced by some fellow agents, while he may be frustrated, handicapped, or even vanquished by others. Similarly, as a personality, he is both a product of his culture and a potential victim of its compelling or conflicting norms and codes.

Anyone may be carried along comfortably in his milieu for a while, only to be torn down miserably after a time as these various environmental components of his life converge and impinge upon him. During long stretches of time, harmful and helpful forces may blend and balance, permitting him a workable and safe equilibrium and amid many minor fluctuations. What is most important for us to realize, however, is the possibility that the scales may be *tipped* critically at a particular time by a clustering of forces from any one area, or from a combination of the triad of environmental pressures, and that, for the individual, a landslide of ill effects is started.

The following represents one possible classification of a few of the many group and social factors that may be related to disease. It is admittedly general and is presented merely to illustrate the variety and to provoke consideration of others:

  I. Factors in the members of the group
    A. Inherent characteristics
      1. Group susceptibility
      2. Tendency to inherent defects
    B. Cultural characteristics
      1. Racial, national, or religious customs
      2. Agricultural customs and methods
      3. Dietary habits or customs
      4. Educational limitations
      5. Linguistic barriers
      6. Traditional family size
      7. Relative status of sexes
      8. Relative status of age groups
      9. Relative importance of family in total social life
  II. Factors in the activities of the group
    A. Political
      1. Stability
      2. Quality
      3. Honesty
      4. Foresight of leadership
    B. Occupation and income
    C. Economy
      1. Basis
      2. Stability
      3. Trade
    D. Leisure behavioral pattern
    E. Mobility
      1. Travel
      2. Migration

    F. Traditional household habits
    G. Traditional purposes of household
  III. Factors in the environment of the group
    A. Geologic and climatic
      1. Severity of winters and summers
      2. Amount of rainfall and available water
      3. Mineral content of soil
      4. Degree of geographic isolation
    B. General environment
      1. Atmospheric pollution
      2. Soil and water pollution
      3. Amount of arable land available
      4. Proximity to detrimental factors (railroads, highways, industries, brothels, bars, fire hazards)
      5. Availability of recreation areas and facilities
    C. Home environment
      1. Size (persons per room)
      2. State or repair
      3. Type of structure
      4. Sanitary facilities
      5. Natural and artificial light
      6. Ventilation

It is well to give constant consideration to these social and environmental influences to emphasize the importance of regarding public health work for what it really is, that is, an applied social science, through which is brought to bear appropriate medical, engineering, nursing, educational, and many other disciplines. It is only by considering the social and environmental conditions under which people live, sleep, work, recreate, procreate, and rear their young that health workers can hope to understand and control disease in the most complete sense. It is only in this way that they can eventually grasp the meaning of total health.

## MODERN DEVELOPMENT

Over a long period social action to combat or remedy the various types of social problems was fractionated into separate, more or less insulated, activities. This was natural, since the recognition of each specific problem and its espousements for public action usually originated with one or several visionary individuals. Sometimes these persons were dedicated to the amelioration of a particular problem because of some personal or familial experience. This was the cause above all causes that motivated them and those they gathered about them. The result was a parochialism of interest and action evidenced by separate health reforms, housing reforms, penal reforms, and so on. Gradually a relationship among all these apparently unrelated social problems became recognized on more or less theoretic and empiric grounds, but attempts to correlate remedial action lagged essentially up to the present generation.

Perhaps the single most significant contribution to this recent development has been the recognition of an emphasis on the family, in contrast to the individual, as the basic social integer. Thus it is now accepted that the individual cannot be considered apart from his family or from the various and many forces in the physical and social environment that may influence his family. Furthermore, it is increasingly recognized as usually futile to attempt to treat an individual problem without taking into consideration the family situation and all the forces that may affect it. This is even recognized to apply to the single individual on the basis of his having come from a family, living in a family substitute, and subsequently entering or establishing a family. In this regard Richardson[24] has written:

The individual is a part of the family, in illness as well as in health . . . the idea of a disease as an entity which is limited to one person . . . fades into the background, and disease becomes an integral part of the continuous process of living. The family is the unit of illness, because it is the unit of living.

It is interesting to consider momentarily the multifaceted functions of the family, which provides, of course, the sole means of continuity and growth of the human species. As Ackerman[25] explains, it accomplishes this by providing a socially supported group pattern for the sexual union of man and woman and a stable situation that encourages a quality of parental partnership essential to the care of the resulting offspring. As he describes it, "The family is literally the cradle for the infant's tender mind as well as his body." The family, when properly established and conducted, presents a circumstance for the provision of food, clothing, shelter, and other materials necessary to life, for the proper emotional development of children and of their parents, for the guided evaluation of personal identities, for the development of normal and acceptable sexual patterns, for the establishment of social and ethical standards and the ability to accept social responsibility, and for the acquisition of knowledge and creative ability.

Children who grow up in a family setting acquire not only the general patterns of the culture of their particular society but also their parents' unique interpretation of it. Thus although children of the same generation of a society develop in a more or less similar manner, the children in each family are somewhat different from those in other families. Part of the role of the family therefore is not only to nurture a new generation that fits into society but also to provide the great variety of personalities necessary for the society and its biologic and cultural evolution.

Many psychiatrists and sociologists have emphasized that one of the greatest values of the family is as a stabilizing force for the individual member, on the one hand, and for society, on the other. It accomplishes this by means of two apparently conflicting mechanisms. For purposes of long-term security the family tends to resist change. However, in times of trouble or emergency it provides a psychic and social cushion, a means for sharing difficulty, and a basis for accommodation to change. Unfortunately, all family structures are not such as to ensure this. As Ackerman[25] states, "In the meeting of new problems and crises, some families are weakened and others grow in solidity and emotional strength. Some families grow and learn from experience; others seem unable to do so because they are too inflexible and tend to disintegrate."

A subject for particular concern is the tendency toward small, urban families. Bossard[26] says, "The very size of the family unit is important to the child . . . for the same reason that the size of the ledge from which we view the precipice below affects our sense of security." In families with one or few children and no grandparents, uncles, or aunts the child has few people on whom he may depend, and a single or at most a few difficulties may spell disaster.

In addition, as Schottstaedt[5] has emphasized, decreasing the number of people in the home tends to increase the frequency and intensity of emotional reactions because there are fewer people to absorb impacts and frictions. Furthermore, support tends to be concentrated in one wage earner, since there are fewer people to contribute to the common family needs. Similarly, household duties and responsibilities of the housewife are increased in a relative sense, since such work must be done whether there is one or a number in the house, and are increased in an absolute sense, since there are fewer or none to share the work with her. Compounding this are the numerous extra-familial distractions and demands on the parents in the urban situation. Schottstaedt also points out how the burden and the risk are greatly increased in the small family when illness strikes one of its members. There are fewer people to perform nursing functions and fewer to assume the customary responsibilities of the one who is ill. As he states, "Available home resources for nursing chronically ill members of the family are therefore decreased and the percentage of people who require hospitalization, nursing home care, or institutional care is increased." With regard to the latter point Parsons and Fox[27] have suggested that the growth and increasing use of hospitals is not merely a result of advances in medical knowledge and its application in an increasingly exacting technology but is also a response to a shift in family structure, which is itself linked to the occupational structure.

Such considerations go far in explaining some of the difficulties encountered in the handling of certain types of illnesses and certain types of individuals. They provide, for example, one reason why in a substantial number of cases medical treatment alone of chronic diseases is ineffective because of tangential relationships to the family economy and other aspects of family and social life. As a result of differences in the amount and type of stress on the male in American society, they explain, in part, the excess of gastric and duodenal ulcers in males. They further provide a logical reason for the recent increase of these conditions among women since their social and occupational emancipation. Also, as has been shown by several investigators, the diabetic individual fares less well in the competitive industrialized urban situation because of frequent and often intense stress. Thus stress threatens security, and the emotional response results in an increase in ketone bodies in the venous blood and fluctuations in blood sugar level. Anyone who has worked with elderly persons is familiar with the frequent difficulty of maintaining their health or, indeed, their interest in it. Left to their own devices because they have passed their biologically and economically productive years, older people tend to feel useless and unwanted. One result is a tendency to neglect themselves. Matters of personal hygiene may not be observed. Nutrition may suffer because of defective teeth, vicarious food preparation, poor eating habits, and lack of appetite caused by feelings of depression. As Schottstaed[5] summarizes the situation, "Many of the diseases of older age are related to three things: nutritional deficiencies, circulatory disturbances, and general disuse."

## INTERRELATIONSHIP OF SOCIAL PROBLEMS

From what has gone before it appears that neither man nor his problems exist in vacuums. By virtue of being a product of a family and a participant in a society, innumerable external factors, both good and evil, impinge on him as an individual. Some act to cause difficulty and problems; others serve to provide support and solution of problems. Thus it is now recognized that the state of personal or familial health or disease is the result of many interacting biologic, physical, and social factors. Depending on the nature of the disease and circumstances, any one of these may be primary and the others contributory. Furthermore, given a state of disease, these same factors are involved in the chances for and mechanism of recovery and rehabilitation. This has led to the consideration of disease in the individual as more and more a social phenomenon, involving several people and especially those immediately related to and around the patient. As Richardson[24] has put it, "Illness is one form of family maladjustment." An attempt to illustrate these relationships insofar as disease is concerned has been made in the previous discussion of man and his environment.

This leads to a still more significant aspect of the subject that requires consideration—the intimate interrelationships among a number of seemingly diverse types of social problems that may affect an individual, a family, and a society. One way to approach the subject is to consider the example of a man suffering from pneumonia who is brought into a hospital. Physical and radiographic examinations may conclusively determine the clinical diagnosis. Sputum examination may clearly implicate *Diplococcus pneumoniae* as the causative organism. However, is it as simple as this? Several questions remain unanswered. It is known, for example, that many more people are exposed to this organism than become clinically ill. Why did this particular individual become ill with pneumonia? True, he could not develop this particular disease in the absence of the organism. Nevertheless, a valid question may still be raised as to what actually caused the illness. Investigation may elicit circumstances such as the following: The patient suffered from overexposure because on the preceding night he slept on a park bench in the rain. He slept on a park bench because he did not know what he was doing. He did not know what he was doing because he was under the influence of alcohol. He indulged in an excess of alcohol because of discouragement and despondency over a bitter argument with a complaining wife. His wife complained because her husband was unemployed and had no income. He may have been unemployed because of inadequate training, intrinsic inability, or some complex interplay of business economics. Which of these factors caused his pneumonia? Obviously they all did.

Similarly, consider the case of an adolescent apprehended by the police as a juvenile delinquent. The immediate circumstance may have involved being caught while breaking into a store. Was the child intrinsically antisocial, and was the fault exclusively his? Investigation may bring out that he is only one of a group of similar adolescents who have formed an antisocial club or gang. It may be discovered that the group is sexually promiscuous, that venereal infections and abortions are common, and that alcoholism and narcotic addictions are present or incipient. In fact, the crystallizing storebreaking incident may have occurred to obtain money for alcohol or drugs. Why did this boy or, for that matter, any of the others belong to the gang and engage in such antisocial behavior? More often than not, discussion with a parent will result in the statement: "I just can't do anything with him." Deeper inquiry and study, however, are certain to bring out several other causative factors, most of them relating to the family and the social environment. Often the family bonds are discovered to be frayed or parted. The home may have only a single parent because of illegitimacy, divorce, separation, illness, or absence of one or both parents due to their employment. In such instances the gang is often a substitute family situation, that is, something to belong to, in which to socialize and to exercise self-expression.

On the other hand, both the parents and the children may live together. However, the home, because of economic stringencies caused by ignorance, misfortune or other reasons may consist of just a few crowded rooms of a substandard quality with little or no privacy, ample

opportunities for bickering and quarreling, and few facilities for cleanliness. Such a situation offers little incentive for the development of a sense of dignity, pride, or responsibility. The most intimate personal and sexual acts may be commonly observed, which encourages a cynical attitude toward them; there is little opportunity or reason to develop respect for the property of others even within the family; education, virtue, frugality, and social responsibility may be derided; dependence on public welfare and public assistance may be the cornerstone of the family finances; parental bouts of alcoholism and physical and verbal abuse may be so common as to establish themselves as the standard of behavior. Under such circumstances one may properly ask: Why did this boy attempt to steal? Why was he sexually promiscuous? Why did he have gonorrhea? Why, perhaps, was he on his way to being an alcoholic or a drug addict? Why had he no respect or use for the concepts of family and society? Obviously none of the answers to these questions can stand alone; they are all interlinked. And they all devolve into the three fundamental questions: Where and how did it all begin? How can this chain be broken? How can similar complex situations be prevented from occurring in others?

One of the conclusions brought out forcefully by such cases is that the primary diagnosis of a situation is not always in the same field as that under immediate or initial consideration. Social problems tend to exist together like different vegetables in a stew, as it were, and occasionally a particular problem erupts on the surface of the simmering stew. Regarded singly and momentarily it gives a limited and fallacious impression. To appreciate the total situation fully one has to stir the stew, sample it, and observe it over a period of time. In terms of such an analogy it is important to realize that although each vegetable when dredged up and examined in the ladle appears to be discrete, it is meaningful only in relation to the total stew and, if spoiled, can affect all other parts of the stew.

Caudill[28] has stated this in more formal terms as the basic conclusion of a presentation in *Effects of Social and Cultural Systems in Reactions to Stress:*

> . . . stress can manifest itself in one or more of a number of linked open systems, and . . . the strain on one system can be transmitted to others so that several become involved in the process of adaptation

and defense. These linked open systems may be thought of as: physiology; personality; relatively permanent meaningful small groups, e.g., the family; and wider social structure, e.g., community and the nation or, variously, economic and political structures. . . .

Following this he points out:

. . . in very few studies [and it might be added parenthetically, in very few action programs] has the research design taken account of more than two of the possible systems as variables. Physicians have found relations between physiological phenomena and conditions that have been conceived as psychological (fear, rage), psychodynamic (unresolved dependency, anxiety), and environmental (cold, imprisonment). Social scientists have shown relations between the structure of the family and its position in the economic or social class system, and have attempted to work with a concept of basic or modal personality in relation to the patterns of child rearing found in a culture. But only a few studies have examined three such variables as more than static background phenomena. . . .

Simmons and Wolff[1] have attempted to present the concept of some of these interrelationships in tabular form. The essential point made by them is that physical, social, or cultural events or forces may constitute either or both sources and consequences of strength or weakness, good or evil. Thus a particular physical source, event, or force may have physical consequences, social consequences, or cultural consequences. This is similarly true of social and cultural sources, events, or forces. It is also important to recognize that the resulting consequences may in turn become sources or forces themselves. This method of presentation is adapted here to illustrate many of the issues raised in the preceding paragraphs.

With regard to the interrelationships among negative or undesirable sources, events, or forces and consequences, the following examples may be considered as *sources:*

1. Physical: Disease, congenital defect, or injury to face
2. Social: Sudden industrialization with an influx of young adult workers
3. Cultural: Development of an urbanized living pattern

Each of these may have undesirable physical, social, and cultural *consequences* (Table 6-8).

In a similar manner sources, events, or forces may be of a positive nature and result in desirable consequences. To illustrate this the following *sources* may be used:

1. Physical: Improved nutrition, public health, and medical care
2. Social: Development of social security and medical care plans
3. Cultural: Provision of improved education

Each of these may have desirable physical, social, and cultural *consequences* (Table 6-9).

## MULTIPROBLEM FAMILIES

Everything that has been said thus far on the subject of social pathology points to the veracity of the common saying, "Misery loves company." This is true in the sense that people and families in difficulty tend to be concentrated geographically, especially in urban situations. It is also true in the sense that difficulties seldom occur singly. In recent years this phenomenon has been described in several ways, one of them by the use of the phrase, disease-

**Table 6-8.** Interrelationships of undesirable physical, social, and cultural factors*

| Undesirable sources or events | Consequences | | |
|---|---|---|---|
| | *Physical* | *Social* | *Cultural* |
| Physical<br>Disease or injury | Facial deformity | Inability to obtain employment | Misanthropy<br>Condemnation of parenthood |
| Social<br>Industrialization | Increased venereal disease | Free sexual relationships and promiscuity | Changes in attitudes toward marriage and family |
| Cultural<br>Urbanization | More accidents and insanitation | Overcrowding<br>Development of gangs<br>Alcoholism | Breakdown of kinship and family bonds |

*Modified from Simmons, I. W., and Wolff, H. C.: Social science in medicine, New York, 1954, Russell Sage Foundation, p. 111.

**Table 6-9.** Interrelationships of desirable physical, social, and cultural factors*

| *Desirable sources or events* | Consequences | | |
| --- | --- | --- | --- |
| | *Physical* | *Social* | *Cultural* |
| Physical | | | |
| Improved nutrition, public health, and medical care | Less illness and longer life | Greater productivity | Stronger family and social responsibility |
| Social | | | |
| Social security plans | Fewer complications | Less pauperization of sick and aged | Changed attitude toward aged |
| Cultural | | | |
| Improved education | Earlier diagnosis, prevention, and treatment | Demand for better public health and medical care | Rational understanding of sickness and health |

*Modified from Simmons, I. W., and Wolff, H. C.: Social science in medicine, New York, 1954, Russell Sage Foundation, p. 111.

delinquency-dependency syndrome. This gives recognition to the fact that at any time in a society there are a certain number of individuals and, more significantly, families who get caught in a vortex of contributory social problems, each of which complicates the others in turn, making it more and more difficult to escape. For some the situation becomes so extreme and hopeless that there results an eventual condition which has been referred to as *cumulative degradation.*

Voiland and Buell[29] provide an interesting and helpful classification of multiproblem, or as they say, disordered families, based on a study of almost 1,000 cases. They describe them as follows:

1. *The perfectionist family.* Their pathologic social functioning is manifested by overemphasis on perfection. Such self-imposed demands for good behavior allow no place for human error; as a result, marital relationships, child-rearing practices, and child development become fraught with anxieties and doubts that distort personal and family living. Prognosis is generally favorable if diagnosed and adjusted early.

2. *The inadequate family.* This is marked by constant dependence on others for encouragement, continued support, guidance, and help in solving problems in social living. They live "hoping for the best," and are incapable of coping with sacrifices or stress. Prognosis is relatively good, provided the situation is diagnosed accurately and agency caseworkers have the time, patience, and teaching ability to build a basis for rehabilitation.

3. *The egocentric family.* The members of this type of family are characterized by self-seeking motives in family interpersonal relationships and social conduct. Its pathology lies in an excess of self-interest and an overemphasis on social status or personal prestige. The prognosis is guarded. Often the husband and wife may consciously recognize the problem and their need for guidance but reject the prospect of receiving advice from "experts."

4. *The unsocial family.* Both partners lack social rapport with other people and their social environment and have strong tendencies toward acting-out behavior, delinquent conduct, and/or regression into psychosis as a pattern of adjustment to problems or dislikes. They lack two essential qualities of good family functioning— a capacity for meaningful personal relationships and normally functioning conscience to guide and stimulate social behavior. This affects marital relationships, parental roles, work habits, and total community relationships. Prognosis is poor. It is noted that from the community's standpoint such families comprise a substantial proportion of its public health and welfare agency loads.

Sometimes and possibly often the type of social pathology indicated in this fourth group passes on through generations. McCulloch and Philip[30] describe a remarkable example in their study of suicidal behavior. They present a dramatic pedigree of 12 members of a family who in three generations indulged in more than 35 suicidal attempts. The grandfather, in whose family there had been much alcoholism and mental illness and who had been treated repeatedly for alcoholic psychosis, was the first to be brought to the poison treatment center. His wife had previously succeeded in poisoning herself. They had 9 children. One died in infancy, and of the rest only one did not attempt suicide. The spouses of two of them also attempted suicide. The daughter of one such couple, at the age of 16 years, shared a man with a violent record with her mother, and during one of many arguments attempted suicide. This family is a classic exhibit of the complex of violence, mental illness, alcoholism, child neglect and abuse, delinquency, and crime. In discussing such situations the authors properly summarize, "In the main, these are people who grow up in an environment in which impulses tend to be acted out. Petty crime, prostitution, and many other forms of degradation have been witnessed as part of their daily lives. They have been reared in a climate where actions speak louder than words, where impulsiveness is dominant, and where people live from day-to-day having weak ties to the past and little investment in the future."

Another way of considering multiproblem families is on the basis of the degree of ability to respond affirmatively to assistance. One type of multiproblem family is self-sufficient under ordinary circumstances and goes along reasonably well until some catastrophe or crisis (medical, economic, or otherwise) sufficient in magnitude to throw the family off balance occurs. This crisis, if unsolved, eventually gives rise to problems in other areas. Unless some assistance is forthcoming, this type of family is in danger of irreparable damage and may become a permanent multiproblem family. If, on the other hand, significant assistance is rendered with regard to the original or to each of the several accumulated and related problems, this type of family is able to rehabilitate itself and assume and maintain its proper and desired role of self-sufficiency.

A second type of family is somewhat similar to the first. It has good intentions and wants to be self-sustaining but lacks good management and staying power. As a result, every once in a while it slips below the surface. If appropriately aided, it is able to climb back and operate on a relatively even keel until some new crisis occurs. Then it slips again and must be helped back again.

The third type of family is the most discouraging to deal with. Either because of overwhelming crisis and catastrophies for which it

has received no help, insufficient help, or, important to this discussion, unilateral help, or because it is an intrinsically defective family, no extent or type of assistance seems to enable it to recover. Often the desire for recovery, that is, for a different way of life, is lacking, unacceptable, or incomprehensible. The roots of the difficulties of these so-called hard-core problem families go very deep. They are almost irretrievably caught in an exceedingly difficult situation that might be referred to as the syndrome of the seven Ds:

| | |
|---|---|
| Disease | Dependency |
| Deficiency (often both | Despondency |
| nutritional and mental) | Delinquency |
| Destitution | Degeneracy |

Williams[31] summarized the same situation with regard to England in the following terms:

... after the Industrial Revolution with its child labor, cheap alcohol, poor wages, and bad landlords, there must have been a much higher proportion of our working-class families living under conditions far worse than anything we see today.

As social amenities become more readily available to the people so the great majority took advantage of the benefits and improved their conditions of life ... Yet one finds a small minority, either through a temperamental instability or a mental defect, who fail to keep pace with the advancing times.

He cites five surveys conducted by the Eugenic Society of Great Britain, which found an average incidence of such hard-core families to be 3 per 1,000 families. He adds, "We find that a large number of these people are in early middle life, able-bodied and capable of regular manual work, who have difficulty in adjusting themselves to the recognized standards of life."

In the United States several significant investigations of this problem have been carried out in recent years. They too have clearly indicated the importance of the family as the basic unit of social significance, the simultaneous or successive occurrence of social problems, and the existence of a small hard core of multiproblem families.

The most comprehensive and illuminating of these investigations was the study of St. Paul, Minn., a more or less typical American city.[32] The study was carried out by a group of consultants from the fields of health, maladjustment, dependency, and recreation, with the cooperation of 108 public and private community agencies. About 41,000 families, representing 40% of the total in the city, had contact

**Table 6-10.** Incidence of social problems, St. Paul, Minn., November 1948

| Type of problem for which assistance was rendered | Percent of families studied | Percent of families in city |
|---|---|---|
| Financial | 17 | 7 |
| Maladjustment | 26 | 10 |
| Health | 38 | 15 |
| Recreation | 46 | 18 |

with one or more agencies during the study month of November 1948. The types of problems for which services were rendered are summarized in Table 6-10.

It should be noted that health problems were among the most common encountered. In fact, during the month studied about 16,000 families, a rate of 147 per 1,000 families, received some services from the 12 public and 18 private health agencies in the community. About one half of these services were in relation to a chronic disease or handicap. With regard to age distribution of those receiving services for ill health, 32% were reported to be under 20 years, 41% were between 20 and 64 years, and 22% were over 65 years. Between one half and two thirds of those who suffered from chronic handicaps or diseases were heads of families; thus their ailments inevitably affected the family income, prospectives, and behavior.

A simple totaling of the figures in the table indicates that several families must have required and received aid for more than one type of problem. On investigation the facts substantiated this beyond expectation. Of the financially dependent families, 77% had problems of ill health and/or maladjustment; 56% of the families with problems of maladjustment had problems of ill health and/or dependency; and 38% of the families with health problems had problems of dependency and/or maladjustment.

The most striking finding of the St. Paul study was that there was a group of about 6,500 families, only 6% of the total in the city, who suffered from such an essentially continuing complex of problems that they absorbed 46% of the health services, 55% of the adjustment services, and 68% of the dependency services. This finding was further refined by the discovery that only 4% of these hard-core multiproblem families were financially dependent because of unemployment. Of

the 6,500 families, 58% were dependent because of ill health and/or maladjustment that rendered them unable to be self-sustaining.

The question naturally arises as to reason for the development of multiproblem families, especially those that form the hard core in a community. Analysis of the reasons is even more difficult than analysis of the problem. Almost all observers agree on one thing: the qualities of family stability and cohesiveness are usually weak in such situations. In connection with concern over the effects of mobility on the family, Foster[33] has itemized four factors that make for family solidarity: (1) stability of location, with the development of an empathy with and a stake in the surroundings; (2) frequent contacts among the members of the family; (3) homogeneity resulting from common or shared experiences; and (4) an intangible dynamic element or life principle within the fabric of the family itself. Foster makes the important point that this appears first as an ideal or common purpose shared by the two people who marry and establish the family. He also expresses the opinion that all four of these basic factors have been subjected to weakening influences during recent years.

It has been observed that multiplicity of problems tends to occur most frequently among recent immigrants to nations or communities. That this would be so is not surprising and is in line with the foregoing. Simmons and Wolff[1] make this observation:

... when peoples migrate, many elements of the new homeland's culture are rapidly adopted while large parts of the original culture survive in the family or small mobile group. Striking examples are found in first and second-generation immigrants ... who because of contemporary patterns of prejudice may be barred from full participation ... and become, in a sense, "marginal men" trapped between two cultures and subject to the conflicts arising from both.

Their statement continues in a sense that gives some hint regarding the development of multiple social problems in another group, that is, the residual aging group:

Furthermore, a person in the same physical surroundings ... may continue to cling to attitudes, habits, and goals acquired in his youth, while the cultural norms are changing rapidly, with the result that he is not in harmony with the newly evolved patterns within his own society. He may be left as one stranded with his own personal and outmoded cultural values and attachments. The sweeping tides of cultural change frequently produce new areas of stress in personalities and not seldom leave their marks on the organism.

All human beings engage to varying extents in a search for status and goals. In recognition of this, Simmons and Wolff[1] present a graphic picture describing the genesis of a third type of individual who tends to become enmeshed in a tangle of multiproblem situations. Approaching the subject from the standpoint of medicine, they describe this person in the following manner:

Clinicians will often find, at the other type-extreme from the creature of culture, the socially deviant individual who also strives, although perhaps unconsciously, for "wayward" goals and who follows his own atypical and partly false clues in response to his life situation. His adaptations are out of harmony with socially approved behavior, as well as inappropriate on a physical basis. Under such circumstances social penalties are added to the physical injuries, and stress may be compounded in a kind of "vicious cycle," for the more the subject reacts the worse becomes his plight. Following his false clues, he simultaneously impairs his body and his social relationships, perhaps even alienating the very persons best qualified to help and support him and whose rejection leads to further deviation.

The last sentence of this statement might well be reread occasionally by persons engaged in social improvement, including those in the field of public health. Too often, it is feared, the natural or emotional reaction to confusion and despondency is hastily grasped as an excuse for taking the easy way out by condemning individuals as intrinsically bad or worthless.

Another interesting possibility that is worthy of consideration, especially in view of recent developments in psychosomatic medicine, is the use of illness as a response to social difficulty or dissatisfaction. It is known that some individuals who cannot achieve satisfaction and fulfillment in positive or socially acceptable channels turn in their search to negative or antisocial channels. These may take the form of alcoholism, drugs, sexual deviation, dependency, or crime. It is possible that for some individuals still another solution is illness, alone or in company with one or more of the other negative forms of behavior. In fact, of these various solutions, sickness used in this sense has the advantage of being the most acceptable and of eliciting the most sympathy and ready assistance. Furthermore, it provides other individuals and groups in society an opportunity for the achievement of their sense of fulfillment and self-satisfaction.

One final aspect of the subject must be mentioned. It is entirely possible that on occasion the exercise of unilateral zeal on the part of public health workers may actually give rise to social problems in families and may contribute to the establishment and continuation of a vicious social cycle. For example, the public health worker knows that tuberculosis is communicable and may insist on prompt hospitalization of a wife and mother if she has this disease. Without question this is scientifically the correct thing to do. It is best for the patient, for her family, and for society—best, that is, from the public health viewpoint. If, however, at the same time that hospitalization of the wife and mother is arranged, the public health worker neglects to work intimately with the total family and with other sources of assistance in the community, good intentions may lead to ultimate greater evil.

Public health workers must recognize that hospitalization of a parent interferes with family structure and relationships. Removal of maternal care and guidance may result in decreased family cohesiveness and supervision, which may lead to delinquency on the part of the children. Prolonged absence of wifely companionship compounded by concern over increased expenditures for medical care and housekeeping may lead to alcoholism and philandery on the part of the husband. This in turn may lead to lowered income. Eventual dissolution of the family with firm establishment of a disease-delinquency-dependency syndrome is by no means an impossibility. If the woman's tuberculosis is successfully arrested or cured, the pleased staffs of the institution and health agency may discharge her to a grim future with an excellent chance of relapse. And worst of all, the undesirable set of circumstances that has been set in motion may well carry over into several future generations.

Therefore at the risk of redundancy it must be emphasized that public health workers should be most circumspect when considering any measure that may interfere with the integrity of the family, its economic base, or its social relationships. Public health workers should always ask themselves if a program or an action might in any way contribute to the disintegration of the family, even though it might aid the family or society in other ways. All such situations call for careful consideration of all possible alternatives, exhaustive attempts to educate those who may be guilty of infractions of sanitary and health regulations, and the use of a multidisciplinary approach to the existing and potential needs and problems of the total family unit.

## POINTS FOR ACTION

Fortunately in most communities a wide variety of resources exist that may be called on for assistance. For some time attempts have been made to provide for some degree of joint planning and action. Usually these take the form of a council of social agencies or a community health and welfare council in which there is membership by many of the agencies active in these fields. However, on the one hand, any joint activity that occurs is often general and on a high level, distant from the family in need; on the other hand, most health and welfare councils are too limited in terms of membership and interests. Not all of the health and welfare organizations in a community are members of the council, and they do not all participate in the joint planning. Furthermore, several other types of agencies should be involved. Among those often absent are agencies for recreation, rehabilitation, public assistance, law enforcement, and the courts.

Another source of partial solution has been the Social Service Referral Center, to which representatives of member agencies (and sometimes others) may refer cases for certain specific investigations or for certain specific services. One common difficulty is that individuals and families sometimes get lost in the referral system. Sometimes they are never referred back to the initiating agency for follow-up or for resumption and completion of care that may have been instituted but interrupted to provide time or opportunity for solution of a secondary or contributory problem. Mention must be made also of an unfortunate practice occasionally indulged in consciously or subconsciously by a few agencies. This is to avoid referral of cases for additional or auxiliary services because of fear that a kind of right of proprietorship over the case might be lost, and this would reflect poorly on the agency when the time came to publish an annual report or to engage in a fund-raising activity based on case load. Obviously such an attitude, however rare, is totally unwarranted and inexcusable if it detracts in any way from the earliest possible and most satisfactory solution of a family's problems.

In England several different approaches have been attempted.[31] In Southampton a rehabilitation committee consisting of heads of pertinent municipal departments has been established. This committee in turn established a subcommittee of principal officers concerned with the operation of various social welfare and relief programs and of representatives of various voluntary agencies. Weekly meetings are held under the chairmanship of the Medical Officer of Health, who acts as coordinator. Any member may bring up specific cases on the basis of their complexity or because inadequate action has been taken. Responsibility for action is clearly placed and followed up. It is believed that this procedure results in consideration of all aspects of the family problem, places responsibility, results in efficient use of home-visiting personnel, and results in action. It is interesting that a committee of experts on delinquency, called together by the World Health Organization and consisting of forensic, general, and child psychiatrists, psychologists, prison directors, criminologists, social workers, and a judge, suggested that jurists, psychiatrists, psychologists, and sociologists collaborate as a kind of "treatment tribunal" to decide the nature of the diagnosis and course of treatment.[34] In many cases a public health worker might also be of assistance. In Bristol, Liverpool, and Manchester, family service units were established after the war. The work is done from hostels by recently graduated social science workers. In addition to using the hostels for clubs, meetings, cleansing, and feeding, the workers help in the homes and gain the confidence of the families so that more effective service and referral is possible. These methods have resulted in about a 10% rate of rehabilitation of problem families. Williams[31] concludes, "Although the methods of dealing with problem families appear at first sight to be fairly costly, is it far cheaper than leaving the problem untackled."

In reviewing the findings of the St. Paul and similar surveys, Kandle[35] concluded that two things were necessary: first, application of the principles and methods of epidemiology to chronic diseases, disabilities, dependency, and maladjustment; second, development by specialists in health, family services, mental hygiene, social casework, and other related fields of more effective means of working together to achieve a sound and complete collective diagnosis and a coordinated form of treatment.

Essentially what is called for is a synthesis

of philosophy, interest, resources, and effort to be applied to total social problems of the community through its families. Certain specific suggestions may be made. Professional parochialism must be broken down. This might be accomplished in part by the provision of more intimate working relationships among the various disciplines and agencies involved. Health departments and health centers should at least provide office space for liaison personnel from certain other public and private agencies and in turn should assign public health personnel to other agencies for the same purpose. Multidisciplinary and multiagency committees or councils for *case* planning and review should be established as well as committees concerned with *program* planning and review. Some of the community agencies and services that might be included or at least consulted are health, welfare, public assistance, hospitals, police, courts, fire protection, voluntary health agencies, and the social service agencies. Beyond this any honest recognition of professional parochialism should lead to the development of some organized means of bringing those who are to be served and who know their problems only too well into the planning of programs. Family reporting and filing systems instead of individual reporting and filing systems should be used whenever possible. All health and other social agencies should participate in a central service referral center established on a family basis as well as on a case basis. Every problem should be studied and handled with the family considered as the unit, and every proposed solution must be regarded in terms of possible undesirable effects.[36]

Since social problems, including health problems, are inevitably family problems and since it is the concensus that most multiproblem situations have their roots in the early period of married life, health and other social agencies should make more use of marriage reports as a means of contact with certain types of individuals and groups before trouble has an opportunity to occur. Undoubtedly some relatively limited assistance in the establishment of a household, alerting a newly married couple as to sources of assistance and counseling, would prevent the unimpeded progression of numerous problem situations. From the overall community standpoint, concentration of multiproblem families in one area, whether the problems are incipient or fully developed, should be avoided if at all possible. Crowded together, they tend

to maintain each other as problem families and groups. Separated, they tend to learn and improve by contact with more stable families.

If by now the reader thinks that he has been led somewhat afield from the basic issue of public health, he might do well to recognize with Koos[37]:

... community organization for health is in no sense an activity divorced from other forms of activity for community welfare ... all community organization is interwoven in a common effort. Health, says modern research, is not to be found apart from a general welfare of the individual and the community. It consists not only of an absence of disease but also of a sense of general well-being, of adjustment to all of the forces that make up the intricacies of the society in which we live.

## ECONOMIC OPPORTUNITY PROGRAMS

The philosophy that the general well-being of society is related to its level of health coincides with that which led to the antipoverty legislation of Congress: the Economic Opportunity Act of 1964 (P.L. 88-452) and the Appalachian Regional Development Act of 1965 (P.L. 89-794). These significant pieces of legislation virtually threw down the gauntlet to the field of public health as well as others. In effect they said, "For years you have been talking about the relationship between poverty and ill health. Yet for years you have been merely treating the signs and symptoms, the diseases, the consequences rather than the root or source of the problem. Now with these new weapons against poverty itself, let us see what can be accomplished!"

The weapons, although obviously insufficient for a truly all-out attack on poverty or the ill health consequences of it, are nontheless formidable. On the basis of multiple causation of social problems the legislation and accompanying appropriations provided significant funds for a multiple attack on the roots of poverty. The areas of assistance included education and training, health services, housing, employment, small business loans, and many others. Several parts of the program were of particular importance to public health workers in that they provided opportunities for health services and accomplishments previously not possible.[38] One program has been Operation Headstart, the chief purpose of which was to provide preschool learning experiences to disadvantaged children destined to enter kindergarten or first grade the following September. In the process, provision was made for a health program so that the children would not begin school with health handicaps.[39] A similar opportunity for extensive health examinations and correction of defects was provided by the Neighborhood Youth Corps program, which was designed to assist young people who dropped out of school and were therefore unprepared for employment. The Community Action Programs allowed, if a community wished, the inclusion of a variety of disease preventive, therapeutic, and rehabilitative activities within the operation of the multipurpose Neighborhood Community Action Centers.

It is of more than passing interest to note that in several cities where large programs of this type were developed, almost no effect was noted on the demand for outpatient services at municipal hospitals, which traditionally serve as the family physician to the poor. In other words the health service needs met at the Neighborhood Community Action Centers appeared to be over and above those customarily met by hospital outpatient departments. Through the Economic Opportunity program several comprehensive neighborhood medical centers have been established in economically depressed areas of various cities. This concept provides under one roof all the outpatient services needed by the poor of a circumscribed area—promotive, preventive, screening, diagnostic, outpatient therapeutic, inpatient therapeutic (in a back-stopping hospital), and rehabilitative—medical, dental, and emotional. Some centers are conducted by health departments, others by university medical centers. For many reasons the most desirable is an operating partnership that involves the health department, the university medical center, and a representation from the neighborhood itself. In places where a comprehensive child health program is being conducted with Social Security funds, it should, of course, be coordinated with the activities of the Comprehensive Neighborhood Medical Center by providing all the services for those under 20 years of age.

During the early 1970s the Economic Opportunity program was gradually dismantled as an organizational entity, and those components that had proved of value were transferred to permanent agencies such as the Public Health Service and the Office of Education.

Truly the opportunity for great advancement in health services appears to be here. The choice to be made was well stated by James[40]:

There are really just two basic strategies for attacking the health problems of poverty:

We can act against poverty itself and raise the standard of living of the poor. We all know that much of the advance of medicine has been due to a general improvement in the basic standard of living.

We can act against disease without doing anything about poverty. We can more or less accept poverty as something that exists and try to do what is medically possible within this framework.

It is to be hoped that workers in public health have the imagination and courage to choose the former. The latter approach has been tried for a long time with limited results and no light at the end of the tunnel. If public health workers do not choose the former, many individuals in other fields of endeavor would then properly push health workers aside and get on with the task themselves.

## REFERENCES

1. Simmons, L. W., and Wolff, H. G.: Social science in medicine, New York, 1954, Russell Sage Foundation.
2. Stern, B. J.: The health of towns and the early public health movement, Ciba Symposium **9:**871, May-June 1948.
3. Buzzard, Sir F.: The place of social medicine in the reorganization of health services, Brit. Med. J. **1:**703, June 6, 1942.
4. Ryle, J. A.: Changing disciplines, London, 1948, Oxford University Press.
5. Schottstaedt, W. W.: Comprehensive medicine in relation to public health, Amer. J. Public Health **44:**1340, Oct. 1954.
6. Steiger, W. A.: Causality and the comprehensive approach, J. Med. Educ. **33:**538, July 1958.
7. Kroeger, G.: The concept of social medicine as presented by physicians and other writers in Germany, 1779-1932, Chicago, 1937, Julius Rosenwald Fund.
8. Ryle, J. A.: Social pathology and the new era in medicine, Bull. N. Y. Acad. Med. **23:**312, June 1947.
9. Galdston, I.: The meaning of social medicine, Cambridge, 1954, Harvard University Press.
10. Rosen, G.: Approaches to a concept of social medicine, Milbank Mem. Fund Quart. **26:**7, Jan. 1948.
11. Grotjahn, A.: Soziale pathologie, Berlin, 1915, August Hirschwald Verlag.
12. Editorial: Social medicine, Lancet **1:**458, 1947.
13. Wolff, G.: Social pathology as a medical science, Amer. J. Public Health **42:**1576, Dec. 1952.
14. Sydenstricker, E.: Health and environment, New York, 1933, McGraw-Hill Book Co.
15. Hass, W.: In Osborne, P. B.: The war that business must win, New York, 1970, McGraw-Hill Book Co.

16. Skeen, C.: In Osborne, P. B.: The war that business must win, New York, 1970, McGraw-Hill Book Co.

17. Allen, F. P.: People of the shadows, Cincinnati, 1954, Public Health Federation.

18. Stockwell, E. G.: A critical examination of the relationship between socioeconomic status and mortality, Amer. J. Public Health **53:**956, June 1963.

19. Chilman, C. S.: Growing up poor, SRS pub. no. 109, Washington, D. C., 1969, U. S. Department of Health, Education, and Welfare.

20. Pond, M. A.:How does housing affect health? Amer. J. Public Health **61:**667, May 1946.

21. Lawrence, P. S.: Chronic illness and socio-economic status, Public Health Rep. **63:**1507, Nov. 19, 1948.

22. Yerby, A. S.: The problems of medical care for indigent populations, Amer. J. Public Health **55:**1212, Aug. 1965.

23. Baird, D.: Social and economic factors affecting the mother and child, Amer. J. Public Health **42:**516, May 1952.

24. Richardson, H. B.: Patients have families, New York, 1945, Commonwealth Fund.

25. Ackerman, N. W.: Psychological dynamics of the family organism, Public Health Rep. **71:** 1017, Oct. 1956.

26. Bossard, J. H. S.: The sociology of child development, New York, 1954, Harper & Row, Publishers.

27. Parsons, T., and Fox, R.: Illness, therapy, and the modern urban American family, J. Soc. Issues **8:**31, April 1952.

28. Caudill, W.: Effects of social and cultural systems in reactions to stress, New York, 1958, Social Science Research Council.

29. Voiland, A. L., and Buell, B.: A classification of disordered family types, Soc. Work **6:**3, Oct. 1961.

30. McCulloch, J. W., and Philip, A. E.: Suicidal behavior, Oxford, England, 1972, Pergamon Press, Ltd.

31. Williams, H. C. M.: Rehabilitation of problem families, Amer. J. Public Health **45:**990, Aug. 1955.

32. Buell, B., et al.: Community planning for human services, New York, 1952, Columbia University Press.

33. Foster, R. G.: Effect of mobility on the family, Amer. J. Public Health **46:**812, July 1956.

34. Psychiatry and the treatment of delinquency, WHO Chron. **12:**330, Oct. 1958.

35. Kandle, R. P.: In modern philanthropy and human welfare, New York, 1952, Grant Foundation.

36. Eller, C. H., Hatcher, G. H., and Buell, B.: Health and family issues in community planning for the problem of indigent disability, Amer. J. Public Health **48:**(supp.) Nov. 1958.

37. Koos, E. L.: New concepts in community organization for health, Amer. J. Public Health **43:**466, April 1953.

38. Kravitz, S. L.: Health aspects of the antipoverty crusade, N. J. Department of Health, Public Health News, Jan. 1965.

39. Editorial: Project Head Start and public health, Amer. J. Public Health **55:**1122, Aug. 1965.

40. James, G.: Poverty as an obstacle to health progress in our cities, Amer. J. Public Health **55:**1757, Nov. 1965.

*Public health is purchaseable;*
*within natural limitations any community*
*can determine its own death rate.*

HERMANN T. BIGGS

CHAPTER 7

# Economics of public health

## INEVITABILITY OF HEALTH COSTS

Two related objections are occasionally heard with regard to public health activities. One is that the establishment and growth of public health agencies and programs have resulted in increasing costs to the public. The other is that public health workers are at a disadvantage in that they cannot point to their successes. This latter statement is made in contrast to the position of the private physician, who with justification can point to the saving of many specific lives by judicious medical and surgical management. Granted that the public health worker can seldom point to specific individuals who have been spared illness and premature death by public health programs, this is more than compensated for by the possibility of measurement in a larger and ultimately more dramatic sense. The fact is that the fruits of public health activities are in essence very different from those of therapeutic medicine and that accordingly the bases of measurement cannot be expected to be the same. Public health work is not fundamentally concerned with the repair of damage already done. Rather, it focuses on the prevention of damage in the first place and the promotion of positive health. Furthermore, by virtue of the fact that although living is expensive, illness is even more so, it should be possible to demonstrate that preventive and promotive health activities offer a sound financial investment to the individual and to the community.

Most intelligent people appreciate the reduction in human suffering that has resulted from the public health movement. It must be realized, however, that the further removed one is by time and space from the threat of personal suffering the less consideration is likely to be given to it. In other words, our very success in public health work tends to mask its value. It is appropriate therefore that the public and its elected representatives be given cause to appreciate the wisdom of expenditures for health from an altogether different viewpoint.

As will be pointed out elsewhere, the costs of all governmental services have persistently increased. Proportionately speaking, the expenditure for public health services represents an area of considerable expansion. This has caused some to point to public health programs as an added economic burden to the taxpayer. It is important to point out and to demonstrate that an increased sum of money spent wisely for health services represents not an increase but actually a decrease in the net bill for personal and community welfare and protection. The construction and maintenance costs of public water purification and sewage disposal plants are admittedly great. The costs, however, do not represent an addition to the taxpayers' economic burden. Their absence would cost a similar if not greater sum for individual facilities, for increased medical care, and for lost earnings resulting from the illnesses that would not be prevented. Single or repeated outbreaks of typhoid fever, for example, would cost a community much more in the long run than would installation of engineering and other measures designed for their prevention. A sound

**113**

financial policy for public health services therefore must take into consideration not only the humanitarian and social gains but also the economic advantages to be derived therefrom. The problem then is to make the public conscious and to organize costs that in any case are destined to occur either as hidden individual expenditures or as socially beneficial public appropriations. Public health is the best form of social and economic insurance.

## WHY LIFE AND HEALTH ARE MEASURED

Beyond the inevitability of these expenditures is the added factor of the economic value of the lives made possible or continued by public health endeavors. To many the thought of placing a monetary value on human life appears to be improper, immoral, or inhumane. Essentially, reactions to life and death are based on emotion and sentiment, and ordinarily people deliberately avoid any thought of placing an economic or cost-value label on a human being. Yet to be realistic it must be admitted that life does have a monetary value. The death of a parent brings to society as a whole as well as to the particular family involved an economic and a sentimental loss that is real and irreparable. This may manifest itself in a lowered standard of living for the family, the necessity of public financial aid, or the loss of a trained worker. Furthermore, governmental recognition is given to the value of a life, and one seldom hears objections to the concept of income tax exemptions.

In addressing himself to this question, Fuchs[1] makes several telling observations:

What, then, is the justification for such an inquiry? The principle one is the fact that the question of the contribution of health services is being asked and answered every day. It is being asked and answered implicitly every time consumers, hospitals, universities, business firms, foundations, government agencies and legislative bodies make decisions concerning the volume and composition of health services, present and future. If economists can help to rationalize and make more explicit the decision making process, can provide useful definitions, concepts and analytic tools, and can develop appropriate bodies of data and summary measures, they will be making their own contribution to health and to the economy.

In the same vein it must be recognized that whereas members of appropriating bodies may be humane and sympathetic, collectively they are becoming increasingly coldly analytic and practical. As a result, it is becoming more difficult to sell public health programs, especially on the basis of sentimentality or intangibles. O'Connor[2] in a discussion of benefits as opposed to risks points this out by saying:

Previously, if any public health proposal could be demonstrated to be in the interests of the public, the health officer was justified in recommending it without examining too critically any untoward or unwanted ecological sequelae which might occur. Not only was the public health official not challenged, but he was armed with the *a priori* assumption that all his goals were in the public interest, and that his responsibility was discharged if his recommendations could be demonstrated to improve health.

It is unfortunate, in a sense, that so many results of public health programs, although of tremendous intrinsic value, are largely of an intangible nature, for example, diseases and deaths prevented, problems avoided, and the like. This makes it all the more imperative that health program planning and evaluative procedures have incorporated in them from the beginning a consideration not only of economic costs but also the anticipated economic return. Such cost-benefit as well as risk-benefit data can be of inestimable value both in obtaining public understanding and support and in budgetary presentations.[3]

In attempting to do so, however, one is immediately confronted with two fundamental problems: (1) problems of definition—What is health? What is incapacitation? etc.; and (2) problems of measurement—How does one measure something that is not there? What base line can one use? The seriousness of these problems varies with time, place, and circumstance, as indicated by Linnenberg.[4] He points out that if a community or nation has a high incidence of a disease, which existing knowledge and methods systematically applied can quickly bring under control, it is possible to make an advance estimate not only of the cost of the methods but also of the likely benefits in terms of worker time not lost and treatment costs avoided. But, he adds, drama of this sort stems only from a sudden breakthrough, as in the case of a new effective vaccine, or from an area being widely afflicted with a serious and especially an economically detrimental disease, such as malaria or yaws, which is anachronistic from the standpoint of modern medicine and which can be brought under control quickly, even though little or nothing is done about other health problems. Our difficulty, he concludes, is that such classic simplicity is absent from most public health work in this country, where public health achievement has progressed so far that our health problems are not so much the yes or no kind as the more or less kind.

## ECONOMIC VALUE OF LIFE

Many have tried to evaluate man or to put a price on his economic worth. One of the earliest attempts was that of Sir William Petty (1623-1687), who originated many ideas later used by the political economist Adam Smith in *Wealth of Nations* and other works. Petty[5] derived his estimate as follows:

Suppose the People of England be Six Millions in number, that their Expense at £7 per head be 42 Millions: Suppose also that the Rent of the Lands be 8 Millions, and the yearly profit of all the Personal Estate be 8 Millions more; it must needs follow that the Labour of the People must have supplied the remaining 26 Millions the which multiplied by 20 (the Mass of Mankind being worth 20 years purchase as well as land) makes 520 Millions as the value of the whole people; which number divided by 6 Millions makes about £80 the value of each Head of Man, Woman and Child and of adult Persons Twice as much; from whence we may learn to compute the loss we have sustained by the Plague, by the Slaughter of Men in War and by sending them abroad into the Service of Foreign Princes.

Later Sir William Farr and Irving Fisher made more scientific computations, using the life table technique, which by their time had been developed. Subsequently this approach was explored more extensively and effectively by Dublin and Lotka.[6,7] Several of their publications have considerable social significance and have been drawn on freely in the following discussion. More recently Weisbrod[8] has combined this approach with several other approaches to place health and expenditures for it in the proper context.

The human body may be considered as being similar to a machine. Like machines its proper function depends on the movement and interaction of various physical and chemical parts, complicated and augmented, however, by a third and much more complex factor—biologic reaction. To resort to a crude analogy the body might be likened to an internal combustion engine with limbs in place of pistons and the organs of internal secretion acting as the carburetor. Superimposed on these is the supervisory function of the human mind, which might be compared with the governor on an internal combustion engine. In a like manner

the human body may be regarded as an economic unit brought into existence for measurable, potential, productive purposes.

A machine designed for the production of ball bearings, for example, is of no intrinsic value in itself, its true value being measurable only in terms of its capacity to produce ball bearings, thereby justifying its existence. Similarly, except in a completely paganistic and hedonistic society, the mere existence of life is of little if any value. It should be realized that life and health in themselves have real value only as they promote efficiency and happiness and that in the final analysis it is the quality of life that counts, not the quantity. Of themselves, life and health are valueless, their true value depending on the activities engaged in by virtue of them.

To return to the example of the machine it must pass through several phases or steps before it is even ready to be of productive value. First, it must be built, which presupposes the existence of a factory in which it may be constructed. Its construction therefore involves from the start a considerable capital outlay for factory site, labor, and tools. On completion the machine is not yet of true value. It must be prepared for use or function. This involves a series of installation expenditures for inspection and checking, for transfer to the site where it is intended to function, and for oiling, tuning up, and other preparations. After this the machine is ready to become productive, and the extent and efficiency of its usefulness depend on its original quality or lack of structural defects, the correctness of its installation, and the manner in which it is routinely cared for while in use. It must be carefully and repeatedly lubricated, fed the proper fuel, inspected, overhauled, repaired, and given proper rest intervals rather than constant grinding use, which would lead to metal fatigue. During this period of use therefore, a certain amount of expenditure and effort is constantly required to maintain the machine, and its ultimate value can be determined only after the value of that expenditure and effort is deducted from the gross value of its productivity.

With man as with machines there are always debit as well as credit items during the period of productivity. It is the hope and goal of the manufacturer that his machine will continue to function with relative efficiency at least long enough to produce sufficient items for sale to offset all of the debits incurred by the capital investment and the installation and maintenance costs. In other words, from the moment the machine is purchased the curve of the cumulative investment in it continues to rise, the curve of cumulative productive value lagging for a considerable period. It is not until these two curves cross that the manufacturer can breathe easily and begin to reap a net benefit from the use of the machine. If any untoward circumstances develop before the two curves cross, the manufacturer stands to lose a considerable investment.

Many things may go wrong after purchase. The machine may have been unsuspectedly defective, it may have been damaged during transportation and installation, or it may have worn out prematurely as a result of improper use or care. These are only a few of the undesirable potentialities the manufacturer must constantly guard against. Even after the two curves cross, all is not necessarily clear sailing because the longer the machine is used the greater is the tendency for parts to wear out and for maintenance and repair costs to increase. Sooner or later a time is reached when these costs become greater than the value of the items produced, and the two curves cross again. Continued use is no longer profitable. The machine has now passed into the phase of obsolescence or, in the case of human beings, senility. More idealistically it may be considered the period of retirement or senior citizenship.

It is of interest to attempt to analyze the items that contribute to the debit and credit

**Table 7-1.** Factors in the socioeconomic value of human life, 1955—summary

| | |
|---|---:|
| *Capital cost** | |
| 1. Economic incapacitation of mother | $    500 |
| 2. Risk of death to mother (prorated) | 12 |
| 3. Risk of injury to mother with immediate or subsequent effect on her economic value (prorated) | ? |
| 4. Immediate costs of childbearing | 488 |
| 5. Risk of infant death (prorated) | 40 |
| 6. Risk of infant illness or injury | ? |
| 7. Interest on capital investment | 30 |
| | $  1,070 |
| *Installation cost†* | |
| 1. Shelter, clothing, and food | $ 11,900 |
| 2. Value of time mother devotes to child care | 15,750 |
| 3. Education—family and community contribution | 4,500 |
| 4. Medical and dental care and health protection | 600 |
| 5. Recreation and transportation | 3,000 |
| 6. Insurance | 100 |
| 7. Sundries and incidentals | 900 |
| 8. Risk of death during first 18 years (prorated) | 250 |
| 9. Risk of disability during first 18 years | ? |
| 10. Interest on installation costs | 23,000 |
| | $ 60,000 |
| *Period of productivity‡* | |
| *Credit* | |
| 1. Earning potential | $ 60,000 |
| 2. Interest on earnings | 50,000 |
| 3. Noneconomic potential | ? |
| | $110,000 |
| *Debit* | |
| 1. Risk of disability during productive period | $    4,000 |
| 2. Medical costs | 6,500 |
| 3. Risk of premature death | 200 |
| 4. Risk of becoming substandard | 5,500 |
| 5. Interest on debit items | 15,000 |
| | $ 31,200 |

*The investment that society has in each infant by the time it is born.
† The investment that society has in each individual by the time he reaches 18 years of age.
‡ The return that society can expect from its investment, with the risks involved during this period.

columns of human life. One such analysis, based on data and crude calculations for the year 1955 as a convenient example, is presented on the following pages. Insofar as possible an attempt has been made to calculate or estimate monetary values for the many factors considered. It must be stressed, however, that *this is done simply to illustrate a general principle,* and the reader should realize that *the values assigned are at best no more than very crude calculations and estimates* that are subject to innumerable influences such as changes in monetary values, wage levels, cost of living trends, and the extent of unemployment, to mention only a few. In other words, *the figures given are not intended to represent true dollar values to be quoted as such but are presented simply to illustrate a concept.* Incidentally, however, the total of the investment in the first two items—capital cost and installation cost—are currently (1972) calculated to average $100,000.[9] The entire picture is summarized in Table 7-1. Rice and Cooper[10] describe a similar recent approach.

## FACTORS ENTERING INTO THE VALUE OF A HUMAN LIFE

### Period of initial capital investment

1. *Value of economic incapacitation of the expectant mother*       −$500

All adult females and males have an economic productive potential. For the majority of women this potential is effected in either or both of two ways: employment for wages or occupation as a housewife. Ordinarily the latter is not thought of in an economic sense, since it rarely involves the transfer of an agreed-on sum of money for services rendered. Nonetheless, the housewife and mother fulfills a function of real economic value. In fact, her absence would necessitate the employment of a paid substitute. The average period of incapacitation for childbearing might be estimated roughly at 3 months, the actual degree of incapacitation varying throughout the period of pregnancy and with individuals. In 1955 the average age of the pregnant woman was 24 years, and the annual value of her real or potential earnings might be estimated at an average of $2,000. This considers her to be in the most typical economic class for her sex, which in 1955 reported a maximum potential annual income of approximately $2,500. Incapacitation for about one fourth of her twenty-fourth year therefore represents about $500 as part of the capital investment in the anticipated child.

2. *Prorated value of the risk of maternal death* −$12

If the efforts of a housewife and mother have an economic value and if, as will be developed, she herself represents a considerable investment, her death as a result of childbearing will constitute a monetary loss to her family and to society. In 1955 there were about 1,950 maternal deaths related to the 4.04 million births that occurred in the United States. The average age of the women who died was 29 years. The average net value of the potential future activity of each of them might be estimated at about $26,000. Therefore the monetary loss as a result of maternal deaths was the product of $26,000 times 1,950 deaths, or about $50.7 million per year, which if prorated among all of the births, amounts to $12 as the value of the risk of maternal death, which should be added to the cost of each child born alive.

3. *Value of the risk of injury short of death to the mother*       −?

As a result of childbearing, many women suffer disabilities or illnesses, which although they do not cause death, have a subsequent effect on their well-being, economic productivity, and length of life. As in the case of maternal deaths, the total economic effect of this should be prorated among all infants born. Although extremely difficult if not impossible to estimate or calculate, its effect appears elsewhere in terms of medical expenditures and shortened lives.

4. *Immediate costs of childbearing*       −$488

Several readily recognizable items are included in the costs of childbearing, such as prenatal and postnatal care, hospitalization, delivery, and expenditures for special maternity clothes, layettes, and the equipment for the care of the newborn infant. There also should be included an item for housekeeping assistance. Although some objection might be raised to this, it may be pointed out that in some households a housekeeper is actually employed for a period preceding and following delivery. Furthermore, since this is not possible for most families, some housekeeping assistance is required and furnished by a relative, friend, or neighbor. Their time and effort has value, and calling on them to assist in the home of the expectant mother ultimately involves their temporary removal from productive enterprise elsewhere. Estimates of these costs for the most typical economic class have been adapted from studies by the Metropolitan Life Insurance Company and the Maternity Center Association, New York City, and are presented in Table 7-2. The average figure may be considered to be about $488.

5. *Prorated value of the risk of neonatal death* −$40

Like their mothers, infants may be subject to injury or death as a consequence of abnormal development or of the birth process. This is analogous to the machine that might be defective in construction or damaged shortly thereafter. During 1955 in the United States there occurred a total of 167,700 known nonproductive deliveries, consisting of 90,000 stillbirths and 77,000 neonatal deaths. Up to this point there had been invested in each of them an average of $1,000, which if multiplied by the number of known nonproductive deliveries, gives $167.7 million

**Table 7-2.** Estimates of average cost of births for women in the $4,500 family income class, 1955

| Type of service | Total cost | Hospital cost | Physician's fee | Housekeeper | Minimum layette | Incidentals |
|---|---|---|---|---|---|---|
| At home | $300 | $ . . . | $ 70 | $150 | $60 | $ 20 |
| Ward | 325 | 95 | . . . | 150 | 60 | 20 |
| Semiprivate | 535 | 150 | 150 | 150 | 60 | 50 |
| Private | 735 | 200 | 225 | 150 | 60 | 100 |

as the annual monetary loss they represent. If this figure is prorated among the year's 4.04 million live births each infant bears as his share of the risk of not being born alive or surviving 1 month a sum of about $40.

6. *Value of the risk of injury short of death to the infant*                          −?

As in the case of mothers, infants may suffer non-fatal damage before, during, or shortly after birth. Again the economic significance of this is difficult or impossible to determine. However, it shows up subsequently in the form of medical expenditures and shortened life.

7. *Interest on capital investment*          −$30

If a man and woman originally considered the advantages and disadvantages of prospective parenthood and, deciding against it, invested the total of the preceding sums for a period corresponding to that of pregnancy, there would accrue at 3.5% compound interest about $30. Although this may sound venal, the fact remains that many people do just this.

*The total capital value of a child at birth in 1955 was therefore about $1,070, which represented the economic interest that the parents and society had in the child by the time he left the human factory.*

**Period of human installation costs**

Although the mechanical contrivance on purchase may be installed and made ready for productive performance in a relatively short time, a rather lengthy period and a considerable cash outlay are required to bring the newly born human mechanism to the point of social and economic productivity. Among the costs involved may be listed the following, the figures for which are in many instances extremely conservative in view of current prices.

1. *Shelter, clothing, and food for first 18 years*
                                           −$11,900

For 1955 a breakdown of this crude estimate was $4,240 for shelter, $1,690 for clothing, and $5,970 for food. Since exception may be taken to the inclusion of an item for shelter, it might be pointed out that from an overall social standpoint, if the addition of a new family member did not result in overcrowding, necessitating an enlargement of living quarters, the family was previously occupying more living space than was fundamentally required.

2. *Value of the mother's time devoted to the care of the child*                          −$15,750

Based on the average value of the potential earnings of a 24-year-old woman at home or at work as $2,500, the value of her time given to the care of the child is estimated to decrease arithmetically from $1,250 for the first year to $400 for the eighteenth year. The cumulative total is about $15,750.

3. *Education*                              −$4,500

It is estimated that the average expenditure for education of a child is $4,500, of which the community bears the major share.

4. *Medical and dental care and health protection*
                                            −$600

This small item of expense if increased substantially, would undoubtedly result in considerably enhanced personal value, productivity, and length of life. It is unfortunate that this is considered to be of the same magnitude as "sundries and incidentals."

5. *Recreation and transportation*      −$3,000

6. *Insurance*                             −$100

Very few children's lives are insured. The average investment was about the figure shown.

7. *Sundries and incidentals*            −$900

8. *Prorated value of risk of death before eighteenth year*                              −$250

Deaths that occur during the first 18 years of life are analogous to irreparable damage of a machine after its purchase and during the process of its installation. During 1955 in the United States there were about 42,000 deaths among persons between the ages of 1 month and 18 years. The average age at death in this group was 9 years. The monetary loss attributable to these deaths might be approximated roughly from the cost items previously listed as 9/18 ($1,070 + $36,750) of the costs of birth and of the installation period, times an annual loss of 42,000 persons, times 18 separate years, during any one of which the death might occur. The product of these figures is about $14 billion, which if prorated throughout the 55.02 million persons in the age group under 18 years, gives about $250 as each individual's share of the risk of preproductive death.

9. *Nonfatal disabilities during first 18 years*      −?

As before, it is impossible to determine or estimate the value of this effect, but it shows up subsequently in costs of medical care and premature death.

10. *Interest on installation costs*        −$23,000

Again, if a decision had been made against conceiving the child in the first place and if all of the installation expenses had been invested instead, at the end of 18 years there would accrue at 3.5% compound interest an additional sum of about $23,000.

*Total installation value in 1955 therefore amounted to about $60,000 for each child who successfully reached the age of 18 years.*

**Period of human productivity**

Up to this point the new human mechanism not only has been constructed but has passed through all of the phases that constitute an installation or get-ready period. Instead of being bolted to a floor, oiled, checked, and tuned as in the case of a machine, the human being has been fed, clothed, educated, and otherwise prepared until he is ready to assume his place as a productive adult member of society. He is now in a position to begin to repay the considerable investment that his parents and society have made in him. From this point on the picture becomes complicated by the necessity of considering both credit and debit items. To make possible an ultimate balancing of the books the individual's cumulative gross earnings must accomplish three things: full repayment of all that has been invested in him, provision of current maintenance costs both personal and community, and provision for future retirement in the postproductive period of life. Added to this is the hope of providing if possible some net surplus to pass on to the succeeding generation. It is on this surplus that all familial and social progress, in contrast to stagnation, depend.

**Credit items.** Three items appear on the credit side of the human ledger. They may be considered as follows:

1. *Net earning potential* +$60,000

In 1955 the most typical wage class into which working adult males fell was that which could look forward to a maximum annual earned income of $5,000. This maximum is approached gradually, beginning with a much lower income at the age of about 18 years, when individuals begin productive work. The maximum is reached as the individual approaches his fortieth birthday, after which the annual net income begins to decline slowly to the time of death or retirement, when a significant or complete drop results. On the basis of his life expectancy the average 18-year-old male in the $5,000 maximum annual income class can look forward to gross future earnings totaling about $100,000. His total future cost of living based on 1955 figures would amount to about $40,000, leaving $60,000 as the net value of the future earnings of persons reaching 18 years of age. Taxes must, of course, be deducted from this.

2. *Interest on earnings* +$50,000

Since interest has been considered in relation to the sums invested in the individual, to be consistent it should be applied also to his net future earnings. Although the individual wage earner does not necessarily receive the interest himself, society as a whole may be considered to benefit, since the mere fact that money is spent means that it has been put to use for

gain. Therefore the $60,000 net future earnings will produce for the working individual or for other members of society to whom it may be transferred through purchases a certain amount of interest. If the interest is compound and the basis of it is scaled from ages 18 to 70 years, it will accumulate to the approximate amount of $50,000.

3. *Noneconomic productive potential* +?

The human mechanism differs from the mechanical contrivance in that it has abilities or potentials to produce value in forms other than material. Thus a human being has a reproductive potential that in light of the foregoing is obviously worth something. One is reminded that the totalitarian dictators of recent European history actually placed a value on the reproductive potential of women and paid the individual cash awards for producing children. Despite this, any attempt to evaluate correctly the reproductive potential of human beings in a monetary sense is pointless. Human beings also have social and intellectual potentials of incalculable value. Who would dare appraise da Vinci, Beethoven, Shakespeare? Yet the world is infinitely richer because of their existence.

**Debit items.** Attainment of the age of productive capacity does not necessarily imply that the individual will actually be able to or will even choose to contribute his share to society's material advancement. Several things may act as deterrents, among which are the forces of disability and premature death and the possibility that the individual, although by now an adult, may be physically or mentally substandard or antisocial.

1. *Value of risk of disability after eighteenth birthday* −$4,000

Various surveys have indicated that in the United States about 2.5% of working time is lost due to absenteeism or inefficiency attributable to illness or injury. Incidentally, a considerable amount of this is preventable. Since the national income in 1955 was about $324 billion, the average economic loss due to disability per potential wage earner, of whom there were about 102.4 million, may be computed as

$$\frac{\$324,000,000,000 \times 0.25}{102,400,000} = \$80 \text{ per worker per year.}$$

With an average working life expectancy of 50 years this would amount to a total of $80 × 50 years = $4,000, which represents each wage earner's prorated share of the nation's economic loss due to disability that must be deducted from his average net productive potential.

2. *Medical costs* −$6,500

The cost of disability in a worker does not merely involve loss of productive power. Since the individual's actual take-home pay is usually affected, there results a loss of family income often necessitating cutting into the future income of the family or into the wealth of society at large. The extent to which this occurs during the average wage earner's life has been estimated by various groups who have studied the problem as about $3,500. In addition, disabilities require expenditures for medical and nursing care and

**Table 7-3.** Potential future earnings of persons prematurely dead, United States, 1955

| Age group (years) | Median age (years) | Deaths (1955) | Individual net future earnings | Total lost future earnings |
|---|---|---|---|---|
| 19 to 24 | 21 | 13,350 | $61,000 | $   814,350,000 |
| 25 to 44 | 35 | 106,360 | 60,000 | 6,381,600,000 |
| 45 to 64 | 55 | 392,800 | 27,500 | 10,802,000,000 |
| 65 and over | 72 | 819,000 | 750 | 614,250,000 |
| | | | | $18,612,200,000 |

Population over 18 years of age in United States, 1955 = 102,400,000.

$$\frac{\$18,612,200,000}{102,400,000} = \text{about } \$200$$

sometimes for hospitalization, drugs, and appliances. The results of studies of these miscellaneous costs place them at an average of about $3,000 during an individual's lifetime. It is significant that one of the chief reasons for borrowing is inability to meet the costs of illness. If the illness happens to be of a communicable nature, there is the added risk of spread of the disease, upon which some value might be placed. The amount is difficult to estimate, but its effect shows up elsewhere in the form of society's total medical bill and as premature retirement and death. Another factor, the value of which cannot be calculated but which shows up later, is the risk of lowering the level of health of an entire family when disability of the breadwinner lowers the standard of living.

3. *Value of risk of premature death of wage earner*
$$-\$200$$

The possibility of premature death of wage earners has been referred to. When this occurs, the worker in most instances has not been allowed to live long enough to neutralize the investment that has been made in him. By prorating the lost potential future earnings of those who prematurely die, each worker's share of this risk of not fulfilling his life expectancy may be crudely estimated as follows at about $200 (Table 7-3).

4. *Risk of becoming substandard or antisocial*
$$-\$5,500$$

A large number of individuals are brought to maturity only to be found defective in one way or another. Many of them require the full-time attention of an additional large group of potential producers in the form of police, mental hospital attendants, and the like.

It is difficult or impossible to determine the total number of such individuals. Estimates vary considerably. For the United States in 1955 some of the estimates were as follows: blind, 330,000; mentally ill or defective, receiving some type of intramural or extramural institutional care, 840,000; attendants of mental institutions, 100,000; physically handicapped, 2,230,000; chronic nonproductive alcoholics, 750,000; narcotic addicts, 60,000; criminals, 400,000 detained and 600,000 at large; police, wardens, etc., 750,000; paupers, 80,000; and prostitutes, 250,000. Some of these figures undoubtedly are overstatements and some of them are duplicative. Neverthe-

less, they have a double significance for the average wage earner. First, he himself shares the risk of becoming substandard. Avoiding that, he finds he must assist in the support of these defectives. The cost is enormous. The annual bill for the care of the mentally ill alone has been estimated at well over $1 billion, and criminals and those who apprehend and guard them must cost about the same. The partially or totally blind, deaf-mutes, the physically handicapped, and some others contribute varying amounts to their own support, and more adequate programs for their training and rehabilitation would increase the degree to which they might be self-sufficient. The cost of support of the handicapped, the substandard, and the anti-social may be put very conservatively at $4 billion annually. Prorated among the wage earners over 18 years of age, this amounts to about $1,000 per wage earner.

In addition, society suffers a loss due to their lack of production. Estimates of this loss prorated among the wage earners over 18 years of age amounts to about $4,500 per wage earner. In toto the prorated share of the cost of the risk of becoming substandard or antisocial might be considered about $5,500.

5. *Interest on debit items*   $-\$15,000$

The total of each individual's share of all the debits that occur during the productive period of life amounts to about $16,000. If this sum were invested instead of being lost, there would accrue at 3.5% compound interest about $15,000 at the end of his productive life, bringing the total loss to about $31,000.

**SUMMARY**

If from the total net productive credit of $110,000 in the admittedly rough example presented, the $1,070 in capital cost, the $60,000 in installation costs, and the $31,200 in debits during the productive period are subtracted, there remains a net balance of about $18,000 per person for the individual's and society's provision for the period of obsolescence, retirement, or senility.

**ECONOMIC RETURN ON PUBLIC HEALTH INVESTMENT**

A previous chapter on world health problems presented several examples of the contribution of public health measures to regional or national economic development and productivity. The economic soundness of expenditures for public health may also be demonstrated by still a different approach. This considers only expenditures saved on hospital bills, medical care, laboratory work, and similar facilities. One example that has been well worked out relates to the control of diphtheria in New York City some years ago, where an attempt was made to prove, among other things, that it is cheaper to prevent than to treat illness. In 1920 there occurred in New York City about 14,000 reported cases of diphtheria. Three thousand people were hospitalized at an average cost of $112, totaling $336,000 for hospitalization. The remaining 11,000 patients were cared for at home at a cost to the city for various medical services of an average of $35 per patient, or a total of $385,000. On the average, public health nurses visited hospitalized patients twice and home patients six times. At 50 cents a visit this cost $36,000. The laboratory work, on the basis of 10 nose and throat cultures examined for each reported case at 5 cents per examination, cost $70,000. Of the patients, 1,045 died from the infection; at an average of $200 each their funerals cost over $200,000. The total cost up to this point therefore was $1,027,000. In other words, the city of New York in 1920 spent over $1 million for the support of the diphtheria organism.

From 1929 through 1931 the city's health department, aided partly by private funds, carried on an intensive, well-organized campaign to secure the immunization of infants and children against diphtheria. The cost of this campaign during those 3 years was $375,000. At the end of the 3 years the program was continued at a cost of less than $10,000 per year. Unquestionably many persons considered these sums an added economic burden. However, what was purchased with that money? During 1939, instead of over 14,000 diphtheria cases, there were only 543 cases, despite known improved reporting. One half of these were hospitalized at $112 each. The total hospital bill therefore was $31,000. The medical bills for those remaining at home at an average of $35 per case totaled $9,625. Nurses' visits to the patients cost $1,100, and the laboratory work was reduced to only $2,750. Instead of over 1,000 deaths, there were only 22 deaths, for whom the funeral cost was $4,400. Even if the cost of $375,000 for the 3-year program is added plus seven times

$10,000 to continue it between 1932 and 1939, the total bill for diphtheria was only $493,875, or one half of the 1920 bill.

Private enterprise has long recognized the soundness of expenditures for health and safety. Between 1911 and 1925 the Metropolitan Life Insurance Company spent over $20 million for health education, early diagnosis, and nursing service among its policyholders. During those 17 years the death rate for policyholders declined more than 30%, which was fully twice the reduction that occurred in the general population. In monetary terms the $20 million spent resulted in a saving to the company and its policyholders during that period of $43 million. This is good business. Whereas the length of life for the general public increased 5 years during the period under consideration, policyholders enjoyed an increased life expectancy of 9 years.

Even more spectacular savings become evident when the economic value of life is considered with regard to such situations. Bolduan,[11] for example, pointed out that in 1935 lobar pneumonia caused the death of 2,039 males in New York City, 809 of them between the ages of 20 and 50 years. He computed that these 809 deaths occurring among working males represented an economic loss of about $20 million. This fact was used in requesting $500,000 to provide adequate pneumonia control work. It was estimated that the expenditure of this amount would result in a saving of $5 million.

Further examples may be found in relation to other diseases. Parran, when Surgeon General, pointed out to the Congress that whereas the $2 million of state and federal funds used in 1937 for the prevention and control of syphilis seems a sizable sum, it is paltry in comparison with the $10 million spent annually for the care of the syphilitic blind and the $32 million spent for the care of the syphilitic insane.

Vaughan, in 1936, while Commissioner of Health of the city of Detroit, requested from the city council an additional $200,000 per year for each of 5 years for early tuberculosis case finding and hospitalization. He was able to demonstrate successfully that the total extra appropriation of $1 million for this purpose would repay itself several times over by the end of that period. In 1930 only 15% of the new cases of tuberculosis were found while still in the minimal stage, 30% were moderately advanced, and 55% were far advanced. By 1943, as a result of the accelerated program for case finding and hospitalization, the figures for minimal and far-advanced cases were literally reversed so that 53% of newly diagnosed cases were in the minimal stage and only 17% had progressed to the far-advanced stage. When it is considered that the average hospital stay for minimal cases in Detroit was 9 months in contrast to 2 years or more for the far-advanced cases, the enormous saving to the taxpayers in terms of hospital costs alone becomes evident. In fact at the time the program began it was calculated that the added annual expenditure of $200,000 saved about $1.4 million each year. The critical importance of careful health planning and appropriations to social and economic development has been emphasized by many, especially in relation to the developing areas of the world,[12-14] as well as in American society. Several examples have also been presented in Chapters 3 and 12. Most who address themselves to this question, however, stress the importance of health improvement measures in such situations being accompanied by advances in as broad as possible social and economic fronts to avoid a rapid increase in dependent people. Ideally the health improvement program should be planned and conducted as an integral component of a country's or region's program for total socioeconomic development and, of course, should include consideration of family planning needs.[15,16]

To further illustrate the magnitude of the savings that have been effected by public health activities, Table 7-4 presents data on several causes of death, the major share of the reduction of which may justly be attributed to organized public health programs. For each cause the number of deaths has been computed that would be expected to have occurred in 1970 if the rates of 1900 had been maintained. It is seen that by the reduction of these causes of death alone 1.57 million lives have been saved each year. Obviously these lives have some value. Even if the investment made in each of them were to be considered as merely $1,000, the total value saved to the nation would amount to almost $1.6 billion each year.

A partial indication of the economic consequences of such improvements is found in an analysis[17] of the benefits that have accrued to the United States as a result of the recent development and use of measles immunization. The key points are shown in Table 7-5. As is seen, through the reduction of deaths, cases of mental retardation, and hospitalization, as

**Table 7-4.** Estimated saving in lives during 1970 as a result of public health measures taken against certain diseases, United States*

| Causes of death | Death rates† | | Deaths | | Lives saved |
|---|---|---|---|---|---|
| | 1900 | 1970 | Theoretic | Observed | |
| All causes | 1,719.1 | 940.4 | 3,493,000 | 1,921,000 | 1,572,000 |
| Infant mortality | 99.9‡ | 19.8 | 371,800 | 73,700 | 198,100 |
| Maternal mortality | 61.0‡ | 2.5 | 22,680 | 920 | 21,760 |
| Typhoid and paratyphoid | 31.3 | 0.0 | 63,500 | 0 | 63,500 |
| Dysentery | 12.0 | 0.1 | 24,500 | 180 | 24,320 |
| Diarrhea and enteritis | 139.9 | 1.1 | 285,000 | 2,200 | 282,800 |
| Smallpox | 0.3 | 0.0 | 610 | 0 | 610 |
| Measles | 13.3 | 0.0 | 27,100 | 120 | 26,080 |
| Diphtheria | 40.3 | 0.0 | 82,000 | 0 | 82,000 |
| Pertussis | 12.2 | 0.0 | 24,800 | 20 | 24,780 |
| Scarlet fever and streptococcal sore throat | 9.6 | 0.0 | 19,600 | 30 | 19,570 |
| Erysipelas | 5.4 | 0.0 | 11,000 | 0 | 11,000 |
| Tuberculosis | 194.4 | 2.7 | 394,000 | 5,560 | 388,440 |
| Syphilis and its sequelae | 17.7‡ | 0.2 | 36,000 | 470 | 35,530 |
| Malaria | 6.2 | 0.0 | 12,600 | 0 | 12,600 |

*Population 1970 = 203,200,000.
†Per 100,000 population, except infant and maternal mortality, which is per 10,000 live births.
‡1915 rates.

well as lost workdays and schooldays, within only a few years a tremendous monetary savings was achieved.

As an example of what needs to be achieved, one notes an analysis[18] of direct and indirect cost implications of the large amount of preventable disease among Indians and Alaskan natives as compared with the general population of the United States. In summary, Indians and Alaskan natives lose 31,470 man years caused by mortality per 100,000 population compared with 14,770 for the United States population as a whole. By whatever measure this preventable difference is of considerable socioeconomic significance.

## POTENTIAL SAVINGS BY PUBLIC HEALTH EXPENDITURES

In a sense, the previous discussion is an accounting of past successes. Consider in addition the potential savings in lives and money that could be made at the present time and in the future if all existing knowledge were completely used. When this reasoning is applied to the total current picture of sickness and death in the United States, the results arrived at are staggering. In 1947 Slee,[19] studying public health problems of the aging population, made a most interesting analysis along these lines. He considered the problem of the thousands of deaths that occur every year in the United States that could be prevented if existing medical and scientific knowledge were effectively used. For each cause of death he estimated the potential percentage of reduction attainable at that time, indicating for each the major factors that would contribute to the reduction (Table 7-6). His figures have been modified to bring them up to date. Each of the theoretic

percentage reductions was then applied to the number of deaths that were attributed during 1970 to each particular cause of death (Table 7-7). The difference between the resulting figures and the number of deaths that actually occurred indicates a total potential saving at the present time of over 600,000 lives per year. This saving, if it had been effected, would have reduced the crude death rate in the United States in 1970 by 31%, from 9.4 to 6.5 per 1,000 population. That this is not a fantastic concept is given testimony by the fact that some American communities and several nations have actually reduced their rates close to that level. If the lives that could theoretically be saved are distributed appropriately by age groups, it is seen that benefits are possible at every point in the life-span. The greatest savings, however, would occur in the adolescent and young adult age groups, in which death involves the greatest possible economic loss. If this analysis were to be pursued further by applying estimated monetary values to each of the 600,000 deaths potentially preventable, the magnitude of the economic loss entailed would indeed appear to be stupendous. Thus if again each life saved was considered to represent an average ultimate net value (lifetime productivity minus capital and maintenance costs) of only $20,000, the total value the nation could save annually would be more than $120 billion.

It is common to complain of high taxes and governmental costs. On the other hand, the average individual does tend to be practical. When it is demonstrated to him that fundamentally the public health program is a matter of common sense and true economy, he will tend to contribute his share of the necessary financial support. Fortunately throughout the

*Text continued on p. 128.*

**Table 7-5.** Summary statement of savings due to immunization against measles

| Type of savings | 1963-1965 | 1966-1968 | Total |
|---|---|---|---|
| Health and resource | | | |
| Cases averted | 1,140,000 | 8,590,000 | 9,730,000 |
| Lives saved | 114 | 859 | 973 |
| Cases of retardation averted | 380 | 2,864 | 3,244 |
| Hospital days saved | 65,000 | 490,000 | 555,000 |
| Workdays saved | 189,000 | 1,435,000 | 1,624,000 |
| Schooldays saved | 3,775,000 | 28,450,000 | 32,225,000 |
| Economic | | | |
| Economic benefits | $63,192,000 | $468,351,000 | $531,543,000 |
| Cost of immunizing persons | 43,500,000 | 64,800,000 | 108,300,000 |
| Net economic savings | 19,692,000 | 403,551,000 | 423,243,000 |

**Table 7-6.** Postulated percentage reductions in deaths, by cause, if all available knowledge were used*

| Cause of death | Reduction (%) | Suggested action |
|---|---|---|
| Typhoid and paratyphoid | 100 | Environmental measures<br>Immunization<br>Epidemiologic control |
| Meningococcal infections | 100 | Control of epidemics<br>Adequate and early chemotherapy<br>Antibiotics |
| Streptococcal infections | 100 | Chemotherapy<br>Antibiotics<br>Antitoxin |
| Pertussis | 100 | Early and thorough immunization<br>Hyperimmune serum, chemotherapy, and antibiotics for secondary infections |
| Diphtheria | 100 | Early immunization and adequate antitoxin |
| Tuberculosis—all forms | 100 | Intensive early case finding<br>Hospitalization and treatment<br>Adequate diet and housing |
| Dysenteries | 100 | Environmental control<br>Chemotherapy |
| Malaria | 100 | Environmental control<br>Chemotherapy |
| Syphilis | 100 | Intensive early case finding<br>Treatment<br>Epidemiologic control |
| Measles | 100 | Immunization<br>Chemotherapy<br>Antibiotics |
| Poliomyelitis | 100 | Immunization |
| Neoplasms | 50 | Early cancer detection and treatment centers<br>Best possible physician and surgeon<br>Chemotherapy<br>Radiation therapy<br>Surgery<br>Circumcision<br>Elimination of smoking |

*Where chemotherapy and/or antibiotics have been listed as the explanations for the reductions in deaths, objection on the basis of the development of drug-resistant organisms will no doubt be raised. Gains possible today might be much less in a few years. It is believed that research will be able to remain one or two drugs, at least, ahead of the organisms.

With the one exception (all other causes), no variation of effectiveness of therapy and other control measures with age of the individual has been postulated. Since any scheme of correction would probably have been as liable to criticism as no correction, the latter course was followed.

**Table 7-6.** Postulated percentage reductions in deaths, by cause, if all available knowledge were used—cont'd

| Cause of death | Reduction (%) | Suggested action |
|---|---|---|
| Rheumatic fever | 95 | Best possible physician |
| | | Prophylactic antibiotics |
| Diabetes mellitus | 60 | Best possible physician |
| | | Intensive early case finding |
| | | Diet |
| | | Insulin |
| | | Applied genetics |
| Diseases of thyroid gland | 100 | Best possible physician |
| | | Newer drugs |
| | | Surgery |
| | | Iodization of all salt |
| Nutritional diseases | 100 | Adequate diet |
| | | Diagnosis and treatment |
| Alcoholism and addictions | 25 | Psychiatry |
| | | Nutritional therapy |
| | | Sociology |
| | | Education |
| Intracranial vascular lesions | 10 | Best possible physician |
| | | Antihypertensive drugs and diet |
| | | Anticoagulants |
| | | Avoidance of infections |
| | | Antibiotics |
| Diseases of the heart | 10 | Best possible physician |
| | | Surgery |
| Pneumonia, broncho- | 75 | Chemotherapy |
| | | Antibiotics |
| Pneumonia, lobar | 90 | Chemotherapy |
| | | Antibiotics |
| Pneumonia, unspecified | 75 | Chemotherapy |
| | | Antibiotics |
| Influenza | 85 | Immunization |
| | | Chemotherapy and antibiotics for complications |
| Peptic ulcer—stomach and duodenum | 50 | Psychiatry |
| | | Best possible physician |
| Diarrhea, enteritis, etc. | 95 | Environmental controls |
| | | Chemotherapy |
| | | Antibiotics |

*Continued.*

**Table 7-6.** Postulated percentage reductions in deaths, by cause, if all available knowledge were used—cont'd

| Cause of death | Reduction (%) | Suggested action |
|---|---|---|
| Appendicitis | 100 | Surgery<br>Chemotherapy<br>Antibiotics |
| Hernia, intestinal obstruction | 95 | Best possible physician and surgeon |
| Cirrhosis of the liver | 25 | Newer nutritional knowledge |
| Biliary calculi | 25 | Best possible physician and surgeon |
| Nephritis and nephrosis | 25 | Chemotherapy<br>Antibiotics<br>Best possible physician |
| Diseases of the prostate | 50 | Best possible physician and surgeon |
| Complications of pregnancy | 87 | Complete elimination of deaths from toxemia and sepsis, and reduction of deaths from hemorrhage by 50% |
| Congenital malformations | 10 | Diet during pregnancy<br>Avoidance of viral infections during pregnancy<br>Surgery (as in recent heart and blood vessel operations) |
| Premature births | 70 | Adequate prenatal care and diet |
| Suicide | 50 | Psychiatry<br>Sociology |
| Homicide | 50 | Psychiatry<br>Sociology |
| Accidents—motor vehicle | 50 | Education<br>Psychiatry<br>Engineering<br>Traffic planning and control<br>Safety measures |
| Accidents—other | 50 | Education<br>Psychiatry<br>Safety measures<br>Engineering |
| All other causes | 50 | Better medical care (except for under 1 year, where deaths from congenital debility, birth injury, and others peculiar to the first year of life could be reduced by 75%), adequate prenatal care and diet, and adequate care during first year of life |

**Table 7-7.** Theoretic savings of lives, United States, 1970, had all available knowledge been effectively applied

| Cause of death | Total deaths 1970 | Theoretic reduction (%) | Theoretic deaths | Theoretic saving |
|---|---|---|---|---|
| Meningococcal infections | 520 | 100 | | 520 |
| Septicemia | 3,140 | 80 | 630 | 2,510 |
| Infectious hepatitis | 1,050 | 100 | | 1,050 |
| Tuberculosis—all forms | 5,560 | 100 | | 5,560 |
| Dysenteries | 180 | 100 | | 180 |
| Syphilis | 470 | 100 | | 470 |
| Measles | 120 | 100 | | 120 |
| Other infective and parasitic diseases | 3,020 | 80 | 600 | 2,420 |
| Neoplasms | 330,840 | 50 | 165,420 | 165,420 |
| Diabetes mellitus | 37,820 | 60 | 15,130 | 22,690 |
| Avitaminoses | 2,740 | 100 | | 2,740 |
| Cerebrovascular diseases | 207,800 | 10 | 187,020 | 20,780 |
| Diseases of the heart | 736,060 | 10 | 662,450 | 73,610 |
| Hypertension | 7,650 | 70 | 2,300 | 5,350 |
| Pneumonia | 58,450 | 90 | 5,850 | 52,600 |
| Bronchitis, emphysema, asthma | 31,450 | 25 | 23,590 | 7,860 |
| Peptic ulcer—stomach and duodenum | 8,450 | 50 | 4,225 | 4,225 |
| Diarrhea, enteritis, etc. | 2,200 | 95 | 110 | 2,090 |
| Appendicitis | 1,380 | 100 | | 1,380 |
| Hernia, intestinal obstruction | 7,390 | 95 | 370 | 7,020 |
| Cirrhosis of the liver | 32,260 | 25 | 24,200 | 8,060 |
| Biliary calculi, etc. | 4,550 | 25 | 3,410 | 1,140 |
| Nephritis and nephrosis | 7,880 | 25 | 5,910 | 1,970 |
| Diseases of the prostate | 2,080 | 50 | 1,040 | 1,040 |
| Deliveries and complications of pregnancy | 920 | 90 | 90 | 830 |
| Congenital malformations | 16,540 | 10 | 14,890 | 1,650 |
| Premature births | 19,580 | 70 | 5,880 | 13,700 |
| Suicide | 22,630 | 50 | 11,315 | 11,315 |
| Homicide | 15,610 | 50 | 7,805 | 7,805 |
| Accidents—motor vehicle | 53,430 | 50 | 26,715 | 26,715 |
| Accidents—other | 57,290 | 50 | 28,645 | 28,645 |
| All other causes | 241,960 | 50 | 120,980 | 120,980 |
| Totals | 1,921,000 | 31 | 1,318,375 | 602,625 |
| Population 1970 | 203,200,000 | | 203,200,000 | |
| Death rate (per 1,000 population) | 9.4 | | 6.5 | |
| Percentage reduction of death rate (actual to theoretic) | | | 31% | |

world it is increasingly realized that parsimony in public health matters is penny-wise and pound-foolish.

## REFERENCES

1. Fuchs, V. R.: The contribution of health services to the American economy, Milbank Mem. Fund Quart. **44:**65, Oct. 1966.
2. O'Connor, R. B.: Benefits vs. risks in public health, J. Occup. Med. **13:**47, Jan. 1971.
3. Hanlon, J. J.: Can accounting sell health? In Economic benefits from public health services, Public Health Service pub. no. 1178, Washington, D. C., 1964, Government Printing Office.
4. Linnenberg, C. C.: How shall we measure economic benefits from public health services? In Economic benefits from public health services, Public Health Service pub. no. 1178, Washington, D. C., 1964, Government Printing Office.
5. Petty, Sir W.: Political arithmetic or a discourse concerning the extent and value of lands, people, buildings, etc., ed. 3, London, 1699, Robert Clavel.
6. Dublin, L. I., and Lotka, A. J.: Length of life: a study of the life table, New York, 1936, The Ronald Press Co.
7. Dublin, L. I., Lotka, A. J., and Spiegelman, M.: The money value of a man, ed. 2, New York, 1946, The Ronald Press Co.
8. Weisbrod, B. A.: Economics of public health, Philadelphia, 1961, University of Pennsylvania Press.
9. Your money's worth: $100,000 to rear a child, Washington Star-News Aug. 14, 1972.
10. Rice, D. P., and Cooper, B. S.: The economic value of human life, Amer. J. Public Health **57:**1954, Nov. 1967.
11. Bolduan, C. F., and Bolduan, N. W.: Public health and hygiene: a student's manual, ed. 3, Philadelphia, 1941, W. B. Saunders Co.
12. Horwitz, A.: Health—a basic component of economic development, misc. pub. no. 66, Washington, D. C., 1961, Pan American Health Organization.
13. Fein, R.: Health programs and economic development. In the economics of health and medical care, Ann Arbor, 1964, University of Michigan Press.
14. Perlman, M.: Some economic aspects of public health programs in underdeveloped areas. In the economics of health and medical care, Ann Arbor, 1964, University of Michigan Press.
15. Ruderman, A. P.: The epidemiologist's place in planning for economic development, Public Health Rep. **81:**615, July 1966.
16. Zukin, P.: Planning a health component for an economic development program, Amer. J. Public Health **61:**1751, Sept. 1971.
17. Axnick, N. W., Shavell, S. M., and Witte, J. J.: Benefits due to immunization against measles, Public Health Rep. **84:**673, Aug. 1969.
18. Reinhard, K. R., Felsman, F. W., and Moody, L. F.: Time loss and indirect economic costs caused by disease among Indians and Alaskan natives, Public Health Rep. **85:**397, May 1970.
19. Slee, V. N.: Public health and old people (unpublished study), School of Public Health, University of Michigan, June 1947.

# PART THREE

# The basis for public health

Public health work, by definition, is carried on mainly under governmental auspices. Despite this, as Kaufman,[1] a political scientist, says in an article that should be studied by all in the health field, ". . . experts whose careers will unfold in the public arena . . . pay little attention to politics in the training of their successors and in the conduct of their own research. Politics is treated as an intrusion to be ignored at best, condemned at worst." He indicates three reasons why such an attitude is wrong. First, specialists such as those in public health all believe that everyone should know more about their field of interest, yet they keep their expertise among themselves. Second, neglect or denunciation of politics threatens the democratic process. "If every apprentice is trained to suspect and despise politics and to dedicate himself to remove his occupation from the political arena, an ever-increasing and more influential segment of the population may acquire a disrespect for the processes which are the core of a democratic policy. Moreover, if every specialty seeking exemption were in fact removed from the arena of partisan contention, the decision-making machinery of the society, deprived of an ultimate adjudicating authority mediating among the specialists, might grind to a stop." Third, politics provides an essential sociological input. As Kaufman strongly emphasizes:

> . . . the neglect of political factors in the study of public health problems and programs omits a critical element in understanding, planning and executing public health services. For whether they like it or not, the practitioners of the public health disciplines are deeply immersed in a political environment. The ones who succeed are the ones who learn to understand it, adjust to it and turn it to their advantage. But few of them, in their formal training or in their professional research literature, receive any assistance in this vital aspect of their work.

The same is even more true of law. Usually the extent of exposure to the legislative process, even of those who reach other professions, is limited to a secondary school or college course in civics, which may include a few paragraphs about how laws are made. The following two chapters on government and on law, with emphasis on their relationship to public health, are presented with the intent to remedy partially these earlier educational gaps.

**REFERENCE**

1. Kaufman, H.: The political ingredient of public health services, a neglected area of research, Milbank Mem. Fund Quart. **44:**13, Oct. 1966.

*Government is a contrivance of human
wisdom to provide for human wants.*

EDMUND BURKE

CHAPTER 8

# Government and public health

## FUNCTIONS OF GOVERNMENT

The particular political system that exists
determines the role of government in relation
to health. Public health programs are financed
and the broad organizational patterns for implementation of these programs are outlined
according to basic policy decisions. In general
a governmental system in a democratic society
performs two distinct functions. The first function is political. The governmental system must
provide a forum for debate on issues that exist
or arise and an appropriate instrument for their
solution. It must provide a structure of laws
and organization that will make possible the
achievement of the aspirations and goals of the
particular society. It must also provide leadership and citizenship if self-government is to
continue to exist. The definition of the role
of government in relation to health is therefore
an important part of the political function of
government. The second general function is the
provision of service and regulatory activities.
Services necessary to a complex society that
cannot be provided by individuals or private
enterprise must be provided by government.
Rules and regulations concerning individual
behavior in relation to personal, group, and
environmental hygiene must be formulated and
enforced by government.[1]

Individuals involved in public health work are
knowledgeable about the service function of
government because this is their field of expertise. Often, however, they have had little
opportunity in their formal education or experience to obtain a first-hand understanding

of the political function of government. Because
the political and service functions of government cannot be separated, it is imperative that
those who work in public health administration
possess an understanding of the political function of government and its relationship to the
service function. This is the major theme of
this chapter.

## POLITICAL SYSTEM

Political science, until recent years, was for
most a description of formal organizational
structures such as legislatures or political parties along with normative political theory. In
recent years political scientists have concep-
tualized politics as a system. Easton[2] defines
the political system as "constituted by the multiplicity of social interactions involved in the
policy making process oriented toward the authoritative allocation of values for society."
Political scientists therefore have attempted to
describe the system in terms of interactions
and goals. Political activity is viewed as the
interaction among governmental institutions
and groups. Governmental institutions are the
vehicles through which the political process
operates and therefore constitute one of the
variables that must be studied to gain an
understanding of the political process. The basic
outline of governmental structure in the United
States is contained in the Constitution. It is
a federal system that is defined as "one where
the governmental powers are divided by terms
of a written constitution between a general
government and the governments of territorial

subdivisions, each government supreme within a sphere marked out in the Constitution."[3]

In this country the states are territorial units that have a traditional fear of the powers of the national or central unit of government. This may be understood in the light of historic background. Some states actually existed as distinct entities. For example, the present state of Vermont was an independent nation between 1777 and 1791. The eastern part of the present state of Tennessee was a separate country, Franklin, between 1784 and 1789. Texas was an independent republic from 1836 to 1845 with its own government, which exchanged diplomats with the government of the United States. Hawaii, prior to becoming a territory of the United States in 1900 and subsequently a state in 1959, also once existed as an independent nation.

It is often overlooked that not until the American Revolution was almost won did the original 13 colonies begin to think seriously about union. During the formative period, numerous influential people insisted that each colony should be a distinct and separate nation similar to the situation on the European continent. In fact, several colonies had plans for importing members of European royal families to form the nucleus of American royal ruling classes. The Continental Congress ultimately solved the problem by settling on the idea of a union of states. The decision, incidentally, was made by a narrow margin of votes.

### The politically dominant state

In so joining themselves into a union the colonies, which were now called states, by no means surrendered their individual rights and prerogatives of which they were already intensely jealous and proud. Instead they took the attitude that most governmental problems would continue to be met and solved best on a separate and independent basis, with only a relatively few matters of common interest and concern requiring reference to the joint overall federal government established by their union.

They recognized, for example, that "in union there is strength," that they had common interests in matters of defense against aggression, and that therefore a single national army and navy should be established, consisting of men from all the states. Each state, however, organized and still maintains its own militia. The expediency of a single agency to deal with matters of international diplomany

was similarly realized, and a federal Department of State was established. To finance these activities of common concern a national treasury and taxing system were instituted. Subsequently, as additional common problems developed or were recognized, other appropriate federal agencies were established.

From the beginning the states were explicit with regard to functions and authorities delegated to the federal government, specifying them, fortunately, in relatively broad terms in the federal Constitution and subsequent amendments. All other activities and powers not so specified were retained by the states. This influenced the development of public health in America to a considerable degree, since no specific mention is made of public health in the Constitution or its amendments. Accordingly, until relatively recently, the federal government has had no explicit authority to establish a federal health department. Furthermore, it was in no way mandatory that the individual states establish state public health agencies unless they wished of their own accord to do so. However, a time was reached when each state recognized the need to do so.

Theoretically the states are fundamental units of government from which the federal and local governments derive. Article X of the Constitution of the United States provides that "The powers not delegated to the United States by the Constitution, nor prohibited by it to the States, are reserved to the States respectively, or to the people." One of the residual powers retained by the states is what is commonly called the police power. The police power may be defined in general terms as the power to protect and promote the health, safety, and welfare of the state and its people.[3] This concept is discussed in some detail in Chapter 9, which deals with law.

## CHANGING CONCEPTS OF FEDERALISM

Operationally, federalism has not remained static. The interpretation of the respective responsibilities of state and national government under the Constitution has changed considerably throughout United States history. Many people today tend to regard the federal government as the ultimate source of power and money. Whereas they do so with increasing justification, this was by no menas always the case. The original concept of state supremacy has been briefly discussed. Suffice to say that in spite of recent trends, the principle is not yet dead, and it is doubtful that its complete demise is inevitable. For a considerable period of United States history the federal government was a somewhat distant or mythical creature to the average citizen. This early relationship has been vividly described by Brogan[4] in the following way:

It should be remembered that is was quite easy for the settler in the Middle West to have no dealings at all with the government of the United States. He paid no direct taxes; he very often wrote no letters and received none, for the good reason that he and his friends could not write. Yet the only ubiquitous federal officials and federal service were the Postmasters and the Post Office. There were no soldiers except in the Indian country; there were federal courts doing comparatively little business. True, the new union had built the National Road, down which creaked the Conestoga wagons with their cargo of immigrants' chattels. It fought the Indians from time to time and it had at its disposal vast areas of public lands to be sold on easy terms and finally given away to settlers. But no government that had any claim to be a government at all has had less direct power over the people it ruled. Politics was bound, in these conditions, to be rhetorical, moralizing, emotionally diverting, either a form of sport or a form of religion. The political barbecue, the joint debates between great political leaders were secular equivalents of the camp meeting and the hell-fire sermon.

Even the inhabitants of the older seaboard states shared this relationship. As Brogan continues:

Few things, on consideration, prove less surprising than the evaporation of federal authority over the South once secession was adopted. Almost the only federal institution that meant anything to the common man was the Post Office—and by a statesman-like turning of the blind eye, the new Southern Confederacy continued to allow the federal government to deliver the mail even after the seceding states had formally broken with the Union.

As time passed, with increasing urbanization, mechanization, travel, industrialization, and interstate and international problems, the national government came more and more into focus in the citizens' eyes. It appears that at the same time there began to develop a blurring of the image of local and particularly of state government. Much of this had to do with increased needs and demands in relation to sources of revenue. There was a period when local governments were in a real sense self-sufficient, but gradually, as the demands made on them increased, they looked more frequently to the state governments for assistance. Up to a point these local appeals were within the financial ability of the states, but gradually they too became inadequate to meet many of the newer, more complex, and more expensive problems. White[5] discusses this accordingly:

The states as instruments of progress are definitely losing ground. Their leadership, with rare exceptions, is mediocre; their administrative organization, again with occasional exception, is inadequate. . . . It seems possible indeed that the future structure of the American administrative system will rest primarily on the national government and the cities, at least so far as the urban population (now approaching 60 per cent) is concerned.

White points out that as early as 1918, Charles E. Merriman made the following suggestion:

Those interested in preserving the balance of powers between the national and local governments might find the urban community a more effective counter weight . . . than the feebly struggling states. . . . A city would not be obliged to climb far to go beyond a state. Already there are seventeen cities of a population over 500,000; nine states with less population than that, and if economic resources and cultural prestige are added to numbers, the contrast is more striking.

In this regard there are (in 1973) 27 cities with populations greater than 500,000, and a significant number of them contain and serve more people than do many of the states.

Originally the powers of the federal government were limited strictly to affairs of interstate and international concern. So intense was the desire to restrict the scope of these powers that they were referred to explicitly in the Constitution and its subsequent amendments. Innumerable aspects of United States social, scientific, industrial, and political development have led in a direction that makes an increasing degree of centralization necessary if not also desirable for survival. To allow for this change and to still maintain the basic principles of this form of government presents a difficult problem indeed.

To accomplish both purposes federal agencies in recent years, with the tacit assent of the states, have increasingly resorted to indirect but constitutionally permissible techniques that have resulted in increased centralization of power in state governments themselves and more significantly in federal agencies. This movement received great acceleration during the 1930s, when the widespread economic depression dealt a devastating blow to local and, to a considerable extent, state finances, rendering them incapable of meeting the demands placed on them. A procession of local governments, having fruitlessly appealed to their state capitals for assistance, turned to Washington as the only source of relief. In light of the underlying social and economic causes these trends toward centralization are certain to continue and increase.

There are many methods short of total assumption of power and function that may be resorted to in order to achieve a practical measure of centralization. Perhaps the simplest is the offering of advice and information by a federal agency to the states or by the states to the local governments. This is so common in the field of public health as to have become one of the prime activities of state and federal health agencies. It takes only a short step to move from the transmission of printed advice and information to occasional visits of state and federal consultants, followed by the loaning of personnel to serve as resident consultants. This occurs especially in the face of local shortages in personnel. Increasingly, officers of federal agencies originally intended as consultants are assigned on a semipermanent basis to serve as directors of divisions of a state health department. Field technical units, developed by state health departments for the purpose of assisting the local units, in many instances assume the position of supervising and even determining the programs of local health departments. Thus activities designed for the purpose of rendering advice and information develop into programs of cooperative or outright centralized administration. A variation is a program of inspection and advice, often without authority, to bring about compliance with recommendations made. The inspecting and advising officials, for example, may merely report their findings to the central authorities, who may then promote additional legislation that often gives them increased supervisory powers. This has occurred, for example, in matters of hospital construction and inspection of sanitary installations.

On the surface the requirement of periodic fiscal and service reports may appear innocuous, and it is certainly justifiable to obtain and share information concerning the general welfare. However, even this may have an indirect centralizing influence of considerable impact. Theoretically a state or local health department has the right to organize its records and reports any way it sees fit to serve its purposes. However, after the right to require certain reports is obtained the next step is to standardize them. Beyond this in more than one instance the requiring of a certain type of report has resulted in an actual change in the local program itself, the local personnel following the path of least resistance, especially if financial grants are involved. This has occurred in varying degrees as a result of requirements for birth and death records, reports of communicable disease, and the standardized fiscal reports of health departments to federal health agencies. An acclerating technique that may be employed is to give the local official a nominal appointment as the local representative of state or federal agency. Thus many local health officers have appointments as collaborating epidemiologists of the Public Health Service.

In some areas local activities are subject to direct supervision and review by the higher government. For example, local assessments often must be reviewed and approved by a state board of equalization or by state tax commissioners. Prior permission may be required and is especially effective when the higher level of government participates in financing. It is rapidly becoming accepted practice to require that plans for city, county, and state hospitals be approved by state and national health and comprehensive planning agencies before allowing contracts to be consummated.

Of a similar nature are approval requirements for the appointment and removal of local officers. Whereas in most states it is theoretically the prerogative of local governments to select their own health officer, in practice this is often not followed for various reasons discussed elsewhere. Not only is approval by the state health officer usually required but often selection is limited to lists prepared by the state health department. In some states local health officers are appointed and removed directly by the state board of health. In one state, employees of health districts are appointed from state civil service lists and, if no eligible individuals are available, from the register of local commissions. The requirement of prior permission is sometimes rendered unnecessary by the determination of standards by a state or federal agency.

The extent to which the average county health officer is affected by these influences may be pictured somewhat as follows: In the first instance he may be recruited by and trained under the auspices of the state health department, using federal funds. His appointment, if not made directly by the state health officer, will probably require his approval. Monthly reports of his activities and those of his staff will have to be made to the state health department on standard forms and a record of all work kept in a form book prescribed by the latter agency. By virtue of his probable designation as registrar he will have to report births and deaths to the state health department on forms, this time prescribed by the National Center for Health Statistics. Since in most instances he is appointed a collaborating epidemiologist, it becomes necessary to send weekly reports of instances of communicable diseases to the Center for Disease Control of the Public Health Service as well as to the state health department. His maternal and child health program may necessitate operation, inspection, and approval of clinics and hospitalization facilities, using standards developed and required by the federal maternal and child health program, which will also ask for reports on standard forms. Arrangement for the use of x-ray equipment and for hospitalization of persons with tuberculosis will in most instances be made by him with the state agency. Finally, he will probably find it convenient if not necessary to obtain education materials, biologics, and even office forms and supplies through the state health department.

Although all this may appear on the surface to result in an effective emasculation of the position of the local health officer, to be fair and practical it should be pointed out that all of these various relationships actually represent effective resources to which he may turn for assistance to develop and conduct a much more effective and satisfying program than he otherwise could. When one considers the limited resources on a local level, one might with justification answer those who declaim any concurrent limitation of local autonomy with the saw, "You can't have your cake and eat it too."

Details of contracts and design of hospitals and health centers have been specified as conditions for approval of plans by state and federal agencies to obtain federal funds. More and more types of licenses are being placed within the jurisdiction of state health departments and through them the federal health and environmental agencies. The Emergency Mater-

nity and Infant Care Program administered by the Children's Bureau through the state health departments during World War II and the many programs authorized by legislation such as the Social Security Amendments of 1965 and 1972 (Medicare, Medicaid, Comprehensive Child Health Services, etc.) provide many examples of the centralizing influence of the right to determine standards. The central agency may be vested with the right to issue general regulations that are binding on the locality or orders that result in a single centralized authority. Both measures are widely resorted to in public health work. Here the initiative passes from the local to the central agency. Although common within states, this type of control is rare in federal-state relationships. The financial aspects of the grant-in-aid program will be discussed later in this chapter.

The federal government cannot dictate to the states the manner in which they should organize their governmental structure, establish their policies, or conduct their programs. However, actual dictation of these matters is not necessary for federal agencies to play a part in the improvement and expansion of public health and other services throughout the nation. The significance of holding the purse strings is well understood by all. "He who pays the piper calls the tune." Among many examples of federal influence on state government organizational structure are the rapid formation of state maternal and child health divisions after the passage of the Sheppard-Towner Act and, more recently, the establishment of separate environmental protection agencies by many states and even some municipalities soon after such an agency was formed on the federal level.

Sums of money transferred may be granted either conditionally or unconditionally; federal grants are usually of the former type, state grants more often of the latter type. Because of this, federal grants are more likely to act as catalyzers than are state grants. In the ideal situation the local taxpayers would constantly exert whatever control might be necessary for the ensurance of the proper use of funds, and it would be unnecessary to attach conditions to grants. When revenue is raised locally, this is more likely to occur than when funds come unfettered from without. By inserting limitations in the form of conditions to grants, therefore, the higher unit of government is in effect substituting for the controls that should ordinarily be exercised by the citizens themselves. There is danger, however, that conditions and standards may become too detailed or rigid to suit the diverse situations existing in a complex nation such as this. As Maxwell[6] pointed out:

Regional heterogeneity is of the essence of federalism, and . . . would seem to indicate that federal grants should be conditioned and closely policed. In practical fact, however, this would be an impairment of state sovereignty. Moreover, any detailed and uniform set of conditions would be unsuited to the diversity of regional and state needs. In a federalism, variation in standards of many governmental functions is common, and therefore the federal government is likely to get into difficulties if it attempts to prescribe common standards in grant programs . . . to surround federal grants with numerous conditions is to assume a homogeneity in state governmental needs which does not exist; to prescribe uniformity where there are deepseated reasons for diversity is an error. Here, then, is a dilemma of federalism.

Usually conditional federal grants-in-aid require adherence to certain steps. First, the state must formally accept the terms of the grant, sometimes by means of legislation. Preparation for use of the grant must next be made by preparing and submitting specific plans and by establishing whatever organizations or agencies are indicated for their fulfillment. Plans are approved centrally by a national administrative agency. Usually, but not always, federal grants must be matched by the state or local government. The program or project itself is carried out by state or local agencies but is subject to central as well as local inspection and audit. Often payment is made to the state only on satisfactory completion of the project or an agreed-upon part of it. Sometimes partial payment is made in advance.

Several means of central influence and control are evident from the steps just outlined. The federal agency may refuse to approve plans or to assist financially in a state program because of unsatisfactory state organization or procedure. Payments may be witheld if conditions of agreement are not observed. Furthermore, the state has little or no recourse beyond the federal agency administering the grant. The application of central influences such as these has occurred frequently in the field of public health. To benefit from grants-in-aid administered by the Public Health Service and some other federal agencies, the states have found it necessary to establish or remodel their

personnel standards and merit systems to the satisfaction of these federal agencies. Record systems, auditing procedures, clinic and hospital construction and maintenance standards, and many other factors have been similarly affected.

The tendency toward centralization has been most evident in the fields of highway construction, education, and social security. It is interesting to study the similarities in the patterns followed in these three areas of public administration. Of particular interest to those engaged in public health work may be a comparison of the history of federal interest in public roads and in maternal and child welfare. The national government first became concerned with highways in 1893, when it established the Office of Road Inquiry, later the Bureau of Public Roads. The original bill establishing this agency included the following statement: ". . . it is not the province of this department to seek to control or influence said action [in building highways] except in so far as advice and wise suggestions shall contribute toward it. . . . The department is to furnish information, not to direct and formulate any system of organization, however efficient or desirable it may be." From the date of its establishment until 1912 the Bureau of Public Roads restricted itself to experimentation, advice to state and local highway officials, dissemination of information, and construction of demonstration roads.

In 1912 an act was passed authorizing construction of post roads, followed in 1916 by a more potent Federal Highway Act that set up a system of grants to the states to assist them in meeting the increased demand for good roads and the increased cost of building better types of roads. Where originally the local county governments had the chief responsibility for the construction and maintenance of highways, this major responsibility and its accompanying authority passed first to the state and then to the federal government. States now receive a large part of their highway funds through federal grants-in-aid, and the Bureau of Public Roads of the Department of Transportation establishes the standards, approves plans, audits the accounts, and inspects the completed work. The effectiveness of these indirect forms of control is indicated by the fact that in 1916, when the Federal Highway Act was passed, 15 states had no highway departments. By the following year every state had a recognized highway department acceptable to the Bureau of Public Roads.

Compare with this the act of 1912 that established the Children's Bureau, directing it to investigate and report "... upon all matters pertaining to the welfare of children and child life, among all classes of people ..." It was designated as a clearinghouse for information on child health and was authorized to carry on research and also field studies. During the first 7 years of its existence, the Children's Bureau adhered strictly to these specified functions. In 1921 with the passage of the Sheppard-Towner Act, the bureau was authorized to participate in the promotion of maternity and infancy programs throughout the nation by means of federal grants to the states. Here the bureau received its first major administrative responsibilities. As in the case of highways, some states anticipated the passage of the Maternity and Infancy Bill and created maternal and child health bureaus or divisions to administer the funds they would obtain if and when the bill became law. Accordingly, by the beginning of 1921, 33 such state agencies had been established, and during the following 2 years 14 more were created. By 1929 maternal and child hygiene bureaus or divisions had been formed and were functioning in the territory of Hawaii and in all the states except Vermont, where the work was carried on under the immediate supervision of the state health officer.[7] In administering the act, the Children's Bureau, as had the Bureau of Public Roads, set standards, approved projects, inspected work within states, and audited accounts. Although the functions involved in the Sheppard-Towner Act came to a halt in 1929, they were essentially reestablished in an expanded degree by the provision of Title V of the Social Security Act of 1935 and by subsequent legislation.

Further comparison is possible by considering the passage in 1942 of the Emergency Maternity and Infant Care Program for wives and children of men in the Armed Forces. This program, administered by the Children's Bureau through the state health agencies, made possible and paid for personal medical care of patients. Although that program was temporary, the principles under discussion were subsequently applied to other program responsibilities of the Children's Bureau.

Concerning roads, White[5] made the following statement:

Related expenditures on highways were thrown out of balance in 1933 and the latter years of the depression as a result of the huge emergency expenditures for public works and the resulting grants and loans to the states. From the fiscal point of view the national government has emerged in the crisis as the senior partner in the firm.

Perhaps this statement was prophetic with regard to the ultimate effect of the grant-in-aid programs on the functional relationship between the local, state, and federal governments. A large part of the considerable opposition to the maternity and infancy program, some of the other grant-in-aid programs, and the various medical care bills has been on this basis.

The foregoing may make those who plan and administer grants-in-aid appear as power-thirsty annelids increasingly draining off the lifeblood of local self-initiative and independence. This view was expressed by Mustard.[8]

Directly, through broad interpretations of the Federal Constitution, and by new laws, or indirectly through grants-in-aid, parity payments, benefits, and rewards, the Federal Government is assuming prerogatives and accepting obligations, particularly in the field of social security, that a quarter-century ago were regarded as lying exclusively within the jurisdiction of the states. Pertinent in this connection is the fact that public health activities are more and more being considered as an integral part of the developing social security program and are receiving increasing federal attention. Thus the Federal Government is at present a potent influence in public health. Perhaps it is more virile than any other area of government for ... many state governments are static in the field, and leadership has focused in the United States Public Health Service. The policy of federal grants-in-aid for state and local health work is becoming increasingly popular, and apparently will be continued in spite of what the opponents of this principle believe it implies sociologically and in terms of state and local autonomy.

However, in fairness to the administering agencies, two considerations should be pointed out. First, it is doubtful that the promotion of bills to provide subsidies for highways, education, and public health programs represented at any stage determined premeditated attempts to transfer power to a central agency. When all aspects of the questions involved are reviewed, it would appear that the acts were passed and the programs developed to meet public demands and needs that could not possibly be fulfilled by the state government, much less by the local government. In other words, they evolved out of social necessity. Maxwell[6] explained this in the following terms:

Local governments have an administrative ability for performance of functions which is greatly in excess of their administrative ability for the collection of revenues. The case of the national government is the other way around: it has an ability to make efficient collection of taxes which is greater than its ability to handle expenditure. . . . It will not be necessary to suppose that all governmental functions are handled by the national government. Local government will have tasks to perform, not because of any defect in the national power, but for the sake of administrative efficiency.

The second consideration is that it must be conceded that these programs have resulted in a considerable improvement of service and facilities for all the people. Speaking of highways, for example, White[5] commented:

It is no exaggeration to state that in the . . . years since the first federal highway act a national highway system has been established at the direction of Congress by the Bureau of Public Roads, and that the standards of construction and maintenance by the states, and their subdivisions have been greatly improved as a direct result of national intervention through the grants-in-aid device. It is impossible to conceive that the transportation needs of the present could be met without coordination, guidance and supervision furnished by the national administration and the support of national funds.

Certainly no one would deny that the same conclusions could be drawn with reference to the extensive developments in public health over the past several decades.

An interpretation of grants-in-aid which is different from that ordinarily made was presented in a study of state aid in New York by Pond,[9] who stated:

American government involves a system of checks and balances unique among the societies of the world. A persistent effort to retain the maximum independence to the individual and preserve to him the minimum of interference on the part of government is clearly discernible. Every state has two opposite evils to avoid, on the one hand overcentralization and on the other, local autonomy run riot. It is often taken for granted that efficiency can be secured by excessive control over localities which largely eliminates the citizen's participation in local affairs. On the other hand, it is quite as frequently believed that local autonomy is something sacrosanct, even when it results in much greater evils than those arising from centralization. Many competent observers believe that England stands alone in achieving both efficiency and a large measure of local self-government. This has undoubtedly been the result of grants-

in-aid. And this is a political mechanism which may fit in perfectly with our own system of checks and balances.

A more complete method of centralization is the partial or total assumption of function. In some states the state health department has direct control of local water and sewage facilities. The department of agriculture in some states has complete responsibility for food inspection. In one state the department of conservation has authority over hotels, resort areas, taverns, and other similar places, including their sanitation. Not infrequently clinics and even complete programs dealing with tuberculosis and venereal and other diseases are maintained and operated directly by the state health department.

A key factor in intergovernmental relations and especially the trend toward dominance by the federal government is the matter of fiscal resources available to or controlled by the respective levels. According to Snider,[3] "The increasing affluence of the national government in matters of policy cannot be seriously questioned. Furthermore, as to its major functions, the national government is free to set up its own complete administration. Its regulation can be made to override states. By its control of the field of taxation and to satisfy its own tremendous needs, it might force the states into progressive diminution of their own revenues and a reduction of their own activities."

Despite the foregoing qualifications and limitations the states today are performing more functions than in the past and are increasing expenditures for domestic programs at a rate actually greater than that of the federal government. Today the United States is essentially an urban society with a population of about 210 million, 74% of whom reside in the 264 Standard Metropolitan Statistical Areas as constituted in 1970. The process of urbanization, which is occurring at an increasing rate, demands that the relationships among the levels of government be redefined. A strict demarcation between the responsibilities of the state and national governments is no longer possible. Today the relationships are unclear and often confused. Meanwhile, creative federalism is in the process of being operationally defined. Whether changes in federal structure can occur rapidly enough to allow the governmental system to perform its two functions adequately in the future is undoubtedly one of the most crucial problems facing American government today.

## ORGANIZATIONAL STRUCTURE

### State and national government

Similarity exists between the organizational structure of the state and national governments. Early in United States history a system of checks and balances was devised that became an important part of the political tradition. Three branches of both the national and state governments exist: the executive or administrative, the legislative or policy making, and the judicial. On the national and, with one exception, on the state level legislatures are divided into two houses. A significant decision of the Supreme Court has held that the districts of both houses of a bicameral state legislature must be apportioned only on the basis of population.[10]

### Local government

All local governmental units are creations of the state. As a result, the character of the various local units varies from one section of the country to another. The state-local government relationship is defined as a unitary system; that is, powers are conferred on subdivisional governments by the legislature of the state government. In other words, the state legislature creates units of government and delegates to them.[11]

The primary units of local government are the city, village, township, county, and special purpose districts. In addition to these units, many special authorities, intergovernmental compacts, and cooperative service arrangements might be considered components of today's local governmental structure. According to the most recent available data[12] there are 81,248 units of local government in the United States. Included are 3,049 official counties, 18,048 municipalities, 17,105 townships, 21,782 school districts, and 21,264 special districts other than school districts. The expenditures of state and local government in 1969 were $132 billion, of which approximately $21 billion was received from the national government.

### Municipal government

Municipal units are incorporated, that is, they are granted separate legal existence by the state to perform functions other than those resulting from state policies. Cities are governed under special charters, general laws, optional laws, or home rule charters. Before incorpo-

ration an area is part of the sovereign state and shares in the benefits and legal exemptions of its sovereignty. On receiving a charter the municipality becomes a corporation and as such can have a corporate name and seal; own and convey real and personal property; raise monies by taxation, borrowing, or issuing bonds; make and enforce its own local laws; and sue or be sued under its corporate name. It differs, however, from other corporations in that it has two kinds of functions. There are, on the one hand, certain public functions in which the municipality acts for the sovereign state and concerning which cannot be sued without its consent. In most states, fire and police protection and public health activities are considered public functions. There are, on the other hand, many activities in which a municipality is engaged primarily or exclusively for its own interests. Examples of these are the construction and maintenance of pavements, municipally owned and operated street railways, and water, gas, and electricity plants. In most instances a municipality is considered subject to suit concerning these activities.

The distinctions between private and public functions are varied. For example, whereas county highways are considered a public function, city streets are usually considered a private function. The construction of sewers is generally considered a public function in contrast to their maintenance, which is generally considered a private function. Frequently the deciding factor is whether or not the individual citizen makes a payment for maintenance such as sewers or for a commodity such as water. The trend has been to make the municipality liable in case of doubt. Even with regard to their so-called public functions, municipalities are being held liable with increasing frequency.

Since the state government creates the municipality, it may also change or abolish it. Certain legal restrictions are involved, however, the complexity and significance of which are well illustrated by the case of Mobile v. Watson.[13] The city of Mobile, Ala., was incorporated by the grant of a charter from the state of Alabama. The city subsequently became financially bankrupt. Chartered private corporations are protected by the federal Constitution against subsequent alteration by a state, but a city charter, as has been pointed out, forms a public corporation that may be abolishd or changed by the state. Accordingly, the legislature of the state of Alabama rescinded the city charter of Mobile, substituted the name "Port of Mobile," and then announced that claims against the former incorporated city were not collectable, since the corporation no longer existed. The United States Supreme Court considered otherwise, however, and ruled that although the city was a state-created corporation with public functions, it also carried out private functions concerning which it could be sued and held liable, and although the state had a right to abolish the city corporation, such an act in no way relieved the citizens of their debts.

Considering cities as the most prominent example of incorporated areas, their governments may take one of several forms. The oldest type is what has been termed the weak mayor-council plan. In this plan the citizens elect by popular vote a mayor and usually a bicameral council of considerable size consisting of councilmen-at-large, plus a number of aldermen from each ward or district of the city. The latter, because of the customary partisanship, generally become designated as ward bosses. The mayor in such instances often holds what might be considered an honorary social office, serving essentially as the officiating representative of the community and little else. Although it is the oldest type of municipal government in America, it is rapidly becoming outmoded because it has been fraught with inefficiency and chicanery, and more efficient plans are being substituted for it. The strong mayor plan of local government is an adaptation of the older form. Here the legislative branch is reduced to a single councilmanic chamber, usually with far fewer members, all of whom are elected at large. The mayor is still elected for a limited term but is given greater executive powers and prerogatives, including increased power of appointment of departmental heads and other officials and greater control over the budget. In most instances the council may reduce budget items proposed by the mayor but may not add or increase items.

The early years of the twentieth century saw the development of two new forms of city government that have attempted to approach the managemennt of civic affairs on a more businesslike basis. The first of these, the commission plan, came about as a result of the devastating earthquake and flood of 1900 at Galveston, Texas. The corrupt and inefficient weak mayor-council government found itself completely incapable of coping with the emergency situation and literally collapsed. Through the efforts of prominent citizens a substitute form of government was established on the basis of the essential services and activities required by the community. Civic affairs were organized in a small number of service departments (such as public safety, public works, public health, and finance) and a legal department. Under this plan a functional commissioner was elected by popular vote for each department. In lieu of a mayor and council the commissioners ran the city government somewhat like the board of directors of a business corporation. Although numerous communities have adopted this form of government, experience has subsequently indicated that although theoretically an excellent plan, it has practical disadvantages. In many instances, for example, agreement among the several commissioners has become impossible, and often competitive departmental cliques have developed, jeopardizing the effectiveness of the total government. In other instances the commissioners in charge of public finance or of the legal department have found themselves in a position to thwart or control the activities and plans of the other departments. As a result, the past three decades have seen a gradual rejection of the commission plan of government.

Interestingly enough the fourth or city manager type of government also developed as an aftermath of another catastrophic flood, this time in Dayton, Ohio, in 1913. The experience of Galveston was duplicated, and in the place of the ineffective weak mayor-council system was substituted a plan whereby only a relatively small council was elected. This council of perhaps 20 to 25 laymen had no administrative duties, technical qualifications being therefore unnecessary. Their meetings usually required little time, their chief functons being the determination of general community policies and the employment of a salaried city manager whose tenure generally depended on satisfactory service. Again this was an attempt to operate a city government like a business corporation, with the employed city manager acting in an administrative capacity similar to that of the general manager of a private corporation. In many ways his position reminds one of the German burgomaster. As with the commission plan of government, the use of this plan has been confined almost entirely to small- and intermediate-sized cities. The extent of its adoption, however, has continued to increase, and already some counties, particularly on the West Coast, have adopted it.

In a few instances an attempt has been made to achieve a mixed or compromise type of approach. Thus the city of Philadelphia has a strong mayor-council form of government, but a key individual in the conduct of the city's services and affairs is a managing director, selected and employed by the mayor with the approval of the council. A certain amount of two-way or even three-way conflict is inherent to such a system in most situations.

**County government**

The county is the one almost universal unit of American government.[14] To some it appears anachronistic. However, counties are convenient areas of administration laid out by the states for the decentralized local performance of certain governmental functions, regarded as primarily of state concern. A significant renaissance has been underway in an increasing number of counties during recent years. This was stimulated in large measure by a grant from the Ford Foundation in 1958 to expand and revitalize the National Association of Counties, which has since been fortunate in having exceptionally able and aggressive leadership. The role of the county is described by Snider[3] as having "greater functional importance today than it had a generation ago." He predicts that further expansion of the services provided by county governments is likely to continue in the future.

The boundaries of counties originally were determined, to a considerable extent, in terms of the distance a constituent could ride on horseback or in a buggy from his home to the county seat and back again within one day. Although at the present time it is possible to traverse several states in one day by automobile and the entire country by plane in several hours, these old established county boundaries are still jealously adhered to.

The entire land area of the United States is divided into counties, 3,049 of them, with spectacular variation in size and population. They vary in size from Kalawao, Hawaii, with a mere 14 square miles, to the 20,131 square miles of San Bernardino County, Calif., which is larger than the states of New Hampshire, Vermont, Massachusetts, Rhode Island, and Connecticut combined. The average county contains about 1,000 square miles. In terms of population at one end of the scale is Loving County,

Texas, with only 164 people, and at the other extreme is Los Angeles County, bulging with over 7 million people. The average county has about 66,000 people. Several states, for example, Georgia, Illinois, Kentucky, Kansas, Missouri, and North Carolina, have 100 or more active county governments. Virginia has 96 counties and 34 independent cities. Texas tops the list with 254 counties. At the other end of the scale are Rhode Island, 5 counties; Hawaii, 4 counties; and Delaware, 3 counties. In Rhode Island and Delaware all powers have been removed from the counties.

In the New England states, county government is of secondary importance. The five counties of New York City are relatively unimportant, having given way to the single city government. City and county governments are merged in Baton Rouge, Denver, Philadelphia, Boston, New Orleans, and San Francisco. This is also true in 34 smaller cities in Virginia. In addition, two legally organized metropolitan governments, Miami-Dade County and Nashville-Davidson County, are essentially reorganized county governments. In South Dakota 5 county areas are attached to other counties for governmental purposes. Alaska, one of the newer states, hopes to overcome some of the organizational difficulties of the older states. By specific mandate of its constitution there are no counties in Alaska at the present time.[15] Instead there are 29 administrative divisions of the state government. Of the counties with independent functional significance, four fifths lack incorporated areas of 10,000 people or more.[16] It is substantially correct therefore to say that the typical county is rural and that its government deals with the government of farmers and small communities.

Certain legal differences exist between rural and municipal governments. County governments are regarded in most instances as *quasi corporations*. This term has little definite meaning. It indicates, however, that although the county may for some purposes have an independent existence, it is primarily an agent of the state and has no private functions. All its functions are public in nature, having been delegated to it by the sovereign state. Accordingly, the rules that govern its negligence or torts of its officials are those that apply to the state rather than to the city governments or to private corporations. A county therefore cannot be sued in the absence of permission from the state. In recent years, however, there has developed a tendency to hold counties liable for contracts or negligence of their officials. At any time a state may extend the degree of county liability by constitution or statute.

County administration has been handicapped by its legal relationships with the state. The flexibility that generally makes it possible for a city to frame a charter and determine its form of government and policies in line with its needs has not usually existed for counties. Instead they have had to accept whatever pattern of government the state legislature allowed, often without regard for the limited financial resources of the counties. As a result, larger counties often must operate through a governmental structure that has long since been outgrown, whereas small counties are burdened by law with a system they do not need and cannot afford. However, county home rule is now provided for in some states. This allows counties to frame, adopt, and change their own charters. County home rule as a general principle has been concerned only with allowing the county to establish its governmental structure and has not increased its ability or freedom to enter fields of activities that have generally been forbidden the county and retained by the state. Often the freedom in determining structure has also been limited, since states constitutionally or legislatively have required that certain county officials be elected even in a county home rule system. At present only 16 counties have framed and adopted charters, and most of these are in California.[17]

Problems of rural areas are simpler than those of an urban area. The economic and social life is geared primarily to agriculture. Life and behavior are more uniform, with less demand for luxury items, although recent trends have been effecting much change in this regard. Improved roads, automobiles everywhere, more convenient shopping centers, and television and radio have tended to make yesterday's luxuries commonplace in many rural areas. Except for the southern states, in most rural situations there are no complex nationality or racial problems, and the customs and inherited attitudes of thought present less variation. This is not meant to imply that the rural population is homogeneous. During the past few decades there have occurred widespread economic depression in the 1930s, World War II in the 1940s, and conflicts in Korea and Vietnam with their concomitant industrial, social, political,

and economic effects in the 1950s and 1960s. These have brought about considerable equalizing among the regions. Nevertheless, distinct and evident regional differences still exist.

With a lesser density of population, people living further apart attend for the most part to their own affairs and self-maintenance, and there is development of considerably less social friction. They have little in the nature of private local interests. Social and economic as well as governmental activities are more in the nature of fractions of larger areas of the state as a whole. For example, whereas city streets exist primarily for the inhabitants of the city, roads in rural areas are necessary for all travelers as well as for those residing locally. True, the difference is one of degree, but it is nevertheless so great as to have received recognition in the courts.

Beyond the problems of the individual household and farm the county seat commands most of the attention of the rural population. To most it represents the prime social, recreational, educational, governmental, economic, and shopping center. The last is perhaps the most significant. Galpin[18] in his studies of life in rural Wisconsin, summarizes:

It is difficult, if not impossible, to avoid the conclusion that the trade zone about one of these agricultural civic centers forms the boundary of an actual, if not legal, community, within which the apparent entanglement of human life is resolved into a fairly unitary system of interrelatedness. The fundamental community is a composite of many expanding and contracting feature communities possessing the characteristic pulsating instability of all real life.

Beyond this, except in unusual circumstances, state and national affairs are of decidedly secondary import except insofar as they affect the county itself.

The results of these differences between rural and urban areas are reflected in the form of local government. Rural governmental machinery is simpler. Fewer officials, boards, and commissions are needed to enforce the simpler local regulations, to carry on the limited administrative work, and to conduct the small number of social welfare activities. Incidentally the officials, boards, and commissions that do exist are usually subject to little or no supervision. Since counties really require for the most part state functions on a smaller scale, much of the administrative work is either performed or supervised by state officials. The interest of the state in local rural affairs differs from its interests in municipal affairs. County boundaries are laid out by the state government with its own administrative convenience in mind and without regard to the special interests, wishes, or needs of any single area or group. The powers of local rural communities likewise are delegated by the state as a parceling out of its own administrative function and not, as in the case of an incorporated municipality, with the idea of creating an independent political entity.

The functions of the county are therefore colored strictly by the circumstances of its origin. In the political field it conducts elections to provide the basis for local representation in the state legislature. Its own legislative powers are almost nonexistent, except for a limited authority to enact certain local ordinances. In the fields of administration and service it serves as the basis for the state financial levy, assessment, and collection, administers public welfare and relief to the poor, directs many school affairs, constructs and maintains roads and bridges, provides public health service, engages in licensing, the letting of local contracts, and the making of local appropriations, and determines salaries of local officials. As will be brought out subsequently, many of these functions are gradually being assumed by the state governments themselves. Reasons for this include the increase in cost of road construction and the increasing professionalization, expansion, and improvement in public health, public welfare, and public school services. In terms of judicial functions the county, through its court, probates wills and registers deeds. It presents a convenient unit of area for the local administration of the state law. As pointed out elsewhere, the local justice of the peace is actually the lowest rung on the state judicial ladder. Counties also serve as the territorial units for the establishment of courthouses, penal institutions, and for the federal post offices.

Perhaps the greatest of all deterrents to good county administration is the almost universal lack of centralized administration. In all but rare instances there is no chief executive to correspond with a mayor or a governor, and the local supply of individuals qualified to serve in the various political capacities is exceedingly limited. Thus Phillips[19] refers to it as the "no executive" form of local government. As he points out:

There are, in general, two principal types of county governmental systems, but modifications are so numerous and sometimes so extensive that generalization is dangerous. The first . . . has a small board of from three to five commissioners or supervisors, which has considerable administrative authority and limited legislative or ordinance-making power. The second . . . has a relatively large board of from fifteen to one hundred and fifty members, with authority somewhat similar to that of smaller boards. The average size of the larger boards is approximately twenty-five members.

The "no executive" type of local government is so called because the board of commissioners or supervisors must share administrative authority with a comparatively large number of separately elected officers, such as the sheriff, coroner, treasurer, clerk, attorney, assessor, surveyor, recorder of deeds, registrar of wills, superintendent of schools, and in a number of cases, auditors, and other officials. Since these officers are elected and are thus directly responsible to the electorate, and since they derive their authority from constitutional or statutory provisions, they are subject to very limited control, if any at all, by the board of commissioners or supervisors.

The voter therefore is faced with the demoralizing task of choosing from a roster of miscellaneous public officials so lengthy that he can hardly know the names of them all, much less their qualifications. The result is an authority and responsibility so diffused and uncoordinated as to make efficient administration difficult or impossible. To a very real degree an official may administer his office simply within the limitations of his own conscience, often with disastrous effects for the public as a whole. This being the case, it is not surprising that partisan politics, inefficiency, and corruption are so rampant in American county government. All too often, appreciable sums of money appropriated for public benefits have found their way into private pockets rather than into their intended purposes.

The basis of county government is a large number of individuals elected from small subdivisions of the county, variously referred to as judicial districts, magisterial districts, militia districts, townships, and hundreds. As might be expected, the majority of those elected are farmers with no legal training or background in government. When meeting together at the county seat, they constitute a body of very local governmental representatives referred to as the county board of supervisors (e.g., Michigan), the county board of commissioners (e.g., New Mexico), the county court (e.g.,

Tennessee), the police jury (e.g., Louisiana), and other designations. Within the limitations imposed by the state they have the authority to levy and collect taxes and to borrow money for the construction and maintenance of county roads, bridges, a courthouse, a jail, and other public property. They have the responsibility of providing relief for the poor and establishing and operating polling places and canvassing the returns. They appoint certain local officials, impanel juries, and carry out numerous other miscellaneous activities. All local executive and legislative functions are in the hands of the county boards, some of which exercise a few judicial functions as well. Except for some counties in New Jersey that have administrative supervisors, the county judge in Arkansas, the ordinary in Georgia, and a few counties with qualified county managers or county administrators (notably in California), it cannot be said that the American county has a chief executive comparable in position to the mayor of a municipality.

The types of other elected county officials vary somewhat in different parts of the country, but certain ones are found in most instances. The county sheriff is elected to protect life, liberty, and property and to carry out the judgments of the court. He has the authority to appoint deputies as needed. The office of county coroner involves the performance of autopsies and the holding of inquests concerning persons who have died suddenly or violently, without medical attention, or under suspicious circumstances. A very important officer is the county clerk, whose function it is to collect and safeguard public records (including in many instances vital statistics), to issue licenses, to open and adjourn court sessions, and to keep a record of court proceedings and the proceedings of meetings of various county boards. If any elected county official is necessary and worthy of his salt, it is the county clerk. In some places a separate recorder of deeds is elected to keep a record of land titles.

A prosecuting attorney is usually elected to prepare evidence for the juries and to prosecute accused persons on behalf of the county. The county treasurer has the responsibility for receiving, recording, and disbursing all funds expended by the county, usually regardless of their source. An assessor is necessary to list taxable persons and property and to assess them at a fair evaluation. In a few states a special tax collector is elected, and in many states a county auditor is chosen to periodically audit county funds and expenditures. In some states this latter function is carried out by the county board itself or by its financial committee. The invitation to fiscal folly involved in the election of an auditor or the execution of this important function by any group of elected officials should be obvious. School boards are generally elected either at large or by district representation separately from the rest of the county government. The superintendent of schools is generally elected by popular vote, although in some states he is appointed either by state authorities or by the county school board. In not a few instances he is the highest paid and most influential official in the county. Many miscellaneous officers may be elected because of provincial need or tradition; among these are county surveyors, fence viewers, engineers, road commissioners, and poor commissioners.

Last but not least among the county officials is the county health officer. In most instances he is unique in not being locally elected. The tendency has been to consider this position the most professional of all local public positions and one that can be entrusted only to a specially trained and well-qualified person. Frequently, local governments experience considerable difficulty in filling this position and increasingly turn of necessity to outside agencies such as state health departments, civil service commissions, or schools of public health for assistance. As a result of this and other factors, a tendency has developed for many local health officers to feel more responsible to the state than to the county government that they serve.

## Township government

Discussion of local government would be incomplete without mention of township government as found in the New England states.[20] This last remaining epitome of democracy functions around the town meeting, which consists of all the citizens entitled to vote. The citizens themselves constitute the true local legislative group. The nominal administrative agents are the selectmen or the township board of supervisors chosen by popular vote at the town meeting. In some places where no regular township meeting is held, they serve also as the legislative agent. Functions and activities of the township and its officers are similar to those carried out elsewhere by county governments. As a result of the vast changes in the forms of transportation and communication, there appears little if any justification for the continued existence of township government.

Within townships are found the governments of smaller urban groups such as villages and boroughs. These are generally organized by means of groups of elected representatives, variously termed councils, burgesses, and boards, that serve as legislative agents. In addition, they usually elect a single executive, who may be designated as mayor, president, burgess, superintendent, or chairman, to serve as the administrative agent. The functions of these governments are those of an embryonic urban community.

### Special districts

Special districts are the most varied of all local units of government. They usually are established to deal with a particular problem such as education, water, sewage, air pollution, and the like. To finance the specific undertaking, special districts have recourse to taxation, assessment, or charging rates based on service costs.[11] Due primarily to the trend of consolidation of school districts, the number of special districts have declined in recent years.

### Apportionment and local government

The question of whether the apportionment standard of populations will be applied to local units of government has not yet been resolved. The basis of representation to a county board was first challenged in a Michigan case, Brouwer v. Bronkema, in 1964.[21] Registered voters of the city of Grand Rapids challenged the apportionment of the members of the Kent County Board of Supervisors among the several townships and the city. It was concluded that "a part of the legislative power of the state is delegated to and exercised by the County Board of Supervisors. That Board, like its parent body, the State Legislature, must be apportioned on a population basis. . . ." The question of apportionment of county boards has been appealed to the United States Supreme Court. In May 1967 the Supreme Court approved unequal districting in the selection of a school board in Michigan and a city council in Virginia. It did not rule on the question of counties.[22] County home rule and reapportionment of county boards may make it possible to establish an organizational structure that would allow county government to function

effectively and therefore be the unit of primary importance in the operation of creative federalism.

### Metropolitan government

From the foregoing it is evident that many reforms are indicated in local government. One of the most pressing is the need for consolidation. It is inevitable that this should come about, and symptoms are already evident in certain fields of public service and in certain parts of the country. The provision of public health services in many areas on a multicounty basis furnishes one example of this trend. Another is the growing interest in the analysis and attack of social problems on a regional basis. The leading role in this latter movement has been taken by the Committee on Southern Regional Studies and Education, with permanent headquarters at the University of North Carolina. Strow[23] has defined the region as "a large area with natural boundaries wherein there are many resemblances among the inhabitants and their culture." Health regions may be considered to be "major areas with distinct health conditions identifiable with the areal limits and caused by the natural and human factors operating within the natural boundaries." The regional approach may be of considerable value in defining and locating public health problems, in revealing causal factors, in creating public consciousness concerning them, and in arriving at methods for their solution.

Attempts have been made to provide a governmental structure for metropolitan areas through a number of mechanisms. In one, intergovernmental agreements and contracts that allow for the provision of a single service on a regional basis are negotiated.[24] Another that has not been used widely consolidates county and city services that are performed under the same administration. In another type of city-county consolidation the limits of the city are extended to the county boundaries. This also results in the elimination of one unit of government.

Possibly the most effective structure for metropolitan government so far is the metropolitan federation. Municipalities in the metropolitan area continue their separate existence. Functions of regional interest, however, are transferred to a new central federated government. Examples of federated government include the Municipality of Metropolitan Toronto, Miami-Dade County, Nashville-

Davidson County, and the Metropolitan Corporation of Greater Winnipeg. Since the formal legal mechanisms for metropolitan government in most areas have been lacking, informal voluntary bodies such as councils of governments have been formed. The membership on bodies such as these includes representatives who participate on a voluntary basis from the various governing units. The weakness of voluntary associations is that they have access to authority only through their member bodies.

Another mechanism that only recently has begun to be utilized in an attempt to resolve the problem of a multiplicity of political jurisdictions in relation to one service area is the nonprofit corporation. Nonprofit corporations, with their boards of directors selected on a regional basis, in a variety of ways may assume effective and efficient administration of publicly financed projects. The result of an increase in the number of such corporations, however, could be a loss of control, manageability, and public accountability. The effect that the utilization of these nonprofit corporations in the implementation of public service programs has on government at all levels is an area that demands the attention of all concerned about government.[25]

It now appears evident that a type of local governmental structure that can adequately meet the needs and demands of an urban society does not exist in the United States today. The incremental changes that have occurred facilitate the performance of the service function of government but hinder the performance of the political function. They do not provide a structure in which regional issues can be debated and resolved. Progress along these lines is necessarily slow. Consolidation of local governmental units presents a most difficult political task with many factions ever alert to oppose it. County voters and county lines as they now exist are important to office holders, local merchants and bankers, political party workers, many property owners, and local newspapers; for patronage purposes they are important to local, state, and federal political factions. Today the inability of the governmental system to respond to demands made of it as a result of outmoded structure contributes in a large degree to the inability of the public health agency to solve health problems with the scientific expertise and knowledge that presently is available.

## THE POLITICAL PROCESS

Political scientists have begun to study politics as a process. Utilizing the new methodologies of social science research, they analyze the political process in a systematic manner in terms of human and group behavior and its social and psychologic determinants.

The role of groups as they affect public policy decisions has been an area of particular interest. Banfield and Wilson[1] discuss city politics in terms of (1) the press, (2) business firms, (3) bureaucracies, (4) civic organizations, and (5) labor unions—the organizational groups that they view as playing a continual role in decision making.

Another political scientist, David Truman,[26] advanced the thesis that everything in the political process can be analyzed in terms of group action. He stated, "Even in its nascent stages government functions to establish order in the relationship among groups for various purposes. What a particular government is under these circumstances, its forms, and its methods depends upon the character of the groups and purposes it serves." The electoral process and the role of political parties are specialized areas of this type of research.

Other political scientists[27] are currently studying voting behavior. "In casting a vote an individual acts toward the world of politics as he perceives the personalities [and] issues . . . measuring perceptions and evaluations of the elements of politics is a first charge in our energies in an explanation of the voting act." The premise of this type of research is that if voting decisions of the national electorate can be understood, one aspect of the total political process will be understood.[27] It would be helpful to public health administrators in understanding politics to become familiar with this type of current research in political science.

## THEORIES OF COMMUNITY POWER STRUCTURE

An increasing number of studies have been carried out in an attempt to describe empirically the decision-making process in a community and thereby provide a model for the American political system. One of the earlier attempts is that of Floyd Hunter[28] in his study of decision making in Atlanta. The conclusion drawn from his study is that an elite, although not monolithic, body does control political decision making. The elitist model of politics that has been formulated by political philosophers such as Pareto and Mosca seems to be substantiated by Hunter's investigation.

The alternative model describes what prevails as a "dynamic system of power interrelationships, involving the interaction of many groups in a contest with each other with policies resulting from their conflict and compromise. . . ." Dahl's[29] famous study of decision making in New Haven advances the thesis of pluralism. By studying three separate decisions on unrelated matters he has found little overlap in the groups of people promoting important programs in the city.

Many criticisms as to the validity of conclusions about the political process that might be drawn from community decision-making studies can be raised on methodologic and theoretic bases.[30] However, these studies, although they may not produce a model of the political system, do provide insights into the political process. As political scientists develop more sophisticated research techniques, more undoubtedly will be done in developing models of political action.

## GOVERNMENTAL REVENUES AND EXPENDITURES

The relative needs of the different levels of government for funds vary considerably. In 1965 and 1966, for example, the federal government was responsible for approximately $129.9 billion, or 57.8% of the $224.8 billion for direct government expenditures. The 50 states accounted for about $34.2 billion, or 15.2%, and the 91,183 (1962) units of local government expended $60.7 billion, or 27%.[31]

**Table 8-1.** Increases in all governmental expenditures, 1913-1961

| Item | Amount (in millions of dollars) | | | |
|---|---|---|---|---|
| | 1913 | 1941 | 1952 | 1961 |
| Payrolls | $1,500 | $7,400 | $29,800 | $50,215 |
| Other current operations | 391 | 9,000 | 26,300 | 91,723 |
| Capital outlays | 722 | 6,200 | 24,900 | 32,320 |
| Public to private cash transfers | 185 | 2,500 | 13,900 | 31,122 |
| Interest on debt | | | 6,600 | 9,710 |

**Table 8-2.** Governmental expenditure, by source and object, 1965-1966*

| Item | Amount (millions of dollars) | | | | Percent | | | |
|---|---|---|---|---|---|---|---|---|
| | All govern-ments | Federal govern-ment | State govern-ments | Local govern-ments | All govern-ments | Federal govern-ment | State govern-ments | Local govern-ments |
| Total expenditure | $224,813† | $143,022 | $51,043 | $60,994† | 100.0 | 100.0 | 100.0 | 100.0 |
| Intergovernmental expenditure | † | 13,115 | 16,848 | 283† | — | 9.2 | 33.0 | 0.5 |
| Direct expenditure | 224,813 | 129,907 | 34,195 | 60,711 | 100.0 | 90.8 | 67.0 | 99.5 |
| Current operation | 130,488 | 70,276 | 16,855 | 43,357 | 58.0 | 49.1 | 33.0 | 71.1 |
| Capital outlay | 39,981 | 17,652 | 10,193 | 12,137 | 17.8 | 12.3 | 20.0 | 19.9 |
| Assistance and subsidies | 13,363 | 9,048 | 2,301 | 2,014 | 5.9 | 6.3 | 4.5 | 3.3 |
| Interest on debt | 12,857 | 9,589 | 894 | 2,374 | 5.7 | 6.7 | 1.8 | 3.9 |
| Insurance benefits repayments | 28,126 | 23,342 | 3,952 | 830 | 12.5 | 16.3 | 7.7 | 1.4 |
| Exhibit: Expenditure for personal services | 72,963 | 32,904 | 10,561 | 29,498 | 32.5 | 23.0 | 20.7 | 48.4 |

*From U. S. Bureau of the Census: Governmental finances in 1965-1966, Series GF, no. 13, Washington, D. C., 1967, Government Printing Office.
†Net of duplicative intergovernmental transactions.
NOTE: Because of rounding, detail may not add to totals.

Total governmental expenditures were $19.3 billion more than the previous year. These figures present only a partial picture, however. If spending is treated in terms of financing rather than in terms of direct final spending, the federal government was responsible for roughly $143 billion, or 63.6%, state government for $39.1 billion, or 17.4%, and local government for $42.68 billion, or 19%.[31] Increases in governmental expenditures for the period 1913 to 1961 are shown in Table 8-1. Expenditures by level of government during the 1965-1966 fiscal year are shown in Table 8-2. Total expenditures for all levels of government broke through the $300 billion ceiling in 1969.

The latest figures available of a breakdown of expenditures by the various units of local government are those for 1962. Expenditures of local government in that year totaled approximately $45.28 million (duplicative intergovernmental transactions excluded); counties, $8.88 billion; municipalities, $17.3 billion; townships and New England towns, $1.7 billion; school districts, $14.9 billion; and special districts, $3.15 billion.[32]

The amounts of money required are influenced chiefly by two somewhat related trends in public administration: first, the changing relationships among and emphasis on different levels of government as previously discussed and, second, the greatly increased demands by the public for more and new types of service.

Most of the increase throughout the period can be attributed to increases in general government expenditures and national defense, with government utilities and other similar enterprises accounting for the remainder. Public to private cash transfers refer to public assistance, veterans' pensions, old age and unemployment benefits, and public employee pensions.

To meet these increasing fiscal demands, units of government on all levels are engaged in a constant search and struggle for additional sources of revenue. Each unit of government, maintaining its own taxation system, finds itself increasingly in conflict with other units of government.

In the early days of American history the most lucrative, stable, and accessible form of taxation was on general property. Since originally most governmental functions and services took place on the local level and because of early fears of federalism, the general property tax was

reserved largely for use by local governments. As a result, even today the general property tax represents the major source of income for local governments, accounting in 1965 for about 87.1% of the total revenue obtained by local governments.[31]

With the great changes that have occurred in social structure and means of earning a living, many new taxable items and activities have appeared. The shift to salaried income by a large proportion of the nation's wage earners has made a tax on earned income practical. The federal government relies primarily on income taxes for the major share of its revenue. No one type of tax is so predominant for state governments, however. Sales and gross receipt taxes, including selective taxes on sales of motor oil, liquor, tobacco products, or other services, provide more than half of all state tax revenues.[31]

Beyond the general property tax, cities and counties have access locally only to fees from licenses, permits, assessments, fines and forfeitures, and institutional funds and earnings. For some time the tendency has been for local governments, both city and county, to give way to the state and federal governments when new revenue sources are discovered or in cases of tax conflict. Tax revenue by type of tax and level of government in fiscal year 1964-1965 is shown in Fig. 8-1.

This dilemma in which local governments now find themselves would not be so acute if the general property tax had remained as useful as it once was. Unfortunately, however, this tax has become increasingly difficult to administer, has been repeatedly subject to personal and political manipulation, and even if correctly applied may sometimes jeopardize individual property owners on whom it is levied. To assess the value of personal property honestly and accurately is in itself a difficult and costly procedure. Added to this is the fact that most tax assessors are local individuals who by virtue of their local election are subject to feelings of indebtedness and favoritism. It is not surprising that the administration of the general property tax not only has been lax and inefficient but often has been used as a political tool.

Since ordinarily the need for revenue increases during periods of economic stress, local governments are faced with the dilemma of having to increase assessments, taxes, and collections on essentially the same people who

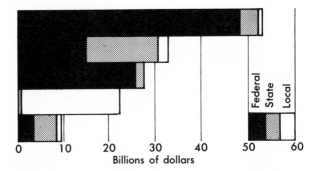

Individual
income taxes

Sales and gross
receipts taxes

Corporation
income taxes

Property
taxes

All other
taxes

Federal  State  Local

0    10    20    30    40    50    60
Billions of dollars

**Fig. 8-1.** Tax revenue based on type of tax and level of government (1964-1965).

**Table 8-3.** Trend of tax delinquency, 1930-1944, median year-end delinquency, 150 cities over 50,000 population

| Years | Percent | Years | Percent |
|-------|---------|-------|---------|
| 1930 | 10.15 | 1938 | 10.70 |
| 1931 | 14.60 | 1939 | 9.25 |
| 1932 | 19.95 | 1940 | 8.70 |
| 1933 | 26.35 | 1941 | 6.80 |
| 1934 | 23.05 | 1942 | 6.00 |
| 1935 | 18.00 | 1943 | 4.70 |
| 1936 | 13.90 | 1944 | 3.90 |
| 1937 | 11.30 | | |

because of general economic stress need the most help. Thus there occurs the real possibility of taking from the right hand to pay the left and the possibility that because of decreased ability to meet tax demands a considerable share of private property will be turned over to government itself by default, thereby eliminating it as a source of tax revenue. As a result, when local tax monies are most needed, collection becomes more difficult. A striking example of this is the state of Georgia, where in 1936 over one third of county taxes were uncollectable. This problem, when it occurs, is not peculiar to rural areas or to the economically unfavored southeastern states. Table 8-3 presents the extent of tax delinquency that occurred in the 150 cities of over 50,000 population during the period of economic depression between 1930 and 1944.[33]

Another factor to be considered with regard to the general property tax is that much property is exempt from taxes. Using Georgia again as an example, the following are not subject to taxation: public property, places of religious worship and burial, charitable institutions, educational institutions, funds or property held or used as endowment by such institutions, real and personal estate of any public library and of any literary association connected with such a library, books, philosophic apparatus, paintings and statuary of any company and association kept in a public hall and not held as merchandise or for sale or gain, farm products grown in the state and remaining in the hands of the producer during the year after their production, and personal property up to the value of $300 and of a $2,000 homestead on application of the taxpayer. In Georgia these account for about one quarter of all real and personal property. As a result, the bulk of real property tax is paid by farmers and small-home owners who as individuals are not organized as are other groups and are therefore unable to exert influence on tax determination bodies.

Netzer[34] summarizes the major defects of the property tax at this time as follows:

1. Its adverse effects on the central city housing stock
2. The difficulty in uniformly assessing business property
3. The horizontal inequity of housing taxes within income classes
4. The regressivity of housing taxes among tenants and among homeowners
5. The lack of neutrality among types of economic activity, particularly in connection with taxes on transportation and public utility property
6. The adverse effects of high central-city business property taxes
7. The effects on urban development patterns outside the central-cities
8. Some part of the regressivity of the tax, in particular that part which results in

**Fig. 8-2.** General expenditure, excluding funds for national defense and international relations, based on level of government and function (1964-1965).

taxing the central-city poor to provide public services designed to alleviate or overcome poverty

The last three of these he regards as defects that relate to local government fragmentation and that might be partially correctable if the tax were levied over broader geographic areas.

The concept of tax or revenue sharing has been discussed frequently in recent years. Basically those who support the concept argue that the federal government, which has an expanding base from which to draw revenue and a highly developed tax-collecting system, should return a percentage to the states.[35] Thus Walter Heller, economic advisor to the President in 1960, proposed that federal revenues be returned to states with few or no strings. Many questions have been raised as to exactly how tax sharing should be implemented: How much money should be shared? On what basis? What should be the relationship of the states to metropolitan areas and metropolitan areas to the federal government in any tax sharing scheme? As described at the end of this chapter, a federal revenue sharing act was passed by the Congress in 1972.

The growing public demand for government services and the resulting increase in expendi-

tures have been referred to. A cursory study over a period of years of itemized expenditures for various specific activities illustrates that the greatest increases have occurred in public service and construction for public use. Looming large among the increased items are those related to social security, including the prevention of illness and the promotion of health, insurance against unemployment and illness, and other similar social prophylactic measures (Fig. 8-2). As a matter of fact, merely over the 25-year period from 1940 to 1965 total expenditures on all levels of government for health and medical services multiplied more than tenfold, from $803.9 million to $9.22 billion (Table 8-4).

To overcome the inadequacies of state and local tax systems it has been necessary to resort increasingly to intergovernmental transfers in the form of grants-in-aid, shared revenues, payments for services, and other types of transfers.[36] Thus in 1965 not only was a total of $11.6 billion transferred from the federal to the state governments but an additional $1.5 billion was transferred by the federal government directly to local governments.[31] In addition, local governments received $16.85 billion from state governments. By 1971 the total

**Table 8-4.** Public expenditures for health and medical care, by type of expenditure, United States, selected fiscal years 1928-1929 through 1964-1965*

| Type of expenditure | Amount (in millions of dollars) | | | | | | | | | | | |
|---|---|---|---|---|---|---|---|---|---|---|---|---|
| | 1928-1929 | 1934-1935 | 1939-1940 | 1944-1945 | 1949-1950 | 1954-1955 | 1959-1960 | 1960-1961 | 1961-1962 | 1962-1963 | 1963-1964 | 1964-1965 |
| Total public expenditures | $509.5 | $558.5 | $858.4 | $2,571.0 | $3,086.0 | $4,358.2 | $6,359.3 | $7,035.1 | $7,619.3 | $8,286.3 | $8,997.5 | $9,949.3 |
| Health and medical services | 410.5 | 517.3 | 803.9 | 2,504.8 | 2,561.0 | 3,947.7 | 5,784.9 | 6,476.5 | 7,046.1 | 7,668.0 | 8,333.4 | 9,216.3 |
| General medical and hospital care | 216.6 | 231.8 | 340.5 | 354.7 | 914.5 | 1,217.3 | 1,952.2 | 2,202.8 | 2,136.4 | 2,274.9 | 2,446.8 | 2,670.3 |
| Defense Department facilities | 29.2 | 28.0 | 99.5 | 1,631.0 | 315.6 | 763.4 | 804.7 | 848.7 | 909.9 | 883.7 | 963.7 | 1,038.9 |
| Medicare | — | — | — | — | — | — | 60.1 | 61.0 | 73.2 | 75.0 | 75.4 | 81.3 |
| Veterans' hospital and medical care | 30.0 | 56.0 | 72.1 | 98.3 | 585.9 | 722.6 | 884.5 | 953.8 | 968.0 | 1,020.3 | 1,069.3 | 1,138.9 |
| Public assistance (vendor medical payments) | — | — | — | — | 51.3 | 211.9 | 492.5 | 588.6 | 812.4 | 1,000.7 | 1,147.6 | 1,375.0 |
| Workmen's compensation (medical benefits)† | 25.0 | 65.0 | 90.0 | 122.0 | 193.0 | 315.0 | 415.0 | 450.0 | 475.0 | 505.0 | 540.0 | 575.0 |
| Temporary disability insurance (medical benefits)‡ | — | — | — | — | 1.4 | 6.0 | 15.6 | 19.6 | 21.5 | 25.7 | 29.3 | 23.0 |
| Medical vocational rehabilitation | — | .2 | .4 | 1.4 | 7.4 | 9.2 | 17.7 | 20.4 | 22.5 | 26.0 | 31.2 | 39.8 |
| Maternal and child health services | 5.0 | 6.7 | 13.8 | 62.1 | 29.8 | 92.9 | 138.8 | 151.8 | 173.3 | 185.2 | 208.3 | 230.1 |
| School health (educational agencies) | 9.0 | 9.9 | 17.9 | 23.3 | 30.6 | 65.9 | 101.0 | 115.0 | 129.0 | 130.5 | 132.0 | 133.5 |
| Medical research | — | — | 3.1 | 17.0 | 72.9 | 138.9 | 471.2 | 603.9 | 819.1 | 964.0 | 1,101.7 | 1,235.2 |
| Other public health activities | 95.7 | 119.7 | 166.6 | 195.0 | 358.6 | 404.6 | 431.6 | 460.9 | 505.8 | 577.0 | 588.1 | 675.3 |
| Medical facilities construction, total | 99.0 | 41.2 | 54.5 | 66.2 | 525.0 | 410.5 | 574.4 | 558.6 | 573.2 | 618.3 | 664.1 | 733.0 |
| Veterans Administration | 4.0 | 2.9 | 14.1 | 16.2 | 156.2 | 33.0 | 57.5 | 53.7 | 52.1 | 69.8 | 76.4 | 84.4 |
| Defense Department | § | § | § | § | § | 33.0 | 40.0 | 44.0 | 24.0 | 23.0 | 42.9 | 34.3 |
| Other | 95.0 | 38.3 | 40.4 | 50.0 | 368.8 | 344.5 | 476.9 | 460.9 | 497.1 | 525.5 | 544.8 | 614.3 |

*Modified from Social Security Administration: Social welfare expenditures, 1964-65, Social Security Bull. **28**:10, Oct. 1965.
†Includes medical benefits paid under public law by private insurance carriers and self-insurers.
‡Excludes medical benefits paid under public law in California and New York by private insured and self-insured plans; such benefits included in insurance benefits under private expenditures.
§Data not available.
NOTE: Totals may not add due to rounding.

amount of federal aid to state and local governments had risen to an estimated $30.7 billion.[12] Health and hospitals represent public services in which significant amounts are transferred ($684 million). The total expenditure for health, hospitals, and sanitation after intergovernmental transfers in 1965-1966 amounted to $10.9 billion, of which $2.45 billion was spent by federal agencies, $2.97 billion by state governments, and the remaining $5.52 billion by local units of government.[31]

## GRANTS-IN-AID

In recent years social problems, of which health is one facet, have increased in scope and complexity. Concurrently, the attitude of the public toward the role of government in the solution to these problems has changed. The public believes that health is a basic human right, that high levels of health are possible, and that health services must be expanded accordingly.[37] The response of government to this demand has been primarily at the federal level. Many factors are relevant in this development, but of particular significance is the previously discussed imbalance of revenue sources among governments. The primary responsibility for the initiation and implementation of health programs, however, still remains at the local level. The mechanism that allows for federal financing and local implementation has been the grants-in-aid. These are defined as sums of money assigned by a superior to an inferior governmental authority.

Grants-in-aid represent one form of transfer of public funds for the purpose of equalizing revenue among the several levels of government and among the states and their contained local areas. They are intended to improve the quality and expand the quantity of governmental programs in less affluent areas and areas of special need by augmenting their revenue with legal transfers of funds from more wealthy regions. No reasonable person would sanction the continuance, for want of adequate funds, of insanitary conditions and inadequate public health programs in some areas that might adversely affect others. This being the case, it becomes necessary to provide some method for assisting the smaller or less favored units of government to meet their obligations.

A second justification for the increasing use of grants-in-aid may be found in the situation previously discussed; that is, the local government units are more restricted as to types of revenue and are administratively in a disadvantageous position for levying and collecting some of the more lucrative sources of funds. Few would deny the right of local governments to share in the fiscal benefits of automobile excise taxes, since the local areas must share in the building and maintenance of the roads over which vehicles travel. It would be confusing, however, to say the least, should each locality attempt to apply and collect its own automobile excise tax. A revenue such as this is obviously applied most efficiently by a higher level of government.

A third purpose of grants-in-aid, as was indicated in the discussion of centralization, is to provide some measure of supervision or control over the activities of the lower units of government. In this regard Snavely and associates[38] have commented that on an intrastate basis, "State authorities, more frequently specialized in their fields and free from local prejudices, can offer valuable suggestions and advice to the communities. Advice, however, even of an official character, is often unwelcome unless an immediate gain can be realized by its acceptance or a loss sustained from its refusal. A double-barrelled gun of this nature, loaded with a reward for compliant counties and with a penalty for recalcitrant districts is available for the central governments in the form of State subventions." What is said here with regard to state and local relationships applies perhaps even more in the federal and state relationship.

Related to this, and arising as a result of it, is a fourth purpose of grants-in-aid: the enforcement of minimum standards upon the recipient of the grant. Undoubtedly, few things have been as influential in promoting the employment of qualified local public health personnel, for example, as have been the conditions attached to grants by both state and federal health agencies.

The idea of grants-in-aid is by no means new, having been first applied in this country in New York State in 1795 for the improvement of schools in the poorer, particularly rural, areas of that state. Federal grants to states began as early as 1808, when Congress instituted an annual appropriation to assist the states in the development of their respective militia.[39] No conditions were attached to these grants, and no federal supervision was exercised. Perhaps the next development of significance was the passage in 1862 of the Morrill Act, which entitled each state to a grant of public lands based on the total number of its members of Congress. States not containing public land were given scrip. The only condition was that not less than 90% of the gross proceeds was to be used for the establishment, endowment, and maintenance of agricultural and mechanical colleges. Subsequent acts added to the original provisions an annual grant of cash to each state. In 1887 the Hatch Act was passed, which provided $15,000 per year to each state for the establishment of agricultural experiment stations. With this act there was instituted the condition of submission of an annual financial report, followed 8 years later by provision for a federal audit. This established a pattern that has never since been altered.

The rising tide of federal influence in state and local affairs is well illustrated by another phase of social security, relief for dependents. Traditionally the care of such individuals in America has been a local and often a private affair. The economic depression of the 1930s changed all this, when because of lack of funds, first private charity, then local governments, and in turn state governments found themselves incapable of meeting the tremendously increased demands. Only one other source of assistance remained—the national government. As a result numerous federal agencies that provided for the first time a basis for a broad system of federal social security were established. These agencies concerned themselves with dependent children, the unemployed, the handicapped, and the aged. This soon crystalized into a permanent legally established program. Again it should be pointed out that this represented not a premeditated design or plan of federal officials but a response to the increasing incapabilities of lower levels of governmental units to meet problems that essentially were those of the nation as a whole. Some writers have pointed out that even if the federal government were to withdraw from this field of activity, a definite change in attitude on the part of the public has occurred and the psychologic loss of prestige by the states is practically irreparable.

The changes that have occurred in the relationship between the federal and state governments have also resulted in some change in the relationship between state and local governments and local and federal governments. Theoretically the national government has no relations with cities. However, even antedating

the depression there had appeared signs to indicate closer contacts between national and municipal authorities. As early as 1925, Anderson[40] pointed to numerous instances in which national agencies played a significant role in the determination and management of municipal affairs. A more detailed study of federal service to cities was made in 1931 by Betters,[41] who commented: "The wide range of activities of the national government which touch intimately on current problems of municipal administration may surprise many." He pointed out that federal agencies had already developed standards in weights and measures, traffic and safety, zoning and building, highway construction, and milk sanitation, and had carried out studies and surveys on local education, finances, crime, vital statistics, and public health. In addition, federal agencies were actively engaged in a cooperative sense in food and drug control, municipal water supplies, sewage disposal, and other fields. Again the economic depression of the 1930s and subsequently World War II accelerated the intimacies of these relationships. Although the federal agencies operated for the most part through the state governments as an intermediary, they did in some instances deal directly with cities. The possible revolutionary consequences of this caused White[5] to comment:

The extent to which actual control of municipal affairs was lodged in Washington as a result of these emergency measures is not easy to define. The federal government did not attempt to weaken the control of the state over its political subdivision, and no change in the legal status of the city was imposed . . . contacts between cities and the national government were broad and in their extent spectacular; but the states were not dispossessed of their traditional constitutional position as guardians of municipal government. The change has been a change in climate rather than a change in topography. Future lines of development are not clear, but it seems likely that the research and advisory services of the national government to cities are destined to increase in importance. So far as the cities enter into debtor-creditor relations with Washington, an element of fiscal supervision may appear. . . . Movement has been rapid since 1933, and a federal bureau of municipal relations is much more within the realm of the practical than it was before the events of the depression. Here is an aspect of central tendencies which in the case of the great urban centers may be of special significance, for they have little to derive from the state capitols as they have much to gain from in Washington.

It is worthy of note that a federal Department of Housing and Urban Development was eventually established by the Congress on November 9, 1965, as an important part of the solution of some of the problems mentioned.

The rural areas of America were not absent from this scene of changing governmental relations. Except for the financing of the county agent program and aid to rural education and agricultural research, contact between the federal government and the rural areas was lacking until the establishment of the Agricultural Adjustment Administration in 1933. The federal government entered into cooperative programs with the farm population, involving the adjustment of farm production to nationally established quotas and the direct payment to individual farmers for compliance with contracts regarding certain crops. County production control associations were established, covering most parts of the rural area of America and including several million cooperating farmers. In the process the state governments were largely ignored. Associated with this program were activities such as the national nutrition program, which had a direct bearing on the health not only of the farm families but of the nation's population as a whole.

Federal grants-in-aid for public health work began with the passage of the Chamberlain-Kahn Act of 1918. Stimulated by the increased threat of venereal diseases during World War I, Congress provided an appropriation of $1 million for each of 2 years to be distributed to the states on the basis of population. The program was administered not by the Public Health Service but by an interdepartmental social hygiene board. After the second year the appropriation was cut and then finally eliminated. As a result, little of a lasting nature continued in any but the wealthier states.

The next use of federal grants for public health purposes was in the field of maternal and child health. Again as a result of increased interest during the war the Sheppard-Towner Act of 1921 was passed. It provided grants of $1.24 million a year to the states for 5 years "for the promotion of the welfare and hygiene of infancy." Contingent on certain conditions, chiefly the existence of a bureau of maternal and child health, each state was eligible for a flat sum of $10,000 and a share of the remainder on the basis of its proportionate population. The share of the remainder and one half of the flat grant had to be matched by the state.

This act was the subject of strenuous opposition, not only on the part of states' rightists but also of the American Medical Association, which as it did later in relation to the Emergency Maternity and Infant Care Program of World War II, viewed it as an entering wedge toward state medicine. Since some professional jealousy existed between the administering Children's Bureau and the Public Health Service, some criticism of the Sheppard-Towner Act was also forthcoming from the latter. After extending the provisions of the act for 2 years Congress terminated the grants in 1929.

Thus the second venture in federal grants for public health programs was short lived and relatively unsuccessful. Despite this, many authorities[38] consider the need for federal and state initiative and aid to be greater in public health than in any other governmental function:

Experience has shown that local governments of rural communities in general will not appropriate sufficient funds for the support of full time health units unless some assistance is forthcoming from outside agencies. Since it is in the rural sections that unsafe water supplies, unsanitary sewage disposal, inadequate medical attention and malnutrition combine to spread disease, it is in these communities that the greatest expenditures should be made. Despite the existing needs, the rural districts, even when aid is offered them, frequently hesitate or refuse to expend their revenue for the protection of health.

Grants-in-aid are intended to promote progress and improvement in lower governmental units by making it possible for them to provide better services and facilities than they can from their own unaided resources. Sometimes, however, this purpose is defeated by the system of distribution. Injudicious methods of subsidization may demoralize a community by fostering overreliance on the higher unit of government with loss of local initiative and sense of responsibility, by causing them to indulge in lavish expenditures, or by allowing them to use the grants as an excuse for unwarranted reductions in local tax rates. Similarly there is a risk of pauperizing communities that happen to be poor in the first instance by enticing them into increasing local taxation and even indebtedness to raise funds for matching purposes. Or there is risk of encouraging them to inaugurate programs and raise public expectancies that cannot be sustained on a long-range basis. Another serious objection has been the tendency for categorical grants to lead to unbalanced state and local programs based largely on financial expediency.

The sound, effective, and equitable distribution of subventions therefore presents a difficult problem indeed. Not infrequently plans have resulted in proportionately and absolutely more aid being allotted to wealthier communities than to those most in need. By distributing grants on the basis of taxable capacity either directly or indirectly through complete matching requirements, by granting equal amounts to all communities, or even by granting on the basis of population alone, there is a tendency, if anything, to increase the inequities rather than to solve the problem.

The great increase in the numbers and types of grant-in-aid programs in the health and health-related fields in the last several years has created serious problems of manageability. The Eighty-ninth Congress alone passed acts that created 21 new health programs, 17 new educational programs, 15 new economic development programs, 12 new programs for cities, 17 new resource development programs, and 4 new manpower programs.[42] Over 170 different federal aid programs exist, financed by over 400 separate appropriations, 21 federal departments, 150 Washington bureaus, and 400 regional offices. The dispersement of responsibility for programs continues to exist on the state level. Funds for programs are channeled for different patterns under a variety of rules and regulations. Effective program implementation at the point where services are given to people (local) is almost impossible because of the administrative confusion that has been created because of the existing grant-in-aid system.

The critical situation that exists with reference to the proliferation of grant-in-aid programs having no effective mechanisms for their implementation has been recognized. Attempts are being made at all levels of government, particularly the federal level, to coordinate efforts. A significant step was taken by the passage of P.L. 89-749, the Comprehensive Health Planning and Public Health Service Amendments of 1966, discussed subsequently.

The circumstances that cause increased needs and high governmental costs are the same as those that result in insufficient resources for meeting the needs and costs. States and communities with proportionately many children and elderly persons, inadequate sanitary facilities, high disease and death rates, and slum conditions have need of more extensive and costly public services than do other states and communities. However, these are the very places that find it less possible to provide them. To accomplish their fundamental purpose, grants-in-aid must be provided, at least in part, in an inverse ratio to the wealth of the various recipient areas. In this way the proportionate amounts received by communities tend to be in accordance with their relative needs.

In distributing grants-in-aid the possibility exists of taking funds from some areas and giving them to others that may be just as able to finance themselves as are those from which the funds were taken. One method of avoiding this involves correcting the apparent taxable capacity of communities to a true common denominator by determining equalized assessments, which is difficult to do, or by using assessment ratios to provide estimated true valuations.

A plan of distribution based on actual financial needs, supplemented by additional grants to encourage compliance with minimum standards, will provide some assistance to all communities and, in addition, will give consideration to those unable to raise sufficient funds of their own to supply the necessary services. If the superior governmental unit allots only a partial share of the maximum possible subsidy to those areas failing to raise the estimated amount of revenue as determined by the use of assessment ratios, this will act as a powerful incentive to provide local funds more in keeping with local financial ability. A plan like this is admittedly more difficult and costly to administer but in the long run will justify itself in terms of greater general improvements, equity, and satisfaction.

The Social Security Act of 1935[43] provided for federal and state cooperation in public health matters on an increased and more or less permanent basis. It provided for annual grants "to assist states, counties, health districts and other political subdivisions of States in establishing and maintaining adequate public health services." The annual appropriation was to be distributed among the states by the Surgeon General of the United States Public Health Service on the basis of three factors: population, special health problems, and financial need. The relative weight to be given these factors was left to the discretion of the Surgeon General after "consultation with a conference of the State and Territorial health authorities."

The failure to specify more exactly the method of distribution of funds appropriated by legislatures has given cause for objection from many quarters. A report of the Municipal Finance Officers Association[44] states:

The federal government has never had a continuing relief policy. The total amount of grants available has hinged primarily upon vacillating concepts of necessity. In addition, allocation of individual grants has been based upon wide administrative discretion. Such a procedure has hardly contributed to predictable municipal budgets. . . . The financial aid of the upper levels of government has undoubtedly saved many localities from complete disaster. Yet the unstable aid policies which have accompanied the greater reliance upon state-collected, locally shared taxes and grants-in-aid have served to accentuate revenue fluctuations for many local governments.

Many health officers also have complained of the difficulty involved in attempting long-range programs due to the uncertainty surrounding the amount of both federal and state funds that might be depended on for budget planning.

Prior to the passage of P.L. 89-749, which altered somewhat the grant-in-aid program as it relates to health, an attempt was made by the Public Health Service to determine indices of financial need and of special health problems. The results were not completely satisfactory, and the relative bases of distribution have been somewhat variable. Other factors, such as the relative cost of rendering health services in each state and the existence of special programs in particular states, have also been tried. Of the amount distributed on the basis of special health problems, one half has been based on mortality, one fourth according to relative costs of services, and one fourth as a remainder. Financial need has been based essentially on per capita income as computed by the United States Department of Commerce.

Matching requirements have been a result of administrative decision rather than of legal specification. Under Section 314d of P.L. 89-749, requirements for state matching were formulated. The requirements for hospital construction funds have varied. In any case the federal share must be not more than two thirds or less than one third. The conditions under which states make grants-in-aid to localities also vary considerably from no specific

predictable basis of distribution to the use of complex mathematical formulas, which, incidentally, are admittedly sidestepped more often than not. No standard formula is applicable to all the states, and each works out its own solution to its own satisfaction. Several state plans that have been used may be of illustrative interest:

*Florida*

Per capita grant varied by population size, with required per capita local contribution (50 cents considered basic) and system of bonus for excess local contribution and penalties for deficiencies in local contributions. One percent is added to or deducted from basic state contribution for each cent above or below 50 cents per capita from the county—not to exceed more than 50% of original basic state contribution. The state retains the right to add or subtract 5% or less of this.

Allocations may be made for special needs not subject to formula.

*Georgia*

Percentage of state participation varies with population with most populous areas receiving 30% and least populous receiving 75%.

*Illinois*

One dollar subsidy for $3 local money or 30 cents per capita, whichever is less. Special need subsidy added in poorer countries to equalize available resources to approximate $1.20 per capita statewide.

*Louisiana*

Total amount available for allocation to local departments is divided by population—this per capita amount is used as general basis and then modified by past progress and health and financial need of area.

*Michigan*

Population, rate of growth, special needs or problems, local tax base, and an indication of local determination in the form of the local appropriation for health.

*New York*

In counties and cities over 50,000 population on basis of 50% of cost of public health services, except where a county health department is established in which event state aid is given in amount of 75% on first $100,000 expended and 50% on balance of expenditure.

*North Carolina*

Based on population, financial needs, and specific program needs.

The most progressive state action in this regard is the Public Health Assistance Law passed by California. This law, which became effective September 19, 1947, provided an annual sum for local health services allocated according to a formula written into the law. Each county receives either a basic allotment or a capitation, whichever is less. The remainder, after subtraction of 7.5% of the total for administrative and consultative services and training, is allocated to health departments that meet standards on a straight per capita basis. It is of further interest to note that this act officially provided for a California Conference of Local Health Officers, which among other things, must approve standards relating to local health service before they can be established by the state department of public health. This plan warrants close study by the federal agencies responsible for the distribution of grants to state and local governments, since it appears to go far in eliminating many causes for dissatisfaction.

## COMPREHENSIVE HEALTH PLANNING AND PUBLIC HEALTH SERVICE AMENDMENTS OF 1966

The Comprehensive Health Planning and Public Health Service Amendments (P.L. 89-749) constituted a highly significant piece of legislation, signed into law November 3, 1967. It provides for comprehensive planning for health services, health manpower, and health facilities on the state and local level. It broadens and increases the flexibility of support for health services in the community and provides for the interchange of federal, state, and local health personnel.

P.L. 89-749 provides for the following types of planning grants: (1) state formula, (2) area-wide project, and (3) training, studies, and demonstration, as well as formula and project grants. However, there are significant differences in how the formula and project grants are administered. Formula grant funds will be available to states and, through them, to local communities on a flexible basis. Until the present time, grants have been given according to defined disease or health problem categories. Under the act they are given to establish and maintain adequate public health services of all kinds, based on a state plan for the planning and provision of public health services that has approval of the Surgeon General. Project grants are awarded to public

or nonprofit private agencies and organizations to focus on priority health targets. The goal of this legislation is to allow for the effective utilization of all available health resources. Under Section 314 of the act states must provide for the establishment of a single agency responsible for the administration and supervision of the state health planning function. For the most part, states have designated the state health department. Some states, however, have created new agencies in the office of the governor. Local and regional areas are also called on to create organizational structures through which comprehensive health planning can be implemented on those levels. The intent is that this mechanism will enable states and localities to allocate resources for problems and areas of highest priority according to their health needs.

The passage of this act has resulted in changes in agency organization at the federal and state levels. An office of comprehensive health planning has been established in the Public Health Service, and a major reorganization of the regional office structure of the Public Health Service has been necessary. Applications for grants under the law must pass through the appropriate regional office. Each regional health director is provided assistance through an Advisory and Review Council, the membership of which must be representative of wide interests, including industry, the medical profession, and universities.[45] Great responsibility rests on public health administrators in the implementation of P.L. 89-749, since this is the first instance of local and state agencies' being given authority and responsibility for the design and implementation of a comprehensive program to be financed federally. Whether local and state health professionals, government and non-government, will be able to meet this challenge successfully will undoubtedly affect the determination of whether this type of a block grant program will be utilized in other service areas. P.L. 89-749 therefore presents a great challenge and opportunity in the development of effective creative federalism. At this writing, serious consideration is being given by the Congress to legislation that will combine the functions and responsibilities of Comprehensive Health Planning, the Regional Medical Program, and the Health Facilities Assistance Program and implement the combination through nonprofit health service area corporations, which would be designed so as to completely cover the nation.

## GOVERNMENT AND METROPOLITAN AREAS

As is evident from this brief discussion of government and public health, the critical problem is whether the governmental system can adapt itself sufficiently and rapidly enough to function effectively under dramatically changing circumstances. Urbanization has resulted in great concentrations of people living and working in what have become known as metropolitan areas and megalopoles. The basic patterns of American governmental structure were designed at a time when the urban phenomenon was essentially nonexistent. A critical concern today is to develop an effective government for urban America. What type of governmental structure can be designed to assure the continuation of representativeness and responsibility to the people yet allow for the financing of services for the burgeoning urban complexes that contain and indeed generate most of the health problems and needs?

Many groups of political scientists, governmental workers, and interested citizens have been formed to study and attempt to arrive at solutions to this perplexing problem. Among them are the National League of Cities, the National Conference of Mayors, Urban America, the National Commission on Intergovernmental Relations, the United States Conference of City Health Officers, and the National Association of County Health Officers. It would now appear that the crucial test of the efficacy of the American governmental system in the late twentieth century will be its ability to operate in an urbanized society.

## REVENUE SHARING

The preceding discussion has pointed out the complaints of state and local governments that in the face of increased population, urbanization, demands for public services, and greater citizen expression they are still hampered by an outmoded system of revenue resources. In addition, whereas they acknowledge the significant increases in federal subsidies and grants-in-aid, they feel tied to the categorical wishes and ideas of the federal government that may not necessarily conform to state or local ideas of problems, needs, and priorities. Although they have the right to apply for federal assistance, state and local decision-making authority is limited.[46] Beyond this is the difficulty of balanced and long-range planning and financing despite the Comprehensive Health Planning Act, which relates only to health, and only to part of that. On top of all this is the considerable amount of red tape, paper work, conferences, and reports required for each of the individual grants by each of the federal offices and agencies involved. An important step was finally taken by the Congress by the passage of the State and Local Financial Assistance Act of 1972. This enables and requires the federal government to share revenue with the states and through them as specified in the law, with local jurisdictions. Such shared funds in the form of block grants replace certain of the previously existing categorical grants-in-aid.

The law provides that the state governments retain one third of state entitlements and that two thirds be distributed to local governments. Distributions are made by formula, which considers population, income, and tax effort, and in some states the proportion of urbanized population and state income tax collections. The local government amount is distributed to county areas based on the ratio that each county area bears to the total area of the state, according to this formula: population multiplied by tax effort, multiplied by its relative income factor. Uses of the initial $6.6 billion allocation to counties, cities, and states have ranged from purchasing much needed equipment, putting the money in the bank awaiting the full effects of federal program cutbacks, reducing property taxes, or developing social programs. In passing the legislation certain "high-priority" areas were recommended. They were public safety, public transportation, libraries, social services, environmental protection, health, recreation, and financial administration.

## REFERENCES

1. Banfield, E. C., and Wilson, J. Q.: City politics, Cambridge, 1966, Harvard University Press.
2. Easton, D.: The political system, New York, 1953, Alfred A. Knopf, Inc.
3. Snider, C.: American state and local government, New York, 1965, Appleton-Century-Crofts.
4. Brogan, D. W.: The American character, New York, 1944, Alfred A. Knopf, Inc.
5. White, L. D.: Introduction to the study of public administration, New York, 1939, The Macmillan Co.
6. Maxwell, J. A.: The fiscal impact of federalism

in the United States, Cambridge, 1946, Harvard University Press.

7. U. S. Children's Bureau: The seven years of the maternity and infancy act, Washington, D. C., 1931, Government Printing Office.

8. Mustard, H. S.: Government in public health, New York, 1945, Commonwealth Fund.

9. Pond, C. B.: Special report of the New York State Tax Commission, No. 3, Albany, 1931, New York State Tax Commission.

10. Reynolds v. Sim, U. S. 533 (1964).

11. Bromage, A. W.: Municipal government and administration, New York, 1957, Appleton-Century-Crofts.

12. U.S. Bureau of the Census: Statistical abstracts of the United States, 1971, ed. 92, Washington, D. C., 1971, Government Printing Office.

13. Mobile v. Watson, 116 U. S. 289 (1886).

14. Duncombe, H. S.: County government in America, Washington, D. C., 1966, National Association of Counties Research Foundation.

15. Local government under the Alaska Constitution—a survey report, Chicago, 1959, Public Administration Services.

16. U. S. Bureau of the Census: County and city data book, 1962 (statistical abstract supplement), Washington, D. C., 1962, Government Printing Office.

17. Ross, R. M., and Millsop, K. F.: State and local government, New York, 1966, The Ronald Press Co.

18. Galpin, C. J.: The social anatomy of an agricultural community, Res. Bull. 34, University of Wisconsin Agricultural Experiment Station, Madison, 1914, University of Wisconsin Press.

19. Phillips, J. C.: State and local government in America, New York, 1954, American Book Co.

20. Gould, J.: New England town meeting, safeguard of democracy, Brattleboro, Vt., 1940, Stephan Daye Press, Inc.

21. Brouwer v. Bronkema, Mich., 1885 (1964).

22. Graham, F. P.: Supreme court limits one-man one-vote rule, The New York Times, May 23, 1967, p. 1.

23. Strow, C. W.: Regionalism in relation to the health of the public, Amer. J. Public Health **37:**898, July 1947.

24. Dyckman, J. W.: Life in super city, Science **138:**1089, Dec. 7, 1962.

25. Smith, B. L. R.: The future of the not-for-profit corporation, The Public Interest **8:**127, Summer 1967.

26. Truman, D. B.: The governmental process, New York, 1951, Alfred A. Knopf, Inc.

27. Campbell, A., Converse, E. P., Miller, W. E., and Stokes, E. D.: American voter, New York, 1964, John Wiley & Sons, Inc.

28. Hunter, F.: In Lockard, D.: The politics of state and local government, New York, 1963, The Macmillan Co.

29. Dahl, R.: Who governs? New Haven, 1961, Yale University Press.

30. Polsby, N. W.: Community power and political theory, New Haven, 1963, Yale University Press.

31. U. S. Bureau of the Census: Governmental finances in 1965-1966, Series GF, no. 13, Washington, D. C., 1967, Government Printing Office.

32. U. S. Bureau of the Census: Census of government—1962, Compendium of government finances, Washington, D. C., 1962, Government Printing Office.

33. Bird, F. L.: The trend of tax delinquency, 1930-1944, New York, 1945, Dunn & Bradstreet, Inc.

34. Netzer, D.: In Mitchell, W. E., and Walter, I.: State and local finance, New York, 1970, The Ronald Press Co.

35. Federal revenue sharing, Research bibliography no. 24, New York, 1967, Tax Foundation.

36. Ecker-Racz, L. L.: The politics and economics of state-local finance, Englewood Cliffs, N. J., 1970, Prentice-Hall, Inc.

37. Barns, E. M.: The role of government in the provision of health services, Bull. N. Y. Acad. Med. **41:**7, July 1965.

38. Snavely, T. R., Hyde, D. C., and Biscoe, A. B.: State grants-in-aid in Virginia, New York, 1933, The Century Co.

39. Annals of Congress of the United States, 10th Cong., 1st sess., 1808.

40. Anderson, W.: American city government, New York, 1925, Henry Holt & Co., Inc.

41. Betters, P. V.: Federal services to municipal governments, New York, 1931, Municipal Administrative Service Pub. 24.

42. Reston, J.: Johnson's administrative monstrosity, The New York Times, Nov. 26, 1966.

43. Social Security Act of 1935, Section 602 (C).

44. Municipal Finance Officers Association: The support of local government, Chicago, 1939, The Association.

45. Cavanaugh, J., and McHiscock, W.: Comprehensive Health Planning and Public Health Service Act of 1966 (P.L. 89-749), Health, Education, and Welfare Indicators, Jan. 1967.

46. Smithies, A.: Government decision-making and the theory of choice, Santa Monica, 1964, RAND Corporation.

*The law is the last result
of human wisdom acting upon
human experience for the
benefit of the public.*

SAMUEL JOHNSON

CHAPTER 9

# Law and public health

## WHY STUDY LAW?

At a conference held in 1961 under the auspices of the American Public Health Association and the United States Public Health Service it was concluded that public health workers were inadequately informed and trained in the legal aspects of public health and the legal framework within which public health programs are designed and activated.[1] This is not surprising, since education about law, for other than law students, is one of the most neglected phases of American culture in the liberal arts curriculum, despite its actual or potential impact on all people repeatedly.[2] The fault is not limited to the health and teaching professions, as Clute[3] brings out in his emphasis of the problem:

As man finds himself beset today with problems that threaten his health and even bring into question his continued existence, it is vitally necessary that he use to the full every possible means of solving his problems. One such means is the law. Yet so far is the law from being used to the full, that it is little understood by health professionals, and, indeed, is hardly even in their thoughts. At the same time, lawyers have little understanding of health matters. In the interests of mankind, it is essential that this gulf be bridged, and without further delay. This will require, among other things, a much more fundamental understanding of the nature of law by health professionals; the establishment of much more solid and durable cooperation between the professionals in health and in law, at every level from education to the solving of problems in the field; and the serious examination of the undeveloped potentialities, as well as the shortcomings, of the law for solving the problems of human welfare.

Fortunately it has become possible to point to the appearance during the past few decades not only of an increasing number of specialists who have bridged the legal and public health fields[4] but also a growing literature and at least a few books.[5] Especially useful have been the series of succinct articles that have appeared routinely in the *American Journal of Public Health* under the by-lines first of Forgotson and currently of Curran. All of these sources, although limited in number, are highly recommended to all health workers. The fact is that it is impractical if not impossible for any health worker, whether in a public or private organization, to attempt to function without at least a general familiarity with the legislative process. This is all that is attempted to present here. Beyond this readers are urged to acquire a familiarity with the legislation, legislative structures, and legislative procedures of their respective communities, states, and nations, especially as they relate to health matters.

The legislative process, in the simplest analysis, consists of the interaction among the three basic branches of government that are usually interlocked by a system of checks and balances. Thus in the United States of America, on which much of the following is based, the *Executive* may veto legislation or sign it into law, the *Legislature* may introduce and enact a law and can override a veto by the Executive, the *Judiciary* may discard a law if it considers it in violation of man's basic freedoms and rights. To these three may be added the operating or enforcement agencies that are held responsible for carrying out the intent of the legislation and also

**159**

may be a significant source of proposed legislative additions or changes. The participation by public health practitioners in the legislative process was encouraged at a World Health Organization Conference of Directors of Schools of Public Health in 1966. The conference report[6] states that "Legislation is an essential element of public health administration, not only for the control of various activities but increasingly as a means of facilitating or permitting the carrying out of certain activities that promote health." Indeed, as several writers[7,8] on the subject have pointed out, everything that is done in a health agency has a basis in law and is subject to legal sanctions of one type or another. As for official health agencies, in addition to their service functions, most other activities involve the enforcement of law.

### DEFINITION OF LAW[9,10]

Many books have been written dealing exclusively with the nature and definition of law. It is interesting that although the average citizen probably considers law as an exact and strictly defined field, its mere definition presents the members of the legal profession with perhaps their most difficult problem. Law, at least in a democracy, depends in the last analysis on the collective wishes of the people, and the type and extent of their wishes vary through place and time. It should be realized that human behavior is subject to a never-ceasing process of evolution, as are also the social factors determining or influencing it. However, law is not unique in this, since definitions are not easily forthcoming in many other fields, for example, literature, art, or public health. Perhaps under such circumstances the essential goal should be to arrive at some reasonably satisfactory definition that will serve as a point of departure for a practical pattern of behavior. An example might even be as simple as the immortal statement of some unknown character who said, "There is plenty of law at the end of a nightstick."

To guide one's thinking it might be well to consider the definitions promulgated by some of the outstanding legal theorists in history. For example, Blackstone[11] considered law as a "rule of civil conduct prescribed by the supreme power in a state, commanding what is right and forbidding what is wrong." It is to be noted in passing that this greatest of all jurists refrained from including in his definition the criteria involved in determining "right" or "wrong" at any particular time. Wilson[12] extended himself somewhat further in his definition by considering law as "that portion of established thought and habit which has gained distinct and formal recognition in the shape of uniform rule backed by the authority and power of government."

### CHARACTERISTICS OF LAW

A law implies an actual or potential command, and a command signifies nothing more or less than a wish or desire. However, the commands and desires of law differ from ordinary personal commands and desires in that they (1) represent community desires or commands, (2) are applicable to all in the community, (3) are backed by the full power of the government, and (4) provide for all people the administration of justice under these laws. Wilson's definition might be considered to be more desirable, since it either states or implies all of the characteristics mentioned.

### PURPOSE OF LAW[13]

The primary purpose of law might be said to be the promotion of the general good by the regulation of human conduct to protect the individual from other individuals, groups, or the state, and vice versa. To effect such protection it must be possible for the individual, the group, and the state to predict within reasonable limits the probable course of judgment in the event of an infringement of the law. Therefore another purpose of law is to assure, insofar as possible, uniformity of action to prevent errors of judgment or improper motives or actions on the part of judicial officers. It is often said that the wheels of justice turn slowly. The rate would be impossibly slow if the accumulative experience of earlier judges were not available to the people and to the courts. This also is a purpose of law.

The most fundamental means by which law endeavors to carry out its purposes is the definition of rights and duties existing between individuals or groups. Legal relationships form the essential subject matter of law, and rights and duties are the most important of legal relationships. A legal right is a power, privilege, or interest of an individual or group that is recognized and protected by law. Simultaneously the law imposes on all others the obligation to refrain from violation of the right. Thus the possession of a right by one person always implies a corresponding duty on the part of some other person or persons to respect that right. For example, A and B enter into a contract. Their legal relationship may be expressed as either A has a right that B perform an act or B owes A a duty to perform an act.

Rights are of two kinds, primary and secondary. Primary rights are those that result merely from an individual's existence as a member of society. A citizen holds these primary rights against the entire community individually and collectively, and the community and each of its individuals owe him a corresponding duty to refrain from violating them. Thus a citizen's person and property are held to be inviolate; that is his primary right, and all others owe him a duty to respect it. Such rights exist not by virtue of any action taken or decision made but are the kind of rights that were termed "natural rights" by eighteenth century legal theorists. They are sometimes spoken of as "rights in rem" and "rights of ownership." Their violation is considered a civil wrong (a tort) or a crime, depending on their magnitude and on whatever statutory law declares them to be. Libel, slander, trespass, negligence, and the like are civil wrongs or torts.

Secondary rights are those superimposed on primary rights as a result of individual action and decision. They are not held against all other persons generally but only against a specified person or group. These rights arise as a result of contract. For example, A and B enter into a contractual agreement. Before the contract their legal relationship, consisting of rights and duties owed each other, was fixed and equal. Now as a result of the contract their legal relationships are different. A's previous primary rights are now increased by a secondary right that B carry out the action agreed upon in the contract. This new right differs in kind from primary rights, first, because it is not due simply to A's existence but results from a mutually agreed upon contract and, second, because it is a right held against B alone and no others.

Remedial rights are sometimes referred to as a third form of rights. They come into existence on the violation of the legal primary and secondary rights just discussed. In other words they are rights resulting from a personal injustice and are held against the individual committing the legal wrong. What they really amount to is a right of reparation, usually in terms of money damages. Thus all that is meant by saying that a person has a remedial right is that if he appeals to the court, he will in all probability be rendered a favorable verdict. As Justice Holmes observed, a remedial right is in the nature of a prophecy.

## SYSTEMS OF LAW

### Development[14,15]

The concept of law has gone through many changes throughout the centuries of recorded history. With primitive man it apparently originated as a combination of gradually developing customs based on tradition and supposedly divine dictates. Perhaps the chief function of the patriarchs of a tribe was to define the practices evolved and followed by their predecessors, and these customs were gradually given the significance of established precedent and law. As to the meaning or reason for such laws, it was the theory of the Hindus and Chinese that laws were an essential necessity of human society, as a result of the innate depravity of man. As evidenced by his nature, laws were necessary to prevent violence and injustice. Therefore it became a primary duty first of the tribal leaders and ultimately of their successor, the state, to formulate and enforce rules of human behavior and conduct.

The Grecian theory of law was somewhat different and followed in general the basic philosophic pattern of their civilization. The Greeks argued that all necessary social laws really existed in nature and were merely waiting to be discovered, similar to the principles of physics. In fact, nature was thought of more or less as an expression of the total of all universal law. This concept that law exists perennially waiting to be discovered as natural truths held sway for over 1,700 years, passing through Stoic philosophy, Roman law, the principles of the Christian Church, and on through the medieval civilizations and governments. It is significant from the present point of view that the men who founded the American Republic and formulated the Declaration of Independence and the United States Constitution with its Bill of Rights had as their legal background the natural theory of law. It is noteworthy that the basic idea of the Declaration of Independence deals with the natural rights of men, which are to be secured rather than granted by government.

Since the establishment of the republic American concept or theory of law has undergone considerable change, especially since the beginning of the twentieth century, so that legislation is now seen merely as a man-made device for the regulation and control of human conduct to assure the ultimate wishes of the greatest number or of the dominant groups in the community.

## STATUTORY LAW

At the present time almost the entire Western world is governed by a combination of two distinct systems of law: (1) statutory law, based essentially on Roman civil law, and (2) the common law of England. Roman law began its development very early in the Roman state. The first authentic legal records were established in 450 B.C. as the Twelve Tables. To these were added innumerable unwritten laws that ultimately as a result of the Institutes of Justinian and others were codified into a system of written law so perfect that even today it operates as the basic law of most European countries. Its geographic adoption was related, of course, to the paths of Roman conquest, which brought the Roman legal code into most parts of the continent. After the decline of the Roman Empire the resulting daughter nations retained the Roman legal system, since they had little other pattern to follow. Later states such as the members of the American Republic provided legislatures to make whatever laws were necessary for government, and the resulting collections of legislative acts constituted the statutory law. For a time the attempt was made to adhere rather strictly to statutory law, but as societies became more complicated, especially as a result of urbanization and industrialization, innumerable additions had to be made in the form of specific interpretations, court decisions, and rules and regulations. The result is that at the present time, for example, in the United States, written or statutory law constitutes only a small part (about 2%) of all existing laws.

## COMMON LAW[16]

It was recognized at an early date that statutory law was in many cases too general to be directly applied to particular cases. As a result, there followed the development of courts, the judges of which were expected to be guided in their specific decisions by the established customs of the community. England took particular strides in this direction. Essentially this recognition of the legal importance of custom represented a practical recognition of the rights of a people to take part in the making of the rules and laws governing their conduct and relationships. This was a great step toward liberty. A custom, in order to be entitled to consideration in law, must meet certain conditions. First, it must have existed for a long time or, as Blackstone put it, "have been used so long that the memory of man runneth not to the contrary." It must be followed continuously, that is, constantly observed and respected whenever an occasion for its observance or respect arises. Second, it must have a peaceful purpose and be reasonable and not inconsistent with the general spirit of the law. Third, it must be definite rather than vague and must be considered binding on all people. Fourth, it must be consistent with all other customs of society.

## STARE DECISIS

With the gradual development and extension of use of the common law courts, another practical procedure soon became indicated. The administration of justice would have become impossibly slow were it necessary to judge every particular controversy directly against existing written law and custom. Therefore the doctrine of stare decisis (the decision stands) developed, whereby a rule of law, whether based on custom or on being recognized by the courts and thereby applied to the solution of a case, formed a precedent that should be followed in all similar cases theräfter unless subsequently deemed absurd or unjust or unless repealed by the legislature. As summarized by Kent[17]:

A solemn decision upon a point of law arising in any given case becomes an authority in a like case, because it is the highest evidence which we can have of the law applicable to the subject and the judges are bound to follow that decision unless it can be shown that the law was misunderstood or misapplied in that particular case. If a decision has been made on solemn argument and mature deliberation the presumption is in favor of its correctness; and the community has a right to regard it as a just declaration or exposition of the law, and to regulate their actions and contracts by it. It would, therefore, be extremely inconvenient to the public, if precedents were not duly regarded and implicitly followed.

The American colonies, having been settled primarily by people of Anglo-Saxon origin, had as their original legal basis the written law existing in England at the time of their migration plus the vast volume of common law which had evolved in England up to that time. It naturally followed that there was superimposed on this an additional and ever-increasing amount of common law based on the social customs that evolved on the new continent. For example, the law governing the state of Indiana consists of the following:

First. The Constitution of the United States and of this state.

Second. All statutes of the general assembly of the state in force, and not inconsistent with such constitutions.

Third. All statutes of the United States in force, and relating to subjects over which congress has power to legislate for the states, and not inconsistent with the Constitution of the United States.

Fourth. The common law of England, and statutes of the British Parliament made in aid thereof prior to the 4th year of the reign of James I (except the second section of sixth chapter of 43rd Elizabeth, the eighth chapter of 13th Elizabeth, and the ninth chapter of 37th Henry VIII) and which are of a general nature, not local to that kingdom and not inconsistent with the first, second and third specifications of this section. *

Added to this is all the common law evolved in Indiana since the inception of its statehood. Statements similar to this are to be found in the constitutions or statutes of each of the American states with the exception of Louisiana, for which the Napoleanic Code provides the legal base.

## EQUITY OR CHANCERY

Up to the time of William the Conqueror (A.D. 1066) the administration of justice was limited to the application of existing laws. However, William the Conqueror assumed the doctrine that the sovereign was the ultimate source of all justice and that he himself was above the law. Hence the well-known saying, "The king can do no wrong," developed. Therefore he and the English rulers who followed him for a considerable period dispensed justice as they considered desirable or expeditious.

Thus if some wrong were committed for which the law offered no true remedy or if the plaintiff believed that the law had not given him complete justice, the king could be appealed to for assistance beyond the power of the courts. As common law courts came to depend more and more on precedents as guides in their dispensing of justice, they became more and

more rigid. Accordingly the king was appealed to with increasing frequency, so much so that the king's chancellor, who was otherwise spoken of as the "keeper of the king's conscience," was made responsible. This was eventually followed by the establishment of separate courts of chancery or equity, the essential purpose of which was to render as complete justice and restitution as possible, going beyond the dictates of existing laws if necessary. As time went on, such courts became strictly limited to situations for which no adequate remedy or solution was offered by the regular law courts. Eventually, however, as chancellors and their courts rendered more and more decisions and judgments, they too, as a matter of course, became more or less bound by precedents, sometimes defeating the original purpose of their existence.

This system of equity as a supplement to the written and common law was also brought to America and established as a part of its legal structure. Separate chancery or equity courts still exist in a few states along the eastern seaboard and in the Southeast. Otherwise, for practical purposes the same court now sits as a court of law, dispensing strictly legal judgments, and again as a court of equity, administering relief in cases for which the law as it exists offers no remedy. Equity serves as the basis for the proper administration of justice in many cases of public health concern, reference to a few examples of which will be made.

Certain principles have been laid down to define the natural sphere of interest and applicability of equity. They may be summarized as follows:

*Equity will not suffer a wrong without a remedy.* This is very fundamental, considering the reason for the development of equity.

*Equity delights to do justice and not by halves.* Thus it is the intention of equity that all interested parties be present in court and that there be rendered a complete judgment adjusting all rights for the plaintiff and preventing future litigation. An example of this is presented by a case * questioning an amendment to a Wisconsin statute relating to the licensing of restaurants. A subsection had been added providing that no permit should be issued to operate or maintain any food-serving business where any other type of business was conducted unless the facilities dealing with the preparation and serving of food were separated

---

*Section 1-101 (244) Burns Indiana Statutes Annotated 1933.

---

*Wisconsin Supreme Court: State ex rel. F. W. Woolworth Co. v. Wisconsin State Board of Health et al., 298 N.W. 183 (1941).

from such other business by substantial partitions extending from the floor to the ceiling and with self-closing doors. The provisions of the subsection were applicable only to restaurants commencing business after the effective date of the subsection. In a mandamus proceeding in which it was sought to compel the state board of health to grant a permit to conduct a restaurant, the complainant contended that the added subsection was void under the federal and state constitutions in that it denied due process and equality before the law. The basis for licensing the business involved, said the court, was for the protection of the public health and safety. "If protection of the public health and safety requires partitions in case of a business subsequently to be commenced, then by the same token it requires them in case of existing businesses; and if one operating an existing restaurant is not required to maintain the partition, and one about to establish a restaurant is required to maintain one, then manifestly the latter is denied equal protection with the former." On this basis the supreme court sustained the contention of the complainant, declared the amending subsection void but allowed the existing statute to remain in force, and instructed the board of health to grant the requested permit, thereby adjusting all rights and preventing future litigation.

*Equity acts in personam.* A law court may merely render a judgment against a person's property rather than against the person himself. For example, the court may command a sheriff to seize and sell enough of the unsuccessful defendant's goods and turn over to the plaintiff sufficient proceeds to meet the money judgment of the court. Equity, on the other hand, commands an individual to perform or to refrain from performing whatever acts constitute the subject of the litigation. Such an action by a court of equity is known as injunction. Failure to obey the command of the court places the defendant in contempt of court and, thereby, subject to personal punishment. Thus if the sewage from the premises of one householder gives rise to an intolerable situation on the property of another, the ordinary court of law can merely render a judgment for money damages in favor of the offended property owner. This, however, does not solve the problem since the original nuisance still exists. In equity, however, not only may there be rendered a judgment of cash restitution for damages already done but, in addition, the court may issue an injunction directing the person responsible to abate and prevent the nuisance from recurring in the future.

*Equity regards the intention rather than form.* This constitutes a weapon against legal decision. Law concerns itself with a strict interpretation of a form of a law transaction, or contract, but equity considers also the intent. This is illustrated by a case* involving the question of whether common-law marriages,

which do not necessitate a license, were included under a state law requiring premarital examinations as a prerequisite for marriage licenses. The superior court said that the act was clearly a public health measure designed to assist in the eradication of syphilis, to prevent transmission by a diseased spouse, and to prevent the birth of children with syphilitic weaknesses or deformities and should be construed so as to effectuate its purpose if at all possible. "Certainly," said the court, "the legislature never intended that such an important hygienic statute could be circumvented by the simple device of the parties entering into a common-law marriage without first obtaining a license."

*Equity regards that as done which ought to be done.* If a contract is broken, the court of law may render a money judgment for damages, whereas equity orders or commands (mandamus) that the contract be specifically performed. This is illustrated by the previously cited case of F. W. Woolworth Company v. Wisconsin State Board of Health et al.

*Equity recognizes an intention to fulfill an obligation.* If an individual promises or contracts to do a thing or if he has done anything that might be regarded as at least a partial fulfillment of the promise or contract, equity assumes that he intends to do it until the contrary is shown. This has sometimes served as a stumbling block to public health officials. For example, a person maintaining a public health nuisance may necessitate numerous fruitless visits and inspections on the part of public health workers. Finally, as a means of last resort the wrongdoer may be brought to court. If he can demonstrate to the satisfaction of the court that in some although inadequate manner he has followed the suggestions or commands of the public health official, the court may dismiss the case, saying in effect: "Why do you bring this man to court when he is taking steps to meet your requirements?"

*Equity follows the law.* In accordance with this maxim an equity court will observe existing laws and legal procedures, insofar as possible, without hindering its own function in the administration of justice.

*Where there is equal equity, the law must prevail.* If both parties to the litigation are judged to have equal rights, the case will be sent back to the law courts where the party with a right in law will have that right enforced.

The logic of this and the previous principle is obvious, considering the purpose for which equity was established. Equity is as an adjunct to law, not a substitute for it.

*He who comes into equity must do so with clean hands.* If an individual claims a wrong, he himself must be free from a related wrong or the equity court will not listen to him. This was a factor in the well-known Chicago drainage canal case,* in

---

* Superior Court of the State of Pennsylvania: Fisher v. Sweet and McClain et al., 35 A 2nd 756 (1944).

* Missouri v. Illinois, 180 U. S. 208, 2 S. Ct. 331, 45 L. Ed. 497 (1901).

which a court of equity refused a judgment against the city of Chicago for the city of St. Louis, partly on the basis that St. Louis itself contaminated its own public source of water.

*He who seeks equity must do equity.* This is similar to the previous principle in that not only must the plaintiff have clean hands but he must be and have been willing to do all that is right and fair as a part of a transaction or a judgment.

*Equity aids the vigilant, not the indolent.* This is known as the doctrine of laches and calls into effect the statute of limitations that fixes definite intervals within which legal action may be instituted after the cause for action has occurred or becomes complete. These time intervals are not the same for all actions and vary further among the states. If a person wishes to receive relief from an equity court, he must be prompt in applying to it. In other words he must not "sleep on his rights."

## ADMINISTRATIVE LAW

In the statutory legislation of an earlier day dealing with comparatively simple social and economic structures the understandable attempt was usually made to include in the written statutes considerable detail with reference to the problem at hand. However, in more recent times, with the accelerating complexity of the social and economic systems and with ever-increasing knowledge in all fields, it has become obviously impossible to include within the statutes sufficient detail to cover adequately all of the situations that might arise in the practical application of the true intent of the law. At the same time United States governmental structure has become more and more complicated and has had more and more demands placed on it in the form of public services and regulatory functions previously undreamed of. The relative recency of the modern public health program provides a good example of this. To meet the situation a considerable and increasing number of administrative agencies have been established by government, on a statutory basis, set up for the purpose of putting into effect the intent of legislation.

The procedure of passing enabling legislation written in more or less general terms was evolved. This legislation included clauses delegating administration and enforcement to a new or existing administrative agency, giving the agency the power and responsibility to formulate whatever rules, regulations, and standards were necessary for carrying out the purpose of the law. It naturally follows that such powers and responsibilities must be in conformity with all existing laws of the community, the state,

and the nation. Thus although the legislative branch of government is the only body that may actually formulate and enact a law and although this power cannot itself be delegated, the legislature may delegate the power to make whatever rules and regulations are necessary to carry out the intent of the law. (In some states even administrative rules and regulations must be reviewed and approved by the state attorney general.) All such administrative rules and regulations, when properly formulated and when not in conflict with existing laws of the state and nation, have all the force and effect of law, even though they arise from an administrative agency and not from the legislature itself. However, their interpretation by the courts tends to be somewhat more rigid than the interpretation placed on the enactments of the legislature itself.

## CLASSIFICATION OF LAW

For purposes of consolidation, a few words on the classification of law may be appropriate. Perhaps the simplest method of classifying laws is (1) by origin and (2) by application.

From the point of view of origin, law may be classified as follows:

*Constitutional law*—law developed by specially designated bodies or legislatures convened for the purpose of framing or amending a constitution

*Statutory law*—legislation that may arise from either representative assemblies or by the process of initiative and referendum

*Decree or administrative law*—rules, regulations, standards, orders, etc. issued by executive or administrative boards or officers within the sphere of their legal competence and responsibility to carry out the intent of statutory laws

*Common law and equity*—decisions made by courts in specific cases

Another approach[8] classifies law into (1) *substantive law,* which provides the rules and requirements of conduct; (2) *procedural law,* which tells how to bring a lawsuit and how to prosecute; and (3) *remedial law* or law of sanctions, which tells what remedies are available for breaches of the law.

From the point of view of application, law may be classified as follows:

*Public law*—law concerned with the establishment, maintenance, and operation of government; the definition, relationships, and regulation of its various branches; and the relationship of the individual or of groups to the state

1. *Constitutional law*—deals with the basic nature,

structure, and function of the state in relation to the powers of the various branches of government; sometimes includes a bill of rights

2. *Administrative law*—as discussed previously
3. *Criminal law*—concerned with offenses or acts against the public welfare and safety, such being considered as offenses against the state and varying from petty offenses and misdemeanors to felonies

*Private law*—law concerned with the rights and duties of individuals and groups in relation to each other; originally based largely on common law but increasingly becoming subject to statutes

## COURTS

American government is based on the wise principle of the separation of powers. Accordingly legislation can be formulated, considered, and ultimately enacted only by the legislative branch. After its enactment the legislature has no further concern with a law except for the possibility of subsequent amendment or repeal. On passage a law is referred to the executive branch of government for its administration and enforcement. However, the constitutionality of the law and the manner of its enforcement are subject to review at any time on the initiative of the citizenry by the third or judicial branch of government, which is manifest by the actions of the courts. It is the duty of the courts to pass upon the constitutionality of laws, to interpret them in the interest of justice and the public good, and to determine their validity whenever controversies related to them are brought before the court in the proper manner.

The jurisdiction of the court may be either original or appellate; that is, the courts may be a place where the merits of a controversy are originally passed upon, or they may be a place to which an unsuccessful and dissatisfied litigant may appeal for a review of the action taken by a court of original jurisdiction. Using the judicial system of the states as a point of departure, their courts may be divided into three categories. At the top are the superior courts, including the state supreme court, the superior court, the court of appeal, or the court of civil appeals. Such courts usually have five to nine justices who hear appeal cases from the lower courts of the state and who have in some instances varying amounts of original jurisdiction. Appeals may be taken from here to the Supreme Court of the United States if the case involves the federal Constitution, federal laws, or treaties. Below the state superior courts are the intermediate courts, including the circuit courts, the district courts, the county courts, and the common pleas courts, the terminology differing in different states. These are courts of original jurisdiction and the first two hear appeals from lower courts in some states. In other states these functions are separated. It is to be noted that a county court, although locally elected and locally responsible for the administration of its verdicts, is actually part of the state judicial system. On the lowest or most local level are the locally elected justices of the peace, who in effect individually constitute the lowest rung on the state judicial ladder.

In addition, a state may set up certain special courts to deal with particular social problems such as juvenile delinquency, domestic relations, industrial relations, etc. On the municipal level of government, by virtue of a charter granted by a state government, an urban community may have the privilege of setting up certain courts of its own to administer justice in cases involving problems of concern limited to the municipality itself. Thus there are police courts with original jurisdiction in minor matters and municipal courts with original jurisdiction in more important cases and also serving as a place of appeal from the police court.

On the federal level is the Supreme Court of the United States, consisting of a chief justice and 8 associates, to which cases may be appealed from the lower federal courts and state supreme courts in instances where the federal Constitution, laws, or treaties are considered to be involved. In addition it has some original jurisdiction in interstate, maritime, and some other matters (see Article III, Section 2, of the Constitution and the Eleventh Amendment). To expedite the federal judicial system a number of intermediate courts have been established. Thus there are 10 federal circuit courts with appellate jurisdiction and below them over 90 federal district courts, which are the principal federal courts of original jurisdiction. There are, in addition, federal courts for special purposes such as the Customs Courts and the Federal Court of Claims. There might also be mentioned the increasing number of federal administrative boards, for example, the National Labor Relations Board, which have a certain amount of delegated original jurisdiction.

## SOURCES OF PUBLIC HEALTH LAW

Public health law may be defined as that body of statutes, regulations, and precedents that has for its purpose the protection and promotion of individual and community health. Although the term *public health* was not entirely unknown to contemporaries of the authors of the American Constitution, its present-day scope and significance were not conceived of. After all, there was no public health profession in existence, and science was not to enter the golden era of bacteriology until about 100 years later. Three quarters of a century were to pass before the need for establishment of the first state health department was to be felt. Still 40 years more were to pass before the formation of the first county health department. The founders of the United States cannot be censured therefore for not considering public health functions specifically in their organization of the new government. They were so remarkably astute and farsighted, however, as to provide for future developments in many fields by the use of certain broad and general phrases that in subsequent periods were to make possible broad interpretations of the Constitution, thereby allowing the introduction and inclusion of certain public health activities in the functions of the federal government.

By far the most important of these broad phrases is that occurring in the Preamble to the Constitution, which includes among the fundamental purposes of the government the intent to "promote the general welfare." This recurs in Section 8 of Article I, which, dealing with the functions of Congress, gives it power "to lay and collect taxes . . . and provide for the common defense and general welfare. . . ." It is the generous interpretation of this by the Supreme Court that made possible the activity of the Children's Bureau in maternal and child health and the subsidization by means of federal grants-in-aid of state and local health programs by the Public Health Service. In fact, these and many other federal agencies owe their existence in large part to the intent that has been read into the "general welfare" phrase.

In addition, the varied and widespread activities of the federal government in fields relating to health have as their legal basis the manner in which numerous other clauses of the Constitution have been interpreted. Thus the direction to Congress "to regulate commerce with foreign nations, and among the several states, and with the Indian tribes" has been construed to include such matters as international and interstate quarantine, sanitary supervision, vital statistics, and direct responsibility for the health of the American Indians. The provision for the establishment of "post offices and post roads" has led to the right of the federal government to bar from the mails material deleterious to the public health. The power "to raise and support armies" and to "provide and maintain a navy" logically placed responsibility for the health of the armed forces (in recent years a not inconsiderable fraction of the population) in the hands of federal agencies. Complete and exclusive jurisdiction over the inhabitants of the seat of the national government (the District of Columbia) is also specified.

The reader may be reminded at this point that the United States, far from being one nation, is in a true sense a federation of 50 separate nations, called states, each with its own history, economic and social problems, and still somewhat jealously guarded intrastate interests. It will be recalled that the members of the constitutional convention carefully guarded the rights of their respective states, jointly turning over to the newly formed federal government only such powers and activities as they considered desirable and necessary for the common welfare and survival of all. Matters that they could adequately handle as individual states were retained by the states. Therefore the federal government truly was and is a creature of jointly concurred action of the several states. Since the beginning it has been inferred that all matters not specifically mentioned in the Constitution and its subsequent Amendments were questions to be dealt with primarily by the states. It is for this reason that the more complete and coordinated organization of public health activities is found on the state and local levels. Each state has developed its own characteristic body of legislation and judicial interpretation as well as its own characteristic type of organization for the implementation of its public health laws, being in a position to do much as it wishes within the limitations of interstate and international conflict. Although there are these 50 differing sets of public health laws and organizations, certain fundamental legal principles, however, are involved in all. A brief discussion of some of these fundamentals is necessary for further consideration of sources of public health powers.

## EMINENT DOMAIN

The first of the basic powers of a state is that of eminent domain, sometimes referred to as the power of condemnation. This is the power or right of a sovereign state to summarily appropriate an individual's property or to limit his use of it if the best interest of the community makes such action desirable. In so doing, however, the state must provide an equitable compensation. In effect the state has the right to demand the sale or limitation of use of private property. The distinction between the exercise of the power of eminent domain and actions on which legislatures may insist without compensation is not clear cut at any given time and varies from time to time. The history of zoning measures to control the height of buildings has been cited as a good example of this. At first the state attempted to control the height of buildings by purchasing from individuals their primary right to build on their own property above the height that was considered most desirable from the community standpoint. Since this action was upheld in the courts, it was resorted to by more and more people in more and more communities until it got to the point where, as Ascher[18] aptly stated, it resembled the economy of the mythical village of Ballycannon, where everyone made his living by taking in his next-door neighbor's washing. In other words, when resorted to on a wide scale, use of the power of eminent domain amounts to individuals' (as taxpayers) purchasing the exercise of a right from themselves as private citizens. Inevitably such a procedure becomes ineffective as a measure of control. Recognizing this, the public through its legislatures may finally say, "We shall forbid this particular action or use by the individual," and the courts more often than not will uphold the action.

In a certain sense the procedure followed by some health departments in the past of paying an allotment to chronic carriers of typhoid bacilli to make sure of their refraining from engaging in food-handling occupations represented the purchase by the state of an individual's primary right. The states in most instances finally simply forbade such activity by these persons.

As pointed out by Ascher, it is interesting to note that those who attempted to bring about a form of building control that eliminated the necessity of compensation deliberately avoided a test case for about 10 years. Finally, when the Ambler Realty Company protested the restriction of its use of land by the village of Euclid,* the United States Supreme Court up-

held this arbitrary use of the police power in a sweeping opinion that had as one of its basic contentions that over 900 cities were already subject to zoning and about one half of the urban dwellers of the nation lived under the benefits of zoning procedures. This is perhaps another way of saying that within a relatively short period of time the social concept of zoning had become part of the custom of American communities and that its requirement could be considered as having become part of the common law.

## LAWS OF NUISANCES
## (NOSCITUR AD SOCIIS)

Long before the United States and its government were conceived the concept was developed by medieval legal theorists that whereas "a man's home is his castle," an individual's use of his private property could be detrimental to others. The use of private property is unrestricted only as long as it does not injure another's person or property. If this occurred, a nuisance was considered to exist, and the individual whose person or property was injured could seek assistance from the courts. Innumerable examples of this exist in the field of public health, especially with regard to the salubrity of the physical environment. For example, an individual property owner has the right to dispose of his sewage in any manner that he may see fit, provided that it cannot actually or potentially affect another. If he allows raw sewage to flow onto the land of another, a social injustice has obviously occurred, and the health and well-being of others have been placed in jeopardy. Legal relief against nuisances may be obtained in the courts by means of (1) a suit of law for damages resulting or (2) a suit in equity to forbid or abate the nuisance.

It is perhaps unfortunate that a large proportion of public health officials still consider the use of the law of nuisances as one of their most important if not their chief legal recourse. The pursuit of this point of view eventually leads to many difficulties and dissatisfactions, since the law of nuisances is subject to increasing limitations, some of which are discussed here.

In the first place there are many things or uses of things that do not intrinsically constitute a nuisance but are merely in the wrong place. An example of this is provided by the case

---

*Village of Euclid v. Ambler Realty Co., 272 U. S. 365 (1926).

of Benton et al. v. Pittard, Health Commissioner, et al.,* in which the plaintiff protested the establishment and operation by a health department of a venereal disease clinic in a residential district. The complaints were that the disease of the patients who would congregate in the neighborhood "were not only communicable but were offensive, obnoxious and disgusting; that the clinic operation would be offensive to the petitioners and that their sensibility would be injured; and that their dwelling would be rendered less valuable as a home and place of residence." The defending health officer and county commissioner filed an answer and a general demurrer, a form of pleading that although admitting all the facts, challenged their legal sufficiency to constitute a cause of action. The judge, after hearing both sides, denied the plaintiff's request for an injunction and sustained the demurrer. On being appealed, however, the Georgia Supreme Court stated that the fact that the clinic was to be operated as a public institution would not alone prevent it from becoming a nuisance if located in a residential section and that the statutory provision requiring the care of venereally infected persons did not imply the right to perform such care in any location. "In other words, a nuisance may consist merely of the right thing in the wrong place regardless of other circumstances." On this basis the judgment of the original trial court was reversed.

Another factor tending to limit the value of the law of nuisances is that a great many of the legal doctrines and decisions dealing with nuisances and their abatement were developed before the germ theory of disease became established scientific fact. During most of its development, no obvious factual or scientific data existed on which to base conclusions, and those appearing in court in such cases were merely pitting their opinions against the opinions of others. This left the court as its only final recourse the expression of its own opinion. As a result, a mass of unsound and unscientific decisions has been built up, which because they are precedents, continue to influence the public health problems of present-day communities. This also partly explains why many supposedly modern health departments are required to expend much time, energy, and funds in activities that have little relationship to public health, for example, garbage and refuse control.

Still another difficulty is caused by the fact that recourse to the law of nuisances does not overcome one of the rules of law. Decision by a law court that a nuisance exists may result in damages being paid to the plaintiff but does not necessarily effect the solution or abatement of the noisome circumstances. There is, of course, the possibility of resorting to a court of equity with the hope of obtaining complete justice. However, here again it is found that a rule of equity may provide a way out for the defendant in that if he can demonstrate to the court's satisfaction his intention or, better yet, partial action to abate the nuisance, the case in all probability will be dismissed from court. The thought might arise that the situation could be improved by trying to bring about more up-to-date judicial interpretations and judgments regarding nuisances. Although theoretically possible, the task involved to accomplish this would be enormous. Furthermore, even if modern present-day standards could be made the basis of definition, these standards and definitions might become outmoded with the passage of time.

## POLICE POWER[19]

There remains another means of legal recourse for the public health official to consider, that is, the police power that the sovereign state possesses. As a matter of fact, public health law owes its true origin and only real effectiveness to this inherent right of the state. Police power originated in the so-called law of overruling necessity, which claims that in times of stress such as fire, pestilence, etc., the private property of an individual might be summarily appropriated, used, or even destroyed if the ultimate relief, protection, or safety of the group indicated such action as necessary. Through time this concept expanded to include even activities designed for the prevention of causes of social stress. The United States Supreme Court has on numerous occasions not only upheld the principle of the police power of the state but also has defined its scope in sweeping terms to include, as did Chief Justice Marshall, all types of public health laws and to acknowledge the power of the states to provide for the health of their citizens.* It should be noted,

---

*Georgia Supreme Court: Benton et al. v. Pittard, Health Commissioner, et al. 31 S.E. 2nd 6.

*Perhaps the best known case is Gibbons v. Ogden, 9 Wheat. 1, 6 L. Ed. 23 (1824).

however, as Justice Brown stated, that ". . . its [legislature's] determination as to what is a proper exercise of its police powers is not final or conclusive but is subject to the supervision of the court."*

One of the best definitions of the police power was given in the case of Miami County v. Dayton,† in which the court defined it as "that inherent sovereignty which the government exercises whenever regulations are demanded by public policy for the benefit of the society at large in order to guard its morals, safety, health, order and the like in accordance with the needs of civilization."

Although the possession of police power is fundamentally that of the sovereign state, the legislature of the state may for practical purposes delegate it to an administrative agency acting as its functional agent. The use of the police power is not a matter of choice when it has been delegated to a governmental agency. The agency has a definite and legal responsibility to use it, but *is accountable for the manner in which it is used*. When the means for action are made available to him, the public officer responsible may be compelled to exercise the police power delegated to him if the public interest indicates such action. Failure to do so makes the public official guilty of malfeasance of office. However, although application of the police power may be indicated and demanded, the manner in which it is employed is usually left to the discretion of the administrative officer; that is, the public officer may select his own methods of enforcement, formulating rules, regulations, and standards as he deems necessary unless the statutes that made him responsible specifically prescribed the method of procedure.

The position of a public health officer in this regard, as related to the summary abatement of a nuisance, was well stated by the Iowa Supreme Court in a case‡ involving such action by a health department in enforcing an ordinance dealing with the improper and indiscriminate dumping of garbage. In upholding the action of the board of health the court stated that although nothing in the statute granted to the officers immunity from the consequences of unfair or oppressive acts, "the particular form of procedure prescribed may vary from the custom-

ary procedure, but essential rights are not violated by granting to the board the right, in an emergency, to proceed in the abatement of a nuisance detrimental to public health, and it is safe to say that most cases calling for action on the part of boards of health are matters requiring immediate action." Of perhaps greater significance, the court went on to say that even though the courts had not been uniform in their holdings, it believed that the weight of authority as well as reason and necessity prescribed that in cases involving the public health, in which prompt and efficient action was necessary, the state and its officers should not be subjected to the inevitable delays incident to a complete hearing before action could be taken.

The careful distinction between the power of inspection and the right of privacy has become increasingly important as a result of a ruling of the California District Court of Appeals.* The court held that the entry by a health inspector into a private residence for the purpose of a routine housing inspection at a reasonable time and on presentation of proper credentials was not a violation of the Fourth or Fourteenth Amendments of the United States Constitution. "The court reasoned that the ordinance in question was part of a general regulatory scheme which was civil in nature, limited in scope, and could not be exercised except under reasonable conditions." The court then defined the conditions in which privacy may be restrained. "In those areas of exercise of the police power where the chance of immediate tangible harm is present, such as in premises which might present fire or communicable disease hazards, the right of privacy most probably will be accorded only that constitutional protection that is given to property or economic rights. In intimate or personal activites not at all likely to cause immediate danger to life or limb, the right of privacy will approach the more protected constitutional position of freedom of expression."[20]

On appeal, however, the Supreme Court† held that administrative searches for housing violations are significant intrusions on the privacy and security of individuals—interests that are protected by the Fourth Amendment against arbitrary invasions by government officials and enforceable against the states

---

* Lawton v. Steele, 152 U.S. 133 (1893).

† Miami County v. Dayton, 92 O. S. 215.

‡ Iowa Supreme Court: State v. Strayer, 299 N.W. 912 (1941).

---

* Camara vs. San Francisco, 277 A.C.A. 136 (1965).

† 87 S. Ct. 1727 p. 1734 ff (1967).

under the Fourteenth Amendment. The court declared that such searches when authorized and conducted without a warrant procedure lack the traditional safeguards which the Fourth Amendment guarantees to the individual. This is true, the court added, whether the discovery of a violation on the initial inspection leads to a criminal conviction or results only in an administrative compliance order.

The court noted the following three significant reservations to its general holdings:

1. Nothing in the opinion is intended to foreclose prompt inspections, even without a warrant, that the law has traditionally upheld in emergency situations.

2. In the light of the Fourth Amendment's requirement that a warrant specify the property to be searched, "It seems likely that warrants should normally be sought only after entry is refused, unless there has been a citizen complaint or there is other satisfactory reason for securing immediate entry."

3. ". . . The requirement of a warrant procedure does not suggest any change in what seems to be the prevailing local policy in most situations, of authorizing entry, but not entry by force, to inspect."[21]

The right of a legislature to delegate rulemaking power to an administrative agency has been questioned many times, but only in one instance has such power been denied to a state or local board of health. This occurred in Wisconsin,* where it was held that the State Board of Health was simply an administrative agency and that no rule-making powers could constitutionally be delegated to it. On the other hand, the Ohio Supreme Court stated "that the legislature in the exercise of its constitutional authority may lawfully confer on boards of health the power to enact sanitary ordinances having the force of law within the district over which their jurisdiction extends, is not an open question."† The question was more or less settled by the United States Supreme Court, which held the following:

(1) That a State may, consistent with the Federal Constitution, delegate to a municipality authority to determine under what conditions health shall become operative.

(2) That the municipality may vest in its efficiency broad discretion in matters affecting the applicability and enforcement of a health law.

(3) That in the exercise of the police power reasonable classification may be freely applied and that regulation is not violative of the equal protection clause merely because it is not all-embracing.*

It is obvious and logical that a municipality or an administrative agency in dealing with questions concerning the public health, for example, can act only when it has been given specific authority for such actions and that the ordinances adopted by the legislative body of the municipality must not only be limited to the subject matter of the power delegated but also must not conflict with or attempt to set aside any provision of the Constitution, of the state law, or of any other sanitary regulations of the state. The same conditions apply to regulations adopted by local boards of health. They can apply only where the subject matter has been placed by law under the jurisdiction of the local board of health.

## POLICE POWER, ADMINISTRATIVE LAW, AND JUDICIAL PRESUMPTION

The delegation to administrative agencies and officers of the right and power to formulate rules, regulations, and standards to implement the intent of legislation has given rise to a relatively new and increasingly important branch of law and source of enforcement powers. It is unfortunate that in the public health profession there are still many who do not adequately realize the great administrative possibilities presented by sound administrative law.[22] There are many communities that although sometimes possessing adequate enabling legislation for various public health activities, have only limited control because of the failure of their health officials to make the rules, regulations, and standards necessary for the proper and adequate implementation of the statutes. By failing to establish a solid legal background based as much as possible on sound scientific criteria and standards, the public health official by his own neglect places himself, his department, and the community at an unnecessary and unwarranted disadvantage.

Even if existing legislation is adequate, something more is needed. The health official must "do his homework" thoroughly. As Grad[8] indicates, "Cases, particularly those to enforce environmental health regulations, are won or

---

* State v. Burdge, 95, Wis. 390, 70 N.W. 347 (1897).
† Exparte Co. 106 O.S. 50.

* Zucht v. King, 260 U. S. 174, 43 S. Ct. 24 (1922).

lost long before they get into court." Samples must be collected, labeled, analyzed, dated, and recorded properly, legally, and accurately. Photographs and dispositions should be obtained if pertinent and helpful. Witnesses should be found, and *facts* must be arranged and presented in a clear and orderly manner. In the discussion of the law of nuisances mention was made of the undesirable possibility of the public health official being in the position of pitting his mere opinion against that of the defendant. The court's only alternative in such a situation would be to express its own opinion regarding the desirability of the action rather than its legality. Ideally it is only the latter with which the courts are essentially concerned, and as much as possible it is preferable that they not have to make decisions regarding the sense or desirability of an action.

When a scientist, a health officer, or another expert is in a position to provide the court with definite regulations and standards based on scientific criteria or group judgment, especially if they have been drawn up with the idea of administering legal advice, the judge of the court is no longer in the somewhat embarrassing position of having to balance what amounts to the personal opinion of the plaintiff against that of the defendant and then being himself forced to make a decision by expressing his own personal opinion. The very existence of sound rules, regulations, and standards serves to pass the burden of proof from the administrative agent to the defendant in the case so that the judge can avoid conflict and save time and face by saying, for example, that the defendant has not presented evidence to show that the health officer did not fairly apply the rules, regulations, or standards that by virtue of their development are more or less accepted without question. Thus there has been established what is termed a *judicial presumption* in favor of the findings, conclusions, and recommendations of the enforcing administrative official.

To obtain the maximum amount of judicial presumption certain conditions are desirable and should be borne in mind. First, laws and ordinances should contain only broad principles with delegation of authority to the enforcing or administrative agency for the development of the necessary details. Second, such rules, regulations, and standards as may be indicated by the law or ordinance should be carefully formulated. Third, they should be based as much as possible on accepted scientific facts or au-

thoritative group judgments. Fourth, it is desirable that they be written with the aid of an administrative lawyer. Fifth, advantage should be taken of the opportunity presented in the process of making the rules, regulations, and standards to lay the foundation for their ready acceptance by the public and the courts of the community. This is meant to imply that the process presents an important opportunity for education and persuasion as well as democratic participation. If those who are to be affected are consulted in the writing of a regulation, they will develop in the process an understanding that is a first step toward voluntary cooperation, acceptance, and self-enforcement. At the same time the public health administrator is provided with an invaluable opportunity to determine in advance how far the community is willing to go.

## LICENSING

A related method of legal enforcement and control is found in the technique of licensing. The legality of the principle of licensing as a method of control and enforcement as well as a source of revenue to meet the cost of the administration of a law has been well established and accepted for a long while. However, intent and methods of licensing are constantly subject to questioning in the courts, as are all other methods of enforcement. Licenses may be granted or revoked under conditions imposed by public health authorities, provided that there is a statutory basis for the licensing and there is no oppressive, discriminatory, or arbitrary action involved in their application.

An example to illustrate the latter is that of a city board of health which voted that after a certain date no more milk distributor licenses would be granted to persons who were not residents of the city. * The plaintiff operated a well-qualified dairy 6 miles beyond the city limits and brought suit to compel the issuance of a license, charging that the regulation was discriminatory. The state law said, "Boards of health may grant licenses to sell milk to properly qualified persons." The court held that the word "may" in the state law should be construed as meaning "shall" so that a local board of health, existing by virtue of state law, had no alternative but to issue a license to any person who satisfied the sanitary requirements. More pertinent to the question at hand,

_____
* Whitney v. Watson, 85 N. H. 238, 157 A. 78 (1931).

it further held that the limitation on non-residents was unreasonable and arbitrary and that if it had been included in a law instead of a resolution it would have been ruled unconstitutional.

On several occasions, licensing has been found useful by health authorities in accomplishing a certain amount of indirect control and prevention of problems not obvious from the primary purpose of the licensing. Several communities, for instance, have found it necessary to institute the licensing of individuals engaged in certain personal service occupations such as masseurs and beauty parlor operators in an attempt to stop advertising by prostitutes operating under the guise of these occupations. This particular use has caused no difficulty, since the right of health departments to maintain sanitary control over individuals engaged in personal services to prevent the spread of communicable diseases has been well established.

However, when an ordinance requiring permits or licenses can be shown to have no public health basis, it will probably be considered an infringement of personal rights by the court and declared invalid. This is illustrated by the case* of a city board of health that passed a regulation providing that no person should engage in the business of undertaking unless he had been duly licensed as an embalmer by the board of health. The Massachusetts Supreme Court held the regulation unconstitutional and invalid, saying, "We can see no such connection between requiring all undertakers to be licensed embalmers and the promotion of the public health as to bring the making of this regulation by the board of registration in embalming or the refusal of a license by the board of health on account of the regulation within the exercise of the police power of the state."

## NECESSITY OF BASIC PUBLIC HEALTH LAWS

In a DeLamar lecture given in 1920, Freeman,[23] who was at that time Commissioner of Health of Ohio, said: "Every thoughtful sanitarian has in his mind the picture of that ideal system of health administration which would be founded on scientific principles, organized on the basis of administrative efficiency, and

manned by a staff of trained workers filled with the spirit of public service. This ideal organization would have behind it a volume of law which, while fully recognizing the principles of individual liberty, would permit no man to offend against the health of his neighbor." Although Freeman added with considerable justification, "However thoughtfully a proposed measure may be prepared by its framers, it has by the time it is enacted into law usually been so altered by ill-considered, hasty or prejudiced amendment as to have lost all semblance of its original form," there may be considered to advantage some of the fields of public health activity in which fundamental legislation is desirable or necessary. The first of these is concerned with the registration or reporting of births and deaths. It is conceded by all to be well-nigh impossible to carry out a public health program in the absence of basic information concerning the circumstances surrounding birth and death. In most parts of the United States it is the public health agency that is charged with the responsibility for assuring the collection of this information. To achieve this it is necessary that each state have the necessary legislation and administrative machinery dealing with mandatory reporting of these biologic events by those in the best position to submit such reports, the attendants at births and death. Related to this is the need for legislation requiring the reporting and control of cases of certain types of illnesses, especially those of a communicable nature. To accomplish this adequately requires careful and exact definition of certain terms such as cases, communicable, isolation, etc., and the listing of the morbid conditions to be included. In accord with what has been said elsewhere, such defining and listing is best accomplished by inclusion in the rules and regulations drawn up by the administrative agency rather than in the body of the statute, which should limit its concern to broad principles, responsibilities, and penalties. The desirability of this is particularly evident on considering the spectacular changes that have occurred in recent years in the areas of diagnosis, treatment, and social management of many of the communicable diseases. If details of reporting and control appear in the law, further scientific advances are certain to result either in the necessity of changing the law or allowing it to become hopelessly out of date.

In the field of food and milk control an

---

*Wyeth v. Cambridge Board of Health, 200 Mass. 474, 86 N.E. 295 (1909).

enormous, confusing, and frequently contradictory mass of legislation and regulation exists.
Undesirable as this situation undoubtedly is,
all will agree that certain types of legal control are necessary. It is obviously important
for a community to exercise some control over
those who produce and handle its food and
milk supplies.[24,25] This has been repeatedly
upheld in the courts. With reference to milk
the Connecticut Supreme Court explained in an
opinion, "The State may determine the standard
of quality, prohibit the production, sale, or distribution of milk not within the standard,
divide it into classes, and regulate the manner
of their use, so long as these standards, classes,
and regulatory provisions be neither unreasonable nor oppresive. The many recorded instances in which the courts have sustained
this power of regulation bear witness to the
liberality of their viewpoint where the public
health and safety are concerned."* Judicial
prejudice in favor of rules, regulations, and
standards dealing with the sanitary quality
of food and milk supplies has been extended
far beyond the actual product itself. It has long
been accepted as proper for the responsible
health authority to formulate rules, regulations,
and standards dealing with the sources of food
and milk, the health and sanitation practices of
all who come in contact with them, the sanitary
facilities provided such persons, and the sanitary nature of all machinery, instruments, or
utensils involved in their transfer from the
source to the ultimate consumer.

In the field of general sanitation, including
the sanitary problems involved in housing and
industry as well as the supervision of water
supplies, sewage disposal, and the like, basic
legislation is necessary to place responsibility
in the hands of the public health agency and
to give it such powers as are needed to activate
the intent of the law. Licensing of certain trades
and occupations has been mentioned briefly.
It is obvious that before such a procedure
can be put into effect the necessary legal
justification must be brought into existence.

Perhaps the most fundamental of all is enabling legislation for the establishment and
development of local work. It should go without
saying that a local area being ultimately subject
to the state must be granted the legal right to
establish official activity dealing with the public
health. The rapid expansion in recent years of

---

* Shelton v. City of Shelton, 111 Conn. 433 (1930).

local health work, especially on the county level,
has developed increasing interest in the proper
formulation of such enabling acts. In the first
national conference on local health units held
in 1946, Mustard[26] summarized the essentials
that should be included in enabling legislation
for local health work. These essentials are included here for their conciseness and inclusive-
ness and because they remain valid:

1. That this volume of law should provide assurance
   that there is a proper balance between local
   autonomy and state supervision.
2. That this volume of law should provide insurance
   that where a local unit of government is too
   small for effective public health administration,
   combinations of local jurisdictions may be made.
3. Insurance that health work locally will not be
   scattered among different elements of the local
   government.
4. Insurance that budgets for local health units be
   sufficient to meet at least a minimum in terms
   of funds, and to meet standards as to personnel.
5. No local jurisdiction will remain in want of
   health service, merely because of unfavorable
   financial position locally.
6. Supplementary to this insurance that even the
   poor areas will be included, there should be
   insurance that there will be adequate state aid.
7. Insurance that the whole state system of local
   health units will not be jeopardized by local
   option.

The actual procedure followed in the enactment of legislation is essentially the same on the
national and state levels of government. Basically there are fifteen steps involved, but they
really boil down to the following: (1) a first and
second reading by title, then referred to a committee (or subcommittee), which may or may
not hold hearings; (2) the bill is placed on the
calendar of the entire chamber for a third reading and debate; and (3) if passed, it then goes
through the same process in the other chamber,
and if passed, it goes to the chief of state for
signature. If he vetos it, a two thirds vote over-
rides the veto.[27]

## WRITING AND PASSAGE OF LAWS AND REGULATIONS

In a discussion of court actions Tobey[28]
stated:

These cases also demonstrate that the actions of
public health authorities must be conducted in a
strictly legal manner, with due guarantee of the
constitutional rights of individual citizens and the
people as a whole. If regulations or procedures are
defective, the courts have no choice but to uphold

the law as it should be, and this they will do despite their willingness to support all reasonable public health measures. Public health officials must bear in mind that prevention applies to law as well as to sanitary science, and they should see to it that legislation and law enforcement comply with adjudicated standards and modern jurisprudence.

More recently Curran[29] also expressed concern about the inadequate attention given to the development of regulations by public health workers. He pinpointed three areas of weakness in most health departments: (1) the departments' ongoing programs tend to operate ahead of the regulations; that is, the regulations have not yet caught up with what the department is actually doing; (2) the current regulations are too broadly worded to be used effectively; and (3) regulations are often based on model codes or the regulations of some other health department without sufficient regard for local conditions.

In accord with this it might be well to consider briefly a few practical considerations with regard to the proper formulation of laws and regulations. Before doing so, it is worth repeating at least two important legislative handicaps to effective administration.[30] The first is that in the formulation and passage of statutes legislatures often attempt to do too much by writing into the law itself excessive detail with regard to administrative responsibilities, organization, itemized appropriations, and procedure. In at least one state, for example, the salaries of the state health officer and others are specifically limited in the state constitution, ignoring economic changes, competition for good administrative personnel, and progress in general. As a result, this particular state, during a period of high living costs and generally increased salaries, finds itself unable to obtain or hold qualified personnel for the administration of its public health program. The thought comes to mind that in the sound administration of a private corporation the board of directors, being somewhat analogous to a legislature, does not attempt to decide on details of procedure, operation, and the like.

The second legislative handicap is the sacrificing of long-term considerations to immediate, local, or personal advantage. It is possible to find many examples of this in the field of public health. In more than one place, legislation and appropriation has been passed, supposedly for the control of tuberculosis or syphilis, but have emphasized the care of the chronic cases

and ignored the all-important factor of early case finding and control of the early infectious phase in the individual. The logical solution to these handicaps may be found in the passage of legislation that considers general policy and leaves the details of procedure and operation to whatever administrative agency the legislature may see fit to hold responsible. This, of course, requires that administrative agencies assume their full responsibility in carrying out the intent of the statutes by adequately and effectively formulating and enforcing whatever rules, regulations, and standards are indicated.

It is customary in the United States for responsibility for the public health to be vested in a board of health that is directed to employ as its agent a health officer and whatever other personnel are needed to carry out its policies. It is much better that rules, regulations, and standards be passed by someone other than the enforcement officer. The public then believes that it is being treated more fairly and that the enforcement officer is not grinding his own axe. In turn the health officer is relieved of the onus of enforcing his own regulations and the risk of repeated personal liability. This alone presents an important justification for the interposing of boards of health between the legislative body and the functioning agency. With these words of introduction the following suggestions are made concerning the formulation of rules and regulations by public health agencies:

1. First is the necessity that they be promulgated by a board of health or whatever other administrative agency in which this authority and responsibility is vested. Furthermore, the agency must have been properly created and legally existing in the eyes of the legislature. If any of its members have been improperly chosen, elected, or appointed, the entire board does not legally exist and all of its actions are considered invalid.

2. The actions of the board must arise by virtue of power and responsibility that has been expressly or impliedly delegated to it by the state legislature.

3. The pronouncements of the board must relate and be limited to its legal jurisdiction and not infringe upon the jurisdiction of another agency or another governmental entity.

4. The rules and regulations must not conflict with the Constitution and laws of the United States or with the constitution and laws of the state of which the agency is a part.

5. The rules and regulations must be reasonable and no more drastic than is necessary.

6. All rules, regulations, and standards must be adopted by a legally constituted board of health

legally convened in an official session. No individual member of a board has power to enact a regulation any more than an individual Congressman has power to enact a statute. Final enactment can result only by a vote at a properly called meeting of the board, notice of which has been given to each of the members of the board and at which a quorum is present. To attempt to act on a regulation by means of telephoning or visiting the office or home of each member individually does not constitute action by a legally convened meeting of the board.

7. Since a board of health regulation is in effect a law, it follows that the same care should be exercised in its formation as is exercised in drawing up a state or federal statute. The first consideration in this regard is proper form (including a title and enacting clause), a series of consecutively numbered articles each related to one subject, a statement concerning the time when the regulation is to become effective, and a statement of penalties involved in instances of proved infraction.

8. The ordinance or regulation must be precise, consistent, definite, and certain in its expression and meaning. The present tense should be used. It should be written for the public and especially for those who will be affected by it. Complicated, high-sounding phrases should be avoided, punctuation used sparingly, and parenthesis almost never used. Foreign or technical terms should be avoided if possible. It has been said that there can be a lawsuit for each extraneous or ill-chosen word and for every ill-advised punctuation.

9. If the legislature prescribes the manner in which regulations and ordinances should be passed, such prescription must be exactly adhered to. If, for example, it is specified in the state law that a proposed ordinance be read and voted on favorably at three successive meetings of a legally constituted and convened board, this cannot be fulfilled as has been sometimes attempted by having the clerk stand and read the ordinance and call for a vote three times during the same meeting.

10. The ordinance or regulation must be enacted in good faith and in the public interest alone and designed to enable the board of health to carry out its legal responsibilities. It should therefore be impartial and nondiscriminatory, applying to all members of the community.

11. In some states it is necessary that actions of boards of health be approved by the attorney general of the state.

12. On legal passage the final step is proper and adequate publication of the rule or ordinance in order that those who are to affected by it shall have ample opportunity to be informed concerning it. This is usually carried out by means of publishing in the local newspapers.

Concerning this last requisite, Gellhorn[22] makes the following comment: "Regarding publication of administrative legislation the situation, especially in the states, is confusing almost to the extreme and eventual reform is certain to be demanded as a result of this disregard of the public interest in knowing what rules and orders they are subject to. Such lack of adequate publication has undoubtedly led to judicial hostility toward delegated legislation and authority."

A final caution might be given concerning frequent practice of adopting or incorporation of rules and regulations by reference. This procedure has the enticement of being convenient and easy but may give rise to legal difficulties in that only existing things can be legally incorporated by reference. Therefore each time the original regulation or law is changed, it is necessary to reincorporate by reference. Furthermore, it is legally impossible, although it is sometimes attempted, to adopt or incorporate a subject by reference on a blanket basis through time because such action amounts to committing the public to regulations that are not yet in existence. It is comparable to asking the public to sign a blank check.

This is not meant to condemn the technique of reference entirely, since its convenience amply justifies its use. However, it should be used with full knowledge of its limitations and potential disadvantages, some of which are illustrated by the case* of a board of health that adopted a regulation dealing with the sale of milk and milk products in accordance with the unabridged form of the 1939 edition of the United States Public Health Service Milk Ordinance. The publication of the new regulation did not contain the ordinance but stated that a certified copy was on file in the office of the board of health. The Ohio Supreme Court in ruling on the case of a defendant charged with violating the regulation, stated: "The effectiveness of legislation by reference has been so generally recognized . . . that no very specific declaration appears in the reported cases." The court added, however, that "no by-law or ordinance, or section thereof, shall be revived or amended unless the new by-law or ordinance contains the entire by-law or ordinance, or section revived or amended, and the by-law or ordinance, section or sections so amended shall be repealed." As long as there was no violation of this section, the court said that it saw no objection to the incorporation by reference in a

---

*Ohio Supreme Court: State v. Waller, 55 N. E. 2nd 654 (1944).

regulation of a district board of health on a duly enacted statute, or a duly enacted ordinance that has been theretofore properly published. However, the Ohio Supreme Court was of the view that the publication of a board of health regulation, which omitted the rules of conduct to be observed and merely referred those who might be affected to a copy of the terms on file in the office of the board of health, did not constitute proper publication as meant by the law and that until proper publication had been made any such regulation was not effective.

## LIABILITY AND AGENCY[5]

To acomplish a desired purpose such as the completion of a contract or the rendering of a public service, practicality usually makes it necessary that the one (the principal) who is legally responsible for fulfilling the contract or for rendering the public service obtain an agent or agents to carry out the details involved. This relationship between a principal and his agents gives rise to an additional series of legal complications, especially in terms of those things for which the principal is liable and those for which the agent is liable. In public health work the citizens of a community as represented by their legally designated board of health may be considered the principal, whereas the health officer acts as the agent of the people and is responsible to the board.

The view has been held repeatedly by the courts, as illustrated by two cases* in which the courts observed that the authority for the appointment of a city health commissioner was precisely the same as that for the appointment of nurses and other employees and that the health commissioner was not a public officer but an employee under the direction, supervision and control of the board of health.

The fundamental rule governing the relationship of principal to agent is that the principal is liable for contractual agreements or other acts of an agent, provided that the agent has acted within the real or apparent scope of his authority. It should be noted from this that the principal is not vested with a blanket liability for all contracts or all acts that might be carried out in his name but is liable only for those acts for which the agent has been given power by him. The most important and difficult

problem is to define or determine the meaning and extent of the agent's real and apparent authority and power.

The powers of an agent have been divided into real and apparent. An agent's real power consists of the authority expressly or impliedly delegated to him by the principal. Expressed powers are given usually in the form of actual and explicit instructions. Thus a board of health may instruct a health officer to control the spread through the community of a communicable disease.

Added to this expressed authority, the agent also has certain implied powers to find it possible to do whatever is reasonably necessary to carry out the instructions given. The health officer, therefore, on being instructed to control the spread of communicable disease, may correctly assume the implied power and authority to include whatever administrative procedures are reasonably indicated, for example, quarantine, contact examination, etc., to accomplish the responsibility given him in relation to the expressed powers.

Over and above his real authority, expressed or implied, the agent has certain so-called apparent powers. In the use of these the agent really exceeds his actual power, and he would be considered liable in many instances were it not for the concept that other persons under certain circumstances are correct in believing that the agent has power to act. The use of apparent power is involved in major part in the solution of individual problems, each with its own peculiar circumstances, and the test of its correct use is the determination of whether or not a reasonably prudent person in similar circumstances would have been justified in acting as did the agent on the behalf of his principal. This may be illustrated by the case of a health officer* who in the face of a smallpox outbreak hospitalized an individual erroneously considered to have smallpox, with the result that the patient became infected with smallpox while in the isolation hospital. The erroneous diagnosis having been made in good faith by the attending private physician and similarly confirmed by the health department diagnostician after exercising due and customary care and judgment, neither the private physician nor the community through its authorized

---

* Ohio Supreme Court: Scofield v. Strain, Mayor, et al., State ex rel.; Reilly v. Hamrock, Mayor, et al., 51 N. E. 2nd 1012 (1943).

* Dillon's Municipal Corporations 771, as quoted by Tobey.[5]

public health agents were held liable. As the court stated, "To hold otherwise would not only invite indifference at the expense of society, but the fear of liability would well-nigh destroy the efforts of officials to protect the public health."

This emphasizes that an agent owes to his principal the exercise of a degree of care and skill which a reasonably qualified and prudent person in terms of the community involved at the time would be expected to exercise under similar circumstances. Therefore the professional agent, in this case a health officer, owes to his principal (the community) the exercise of a reasonable degree of care and skill as judged by the time and place. It should be noted that except where a contract exists to the contrary, no guarantee is involved that a certain result will be effected. All that is required by the law is the exercise of that degree of skill, knowledge, and care usually displayed by similar members of the profession under similar circumstances.

In the absence of malice or corruption or a statutory provision imposing the liability, health officers generally are not liable for errors or mistakes in judgment in the performance of acts within the scope of their authority where they are empowered to exercise judgment and discretion. Personal liability therefore depends on proof of bad faith, which "may be shown by evidence that official action was so arbitrary and unreasonable that it could not have been taken in good faith."[31] Although obviously difficult to ascertain, bad faith has been demonstrated to the satisfaction of the courts, as in the case* of a smallpox patient who was forcibly transferred from her home to a dirty, insanitary cabin, for which action a health officer was understandably held liable.

It logically follows, however, that if reasonable and legal instructions have been given to an agent by his principal, it is the agent's duty to obey them or think that he knows a better way in which to accomplish the purpose desired. In such an instance should the agent willfully disobey the principal's instructions or laws, and injury or any other undesirable result follow, the agent is liable for whatever damage have been sustained as a result of his disobedience.

With regard to liability of the principal if it is a government, it must first be reemphasized that the state is sovereign and, as such, cannot be sued or held liable by its individual citizens except where it grants permission. Since county governments are essentially local administrative and political units of the sovereign state, the same rule tends to be applied to them. However, there is an increasing tendency on the part of states to allow counties to be sued and to hold them liable whenever there is question or doubt. Municipalities are somewhat different in that they are corporations carrying on various functions and services. Some of these functions, for example, the operation of a transportation system or a water works, are considered private, and the city may be sued concerning them; however, other functions and services such as the maintenance of police and fire departments are public functions, and concerning these the city cannot be readily sued. Public health activities fall into this category. Some states have been highly specific in this regard, as evidenced by a Michigan Supreme Court decision that said, "The matter of public health is not local; it concerns the State. In matters relating to public health the city acts as an arm of the State, and the property whose use is devoted to the public health is used in the discharge of a governmental function."*

## EXTENT OF USE OF LAW IN PUBLIC HEALTH

Seen in its proper relationship, legal enforcement represents only one of several ways by which an administrator acting as an agent of the community may bring about desirable results and effect conformity to the socially desired standards of the community. In effect, the administrator has three main tools or methods of approach at his disposal—education, persuasion, and coercion—and the extent to which he successfully blends and balances them is one of the best measures of true administrative ability. As Tobey[5] has warned, "A health officer who is constantly involved in court actions, either as plaintiff or prosecutor or as defendant, would hardly be classed as an efficient public officer since he should be able to administer the public health of his community or State and enforce the public health laws in the great majority of cases by means of persuasion and education and by suitable action

---

*Moody v. Wickersham, 111 Kan. 770 (1922).

*Michigan Supreme Court: Curry v. City of Highland Park et al., 219 N. W. 745 (1928).

before the board of health." The efficient and reasonable health officer must be ready to recognize sincere and honest attempts to meet the standards set up by society when such attempts are within the range of social tolerance, and he must be able to explain the tolerance point to the average citizen, the legislature, and the courts. On the other hand:

Many of the most important achievements of public health have had the support of laws and ordinances requiring conformity to specified sanitary standards. Without this support movements for the extension of public health work would have evolved more slowly and would still be far from their present state of development. Informed public opinion would have brought about great improvement, but more slowly. The coercive power must, therefore, be considered a powerful factor in the development of effective public health work, but it has definite limitations.[32]

The early history of public health in America might be characterized by almost complete dependence on legislation and its enforcement.

During the past generation the student of public health has witnessed a rapid shift in emphasis away from the doctrine of direct control toward that of education. This change has been due in no sense to the failure of the regulatory theory but rather to the broadening scope of public health that now includes problems of personal hygiene. . . . Even the exercise of the regulatory authority must rest on education, for an uniformed legislative body will not enact proper laws or appropriate funds for their enforcement, and an uninformed public will not tolerate regulations it does not understand or appreciate.[32]

In most instances, social legislation is framed by persons who are somewhat more advanced in their social thinking than is the average citizen. Only relatively recently has the realization come about that legislation dealing with social concepts that are too far ahead of the citizenry as a whole is almost inevitably doomed to failure.. Many tragic examples of this nature may be found in the history of public health; one of the best known is the fate of the General Board of Health of England, established in 1848, which failed as a result of overenthusiasm due to Edwin Chadwick's social thinking and planning, which was too far ahead of the people of England at the time. At least one local health officer in America was literally tarred and feathered because of his persistent attempts to institute complete pasteurization of milk when the strongly opinionated citizens of his area were not intellectually prepared or ready for it.

As a result of the relatively recent realization that social progress of all types must be based on an understanding and acceptance by the majority of those involved, leaders in the field of public health administration have turned increasingly toward emphasis on educational and persuasive action, minimizing the legal and enforcement approach. Boyd[33] pointed out that permissive legislation for the establishment of local health units in Illinois existed for 25 years, but as a result of the legislation alone, only 6 county health departments came into being. As a result of subsequent public educational methods, however, the citizens in most parts of the state expressed their desire for local health departments with almost no opposition. The place of legal enforcement in present-day public health activity has been well stated by Lade[34] in discussing the control of venereal disease:

Now compulsion is not the only recourse in these cases—not even the first recourse. A substantial number of contacts resistant to examination and patients delinquent from treatment will respond to information, reassurance, persuasion, or assistance when unable to pay for examination or treatment. Indeed, the extent to which these measures are successful is to a degree a measure of the efficiency of a health department, and a demonstration of the superiority of our democratic government over a dictatorship. But there will always be a residue of cases resistant to all of these measures who are the kernel of the venereal disease problem. Here a show of force is frequently all that is necessary. Nevertheless, behind the facade there must be a solid structure of duly constituted authority, lest we have government by the whim of officialdom. Hence, law is necessary as an expression of sound medicolegal thinking in a problem which concerns all the people.

Obviously a balance is necessary. No single approach meets all situations, and not infrequently firm action must be taken. Curran[35] recently took health professionals to task in words worth careful attention: "Professionals in the health field have traditionally downgraded the use of legal sanctions. They have preferred to achieve their goals of better health for the American people through education. . . . Many professional public health people have forgotten that their basic responsibility is to protect and to improve the health of the masses of people and to use all effective public means to achieve it." Then in noting an increasing legal activist role of health workers in company with the poor and with consumer groups, he adds, "In the future, we may look for greater participation in this field by 'traditional' health professionals and their 'traditional' professional organizations. Otherwise," he warns, "this will be another growing number of health fields taken our of the hands of the old-line health groups."

## COURT PROCEDURE

Since despite all wishes to the contrary every active health officer will sooner or later find himself in court, it may be well to include a few words concerning court procedure. When court action appears to be necessary, all other efforts for the conformance to social standards and for the enforcement of a law or ordinance relating to them having failed, the first step is to bring charges against the offender. The party who initiates the action is called in law the plaintiff and in equity the complainant. The individual against whom action is brought is known as the defendant in both law and equity. In bringing charges against the defendant, the first step is to determine which court has jurisdiction. The same action may be interpreted as constituting any one of several different criminal acts, depending on the intent, the circumstances, the existing laws, and the consequences. Thus to give dangerous, contaminated material to an individual is considered an assault, to make it available to the public at large results in a criminal nuisance, and if sent through the mails, it is a breach of the postal regulations. The first two offenses are crimes under the common law or statutes of a state; the third offense is a crime under the acts of the Congress of the United States. As pointed out previously, violations of public health laws or regulations usually are considered misdemeanors. In any case infractions of these laws constitute a criminal act so that the case is within the jurisdiction of a criminal court such as a police court.

The plaintiff then files with the court a complaint (sometimes referred to as declaration, information, petition, bill, or statement of claim) that he has drawn up himself or preferably with the aid of a municipal, county, or state attorney. This should consist of a detailed statement by, for example, the health officer of the facts and circumstances leading up to the controversy and including the terms of any regulation or ordinance violated, the plaintiff expecting to prove the facts and circumstances beyond reasonable doubt in court with the aid of

creditable witnesses to obtain a favorable judgment. The magistrate of the court then issues a summons ordering the defendant to appear in the particular court on a certain stated day and hour, and the summons is served in person to the defendant by an officer of the court. The purpose of the summons is to give actual written notice to the defendant that legal action has been instituted against him. Its personal service is essential, since a court is powerless to render a judgment against a defendant who has not been so notified. Each individual is entitled to his day in court to have the opportunity to bring out whatever defense he may find possible. The defendant now has a choice of six procedures:

1. He may ignore the proceedings, placing himself in default and inviting judgment against himself.

2. He may confess to the accusation of the plaintiff and again invite a judgment against himself.

3. He may enter a plea in abatement, questioning whether the court has power or jurisdiction to act against him and whether proper procedure has been followed.

4. He may file a demurrer, stating in effect that although he admits the truth of what the plaintiff states as a matter of law, the facts do not entitle him to recover.

5. He may file an answer or a plea consisting of a denial of the facts stated in the plaintiff's declaration.

6. Again the defendant may admit the facts brought out by the plaintiff but bring out still other facts in avoidance or in excuse of those alleged by the plaintiff. Pleading continues until one side denies the facts claimed by the other, thereby raising an issue calling for a decision and the case is then ready to go to trial.

Most public health legal controversies do not take place before a jury, although either side is entitled to a trial by jury if it so wishes. The first step in such instances is the impaneling of a jury, consisting of the calling of prospective jurors from an approved list and questioning them individually concerning prejudices for or against either litigant. The function of the jury is to decide questions of fact, in contrast to the judge's function of deciding questions of law. When the court proceeding gets under way, counsel for each side may make an opening statement that explains briefly what he expects to prove. After this each side introduces its evidence.

All offenses consist of two factors, that is, the criminal act and the criminal intent, and both must be proved beyond reasonable doubt to demonstrate the commission of a crime. A criminal act is an action or omission that the law forbids. To be considered criminal the act must be defined by a law or regulation forbidding its commission. The rule of law is strictly interpreted in favor of the accused so that the act is not considered criminal unless it corresponds exactly with the definition contained in the law. The criminal intent is the state of mind of the accused at the time when the criminal act was committed. It involves a conscious recognition of the unlawful nature of the act, followed by a determination to perform the act. The courts presume the existence of criminal intent on the basis of the actual commission of the act, and it is usually unnecessary to produce evidence of criminal intent unless the accused attempts to prove that at the time the criminal act was committed he was incapable of determining or understanding its nature and unlawfulness or that the act was involuntary. Such proof must be based on (1) youth, (2) insanity, (3) mistake of fact, (4) accident, (5) necessity, or (6) compulsion. If he is able to do so to the satisfaction of the court, although the commission of a criminal act is recognized, the proved lack of criminal intent causes the court to consider that he did not perpetrate a crime and he will be declared innocent.

When all evidence has been brought forth, the judge instructs the jury concerning the law involved in the issues raised, and the jury then retires to decide on a verdict. When the jury renders its verdict but before the court pronounces judgment, the losing party may make a motion for a new trial. This may be granted if the court believes that there has been made an erroneous ruling concerning the admission or rejection of evidence, if an erroneous instruction has been given to the jury, or if the verdict is obviously contrary to the weight of the evidence given. If the motion for a new trial is refused, the court renders its judgment. If the losing party still believes that there was a substantial error in the conduct of the trial, he may thereupon take the case on appeal to a superior court of appeal, in which case he is termed the *appellant* and the other side is the *appellee*. The court of review or appeal is exactly what its name implies, since it does not conduct a new trial. It simply considers the record of the proceeding that took place before the inferior trial court, the exceptions taken to ruling of the trial judge with regard to procedure, pleading, admission of evidence, instructions, etc. If the court of review or appeals decides that a substantial error prejudicial to the losing side was made by the lower trial court, the judgment of the lower court is reversed, and the case is remanded for a new trial.

## EXPERT WITNESS [36]

Occasionally the public health worker takes part in a court proceeding, not as a plaintiff or defendant but as an expert witness for either side or for the court itself. Whereas ordinary witnesses are restricted in their testimony to exact statement of facts, expert witnesses are called on to give opinion testimony. Before being considered an expert witness, evidence of competency must be presented to the satisfaction of both sides. In general any licensed physician is considered to qualify as an expert witness in controversies dealing with medical questions. Specialization is not necessary, and the expert witness may give an opinion even if he never before saw either litigant and even if he never before observed a similar case. Expert witnesses are customarily compensated for their services, but compensation can never be contingent on the winning of the suit by the side for whom the individual appears as a witness.

Courts in general tend to be suspicious of any opinion or expert testimony, and its acceptance by the court depends largely on the manner in which it is given.[37] With this in mind the expert witness should prepare himself well for whatever questions he might anticipate will be presented to him. He should be serious and unassuming and present an attitude of wanting to assist an intelligent jury in their rendering of a verdict by offering whatever special knowledge he may possess. The expert witness should be free of partiality and bias, frankly and honestly admitting a fact even if it injures the side that employed him as a witness and honestly admitting lack of knowledge on a particular item if he does not have it. He should listen carefully to all questions and answer clearly, directly, and concisely in language understandable to the jury (with a simple yes or no whenever possible). The wise witness never volunteers information when on the stand, assuming that, if significant, counsel will bring it out. Perhaps the most fatal mistake that might be made by an expert witness or any witness for that matter is to allow himself to be successfully prodded into losing his temper.

Finally, health workers would do well to heed the dictum of the famous French expert in forensic medicine: "If the law has made you a witness, remain a man of science; you have no victim to avenge, no guilty or innocent person to save."

## REFERENCES

1. Grad, F. P.: Public health law manual, Washington, D. C., 1970, American Public Health Association.
2. Freund, P. A.: The legal profession. In Lynn, K. S.: The professions in America, Boston, 1965, Houghton Mifflin Co.
3. Clute, K. E.: Law and health, some current challenges, Milbank Mem. Fund Quart. **50:**7, Jan. 1972.
4. Curran, W. J.: Public health lawyers, Amer. J. Public Health **59:**854, May 1969.
5. Tobey, J. A.: Public health law, New York, 1947, Commonwealth Fund.
6. Report of Conference of Directors of Schools of Public Health, WHO Tech. Rep. Series no., 351, Geneva, 1967, World Health Organization.
7. Hamlin, R. H.: Public health law, or the interrelationship of law and public health administration, Amer. J. Public Health **51:**1733, Nov. 1961.
8. Grad, F. P.: An effective legal enforcement program, Amer. J. Public Health **59:**947 June 1969.
9. Gray, J. C.: The nature and sources of law, New York, 1909, Columbia University Press.
10. Cardoza, B. N.: The nature of the judicial process, New Haven, 1921, Yale University Press.
11. Blackstone, W.: In Lewis, W. D., editor: Commentaries, Philadelphia, 1897, Rees, Welsh & Co.
12. Wilson, W.: The state, elements of historical and practical politics, Boston, 1918, D. C. Heath & Co.
13. Gurvitch, G.: Sociology of law, New York, 1942, Alliance Book Corporation.
14. Cardoza, B. N.: The growth of law, New Haven, 1942, Yale University Press.
15. Seagle, W.: The quest for law, New York, 1941, Alfred A. Knopf, Inc.
16. Holmes, O. W.: The common law, Boston, 1881, Little, Brown & Co.
17. Kent's Commentaries, Lecture 21.
18. Ascher, C. S.: The regulation of housing, Amer. J. Public Health **37:**507, May 1947.
19. Freund, E.: The police power, Chicago, 1904, Callahan.
20. Forgotson, E. H.: 1965: the turning point in health law—1966 reflections, Amer. J. Public Health **57:**934, June 1967.
21. Edelman, S.: Search warrants and sanitation inspections—the new look in enforcement, Amer. J. Public Health **58:**930, May 1968.
22. Gellhorn, W.: Administrative law—cases and comments, Chicago, 1940, Foundation Press, Inc.
23. Freeman, A. W.: Public health administration in Ohio, DeLamar Lectures, Johns Hopkins University School of Hygiene and Public Health, Baltimore, 1921, The Williams & Wilkins Co.
24. Tobey, J. A.: Legal aspects of milk control, Washington, D. C., 1924, Reprint 939, U. S. Public Health Service.
25. The legal phases of milk control, Washington, D. C., 1929, Reprint 1343, U. S. Public Health Service.
26. Mustard, H. S.: Legal aspects of planning for local health units, Amer. J. Public Health **37** (supp.):20, Jan. 1947.
27. Fischer, J.: How our laws are made, Washington, D. C., 1971, Government Printing Office.
28. Tobey, J. A.: Recent court decisions on milk control, Washington, D. C., 1933, Reprint 1555, U. S. Public Health Service.
29. Curran, W. J.: The preparation of state and local health regulations, Amer. J. Public Health **49:**314, March 1959.
30. White, L. D.: New horizons in public administration, Tuscaloosa, 1945, University of Alabama Press.
31. Kirk v. Aiken Board of Health, 83 S. C. 372 (1909).
32. Anderson, G. W.: In Graham, G. A., and Reining, H., editors: Regulatory administration, New York, 1943, John Wiley & Sons, Inc.
33. Boyd, R. F.: Legal aspects (of local health units) from viewpoint of a state health department, Amer. J. Public Health **37**(supp.):31, Jan. 1947.
34. Lade, J. H.: The legal basis for venereal disease control, Amer. J. Public Health **35:**1041, Oct. 1945.
35. Curran, W. J.: Making new health law: "sue the bastards," Amer. J. Public Health **60:**2016, Oct. 1970.
36. Curran, W. J.: The doctor as a witness, Philadelphia, 1965, W. B. Saunders Co.
37. Association of the Bar of the City of New York: Impartial medical testimony, New York, 1956, The Macmillan Co.

# PART FOUR

# Management of public health programs

The knowledge and abilities expected in modern public health work are many and varied. Ordinarily the basic professional training prepares for only a small part of the duties required. Society and its health problems have become increasingly so complex that the functions of the health officer and of many of his staff are now primarily those of public administrators and only secondarily related to their original professions.

A department of health is a public agency created to perform several types of public tasks. Like most other public agencies its functions may be categorized as (1) provision of health leadership in the community; (2) service, for example, the operation of a tuberculosis clinic or of a laboratory; (3) control of certain human activities, for example, the isolation of communicable disease cases or supervision of food and industrial establishments; (4) education of the public concerning healthful behavioral patterns, for example, immunization, diet, and proper care of infants; and (5) guardianship, for example, the collection and safeguarding of certain public records, especially those relating to birth, illness, and death.

To perform these functions successfully requires the adequate application of all facets of administrative practice. Gulick[1] invented the acronym *posdcorb* to indicate the component functions or activities involved in administration. The meaning of this word is as follows:

Planning what needs to be done
Organizing the structure of the agency
Staffing the agency
Directing the work of the agency and making decisions relating thereto
Coordinating all staff activities
Reporting to the executive and through him to those to whom he is responsible
Budgeting and all other aspects of fiscal management and control

In a similar sense Litchfield[2] characterized the administrative process as a cycle that includes (1) decision making, (2) programming, (3) communicating, (4) controlling, and (5) reappraising.

Much progress has been made in the art and science of administration during recent decades. Public health organizations have contributed to and benefited from these changes significantly. In a relatively brief period of time a considerable amount of long-range planning has been done in public health. Of particular importance was the passage of the Comprehensive Health Planning Act, the Regional

Medical Programs Act, and other laws and their subsequent amendments. With regard to structural organization there is much interest and activity in the consolidation of public health agencies and the integration of internal administrative responsibility. This has brought about a new interpretation of the function of executive personnel of health agencies. In the field of agency staffing there have been developed new and more effective techniques of job classification and examination of prospective employees, increasing adoption of merit systems, and pre-service and in-service training programs. This has resulted in a notable decline in political patronage and an increasing employment of professionally qualified individuals for executive and technical positions.

The internal organization of many agencies has undergone constant experimental change, and administrative analysts, functioning first as consultants and later as employees of health agencies, have accelerated the development and acceptance of greatly improved procedures. These changes have also brought about better coordination of staff activities within organizations and, in addition, have resulted in greatly expanded interagency coordination. This incidentally has been one of the many factors involved in the expansion of national administrative power and influence at the expense of the states, and of the states at the expense of the local governmental units. During this same period, there has come about a more practical attitude toward the establishment and use of budgetary procedures. Administrative and service functions of health departments have expanded greatly. In this category are included responsibility for standards, construction, supervision, and sometimes operation of various types of health-related facilities. There has been a steady shift away from law enforcement by court action to law enforcement by administrative regulation, with further concurrent shift away from the use of laws and regulations for health promotion to the educational approach wherever possible. Each of these many factors has placed increasing burdens on public health officials and has forced them to adopt a broader view of their responsibilities and functions. The important developments in this field have led to an emphasis on pre-service and in-service training in the various aspects of administration by schools of public health, health agencies, and professional associations. These fundamentally important organizational, personnel, fiscal, planning, evaluative, and public relational aspects of public health work are discussed in this section.

### REFERENCES

1. Gulick, L.: Notes on the theory of organization. In Gulick, L., and Urwick, L., editors: Papers on the science of administration, New York, 1937, Institute of Public Administration.
2. Litchfield, E. H.: Notes on a general theory of administration, Admin. Sci. Quart. **1:**12, June 1956.

*In good administration, every decision should
be made at the lowest possible level of command.
Otherwise, there is little or no use for the
creation of a pyramid of organization.*

LENT D. UPSON

CHAPTER 10

# Principles of organization

## PURPOSES OF ORGANIZATION

The field of administration consists essentially of two parts: (1) organization, which deals with the internal structure and the disposition of the personnel and other resources of the agency, and (2) management, which is concerned with the direction of the personnel, fiscal control, and other techniques related to operation. It is the former that is of concern at this point. Subsequent chapters will discuss the various phases of management. Some overlapping, however, is unavoidable. Generally speaking, the aim of organization is to arrange people into working groups, associating those with similar functions or purposes to more efficiently obtain a desired result from their group action. Gaus, White, and Dimock[1] state this in more detail, "Organization is the arrangement of personnel for facilitating the accomplishment of some agreed upon purpose through the allocation of function and responsibilities. It is the relating of the efforts and capacities of individuals and groups engaged upon a common task in such a way as to secure the desired objective with the least friction and with the most satisfaction for those for whom the task is done and those engaged in the enterprise." Although illustrating the difference between organization and management, this definition also points out the relationship between the two, indicating that organization consists of more than the placement of groups of personnel as if they were building blocks. The process of organization, by virtue of the nature of those involved, is forced to consider personalities to a certain degree. However, the extent to which this is allowed should best be limited as much as possible. It should be remembered that in the long run the organization is expected to outlast any individual in it and accordingly, it is better to fit the personnel to a sound structure rather than to sacrifice sound structure to individual whims of personality.

## GENERAL PRINCIPLES OF ORGANIZATION

In launching an organization there are certain basic questions that must be asked by the person who finds himself in the responsible executive position: What is expected of him? In what direction are he and the organization headed? What is the logical order of initiating activities? There is likely to be great temptation to try to develop simultaneously on all fronts. To avoid this requires self-control, careful and continuous analysis, a sense of timing and strategy, patience, and deliberateness. Unless this is done, the executive soon finds himself and his organization involved in a confusing, meaningless series of uncoordinated moves.

The steps involved in the development of an organization or a program have been well and succinctly described by Dimock[2] as follows:

First, you must know what the job of your agency is—if in business what the product and the market are to be; if in government, what the statutory authority and the executive mandate indicate. Second, you must select and appoint at least two or three key men to your staff so that the organization may begin to unfold. You can now formulate your plans somewhat more in detail because you have additional principle power on which to draw. Third, recognizing

**185**

the size of the task, you interpret your plans into financial terms which means budget and work planning. You can now begin to fill in the gaps in your organization with the necessary personnel, thus continuing the biological process of cell division already started when you picked your right hand man. And finally, you must prepare to expand, to gear your enterprise in such a way that you can take on new functions, new activities and emphasis without losing your stride.

Many executives of new organizations feel themselves torn between two extremes: a wish just referred to, to start immediately on all fronts, regardless of possible inadequacy of preparation, personnel, or facilities, and a wish to defer any action on a program until all desirable, adequate personnel and facilities are available. Both approaches, of course, are unwise. Every organization, including new ones, must function and produce to some extent and in some direction even at the start. However, it is far better to engage in one or a few activities that offer a reasonable chance of acceptance and success than to move inadequately in all directions at once. Careful study of any community will reveal certain problems that are sensitive and others that are not controversial. Thus an attempt by a new health department or executive to push an effective industrial hygiene program in a mining community may bring about disastrous consequences. Both labor and management may regard the activity with suspicion and do everything possible to prevent its acceptance and success. Under ordinary circumstances neither faction will have any objection to a maternal and child health program or efforts to secure protection against disease. In the long run it may be advisable for the public health agency to establish a foothold and to gain community acceptance and support by beginning along these lines with the hope of subsequently moving on to other fields. In other words, the planning and organization of the public health program may often best be done on a gradual selective basis, even when this involves the sacrifice of immediate benefits for long-range progress. Both the new and the well-established organization must continually move and grow. Stasis actually represents retrogression in these dynamic times, and a program based solely on the status quo has already begun to decay and die.

In his classic *Organization as Affected by Purpose and Conditions,* Robb[3] emphasizes the following:

Most organizations have grown gradually, and the conditions surrounding this growth often influence greatly the form that the final organization takes. Long existence of customs and methods, and the consequent knowledge of the plan throughout the organization, may be of more importance than the features that might be secured by a theoretically better structure.

This concept is emphasized even more dramatically by Frank[4] in his thesis that there are three types of administrative organization rather than merely one. He lists them as "(1) *under-defined,* in which role expectations of administrative behavior are not well spelled out; (2) *well-defined,* in which administrative roles are explicitly and coherently defined; and (3) *over-defined,* in which role expectation cannot be satisfied, by role incumbents." In his discussion of how these three types of organization differ in their implications for vitality and change, he points out the desirability and advantages of the first, or under-defined, type of organization in fluid or changing circumstances. It provides the greatest opportunity to exercise imagination, initiative, and innovation on the part of employees rather than to fix or freeze them and their abilities. He tops this with a statement that should be rethought frequently by all public health workers:

All of us who have ever been clients of an organization, bureaucratic or otherwise, which resembles the (so-called) ideal type of well-defined roles, have noticed and I venture to say suffered and denounced the conformity and ritualism in role performances to which type 2 organization gives rise.

To a considerable extent, organizational theory stems from military experience because of its example of the value of discipline, the exact definition of functions, and the clear placement of responsibility. Early attempts to transfer these principles to government, business, and industry and later to public service appeared initially to be appropriate and successful. Eventually, however, they were found to result in problems and mistakes when the ends sought were different from military victory, requiring acquiescent obedience. Nevertheless, some type of organization is necessary, and as has been indicated, the problem is which type. The choice depends much on purpose and circumstance. As Sayre[5] points out, "Organization theory in public administration is a problem in political strategy; a choice of structure is a choice of which interest or which value will have preferred access or greater emphasis. Organization is, therefore, a determinant in bargaining."

The approaches to organization theory, according to Sayre, may be identified as "(1) organization as a technological problem in scientific management; (2) organization as a social process emphasizing human relations, informal organization, face-to-face relationships, etc.; (3) organization as the anatomy of decision-making, explored by an analysis of formal and informal decision-making patterns; and (4) organization as the concept of an entity which can and should be held accountable for something and responsible to someone."

Certain well-established principles of organization are applicable equally to public and to private enterprise. In the final analysis they consist essentially of the application of common sense to the management of a group of people working toward a common goal: the maintenance of a balance between responsibility and authority, a consideration of the limits of human capability, and the relationship between ultimate productive action and the supplementary needs related to it. The outstanding principles may be summarized in the following adaptation of an outline by Pfiffner and Preshus[6]:

1. An organization should have a hierarchy, sometimes referred to as the "scalar process," wherein lines of authority and responsibility run upward and downward through several levels with a broad functional base at the bottom and a single executive head at the apex.

2. Every unit and person in the organization without exception should be answerable ultimately to the chief executive officer who occupies the supreme position in the hierarchy.

3. The principal subdivisions on the level immediately under the chief executive officer ordinarily should consist of activities grouped into divisions or bureaus on the basis of function or general purpose.

4. The number of these departments should be small enough to permit the chief executive to have an effective "span of control," yet large enough to provide effective contact with all of the major functions of the organization.

5. Each of these departments should be self-contained insofar as this does not interfere with the necessity of integration and coordination.

6. Provisions should be made for staff services, both general and auxiliary in nature, to facilitate overall management of the organization as a whole and coordination and function of its component divisions.

7. In organizations large enough to warrant it certain auxiliary activities, such as personnel and finances, should be directly under the chief executive officer and should work closely with similar units in each of the line departments.

8. The distinction between staff and line activities and personnel should be recognized as an operating principle and be made clearly understood to all concerned.

## LEVELS OF ORGANIZATION
### Policy making

From the standpoint of organization public agencies such as those dealing with public health may be divided into three distinct levels: policy making, administrative, and functional. Policy making is primarily a function of legislative bodies concerned essentially with the overall or broad aspects of public responsibilities and programs. Thus the legislative branch of government determines the areas in which a public agency must act and the boundaries limiting that action. The details of policy are usually left or delegated to boards, the members of which are generally appointed rather than elected. Thus it is customary in the United States for the public health law to be promulgated by the legislature and for the detailed rules and regulations necessary for the practical implementation of the mandate of the law to be stated by a board of health. The actions of both the legislature and the board are of course subject to adjudication by the courts.

### Boards

Boards of health preferably consist of an odd number of members, neither too many nor too few (usually 5 or 7 members), appointed by the elected executive head of the government, the chairman of the county board of supervisors, the mayor, or the governor, for overlapping terms. Thus members of a 5-person committee may serve for 5 years each, with one appointment expiring each year. In practice there is considerable variation in the manner of appointment of board members, in their characteristics, and in their constituent number. Using state boards of health as an example, the number of members appointed varies from 3 in several instances to 14 in one state. With a few exceptions members of state boards of health are appointed by the governor, whose selections are subject to senate approval in about a dozen states. In several states the appointment must be made from a list of nominees submitted to the governor by the state medical association, and in one state members actually are appointed directly by the state medical association. In another state it is specified that the "Medical Association together with the Comptroller General shall be known as the State Board of Health." In this case the executive committee of the state board of health (7 members of the medical association) performs the functions usually delegated to state boards of health. The usual period of service on boards varies from 2 to 7 years, with 6 years being the most common. In about three fourths of the states the terms of the members of the state board of health are overlapping.

Referring for descriptive purposes to state boards of health, few states specifically require lay representation. Most states stipulate that a certain number (and in a few instance all) of the members must be physicians. Other specifications include a dentist, a civil or sanitary engineer, a pharmacist, an attorney, a veterinarian, an osteopath, and a woman. In one state the board of health consists of 3 ex officio members: the governor, the attorney general, and the superintendent of health, who in this instance is appointed by the governor. The inappropriateness of such an arrangement as well as of a completely medical board is obvious. It is desirable that there be represented on a board of health the interests and points of view of various key groups in the community. The most important of these but the most commonly overlooked is the public itself.

Elling and Lee[7] provide an interesting and provocative analysis of community leadership and health board membership. They classify community leaders into three occupational types: (1) economic dominants—business executives and men of wealth; (2) elective leaders —elected labor officials, politicians, and government officials (all of whom depend for their position on some kind of popular support); and (3) knowledge specialists—professionals and executives of community organizations, for example, religious, civic, educational, law, and other groups. They note that voluntary health agencies and hospitals, as might be expected for fund-raising purposes, have a predominance of the first category (business executives and men of wealth) on their boards. This is in contrast with governmental health boards, the majority of whose membership is drawn from elective leaders and knowledge specialists. Perhaps of greater significance is the authors' observation that in neither case does the leadership tend to be representative of the population. They maintain, "This situation may not be bad if the leadership for whatever reason . . . has pursued a benevolent policy and sought to raise the level of living in the community. This is a matter of personal judgment. Extensive benefits have apparently derived from the leadership's decision to focus on and rejuvenate the local community. Those who have not fared well in the process and those who have not yet had their turn at 'the table'—for example, the deprived Negro and other families in Pittsburgh's notorious 'Hill District'—will perhaps judge otherwise." Goodenough[8] also points to this as a major error in representation at the policy level. As he indicates, the higher levels of the health organization have their closest associations with the *sponsoring public* (those who provide the financing) and some of its *entailed publics* (those whose interests are likely to be affected by the agency's activities). They tend to have the least association with the *target public* (the object of the sponsoring public's and the agency's program). By contrast, the agency's field staff has its closest association with the target public but has limited power or incentive when major decisions are made regarding the agency's programs. As a result, the target public—the one for which the agency is supposed to exist—is relatively unrepresented in problem analysis and policy decisions.

This pattern now appears to be undergoing rapid change largely as a result of insistence by various civil rights groups, consumers' organizations, labor unions, and some other organizations. Increasingly there is pressure and action to seat representatives of those to be served on various types of boards and committees that deal with health and other social questions. This trend will hopefully improve the heretofore restrictive and preferential situation.

Certain objections to the policy of having boards consist of ex officio members should be indicated. Sometimes boards are so formed to reduce or avoid administrative costs. Although it is true, as claimed by some, that ex officio membership provides contact and understanding among several agencies of government and government officials, there are other ways of accomplishing this desirable end. Unfortunately such members are often appointed to the board without any consideration of their ability to be of service. Furthermore, this added responsibility, if taken seriously, consumes either much personal time or time that might better be devoted to the duties of the individual's primary office. Not infrequently the health officer is added as an ex officio member of the board of health. This defeats some of the basic purposes of the board, which will be discussed later. No objection is raised, however, to the health officer's meeting with the board as a nonvoting participant and perhaps acting as its secretary. In fact this is to be recommended.

Generally speaking, therefore, boards of health should be more equitably representative than ordinarily is found. There are many advantages. Policies will be developed with a better understanding of the opinions and preferences of those most directly concerned and affected as well as of the probable receptivity and results. Policies are thereby more likely to be realistic and acceptable and therefore more easily enforced. When the primary groups affected are represented on the board, an opportunity is provided for them to be educated and to understand the viewpoints of others in the community and of the responsible public authority. Opinions that tend to be hidden or overlooked are brought out into the open and given a fair opportunity to be heard. Finally, the determination of policy by a reasonably representative board is a much more democratic procedure than is administrative dictation by either an elected or appointed official.

A legally established board has still other advantages for the health officer and his department. It provides for a nonpolitical method of appointment and removal of the executive health officer, who should be a professionally trained career person and, as such, protected from political interference. By virtue of its delegated responsibility a board also protects the health officer from many legal involvements. Finally, if provision is made for overlapping terms, the board provides for continuity of community public health thought, direction, and action from one political administration to another or when a change of health officers occurs.

It is only fair to state that under certain circumstances, boards may have disadvantages that arise in either or both of two ways: conflict among the members of the board itself or conflict between the board and its executive officer. Although it is generally desirable for boards to be representative of the constituency they serve and of outstanding interested parties and groups therein, conflict within boards is

more likely to occur when the membership represents many diverse groups. Occasionally board members may choose sides, with the result that agreements can seldom be reached; as a consequence, effective administrative action by the executive officer is weakened or paralyzed. The actions of the board in instances such as this may consist of a series of majority or minority decisions and bitter charges that one side or the other is attempting to steamroll policies through or to capture imparital members. In such situations what real progress may be made depends, largely on the joint action of any impartial board members and a wise executive officer. Working together for commonsense mediation, they may sometimes bring about conciliation or at least effective compromise.

Conflict between the board members and the executive officer may develop in several ways. The executive officer, either because of dogmatic personal forcefulness or preoccupation with his daily work, may ignore his board, fail to consult or give it work to do, or disregard its recommendations. If the board and its traditions are weak, he may get away with it. Not infrequently, on the other hand, there may be one or more particularly active and forceful board members who because of overenthusiasm or a wish to express power and influence may step beyond their prerogatives and attempt to enter the field of operations. In doing this they encroach on the functions and responsibilities of the executive personnel. In addition to these situations there is the type of executive who because of personal weakness or of particular confidence in his board may try to pass his responsibilities to it. Fortunately this is observed relatively infrequently. From the foregoing it is seen that the ideal relationship between an executive officer and his board is a delicate one wherein each party must be constantly alert to his own responsibilities and prerogatives and those of the other party. Board members must always bear in mind that the field of operation belongs to the administrative or executive officer, who in turn must respect the functions and responsibilities of the board by keeping them informed, asking their advice, and including them in his professional plans.

Boards have certain specified responsibilities and functions. In a very real sense a board of health should be the health conscience of the community. In the final analysis the board of health is the legal representative of the community's public health program and agency. As such, it has certain semilegislative powers, particularly with regard to the promulgation of rules and regulations that may be deemed advisable for the community. Related to the semilegislative powers are certain limited semijudicial powers in that a board of health may hold hearings on some matters relating to the public health. Perhaps the most important administrative responsibility of a board of health is its customary power to appoint the executive health officer and if necessary, to dismiss him. Boards of health sometimes have responsibilities relating to determination of general administrative and program policy, approval of major appointments, and budget review and approval. Except in unusual circumstances, such involvement in the details of operation are generally considered undesirable. A board of health should meet at regular intervals, at least once each month, at the request of the health officer, and at times of emergency. Board members should be free to advise the executive officer either on his request or on their own initiative. They are entitled to be kept informed, should have access to all health department records, and when their suggestions and recommendations are not followed, are entitled to an explanation.

It cannot be denied that an organizational pattern that includes a board of health may sometimes appear to be less efficient and slower in action than one operated along more dogmatic, bureaucratic, or dictatorial lines. The design of an organization is necessarily of great importance in the search for an efficient instrument of action. In a democratic society, however, the organizational mechanism must correspond, at least in its fundamental form, to a pattern that is acceptable to the people who are to be served. It is often necessary to sacrifice some measure of efficiency in deference to the public wish for freedom of action and even to their prejudices and lack of understanding. A realization of this serves to emphasize the basic importance of public education in the public health program, which in the final analysis bears the most satisfying and lasting fruits.

### Advisory committees

Because of the numbers involved, complete interest representation is impossible to achieve on the policy-making board of health. To offset this many public health agencies have formed advisory councils or committees as an additional means of obtaining broader community contact and participation. Often the existence of advisory committees enables civic-minded individuals and citizens with specialized knowledge or interest to render services of great value to the community.

Advisory committees are of two general types —constituent and technical. Members of constituent advisory committees may be chosen for their personal qualifications or because they represent social, professional, or other groups in the community. The chief advantage and use of constituent advisory committees is to act as a channel through which the community, on the one hand, and the health department, on the other, are kept aware of each other's thoughts, plans, and action. They are of considerable value in the health education program as well as occasionally serving as a line of defense for the functional public health agency. Members of technical advisory committees assist the administrative officers of the public health agency in the formulation of plans and in the development and application of various techniques of value in the public health program. Naturally the larger and more complex the community the greater will be the number of technical advisory committees that might be indicated. Thus a large city or state health department may have advisory committees dealing with problems of pediatrics, maternity, engineering, law, and the like. Advisory committees should have no powers, of course, and the executive officer must be constantly on guard to thwart the assumption of power by overenthusiastic advisory committee members. A mitigating technique in this regard is for advisory committees to be established on a temporary basis, the need to be determined by the executive officer of the health department. This is generally considered to be good practice, since it is pointless to have a permanent committee for needs that arise only occasionally.

### Administrative level

On the executive or administrative level of organization is what is often referred to as the hierarchy, built on a scalar plan (Fig. 10-1). At the apex of the pyramid is the chief executive who, for this purpose, is the health officer or health commissioner. Although an employee, he is in a somewhat different position from the rest of the employed personnel of the agency. It is he who is responsible for the overall management of the agency and for the planning and implementation of its program 24 hours of every day. Whereas the remainder of the personnel may be subject to civil service or merit system status, he usually is not. The activities of the chief executive are usually defined and limited by the terms of the corporate charter or state law. He has the privileges of what has been called an economic royalist, which means that he has been entrusted with a considerable sum of other people's money and is expected to find ways to put it to as profitable use as the law allows and his board approves. On the other hand, his position differs from that of a private executive or administrator in that although the latter may do anything except what the law forbids, the public administrator may do only those things that the law specifically allows.

The functions of a chief executive are threefold: political leadership, administrative management, and ceremonial representation. It is with the second of these that this section is chiefly concerned. In fulfilling his managerial duties the health officer should first acquaint himself thoroughly with the most minute details of certain aspects of his position. The first of these are his rights, prerogatives, and responsibilities. This becoming acquainted involves a careful study and analysis of the public health law and sanitary code under which he is to operate. Next he must familiarize himself with the resources actually and potentially available to him, including funds, personnel, and materiel. To exercise his rights, meet his responsibilities, and properly use the resources available to him the health officer must next perform a careful and thoroughgoing analysis of all his evident and potential problems. These problems are not necessarily restricted to matters requiring professional or technical knowledge. Many of them may be in the realm of personnel management, public relations, or finances.

Beyond this initial stocktaking, which of course should be frequently repeated, the public health administrator has several duties of a managerial nature. Some of these are imposed by charter, constitution, or statute, some are defined in executive orders, whereas others may be merely customary or attributable to the administrator's personal wishes and interests. The most important of these is the determination of the basic administrative policy of the agency. It is the health officer's right and duty to decide in what direction the program should move, when each move should be made, and the manner in which progression is best achieved. He is usually wise, however, to exercise these rights and duties in concert with the various wishes and forces in his jurisdiction. Otherwise he may find that he has pushed programs that conflict with the values and positions of professional, civic, or political groups that are pursuing their interests and goals by more traditional methods.[9]

The administrator should next issue the necessary oral or written orders, directions, and commands to his subordinates to put his administrative policy into effect. This necessitates that he work out the details of organization of the agency and its internal structure, subordinate leadership and responsibilities, and organize whatever committees are needed to solve controversies, adjust relationships, or establish policies and techniques to meet emergencies. This leads to the need for coordinating the activities of the subdivisions of the agency. Most of this is best accomplished at lower levels, but the chief executive has a clear responsibility for overall coordination. He must arbitrate claims of conflicting action and overlapping jurisdictions. Within the agency he serves as the court of last resort.

In the financial field he must develop a fiscal program for the agency, prepare and submit a budget, and supervise the expenditure of the appropriations. He should have direct responsibility for the appointment, supervision, and discharge of all personnel in the level immediately below him, usually consisting of division and bureau heads and certain staff and auxiliary personnel. Discharge, however, should be subject to review and approval of a civil service board. Although in large agencies choice and supervision of line personnel should be a prerogative of the appropriate division or bureau chief, decisions should be subject to the approval of the chief executive. The executive health officer by virtue of his position bears the ultimate responsibility for supervision, facilitation, and control of administrative operations. He is not expected to perform all or even part of the many jobs or services of the agency, but it is his responsibility to see that they are done properly and effectively. This means that to be effective he must pass down or delegate some of his authority and responsibility. This frequently ignored fact will be later discussed in more detail. Another duty of the chief executive relates to public relations, which is discussed in Chapter 14. In addition, general policies must be established and disseminated throughout the structure of the organization. Management planning must be carried on continually and must include job analyses, organizational studies, budget planning, work flow studies, and insofar as possible, standardization of systems, techniques, and procedures. Internal checks must be established to show danger signals automatically when responsibilities are not met or when authority is overstepped. Finally, provision must be made to assure this flow of management up, down, and across the hierarchy of the organization.

Although the foregoing rules are sound and are based on the experiences of many, one of the commonest organizational mistakes is to assume that a position or function can be established according to hard-and-fast specifications and that any one of several people can be found to fill it satisfactorily and equally well. Human beings are not made to fit into precise patterns. According to Pfiffner and Preshus,[6] "The functions delegated to each man can be performed only within the limits of his individual capabilities. The best procedure for preparing an outline of responsibilities is first to draft an ideal organizational chart, then to sit down with the individuals whose names appear on the chart, discuss specific responsibilities with them at length and with infinite patience, and then to allocate responsibilities wherever common agreement dictates."

## GENESIS OF THE PUBLIC HEALTH ADMINISTRATOR

At this point it may be of value to consider the nature of the public health administrator to obtain a better understanding of him and his function. Is he merely the individual in nominal charge of the organization or program component thereof? It is not necessarily that simple. It is unfortunately true that some public health administrators are little more than the individual whom circumstance happens to have placed in the top position in an organization. In a real sense, however, the term *public health administrator* may be a misnomer. Although it is true that those who are called on to direct public health programs have usually come up through the ranks, accumulating in the process experience in many program aspects of public health activitiy, by

the time they reach the point of being placed in a position of high authority and responsibility they are often no longer primarily public health workers. By this time they may be only secondarily public health workers and have become primarily public administrators with speical interests in and responsibilities for the management of activities related to the public's health.

This is not meant to imply that such individuals need not have a solid background in public health work. In fact, it is difficult to think of anyone's successfully understanding and directing a group of public health specialists without knowing, through past training and experience, what kinds of people they are, their abilities, their potential contributions, and what it is that they are attempting to do. The essential point is that the individual commonly referred to as a public health administrator typically finds himself called on to make fewer and fewer decisions in the technical, professional, and scientific aspects of public health, since he is too busy, or should be, with broader policy matters. Besides, he has or should have working for him many other experts who are better able to handle the strictly technical details. To the contrary, more and more of the public health administrator's time must be devoted to strictly administrative and managerial problems—how to obtain funds, how to get people to work together, how to deal with other parts of the government and with the public, and similar nonpublic health or nonmedical matters. It should be noted that all these activities in one way or another involve *relationships*. Indeed, executive or administrative work is essentially a relationship type of work. The executive or administrator is always relating to someone else. If he is not, he is wasting his time on something that a clerk could do much better.

The genesis and fate of individuals in such positions are interesting. The term *spiralist* has been suggested by some British writers to depict the shift in role that certain individuals such as public health administrators and similar managerial officials undergo. Their development or evolution is somewhat as follows. An individual obtains some extremely specific education. He begins to put his acquired specialized knowledge to work in a particular field. At that point he is at the direct center of a potential spiral. If he succeeds, he acquires in the process more knowledge and experience not only in the area of his original specialized interest and its efficient application but also in related fields. His concepts, imagination, and interests begin to move laterally outward in ever-widening circles. Because of this, he becomes more ambitious and more valuable to his organization. Therefore he begins to progress upward as well as laterally into positions of greater and greater responsibility. Each of these in turn widens his horizons even more. Up to a certain point, as he progresses outward and upward in this spiral, he still continues to work in his original field. However, he may eventually reach a point where his interests and value have become so broad as to cause the centrifugal force of the outward and upward movement to throw him out of the orbit of the spiral in whose center he originated. In such an eventuality he is by no means lost to his original field. He has, in fact, become part of a much larger enterprise of which his original spiral was only one of several parts. When this happen, therefore, although he does not cast off the influences of his original field of interests, they become somewhat secondary to an even greater and more significant interest.

Thus it is with the public health administrator who begins (perhaps as a clinic physician, field nurse, or field engineer) performing some specialized service, then progresses to become the chief of a particular specialized program, later becomes perhaps the director of a small generalized health unit from which he may be called into a central office for broader program planning and direction, and eventually is placed in charge of all the many activities involved in a broad-based, multidisciplinary public health program. In the medical field he may even progress to appointment as a health officer, commissioner of health, surgeon general, or a minister of cabinet rank with overall responsibility for the conduct and representation of all aspects of his chosen field of interest. By this time he has progressed far from the specialized clinic physician that he originally was, and the demands on his time and energy are such as to preclude involvement in the minutiae of clinical or specialized affairs. He has now passed out of the orbit of the specialized public health spiral and has entered the larger orbit of public administration. He has become a public administrator with particular interest in health matters.

Despite this, not infrequently one sees individuals who have achieved or have been appointed to positions of high managerial and administrative responsibility who apparently cannot overcome their nostalgia for their initial specialized interest. They continually want to crawl back into their original professional womb. Although they may have working under their direction individuals with great competence and more current specialized knowledge, they find it impossible to believe that anyone can handle the detail as well as themselves. They erroneously consider it a sign of weakness to behave otherwise. They simply cannot keep their fingers out of the minutiae of the specialized activity. Such an individual can never be a good administrator. He cannot have it both ways, no matter how sincere or capable he is. If the individual in high authority insists on personal involvement in detailed specialized decision and activities, obviously he will have insufficient time or energy for the requirements of his administrative and managerial duties and responsibilities. If he cannot think and act differently, he had better vacate his top policy and administrative position to allow someone else to function in it more adequately. On the other hand, if he remains and attempts to play both roles, the price will be chronic exhaustion and the loss of good personnel.

It is appropriate to ask why many public health administrators concentrate on professional and technical matters rather than on their administrative and managerial responsibilities. It is perhaps because, having begun as professionals, they feel competent, comfortable, and secure in the former, whereas they are not absolutely sure that they know how to do the latter and are therefore really afraid of the job.

The behavioral and psychologic aspects and implications of these sets of circumstances have been explored and presented by Lefcowitz,[10] who also indicates that "the public health professional is marginal in his movement into the field, in his structural location with respect to his profession, and in terms of his activities as a public health official." As a consequence, he concludes that "the public health worker is beset by pressures, sometimes opposing, from his fellow professionals and the public or its representatives."

## THE ADMINISTRATOR'S ORGANIZATIONAL ROLE

What then are the roles of the public health administrator? They are many. The public health administrator may be regarded in a variety of ways by a variety of people or groups, depending on the circumstances of the contact or relationship. There are the viewpoints of his family and friends, the members of his board of health, the political hierarchy, his subordinates and superiors, the private practitioners of medicine and other healing arts, the irate citizen, the businessman and industrialist, and his own viewpoint of himself. Sometimes in the privacy of his own thoughts he can feel lonely, confused, disillusioned, and sorry for himself. *But* he must never show it. This is perhaps the first and most important lesson to be learned.

In general, however, his roles may be considered as fourfold: (1) a technical professional specialist, (2) a public official, (3) an administrator, and (4) a community leader.

With regard to his role as a technical professional specialist, it has already been indicated that by the time he gets into his administrative position his personal expertise is already somewhat diluted by his broader responsibilities, not to mention the passage of time and scientific advances. Accordingly, perhaps his wisest and most practical recourse is to be thoroughly aware of sources of technical and professional expertise around him and not to be too proud or afraid to use them. After all, no one can expect him to be all things to all men.

As far as his role as a public official is concerned, he has certain commonly expected responsibilities. Predominant among these are (1) to represent the community's overall interests and leadership in all matters relating to health in its broadest terms, (2) to engage in certain ceremonial activities, both as a figurehead and as a personality, (3) to assure that the laws governing his jurisdiction and organization are faithfully and equitably enforced and complied with, and (4) to make known to his superiors changes in goals, laws, and resources that in his judgment are desirable or necessary.

In his role as an administrator he must be a program planner, a program builder, a program organizer, a program staffer, a program leader, and finally, a father image. He must develop a capacity for making things happen, for getting things done through his organization and the efforts of those who are involved.

To paraphrase the words of the International City Managers Association[11] he must become adept at guiding human and physical resources in the form of dynamic units of organization to the satisfaction of those served and with a high sense of morale, achievement, and satisfaction on the part of those who render the service.

Attention should be directed to a few personal details. In filling this administrative role the public health administrator should have three outstanding characteristics: (1) a genuine inherent interest in and affection for people (including his staff), (2) a strength or power of personality that gives an impression of considerable reserve force power and ability (i.e., a sense of determination and sincerity), and (3) a scientific and analytic type of mind that aims at winning or achieving by means of prevention rather than by means of remedying health or administrative errors that have been allowed to occur.

To assist him in the demonstration of these the good administrator should consciously develop and exercise certain important personal traits:

*For staff stimulation*—enthusiasm, cheerfulness, unselfishness, resoluteness

*For organizational stability*—calmness, consistency

*For efficiency and time saving*—receptivity, simplicity, directness, and frankness

*For conformity*—firmness, tact, toleration, patience

*For restraint*—dignity (to assure that responsibility is not regarded lightly)

*For staff loyalty*—courtesy, consideration, kindness

By virtue of his role as a community leader, the considerable power and resources at his disposal, and the fact that he is now part of a larger sociopolitical spiral or galaxy, the public health administrator at this point has become an *agent of social change*. Unfortunately many public health administrators do not appear to recognize this fact, much less to realize the full significance of it. All too many administrators of public health programs seem content to drift along from day to day and year to year merely attempting to solve problems as they arise by the forces of chance and circumstance rather than to plan and function forcefully to determine or to circumvent chance. They are content to ride in or even to follow the wagon instead of driving or leading it down the road they think it should follow. They are content to be passive participants rather than deliberate contributors to the determination of public health and social progress. They do not recognize the great chal-

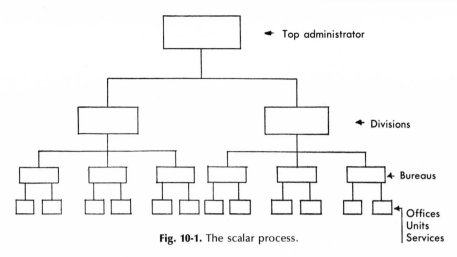

Top administrator

Divisions

Bureaus

Offices
Units
Services

**Fig. 10-1.** The scalar process.

lenges presented to them for the achievement of broad social and economic progress.

## THE SCALAR PRINCIPLE

The term *scalar principle* has been referred to in the preceding discussion of the hierarchy and the executive officer. It consists of the administrative arrangement of the functional groups or units in steps as in a scale (Fig. 10-1).

This involves the three considerations of leadership, delegation, and functional definition. There must be a single supreme leader of the organization, but as has been discussed, to exercise his leadership effectively it is necessary that he delegate both authority and responsibility to subleaders on the various subordinate steps in the organization. Each of the primary steps, usually referred to as divisions or sections, is determined on the basis of secondary constituent purpose or function, such as water control, food control, or milk control. The looseness of and the resulting confusion from different terminologies are somewhat unfortunate; department, division, bureau, service, and office often are used interchangeably if not haphazardly in the structural plans of many organizations. Actually it matters relatively little how the terms are used as long as they are used in a consistent manner are are understood.

The fundamental concept of the scalar principle is unity of command, with lines of authority and responsibility going both up and down so that every individual in the organization is directly responsible to only one superior and through him ultimately answerable to the head of the organization. These lines are sometimes referred to as organization lines or channels. In theory all intraagency communications and actions are supposed to follow these lines and should never cross or short-circuit them. Daily practice tends to produce many exceptions to this rule. Although some kind of formal organization with its hierarchy is obviously required and although employees are accustomed to working within it, such organization is not necessarily well liked. Many employees, professional and otherwise, are in a constant state of conscious or subconscious rebellion against it. Rebellion may not be overt or manifest by subversive action. Usually it consists of subtle resistance such as refusing or being unable to meet officially established performance standards.[12]

Under any circumstance lines of authority and responsibility should never be considered permanent, since good organization, as well as progress, depends partly on the skills and personalities of the individuals involved and partly on the nature of the functions to be performed. "If the organization doesn't permit a man to go directly to anyone who can help him with a problem, it may retard rather than help him. If you insist that a man must always follow a strict organizational hierarchy, you may have simply installed red tape. To put it another way, you have set up an obstacle to action."[13] Clarence B. Randall,[14] former President of Inland Steel Corporation and Special Advisor on Foreign Economic Policy to President Eisenhower, has dealt with this practical issue in his fascinating book *The Folklore of Management.* He stresses the importance of flexibility of mind and method to achieve good administration, pointing to the infinite variety of changing circumstances. An organization or organization chart that may be precise today may be of little use tomorrow. Then he makes the following statement:

There is one further difficulty with overemphasis on the formalizing of relationships, which is this: a chart which suits one group of persons will need revision just as often as there are personnel changes. Jobs have no vitality of their own. . . .Take the man away and the job will never be quite the same again. A relationship which functions smoothly under a particular chart and the one set of job descriptions, so long as the original incumbents remain, will begin to show stress when promotion, death, resignation, or retirement intervene. No two individuals will ever bring successively to one job the same complex of strengths and weaknesses, and when a new teammate arrives, some compensating adjustments must be made by those around him. No chart can ever do this for them.

The wise administrator therefore "will remember that the organization chart is a useful scaffold with which to build a house but will know that it is not the house."

An organization, in other words, is a living thing that continually grows and changes, and its structure, accordingly, must be adaptable. The administrator must set up the best structure possible but should never hesitate to change it for a good reason. The units to be headed by subleaders should be established or differentiated on the basis of functional definition. The trend has been to provide a small number of relatively large major divisions, each with a single major purpose or function and each further subdivided into bureaus, if necessary, on the basis of subfunctions.

Although sound in theory, this is often more easily said than accomplished, since many instances arise in which two or even more departments or other organizational units are involved and appear to have valid claims. Should the industrial hygiene program be placed in a state health department or in a state labor and industry department? If the former is decided on, should responsibility for the program be delegated to the division of environmental health or the division of medical services; or should it be set up as an entity in itself? Should the school health program be in the department of health or in the department of education? Whether assigned to one or the other, the school health program involves safety, sanitation, medical services, and educa-

tion, each of which extends into other fields. With these problems in mind White[15] asks the question: "When is a function of sufficient major importance to warrant organization as a division rather than as a bureau with other related functions in a broader unit? Decisions on such cases usually flow from other considerations than abstract plan, the pressure of interest groups, the capacity of those who possess to resist change, bureaucratic and political bargaining. The concept of function itself is not entirely precise, although it is a genuine guide. The fact that no division can be functionally self-sufficient and must inevitably have frontier problems with its neighbors is itself a further guide to the necessity for general staff and strong overhead management."

Although it is best for the individual division or bureau to be concerned with a particular function, each should contribute to an overall major purpose of the department as a whole and not be allocated to the department as a result of a search for a roosting place. At least one department on the federal level, the Department of the Interior, has been referred to as a federation of unrelated bureaus rather than a department. Occasionally it is found expedient and practical to form administrative units on bases other than functional. Thus they may be determined by geographic area, such as the Tennessee Valley Authority, or by type of clientele, such as the Department of Public Welfare or the Veterans Administration.

The question frequently arises in relation to public service organizations such as health departments concerning whether the unit of organization should conform geographically to already existing boundaries, such as corporate limits and county lines, or whether altogether new boundaries should be established based entirely on the nature of the problem to be met or the distribution of the public to be served. This latter concept is what the British refer to as problem or service *catchment areas*. Theoretically at least much can be said in favor of this type of administrative district. The size and limits of an administrative district, being divorced if necessary from political boundaries, may be determined on the basis of groups of population, trading or economic areas, topographic considerations, or convenience of officials and citizens. They are relatively easy to readjust with little or no friction, in contrast with service areas whose boundaries conform to those of established political units. The effect of the latter is commonly seen when attempts are made for purposes of efficiency to expand the jurisdictions of local health departments either by combining a city with its surrounding county or by combining two or more counties for health service purposes. Vested political interests are disturbed. Conflict arises between city and suburb and between village and farm.

Nevertheless, the administrative district based on problem or service needs has limited governmental status, no independent existence, and usually no power to raise revenue in its own right and by its own action. It can easily find itself standing alone and helpless. Hence, public health units in the United States are based on politically defined units of government: municipalities, counties, combinations of counties or combinations of counties and municipalities, and states. The characteristics of such units of government have been outlined by Anderson[16] in the following manner:

1. The unit has its own separate continuing governmental organization, either a board or a council, or in some cases a single elective or appointive official.

2. This governing body has the power year after year to provide some governmental service, or some quasi-governmental service like a public utility on its own responsibility and subject to its own control.

3. This governing body is independent of other local governments and is not a mere board handling some function on behalf of, or as a department of, another local corporation.

4. The area covered by a unit of local government may or may not coincide with the area of some other local government. If the areas coincide, the test is whether the corporate existence is separate for the two or more units occupying the same area. There can be separate public corporations in the same area, of course, if they are organized for different purposes.

5. Among the important powers of any unit of local government the power to raise revenue by taxation, or by special assessment, or by fixing rates for service rendered must be considered one of the most important. When other tests fail, this test may decide the case.

Returning for a moment to the internal structure of the organization, it is not possible to make a single rule concerning the number of subdivisions or bureaus that should be established. The decision varies with individuals, time, place, and circumstances. Some agencies, such as health departments, with many professional types (engineers, physicians, nurses, veterinarians, health educators, etc.) may justify a larger number of subdivisions than will an agency with a more or less homogeneous personnel, such as a fire department. Furthermore, some executives believe that they must have, and are capable of maintaining, more effective and frequent contact with the workers of their organization through many division chiefs.

The smaller the organization the greater are the tendency and reason for the chief executive

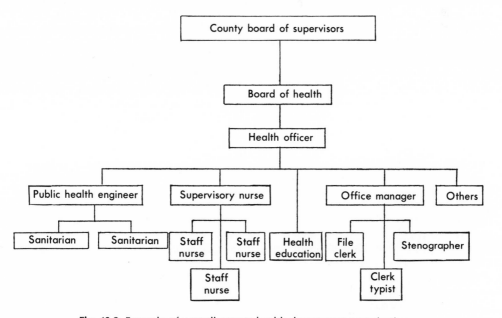

**Fig. 10-2.** Example of a small county health department organization.

to have personal contact with all phases of activities. This is most completely seen in the small county health unit, where the limited staff makes much subdivision unnecessary. The typical result is a structure such as illustrated in Fig. 10-2.

In this situation the health officer, in addition to performing the medical activities of the agency, personally carries out all the staff and auxiliary functions and directly supervises the rest of the personnel, except in the case of staff nurses, who when sufficient in number, are supervised directly by a chief nurse and indirectly by the health officer.

## ORGANIZATIONAL STRUCTURE

The problem of structural organization is an important one because its solution depends on whether the chief executive is actually in command of or at the mercy of his organization. The more widely dispersed his direct organizational contact the further away he gets from the functions of top administration. Generally speaking, a small number of divisions is desirable, giving a quantitatively limited but qualitatively strong span of control. Too fine a structural breakdown tends to bring about several undesirable effects. The number of fields or directions on which the average capable human being can effectively focus attention is limited and has been estimated to be not more than six to eight. The type of structure unfortunately found so frequently in large health departments with a dozen or more divisions strung out across the line makes it impossible for the administrative health officer to grasp and to hold in his span of attention and control all phases of the program. He finds it difficult to see the activity of each division in relation to all the others, and this results in unbalanced decisions and a field day for pressure groups or a few forceful division chiefs.[17]

An example of this horizontal type of administration is shown in Fig. 10-3, which presents the structure of the health department of a moderate-sized state with a relatively small and homogeneous, predominantly rural population (State A). Interpreting the organization chart literally, it appears as if 17 division directors report directly to the chief executive officer. That an arrangement of this nature could actually function as depicted is improbable. In practice, in most instances of this type, there is usually some division of responsibility and

authority between the state health officer and his one or several deputies.

Fig. 10-4, which presents the plan of organization followed for many years by the health department of State B, illustrates a particularly poor structure. The Commissioner had a dual responsibility to the Governor and to the Public Health Council, the members of which were also appointed by the Governor. Directly responsible to the Commissioner in turn were the directors of nine separate divisions, a number considered somewhat excessive for effective span of control. Attention should be called further to a number of incongruities within the line structure. Altogether there were four separate laboratories, not counting those that for good reason were located in and served the hospitals. The laboratory designed to serve the Division of Sanitary Engineering was itself set up as a divisional entity. Although the Cancer Section was within the Division of Adult Hygiene, the Cancer Hospital was placed in the Division of Tuberculosis. Public Health Education was effectively provincialized in the Division of Child Hygiene. A final point of wonder was the placement of responsibility for Health Districts in the Division of Communicable Diseases. Interestingly enough this particular state health department had a long and honorable record of effective service, perhaps, one might say, despite its form of organization. It was eventually reorganized into five sections: general services, preventive medical services, hospital and medical services, environmental sanitation, and local health service. Each contains a reasonable number of logically related divisions, the directors of which are responsible to a deputy of the Commissioner. Since being reorganized, it has operated even more effectively and with greater coordination and smoothness.

A particularly satisfactory and workable arrangement is presented in Fig. 10-5, which shows the structure of the health department of one of the largest and most complex states. In this organization the span of control for the chief executive and for each of those directly responsible to him has been limited to a reasonable practical number. Futhermore, services and functions have been combined in as logical a manner as possible. Lines of direct responsibility and reciprocal relationships are clearly indicated.

There are three types of organization charts: skeleton, personnel, and functional. Skeleton charts, of which the foregoing are examples,

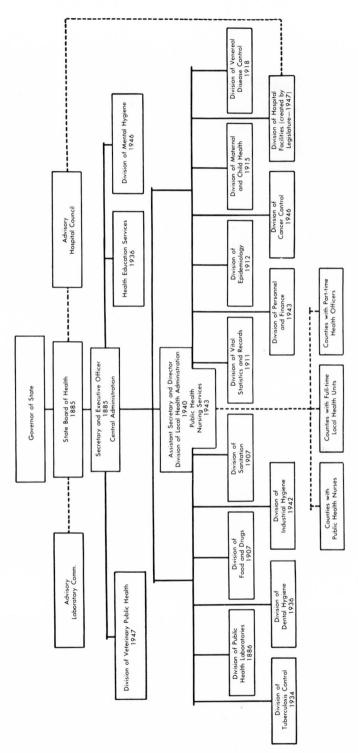

**Fig. 10-3.** Organization of State A health department.

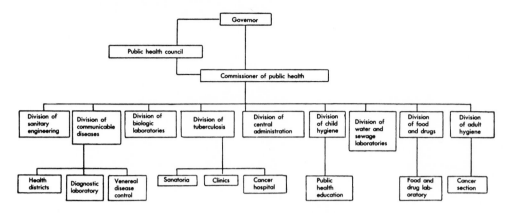

**Fig. 10-4.** Former organization of State B health department.

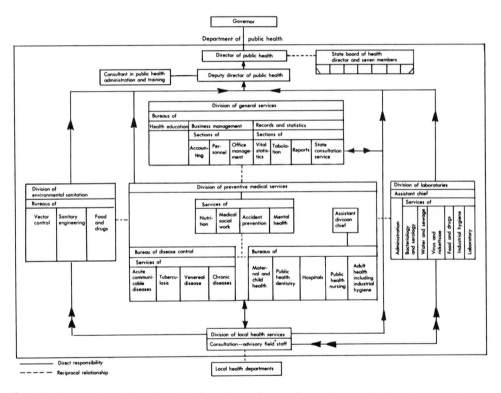

**Fig. 10-5.** Organization of State C health department showing lines of responsibility and relationship.

merely present the major units of the organization. Personnel charts show, in addition, the major positions and often the names of those persons occupying them. Functional charts not only depict the major units but also describe briefly the functions, purposes, duties, and activities of each.

A small number of divisions does not necessarily free the chief executive from details, since there may easily develop several layers of administration that block him off from the rest of the organization, as illustrated in Fig. 10-6. However, the facts of life are that such an arrangement may be necessary under certain circumstances.

A final warning with regard to number and type of divisions or bureaus relates to the danger of statutory definition of an organization's

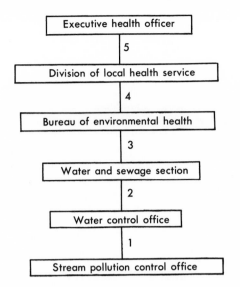

```
┌─────────────────────────────────┐
│     Executive health officer    │
└─────────────────────────────────┘
                │
                5
                │
┌─────────────────────────────────┐
│  Division of local health service │
└─────────────────────────────────┘
                │
                4
                │
┌─────────────────────────────────┐
│  Bureau of environmental health │
└─────────────────────────────────┘
                │
                3
                │
┌─────────────────────────────────┐
│    Water and sewage section     │
└─────────────────────────────────┘
                │
                2
                │
┌─────────────────────────────────┐
│      Water control office       │
└─────────────────────────────────┘
                │
                1
                │
┌─────────────────────────────────┐
│  Stream pollution control office │
└─────────────────────────────────┘
```

**Fig. 10-6.** Undesirable organizational stratification.

internal structure and the functions of each division or bureau. When this is done, as has occurred in several instances in public health, there invariably develops a group of inflexible and unmanageable principalities.

The bureau is the basic functional unit of the department. Generally speaking, it has a homogeneous structure intended to perform a particular task or a series of closely related tasks, in contrast with the division, whose function it is to coordinate, to maintain effective working contact between the functional bureaus, and to channel the basic functional units communicating with the chief executive. Ordinarily the bureau is a highly stable unit of organization. It may be moved within or even without the total organization into new relationships with others of its kind, but it is seldom torn apart or abolished. Although the direction of a bureau involves some problems of general management, the outstanding problems are usually technical in nature, dealing with the most effective manner in which to perform the specific task at hand. Work is assigned to divisions and bureaus generally on the basis of the character of the work itself. Not infrequently, however, other circumstances, such as an unfilled supervisory position or the personality of a particular bureau chief, may affect the distribution of activities. A particularly aggressive bureau or division chief, wishing to become a minor empire builder, may extend his jurisdiction in as many directions as possible,

usually along the lines of least resistance. The units of organization supervised by less forceful persons thereby tend to lose their functions and in the long run to pass into oblivion.

Even within the functional unit, workers should be grouped unofficially, if not officially. As Sartain and Baker[18] indicate, proper organizational processes are as important on the supervisory level as on the higher management level. This is often overlooked. They emphasize that "Careless, inefficient, or unethical assignments of duties, authorities and responsibilities to subordinates can result in a loss of leadership, with disastrous consequences." Interestingly enough, even if management should fail to do so, workers eventually arrange themselves into the ultimate functional units of activity. Naturally it is best for all concerned if such arrangements are a matter of organizational policy and planning. To bring this about each employee in each position should be characterized from several points of view. Gulick[19] suggests that proper grouping must be based on a consideration of five factors, which for purposes here may be illustrated as follows:

1. Major *purpose* or service, such as milk control, operating a treatment clinic, or education
2. *Process* used, such as laboratory analysis, administration of therapy, or home visits
3. *Persons* or *things* dealt with or served, such as expectant mothers, tuberculosis patients, or restaurants
4. *Place* where service is rendered, such as the Eastern Health District, Macomb County, or Central High School
5. Knowledge, skill, and facilities available and procedural convenience

## STAFF SERVICES

For a considerable period, almost all bureaus and divisions of public agencies were more or less self-contained units performing all of the activities and functions necessary for their operation and maintenance. Beginning about 1900, with the expansion of public service and its increased specialization, there developed the trend of splitting off from the various functional units of organization all operations of a staff or housekeeping nature. Activities of this type were then brought together to form what are referred to as staff and auxiliary services. They are usually aligned structurally in close relationship with the chief executive officer of the organization. Still more recent has been the tendency to develop these staff agencies into a combination of service and control units.

Staff agencies do much more than study, plan, and advise. Their ultimate purpose is to facilitate the work of administration. They frequently are called on to assist the line or functional units by working with them but without infringing on their authority or responsibility. The executive staff agency is not in the direct line of the administrative hierarchy. Lines of authority, command, and responsibility should not pass through them. Instead, they are situated somewhat apart, on the sidelines so to speak, as adjuncts to the office of the chief executive. Because of this rather special status, their purpose and value often tend to be misunderstood. Occasionally the staff person may have a certain amount of specially delegated authority, but when this is so, it must be made clear to all concerned that the authority has been delegated and that it is definitely limited as to time and extent.

Staff agencies are of three types: administrative, service or auxiliary, and technical. General or administrative staff functions are usually concerned with problems of overall management, such as budgeting, program planning, personnel management, and structural organization. They are designed to assist the chief executive in handling important management matters without his becoming entangled in a mass of details. This is accomplished through personal secretaries and in larger organizations through administrative assistants and economic advisors. The functions of administrative staff personnel vary considerably. The staff officers in most instances receive reports and investigate the efficiency and administration of the units making up the organization; they look for duplication of work, formulate and suggest plans for the coordination of the units, and handle the route work of the executive. In collecting documents and information and in planning a course of action they advise the chief executive with reference to problems and proposals, and when a decision is made, they may transmit and explain the orders to the line officers concerned and follow up by observing and reporting the results. In theory they have no independent power or authority apart from the chief.

An administrative staff officer usually finds himself in the peculiar situation of having an interesting, important, and fruitful job but one in which his intentions are frequently misunderstood. He therefore must possess certain special characteristics to carry out his duties properly. First of all, he must have negotiating ability rather than a highly developed capacity to command. This requires great patience and persistence rather than a tendency toward making quick and fixed decisions. He needs a broad range of practical knowledge rather than extensive specialized or technical expertise in one or a few fields. He must be loyal to the policies and views of his superior rather than concerned with the promotion of his own plans or recommendations. Finally, he must have an honest willingness to remain more or less in the background rather than a wish for personal prominence and publicity. As aptly stated in the report of President Roosevelt's Committee on Administrative Management, "He must be possessed of high competence, great physical vigor and a passion for anonymity."

Service or auxiliary staff functions usually deal with the more strictly housekeeping activities of the organization, including the facilitation of office services such as the operation of a stenographic pool, statistical services, legal aid, central purchasing and supplies, and accounting. Although usually referred to in terms of services, many of these activities relate, at least in part, to control of line units.

One of the auxiliary services that sometimes gives rise to controversy is that of central purchasing and supplies. Whereas this office is intended to assist the line or functional units in the most efficient and economic manner possible, there is an implied division of responsibility and authority between the unit which uses and that which purchases. Theoretically the procedure should operate in about the following manner: The functional or line unit, perhaps a bureau or a division, takes the first step. It decides on the articles or material needed and describes them on a standard form, specifying the quantity required, the desired time and place of delivery, and any special considerations of the purchase in question. This requisition may even include the names of preferred manufacturers when one commercial product is considered superior to those of other companies. The requisition is sent to the central purchasing office usually after it has been examined by the comptroller or fiscal officer to be certain that sufficient funds are available. Actual purchase may then be made by the central purchasing officer, if possible on the basis of open competitive bids. The authority to purchase is vested solely in him. On delivery, inspection and maybe even laboratory tests are carried out to ascertain the proper quality and quantity of the materials supplied.

The point of possible controversy revolves primarily around whether the purchasing officer should have the right to modify a requisition either quantitatively or qualitatively. The extent to which he has this right essentially depends on the policy of the particular organization and occasionally on legally specified authority. Another objection concerns the delay encountered in obtaining the materials. Functional units not infrequently complain that by the time delivery is made the need has passed. Many organizations have attempted to solve this problem by allowing direct purchase of emergency material and specialized equipment under specified circumstances.

Technical staff service, as the term implies, is primarily concerned with methods, planning, and technical aspects of the operation. The technical personnel are functional specialists, such as are found in technical field staffs of state health departments, and skilled specialists loaned to states and localities by various national or other similar agencies. Whenever such technical specialists are loaned or seconded to work in line units, they should be answerable to the director of those line units rather than to some technical headquarters or to the top executive.

The relationship of the technical field staff to the functional line unit poses several problems. The situation in which they are perhaps most clearly seen is the functioning of a technical field staff of a division of local health service in a state department of health. The objective, of course, is to provide a smooth effective channel along which the knowledge and facilities of the central organization can flow to and through local units without destroying the initiative of the local personnel or impairing the authority that the director of the local unit must possess if he is to administer his program successfully.

Complete autonomy of the local units tends to inhibit the flow of technical service and advise from specialists in the central office to their counterparts on the local level. On the other hand, for central office specialists to have directing authority over corresponding specialists or technologists on the local level interferes with or destroys the proper coordination of the various activities of the local organization. When this occurs, the director of the local unit is reduced to little more than an administrative clerk. This is an unfortunate occurrence, since the local health officer is the only person with local personnel and facilities who is in a position to know where, when, how, and to whom local service should be rendered.[12]

As in the case of the administrative staff, care must be taken on the top level to assure complete understanding, both on the state and on the local level, of the purpose and function of the technical field staff. In turn the members of the field staff must do everything possible to deserve and gain the trust and confidence of the local personnel. The first and perhaps most important step toward this goal is for the top executive of the state or central agency to choose the members of the field staff as much on a personality basis as for their technical knowledge and ability.

Much depends on the organizational arrangement by which the aid of the technical experts of the central agency is channeled to the local unit. A mistake that has been made occasionally is to follow the pattern illustrated in Fig. 10-7. In this situation each functional division of the state agency independently sends its expert consultant directly to the personnel of the local agency. Even if this pattern is improved to the extent of channeling all the state technical field consultants through the county health officer, confusion and annoyance will still result. Coordination of the policies, activities, and methods of approach is extremely difficult, if not impossible, to attain. A given worker on the local level is likely to have several consultants from the state agency on his hands during the same period. In fact, the meeting of the state consultants in the field may be unexpected to them. The waste and inefficiency inherent in such a situation is obvious.

Experience has indicated that a much better approach to the problem is that illustrated in Fig. 10-8. By this pattern all technical field consultants who go into the local units originate from a single coordinating division or headquarters. Duplication of efforts and multiplicity of visitors are avoided. All requests or plans for field consultation are channeled through the director of the local unit, on the one hand, and the director of the division of local health service, on the other, the latter usually designated as deputy state health officer.

One of the potential dangers involved in the use of staff agencies is that the chief executive

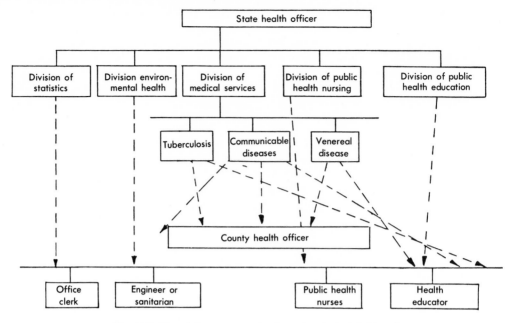

**Fig. 10-7.** Unsatisfactory organization of technical field staff.

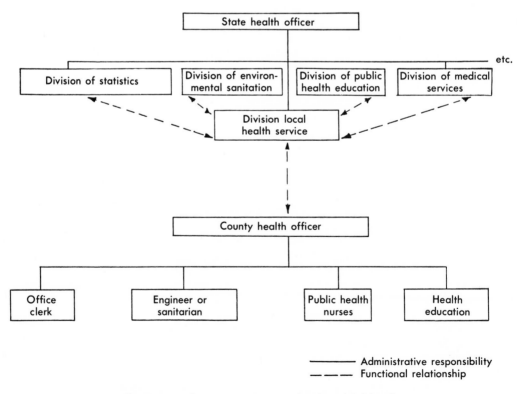

——— Administrative responsibility
— — — Functional relationship

**Fig. 10-8.** Satisfactory organization of technical field staff.

may become overenthusiastic or impatient with his functional subordinates and direct a staff assistant in whom he may have personal confidence to take a line situation in hand and straighten it out. Invariably this results in divided responsibility, with the personnel in general not knowing exactly whose orders they are expected to follow. Naturally this tends to cause resentment on the part of the division or bureau head. Furthermore, the personnel of the unit frequently adopt an interesting protective attitude toward their division or bureau chief even if they know him to be weak or to have other faults. The staff officer more than anyone else then finds himself in the unenviable middle position between the chief executive, on the one hand, and the functional personnel, on the other. Operating units are understandably jealous of their integrity and authority and resist any interference by an outside person, whom they may consider an administrative spy, stooge, or snoop. In any case they can easily thwart the work of a staff officer by following a policy of noncooperation and passive resistance of a degree short of insubordination. The staff officer in such cases must move warily, taking the time to win over not only the director of the operating division but also his personnel, demonstrating that he is there to assist rather than to criticize or undermine. The most desirable approach is to study the situation in cooperation with the division and with its assistance to seek a remedy. New findings or recommendations should be reported to the chief executive, preferably in company with the head of the operating unit involved, to whom should fall the responsibility for issuing whatever orders or taking whatever steps are considered necessary for correction or improvement of the particular situation.

## DECENTRALIZATION

A problem somewhat similar to the relationships between a county health department and the technical field staff of a state department of health exists when an agency attempts to decentralize its operations for purposes of greater efficiency and service. As has been said elsewhere, one of the chief characteristics of public health work is that it deals essentially with people rather than with things. Even in the sanitary control of inanimate material such as food, milk, or water it is the attitude, understanding, and cooperation of the producer, the handler, and the purveyor that are the important

factors. Most of a health department's budget is devoted to the salaries of professional workers who work with or serve the public or groups thereof. Nothing is manufactured. Practically speaking, the sole product is interpersonal relationships. This being the case, it is only good sense to attempt the delivery of these personal services and interpersonal relationships as close to and as convenient for the consumer as possible.

In a very real sense no one really lives in a city, state, or nation. As far as actual living is concerned, it occurs in neighborhoods. This is particularly true of large cities, where only a relatively few blocks are meaningful in the daily life of the average individual, that is, the area around the home, the school, the church, the shopping and recreational centers, and for the breadwinner the area around the place of employment. Certainly a city hall or a state capitol building is relatively meaningless to the average person, and if he has any feeling for them at all, the chances are that they are not particularly friendly. Attempts have been made in some places to carry out public health programs from city halls or state capitals. None has really succeeded. Increasingly, therefore, attention has been given to the decentralization of personnel, activities, and services to the maximum extent practical and possible.

In such situations, large cities for example, it is customary to divide the total area into districts each with a population of from 100,000 to 200,000 persons. In defining the district boundaries attention should be given to factors that may limit movement, such as streams, ridges, or railroad tracks, to concentrations of industries, to socioeconomic concentrations, to public transportation facilities, to boundaries of other departments and agencies, and to numerous other considerations. A district health center is usually established in each district, with perhaps a number of satellite clinic facilities, preferably near shopping centers, serviced from the district health centers. The health centers serve as the headquarters of the district health staffs and as the location of the more important activities of the district health program.

Mere physical decentralization alone, however, does not result in a decentralized program. It must be recognized and accepted that the public health personnel who work in a particular district are in the best position to be familiar with the problems, needs, and resources within

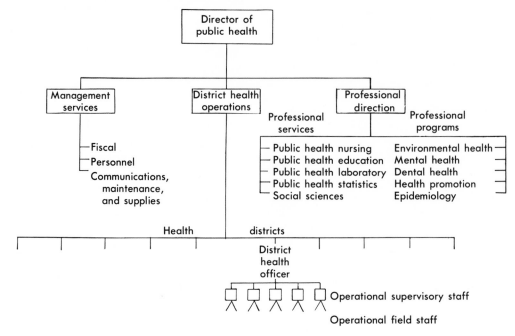

**Fig. 10-9.** Example of a decentralized city health organization.

that district. Therefore insofar as that district is concerned the district personnel should have the responsibility and the authority for determining and carrying out the details of the daily operations and activities, consistent, of course, with the overall policies and goals of the organization as a whole. Furthermore, to assure a well-coordinated district program all personnel assigned to a district should work under the administrative or *operational* direction of a district health officer. Some measure of administrative authority and responsibility must also be decentralized, or the intent will be defeated by red tape and delayed communications or starved by bureaucratic anemia. An important consideration therefore is to obtain capable individuals for the positions of administrative leadership in the decentralized units, and to allow them, organizationally and functionally, to determine and carry out their local programs to the maximum extent feasible. So that they can do so, of course, provision must be made for obtaining and dispensing funds, personnel, and materiel. Also a communications system must exist among the decentralized units and between them and the central offices. These are management functions that can only be carried out centrally. In addition, the central administration's program divisions must be concerned

with the establishment of standards and qualifications, with performance or quality control, and with the *professional* and *technical* aspects of program conception, planning, supervision, and evaluation.

It would appear therefore that, except in very small agencies, organizational activities and responsibilities divide themselves naturally into three functional areas: management, field operations, and professional or technical direction. One of the most difficult administrative problems is to bring about a method of organization and a degree of personnel understanding that will allow each of these three functional areas to perform adequately and satisfactorily both unto itself and in relation to the other two. Fig. 10-9 is an example of this type of organization that has proved to be successful.

## COORDINATION AND CONTROL MEASURES

To devise a sound organizational structure and to staff that structure with qualified personnel under a capable chief executive does not necessarily guarantee continued successful function. Certain measures and techniques must be put into operation and constantly maintained to make sure that principles and policies set down are adhered to, that the plan which has been adopted is followed, that the responsibility delegated has been met, and that the orders and work which have been assigned have been fulfilled. The general purposes of these measures are (1) to keep the activities of the total organization and each of its component parts in line with established policies, (2) to maintain a proper balance among the various divisions and bureaus of the organization, (3) to maintain efficient work standards and performance, (4) to assure consistency of action, and (5) to prevent the development of personnel stresses and strains through the promotion of harmonious and satisfactory work relationships.

The tendency for certain aggressive subexecutives to magnify the importance of their work and to become empire builders has been referred to. Usually every unit in an organization is imbued with the essential value of its work and can present arguments to justify its expansion in terms of jurisdiction, appropriations, and personnel. However, the resources available to the total organization are limited and must be carefully and logically distributed among all the functional units on a basis determined by the overall purpose and program of the organization. To accomplish this successfully involves continuous efforts for the coordination of all parts of the organization.

Coordination has been spoken of as the dynamics of organization. It is a broad term that includes a wide variety of activities, the aim of which is to have related workers or groups of workers function harmoniously and effectively together where and when they are needed to avoid duplication and conflict. Pfiffner and Preshus[6] have presented an excellent example of automatic administrative coordination in terms of what occurs when a fire alarm is sounded. When the police and firemen answer the call, "upon their arrival they are likely to meet repair crews from the telephone company, the gas company, and the electrical company. The high pressure pumps of the water company are already in action. All of these coordinated activities have been set in motion through the alarm system." In public health work this type of situation can be observed perhaps most dramatically in the teamwork of a well-trained epidemiologic staff working to control an outbreak of a communicable disease. Diagnosis and control of the problem requires the smooth, well-coordinated interaction of many types of personnel. Medical and nursing personnel provide care for those already afflicted to speed their recovery and to prevent the further spread of disease from them. Field investigators obtain personal histories and make whatever other inquiries and examinations are necessary to trace the original source of the epidemic. Here the sanitarian and the engineer may play a most important role. Working with them may be a staff of laboratory workers. Meanwhile the cooperation of the public and the professions is solicited through the efforts of health educators.

There are many techniques that may be used to assure effective control of the activities and program of an organization. Much could be written about each, and the following is intended as merely a brief outline. The most elementary step that can be taken is the development of an organization chart. Several aspects of this have already been discussed, and little more will be added at this point. Suffice to say, the concept of the use of organization charts has been a subject of controversy. Some authorities in administration have warned of danger in the mere existence of charts, since there may easily develop a tendency to tie the future of the program to the chart, thereby hampering growth and development, rather than to constantly adjust the chart to the program. True as this potentiality may be, it is believed that to attempt to administer a program and to supervise an agency of any but the smallest size without some form of organization chart showing channels, responsibilities, and authority is like trying to steer a ship blind without a chart to show passages, reefs, and shoals, on the one hand, and without established connections with the engine room, on the other.

Once the structure is established, many methods of overall management and control of the activities of the agency become possible. Various types of manuals have been found to be of value even in small agencies. Worthy of particular mention are administrative manuals that present the legal and other policies to be followed and technical or work manuals that describe in detail the steps to be taken in the performance of particular functions. Standing orders for the nursing personnel may be considered a special example of this category. Manuals are especially useful for the orientation of new personnel and are indicated particularly in larger organizations. As is the case with many similar types of materials, they must not be allowed to become stale but must constantly be reviewed and updated. Of like nature are written executive and administrative orders, information circulars, and special instructions and directives. These should be numbered, codified, indexed, and routinely channeled throughout the organization.

One of the chief means of administrative contact with and therefore control of the functional units of the organization is through written records and reports that may be required to flow upward. Generally speaking, these are of two types: financial and service. In the typical large health department, for example, the staff nurses routinely submit daily or weekly reports of visits and services with costs of transportation or mileage noted. These are summarized, first, for the individual nurse's service and payment records and, second, for the monthly and annual report of the nursing division. When correlated with salaries, overhead, and transportation costs, the ingredients of service cost accounting become available. Records and reports should not be relied on entirely for contact with the functional units. Those in executive positions do well to get out occasionally to the level where the work is being done and the service is being rendered.

It is important to review at least periodically the purpose of and need for each record or report. Two examples may illustrate the point. In one large health department a request was made for a temporary review of certain office procedures. Subsequently an organizational analysis found that one clerk-typist was devoting her entire time to the compilation and typing of a highly detailed monthly report, referred to as Dr. X's report. When each report was completed, it was sent to another office, where it was immediately and permanently filed. Inquiry brought out that Dr. X, who had originally requested the information, had left the organization about 8 years before. A similar instance was discovered in the progress of a community health survey. Here a certain record flowed through a small office with a single typist, who carefully made a copy of each record before sending it on its way. The copy was filed by her with equal care, but in response to questioning she stated that to her knowledge no one had ever referred to her file of copies. The origin of this strange ritual was never discovered.

To a considerable extent the program and activities of a health department are imple-

mented by means of correspondence. The handling and routing of correspondence therefore becomes important. One occasionally finds chief executives, such as health commissioners of even large cities and states, who for reasons of vanity, distrust, or uncertainty insist that all incoming and outgoing mail pass through their hands. This procedure, of course, is foolish and wasteful and indicates questionable administrative ability. A practical screening procedure should be developed to conserve the time and energy of those in the hierarchy of the organization. Thus bureau chiefs may read or scan most or all of the dictated correspondence arising within their units, and division chiefs may read a great deal, whereas the chief executive may limit himself to letters involving complex issues, controversial cases, new policy, or important persons.

Before the close of this discussion on the higher level of the organization mention should be made of staff conferences and special committees. Staff conferences serve the dual purpose of administrative control and promotion of good personnel relations. They are best held at definitely stated intervals, neither too long nor too short. Some health departments find it advantageous to have staff meetings weekly, others biweekly, and still others monthly. In times of emergency or when developing a special program, they may, of course, be held more frequently. Although the chief executive should preside over the meetings, he should not monopolize the discussion. Each division and bureau head should be provided with an opportunity to present his problems or contributions. The designation of a staff secretary and the keeping of minutes are sound policies to be strongly recommended. Pro tem staff committees often serve important purposes. They may be formed for the purposes of inspection, survey, investigation, planning, coordination, or technical study. It is often advantageous to include one or several representatives from whatever unit or service is involved, and they should report back to the executive or to the staff.

Closer to the functional line employees are several procedures that facilitate control. Important among those that might be mentioned are work-flow charts, cross-checks, job analyses, and descriptions and standardization of methods and procedures. The use of internal cross-checks is frequently possible. These are arrangements for checking the work of one employee, unit, or agency against that of another. Examples that may be cited in the field of public health are the routine or spot check of reports of inspections against related laboratory reports and the check of supplies of biologics furnished against therapeutic or immunologic services rendered.

The classification of positions is valuable but merely as a first step. It is important that there be developed careful and accurate job or position analyses and descriptions, which should, of course, be updated periodically.[20] Not only do they make possible more logical employment standards, qualifications, and placement policies but they encourage career development and help to improve curricula. The public health profession has progressed considerably with regard to the establishment of personnel qualifications. They have been formulated for both the quality and quantity of various professional types of personnel. In addition, an extensive array of standards have been developed by committees of experts for programs, for goals, and for many technical procedures. Much of this has been a result of the efforts of the American Public Health Association, the United States Public Health Service, and the World Health Organization, especially those concerned with laboratory methods and administrative practice. Out of them have come, for example, the widely accepted and used reports on *Standard Methods of Water and Milk Analysis, Control of Communicable Diseases, and Evaluation of Health Practices.*

## REFERENCES

1. Gaus, J. M., White, L. D., and Dimock, M. E.: The frontiers of public administration, Chicago, 1936, University of Chicago Press.
2. Dimock, M. E.: The executive in action, New York, 1945, Harper & Row, Publishers.
3. Robb, R.: Organization as affected by purpose and conditions. In Merrill, H. F., editor: Classics in management, New York, 1960, American Management Association.
4. Frank, A. G.: Administrative role definition and social change, Human Organization **22:**238, Winter 1963-1964.
5. Sayre, W. S.: In Sweeney, S. B., and Davey, T. J., editors: Education for administrative careers in government service, Philadelphia, 1958, University of Pennsylvania Press.
6. Pfiffner, J. McD., and Preshus, R.: Public Administration, New York, 1967, The Ronald Press Co.
7. Elling, R. H., and Lee, O. J.: Formal connections of community leadership to the health system, Milbank Mem. Fund Quart. **44:**294, July 1966.
8. Goodenough, W. H.: Agency structure as a major source of human problems in the conduct of public health programs, Amer. J. Public Health **55:**1067, July 1965.
9. Rosen, G.: Some substantive limiting conditions in communication between health officers and medical practitioners, Amer. J. Public Health **51:**1805, Dec. 1961.
10. Lefcowitz, M. J.: The public health professional: a marginal man, Amer. J. Public Health **54:**1125, July 1964.
11. Confrey, E. A., editor: Administration of community health services, Chicago, 1961, International City Managers Association.
12. Weber, M.: The theory of social and economic organization, New York, 1947, Oxford University Press, Inc.
13. Schleh, E. C.: Successful executive action, Englewood Cliffs, N. J., 1962, Prentice-Hall, Inc.
14. Randall, C. B.: The folklore of management, New York, 1962, Mentor Executive Library Books.
15. White, L. D.: Introduction to the study of public administration, New York, 1955, The Macmillan Co.
16. Anderson, W.: The units of government in the United States, Public Administration Service pub. no. 42, 1934.
17. Editorial: Vertical versus horizontal administration, Amer. J. Public Health **32:**86, Jan. 1942.
18. Sartain, A. Q., and Baker, A. W.: The supervisor and his job, ed. 2, New York, 1972, McGraw-Hill Book Co.
19. Gulick, L.: Notes on the theory of organization. In Gulick, L., and Urwick, L., editors: Papers on the science of administration, New York, 1937, Institute of Public Administration.
20. Donovan, J. J.: Career development classification, Amer. J. Public Health **51:**591, April 1961.

*If your company is run "by the book,"*
*If the job description is more important than the man,*
*Your organization is in danger of creeping paralysis.*

CLARENCE B. RANDALL

# CHAPTER 11

# Personnel management

## PEOPLE MAKE THE PROGRAM

"The tripod upon which the public health structure of any country rests is (1) a force of well-trained personnel, (2) the appointment, promotion and retention of personnel on a merit basis, and (3) adequate financial support, evidencing public understanding of the problems involved."[1] These considerations plus the fact that the management of personnel and their problems is one of the health administrator's first, continuing, and most difficult tasks require attention to this field.

In many places, personnel management in public health has been influenced by factors not always desirable. Among those that may be cited are unfavorable attitudes toward public service, acceptance if not support of the practice of political patronage and of the spoils system, a tendency to expect and to tolerate some degree of inefficiency or even dishonesty in public affairs, and a heritage of relatively low salaries. Fortunately in many places and in many nations these factors are well on their way to disappearance. The word *politics* has been used. It should be recognized that the word is often misunderstood or misinterpreted. What is meant most often is a type of selfish, pernicious partisanism. Politics in this sense has been passing out of the American scene as a result of a greatly broadened educational base, the growth in demand for good and efficient public services, the development of civil service and merit systems, and the appearance of a more dedicated and sophisticated type of political leader.[2] Furthermore, it should be realized that

there may be many forms of pernicious politics other than those stemming from political parties and that all of them are deterrents to efficient service. The public health worker, in the course of his work and contacts, may find himself involved in personal politics, fraternal politics, racial politics, religious politics, professional politics, labor politics, economic and social politics, and politics of many other types. It must be realized that political activity is a necessary part of any system of representative government and indeed of sound responsive public health practice. Politics has been described as the art of the possible. The manner and extent to which the latter is true has been well presented by Mattison,[3] who described and compared the model of a public health program from the viewpoint of a politician in contrast with that of a health director and indicated points at which their common interests and goals may come together for the public good. A symposium on *The Politics of Public Health*[4] stated that "Politics has a depth and complexity encountered in no other human pursuit. Einstein perceived this and succinctly summed it up when he was asked why it was that men who can develop wonder drugs and stamp out epidemics cannot understand politics. The wise old man answered, 'Politics is more difficult than medicine.'"

The field of public health has certain characteristics that give rise to some special personnel problems. It is a curious mixture of public and social responsibility and service. It is notable, however, that public health as a social obligation has only recently been accepted by government and that much public health service is still provided by private voluntary organizations. Furthermore, it is still common for the budgets of official health agencies to be augmented by funds from private sources. In a real sense the field is still largely in the process of organizational development. The major component of public health expenditures is for personnel. A complex spectrum of ability and function is required that necessitates the activity of many different specialized types of personnel. Involved are physicians, dentists, veterinarians, engineers, sanitarians, chemists, nurses, bacteriologists, educators, social scientists, management specialists, and many others, each with particular pride and interest in his specialty.

Not only are the activities of many types but they are continually undergoing change, adaptation, and evolution. What is appropriate and adequate practice today may be inadequate or outmoded tomorrow. Furthermore, the field is constantly and rapidly expanding, having begun with the barest essentials of sanitation, added preventive medicine and health promotion, and now extended into the entire complex of medical and health institutional care and management. In contrast to many private and public enterprises there are relatively few activities in public health that are subject to formalization or exact quantification. In most instances the product to be sold tends to be intangible, and the consumers are all the people, with their varying types and degrees of need, pride, prejudice, reticence, and intelligence. Often the selling literally involves a change in the habits, desires, and customs of people so that a successful approach in one instance, time, or location may fail in other circumstances.

## HEALTH MANPOWER PROBLEMS

Because of the relative newness of public health work and the great recent demand for services, additional difficulties have arisen, many of them involving personnel. For a considerable period there were no special facilities for training individuals for this field. In the absence of trained specialists it was considered satisfactory to employ a wide variety of generally unqualified individuals, including retired or unsuccessful practicing physicians and political appointees. Related to this was the inability to attract and retain capable personnel because of insecurity of tenure, low salaries, and competi-

tion from other fields and also because the profession of public health was not yet well enough known to be attractive. The problem was summed up by Rosenau,[5] who commented:

The time has long since gone by when the physician can spend a few hours from his busy day to look after the duties of the health office. The situation demands the entire time and energy of those who consecrate their lives to the public welfare. In order to attract capable men to the new profession it is important that the health officer should have an assured tenure of office with adequate pay and freedom from politics.

To complete the circle, as a result of the previously mentioned inadequacies, there was a corresponding lack of established, well-organized agencies in which at least practical field training experience might be obtained.

As time went on, however, the public health profession undertook to solve these problems on many fronts. Through the efforts of those concerned with public health work as a career a fairly rapid maturing of the profession occurred, which resulted in widespread public and professional acceptance, accumulation of sound experience, and the application of more scientific procedures. Gradually medical schools began to include preventive medicine and public health in their curricula. The recency of this, however, is emphasized by a prophecy by Rosenau[5] in an article written in 1915. "The modern practitioner of medicine is fast adding prevention as one of the tools of his equipment. The future student of medicine will make a study of health and how to maintain it, as well as a study of disease and how to cure it."

The fact is, however, that even to this day it is a rare medical school that does even a reasonably competent job in this respect. Medical curricula are still almost completely illness oriented, and most medical schools and teaching hospitals are more interested in clinical departments that bring in sick patients, for most of whom someone or some agency pays, than in a department that strives to prevent illness and promote positive health. A significant trend for the better should be noted, however. An increasing number of medical schools are discovering that patients originate from some place—the community with all its complexities—and that the genesis of most illness, hence the more complete handling of the case, is to be found in the community and not merely within the walls of the hospital or the physician's office. As a result, experimentation is occurring in several of the more progressive centers of medical education in the teaching of comprehensive medicine, community medicine, or social medicine.

## TRAINING IN PUBLIC HEALTH

Because of the rapidly evolving scope of public health, medical training alone was soon recognized to be inadequate preparation for a health officer as well as failing to serve the needs of the nonmedical personnel in public health work. In pleading for specialized training and degrees for public health workers, Rosenau[5] said:

> Public health work is becoming, in fact, has already become, a separate profession. It has split off from medicine just as medicine long ago split off from the priesthood. Public health service, as a career, must be an end in itself. It is often difficult and sometimes impossible to bend the physician into a health officer. The ordinary medical training does not qualify a person to be a health officer.

In 1912 a program of basic training in the biologic sciences was established at Massachusetts Institute of Technology in cooperation with Harvard University similar to the first 2 years of medical school, followed by courses in public health science instead of the usual clinical courses pursued by medical students. In 1914 a conference of leaders of education, medicine, and public health called by the General Education Board recommended that public health schools of high standards be established as separate entities affiliated with universities and their schools of medicine. The first distinct school of this type was established in 1916 at the University of Pennsylvania. This school is no longer in existence. However, the university still awards occasional public health degrees in certain specialized areas. As time passed, additional schools were established.

An additional complication arose. Due to the acceptance of the value of public health programs and the demand for personnel, a large number of educational institutions of varying quality began to grant degrees in public health, more often than not on the basis of grossly inadequate training. By 1939 a total of 45 schools and universities were listed as granting 18 different kinds of degrees in public health.[6] The situation became so undesirable and confusing that finally in 1941 there was established an Association of Schools of Public Health, consisting of schools later accredited by

a system developed by the American Public Health Association.[7,8] As a result, there are now in the United States 18 schools accredited to grant acceptable professional degrees in this field. These are the University of California at Berkeley, University of California at Los Angeles, Columbia University, Harvard University, University of Hawaii, Johns Hopkins University, University of Illinois, Loma Linda (Cal.) University, University of Michigan, University of Minnesota, University of North Carolina, University of Oklahoma, University of Pittsburgh, University of Puerto Rico, University of Texas at Houston, Tulane University, University of Washington, and Yale University.[9] In Canada the University of Toronto and the University of Montreal are also accredited. In Latin America a similar Association of Schools of Public Health was formed at a conference of deans in Mexico in 1959. As yet no accrediting system has been established, but biennial meetings that have been held since with the assistance of the Pan American Health Organization have gone far to enhance professional education in public health in Central and South America.[10-13]

To establish criteria for the accreditation of schools it was logically necessary to first determine qualifications and standards of function for prospective personnel of public health agencies. In other words, what should the final product of the schools be? Efforts toward this end were begun in the late 1930's by the Committee on Professional Education of the American Public Health Association, with the result that educational qualifications have been established for the majority of the various kinds of professional personnel who might be employed by an official or nonofficial public health agency.[14]

Although each specialty is of necessity dealt with separately, those usually considered to represent the basic personnel of a health department, that is, health officers, public health engineers, and public health nurses, have certain requisites in common. These may be summarized as follows:

1. Graduation from an approved professional school (medicine, nursing, etc.)
2. An academic year in a school of public health or, in the case of nurses, a school approved by the National League for Nursing, leading to a degree
3. A period of practical supervised experience in a health department

4. The customary desirable personal qualifications

It was soon realized that just as an internship was necessary to round out the academic training of the medical graduate, so a period of practical field training should supplement study at a school of public health. Therefore a special Subcommittee on Field Training analyzed the types of field training desirable for public health personnel, dividing them into the following five categories[15]:

1. Observation—duration: 1 day to 1 week. The individual takes no direct part in the activities of the health department. It is best suited for a well-trained, experienced person who simply desires to learn of new procedures or to discuss new policy.

2. Orientation—duration: 1 to 2 months. This is training to prepare an individual for a specific position in a specific place. It is intended to familiarize a skilled person with the particular problems, laws, codes, customs, and procedures of that area or state in which he is about to work.

3. Field experience—duration: 3 to 6 months. This training is supplementary to a theoretical, academic training in public health. It is comparable to an internship which follows medical training. The training areas should be carefully selected and require teaching personnel, in addition to standard personnel.

4. Apprenticeship—duration: 3 to 12 months. This training is given before the candidate has had his academic year of work at a school of public health. It has special advantages in the selection and training of medical health officers. The individual is employed as an apprentice by the health department, and if he likes the work and proves to be capable he is then given a period of academic training by the state and returns to his official sponsor at the completion of the theoretical work.

5. In-service training—This is simply a continuous educational program for all types of personnel in the health department, in order to keep them abreast of the times. It is a special function of the local health department, with aid from the state health department.

The next step taken was the development of accredited field-training areas to supplement the academic training received in a school of public health. This began in 1950 and has been carried forward under the tripartite aegis of the Committee on Professional Education of the American Public Health Association, the Council on Medical Education and Hospitals of the American Medical Association, and the American Board of Preventive Medicine and Public Health.[16] By now about one half of the states and through them a number of localities have programs approved for residency

training.[17] The program is analogous to the approving of hospitals for internships and residencies. Still another step was the establishment in 1949 of the specialty board, the American Board of Preventive Medicine and Public Health, by the Council on Medical Education and Hospitals of the American Medical Association assisted by the American Public Health Association. The purpose of this board was "1. To encourage the study, improve the practice, elevate the standards, and advance the cause of preventive medicine and public health [and] 2. To grant and issue to physicians duly licensed by law to practice medicine, certificates of special knowledge in preventive medicine and public health."[18]

In addition to these activities that relate only to physicians, several other professional disciplines engaged in public health work, notably environmental health and public health nursing, have also developed programs for approved field training and accreditation.

Further trends toward the solution of personnel problems in public health are the increasing adoption of merit systems, in which the American Public Health Association, the United States Public Health Service, and the Children's Bureau have taken leading roles,[19,20] and the gradual improvement of salaries resulting from several circumstances, including personnel demand in relation to supply, improved training, and recognition of the value of public health work. In relation to the health manpower shortage and training needs has been the important recognition that the problems are of national scope rather than simply state or local. An increasing number of fellowships for professional public health training have been made available to the states through federal grants; and in 1958 Congress passed the first bill to subsidize accredited schools of public health to a modest extent, partly on the basis of their representing regional training centers for the nation. Since that time several national conferences on health manpower and public health training have been held, leading to increased federal efforts to improve the situation.[21]

The need for these steps was indicated by the fact that as recently as 1951, although the majority of physicians employed in public health agencies had attended various short courses and institutes on specialized subjects, only about one third had formal training leading to a degree in public health. About 36% of staff nurses employed in state and local health agencies had 1 year or more of study in public health or public health nursing. Of sanitation officers, approximately one third had no public health training.[22] This situation has improved somewhat since then, but there are still significant numbers of individuals in all categories working in public health with inadequate specialized training backgrounds.

## HEALTH MANPOWER NEEDS

Because of the persistence of the health manpower shortage combined with the rapid development of new knowledge and techniques, the field of public health has been experimenting with several additional approaches. Among these have been not only programs for updating existing personnel[23] and many programs for the training of volunteer and ancillary workers but also more recently special programs to take advantage of the special cultural knowledge and abilities of individuals recruited directly from socioeconomically depressed neighborhoods.[24]

The generally accepted minimum staffing requirements for basic health services are as follows:

One public health physician for every 50,000 persons (or one for every local health unit, whichever is less)

One public health nurse for every 5,000 persons if bedside nursing is not included; otherwise, one for every 2,500 persons

One supervising nurse for each 6 to 8 staff nurses

One sanitary engineer or sanitarian for every 15,000 persons

One clerk for every 15,000 persons

The adequacy of such a staff depends, of course, on the nature or degree of comprehensiveness of the services that they are called on to render. Obviously, if a health service facility is involved in the delivery of comprehensive health care, the ratios presented would be completely inadequate.

One of the most complete analyses of the quantitative needs for public health personnel at a point in time was that presented by the Emerson report over 30 years ago.[25] Although now obviously out of date, it does give perspective to the problem. It indicated that in 1942 there were 40,782 persons employed in providing local public health services under the auspices of the local, state, or federal governments. One fourth were part-time workers, three quarters of whom were health officers

and clinic physicians. It was estimated that at least 23,000 additional trained individuals were needed to provide the minimal public health services on the local level alone. Greatest needs were for public health nurses, dentists and dental hygienists, health educators, and environmental workers.

The interval since has seen slow improvement. By the end of 1949 the number of full-time personnel employed by full-time official local health agencies totaled 33,555. Fewer than half of the local units had sufficient physicians to meet minimum requirements. Approximately one fourth of all units reported no physicians employed on a full-time basis. Shortages were still much more pronounced for nurses than for any other types of personnel. Only 6.5% of local health units had enough nurses to meet the minimum standard. With regard to environmental health personnel, that is, sanitary engineers, sanitarians, and veterinarians, nearly 63% of cities but only about 31% of counties met minimum standards. About 50% of units had adequate clerical and office staffs. According to accepted requirements, there were needed an additional 1,223 physicians, 11,826 nurses, 1,982 environmental health personnel, and 1,587 clerks.[26]

For other specialties approximately 20% of budgeted positions for health educators, public health dentists, and medical social workers were vacant at that time. For nutritionists the figures was 16%, for laboratory workers about 10%, for veterinarians 10%, and for statisticians and analysts 15%.[27]

By 1965 the situation appeared on the surface to have improved somewhat with a total of 51,632 full-time workers of different categories reported employed by local health departments. This represented a 50% increase since 1949. Gains, however, have been uneven. Thus full-time public health physicians increased only from 1,609 in 1949 to 1,668 in 1965, and laboratory personnel from 1,391 in 1949 to 1,546 in 1965. The greatest gains made over this period were in environmental health personnel (from 6,531 to 10,369), in medical and psychiatric social workers (from 111 to 688), and in public health nurses (from 11,251 to 16,058). Despite this, when the increase in population during the 16 years is taken into consideration, it is found that with the exception of social workers and dentists, no net gains were achieved and some significant decreases in relative numbers had occurred.[28] To evaluate the situation adequately one must also consider the significant increase in general earning power and the standard of living with a resultant greatly increased expectancy and demand for public health services on the local and especially urban level. It is interesting but not surprising to note that although in absolute numbers the need is greatest in the larger, more populated communities, the proportionate need is greatest in the smaller, less populated areas. Undoubtedly this is attributable to the many attractions of work and life in urban and suburban as against essentially rural or small-town circumstances.

In summary it might be stated that at the present time the two intimately related factors that contribute the most to retarding the development and expansion of public health work are (1) inadequate competitive salaries and (2) inadequate numbers of trained personnel.[29]

## PERSONNEL MANAGEMENT

It has been stated that one of the health administrator's chief responsibilities is the direction and supervision of the function and activity of the other members of the health department staff. This is important in any organization, but its relative importance is perhaps accentuated in public health practice because to an unusual degree the personnel literally are the health department, and furthermore, the successful function and behavior of the members of the health department's staff determine in the last analysis the acceptance and success of the organization's work. This is true because acceptance and success depend on the reaction of the public, and it is through personal contacts of the department's staff with the public that the health program operates.

Despite this, several health officers and other health administrators unfortunately neglect the personnel aspects of their programs. Too often the health officer regards himself merely as the source of medical knowledge and activity in the department, with essentially a nominal responsibility as the representative head of the agency. Common as this attitude may be, it is certainly not good practice and is naive from the viewpoint of legal and executive responsibility. The capable administrator, in public health work as elsewhere, must assume an active interest and responsibility for every phase of personnel management, from recruitment and employment to dismissal if necessary.

## RECRUITMENT AND EMPLOYMENT

### Merit systems

Recent years have seen the development and wide acceptance of the merit system principle for the purpose of recruiting and selecting capable individuals to fill specific positions in the civil service. It is curious to find occasionally among administrators of public health programs a certain amount of conflicting resentment toward the civil service or merit system idea and at the same time complaint against political patronage pressure as a handicap to efficient service. This dissatisfaction may perhaps be attributed to three things: (1) lack of understanding by the executive of the essential purposes and potentialities of the merit system; (2) the unfortunate fact that some civil service agencies still think of their original "fight the spoilsman" slogan and consider themselves more as policemen than as program facilitators; and (3) lag in the development of new personnel techniques to aid effective administration. Despite these attitudes and difficulties, it is obvious that merit systems are here to stay and generally speaking have already resulted in considerable improvements in public service.

By now the majority of governmental employees in the United States serve under merit systems, and each year sees more added to the list. In 1955 White[30] correctly predicted:

> . . . the basic conditions of government are such that the eventual triumph of the merit system seems inevitable. The ever-increasing technological aspects of governmental operations; the greatly intensified social responsibility of government, making the risk of administrative failure equivalent to the risk of social catastrophe; the emerging professional point of view in many branches of administration; and the expansion of civil service unions intent on protecting their own interests by the steady application of the merit system, these and other circumstances forecast the certain destruction of patronage in due course of time.

Civil service systems and merit systems have had a long and slow history, and only recently has there occurred accelerated adoption of the idea. Although the first but unsuccessful measures were taken by the national government as early as 1853, it was not until the assassination of President Garfield in 1881 by a disappointed office seeker that increasing sentiment was crystallized. As a result, Congress reluctantly approved the Pendleton Act, which serves as the basis of civil service regulations in effect today. Originally the Pendleton

Act included only about 14,000 federal positions, chiefly those in the postal and customs services. Successive presidential orders have increased the number of federal employees included under the merit system to about 90% of the total at the present time. Of particular effect has been the Ramspeck Act of 1940, which gave the President wide authority to extend the scope of the civil service act and the classification act. The first state civil service law was passed by New York in 1883. Two years later Massachusetts followed suit. Twenty years passed before any other states took action (Illinois and Wisconsin in 1905). More widespread adoption continued slowly until the late 1930s. By 1937 only 10 states had adopted merit system legialstion. When many states finally introduced the principle, it was due largely to pressure from federal agencies rather than to an appreciation on the part of the state themselves of the value of civil service or merit systems.

Concerning public health agencies, with rare exceptions states that established civil service or merit systems did so because of restrictions in the federal laws and regulations governing financial payments to the states for the much needed grants-in-aid programs of the United States Public Health Service and the Children's Bureau under the Social Security Act. The effect of the federal requirements is dramatically indicated by the fact that in 1940 alone, the year after their adoption, 12 states established merit systems affecting public health personnel! The purpose and method were described as follows[31]:

In the interests of promoting and maintaining sound personnel policies, Federal administrative agencies are authorized to examine civil service or merit systems of states and territories receiving "grants-in-aid" funds. Such systems when submitted by the state and territories are considered by Federal agencies under two headings and approval or disapproval is given either or both of these. The parts thus examined are: (1) the basic or rule, (2) the classification and compensation plan. The score by 1945 for 51 states and territories with the United States Public Health Service is:

| | Reviewed | Approved |
|---|---|---|
| Law or rule | 50 | 45 |
| Classification and compensation plans | 46 | 20 |

By now less than 10% of local public health workers are not included in some type of merit system.

The terms *civil service system* and *merit system* are often used interchangeably as if they were synonymous. There is a difference, although the distinction is slight from a practical standpoint. Both are nothing more or less than organized methods of selecting and advancing employees on the basis of their qualifications in relation to the aptitudes required by a particular job, together with relatively assured permanency of tenure, prescribed personnel benefits, and equal pay for equal work. If the plan exists by virtue of a statute, it is usually referred to as a civil service system. If it originates from an administrative ruling, it is called a merit system. A merit system therefore might be considered a civil service system without benefit of legislation. However, as this newer term gained in popularity and generic use, it appeared also in legislated plans so that one cannot automatically infer the structure from the name. Neither term has yet been supplanted by the preference of personnel administrators to speak of public personnel programs in which the merit principle is assumed.

To accomplish the purposes outlined several prerequisites are indicated. In a civil service system the first essential is the necessary enabling legislation accompanied by adequate appropriation for the satisfactory operation of the program. The legislation should provide the necessary authority to the civil service agency so that its activities may not be circumvented or ignored. If a number of agencies are involved, of which the health department is only one, provision should be made for uniform policies and procedures inasmuch as possible. The law itself should give attention to the removal of the system from the influences of local politics. This is desirably accomplished by providing for a separate personnel agency administered by a career executive under a nonpartisan advisory, regulatory, and appellate commission whose members serve for overlapping terms.

Of more recent origin is the trend toward professional personnel units[32] within large functional agencies such as health departments of states or large cities. This unit reports to the agency administrator, assisting him in carrying out his personnel responsibilities, and provides liaison with the civil service agency. To provide for the selection and promotion of employees on the basis of their qualifications or merit a civil service agency is faced with the preliminary problem of position analysis and classification. This is further necessary to make possible the desired uniformity of policy previously mentioned and to prevent several individuals doing essentially the same type and amount of work from getting widely varying compensation. Needless to say, position analysis and classification and the resulting qualifications for prospective personnel should be carried out jointly by the administration of the functional agencies and the civil service agency, or a personnel department under the latter's control, with an attitude of helpfulness. It should be revised periodically to reflect changes occurring in the content of positions.[33]

Once position classifications and personnel qualifications have been established, the next step is to provide for the recruitment and examination of applicants. In the field of public health more recruiting activities are carried on by the public health agency itself than by the civil service agency, since in most instances the health officer is in a better position to know the type of individual he wants and where he might look for him, and candidates usually do not abound. Examination may consist of one or all of the various approaches, including substantiated records of training and experience, written examinations largely for the purpose of determining technical knowledge, and personal interviews chiefly to get an insight into the personality of the applicant. Since achievement of a high grade is not invariably indicative of desirable personnel and since, as will be discussed, an important phase of operation is the interplay between the personalities of the executive officer and his subordinate personnel, it is only reasonable to allow the executive officer a choice among the top two or three candidates who were successful in the examination.

When circumstances result in a surplus of desirable applicants, it becomes an added function of the civil service agency to maintain a register of qualified personnel. Where retirement plans have been put into operation, responsibility for them has often been given to the civil service agency. In addition they frequently serve as places of appeal and review in instances involving disciplinary measures, dismissal, or overt employer-employee conflicts.

**Compensation, tenure, and promotion**

As previously stated, one of the essential purposes of a compensation plan based on position classification is equal pay for equal work. In the absence of such a plan the weak executive tends to be unconcerned or ineffective in obtaining increases for his personnel in general. At the other extreme is the executive with a strong and aggressive personality who may tend to secure increases for favorite employees without consideration of the absolute or comparative value of their services. Compensation in such instances may then depend largely on political influence, friendships, favoritism, and nepotism. Needless to say, the morale of the employees of either of these types of administrators rapidly degenerates.

The position in an organization having been classified and a general policy of compenstion having been decided on, the next step is the allocation of pay rates to the various position class titles. Usually this is done by establishing a range from the minimum rate to be paid to new employees up to a maximum that may be paid to anyone in the particular position class. In setting this salary scale consideration should be given to numerous factors, among which are payment for comparable work elsewhere in the same locality, cost of living, wage trends, the financial condition of the community and agency, legal restrictions that may exist, and recognition of union rates. In many professional health classes the national mobility and recruitment of personnel cause salaries for comparable work in agencies across the country to become a significant factor. Once set, salary scales should be reviewed regularly to maintain currency.

It is generally desirable that the minimum rate of a position class should not be less than the maximum rate of a lower class. Between the minimum and maximum there should be one or more intermediate steps. A usual compensation policy is to start the new employee at the minimum of the rage, granting the first increase at the end of an introductory or probationary period, followed by further increases annually thereafter until the maximum salary for the particular position class has been reached. It should be clearly understood, however, that compensation advancement is not automatic but only follows demonstrated and continued proficiency. Whenever possible the decision concerning an increase should be made by more than one person. For example, in larger organizations the decision might involve the combined judgments of the executive health officer, the immediate supervisor of the employee in question, and the personnel officer.

Of considerable assistance in making decisions concerning compensation increases is the use of efficiency and service ratings. It is recommended that the administrator periodically and systematically survey or study the efficiency of his employees and that the results be made part of a permanent personal history file of each employee. Inasmuch as possible the evaluations should be based on factual data, measurable performance, and work records rather than on purely personal judgments, although the latter should be included as auxiliary information. An important personnel function of the administrator therefore is an attempt to develop practical and equitable standards of measurement or evaluation. There should also be included in the employee's personal history file memoranda concerning specific and noticeable changes in behavior, attitude, or efficiency. Contrary to all too frequent practice,these memoranda should relate to changes for the better as well as for the worse. Furthermore, they too should consist of statements of fact rather than mere supervisory deductions, impressions, or opinions, which not infrequently are biased.

The factors involved in determining tenure and promotion are essentially the same as those that determine the granting of step increases in compensation. It is customary and proper that an employee expect to hold a position as long as he adequately fulfills its purpose and as long as his behavior is not detrimental to the interests of other employees or of the organization.

Vacancies in the organization may be filled in essentially two ways: promotion of an employee already working in the organization or employment of someone new from outside. If the position is other than the lowest in the scale and if it is filled by promotion from within, the executive is faced with the possibility of having to carry out promotions all down the line, involving considerable reshuffling, readjustment, and retraining.

Although on the surface this may appear to have the disadvantage of upsetting the work of the organization to a considerable extent, it also has definite advantages. First, if it is wished that employees approach their work from the point of view of possible careers in public service, promotion from within can be considered a fundamental premise and is conducive to desirable organizational morale and loyalty. It also develops a staff with wider interests and abilities than is otherwise possible. Furthermore, to follow a policy of filling upper positions from outside discourages the really capable individuals from remaining in the organization, with the result that over a period of time there is built up a residue of predominantly disappointed, disillusioned, and mediocre employees. Once this occurs, the responsible executive, or one so unfortunate as subsequently to take his place, finds himself with no choice but to go outside for capable personnel. Finally, if there is any reason for employees to suspect that an outsider has been brought in because of personal or partisan favoritism, a disastrous lowering of morale is sure to follow.

It must be realized, of course, that some positions must be filled from the outside, especially during a period of organizational growth or when there is no one within the agency truly capable of filling the vacancy. Occasional problems of intraagency frictions, favoritism, and cliques may be effectively solved only by the reallocation of certain of the present employees and the introduction of one or several new employees. In general, perhaps the best course to follow is in the middle, filling positions from within as much as possible but always keeping in mind the basic interests and purposes of the organization. Accordingly many capable administrators follow a policy of occasionally introducing a few new, particularly well-qualified leaders in key positions made available by retirement of older employees or by their reassignment to other duties, in conjunction with the development as rapidly and as extensively as possible of a group of promising younger employees well trained from within.

Some ill-advised executives avoid the advancement of younger capable employees either from fear of their possibly presenting eventual competition to themselves or from fear of losing them to another agency. Such an attitude is absurd, of course, since the truly capable administrator need have no fears of competition from loyal staff members, and should his capable assistants advance into other fields or agencies, that might be considered a measure of the successful nature of the administrator's policies and leadership. In fact the wise executive should derive considerable satisfaction from seeing individuals trained by him go out and spread his philosophy and viewpoint much farther than he could every hope to do by himself.

## THE EXECUTIVE AND HIS PERSONNEL

Administrative management is essentially a question of the organization of manpower, materials, resources, and strategy for the accomplishment of a desired goal. This is impossible unless the administrator has successfully organized himself so as to intelligently understand the causes of the problems he meets in his day-to-day work and the remedies for their adequate solution. It requires therefore an intimate knowledge and understanding of a great many factors, including people as well as materials, plus a great deal of curiosity, imagination, determination, integrative ability, and good judgment. In a field such as public health there also is required a greater than usual social consciousness and understanding. Accordingly the work of the public health administrator becomes much more than a matter of writing rules and regulations, issuing orders, or establishing clinics. In effect it involves the power and ability to influence if not to determine the happiness, welfare, and even the lives of a large number of people, beginning with the staff of the agency and extending out to include every member of the public. This is statesmanship in the correct sense of the word in that the executive health officer, in keeping with executives of other fields, plays an active and significant role in shaping the future not only of his organization but also of a community and of a society as a whole. This represents a truly great responsibility.

To be successful the executive officer must be well balanced. He should possess the type of personality that marks him naturally for a position of leadership and inspires the confidence of others because of a mature interest in them rather than using them for his own selfish purposes. He should demonstrate a constant sense of fairness, giving his employees the assurance that their individual and collective welfare and interests are safe in his hands and that they will not be subjected to the undesirable influences of prejudice, favoritism, or arbitrariness. Sartain and Baker[34] put this well in saying "There is a finesse associated with effective supervising that is somewhat analogous to the expertise which makes a knowledgeable physician a gifted surgeon. Regardless of the scientific advances made in management, the value of its art form will never be diminished. The acquisition, recording, and distillation of human experience will always be a pertinent part of the management process." On the other hand, they warn that "Management is in transition from an art, based only on experience, to a profession, based on an underlying foundation of principles and science."

The most effective administrator is one who is not specialized in any particular field, which would make him a technologist and would result almost certainly in an unbalanced program. He should, however, gain enough knowledge and understanding of the various technical phases and activities of the organization to enable him to coordinate them intelligently and assist administratively in their development.

It therefore follows that the administrative health officer, like executives in other fields, must establish his goals, make plans for their attainment, create a sound organization providing for practical levels of authority and coordination, recruit and manage good personnel, delegate responsibility and its concomitant authority, establish whatever rules and regulations are needed for smooth operation, develop a sound financial policy and an efficient work plan, provide continued leadership, education, and inspiration, maintain good morale, secure cooperation, and keep the plans and programs of the organization constantly in tune with the social forces on which depends its success and survival. To accomplish all this he needs personal characteristics such as those summarized by Dimock [35]:

The successful executive, therefore, is he who commands the best balance of physique, mentality, personality, technical equipment, philosophical insight, knowledge of human behavior, social adaptability, judgment, ability to understand and to get along with people, and a sense of social purpose and direction.

This sounds as if some type of superman is required. However, this does not necessarily follow, since, stripped to the essentials, what is required is a determination to carry out a certain few proved administrative principles, for example, that authority should equal responsibility or that functions should be defined, plus a genuine liking and understanding of human nature. The administrator's function is to maintain a sense of goals, strategy, and timing and to supply specific encouragement, instruction, and pressure at the right point and time. The executive is most effective when, having delegated as much detail as possible to his subordinates and their having contributed everything of which they are capable, he provides the extra 5% of knowledge and leadership with which to turn out a completed and workmanlike job.

The executive health officer should always bear in mind that he is placed in a managerial position for a social purpose and not because of any personal interest in him or his welfare. He is employed for more than routine management and housekeeping. He is expected also to be a tactician and social philosopher, using his wits, his ability as a leader, and his understanding of social forces to improve the state of society. Since society and the forces influencing it constantly fluctuate, he never operates in a fixed environment. He must constantly adapt himself, his program, and his organization to these environmental changes and, furthermore, must try to influence the environment in any way that might seem indicated for the accomplishment of the ultimate purpose of the program.

With this in mind there should be mentioned a not unfamiliar type of administrator commonly referred to as a promotor, who, although possessing great imagination, enthusiasm, and salesmanship, lacks the ability or momentum to follow through. He finds it difficult to sustain an interest in any one thing for long, dislikes routine, and is constantly searching for new worlds to conquer. Accordingly his interest and energy jump unpredictably from one thing to another, with the result that his personnel never know in what direction they are going next or what their relative positions will be. Particular subordinates may receive concentrated attention and support one day, only to be ignored and forgotten the next. That this is conducive neither to a sound balanced program nor to high morale is obvious.

There are others, however, who achieve a balance between promotional ability and executive leadership. They, although never satisfied with the status quo, realize nevertheless that "the show must go on," that all parts of the program must be continuously sustained. Possessing strong imagination, they are ever on the alert to new problems and methods of attack, carrying a promotional activity to the point where it has been established and accepted and may be turned over to a capable subordinate for its complete development, without at any time unbalancing or confusing the program as a whole. This is the difference between the will-o'-the-wisp promoter and the executive with promotional ability.

Whereas the latter type of leadership is desirable in every organization at all times, it is of particular importance in the initiation and development of a new enterprise. Such circumstances require an unusual amount of imagination, courage, exploration, self-confidence, and planning ability, plus a sense of good timing and an ability to combine what is in the process of creation with what already has been brought into existence. In this regard it should again be realized that public health work, being a rapidly expanding field, requires that to be effective the executive health officer must constantly face the problem of initiation and promotion of new programs.

It is therefore clear that the health executive of a functioning agency must be three things: a trouble shooter constantly expecting the unexpected and always ready to deal with crises, a supervisor delegating everything he can to those working under him, and a promoter of new programs to increase the usefulness and effectiveness of his organization. As pointed out by Dimock,[35] this order is reversed in the formative stages of a new organization. Many executives successfully carry out one or two of these, but the test of a truly competent administrator is if all three can be accomplished.

It may be appropriate to give some consideration to what makes an effective chief executive officer. Perhaps the most comprehensive general statement which could be made is that the characteristics of a good administrative officer are in many ways similar to those required for good parenthood. A primary function of the executive health officer is to provide leadership. His usual problem is how to lead his organization in the face of the limitations and obstacles found in most situations. There is no standard answer to the question. Solution depends to a considerable degree on the individual and his personality rather than on his technical knowledge. This explains why capable technologists are often unhappy failures when placed in administrative positions. The answer to the question varies by place and time. The problems encountered in a new organization are different from those of an old established agency. It should also be recognized that different organizations have different backgrounds of development that condition the rate and manner in which they move. Executive manner and action are certain to differ under emergency conditions, in contrast with normal circumstances.

Perhaps the most important philosophy for the executive to adopt is that the end results are the products of the organization, not those of any one individual, even himself. In the long run any effect he has is due to his influence and not to his command. Whether or not he wants to, he must rely on his subordinate staff to accomplish the purposes of the agency. Even if this were not true, the executive should not attempt to take over the tasks of those on lower levels. To do so invariably confuses and antagonizes the personnel in general and the division and bureau heads in particular. The executive health officer's position is that of a catalyst dealing with people, assimilating their ideas, evaluating them, and determining lines of action and seeing that action is taken. He should do everything possible to conserve his time and energy for these higher level administrative functions by adopting the policy of Andrew Carnegie, who never did anything he could hire someone else to do for him. The executive health officer should approach his position with a long-range view, recognizing that most administrative changes and advances take a long time. This means that he must balance his type or method of action to fit particular situations, slackening the line at this point and at this time and reeling in or striking out at other places and at other times.

A popular picture exists of an executive austerely established behind a shiny desk in a comfortable office, granting a series of interviews to a parade of subordinates and others who appeal for advice and guidance. This presents a poor picture of administrative practice. As in any other field, the chief executive in public health is neither the ultimate fountainhead of all knowledge nor physically capable of personally directing the activities of a large number of individuals. The numbers of those within his agency with whom he has intimate working relationships should be limited, otherwise he misses the forest for the trees. This is not meant to imply that the executive should confine his contacts or relationships to those who voluntarily come to him; rather he should actively seek out those who need his help and who can be of assistance to him.

## Delegation

An organization functions most effectively when a capable executive officer, rather than attempting to control and supervise intimately each of the various activities that make up the total program, is able to delegate control and supervision to responsible subordinates. Second perhaps to recruitment of best possible personnel, this is probably the most important single factor in successful administrative practice. The executive has to decide what part of his responsibilities and authority he will entrust to those immediately below him and what he will withhold for himself. Each of these key subordinate executives should be allowed to choose those who will work under him, or he cannot fairly be held responsible for results. The subordinate executives in turn delegate to those next in rank such parts of their own specified responsibilities as they may choose, and so on down the line. As Dimock[35] has described it, the executive in effect says to his department heads, "You know our objective. You know the plans. You know the policy. Now the job is to see that this part of the work is done. I am holding you responsible for it. It is up to you to get results."

This type of leadership almost certainly pays dividends, since it gives competent individuals pride in their work and encourages initiative, self-confidence, and ability. The opposite and usually unsuccessful approach is that of the executive who insists that all actions and decisions originate with him and that everything go in or out over his desk. Indeed, Sartain and Baker[34] point to studies which indicate that supervisors who give the greatest amount of instruction and direction tend to achieve the poorest record. This approach inevitably causes division heads either to leave the organization for more reasonable and stimulating fields or to lose interest and initiative, thereby becoming intimidated "yes men" of little real value to the organization. The latter, whereas they may appear to be obedient, gravitate into a sullen rut, secretly delighting in the event of administrative errors. Equally inevitable in such cases is the puzzlement of the executive over the apparent lack of cooperation, understanding, and support from his subordinates.

It is not to be inferred that the job of the executive is merely to find capable subordinates, to delegate authority to them, and then to sit back in ease and watch the wheels go round. The real test of sound leadership involves the ability, after delegating authority, to step in unobtrusively at appropriate times to give suggestions or directions on the basis of greater knowledge and a more complete understanding of overall strategy. Pfiffner[36] has listed certain rules and prerequisites for the successful delegation of authority and responsibility. The first, most important, and most frequently overlooked of these is simply that the executive must honestly want to delegate. If responsibility is to be delegated, subordinates must be carefully chosen and must be capable of bearing responsibility. Their responsibility must be defined for them, and they must be trained to carry it. Furthermore, if responsibility is delegated, there must also be delegated with it the appropriate type and amount of authority. Failure to do so is the second most common error. If subordinates are good enough to employ in the first place and to assume responsibility, they are good enough to trust.

Delegation has been referred to as fundamentally necessary for successful administrative management. In fact administration might with considerable truth be defined as getting things done through others. In present-day public health organizations as well as in other organizations it is impossible for one person to do the whole job. The head of an organization should not try to handle all of the details himself; it is a physical and mental impossibility and it is not expected. Decisions should be made at the lowest possible point in the organization's line of command. Were this not true, there would be little use or justification for creating an organization in the first place. The wise executive will employ as subordinates individuals who are more capable than he is in each of the various functions of the organization and will let them take care of the details. Far from indicating weakness, it is a sign of a good administrator for subordinates to be called on to present detailed information to outsiders as well as to the executive himself. Furthermore, to do so boosts the ego, job interest, and loyalty of the subordinate.

Probably the average executive does not adequately understand the basic principles involved in delegation. Not uncommon is the pitiful spectacle of an executive who, feeling that only he can do each job correctly, is trying to face all points of the compass at once and has become a slave to nonadministrative minutiae with which others are better fitted to cope. He lets the job run him instead of the preferred and intended reverse. Meanwhile his subordinates must helplessly stand by, losing interest and initiative, merely nodding assent to the wishes and actions of their superior.

On the other hand, there are the many executives who, apparently lacking the courage of their convictions, delegate responsibilities to a greater or lesser extent but avoid establishment of clear-cut lines of command and neglect to invest the employee with the corresponding authority needed for adequately meeting the added responsibility. They thereby tend to expect more from their subordinates that they have a right to, expressing great surprise and disappointment when their subordinates appear not to stand up fully to their responsibilities. They appear not to realize that a subordinate under such circumstances, in addition to feeling a lack of recognition and trust, is in great danger of being left out on a limb, caught between an employer who demands that he carry out a delegated responsibility and other employees who understandably question his right to make requests or issue orders.

Failure to delegate therefore has many undesirable consequences. First, and probably of least importance, is that the executive tends to drive himself toward a physical or mental breakdown, following never-ceasing, high-pressure workdays coping with annoying details and sleepless nights fed by bulging briefcases. Inevitably the organization suffers because the executive himself is the chief bottleneck and the work is incompletely and inefficiently done. The agency loses the benefit of whatever abilities exist in the rest of the personnel, capable potential employees shy away from the uninspiring environment, and those within the organization soon ask themselves either, "Why stay?" or "What's the use of working or trying?"

All who have studied the problem agree that in almost all instances of "one-man shows" with the absence of delegation, the essential difficulty is one of psychologic inadequacy on the part of the executive. This masquerades in many forms: conceit, boorishness, false pride, false interest, fussy perfectionism, or obvious lack of self-confidence. As Dimock[35] has said: "Show me the man who does not delegate and it will frequently be found that he is a bundle of fears and misgivings. He is afraid to make mistakes. He is afraid that he will be tricked or embarrassed. He is afraid that others would not do it his way." This gives a sadly accurate word picture of more than one executive officer in the field of publc health.

Successful and effective delegation therefore requires a few simple considerations. The first as noted is that the executive must truly and consciously want to do it. It is never a subconscious action. The executive must look on his function as essentially that of a coordinator of the activities of many others, each of whom has been entrusted with specific responsibilities and authority. He must consider his position akin to that of the conductor of a symphony orchestra through whose coordinating activity inspiring music results where there might otherwise be cacophony.

The organization must be set up with clear-cut and well-understood lines or channels. In delegating, these lines must be respected, never making one person responsible for a job only to give the job or the authority for it to someone else. Perhaps the most important consideration involved is the realization that delegation properly involves a multiple action. The key setting off the chain reaction is the necessity of delegating work load or function. This implies a delegation of responsibility. In turn, to make the fulfillment of the responsibility possible, delegation of an appropriate additional amount of authority is necessary. In some instances a change in the title or rank of the employee is indicated as part of the delegation of authority in order to implement it.

In discussing the relationship between delegated responsibility and authority most writers speak in terms of equality. Actually what is called for is an even more delicate adjustment. The good executive has a real interest in the development of his subordinates as well as in getting the work done. Accordingly, he will grant to the responsible subordinate the amount of authority required by the responsibilities plus just enough to allow expanded opportunity for experience and improvement without risking considerable difficulty and a sense of failure.

It must always be understood that delegation is in effect a loan that is never permanent and that it can be recalled at any time. Delegation is most effective in an atmosphere of mutual understanding and respect. The executive has the right to expect that his trust will not be abused. He should, however, be constantly alert to the possibility that his trust as manifest by delegation might not be justified. Unfortunately he will occasionally find this to be the case. Such instances are not always easy to handle, as Dimock[35] has emphasized:

The worst kind of a person to deal with in any organization is the slippery evasive individual who gives the appearance of a good fellow and a square shooter, who pays a sort of obsequious deference to the wishes of his superior, but who goes contrary to known policies and abuses his authority to the extent where it cannot help but be noticed, but not quite to the point where the official is justified in chopping off his head. It is this kind of person more than any other who gives the executive pause when it comes to delegation, and who is most likely to damage the morale of the organization as a whole. The egoist is soon discovered and can be eliminated. The man with an inferiority complex can be built up and restored to normalcy. The devious person is the hardest to handle on all scores, but especially in any situation requiring a delegation of authority.

Another important aspect is the power relationships of the head of an organization. The successful leadership of an organization involves a constant struggle with those in other organizations or groups who also possess power. The executive health officer must recognize this and be ever ready and able to engage in a struggle for proper power. This is vital if his organization is to survive and if he is not to betray it, its employees, and those it serves. He should not allow himself to be deluded or deterred in this by false modesty, weakness, or complaisance. Of course a struggle for power should never be simply for the accumulation of power for its own sake or for self-aggrandizement but should be engaged in to assure that no important or essential part of the organization and its program will be lacking or misplaced.

A most succinct summary of the approach to such situations was presented by Upson[37]:

As an executive, you must expect some people to disagree with you—some who are smarter than you are and honestly object to both your methods and objectives; some who are less smart than you are and out of that inadequacy damn what you are doing in an effort to make themselves appear big; some, who dislike or misunderstand your motives and who will fight everything you try to do simply because you are doing it. Of these groups, respect the first, ignore the second, and fight the third—and fight them without compromise, winner take all.

## Morale and discipline

In every organization some rules or regulations will be necessary, but if they are to be effective, they must be few, simple, readily understood, and inflexible. Items that may be effectively included are limited largely to such matters as the hours of work, the length of the lunch period, the handling of certain records and correspondence, and holidays and leaves. The administrator's real difficulties begin at the point where objective inflexibility ends.

He cannot hope to constantly police the work and behavior of all of his subordinates and even if he could, it would preclude the possibility of good leadership. The best he can hope for, and what is probably most desirable in the long run, is to develop inasmuch as possible an almost subconscious self-discipline within the group itself so that improper behavior of a particular employee is considered by his fellows as an infraction against their self-developed and self-enforced code of working ethics.

The executive and his supervisors should always bear in mind that although most people are willing to be subordinate to good leadership, they are not willing to be subservient. Sartain and Baker[34] say, "Within the last few decades, management is said to have discovered its employees and to have succeeded, at least partially, in ending the costly waste of human assets . . . much of the secret of good supervision depends on an understanding of and a respect for the dignity of the individual." Even though the person in authority may have the legal or financial power to demand obedience, the subordinate similarly has the power to refuse to obey or, what is more practical from his standpoint, the power to circumvent orders while appearing to obey.

Individuals in an organization may often with relative ease find it possible to chronically arrive late and leave early or to spend considerable time visiting with fellow workers. If promptness and attention to work has become part of the organization's code of working ethics over a period of time, in most instances the administrator will find it unnecessary to deal with the individual situation himself. The other employees by virtue of their own interest in the matter will handle it for him. They will take the attitude that the individual is trying to get away with something that is contrary to the best interests and welfare of the group. If, on the other hand, there is a tradition of slipshod management and administration, the affairs of the organization will tend to assume the atmosphere of a routinized semisocial event to the detriment of the program and the morale of all concerned.

The question of attendance control is only one example of a great many problems of administrative management for which there is more than one answer. Depending on the type of activity in which the organization is engaged, attempts to obtain strict adherence to the scheduled hours of work may be a deterrent to wholehearted cooperation and high personnel morale. This probably applies to most phases of public health work, where a reasonable degree of latitude allowed by a good leader will in most instances result in greater loyalty to and interest in the work than would otherwise be attained. An organization is recalled where unusually high morale, evidenced by interest, willing overtime, and loyalty, was definitely jeopardized by the installation of a time clock for the professional personnel by an overenthusiastic efficiency expert from the mayor's office.

In terms of what has been said, therefore, the goal for which the good administrator will aim is a cooperative team, which is probably most successfully achieved by the development of a logical organizational structure with well-defined and understood lines of authority and responsibility and a well-established tradition of good self-discipline. Good personnel management depends partly on sound organization and partly on sound individual guidance, correction, reward, and punishment. It has been said that the administrator must understand people and be a leader. There are two kinds of leadership, the first demonstrated by a person with superior ability whom people gladly follow, the second consisting of mere possession of authority. Authority in itself is of limited value. It is well to remember the adage, "You can lead a horse to water but you can't make him drink."

The wise executive will understand the difference between a well-balanced person and one who is emotionally disturbed, and he will be conscious of the gap that may exist between ability and achievement. He will recognize that these characteristics apply to himself as well as to his subordinates. He will realize that an emotionally immature person will tend to measure accomplishments against those of more gifted or more fortunate people or against some unreasonable standard he has set for himself. Such a person remedies failure by daydreaming, rebellion, self-pity, bullying, bragging, or even by deliberate failure, a form of overcompensation. The well-balanced person, on the other hand, will measure his accomplishments against his honestly recognized aptitudes and share of luck. His aim is to seek a cause worth serving, one for which he has an aptitude and in which he can find mental and emotional satisfaction. In dealing with personnel, therefore, the executive should be aware of the various types of behavior defenses that may arise from a feeling of failure or dissatisfaction. These are of many types: "If I give in, you won't need to hurt me." "If I am humorous, you won't think to hurt me." "If I flatter you, you will be deterred from hurting me." "If I am sick and unfortunate, you will be ashamed to hurt me." "If you love me, you won't want to hurt me." "If I hurt you first, you won't be able to hurt me."

This leads to the question of discipline. As White[30] has indicated:

> In a healthy organization the staff possesses a high morale which relegates discipline of any type to a position of secondary importance. For most persons the attitude and morale of the group are a sufficient guide to conduct; and where effective leadership and good supervision exist, problems of discipline largely disappear. The basic attack on disciplinary problems is therefore an indirect one, rather than the search for new forms of action or the imposition of heavier penalties.

Almost every instance requiring discipline comes after a failure of some kind on the part of management. This applies even to cases of "born troublemakers," since an effective personnel program would preclude their employment in the first place. It should always be realized that a disciplinary act deals with much more than the immediate present and the individual directly involved. The case at hand merely concentrates in the present the results of the past and possible consequences of the future. Futhermore, literally every other member of the organization is alert and watching for the outcome because the solution will show him what to expect under similar circumstances. Magoun[38] illustrated this point with the story of the office boy who was disciplined for absenting himself from work to attend a family funeral after having been refused by the boss, who suspected that he went to a baseball game. Needless to say, such an employer would never be forgiven by those working under him for his bad judgment and ill-considered disciplinary action.

Whereas avoidance of conditions requiring discipline is much better than successful discipline, failure to discipline when it is indicated is demoralizing to the group. There are several behavior patterns that require action of some sort on the part of the administrator or supervisor. Among these are inattention to duty, including chronic tardiness, laziness, carelessness, breakage or loss of property, inefficiency, insubordination in the form of violation of an order, regulation, or law, or disloyalty to the organization. Certain personal behavior such as continued and overt intoxication, immorality and lack of integrity manifest by violation of a recognized code of ethics, soliciting, accepting a bribe, or deliberately neglecting to enforce a law also requires action.[39]

A poor executive, in approaching disciplinary problems of this sort, will tend to rely merely on his power to coerce and command. In so doing he is actually attempting to reassure himself for his own feeling of inadequacy and weakness, refusing to recognize that perhaps he and his lack of leadership had something to do with the development of the problem at hand. The capable executive, on the other hand, sees unbalanced behavior as a symptom of wrong conditions either in the way the employee has been handled or in some external situation such as the work, social, community, or home environment. He will recognize the importance of the employee's stage of emotional development and even consider the possible influence of frustrations and insecurities of earlier origin along with those developed in the recent past.

In dealing with a dissatisfied or rebellious employee the executive should ask himself several questions of a psychologic nature. What accounts for the emotional insecurity that resulted in the employee's decision to press the rebellion, to sidestep the basic difficulty, instead of consciously and honestly recognizing his feelings and responding to them in an intelligent manner? What opportunity can be given him to gain self-assurance so the solution will be permanent rather than temporary?

Some may consider an approach such as this as being unwarranted, patronizing, and out of place in business, industry, or public service. It might be pointed out, however, that considerable attention is paid to inanimate machinery, and if something goes wrong in its mechanism, those in charge go to great lengths to discover the seat of the trouble rather than to discard the whole machine or to rely on makeshift repairs. It is high time that administrators or supervisors realize that the animate mechanism, the human employee, merits this and much more attention and consideration.

The actual approach to a disciplinary action should never be casual or momentary. A series of steps should be taken. The executive officer should first study himself to discover and eliminate personal bias and to discover any personal responsibility for the situation. He should make a many-sided approach to the problem, looking at it through the eyes of the employee himself, his family, his fellow employees, and his immediate supervisor. The entire situation should be investigated, giving consideration to the condition of work at the time, the employee's past record, the morale and behavior of the employees as a group, the type and degree of infraction, the organization's tradition in such cases, and any outside conditions that may have influenced the employee. An attempt should be made to discover whether the failure was due to misunderstanding, an emotional upset, lack of experience, some irregularity in working conditions, or poor leadership. Throughout the whole process the executive should look on his function as that of a counselor rather than that of a judge and should be alert to opportunities to solve the problem from the point of view of the welfare of the organization while enabling the employee to save face.

Magoun,[40] in teaching human engineering has used the case analysis method to considerable advantage. The approach to disciplinary situations that he suggests is outlined in some detail because of its value as an exercise in the solution of personnel problems.

*Prepare*

I. Study the situation until you feel completely clear as to
   A. How your habits and emotions color what you see in it
   B. How the other people concerned are affected by it
   C. All the significant facts
   D. Exactly what the problem is that requires solution (problems in human relations are almost never what they seem to be on the surface)

II. Write down the essential facts of the problem
   A. Be sure to avoid any interpreting and include only accurate concise statements of fact
   B. Be sure to include material other people recognize as facts, even though you may not

III. Write down the emotions involved in the problem
   A. What desires created the situation?
   B. What desires are maintaining the situation?
   C. What long and short term goals are desired by you and others and why?

IV. Check by making believe you are each person involved, and see whether you have made a valid presentation of his facts, problems, and desires from his point of view

*Analyze*

I. Separate the fundamental from the trivial (beware that your emotions do not fool you in this)

II. What are the key logs in the jam?
   A. Make a careful and exhaustive analysis of each person's acts and reactions, step by step. Begin by finding out first, in detail, all the consequences each person's attitude has for him and what satisfactions it fulfills. Then be sure to get to the bottom of what actually happened, and work out an exact explanation of why. Does it make psychologic sense? Common sense?

III. Write all of this out in its proper relationship
   A. So that you can see the problem as a whole
   B. So that you can see where the situation is going and how fast

IV. Write out in significant detail the requirements for a total solution
   A. What are the things it must accomplish—can accomplish? Why is any given goal desirable? Why are there only certain ways of achieving it?
   B. Check for the immediate and total satisfaction of each person involved
   C. Note conflicting desires that must be harmonized by a successful solution

V. Contrive a total solution
   A. Write out every possible alternative showing how you derived it, and choose the best one (usually the simplest) that offers the interweaving of interests

*Handle*

I. Once the goal has been determined, the means become the most important thing; now that you have decided what to do, plan to do it
   A. With a minimum of self-assertion or disturbance to habit patterns
   B. With careful consideration of time, place, and individuals
   C. With reference to the various possibilities that may arise

II. Write out your plan concretely, accurately, and in detail

III. Rehearse your plan as one would familiarize himself with a detailed map

    A. Go through it step by step, with the help of someone else, looking for flaws in your plan, flaws in your attitude, ways of bettering your presentation in terms of the individual involved and places where you might meet failures due to the unexpected

IV. Wait for the appropriate time and conditions, then try out your plan

    A. Be thoroughly sincere and keep voice, eyes, posture emotionally calm

    B. Begin by getting the facts understood

    C. Present your case in terms of his intelligence, viewpoint, and emotional responses

    D. Listen to his case so that you can express it to him better than he did to you; then he knows you understand it; you may also catch any new evidence that you overlooked

    E. Together come to a decision based on the facts

*Evaluate*

I. Review the entire case

II. Write out its lessons

    A. What almost failed and why?

    B. What almost succeeded and why?

    C. What did you do for yourself and others?

    D. What did you do to yourself and others?

The types of disciplinary action that may be taken in specific situations can be divided into several categories. First, there is what might be termed the indirect or informal approach. Here there is no specific or explicit reference made to dissatisfaction, and reliance is placed on inference by the employee as a result of a change in attitude in the executive officer or supervisor. There may be developed, for instance, a more or less obvious chilling of the atmosphere, closer supervision of work, a failure to invite the employee to confer or consult with reference to relevant matters, a rejection of proposals, or a reduction in estimates. The employee might further experience some loss of privileges, a curtailing of authority and responsibility, or actual reassignment to less desirable work. The assumption of this approach is that the employee will be intelligent enough to "get the point" and without further action spontaneously undertake a program of self-improvement.

A more explicit approach may be the application of what are sometimes referred to as direct or formal penalties of the first degree. Usually these are imposed and enforced by the head of an office or division on his own responsibility and without review. They may take the form of formal notice and warning, reprimand, delay in salary increment, loss of seniority, or requirement of overtime. The use of the last two disciplinary actions is somewhat open to question. The employee may with considerable justification and support object to unpaid overtime as a means of getting some work done for nothing. With regard to seniority the supervisor or administrator may find himself involved in a controversy, frequently with the employee and the civil service agency on one side and himself on the other, since for some reason it is not rare to find civil service agencies considering as one of their functions the protection of the misunderstood employee from an overbearing or malevolent supervisor or administrator.

The transfer of an employee might be considered a penalty of the first degree and in many instances solves the difficulty to everyone's satisfaction. Not infrequently the problem employee may cease to be a problem if he is reassigned to work under another supervisor, put in a new social or physical environment, or assigned a different type of work. This is understandable, considering that personnel problems involve much more than the employee, that is, fellow employees, the physical environment, the supervisor, the type of work, and so on. The surly and careless file clerk may turn out to be an excellent receptionist. The inefficient and unproductive field nurse may develop into an exceptional clinic assistant. Although often effective, there is one objection to this approach: it encourages some supervisors and executives to feel justified in dodging personnel problems, to the development of which they have often contributed, simply by transferring them to others. Much more than a transfer is needed in every instance—a complete study of the circumstances of the problem is indicated.

If more drastic disciplinary action is indicated, what have been referred to as penalties of the second degree may be applied. They usually require the action of the head of the department or organization itself, and sometimes the employee has the right to appeal to a board, a civil service commission, or occasionally to a court. The first penalty in this category is temporary suspension. It is questionable if this is ever sound or justified. The fact that the employee is subjected to enforced although temporary absence from work and therefore loss of salary inevitably results in his return to work in a more disgruntled, defensive, and vengeful frame of mind than when he left.

The same objection may be raised to the use of demotion as a penalty. Occasionally, however, if the employee has great intrinsic desirability for the organization, a temporary demotion, with the clear understanding that reinstatement will readily follow demonstration of good intentions, may be indicated. One might well raise the question, however, whether some of the less drastic methods of approach would not be equally or more effective in such instances.

Dismissal or removal for cause is, of course, the extreme and final measure. A word of caution is indicated here and applies to all types of disciplinary action. When it first appears that an employee may be a problem, a detailed documentary record should be made of pertinent instances and facts for possible reference and use in the event that subsequent disciplinary action may be appealed. It is a good policy to keep the employee in the case informed at every step concerning his status rather than to subject him, as too often happens, to a sudden release of pent-up managerial objections. This always should be and can be done with an atmosphere of counseling, which shows a genuine concern for the employee's welfare as well as for that of the organization. True, this often takes much time, but in the long run it pays great dividends in the maintenance of high morale. In the past and to a considerable degree in the present the attitude of executives toward dismissal has been that it represents merely a disagreeable experience for the employer, involving simply the summary discharge of the employee. If dismissal is necessary, the employee should be made to realize that it is in his best interest as well as that of the organization and, in effect, presents an opportunity for his rehabilitation elsewhere.

One final word of caution: Under no circumstances should a worker be subjected to any active form of disciplinary action in the presence of his fellow employees. Whereas superficially some of them may appear to enjoy it, they will all resent it.

## CONDITIONS OF WORK

### Job appeal

A high level of employee morale has been referred to repeatedly as a prime essential for the satisfactory and efficient operation of a public health program. Good morale is difficult if not impossible to define. Perhaps, like health, the best way to recognize it is when it is absent. If the state of mind and the working relationships of a group of people are satisfactory, the administrator seldom finds himself even thinking about the problems involved in the development and maintenance of good morale. In contrast, he becomes acutely aware of the problem if things are not what they should be.

The nature of high morale might be better understood by some of its symptoms, such as a pride of the employees in being identified with the organization and their pleasure in working for it. There are health departments, unfortunately, in which the employees look on their activity as merely a means of earning a wage or salary. On the other hand, health organizations exist in which everyone, including the office boy, the elevator operator, and the lowest clerical worker on the staff, believes that the organization is his health department and that he is contributing something essential to its activity; he thereby derives considerable happiness and satisfaction from his daily work.

Although morale is determined by a great many factors, unquestionably the most important is the quality of leadership of the "line officers," that is, the immediate supervisors of the workers and the amount of inspiration and job interest they can impart to the personnel. The concept that once prevailed with regard to subordinates was, "If you don't like the orders or the work, you can quit or be fired." The ultimate futility of this approach is exemplified by the attempts of the Nazi conquerors to force the people of the countries they overran into productive labor. The whole world knows the devastating and significant effects of the slowdowns to which these conquered workers resorted.

Now, instead of trying to prod or drive the employee into doing work, the approach is based on good leadership, example, and respect, job and employee analysis, and employee training. From this is seen the great importance of the specific job in relation to the specific worker. Frequently both an employee and a job are individually desirable and important but simply may not mix. As previously mentioned, an unsatisfactory file clerk may on reassignment turn out to be an excellent receptionist. Very few situations in life work only in one direction. If an employee is expected to give his best effort to his job, the job should be expected to give him something in return. The activity must appear to be something more than busy work or dull routine. The worker must have the opportunity to realize its significance and its contribution to the attainment of the total goal.

An excellent example of this was found in the attitudes of the large number of clerical workers who were engaged by state health departments during World War II to handle the routine paper work of the Emergency Maternity and Infant Care Program for the wives and infants of servicemen. Unfortunately most state health departments simply employed clerks, assigned them to tables and desks, distributed pens or rubber stamps, and subjected the clerks to a continuous rapid flow of inanimate sheets of paper. This gave them no real understanding of the significance of the program and the vital part they were playing in it. It was not surprising that these organizations experienced considerable difficulty, not merely in obtaining personnel but also in holding them. In fact in many instances personnel turnover was truly appalling and seriously hampered the effectiveness of this important program. In a few states, however, some consideration was given to the worker, his intelligence, and the possible monotony of the job and the relation of it to the employee's morale. It was refreshing to visit these few state health agencies and to notice the alert and satisfied expressions on the faces of the workers. In discussing the work with them, the same interpretations were repeatedly encountered. They were not working with pieces of paper and rubber stamps; they were making it possible for a large number of women and children to obtain necessary medical attention. They looked on the beneficiaries involved as "their mothers and their babies" and thereby received considerable satisfaction from the work they were doing in helping them. As might be expected, although these latter organizations had the same difficulty in obtaining new personnel, having done so they kept them, and in a highly satisfactory state of morale.

The administrator's responsibility for seeing that his staff is well informed of the agency's current goals, its progress toward them, and the importance of every job in their achievement is too often overlooked or is exercised casually. Whereas free communication may be conducted best on an informal personal basis, there must be planning to assure that it does occur. In large agencies use of mass communication techniques is often a necessary and desirable supplement to building a staff that knows what is going on and feels that it is part of the organization.

Dimock,[35] in the course of management studies, asked several businessmen for their views concerning factors that determined employees' activities. In other words, for what reason do men and women put forth their best efforts? The replies received were so consistent that he felt justified in suggesting the incentive scale shown in Fig. 11-1. Up to a point the chief incentive is increased income to give a sense of security. At some point there is superimposed on this financial urge a desire for power and position, an opportunity to determine policy and to make one's own work. This in turn is eventually replaced by a desire for recognition and prestige, and eventually when these three urges or appetites are appeased, there is added a spirit of altruism and a desire for public service. Dimock concludes that the latter is the ultimate and most rewarding of all incentives.

The question of job appeal might be summarized therefore as including serious consideration of two factors: the assignment of the right employee to the right job, and the provision to the worker of an opportunity to realize

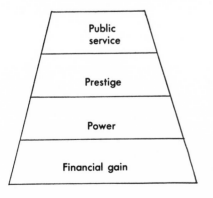

**Fig. 11-1.** Personnel incentive scale. (From Dimock, M. E.: The executive in action, New York, 1945, Harper & Row, Publishers.)

and understand the significance of the work he is being called on to do and to obtain a fair measure of personal reward and satisfaction.

Certain physical factors should not be overlooked in considering job appeal. It is a definite responsibility of administrators and supervisors to be constantly alert to needs and methods for the improvement of the physical environment in which their personnel must work. It has often been said, and with considerable justification, that health departments traditionally are relegated to the least desirable rooms in the basement of a city hall, county courthouse, or a state capitol building, preferably as close as possible to the public comfort station. Unquestionably there have been many instances of progressive public health personnel leaving positions because of an undesirable working environment. A health officer should always attempt to make his department an outstanding physical example of the cause for which it works. It is illogical to expect the public to respond to the educational efforts or even to the statutory measures of an organization that tolerates itself being housed in quarters that exemplify all the circumstances it criticizes and condemns.

A satisfactory working environment is in reality a sign of administrative efficiency. It has been shown repeatedly by industrial and other studies that the improvement of lighting, ventilation, and attractiveness is invariably followed by a significant increase in work output, a decrease in physiologic fatigue, and greatly improved employee satisfaction and morale. Unquestionably public health officials in the past have been guilty of unwarranted complaisance and timidity in competing with other public officers for desirable quarters and in the promotion of attractive and efficient health centers. The health officer should realize that few things are truer than "Do not ask and you shall not receive."

## Overtime

In every organization work during time other than the regular working hours is occasionally necessary. Emergencies and pressure periods are certain to occur, especially in a field such as public health. It is reasonable to expect the personnel to have sufficient interest in the program of their organization to do their part willingly in meeting emergency situations, and if the personnel relationships are satisfactory, no difficulty or opposition will be encountered. However, the amount of overtime work should be kept at a minimum and should be engaged in only after careful study and with adequate reason.

Continued or repeated overtime is administratively unjustifiable. A habit of overtime indicates either inefficient work methods or personnel, either of which signifies inefficient administrative management. It is patently unfair to expect effective work and satisfactory function during the regular workday when the employees have been mentally and physically fatigued by chronic overtime requirements. When overtime is necessary, provision should always be made for compensation either in time off or in additional pay at the rate of time and one half. Whenever possible, the latter method should be followed. Generally speaking, to allow addition of accumulated overtime to the annual vacation is undesirable, since it encourages deliberately sought for overtime and may result in considerable personnel depletion for part of the year.

## Leaves

Annual vacation leave with full pay of the personnel should always be planned for and encouraged. This bears many advantages for the organization and for the employee himself. The physical and psychologic need for weekend rest and for an annual vacation has been well established by social custom and proved by scientific investigation. An organization should have a definite policy concerning vacations. Usually an employee is not entitled to vacation until he has rendered at least 6 months of service. Many organizations, however, allow 1 day of cumulative vacation time per month of service, which is due the employee regardless of the date of his employment. It is most common at this stage of social and economic progress to allow for an annual vacation period of 2 weeks. This applies particularly to office and other nonprofessional personnel. Scientific, professional, and educational workers often are allowed longer vacations, perhaps in consideration of their greater period of training or in relation to the vacation time of their professional brethren engaged in teaching. Justification of this distinction is somewhat vague and untenable; undoubtedly the ideal would be an annual leave of about 1 month for all.

It is decidedly undesirable to allow employees to work for additional pay instead of taking their vacation, since this defeats the purposes of the vacation idea and generally results in employee regret and inefficiency. Similarly it is unwise to allow the addition of unused sick leave to vacation time, since this defeats the purpose of sick leave. If a holiday occurs during the vacation period of an employee, it is only fair to allow him an extra day off. However, the additional day off usually should be taken at a later date and not added to the vacation period, since this tends to cause difficulty in scheduling the vacations of the other employees.

Provision for sick leave should be considered a protection or insurance against a time of potential future need and not simply an added benefit to which the employee is entitled whether or not he becomes ill. In an increasing number of public agencies it is supplemented by various forms of disability and hospitalization insurance. Policies with regard to sick leave vary considerably. In smaller organizations there are often no specific provisions made, illness among the personnel being dealt with on an individual basis as it occurs. In other organizations, especially in larger agencies, a specific number of days per year is allowed for sick leave.

This frequently gives rise to several difficulties. Some workers look on the total number of sick leave days as their inevitable due whether or not they become ill. If no administrative controls are applied, there may develop considerable abuse of sick leave privileges, causing resentment by conscientious employees and an undesirable state of morale in general. Some organizations attempt to solve this by requiring a visit by a physician or a report from a private attending physician. However, this is an administrative and personal nuisance, necessitates added expense, and develops a not unjustified feeling of resentment among employees that they are not being trusted. It has been suggested by some that the solution is to make sick leave cumulative. This encourages employees to regard it as a saving or an investment and is a sound policy considering the occasional but inevitable occurrence of prolonged and catastrophic illness.

Of course the ideal approach to the problem is one that is aimed at the reduction of the need for absence due to illness. This is desirable from the point of view of both the organization and the employee. A number of simple principles are involved. The first is provision for preemployment physical examinations and periodic reexamination. Although essentially most benefit accrues to the employee, the fact that an organization requires these examinations makes it duty bound to bear whatever cost is involved.

Those returning to work after a period of illness should undergo careful examination, both from the point of view of protecting the other employees and of preventing premature return to work followed by a more serious and prolonged breakdown. If necessary, provision should be made for the follow-up and correction of physical defects, and employees with physical handicaps should be assigned to work with this in mind and supervised with particular care. The importance of a desirable working environment was previously referred to in relation to morale. This factor is of significance also in the prevention of illness and accidents. Many studies have demonstrated significant reductions in illnesses and accidents after improvement of the physical circumstances in which people must work. In-service training will be discussed in the next section, but here might be emphasized the importance of including education in personal health and safety practices.

Provision should be made for certain other types of leave. If an employee is asked to serve as a witness or as a member of a jury, it represents a citizen's responsibility about which he has no choice. It is therefore only right that the meeting of this responsibility be made possible. Of similar nature are leaves for military purposes. In no sense should absence from work for these reasons handicap the employee's reinstatement or opportunities for advancement.

Several strictly personal matters that require consideration are perhaps best dealt with on an individual basis. If illness or death occurs in the family of an employee or if it is necessary for him to move during a working day, it is justifiable to grant a reasonable time away from work. Not infrequently employees request the privilege of extended leave without pay. If a sound reason exists, it is usually well to grant the request. However, it is administratively unwise to allow repeated or extended leaves without pay for personal activities that are strictly matters of choice, such as extra vacations, fishing trips, and the like. It is recommended that this be avoided as much as possible, since it serves to interrupt and confuse the work of the organization and since some other employees and possibly the public are likely to misunderstand the situation and consider it evidence of favoritism.

Certain types of personnel, particularly those who are members of professions, are entitled to leaves within reasonable limits for the purpose of educational and professional improvement. Everything possible should be done not merely to allow this but to encourage their attending and taking an active part in the meetings of the professional societies and associations to which they do or should belong. Here again there is a reasonable extent to which time away from the job should be allowed to any one person. There are occasional individuals who tend to be professional conventioneers and who unless restrained will spend the majority of their time attending meetings and conventions away from the job for which they are presumably employed. Not only does the work of the organization suffer but the other employees are thereby prevented from obtaining their fair share of this privilege.

**In-service training**

The process of learning should stop only with the last breath of life. The knowledge and ability that the public health worker brings to his job in the first instance should represent at most only the beginning of an ever-growing fund of ability on which he may base professional action. An organization that does not aid and abet continued improvement of its employees is remiss in its responsibilities and in the long run handicaps itself. There are many ways of accomplishing the desired purpose, all of which may be included in the term *in-service training*. The purposes of an in-service training program have been well summarized by Palmer[41] as follows:

1. To make up for deficiencies in technical and scientific information required for the job generally
2. To enlarge the outlook and understanding on the specific job
3. To acquaint the staff with the fundamentals of personal and public relationships in order to encourage smoother functioning of the day-to-day job
4. To keep the staff abreast of newer technical, procedural, and administrative developments as derived from experience in other jurisdictions

A good program will follow many different approaches and most desirably will involve in one way or another all of the personnel from the administrator himself to the custodian. The methods used may consist of a formal orientation course or a field orientation in a well-organized health department. Of importance are conferences, both individual and group, institutes, staff meetings, and refresher courses. There is a growing feeling of a need for a more intensive practical experience comparable to an internship. Often visits to other health departments are worth while in order to acquaint the personnel with problems and procedures in other areas. As mentioned previously, attendance at business and professional meetings and conferences should be encouraged. If an employee has enough interest and ambition to cause him to attend a school while continuing to work, particular consideration during the period of time involved is often justified. A policy of granting full-time leaves for professional education is a highly desirable adjunct to the effective development of a staff in a career service. An in-service training program is as important and as possible in a small organization as in a large one and in a rural area as well as in a city with many facilities available. Successful and worthwhile programs have been carried out on all levels of government. Often valuable assistance is available from state and federal agencies, universities, various professional organizations, foundations, or private corporations.

**Retirement**

Retirement systems have become increasingly important in public health recruitment. Security is a basic desire, especially in a person's later years. Even though retirement systems have multiplied in recent decades, they are still not available to about one third of local employees. A good retirement system does at least four things: (1) it aids in organizational efficiency by making it possible to replace older personnel with younger people who possess more recent training and greater physical ability; (2) it does justice to all existing or prospective employees; (3) it aids in the solution of one of the greatest social problems that exists, that of dependency of the elderly; and (4) from the individual's point of view a sound system coupled with preretirement counseling represents good gerontologic practice by making possible a gradual tapering off of activities as physical stamina decreases.

If a retirement system exists, it is fundamental that payments be adequate, because if they are too small, there will develop a tendency to refuse the pension and to remain on the job at a salary for as long as possible, thereby defeating the purposes of the plan. For the same reason and to conduct the retirement system on a sound insurance basis it is equally fundamental that participation in the plan be compulsory. In addition, provision should be made for adjustment of the amount of the pension payments in relation to increases in the cost of living. The equity and importance of this is self-evident.

There are two principal types of retirement plans. The first is a simple cash disbursement plan that consists essentially of including an item in each budget to provide for pension payments. In this system total payments are small at first when few are entitled to benefits. As time passes, however, and more employees become older and eligible it becomes necessary to budget and therefore to tax for greater and greater amounts, resulting in a large proportion of the budget being for the payment of pensions rather than for actual services. Repeatedly organizations that have used this plan have become insolvent and in many instances have had to decrease or completely stop pension payments to which they had committed themselves and to which they had led their employees to look forward.

The second and more sound approach is through the use of an actuarial plan. Here future retirement objectives are calculated and planned for in advance for each employee. Such a program begins with larger payments than does the cash disbursement plan, but it builds up a reserve, the compound interest from which considerably lightens and in some instances completely absorbs the immediate financial burden.

The retirement plan may consist of contributions from employees alone, from the organization or government alone, or from the employees and the organization or government jointly. Typically, Social Security retirement benefits are part of the plan. The actuarial plan is the best method, since it gives both the employee and the organization an interest and a stake in the solution of the problem. For the employee it represents enforced savings with interest, plus reward for continued good service. For management it represents an orderly and socially responsible system for extending security to the current employee and separating the superannuated employee. If an employee leaves the organization before becoming eligible for pension payments, he should have the right to receive the total of whatever contributions he has made to the plan, plus whatever interest has accrued to that total. Under such circumstances, however, he should not expect to receive any of the contributions made by the organization or government, since that too defeats the purpose for which the plan has been established.

The fact that public health personnel tend to move from job to job and from one state to another in improving and advancing themselves professionally indicates the desirability of some type of interagency and interstate reciprocation with regard to retirement plans. In fact, in view of the characteristics of the function, which is clearly in the national interest, a federally managed retirement system for public health workers is clearly justified and long overdue. Such a system is still lacking and represents one of the most serious gaps in personnel management in public health. No one would question the desirability of workers in a field like public health obtaining many and varied experiences. Dependence on a jigsaw of scattered and disparate retirement plans and sometimes on none at all serves as an effective deterrent to this goal.

## REFERENCES

1. Parran, T.: Public health schools and the nation's health. Dedicatory address, School of Public Health, University of Michigan, Sept. 19, 1944 (official publication).
2. Bailey, S. K.: Ethics and the public service, Public Adm. Rev. **24:**234, Dec. 1964.
3. Mattison, B. F.: Political implications in good public health administration, Amer. J. Public Health **55:**183, Feb. 1965.
4. Tucker, R. R., Richardson, E. L., Lifson, S. S., and Aronson, J. B.: The politics of public health —a symposium, Amer. J. Public Health **49:**301, March 1959.
5. Rosenau, M. J.: Courses and degrees in public health work, J.A.M.A. **64:**794, March 6, 1915.
6. Committee on Professional Education of the American Public Health Association: Public health degrees and certificates granted in the United States and Canada during the academic year 1939-40, Amer. J. Public Health **30:**1456, Dec. 1940.
7. Editorial: Accreditation of schools of public health, Amer. J. Public Health **35:**953, Sept. 1945.
8. Criteria and guidelines for accrediting schools of public health, Amer. J. Public Health **56:**1308, Aug. 1966.
9. The school of public health: past, present, future, Public Health Rep. **78:**867, Oct. 1963.
10. Conferenciá sobre escuelas de salud publica, Bol. Ofic. Sanit. Panamer. **48:**4, April 1960.
11. Conference on schools of public health, Mexico, Amer. J. Public Health **50:**1039, July 1960.
12. Recommended norms, schools of public health in

Latin America, Washington, D. C., 1965, Pan American Health Organization.

13. Directory of schools of public health in the Americas, Washington, D. C., 1966, Pan American Health Organization.
14. Committee on Professional Education of the American Public Health Association: Individual reports, Amer. J. Public Health.
15. Proposed report of field training of public health personnel, Amer. J. Public Health **37:**709, June 1947; **45:**1351, Oct. 1955.
16. Editorial: Field training for public health personnel, Amer. J. Public Health **36:**178, Feb. 1946.
17. Guide for residencies in public health, Amer. J. Public Health **48:**1407, Oct. 1958.
18. The American Board of Preventive Medicine and Public Health Inc., Amer. J. Public Health **39:**425, March 1949; **49:**561, April 1959.
19. Burney, L. E., and Hemphill, F. M.: Merit system in public health, Amer. J. Public Health **34:**1173, Nov. 1944.
20. Mountin, J. W., Cheney, B. A., and Simpson, D. F.: Merit system administration in official health agencies, Amer. J. Public Health **37:**23, Jan. 1947.
21. Peterson, P. Q., Murray, L. J., Crabtree, J. A., and Amos, F. B.: The 1963 national conference on public health training, Amer. J. Public Health **54:**1049, July 1964.
22. Flook, E.: Public health service, personal communication, 1955.
23. Weiss, R. L., et al.: Retreading public health workers through training, Amer. J. Public Health **55:**242, Feb. 1965.
24. Bellin, L. E., Killeen, M., and Mazeika, J. J.: Preparing public health subprofessionals recruited from the poverty group, lessons from an OEO work-study program, Amer. J. Public Health **57:**242, Feb. 1967.
25. Emerson, H.: Local health units for the nation, New York, 1945, Commonwealth Fund.
26. Report of local public health resources, 1951, Public Health Service pub. no. 278, Washington, D. C., 1953, Government Printing Office.
27. Building America's health. Report of the President's Commission on the Health Needs of the Nation, Washington, D. C., 1952, Vol. 3, Government Printing Office.
28. Health resources statistics, 1973, DHEW pub. no. (HSM) 73-1509, Washington, D. C., 1973, Government Printing Office.
29. Health manpower—Report of National Commission on Community Health Services, Washington, D. C., 1967, Public Affairs Press.
30. White, L. D.: Introduction to the study of public administration, New York, 1955, The Macmillan Co.
31. Mountin, J. W.: On making public health positions more attractive, Amer. J. Public Health, **35:**1150, Nov. 1945.
32. Albouze, A. R.: Functions of the departmental personnel office, Personnel brief no. 23, Chicago, 1962, Public Personnel Association.
33. Donovan, J. J.: Career service classification, Amer. J. Public Health **51:**591, April 1961.
34. Sartain, A. Q., and Baker, A. W.: The supervisor and his job, ed. 2, New York, 1972, McGraw-Hill Book Co.
35. Dimock, M. E.: The executive in action, New York, 1945, Harper & Row, Publishers.
36. Pfiffner, J. McD.: Public administration, New York, 1946, The Ronald Press Co.
37. Upson, L. D.: Letters on public administration from a dean to his graduates, Detroit, 1947 (privately printed by the author).
38. Magoun, F. A.: New phases in personnel training, Public Health Nurs. **38:**592, 1946.
39. Allen, F. E.: Remedies against dishonest or inefficient public servants, Annals **169:**172, 1933.
40. Magoun, F. A.: Personal communication, 1948.
41. Palmer, G. T.: Quoted in Bearg, P. A., and Stockle, R.: Inservice training in a rural health department, Amer. J. Public Health **36:**1304, Nov. 1946.

Is it that some high Plan betides,
As yet not understood,
Of Evil stormed by Good,
We, the Forlorn Hope over which
Achievement strides?

THOMAS HARDY

CHAPTER 12

# Planning and evaluation<sup>*</sup>

## EVOLUTION OF PLANNING

During most of public health history, programs and activities developed in a generally unplanned manner. Several phases may be identified. For a long while much of the effort proceeded on the basis of crises—an epidemic, a flagrantly unsalubrious situation, or a natural disaster. The carry-over of this approach is still observable to an unfortunately common extent. Next, due to the efforts of the American Public Health Association's Committees on Administrative Practice and Evaluation, dating from the early 1920s, and coupled with the development and increasing sophistication of professional public health training, increasing numbers of health officers began to give serious attention to better planning. To no small degree this depended on their personal interests and former experience, but gradually their staffs and even members of the community began to be involved. This led in recent years to the development of special short training courses, sometimes in schools of public health and sometimes within operating agencies, on the planning and evaluative aspects of public health. Particular mention should be made of the numerous excellent seminars sponsored during the 1950s and 1960s by a Joint Committee on Executive Development of the Association of Management in Public Health and the Health Officer's Section of the American Public Health

Association as well as by the Center for Disease Control of the Public Health Service.

As funds became more plentiful for public health work, as the perimeters of the field were extended by legislation, as public demands and expectancy for service increased, and as government and management in general became more sophisticated, health agencies became more visible and began to be held more accountable for their stewardship. This of course brought about a greater consciousness of the importance of more careful planning and programming. Two events served to crystallize this trend and caused more interest and activity in health planning on the part of a wide variety of individuals and organizations during the past decade than any time in the past half century. The first was the development and refinement of certain planning techniques designated as PPBS (Planning-Programming-Budgeting Systems) by the Department of Defense.[2] The success of this prompted the President in August 1965 to direct his Cabinet members to apply the approach to the activities of the departments and agencies under their direction. The second event was the enactment by Congress in 1966 of P.L. 89-749, The Comprehensive Health Planning and Public Health Services Amendments.[3] The significance of this act has been threefold in that (1) it tends to move federal health assistance away from categorical grants toward block grants to make possible greater state and local program determination, (2) it encourages and requires more deliberate and hopefully more efficient program planning, and

---

*For an extensive bibliography see Strauss and de Groot.[1]

**235**

(3) it recognizes the breadth of social concerns and potential involvement by requiring the establishment of state and local or regional (so-called "area-wide") planning commissions consisting of a broad spectrum of professions, agencies, institutions, and citizen groups. These have become known as 314 (a) and (b) agencies, after the section of the legislation that created them.[4]

In his analysis of the Comprehensive Health Planning Act, Curran[5] refers to it as audacious, not only for its great breadth and implications but also because of its meager constitutional authority. He depicts it as "public policy executed with great *elan*." For one thing, he indicates, the Constitution does not provide for federal involvement in private as well as public planning, and legal means of enforcing such an interest is limited. The indirect means developed was to condition receipt of federal funds on development of acceptable planning agencies. He points out further that the legislation actually gives the local or area-wide planning agencies no power or authority. Any they may receive is from the legally constituted state or local governments. There is neither provision for representation on state health planning agencies of local health planning agencies nor for review by local planning agencies of federal health funds that come into their communities. Curran finally points to the irony of the fact that the act's legislation sets out far more requirements, conditions, and encouragements for comprehensive health planning (hence function) on the state and local level than on the national level, where for all practical purposes it is notable by its absence. As he says, "Comprehensiveness and coordination is much easier to order in some else's jurisdiction than in one's own."

## PROBLEMS IN PLANNING

The trends described have generated problems for some public health administrators. As indicated at the opening sentences of this chapter, some still strive mightily to maintain the status quo. But that is a losing game, as bluntly indicated by Mathewson.[6] As a successful public manager, in no way unsympathetic with public health workers and their goals, he comments:

To be completely frank, I must say that many of the public health officials with whom I have come into contact have played a very limited role or have stayed completely outside of the dynamics of the community decision process. Of course, there are several understandable explanations for this. Many public health technicians who live with human suffering and whose days are filled with unending efforts to alleviate the suffering cannot conceive that the rest of the world needs more than a call for help to galvanize it into appropriate action.

And he cannot help but conclude that:

. . . most public health officials . . . fail to take a full part in the political process—in assuring the implementation of their proposals—because they simply do not understand the dynamics of community decision making. They do not know why proposals for some absolutely essential public health activities are cancelled, postponed, under-financed, watered-down, or even ignored. And not knowing, they pass the baton to others, satisfied with the technical adequacy of their contribution and hopeful that someone else will transform their dreams into reality.

The fact that this has actually come about in many places and has had far-reaching implications not only for the determination of health policy but also for the control of health care systems is now the cause of considerable frustration for many public health administrators who let a unique opportunity slip away.[7]

Gorham,[8] who had much to do with the development of PPBS in the Department of Defense and who subsequently moved to the Department of Health, Education, and Welfare for the same purpose, has commented on the limitations of planning techniques. "Anyone in government knows that most decisions on spending emerge from a political process and are most heavily influenced by value judgments and the pressures brought to bear by a wide range of interested parties." He pointed out that the leaders of government may have preferences about programs, unrelated to costs, benefits, or efficiency. One may be interested in a particular program because its beneficiaries are numerous or politically powerful or vocal. Another may have experienced a heart attack or have a crippled child and therefore tend to favor programs aimed at these conditions. A program conducted as part of Social Security benefits financed from a payroll tax may be favored over another perhaps more important program that would necessitate increased tax revenues. Hilleboe and Schaefer[9] also have indicated the problems imposed by inadequate data, insufficient attainable resources, the current rapidity of scientific and technologic changes, and the scattered responsibility and authority in health matters.

Evidence that more than a plan for planning

is needed is provided by Roseman's[10] review of the first 5 years' experience with the comprehensive health planning program. Among the problems he noted were the following: (1) a pattern of conflict-avoidance in policy formulation and goal establishment; (2) a failure to deal with root causes of health problems; (3) a lack of political influence, leadership, or expertise, coupled in some states with a naive supportive clientele inside and outside of the health field; and (4) grossly inadequate funding to provide plans for comprehensive health care delivery in the light of anticipated national health insurance. On the other hand, as challenges he sees the following: (1) the development of plan implementation procedures and (2) overcoming the undue emphasis placed on traditional objectives such as cost reduction, coordination, and resource reallocation. He believes the prospects for comprehensive health planning survival as a bureaucratic entity are good but its innovative planning role limited, based on performance so far.

Nevertheless, as Gorham[8] concluded, whereas

. . . the tools of analysis are still fairly primitive —we are learning as we go along—and the best they can now do is to clarify some of the consequences of choices. . . . But the very process of analysis is valuable in itself, for it forces people to think about the objectives of Government programs and how they can be measured. It forces people to think in an explicit way. It is an important tool in the fight against creeping incrementalism—"ten percent to those with the most bureaucratic or political muscle, five percent to all others."

With reference to the comprehensive and total community approach to planning this too has its inherent problems. Public health workers, prideful of their educations, experiences, and professionalism, cannot be expected to be entirely pleased with situations in which their ideas, proposals, or decisions are subjected to the scrutiny and even veto of "the uninformed," be they from the governmental or community agencies or from the public at large. However, "the increased community involved, always sought but seldom attained, will more than make up, in the long run, for the transient confusion or the few moments lost while these new elements become familiar with the facts and figures and gear themselves to the mechanics and procedures essential to sound program planning. Given the motivation and a blueprint, the effective delivery of the requisite health services will not be far behind."[11] This

viewpoint is emphasized more strongly by the National Commission on Community Health Services.[12]

The nature of today's society and the complexities of health and other community services require a broad approach to planning and action which can be fitted to each particular community situation, yet is in harmony with broader trends and is capable of further development and change. The Commission believes that planning is an action process and is basic to development and maintenance of quality community health services. Action-planning for health should be communitywide in area, continuous in nature, comprehensive in scope, all-inclusive in design, coordinative in function, and adequately staffed.

The responsible participation and involvement of all sectors of the community, coordination of efforts, and development of cooperative working arrangements are fundamental to effective action-planning. Health service objectives can be met through processes which provide opportunity for citizens to work together to understand, identify, and resolve problems, to set intermediate and long-range goals, and to act to achieve the goals.

The readiness and ability of communities to respond to health needs and problems are dependent, in large part, on the presence of effective mechanisms for planning.

In a pluralistic society, wise and acceptable decisions and policies can be made less and less by the single channel approach. This is why interorganizational and community planning approaches and the systems analysis devices are becoming ever more important. Already, for example, several state governments specify that certain policies, such as those relating to water use and conservation, be made by a cabinet rather than by a single departmental director or board. In other words, it is becoming increasingly important to find the multiple interfaces among organizations, programs, and groups that have some commonality of interest, concern, responsibility, or action.

## OBJECTIVES OF HEALTH PLANNING

In recognition of the growing importance of improved planning by health agencies the Program Area Committee on Medical Care Administration and Public Health Administration of the American Public Health Association addressed itself during recent years to the development of a formal statement on the subject.[13] The statement as adopted presents the following useful list of the purposes or objectives of careful health planning:

1. Improve organizational patterns for health services

2. Speed development of needed new health services, strengthen existing services, and improve utilizations
3. Discourage programs not needed in the community
4. Improve the quality of health care through better coordination
5. Eliminate duplication of health services among official and voluntary agencies at all levels
6. Reduce fragmentation of health services at the state and community levels
7. Help to achieve better geographical distribution of health services, with optimum utilization
8. Establish priorities among new health programs and services, develop better balance among health programs, and provide services more responsive to the special health needs of the area
9. Foster better use of scarce health manpower and more effective development of training resources
10. Identify health needs and problems and help to set realistic goals, keeping expected changes in the area's characteristics in mind
11. Spur faster application of new health knowledge
12. Encourage closer relationships among health services, research, and training
13. Help to integrate health needs into physical, economic, and other areas of planning for community development

Particular attention should be directed to the last of these objectives, since it is so often overlooked or ignored. Earlier, public health administration was defined as "the planned and organized social application of the knowledge and techniques of various and varying disciplines to the biological, physiological and sociological advantage of man." In this definition emphasis is placed not only on the importance of planning but also on planning within the total social context. In other words it is important at the outset to regard planning in the field of public health as only one facet of total social and economic planning.[14] This was emphasized also by Seipp[15] in a discussion of health planning and economic development:

While program planning continues to be of major importance to health workers in the developing countries, there has emerged today an essentially new emphasis to plan for health as part of the totality of developmental effort. In this context, health measures are evaluated in terms of their significance for the process of development as a whole. The essential planning problem is to maximize the contribution forthcoming from the provision of health services to the total nation-building efforts of society. Planning within the health sector thus is undertaken in the terms of the larger framework of national developmental planning. . . . Health, it is obvious, cannot be overlooked as an end in itself. At the same time, the improvement of the health of a population represents an essential means or instrument for the developing society to attain its social and economic goals. It is when health measures are assessed from this instrumental point of view that they can be recognized as productive in character. They represent a necessary element in the total process of development, facilitating the attainment of the general goals of a society.

The World Health Organization understandably has also addressed itself to this aspect of planning of public health services and urges more attention to it by economists, political leaders, and health workers.[16,17]

At one time I was asked to advise a developing nation whose economy was based primarily on mining under exceedingly poor conditions. At the time the government was also encouraging the settlement of potentially good agricultural areas. After careful study the primary recommendations were for the establishment of a strong occupational health program and an intensive antituberculosis program based essentially on almost universal ambulatory prophylactic and therapeutic drug administration to miners and their families, among whom the incidence of tuberculosis was tremendous. The intent was obvious—to shore up the immediate economic producers on whom the nation depended almost entirely at the moment. Next, emphasis was placed on malaria eradication and the establishment of effective health posts along the routes of forest clearance and settlement. The intent here was to protect the health of the new group of producers on whom the nation would depend more as time passed. It was thought that other activities could and indeed would have to wait their turn.

A number of subsidiary recommendations might be of interest: (1) a thorough hydrographic survey of the rivers to determine appropriate sites for dams; this would assure a constant supply not only of water but also of electricity important to community development, education, food preservation, etc.; (2) the construction of refrigeration plants for the preservation of meat and other foods; cattle raising had already begun to prosper, and meat spoilage was becoming a problem; (3) the construction of some chicken-packing plants; this was aimed particularly at providing a year-round source of low-cost poultry protein in a protein-deficient society; (4) a celotex factory adjacent to one of the large sawmills that had already been constructed to process lumber for export; housing had already become a severe problem to the solution of which inexpensive celotex could contribute; and (5) the pavement of certain feeder roads in the area being settled; this would make the settlements more accessible year round for health, educational, and other purposes. These and some other recommendations for planning may appear remote from health interests, but in each case they would eventually contribute in some way and to some extent to the attainment of good health. By like token each of the health measures recommended clearly would contribute to the social and economic development of the area.

## TERMINOLOGY IN PROGRAM PLANNING

Already a considerable number of source and reference materials have developed on the subject of planning.[1,9,18] Terminology in this relatively new field has already become somewhat confusing. A variety of names, achronymic or otherwise, have been invented and applied to the analytic methods involved by various writers, teachers, and practitioners. Among those encountered are program development, program planning, program analysis, decision trees, program cost accounting, cost-benefit analysis, operations research, systems analysis, PPBS (Planning-Programming-Budgeting Systems), PERT (Program Evaluation and Review Technique), and ASTRA (Automatic Scheduling with Time Integrated Resource Allocation). Many of these names and methods are synonymous, some represent parts of others, and many overlap. The more encompassing are PPBS, operations research, and systems analysis. Essentially these are synonymous and are concerned with the complete spectrum, from fact finding, problem definition, goal setting, programming, controls and evaluation with proper feed-ins and feedbacks of information, resources, and results to subsidiary or final outputs or solutions. An example of this systems approach is shown in Fig. 12-1, which represents the elements of a research procedure and the ways they may be systematically interrelated.[19]

**PPBS (Planning-Programming-Budgeting Systems).** PPBS is a procedure intended to make possible the better allocation of resources among alternate ways to attain a desired objective.

Its essence is the development and presentation of information as to the full implications, the costs and benefits, of the major alternative courses of action relevant to major resources allocation decisions. . . . Such problems as budget and implementation, manpower selection, the assessment of the work efficiency of operating units and cost control of current operations are generally considered to be outside the purview of PPBS. Cost accounting and non-fiscal performance reporting systems are very important in providing basic data required for PPBS analyses (as well as for fiscal accounting and management control purposes). However, such systems are usually considered complementary to PPBS rather than directly part of it. . . . The main contribution of PPBS lies in the planning process, i.e., the process of making program policy decisions that lead to a specific budget and specific multi-year plans.[20]

Michael[21] considers the PPBS to enable an agency or organization to plan programs in terms of the best choice among alternatives of action, based on sound knowledge and careful analysis of the implication of each alternative. He describes the process as involving the following:

1. Appraisal and comparison of health and various other activities in terms of their relative contributions to health objectives
2. Determination of how given objectives can be attained with minimum expenditure of resources
3. Projection of health activities over a long enough time period to provide proper perspective
4. Consideration of the relative contribution of private and public activities toward health objectives
5. Revision of objectives, programs and budgets in the light of experience and changing circumstances (i.e., feedback)
6. Explicit recognition of the need to demonstrate results for effort expended
7. Application of new analytical techniques as an aid to, but not a replacement for, leadership judgment at all levels

**Operations research.** Operations research originated from the efforts of scientists of many disciplines to solve military operations problems during World War II.[22] It is a term applied to "research into some or all aspects of conducting or operating a system, a business, or a service, while treating the system as a living organism in its proper environment. . . ." According to Andersen,[23] its major phases are as follows:

1. Formulating the problem, including definition of the objectives
2. Collection of data relevant to the problem

3. Analysis of data to produce a hypothesis and a mathematical model to represent the system under study
4. Deriving solutions from the model
5. Choosing the optimal solution and forecasting results
6. Testing the optimal combination of interventions, with controls built into the system to keep continuous check on the hypotheses
7. Recommending implementation of the solution, including the control system

**Systems analysis.** Systems analysis is primarily focussed on the first phases or parts of

**Fig. 12-1.** Example of systems approach—the research context. Boxes represent activities; solid lines, flow of information, influence, or funds; dotted lines, feedback. (From Blumenthal, M.: Traffic accident prevention as a system component, Public Health Rep. **81:**569, June 1966.)

PPBS or operations research procedure; that is, ". . . the interpretation of broad objectives and guidelines, and the structuring of information in such a way that the decision maker can see and evaluate the options available to him. . . . The realistic goal of systems analysis is the improvement of the decision-making process, not the creation of a mechanism that automatically produces ideal decisions."[20] Hopefully the method provides the decision maker with more accurate or dependable information with reference to the cost and value of potential programs. The process involves the following steps:

1. Definition of the problem
2. Projection of determinants of the problem
3. Generation of alternative approaches to solving the problem
4. Evolution of the cost-effectiveness of the alternatives
5. Interpretation of the qualitative results

**PERT (Program Evaluation and Review Technique).** PERT is adapted from the work-flow studies long used in industrial management. Proceeding on the basis that the relations within the planning process are dynamic, it provides a graphic detailed representation of the components of a program. "It is most useful when planning the implementation phase of a program. Essentially, it is a method of mapping future activities so that anyone can visualize the total plans of action for a program."[24] However, it is useful in planning only objective-oriented programs with specific measurable end results. The characteristics of the technique are as follows[25]:

1. A work breakdown structure, beginning with a final objective subdivided into a series of smaller subobjectives.
2. A network including all activities and events necessary to reach each subobjective. Activity is an effort required to move from one event to another. An activity may also indicate simply a connection or interrelationship between two events which does not require any effort. In the latter instance, estimated time for the activity would be zero. Specific and definable program accomplishments that do not require time or resources are events.
3. Identification of time estimates for various activities as well as the total process, including a critical path. The longest path, in terms of time, through the network from the beginning to the ending event is the critical path.
4. A method of network analysis that provides continuous evaluation of program status and identification of problem areas so that preventive action can

be taken. The network is a diagram of activities and events necessary to reach a program objective. It shows sequences of accomplishment, interrelationships, and dependencies. Analysis of the network by the administrator at any stage of the program permits him to determine whether anticipated progress is being made and if not, specifically where the bottleneck is occurring.

## APPROACHES TO PLANNING

With this general background, what types of problems and factors must be considered when health administrators attempt to develop programs for the achievement of public health purposes and goals? Generally they appear to fall into three categories:

Plan—including programming, control, and evaluation

Money—including its acquisition, management, and accountability

People—including recruitment, training, organization, and management as well as relationships with other parts of the government and with the public in general

For purposes here it should be pointed out that although planning appears to be only one of the three considerations, everything in each of the other two factors is in fact involved in program planning. In other words, a plan is incomplete if it does not include consideration both of what resources exist and how best to use them and also of what methods of evaluating results it is hoped will be obtained. It might also be worth indicating that the plans of an organization, to the extent that they exist, are usually illustrated in a general sense by (1) the organization chart, (2) the staffing pattern, and (3) the budget.

In modern public health administration it is becoming evermore necessary to develop and use effective and objective approaches to program planning, establishment of program priorities, program control, and program evaluation. This is important in order to know (1) What are the goals and standards? (2) What should be done? (3) What is being done? (4) What does it cost? (5) Is it being done efficiently and effectively? (6) Is it worth doing?

### Goals and standards

One of the most serious limitations of public health agencies in the past and one of the chief reasons why they have often found themselves ineffective and in difficulty is that often the agencies have not defined their goals and standards in sufficient detail, with adequate enough precision, and with consideration of all the community's interests or needs.

The determination of goals and standards depends on several factors, each of whose relative significance varies through time. The initial approach is to find out what the government and the people that it represents had in mind as their purpose in establishing and continuing the health agency. This is important, regardless of the amount of agreement with that purpose. To ignore it may doom one's best intentions and efforts to failure. A more familiar approach to the determination of goals and standards is the collecting and analyzing of statistics, reports of births, illnesses, and deaths, or the conducting of special surveys and studies. Information from such sources, if properly obtained and logically analyzed, points to problems that suggest desirable goals to be attained or desirable standards to be established, achieved, and maintained. Obviously the problems indicated by such data should be studied in relative terms, that is, in relation to other times, in relation to other places, and in relation to each other.

**Priorities**

The relation of possible goals to each other is of particular interest and concern to public health administration because it necessitates the development of some means of determining the relative importance of various health problems and hence various public health activities. In other words it involves the establishment of *priorities* in relation to goals. At any given moment or place there are many different public health problems, always many more than can be attacked adequately with available resources. Some problems obviously must take precedence over others. As previously indicated, it is unfortunately frequent that the decision is made on the basis of whim, on some personal interest of the public health administrator, or in deference to particular political or public pressure groups rather than as a result of careful study and analysis.

How may this important early step in program planning be approached? There are certain fundamental factors that should be considered in program priority determination. For example, a problem that affects a large number of people ordinarily should take precedence over one that affects relatively few people, but not if the former is the common cold and the latter is endemic smallpox. A disease that kills or disables should take precedence over one that does not, but only if an effective method of scientific attack is at hand. There are many such factors that should be taken into consideration: existence of scientific knowledge and techniques, economics, cultural acceptability, availability of suitable personnel, and propriety and legality of the contemplated action, to mention only a few. In addition, as Nathan[26] has pointed out, one should consider pressures and interests of special and local groups, expressed views of the chief executive, editorials in the local newspapers, official policy expressed by the legislature, opportunism when funds are made available with regard to a particular problem, sudden advances in knowledge or techniques, and the need for research and demonstration. Further exploration, experimentation, and trial are needed in this field.

A somewhat detailed and complicated approach is one first developed as an administrative aid in connection with the International Technical Assistance Programs of the United States Government. It has subsequently been refined for provocative, experimental, and in-service training purposes.[27] It is presented here for the possible interest it may have. Actually the process of its development by the staff of an agency, rather than its end products, is perhaps its most valuable characteristic. The first step is for the key professional and management personnel to meet together and to list every conceivable type of activity and program that is being engaged in, might be instituted, or has ever been requested. The number of items may easily number in the hundreds. Following this listing down one axis, across the other axis is listed every conceivable factor that might be considered in judging whether or not a particular activity or program should or could be engaged in at the moment or in the near future. Then there is discussion of each possible activity or program in terms of these many factors, resulting in a rating of each from 0 to 4+. By this means it becomes possible to consider existing or potential activities or programs from a broad overall objective yet relative point of view. From the concensus that develops the results usually fall into three broad priority categories:

1. For activities or programs that are consistently rated 3+ or 4+ for every qualifying factor the conclusion is that under all circumstances these particular activities should be carried out.

2. Of secondary importance are certain activities or programs that ordinarily might not merit attention without special precise explanation and justification because of reservations with regard to one or several of the qualifying criteria.

3. In the third category are certain activities or programs that are not justified and should not or cannot be engaged in. It is recognized, however, that in unusual instances certain nonhealth considerations might result in a decision to engage in one of these activities.

Repeated trial of this procedure appears to indicate the existence of a dynamic formula consisting of four components as follows:

Component A = Size of problem
Component B = Seriousness of problem      } Public
Component C = Effectiveness                  health
Component D = PEARL                          need

The formula then appears as:

$$\text{Basic priority rating (BPR)} = \frac{(A + B)C}{3}$$

$$\text{Overall priority rating (OPR)} = \frac{(A + B)C}{3} \times D$$

The range of scores for each of the four components is decided on as follows:

A = 0 to 10
B = 0 to 20
C = 0 to 10
D = 0 *or* 1

The maximum obtainable product of the four components (A, B, C, and D) is therefore 300. By an arbitrary division of this maximum product by 3, the maximum score becomes 100. Every computed rating will then be in the range 0 to 100.

It now becomes necessary to consider certain fundamental qualifying factors. These are shown as PEARL, explained on p. 244.

As in the case of many evaluative procedures, a large so-called subjective element enters into this exercise. The choice and definition of the components in the formula and the relative weights assigned to them are based on group concensus. Application of the formula in the rating of programs and activities involves the judgments of individual raters. However, some scientific control may be achieved by the use of a representative sample of qualified raters, a precise definition of terms, the delineating of exact rating procedures, the utilization of statistical data to guide ratings when feasible, and a statistical averaging of scores derived by

raters working independently. However, some further detail on the components of the formula is necessary.

**Component A—size of problem.** For purposes of assignment of priorities, size of problem is defined as the *total number of persons having the problem or being directly affected by the problem expressed in rates per 100,000 population.* Qualifying within this population are those persons who reasonably may be expected to receive services if the services were available. Not qualifying within this population are those persons who have the problem or are directly affected by it but for whom public health services are inappropriate.

Since there are many problems that will be defined in terms of comparatively small demographic groups, it was arbitrarily decided that size of problem be scored according to the following scale:

| Units per 100,000 population (component A) | Score |
|---|---|
| 50,000 or more | 10 |
| 5,000 to 49,999 | 8 |
| 500 to 4,999 | 6 |
| 50 to 499 | 4 |
| 5 to 49 | 2 |
| 0.5 to 4.9 | 0 |

Thus if a problem is defined in terms of the population of a large city, it is obvious that the following scale would result and apply:

| Population in city (component A) | Score |
|---|---|
| 1,000,000 or more | 10 |
| 100,000 to 999,999 | 8 |
| 10,000 to 99,999 | 6 |
| 1,000 to 9,999 | 4 |
| 100 to 999 | 2 |
| Less than 100 | 0 |

**Component B—seriousness of problem.** Seriousness of problem is defined in terms of four factors: *urgency, severity, economic loss,* and *involvement of people.* The component "seriousness" is assigned a range of 0 to 20 in the formula. Each factor of seriousness is assigned a range of 0 to 10. Thus it is possible to obtain the maximum score of 20 for seriousness even though only two factors contribute to it. However, if all four factors rate 10, the maximum for all four would still be limited to 20.

| Factors comprising seriousness | Range of score |
|---|---|
| Urgency | 0 to 10 |
|   Public concern | |
|   Public health concern | |

| *Factors comprising seriousness* | *Range of score* |
|---|---|
| Severity | 0 to 10 |
|   Mortality | |
|   Morbidity—degree and duration | |
|   Disability—degree and duration | |
| Economic loss | 0 to 10 |
|   To individuals | |
|   To community | |
| Involvement of people | 0 to 10 |
|   Potential—number of persons who may acquire problem or be affected by existing problem, and relative degree of involvement | |
|   Indirect—number of persons affected socially, economically, psychologically, etc. and relative degree of involvement | |

**Component C—effectiveness.** Effectiveness is yet to be studied comprehensively. It involves the difficult field of evaluation, for which valid measuring devices are largely yet to be developed. It is believed that this component should be assigned two values:

$C_1$ for the program or activity as it is now being carried out

$C_2$ for the program or activity as carried out optimally

**Component D—PEARL.** PEARL consists of a group of factors not directly related to the actual need or effectiveness but which determine whether a particular program or activity can be carried out at a specific time.

$$P = \text{Propriety}$$
$$E = \text{Economics}$$
$$A = \text{Acceptability}$$
$$R = \text{Resources}$$
$$L = \text{Legality}$$

Each of these qualifying factors is given a value of 0 *or* 1, and since together they represent a product rather than a sum, if any one of them is rated 0, it not only gives PEARL a total rating of 0 but also makes the OPR score 0. Therefore although the BPR might be high, the proposed activity or program is impossible or impractical at the moment, and certain intermediate steps are indicated.

**Program inventory
and performance reporting**

The question, What is being done? is less simple than it sounds. It is essentially a matter of *program inventory*. Fundamental to a useful program inventory is an adequate *performance reporting system* in which the various activities engaged in are reported in terms of the nature of the work performed. An important distinction

must be made here. Whereas the more usual type of reporting is focussed on personnel function, activities carried out, or services rendered (e.g., number of inspections made, laboratory specimens examined, or homes visited by public health nurses), to be of true value, performance reporting should be focussed on a program purpose such as food establishments supervised or individuals immunized (in other words results actually achieved). This has been emphasized by Flook[28] in the following statement.

There is a fine distinction between the traditional activity counts—enumerations of nursing and clinic visits for various purposes or of sanitary inspections of different types of establishments—and the kind of statistics which focuses attention on numbers of persons served and types and amount of service received. With the traditional counts, quantitative evidence is being accumulated to describe how each public health worker spends his time—how much effort is being expended for each separate program. With the latter type of statistics, information is being collected on the results of that effort.

Measurement of results then, is the key to what we want to achieve with service statistics. The term service yield indices is an apt phrase. Just as a farmer finds it necessary, if he is to know whether he is operating at a gain or loss, to reckon the number of bushels of wheat or bales of cotton he gets per acre in return for the labor and expense of production, so the public health worker must calculate the service being rendered to the community in relation to the need for service.

Nathan[26] has commented on this important point from a slightly different viewpoint:

There is not enough known about methodology to make such a broad, sweeping statement. Perhaps a case in point may help to illustrate: Let us consider inspection of pasteurizing plants. We know that certain communicable diseases may be transmitted through milk. We know that proper pasteurization of milk will establish a barrier preventing the transmission of the organisms causing these communicable diseases. We therefore require the pasteurization of milk and establish a procedure of inspection of pasteurizing plants. To assure proper pasteurization we say that a certain number and type of inspections are necessary. Is our goal in this instance the prevention of communicable diseases, the carrying out of a certain number and type of inspections, or is it to make sure that the pasteurizing plants adhere to standards?

**Performance budgeting**

The development and availability of a program inventory based on valid performance reporting makes possible an approach to the fourth and fifth questions: What does it cost? Is it being done efficiently and effectively? This is the realm of performance budgeting, which will be discussed in Chapter 13. As stated there in its simplest terms it is nothing more than the application of benefit-cost accounting to a performance report. It summarizes the program activities performed in terms of unit cost, telling the total cost of achieving immunization of an individual or the cost of obtaining compliance with a food ordinance. With this available for all parts of a program a further step becomes possible, the determination of the cost of total program in relation to what it achieves. One then has a true program budget that measures the total impact of a program in terms of its cost. With this, in relation to the first question listed (What are the goals and standards?), it is then possible to answer the sixth and final question, Is it worth doing?

Grosse[2] presents a timely and clear illustration of this procedure (Table 12-1) and the value it may have in sound decision making. The cost-benefit analysis brings clearly to the surface several important considerations. More deaths from uterine-cervix cancer can be prevented than for any of the other types of cancer considered. Furthermore, the cost per case found and the cost per death averted were both significantly lower than for the other types of cancer; also the cost per examination was reasonable. By all counts, with a fixed amount of funds, a program to detect early uterine-cervix cancer would be both the most efficient and produce the greatest success.

## EVALUATION

The subject of evaluation and the many ways in which it may be and has been approached are large, complex, and dynamic. The ap-

proaches have been summarized in an especially worthy manner by Hilleboe[29] in his address at the Second Annual Award Lecture on Public Health at the Fifty-Ninth Annual New York City Health Conference on June 12, 1963. The subject has also been dealt with extensively in the Proceedings of the First and Second National Conferences on Evaluation in Public Health.[30] There are certain subjective and philosophic determinations necessary before one proceeds to the details or mechanics of evaluation. Thus what is to be evaluated—services, activities, results, or qualifications? If performance or services are to be measured against certain standards, as they must be in the final analysis, how firm, objective, valid, or applicable are the standards? Who develops them and on what basis? If an activity or program is to be evaluated, for what purpose, toward what end is it to be evaluated?

Earlier there was brief discussion of the importance of measuring end products or end results rather than motions by employees. At the same time it was emphasized that, cruel though it may seem to some, programs designed to benefit certain individuals or groups may be much more valuable in the long run than certain others. Sanders[31] emphasizes this further by saying, "To answer the question of what constitutes adequate health care for a community, we must be able to identify the contribution which that care makes, and the extent to which a reallocation of resources is required to maximize productive man-years per life. This should be the acid test in appraising the efficacy of health services, and in determining whether a community is making optimum outlays for health care. The goal is difficult of attainment, but the stakes are enormous for our nation and for mankind."

**Table 12-1.** Cost-benefit analysis, cancer control program, 1968-1972*

|  | Uterine-cervix | Breast | Head and neck | Colon-rectum |
|---|---|---|---|---|
| Grant costs ($000) | 97,750 | 17,750 | 13,250 | 13,300 |
| Number of examinations (000) | 9,363 | 2,280 | 609 | 662 |
| Cost per examination | $10.44 | $7.79 | $21.76 | $20.10 |
| Examinations per case found | 87.5 | 167.3 | 620.2 | 496.0 |
| Cancer cases found | 107,045 | 13,628 | 982 | 1,334 |
| Cost per case found | $913 | $1,302 | $13,493 | $9,970 |
| Cancer deaths averted | 44,084 | 2,936 | 303 | 288 |
| Cost per death averted | $2,217 | $6,046 | $43,729 | $46,181 |

*From Grosse, R. N.: Planning, programming and budgeting, Bull. N. Y. Acad. Med. **44:**125, Feb. 1968.

The meaning of evaluation is of great importance in relation to any efforts to achieve it. The American Public Health Association has defined evaluation as it relates to health as "the process of determining the value or amount of success in achieving a predetermined objective. It includes at least the following steps: formulation of the objective, identification of the proper criteria to be used in measuring success, determination and explanation of the degree of success, recommendations for further activity."[32] Although each of these steps is of obvious importance, particular attention is directed to the last, the feedback aspect of evaluation, the recommendations to be derived from the evaluation process that may serve to alter or improve the program or activity that has been evaluated. James[33] stated this well in saying that evaluation ". . . differs from research primarily in that it does not seek new knowledge, but attempts to mark progress toward a prestated objective. While research can end with the presentation of results, evaluation is viewed as part of a circular process. Its findings are reincorporated into the specific program from which they came."

It is also important to distinguish between evaluation and the mere development of indices of health or of health practice and the surveys necessary to obtain them. Indices and surveys of this type can be of great value in several ways—problem identification, need definition, public relations, and statistical comparison[34,35]—but they must not be confused with true evaluation. Brief descriptive reference has been made earlier in this chapter to PERT. This systematic approach to problem solving or goal achievement illustrates very well the most desirable and useful approach to evaluation. Here evaluation is deliberately built into the planning process not only at the beginning but as one of the major phases or purposes of the planning process. Then to justify having done this the products or results of evaluation, that is, the evaluative output, is fed back into the dynamic system as it proceeds.

Another interesting way of evaluation of health services has been developed by Greenberg,[36] who also emphasizes that evaluation is not an assessment of need or community diagnosis but a follow-up procedure to ascertain effectiveness or goal fulfillment among the recipients of service in a program. After considering the components of program input, for example, organization, personnel, funds, data,

etc., he visualizes evaluative output as follows:

*Immediate goals*
Increase in knowledge; improved attitudes and practices
Reduced *d*isinterest; reduced *d*issatisfaction
*Intermediate goals*
More positive health; improved status
Reduced *d*iscomfort and *d*eprivation; reduced disease
*Long-range goals*
Reduction in morbidity and mortality
Reduced *d*isability; reduced *d*eath

Other types of output may take the form of accompanying favorable effects in the community other than among recipients of service or of untoward side effects. Overall efficiency may then be expressed as

$$\frac{\text{Output (in terms of goal fulfillment)}}{\text{Input (in terms of dollars, services, and/or personnel time)}}$$

**Evaluation aids.** The *Evaluation Schedule For Use in the Study and Appraisal of Community Health Programs*,[37] developed over many years by the American Public Health Association, deserves particular mention, since it provided an admirable, stimulating incentive and method for administrative control and coordination as well as for appraisal. Referring to this study, Pfiffner and Preshus[38] made the following statement:

Probably no administrative field has gone further than public health in developing criteria to judge the effectiveness of its work. Since public health administration in its present form is so young, this fact becomes especially significant. The standards and measurement referred to are the results of experiences growing out of a number of public health surveys covering a period of years. . . . The criteria are so objective that little is left to the opinion of the appraiser. . . . Indeed, it has been shown quite conclusively that there is a very direct relation between the amount that is spent for public health administration, score achieved, and the health of the community as shown by the mortality and morbidity rates.

Rating was based on performance rather than results. In other words the schedule took cognizance of the administrative organization and facilities of the health administration rather than sickness and death statistics. It considered in spearate detail the following 16 phases of the public health program:

1. Personnel, facilities, and services
2. Public health problems

3. Community health education and staff training
4. Communicable disease control
5. Tuberculosis control
6. Venereal disease control
7. Maternal health
8. Infant and preschool health
9. School health
10. Adult health
11. Accident prevention
12. Water supplies and excreta disposal
13. Food control
14. Milk control
15. Housing
16. Financial support for local health work

For a period the American Public Health Association also published a document entitled *Health Practice Indices*, which consisted of an extensive series of line charts relating to the particularly significant items in the *Evaluation Schedule*. Each chart presented the reported experience of several hundred investigators. It had value in allowing a health officer to insert the position of his community in each chart. Concurrently the association published a summary scoring sheet that made it possible to obtain an overall view of the strengths, weaknesses, balance, and coordination of the program of a public health agency. Certain items were graphically emphasized, being considered of such great importance that a poor score for them outweighed any benefits that might result from other activities. Thus an approved water supply, a satisfactory sewage disposal system, and pasteurization of milk were considered fundamental to the health of a community regardless of whatever other accomplishments were achieved.

The American Public Health Association has also developed a *Guide to a Community Health Study*[39] for use by community organizations and agencies in studying and improving all aspects of their community's health structure and program, both official and nonofficial. Every public health worker should become thoroughly familiar with this valuable document.

The use of administrative control tools such as these is of great importance in measuring success and progress toward the goals and objectives that should always consciously exist. Generally speaking, once the administrator determines the needs, goals, obstacles, facilities, and abilities, failure to reach the goals can be due only to poor administration and inattention to duty.

This brief and general discussion of program planning and evaluation can have no better closing than a comment by Crabtree[40] when he was Dean of the Graduate School of Public Health of the University of Pittsburgh:

Perhaps today's greatest challenge to public health administration is to advance and accelerate the pace of research aimed at the establishment and validation of a body of administrative theory applicable to its broader dimensioned problems and issues. To take the attitude . . . that administration is only an art and will never become a science is to say that every outcome of any administrative action is altogether unique, and therefore there can be no transferable knowledge or understanding of either the administrative process or the phenomena involved therein.

That administration can become a science rests on the assumption that regularities can be detected and identified in the phenomena involved in the administrative process and that there must be an orderly arrangement of the elements of the process itself. The administrative process basically is a systems process. . . . There is encouraging evidence today that public health is becoming alert to these possibilities.

## REFERENCES

1. Strauss, M. D., and de Groot, I.: A bookshelf on planning for health, Amer. J. Public Health **61:** 656, April 1971.
2. Grosse, R. N.: Planning, programming and budgeting, Bull. N. Y. Acad. Med. **44:**125, Feb. 1968.
3. Fact sheet on partnership for health, Washington, D. C., 1968, U. S. Department of Health, Education, and Welfare.
4. Colt, A. M.: Elements of comprehensive health planning, Amer. J. Public Health **60:**1194, July 1970.
5. Curran, W. J.: Comprehensive health planning: audacious law-making, Amer. J. Public Health **58:**1100, June 1968.
6. Mathewson, K.: Program planning in relation to the total community. In The executive process in public health administration, Ann Arbor, 1968, University of Michigan School of Public Health.
7. Brown, D. R.: Community health planning, or who will control the health care system, Amer. J. Public Health **62:**1336, Oct. 1972.
8. Gorham, W.: PPBS, its scope and limits, The Public Interest **8:**4, Summer 1967.
9. Hilleboe, H. E., and Schaefer, M.: Papers and bibliography on community health planning, Albany, 1967, Williams Press.
10. Roseman, C.: Problems and prospects for comprehensive health planning, Amer. J. Public Health **62:**16, Jan. 1972.
11. Editorial: Planning for healthful communities, Amer. J. Public Health **56:**1987, Dec. 1966.
12. National Commission on Community Health Services: Health is a community affair, Cambridge, 1966, Harvard University Press.

13. Guidelines for organizing state and area-wide community health planning, Amer. J. Public Health **56:**2139, Dec. 1966.

14. Hanlon, J. J.: Can accounting sell health? In Economic benefits from public health services, Public Health Service pub. no. 1178, Washington, D. C., 1964, Government Printing Office.

15. Seipp, C.: Health planning and economic development. Address given at the John Grant Memorial Session, Ninety-First Annual Meeting, American Public Health Association, Kansas City, Nov. 13, 1963.

16. Planning of public health services, WHO Techn. Rep. Series no. 215, 1961.

17. Hilleboe, H. E., Barkhuus, A., and Thomas, W. C.: Approaches to national health planning, Geneva, 1972, World Health Organization.

18. Anderman, R. C.: Bibliography on program planning, budgeting and evaluation in public health, Philadelphia, 1967, Fels Institute of Local and State Government (mimeographed).

19. Blumenthal, M.: Traffic accident prevention as a system component, Public Health Rep. **81:**569, June 1966.

20. Hatry, H. P., and Cotton, J. F.: Program planning for state, county and city, Washington, D. C., 1967, George Washington University Press.

21. Michael, J. M.: Planning-programming-budgeting and health program planning. In The executive process in public health administration, Ann Arbor, 1968, University of Michigan School of Public Health.

22. Flagle, C. D.: Operational research in the health services, Ann. N. Y. Acad. Sci. **107:**748, May 22, 1963.

23. Andersen, S.: Operations research in public health, Public Health Rep. **79:**297, April 1964.

24. Arnold, M. F., et al.: Health program implementation through PERT, San Francisco, 1966, Western Regional Office, American Public Health Association.

25. Merten, W.: PERT and planning for health programs, Public Health Rep. **81:**449, May 1966.

26. Nathan, M. R.: Some steps in the process of program planning, Amer. J. Public Health **46:**68, Jan. 1956.

27. Hanlon, J. J.: The design of public health programs for underdeveloped countries, Public Health Rep. **69:**1028, Nov. 1954.

28. Flook, E.: The value of good service statistics in a modern health department, Public Health Rep. **68:**811, Aug. 1953.

29. Hilleboe, H. E.: Improving performance in public health. Second Annual Award Lecture on Public Health presented at the Fifty-Ninth Annual New York City Health Conference, June 12, 1963 (mimeographed).

30. Proceedings of the First and Second National Conferences on Evaluation in Public Health, Ann Arbor, 1955 and 1960, University Publications Distribution Service (mimeographed).

31. Sanders, B. S.: Measuring community health levels, Amer. J. Public Health **54:**1063, July 1964.

32. Glossary of administrative terms in public health, Amer. J. Public Health **50:**225, Feb. 1960.

33. James, G.: Evaluation in public health practice, Amer. J. Public Health **52:**1145, July 1962.

34. Conceptual problems in developing an index of health, Public Health Service pub. no. 17, Series 2, Washington, D. C., 1966, Government Printing Office.

35. Measurement of levels of health, WHO Techn. Rep. Ser. no. 137, 1957.

36. Greenberg, B. G.: Goal setting and evaluation: some basic principles, Bull. N. Y. Acad. Med. **44:**125, Feb. 1968.

37. American Public Health Association: Evaluation schedule for use in the study and appraisal of community health programs (reprinted), New York, 1937, The Association.

38. Pfiffner, J. McD., and Preshus, R.: Public administration, New York, 1967, The Ronald Press Co.

39. American Public Health Association: Guide to a community health study, New York, 1961, The Association.

40. Crabtree, J. A.: Plans for tomorrow's needs in local public health administration, Amer. J. Public Health **53:**1175, Aug. 1963.

CHAPTER 13

# Fiscal management

## GENESIS OF FISCAL CONTROLS

Since public health activities are usually performed by governmental agencies, it necessarily follows that public revenues must furnish the most stable and largest part of the funds supporting them. This being the case, it is important that public health personnel and especially the administrators of official public health agencies constantly bear in mind that the handling and administration of these funds represent a public trust. It is obviously impossible to separate public health administration and public finance. Each act performed for the promotion of public health involves an expenditure of money, whether for supplies, transportation, or salaries of personnel. In fact the very nature and extensiveness of the public health program is determined in the final analysis by the amount of the funds available for its conduct. Accordingly an understanding of the sound management of the public financial program forms one of the most important responsibilities in public health administration.

It is surprising to realize that until 1910 no executive budget existed on any level of government in the United States. Until that time, operating bureaus and departments approached appropriating bodies individually and directly requested and received for the most part "omnibus" appropriations for support of their respective activities. The following item from the budget of the city of Chicago for 1909 may serve as an example of this highly undesirable procedure and make evident the opportunities for inefficient if not dishonest public administration under these circumstances.

For repairs and renewals of wagon and harness, replacement and keep of livestock, identification, police telegraph expenses, repairs and renewals of equipment, hospital services, printing and stationery, secret service, light and heat, 25 more horses for mounted police, and for repair of Hyde Park station; also other miscellaneous expenses . . . $205,000.

Since about 1910 the trend on all levels of government has been toward decentralization of the responsibility for public financial management. In the larger units of government, that is, federal, state, and large cities, separate fiscal departments have been established to meet the need. Thus on the federal level there is the Office of Management and Budget, directly under the President. Similarly every state and local government of consequential size has a similar unit to oversee fiscal affairs. It is notable that increasingly their functions are being expanded to include management, planning, and evaluation. Some aspects of this have been discussed in Chapter 12, but a few points may be emphasized to advantage here, however. The trend began with an effort to coordinate the accounting function with revenue administration, budgeting, purchasing, and in some instance, treasury management.[1] White[2] accounted for this trend in terms of ". . . loss of confidence in legislative bodies as agencies for fiscal management; realization of the desirability for fixing responsibility for the management of fiscal affairs; rapidly rising governmental expenditures and debts which emphasized the necessity for fiscal reform; and the studies of research bureaus, which made apparent the waste due to disorganized

**249**

fiscal management and which offered promising, reasonable alternatives."

It is interesting to trace the development of what is now referred to as PPB, or Program Planning and Budgeting. As indicated previously, the United States like many countries entered the twentieth century with no budget system. The amount of waste and chicanery is not to be wondered about. In the 1920s the idea of expenditure control was under way with emphasis on accountability. As a result of the Hoover Commissions of the late 1930s and early 1940s, a shift developed toward improved management as the focus and with more efficient expenditure as the goal. The 1950s saw the real development of the idea that the budgeting system had potentials beyond accountability and efficiency. Accordingly the concept of program planning and budgeting was developed to tie sound planning to the expenditure control and management part of the budget process. Such a system defines objects of expenditure and determines the input and output in absolute and relative terms. This makes it possible to answer such questions as what is the payoff or what is being obtained for the expenditure and effort, what does it cost to perform a certain act or to provide a certain service, and what are the alternatives and are they more efficient and effective. This latter especially provides a basis for adaptation and alteration through time and makes it more logically possible to shift emphasis when goals are achieved.[3]

This trend toward centralizing fiscal activities in no way removes the need for interest and responsibility on the part of public health officials in these matters, since of necessity part of the responsibility for fiscal matters must rest with the operating department as well as with extra departmental budget offices, comptrollers, finance directors, and others. Indeed, in a sense the past has caught up with the present-day health official. Very early, sanitary laws empowered boards of health to establish a fee for the issuance of licenses for certain activities. Usually it was specified that the fee must not be greater in amount than the cost of administering the enforcement —cost of inspections, amount of overhead, and the like. In effect, cost-benefit analysis and performance budgeting were required without thinking of them as such.

Program budgeting involves a series of relationships that constitute one of the most important aspects of public health administration. In general the functions are divided in somewhat the following manner. The health administrator is responsible for estimating the needs of his organization, which the budget office has the right to review and modify. Expenditures are initiated by the health department, but they may require approval by the central comptroller. The health department is responsible for the preparation of reports indicating and justifying expenditures to provide accountants and auditors from central fiscal offices with information necessary for their analyses. Within the functional health department responsibility for financial matters rests nominally with the administrative health officer. Usually he is the one authorized to incur expenditures, as indicated by his signature on payrolls, requisitions, and other financial documents. In large organizations this authority is sometimes delegated to division or bureau heads. The tendency has been to establish a fiscal officer under the health officer to assume immediate concern for the financial aspects of the operation of the department as a whole.

## FISCAL POLICY MAKING

There are important fiscal policy differences between the public and the private sector. In the latter, decision making can be guided and implemented by considerations that are subject to reasonably accurate evaluation. Commodities produced and services rendered in the private sector are sold at prices controlled by cost, demand, and competition in the market. Profit is the basic and controlling motivation. Market and cost analyses are utilized as criteria in fixing prices and projecting demand; accounting methodology and financial analysis provide bases for the measurement of profit. These are valuable tools in decision making. A private enterprise obviously cannot continue for long if it does not operate at a profit. Therefore if original decisions are based on erroneous conclusions, this soon becomes evident.

Unfortunately, public affairs do not provide this degree of predetermination and control. Most of the enterprises in the public sector are not subject to such ready solution. The criteria that provide relatively definitive guidance in the private sector have little or no validity in the public sector. Taxes are mandatory, and the impact of public services is largely coercive. There is no essential relationship between the amount paid by and the service performed for any individual or group of individuals; need for service is likely to be as great as or even a greater determinant factor than desire for service. Under any circumstances, however, fiscal considerations must be involved. It is important, nevertheless, that they be viewed in proper perspective, since in most cases the ultimate decision will be, or should be, made in context with other significant considerations. This is to say that the decision-making process normally involves the consideration and evaluation of a complex combination of factors and that whereas no ultimate decision should be made without carefully weighing its fiscal aspects, neither should it be made with undue or exclusive emphasis on them.

Before either the health officer or the various fiscal officers may function it is necessary that legal policies be established governing the operation of financial matters. Traditionally this responsibility for determining fiscal policies and objectives has rested with the legislative branch of government, which must provide the legal framework for the creation of a sound financial structure to implement the public health and other objectives that the legislature as representatives of the people outlines. Therefore it is the legislative branch that must decide on the general nature and extent of the public health services to be provided, appropriate whatever funds are necessary to meet their cost, and put into effect whatever revenue measures are necessary for financing the appropriations made. It must fix the authority and responsibility for the collection and expenditure of these revenues, establish the operating units, organize the machinery through which the operating units are financed, and account to the public for the revenue measures enacted, the expenditures incurred, and the services rendered. The progressive health administrator might well assume an honest responsibility for providing inasmuch as possible information and advice for the guidance of the legislators in the performance of these functions.

## FINANCIAL OPERATIONS

Financial operations, the second phase of the public financial program, is concerned with implementation of the policies and plans of operation that have been outlined by the legislature. It includes revenue administration, treasury management, budgeting, accounting, and purchasing. The first two of these are seldom of direct concern to the health officer and are mentioned here merely so that the public health worker will be acquainted with their general content. Revenue administration is concerned with the assessment, levying, and collection of taxes; the study of proposed tax measures; advice to the legislature, the executive head of the unit of government, and the budget officer on problems relating thereto; the preparation of revenue estimates and proposed revenue measures for the executive; and the maintenance of records and accounts of all revenue assessed, levied, adjusted, collected, and deposited with the treasury. Treasury management is concerned with the custody and disbursement of public money and the custody of whatever securities are held in trust by the governmental unit. The treasury accepts money and gives receipts, assures that a cash reserve is constantly maintained, and disburses money on the presentation of legally authorized warrants or disbursement orders.

### Budgeting

Of direct concern to the health administrator is the budget process. Since he is responsible for the public funds provided to him for the operation of his department, it is only reasonable and logical that he conduct some system of financial bookkeeping that will give a continuous, accurate, and verifiable account of his stewardship. A departmental budget provides such a system.

The question might be raised concerning the fact that frequently many of the funds that are made available, especially to local departments of health, come from sources outside the local governmental unit, some even from private sources. Among these are the increasing number of grants-in-aid from the state and federal governments, private foundations, and various voluntary health agencies.[4] For administrative purposes all monies, regardless of their source, should appear in the budget and be placed in the custody of the state or local treasurer. This of course does not preclude their being credited to a health department account or fund to assure their being used only for the purposes for which they were granted. A single operating account may be viewed in two ways. Among its advantages are a reduction in the number of original entry accounts to be maintained; simplification of fiscal document processing; easier fiscal adjustments as programs change; and more meaningful reporting from a program standpoint. Disadvantages are encountered in locating errors; more work is required in preparing reports for fiscal accountability; and budgetary adjustments are more difficult. Many states and localities have experimented with variations and combinations in an attempt to find a method satisfactory to most needs.[5]

A fund may be established by the legislative body of the government, by a contractual agreement, or by an executive order, and may be abolished only by the agency establishing it. The number of separate funds should be kept at a minimum, since a multiplicity of them effectively hampers the development of broad, well-balanced programs. In general, the following funds may be considered:

**Expendable funds**

*General fund*—this usually contains most of the available funds. It represents the unrestricted fund of the organization as far as budgeting and expenditure are concerned. It can be spent for any legal purpose for which the organization may wish to use it and may be drawn on for the replenishment of other funds.

*Special funds*—these are restricted as to use, since they are established for specific purposes. They cannot be transferred to other funds. Some originate by means of the government levying a special millage tax to pay for a particular function. This forms a kind of special appropriation and is usually not considered in the budget, thereby confusing budget planning. Special levies as a whole are undesirable. Much more preferable is a general levy adequate to cover all the needs of a government with the exception of sinking funds, the proceeds of which, however, should go into the general fund.

*Sinking funds*—these are a form of special expendable funds set aside for the redemption of bonds or other similar obligations. They are nontransferable.

**Working capital funds**

The purpose of these is for conducting the many organizational and institutional activities. They are usually replenished by means of transfers from other funds.

**Endowment funds**

The principal of these funds cannot be expended, but the income accruing their investment may be spent for the purposes specified in the conditions of endowment.

**Suspense funds**

These are not funds in the true sense of the word. They consist of sums of money made available for special purposes, their distribution and use pending transferal to other funds.

The average person interprets the word *budget* as meaning a complicated scheme devised for the purpose of saving money, a scheme he wishes he had followed when the income tax form arrives. In one sense this interpretation is correct; in another it is not. Although it is true that a budget may help in saving and planning for future needs, that is not its primary purpose. To the contrary, in public service a budget is most concerned with the manner and rate at which available resources are to be expended. In brief, therefore, a budget may be defined as an administrative tool for the purpose of (1) estimating future needs and future resources and (2) the wise apportionment and systematic expenditure of the resources that are available during a given period of time.

The public health administrator should realize that the construction of a budget not only fulfills the demands of the agencies providing the funds but also may hold many advantages and uses for him in his management of the health department. It has a considerable influence on the economical use of working resources, since it is intended to make possible the maximum use of the facilities and current assets of the organization. It prevents waste and conserves resources by regulating expenditures for definite purposes and in accordance with appropriations established by the administrative head of the organization. A well-constructed budget places definitely, exactly where it belongs, the responsibility for each function of the organization. It makes for coordination by causing all individuals and departments of an organization to cooperate in attaining the goals fixed by the budget. A budget presents in cold figures the best judgment of the executive responsible for a definite organizational objective and thus guards against both undue pessimism, which leads to underactivity and poor work, or undue optimism, which leads to overexpansion. By indicating variance between estimates and actual results obtained it may serve as a danger signal for the administrator and thereby show when to proceed cautiously and when expansion may be safely undertaken.

Similarly it is valuable in determining the relative effectiveness and cost of activities and procedures, since it tests the ability of the organization to make things happen in accordance with a well-ordered plan. A highly important benefit is that it compels the organization to study its market (the people) and its own methods and services, thus disclosing ways and means for strengthening and enlarging the organization. It provides the only means for predetermining when and to what extent financing will be necessary and serves as a guide to future needs, possibilities, and sources of revenue. Finally, organizations that develop and follow a well-ordered budget plan find greater favor from their administrative superiors or boards of directors, business associates, and potential sources of income.

Once the decision is made to use the budget idea, certain principles should be followed to assure its success and helpfulness. Perhaps most important, and so often overlooked, is confidence in the idea and willingness to cooperate with it. Nothing will ensure its failure more effectively than skepticism of its value, apprehension of the work involved, and a feeling that it is simply a red-tape requirement to which adherence after completion is not necessary. Related to this is the importance of enlisting the interest, aid, and cooperation of all subordinates in the preparation of and adherence to the estimates relating to their work. Estimates should be based on past performances and existing assets as well as on plans for expansion and anticipated assets. The amount of estimates should be based upon the total probable assets available rather than upon that which is desired or ideal. All sources of income as well as all anticipated expenditures should be included in the budget, which should indicate clearly where the funds come from, since this in itself has an educational value and paints the total financial picture. To indicate all sources of funds may also serve to cause awareness of future budgetary problems. This is always an important consideration in any future program planning. It follows that the interval over which a budget is to be effective should be restricted to a period for which dependable estimates of sources and expenditures may be prepared.

## Budget preparation

The mechanical procedures involved in setting up the budget should be kept as simple yet as useful as possible; this necessitates the attainment of a practical balance between the two. The items might best be classified primarily by units of organization, for example, division of preventive medical services, division of environmental sanitation, bureau of vital statistics, etc. Such a classification requires a sound or-

ganization with well-defined lines of authority and responsibility. Beyond this, provision should be made for reasonable flexibility within the budget with a not too detailed breakdown of items. With regard to the relative advantages and disadvantages of a lump-sum budget as against a more detailed budget, it may be pointed out that although the former provides more administrative leeway, the latter makes possible more effective control and planning and has an educational value entirely lacking in a lump-sum type of budget. For further breakdown, analysis by function or type of service is one of the most convenient and useful methods. This is particularly true in public health agencies, since the units of organization (bureaus, divisions, etc.) are essentially functional, for example, vital statistics, sanitation, health education, communicable disease control, and others.

Expenditures may be broken down to administrative advantage in terms of, for example (1) operating expenses, that is, salaries, travel, supplies, repairs, etc.; (2) capital costs; and (3) fixed charges, for example, interest on bonds, etc. Figs. 13-1 and 13-2, which show portions of the budget of a large city health department, illustrate this.

In most instances it is desirable to include a contingent fund, which should be kept small (3% to 5%), a large contingent fund being indicative of poor planning and management. It should be used as sparingly as possible and should be applicable to all items in the budget with one exception; that is, salaries should never be augmented from a contingent fund for any reason. A final requisite, and perhaps one of the most important, to a successful budget is placing the responsibility for its maintenance in the hands of one capable individual. Since a budget is essentially an estimate of future needs and activities, its construction should take into consideration the following: the cost of operation on the present scale, including administrative, functional, and depreciative costs; the anticipated cost of operation of expanded activities; and the need for coordination of the existing and anticipated activities into one well-balanced whole so that the expenditures of money, time, and effort for the various activities will be in a proper and balanced relationship to one another.

Concerning the detailed steps involved in drafting the budget, no single method or technique exists that will satisfactorily fit all

**GENERAL FUND— Health—General**

| | Account code Function | Account code Object | Items numbered are the appropriations. Items following in detail are explanatory of the appropriations—see city charter title VI, chap. 1, sec. 7. | Expended 1966-67 | Budget allowance 1966-67 No. | Budget allowance 1966-67 Amount | Adjusted allowance Dec. 31, 1966 No. | Adjusted allowance Dec. 31, 1966 Amount | Expended July 1, 1966 to Dec. 31, 1966 | Requested 1967-68 No. | Requested 1967-68 Amount | Revision by the Mayor No. | Revision by the Mayor Amount | Revision by the Council No. | Revision by the Council Amount |
|---|---|---|---|---|---|---|---|---|---|---|---|---|---|---|---|
| 1 | 3010 | 111 | ADMINISTRATION: | | | | | | | | | | | | |
| 2 | | 111 | Salaries | 66,439.72 | 19 | 73,835.00 | 19 | 74,287.00 | 32,707.25 | 19 | 74,182.00 | | | | |
| 3 | | 301 | Duplicating and Office Supplies | 3,475.74 | | 4,000.00 | | 4,000.00 | 1,436.39 | | 4,000.00 | | | | |
| 4 | | 302 | Postage | 10,000.00 | | 9,000.00 | | 9,000.00 | 4,200.00 | | 10,000.00 | | | | |
| 5 | | 303 | Reimbursement, Purchase, and Repairs of Badges | 67.25 | | 300.00 | | 300.00 | 52.50 | | 250.00 | | | | |
| 6 | | 405 | Telephone and Telegraph Services | 6,925.60 | | 7,300.00 | | 7,300.00 | 3,546.56 | | 7,200.00 | | | | |
| 7 | | 414 | Rental of Buildings and Space | 23,500.00 | | 23,500.00 | | 23,500.00 | 11,750.00 | | 25,000.00 | | | | |
| 8 | | | | | | | | | | | | | | | |
| 9 | | | | 110,408.31 | | 117,935.00 | | 118,387.00 | 53,692.70 | | 120,632.00 | | | | |
| 10 | 3020 | | Health education | | | | | | | | | | | | |
| 11 | | 111 | Salaries | 24,416.59 | 15 | 43,861.00 | 15 | 44,163.00 | 12,631.96 | 15 | 44,724.00 | | | | |
| 12 | | 301 | Purchases and Rental: Educational Films, Publications, and | | | | | | | | | | | | |
| 13 | | | Displays | 138.00 | | 600.00 | | 600.00 | 53.20 | | 600.00 | | | | |
| 14 | | | | | | | | | | | | | | | |
| 15 | | | | 24,554.59 | | 44,461.00 | | 44,763.00 | 12,685.16 | | 45,324.00 | | | | |
| 16 | 3030 | | Vital statistics: | | | | | | | | | | | | |
| 17 | | 111 | Salaries | 33,896.72 | 15 | 38,013.00 | 15 | 38,887.00 | 18,174.59 | 15 | 39,032.00 | | | | |
| 18 | | 113 | Salaries—Issuing Birth Certificates | 11,161.64 | | 19,550.00 | | 19,734.00 | 4,535.66 | | 15,000.00 | | | | |
| 19 | | 301 | Supplies | 1,759.00 | | 1,770.00 | | 1,770.00 | 627.83 | | 1,770.00 | | | | |
| 20 | | | | | | | | | | | | | | | |
| 21 | | | | 46,817.36 | | 59,333.00 | | 60,391.00 | 23,338.08 | | 55,802.00 | | | | |
| 22 | 3041 | | Sanitary engineering: | | | | | | | | | | | | |
| 23 | | 111 | Salaries | 94,617.99 | 31 | 106,420.00 | 31 | 106,940.00 | 48,568.74 | 31 | 107,210.00 | | | | |
| 24 | 3042 | | Sub-standard housing inspection: | | | | | | | | | | | | |
| 25 | | 111 | Salaries | 39,509.83 | 18 | 53,605.00 | 18 | 53,927.00 | 19,563.22 | 18 | 54,397.00 | | | | |
| 26 | | 301 | Supplies | 90.79 | | 200.00 | | 200.00 | 17.27 | | 200.00 | | | | |
| 27 | | | | | | | | | | | | | | | |
| 28 | | | | 39,600.62 | | 53,805.00 | | 54,127.00 | 19,580.49 | | 54,597.00 | | | | |
| 29 | 3043 | | Food inspection: | | | | | | | | | | | | |
| 30 | | 111 | Salaries | 289,923.92 | 97 | 325,294.00 | 97 | 325,900.00 | 147,882.28 | 97 | 321,102.00 | | | | |

**Fig. 13-1.** Example of budget form for a city health department, presenting data based on unit of organization and purpose.

GENERAL FUND—HEALTH—GENERAL

| Account code | | Items numbered are the appropriations. Items following in detail are explanatory of the appropriations—see city charter title VI, chap. I, sec. 7. | Budget allowance 1966-67 | | Adjusted allowance Dec. 31, 1966 | | Request for 1967-68 | | Revision by the Mayor | | Revision by the Council | |
|---|---|---|---|---|---|---|---|---|---|---|---|---|
| Function | Object | | No. | Rates | No. | Rates | No. | Rates | No. | Rates | No. | Rates |
| | | 1 Public Health Nurses | 4 | 6,595 to 6,967 | | | 4 | 6,595 to 6,967 | | | | |
| | | 2 | | | | | | | | | | |
| | | 3 | 15 | | 15 | | 15 | | | | | |
| 3030 | 111 | 4 Vital statistics: | | | | | | | | | | |
| | | 5 Deputy Registrar of Vital Statistics | 1 | 7,651 to 8,285 | | | 1 | 7,651 to 8,285 | | | | |
| | | 6 Junior Statistician | 1 | 6,657 to 7,095 | | | 1 | 6,657 to 7,095 | | | | |
| | | 7 Technical Aid (General) | 1 | 5,327 to 5,459 | | | 1 | 5,327 to 5,459 | | | | |
| | | 8 Senior Clerk | 1 | 6,525 to 6,936 | | | 1 | 6,525 to 6,936 | | | | |
| | | 9 Intermediate Clerks | 9 | 5,261 to 5,393 | | | 9 | 5,261 to 5,393 | | | | |
| | | 10 Intermediate Typist | 1 | 5,261 to 5,393 | | | 1 | 5,261 to 5,393 | | | | |
| | | 11 Junior Stenographer | 1 | 5,327 to 5,459 | | | 1 | 5,327 to 5,459 | | | | |
| | | 12 | | | | | | | | | | |
| | | 13 | 15 | | 15 | | 15 | | | | | |
| 3041 | 111 | 14 Sanitary engineering: | | | | | | | | | | |
| | | 15 Sanitary Engineer and Secretary | 1 | 10,613 to 11,441 | | | 1 | 10,613 to 11,441 | | | | |
| | | 16 Associate Sanitary Engineers | 2 | 8,761 to 9,476 | | | 2 | 8,761 to 9,476 | | | | |
| | | 17 Head Health Inspector | 1 | 8,047 to 8,761 | | | 1 | 8,047 to 8,761 | | | | |
| | | 18 Senior Assistant Sanitary Engineer | | | 1 | 8,047 to 8,523 | 1 | 8,047 to 8,523 | | | | |
| | | 19 Principal Health Inspectors | 7 | 7,492 to 7,809 | 6 | 7,492 to 7,809 | 6 | 7,492 to 7,809 | | | | |
| | | 20 Senior Health Inspectors | 10 | 6,859 to 7,174 | | | 10 | 6,859 to 7,174 | | | | |
| | | 21 Junior Health Inspectors | 2 | 6,459 to 6,723 | | | 2 | 6,459 to 6,723 | | | | |
| | | 22 Senior Sanitary Engineering Aid | 1 | 7,095 to 7,571 | | | 1 | 7,095 to 7,571 | | | | |
| | | 23 Junior Cartographic Draftsman | 1 | 5,723 to 6,174 | | | 1 | 5,723 to 6,174 | | | | |
| | | 24 Intermediate Clerks | 4 | 5,261 to 5,393 | | | 4 | 5,261 to 5,393 | | | | |
| | | 25 Junior Stenographer | 1 | 5,327 to 5,459 | | | 1 | 5,327 to 5,459 | | | | |
| | | 26 Junior Typist | 1 | 4,752 to 4,980 | | | 1 | 4,752 to 4,980 | | | | |
| | | 27 | | | | | | | | | | |
| | | 28 | 31 | | 31 | | 31 | | | | | |

**Fig. 13-2.** Example of budget form for a city health department, presenting data based on unit of organization and function.

situations. It is strongly suggested that the newly appointed public health official assume as one of his earliest duties the acquiring of an intimate acquaintance not only with his own budget but also with the total budget of the governmental unit with which he is identified and the budgetary methods and forms being used. However, since the budgets of all governmental agencies have the same general purpose, certain similarities exist in their form. Geiger[6] summarized these well-accepted basic principles as including the following eight factors:

1. Expenditures of a preceding period equal in time to that for which the budget is being prepared. The period should be closed, so that actual expenditures as they occurred are stated in this column.

2. Budget of the present period. These figures can include only the budget as it was set up, since expenses thereon are still being incurred while a budget for the future is being prepared.

3. Changes in the present budget period. These figures should include any significant changes in the present budget that have occurred or that may be anticipated, such as changes in salaries or in departmental organization, which will have the effect of modifying the present budget. This column thus has the effect of bringing the present budget up-to-date.

4. Expenditures of the present period, given as actual expenditures to the time the next budget is being made, and as estimates of the expenditures to the end of the present period. The actual expenditures and estimates are totaled.

5. Object of expenditure. This column designates each item for which expenditures have been made or are requested. This should include the salary group, classed as permanent, as temporary, or as services secured on a contract basis. Other groups will include materials and supplies, fixed charges, foodstuffs, equipment, and any other divisions of expenditures.

The remaining columns refer to estimates and requests for future activities, for which the preceding columns have provided a basis.

6. Budget request for the next period. Each item should be arranged in such a manner that comparison with the present budget will be as simple as possible.

7. Comparison between the present and anticipated budgets. Since comparison of present and requested budgets (items 2 and 6) is crucial in the consideration of new budgets, this column should indicate all items for which an increased expenditure is desired, items which are not changed from the present budget, and items which are dropped or in which a decrease in allotment of funds is desired.

8. The adopted budget. At least one column will be necessary for the budget adopted. As many additional columns should be provided as may be demanded in accordance with the number of official approvals required. This greatly facilitates the recording of recommendations by different officials empowered to approve one or all phases of the budget previous to its final adoption.

The budgetary process is implemented by a highly complex system of communications, and its effectiveness depends largely on the extent to which and the manner in which the system of communications is used in policy determination, program decision making, and all aspects of administration, including public and professional relations. In effect, the ultimate success of the entire program or operation depends on this. The health official who attempts to determine and obtain his budget single-handedly is certain to be disappointed not only in what funds he obtains but also in the understanding and support of his program goals and efforts. Among those involved to varying degrees in the budget process are the following:

1. The interrelated but frequently divergent interests and views of the legislative, executive, and administrative branches of government
2. Individual functional agencies of government
3. Various other levels of government
4. Geographic, neighborhood, or ethnic groupings
5. Political parties and organizations
6. Citizens' organizations—general (citizens' leagues, leagues of women voters, etc.)
7. Citizens' organizations—special interest (parent-teacher associations, bar associations, medical societies, health societies, property owners' associations)
8. Labor organizations and other groups representing employees
9. Industrial and business organizations
10. Organizations of governmental agencies and officials

The budgetary process is continuous and overlapping in that preparation of the budget for the forthcoming fiscal year must begin while the budget for the current year is being executed. The following comprise the four major phases of the budgetary cycle:

1. The preparation of departmental requests, the evaluation of revenue potential, executive review, the formulation of the budget

document and its transmission to the legislative body

2. Legislative review and authorization (This may or may not involve executive veto or approval.)

3. Execution of the budget in accordance with legislative authorization (This involves translation of the fiscal program into an operational program by the various departments and agencies of government under the general direction and control of the executive.)

4. Postaudit evaluation and review to determine whether expenditures have been made and operations conducted in accordance with legislative intent in conformity with law

The preferred steps that lead toward the development of a final budget for a public agency are generally as follows. The date on which the department must submit its budget request to the bureau of the budget or budget officer is usually fixed by custom in relation to the fiscal year. With this date as an anchor point, about 2 months prior to this time the department director should send out to the director of each division or other unit of organization in the department a memorandum concerned with the approaching budget exercise. It should include a calendar of events or deadlines that indicates what steps are to be completed as of certain dates. It should also direct each division director to develop the budget request for his division preferably in consultation with his chief program aides. Any general statements or special policies relating to the budget year under consideration should be included in the memorandum. All divisional budget requests should be submitted to the departmental director (or his departmental budget officer) by a specified date. The department director, preferably in company with his budget director and any other pertinent staff members, should then carefully review each divisional budget proposal, annotating items to be deleted, altered, or added. The departmental director should then schedule a series of departmental budget hearings to provide each divisional (or program) director with an opportunity to explain or defend the proposals he has put forward. On the basis of these hearings the departmental director should then refine the budget further, add his own ideas and provisions for the needs of his office, and submit the final departmental budget proposal to the director of the bureau of the budget or the budget officer of the jurisdiction. This officer in turn should schedule a hearing at which the departmental director may defend or explain his budget.

**Budget presentation**

It is not enough to prepare even the best of budget documents. Its contents must be thoroughly understood and presented in appropriate fashion to those in a position to influence its fate. The process therefore involves a good deal of art and psychology as well as knowledge. All possible information should be obtained with reference to factors that may have affected the health program in the past and that might affect it in the future. The personal and political interests and biases of those to whom it must be presented should be determined. Biographies and the voting records of members of pertinent committees are encouraged. Even before reaching the legislature one's superior, as Draffin[7] points out "Unfortunately . . . may, for good reason as far as he is concerned, recognize other proposals in preference to yours. The chances are that you have knowingly failed to provide him with the kind of information he expects." He suggests that anyone with budget approval authority who shows interest in health, health programs, or the health agencies should be cultivated by providing them with interesting and meaningful information and data not merely in relation to the budget process but especially between budget periods. They should be invited to attend and if possible participate in various meetings of the agencies, and their ideas and opinions should be solicited.

The budget presentation itself should be clear, succinct, and factual. Questions should be invited, and if answers are not readily available, an offer should be made to provide them subsequently for the record. Increasingly legislative bodies have available to them highly competent staffs who are concerned with measurable program goals and accomplishments and are dissatisfied with broad generalizations to specific questions. It is suggested that the individual who anticipates being involved in budget presentations take advantage of prior hearings by the official or legislative committee before which he must subsequently appear to be cognizant of their tone.

The department director should be allowed to be accompanied by whichever divisional or program directors and administrative staff he wishes. On the basis of the preliminary administration or executive hearing, the budget officer will readjust the departmental budget request and submit it to the chief of government (e.g., the mayor or governor) and the comptroller. They in turn review the proposed departmental budget as readjusted by the budget officer. The departmental director is again scheduled for a budget review session, this time with the chief of government and his comptroller, who subsequently accept the proposed budget or revise it according to their views. It is then sent to the legislative branch of government (the city council or the state legislature), where still again the departmental director has an opportunity to defend it or to express his needs in relation to whatever might have been eliminated by the budget officer or the chief of government and his comptroller. The legislature then takes it under advisement in relation to the budget requests of all parts of the government, fiscal resources, and their own interests. The result is the final approved budget.

Increasingly another step is being added to the process. It takes the form of an interim or preliminary budget hearing much earlier in the year at which department heads have an opportunity to discuss their existing and anticipated needs with the budget officer and sometimes with other officials. This has the advantage of giving everyone a preview of what in general to expect during the actual subsequent budget exercise.

In counties without a chief executive or comptroller the procedure varies.[8] Preferably it involves hearings before the county budget officer, the county board of auditors, and the county ways and means or finance committee. The latter might be regarded as the counterpart of the legislature or city council, and the board of auditors as the counterpart of the chief of government and his comptroller.

In the construction and operation of his budget the health officer should make it a practice to maintain contact with the budget director and the finance or ways and means committee of his government. He should keep them constantly informed and call on them for advice, causing them to realize that the financial problems are theirs as well as his. This may present a delicate problem in personal relationships but usually results in benefits that are well worth the effort. There may be a tendency

for some health officers to take the attitude that it is necessary to work on the budget only as budget time approaches. To so restrict one's use of this valuable administrative tool eliminates most of the possible benefits that might be forthcoming from its existence. The wise administrator works closely and constantly with his budget the year round and on a long-term basis, using it as one method of continuously feeling the pulse of his organization. Trial balances should be run as often as is indicated. He should regard the budget as inviolate and as one of his most important administrative tools. He should adhere to its contents as strictly as possible, deviating from it only as a means of last resort. A certain amount of transferring of funds is inevitable but should be kept to a minimum, since it is a sign of poor management and again defeats the purpose for which the budget was originally brought into existence.

If an emergency or other situation that requires an unexpected and unpredictable expenditure of funds should arise, the health officer should feel free to appeal to the appropriating body for an emergency appropriation rather than attempt to meet the situation by transference of monies that have been set aside for other predictable expenditures. It is believed that in most situations if an honest and understandable explanation of the need is given, an additional allotment will be forthcoming. In this connection it might be well to point out that a good administrator will not attempt to use emergency situations as leverage to increase his general budget or to make up deficiencies arising out of poor management.

In the process of obtaining the appropriations requested in his budget the health officer should not assume the entire burden himself but should share it with others in the community such as his health council and other groups of interested and influential citizens. By convincing them of the need for the services for which the money is requested, the health officer may increase the forcefulness of his requests and arguments manyfold with greater assurance of the appropriation being granted.

The efficient health officer will be constantly alert to discover new ways in which to use the budget. He may use it to demonstrate the public health activity in his own area or to show what is being done elsewhere in comparable situations. The use to which the taxpayer's dollar is being put is always of public interest and can be used for effective publicity and educational purposes. A budget may be used as the starting point for requests for state and federal grants-in-aid for the health program and also furnishes a fundamental source of information for self-evaluation and appraisal. It may furnish the key to the determination of the efficiency of various public health procedures and show the way to the achievement of better results per dollar of tax money spent.

It has been pointed out that the budget should be based not on a series of guesses but rather on estimates arrived at inasmuch as possible from the past experience of the organization. It is obvious therefore that to be satisfactory the budget should result from a careful analysis of accounting data, including actual previous experiences and current cost and price trends. Most states provide for the installation and maintenance of a system of uniform accounting by local governments and often provide further for periodic audits by a central state fiscal authority. However, legal provision does not necessarily imply action, and effective enforcement of these provisions appears to be the exception rather than the rule. The lack of an efficient system of accounting makes sound budgetary methods impossible and often results in expenditures that comply with only the barest minimum requirements that may be specified in the law.

### Accounting

A sound system of accounting serves many purposes. It provides a financial record of the activities of an agency, reveals its financial condition at all times, provides necessary data on which the departmental administrator may base plans for future action, gives substantive protection in case of question, and provides the fundamental starting point for audits. White[2] states this as follows:

From the point of view of the department head or the chief executive early and accurate accounting reports are necessary in order to direct the course of the work and future expenditures. They also provide the essential record to demonstrate the appropriate and legal use of funds, making certain that each subdivision of an organization is actually using money for the purposes for which it was appropriated. The accounts and supporting financial documents provide the evidence on the basis of which each spending officer justifies his expenditures, either to the finance director or to the auditor. While the accounting system is thus essential as a means of preventing the wrongful uses of funds, it also underlies all other types of executive control of fiscal operations. It is the basis on which executives act to prevent deficits as well as the documentary foundation for questioning the care and wisdom with which the funds have been used.

Health departments should maintain at least the following basic accounting records: (1) general ledger and (2) complete and detailed record of receipts and expenditures. The general ledger (Fig. 13-3) is the record of the various accounts or controls pertaining to assets, liabilities, and types of revenues and expenses of the health department. Posting to these accounts or controls are made from the books of original entry, namely the cash receipts and expenditure record (Fig. 13-4) and the book of transfer vouchers (Fig. 13-5). All departmental receipts and warrants, including their amounts, should be recorded in the combination cash receipts and expenditure record in their respective numerical order and classified as to source and type of expenditure. Receipts should be posted in the treasurer account-deposits column and classified under the miscellaneous accounts-credit column (Fig. 13-4). Similarly the amount of each warrant should be recorded in the column entitled treasurer account–amount of warrants and classified in further columns according to the monies used and type of expenditure. The code number of the general ledger control account should be used to designate proper postings to the general ledger. Great care should be given to using the proper code number, since this governs the final classification of expenditures.

During the course of recording and posting items to the general ledger controls and accounts, numerous errors will arise that if left unchanged will not reflect a true statement of revenues and expenditures. For this reason the record of transfer vouchers is used to correct erroneous postings to accounts and to adjust and close out revenue and expense accounts at the close of each year's business. For future audit and reference purposes full explanation for each transfer should be recorded in the space provided.

An important accounting procedure increasingly used by public health and other agencies is encumbrance control. This is designed to ensure adequate funds for future payment of obligations made in the present. The Emergency Maternity and Infant Care Program, which operated during World War II, provides a convenient example. Lump-sum allotments were made to the states each month on the

**Fig. 13-3.** Example of general ledger form.

basis of the estimated number of births that would occur during the following month. To forestall the great possibility of committing itself to future payments in excess of the sums allotted to it for the purpose, each state was encouraged to set up an encumbrance control procedure that simply deducted on paper from the total funds made available the amount of money that eventually would be required for payment of physicians and hospitals. It was somewhat as if payment were being made before the services were actually rendered rather than on their completion some months in the future. In this way the state could ascertain at any time the total amount of non-obligated funds available with which to provide care for additional individuals. In addition it provided a basis on which to apply in advance for deficiency allotments.

The program involved various types of services, for example, obstetric, medical, surgical, hospital, and nursing. With cases of uncomplicated pregnancy and delivery the procedure was relatively simple; a standard fee was agreed on by the medical profession and each state

health department. Similarly per diem bed costs were determined and agreed on for the participating hospitals. When a private physician notified the health department that he was assuming the care of a woman who was expected to deliver normally, 6 months hence, for example, it was a simple matter to immediately set aside or encumber a sum of money sufficient to cover the physician's standard fee and the anticipated hospital bill. The latter could be rather accurately estimated as the product of the hospital's per diem bed cost times the average number of days that patients in the locality or state stayed in the hospital after delivery.

The procedure for encumbrance control becomes slightly more complicated when dealing with a service that is not as predictable as to time and cost as a normal pregnancy. Success depends on standardized fees and costs for services and materials. Insofar as possible, estimates of the probable extent of the services needed should be based on averages for the particular condition and/or type of patient in the particular area, and large sums should not

**Fig. 13-4.** Example of combination cash receipts and expenditure form.

**Fig. 13-5.** Example of transfer voucher form.

be encumbered over long projected periods for the care of patients the cost of which is impossible to estimate with reasonable accuracy. An example of the manner in which a case of illness in an infant would be satisfactorily handled is given in Table 13-1.

The Children's Bureau, which was responsible to Congress for the program, naturally did not wish large unused and unencumbered sums accumulating in the individual states. On the other hand, it wanted to give assurance to each state that sufficient funds would be available at all times for payment of statements received. The states therefore maintained a summary record of encumbrances and unobligated balance such as that presented in Table 13-2. In addition to using it for their own guidance the states submitted their totals each month to

the Children's Bureau to serve in determining the amount of money that should be sent to each state for the forthcoming month from the United States Treasury.

**Performance budgeting**

In Chapter 12, which deals with planning and evaluation, brief mention was made of cost-benefit analysis leading to the development of a program performance budget. Performance budgeting has been well described by Klepak[9] in his discussion of its application to public health. In effect it summarizes the program activities performed in terms of unit cost. Thus performance budgeting tells what it costs to immunize the individual against a specific disease or to supervise the average food-handling establishment. When such detailed cost analysis or inventory is available for all components

**Table 13-1.** Maternity and infant care encumbrance control record*

| Date | Description | Transactions: increase-decrease | | | Totals to date | | Balances | | |
|---|---|---|---|---|---|---|---|---|---|
| | | Allotment | Expenditures | Purchase orders—requisitions | Total allotment | Total expenditures | Unexpended balance | Accounts payable | Unencumbered balance |
| 2/ 8/45 | ( 1) Medical | $24 | | | $ 74 | | | | $74 |
| 2/ 8/45 | ( 2) Hospital | 50 | | | 84 | | | | 84 |
| 2/18/45 | ( 3) Hospital | 10 | | | 84 | | | | 84 |
| 2/22/45 | ( 4) Hospital | | $60 | | 84 | $ 60 | | | 24 |
| 2/23/45 | ( 5) Medical | | 24 | | 84 | 84 | | | 24 |
| 5/ 8/45 | ( 6) Medical | 24 | | | | | | | |
| 5/ 8/45 | ( 7) Hospital | 50 | | | 158 | 84 | | | 74 |
| 5/26/45 | ( 8) Medical to adjust | −24 | | | | | | | |
| 6/26/45 | ( 9) Medical | 36 | | | 170 | 84 | | | 86 |
| 6/ 3/45 | (10) Medical | | 36 | | 170 | 120 | | | 50 |
| 6/ 3/45 | (11) Hospital to cancel | −50 | | | | | | | |

*Explanation: Child becomes ill, and mother applies to participating physician for care. Physician decides hospital care needed, so sends in applications for medical and hospital care. These are both authorized and funds encumbered (1) and (2). (Maximum of $24 for first medical authorization and 10 days at $5 per day for hospitalization.) Two additional hospital days are needed, so reauthorization for them is made and $10 additional encumbered (3). After hospital service is rendered the hospital submits a bill for $60 (4) for which a check is made and sent. The physician, having completed care, submits a bill for $24 (5) for which a check is made and sent.

Several months later the child again becomes ill, and the standard amount of funds for hospital and medical care are encumbered as before (6) and (7). The physician requests further authorization to provide for a minor operative procedure for which funds are then encumbered by canceling out the previous medical authorization (8) and encumbering the new amount necessary (9). The physician subsequently submits his bill, which is paid (10), and notifies that the care was rendered at the patient's home so that the allotment for hospitalization is canceled (11), bringing the unencumbered balance to zero.

**Table 13-2.** Record of encumbrances and unobligated balance for maternity care

| Date | Authorization numbers | Amount encumbered | Amount paid | Adjustment | Unencumbered balance |
|------|-----------------------|-------------------|-------------|------------|----------------------|
| 6/30/43 | (Received from U. S. Treasury $50,000) | | | | |
| 7/ 1/43 | 1-50 | $ 3,750 | | | $46,250 |
| 7/ 2/43 | 51-125 | 5,200 | | | 41,050 |
| 7/ 3/43 | 126-300 | 12,200 | | | 28,850 |
| 7/31/43 | 301-499 | 14,000 | | | 14,850 |
| Total for July | | $35,150 | | | |
| 8/ 1/43 | (Received from U. S. Treasury $35,000) | | | | $49,850 |
| 8/ 5/43 | 500-650 | $13,000 | $ 2,500 | $ 500* | 37,350 |
| 8/10/43 | 651-675 | 1,750 | 5,000 | 200 | 35,800 |
| 8/20/43 | 676-801 | 5,715 | 5,000 | 250 | 30,335 |
| 8/31/43 | 801-950 | 14,235 | 7,500 | 50 | 16,150 |
| Total for August | | $34,700 | $20,000 | $1,000 | |

*The first entry in this column ($500) is based on the assumption that authorizations totaling $3,000, issued early in July, were paid on August 5 in the amount of $2,500, or $500 less than the amount encumbered. This amount is therefore released for the commitment and added to the unencumbered balance in the last column.

or functions in a program, the determination of the cost of the total program becomes possible. One then has a true program performance budget that provides a measure of the total impact of a program in terms of its cost.

The advantages of a program inventory and the resultant performance budget that it makes possible may be summarized as follows:
1. Provide effective tools in planning a well-balanced program
2. Assist in developing short- and long-range program objectives
3. Provide elements for the control of programs and their costs
4. Provide detailed information concerning work volume and unit costs
5. Provide a sound basis for comparing past, present, and future activities, programs, and performance
6. Aid greatly in supporting requests for funds on a demonstrable and realistic basis
7. Discourage "padding" of the budget by program directors
8. Aid in the sound expansion and contraction of program activities
9. Permit personnel to see relationships among activities and programs
10. Provide qualitative and quantitative measures of personnel and departmental efficiency

This is the theory. However, certain general precautions are necessary.[10] The program inventory, the performance report, the performance budget, and the program budget are only administrative tools. They must be used properly as aids to administrative evaluation—not in place of it or as ends in themselves. The performance budget specifically must be regarded as a classification of proposed expenditures in terms of things to be done or accomplishments to be achieved rather than things to be bought. Furthermore, yardsticks of performance standards have not yet been developed in many important areas. Ideally there should be standard cost tables and quantitative measurement devices for every important element of the health program.

Michael[11] bears these points in mind in his comprehensive itemization of the steps required in the development of a performance budget based on careful planning as follows:
1. Determination of health status (This involves identifying and measuring health problems and comparing them with one another.)
2. Establishment of an ultimate goal for each of the problem areas established above (These goals must be stated in measurable terms but may be as idealistic and ambitious as good judgment dictates.)
3. Determination of attitudes, value systems,

and resources of the community for whom the program is designed

4. Analysis of health problems, their causes, and contributing factors
5. Development of alternative plans of action to eliminate or modify the problems
6. Conduct of cost-benefit and cost-effectiveness studies for the alternative plans of action
7. Establishment of comprehensive health objectives and plans of action on a short- and long-range basis
8. Analysis of all program areas, including cost-benefit and cost-effectiveness studies to ensure an integrated program designed to make maximum progress toward established goals and objectives
9. Institution of continuing evaluation

Performance budgets cannot be used in every organization and program. If activities are of a highly routinized and objective nature and large numbers of people and objects are involved, a performance budget can be an invaluable aid to an administrator in learning not only what may be accomplished but also how well it is accomplished. In smaller organizations, dealing with less tangible objectives as, for example, a small local health department concerned with total health conditions, there are better ways of determining efficiency and more simplified methods of expressing end products in budgetary terms. In such instances supervisory impressions, reporting, inspection, and other subjective approaches may be useful and dependable.

A basic problem is that by their very nature preventive medicine and public health deal with negatives—cases and epidemics of disease prevented, home or industrial accidents guarded against, disasters avoided, and the like. To attempt to measure the value and efficiency of the efforts applied to such ends is completely different from measuring the cost of gallons of water processed, miles of streets paved, or radios manufactured. To place a monetary value on the prevention of an epidemic is largely conjectural. Public health programs are actually a form of investment. When one deals with investment as a primary consideration in the performance of a function, the ordinary accounting rules do not apply. In the final analysis the only rule that is possible is that of the net return, which is the net of the benefits over costs otherwise incurred.

Many examples might be cited to illustrate these reservations. A few may be worth noting. Public health is an organized endeavor involving constant dynamic change toward improvement of the social and environmental scene. The more effective and efficient its performance the higher the relative unit costs tend to be. The elimination of each remaining case of tuberculosis is necessarily increasingly costly. As communicable diseases are conquered and the age distribution of the population shifts upward, there occurs a shift from low-cost mass communicable disease laboratory examinations to the more time-consuming, hence more expensive, laboratory examinations for the more individualized cases of chronic diseases. In this dynamism increasingly is observed the sudden availability of newer, more effective, and often less expensive methods of diagnosis and treatment. Tuberculosis provides a good example. Within a few years it has become possible to treat patients effectively at a much lower cost and for a shorter period of time than before. The effect of such changes on comparative performance budgeting systems is obvious. Then there is the example of two child health clinics, in one of which each physician examines an average of 10 children per hour, in contrast with the other clinic, where each physician examines an average of 4 children per hour. How does one properly evaluate the efficiency of these two clinics on the basis of costs per child examined? A final example relates to food sanitation, where the obvious ultimate goal is a uniformly sanitary food service. If, as often suggested, function and efficiency were to be measured in terms of violations investigated and corrected, the best program would appear to be the least effective or efficient in terms of costs.

Although the foregoing qualifications and examples are proper and valid, they do not justify an attitude of defeat or an unwillingness to search for some useful measures of achievement and efficiency in public health practice. Within the inherent limitations it is believed that some practical measures exist. Perhaps the problem is not so much the discovery and development of such measures as is their interpretation and use. If these measures are considered only as stable as the activities and programs they measure and are subject to parallel change, no serious difficulty should ensue. Any attempt therefore should be based on the following premises:

1. All costs should be accumulated, if pos-

sible, to reflect major functional activities or programs. (Compromises are necessary because the broader the program category used the more difficult it is to find a common performance unit to reflect the total activities of the program.)

2. Fixed costs should be separated from variable costs. (This is especially important when dealing with a declining problem and program with a declining work load situation, such as tuberculosis.)

3. Variable costs should be related to work load and accomplishments. (These costs, although not including all direct and indirect expenditures devoted to the achievement of a particular goal, do provide the best and perhaps only real reflection of operational efficiency.)

4. Cost standards thus established can be used to appraise program and activity performance.

5. Since by their nature public health activities involve for the most part interpersonal action, the costs of materials in most instances are considered to represent a relatively insignificant proportion of the total cost. In many instances therefore the cost of materials may be ignored. In certain other instances, for example, laboratory work or immunizations, materials do add substantially to the total cost of the function or activity and should be included.

6. Whereas attention should be focused primarily on specific program areas, there is some value in attempting to develop cost centers in certain broad across-the-board service areas, for example, laboratory work, public health nursing, and district health operations, to attempt to obtain some overall operational cost and efficiency figures.

The following are a few examples of the many cost centers that actually or theoretically may be measured. It must be recognized that the best of them are subject to many intrinsic and extrinsic influences over which a public health organization and its staff has limited or no control and that may cause considerable fluctuation.

**Food protection**

$$\frac{\text{(a) Cost of manpower per year}}{\text{(b) No. of establishments supervised per year}} =$$
$$\text{Cost per establishment supervised}$$

Here the numerator (a) should include the total number of man-years of time devoted by inspectional staff to routine complaint, violation, and follow-up inspection of establishments in which food is received, stored, processed, sold,

or served. It also includes the time devoted by clinicians, public health nurses, disease control investigators, and laboratory personnel involved in the examination and follow-up of present and prospective food-handlers to the point where they might be diagnosed as having some communicable disease, under which circumstances the problem becomes one of epidemiology. Since all these categories of personnel are generalized, it is necessary for each staff member to record the number of hours devoted each workday to travel, inspection, office and clinical work relating to the foregoing purpose. The total man-years that results is multiplied by the average actual salary of currently employed personnel to obtain the numerator. The denominator (b) is the total number of separate establishments in which food is received, stored, processed, sold, or served with which the division of environmental health of a community health organization has direct or indirect contact in relation to supervision, inspection reports, complaints, violations, or follow-up.

**Epidemiology.** Several cost centers are possible in this area. The first example relates to the general efficiency of the overall program as follows:

$$\frac{\text{(a) Cost of manpower and materials per year}}{\substack{\text{(b) No. of cases, contacts, and suspects} \\ \text{investigated per year}}} =$$
$$\text{Cost per individual investigation}$$

This is a general index that interprets investigation in its broadest sense to include routine and special case finding based on x-ray examinations, blood tests, and clinical or laboratory examinations in health centers, central diagnostic units, mobile diagnostic units, street-corner campaigns, etc. It also refers to both endemic and epidemic situations. The justification for so doing is based on the premise that in the final analysis most of the time of an epidemiologic staff is devoted to investigation of cases, contacts, and suspects toward the end of getting them under treatment. To be valid, however (a) must exclude the time of physicians, nurses, and clerical personnel who work in relation to treatment. Also it must include the value of the man-years of time devoted by generalized public health nurses and by disease control investigators. This necessitates their keeping a daily log of the amount of their field, travel, and office time devoted to this purpose. The denominator (b) is the total number of individual cases, contacts to, or suspects of acute communicable diseases, venereal diseases, and tuberculosis that are investigated throughout the year by the community health organization.

An example of a cost center of a more specific nature is in relation to the cost of finding a new case of tuberculosis. The same procedure applies to a long series of disease-related activities. It must be recognized that the more successful the activity the more the cost per case found will rise.

$$\frac{\text{(a) Cost of manpower and materials per year}}{\text{(b) No. of new cases of tuberculosis}} =$$
$$\text{Cost per new case of tuberculosis found}$$

The numerator (a) is based on the man-years devoted by physicians, radiologists, x-ray technologists, clinic nurses, clinic clerks, field public health nurses, field disease control investigators, and clerical personnel to the discovery and investigation of new cases of tuberculosis and the placing of new patients under treatment. It is necessary for each worker to keep a daily log of the time devoted to the clinical, travel, home visit, and office aspects of this activity, which multiplied by their respective salaries and totaled provides the cost of the manpower per year for this purpose. Added to this is the cost of expendable materials requisitioned and used by such personnel for this specific purpose. The sum of these two figures provides the cost of the activity. The denominator (b) is the number of new cases of tuberculosis diagnosed and brought under care during the year by staff of the community health organization. Not included in this sum are cases of tuberculosis diagnosed for the first time after death of an individual.

### Maternal health

$$\frac{\text{(a) Cost of manpower in maternal health clinics per year}}{\text{(b) No. of patient visits per year}} =$$
$$\text{Cost per maternal patient visit}$$

The numerator (a) is the number of man-years of each physician, nurse, and clerk working in relation to maternal health clinics, including field follow-up by public health nurses, times the sum of their salaries. The denominator (b) is the number of patient visits to maternal health clinics during the year.

### Vital records

$$\frac{\text{(a) Cost of manpower per year}}{\text{(b) No. of certified records processed per year}} =$$
$$\text{Cost per certified record processed}$$

The numerator (a) consists of the sum of the salaries of the individuals employed in the vital records office. The denominator (b) is the number of vital records for which certified copies are requested and delivered.

### Laboratory

$$\frac{\text{(a) Cost of manpower and materials per year}}{\text{(b) No. of laboratory examinations per year}} =$$
$$\text{Cost per laboratory examination}$$

The numerator (a) consists of the cost of all salaries in the public health laboratory plus the cost of all expendable materials requisitioned by the laboratory, including the value of all specimen kits distributed to physicians, hospitals, and others, and any postage or other transportation costs involved. The denominator (b) includes the total number of all laboratory examinations performed (not specimens received) during the year.

### Public health nursing

$$\frac{\text{(a) Cost of PH nursing time for each type of program per year}}{\text{(b) No. of nursing visits for each type of program per year}} =$$
$$\text{Cost per visit}$$

This example provides a series of figures, one for each type of program, for example, tuberculosis, maternal health, child health, etc. The numerator (a) is based on the total number of man-hours devoted by members of the field public health nursing staff to various types of programs. This necessitates each field nurse's keeping a detailed record of her time and activities throughout each day, which separated into program categories and each multiplied by her individual salary provides the value of her time devoted to each program. This sum combined with similar data from all other field nurses provides the cost of the field nursing component of each major program. The denominator (b) is the number of nursing visits for each type of broad program area per year.

### Air-pollution control

$$\frac{\text{(a) Cost of manpower per year}}{\text{1}}$$
$$\frac{}{\text{(b) Amount of air pollution}} =$$
$$\text{Efficiency quotient of program}$$

This represents a more difficult type of activity to measure. Air pollution is obviously less tangible than a person immunized or a visit made. Here the numerator (a) includes the total man-years of time devoted by field, environmental health laboratory, and central office staffs to routine, complaint, violation, and follow-up inspection of residential, industrial, and dump sites that may or actually contribute to controllable contamination of the atmosphere. Some of these individuals devote all of their time and others devote part of their time to this purpose. It is necessary for each of them to keep records of this time to be accumulated and translated into man-years or fractions thereof, which when applied to their respective salaries and totaled, provides the total cost of personnel time devoted to this activity. The reciprocal (b) is of the amount of air pollution. The reciprocal is used, since otherwise the more effective the program the higher the apparent cost would be to the limit of infinity. Air pollution can be measured by instrumental determination of the total amount of suspended particulate air pollutants (in milligrams per cubic yard) times an appropriate standard number such as 1,000. A reading may be made once each month and the 12 readings averaged.

It is recognized that this quotient is not a cost figure. However, it is desirable to begin exploring the development of the true indicators of program usefulness and efficiency. It must be recognized that this efficiency figure is subject to alteration by nonprogram factors such as meteorologic changes, fires, emergencies, and especially by an increase in industry or in the use of motor vehicles.

### Purchasing

Related to accounting or expenditure control is the obtaining of materials and supplies involved in the operation of public agencies. Until relatively recently the pattern followed was largely the provision to each individual operating department of lump sums of money for operation or maintenance. There existed also a general belief that purchases and contracts should be distributed as widely as possible throughout the various business concerns existing in the area served, apparently with the end in view of obtaining their goodwill and support of the government and its program. Why this was believed necessary is somewhat difficult to understand, since business and industry has always followed a more progressive and efficient course.

The recent trend therefore has been toward the development of central public purchasing agencies with the authority to purchase or to formulate regulations governing the purchase of all materials, equipment, supplies, and contractual services for all of the public agencies in the particular unit of government. As this approach developed, to promote their effectiveness public purchasing agencies have generally been given the authority to inspect all goods delivered, to test samples submitted with bids or deliveries, to transfer or dispose of any materials, supplies, and equipment from operating agencies, and to maintain a central warehouse. Centralized purchasing has many advantages, including lower unit costs, better delivery service, reduction of overhead costs, standardization of products and of purchasing and expenditure documents, more efficient accounting control over expenditure, and simplification of the ordering, delivery, and storage problems of both vendors and operating agencies.

Complaints are frequently raised against central purchasing agencies, usually to the effect that they hamper the activity of the functional department by causing delays, red tape, and the acceptance of substitute or unsatisfactory materials. The subject of most controversy is whether or not the purchasing agent should have the right to modify the requisition sent to him, to substitute for a specified material or brand, or to refuse to place an order for materials requested by a functional agency. The statutes of some states specifically allow this right, some imply it, others deny it, and worst of all in several states the issue is entirely ignored. It is thought that most or all of these objections may be easily avoided, provided the purchasing agency, on the one hand, constantly considers that its existence is justified only in terms of the auxiliary service it finds possible to render to the functional agency and if the latter, on the other hand, takes pains to make clear to the purchasing agency its exact needs and the reasons for them. The problem therefore is essentially one of proper interagency relationships and understanding.

Although a system of continuous expenditure control assures the efficiency of operation and expenditure, only an audit following the completion of the budget period can determine their legality. Therefore it is necessary in the public interest that there be some method of assuring not only that the public money is being legally spent but that the public is receiving reasonable value for it. The auditor is in effect an arm of the public's legislature, which not only has established a public program but has provided appropriation for its fulfillment. A system of postauditing involves the examination and appraisal of accounts, records, and statements as well as accounting and operating procedures. It provides the legislature with information and analyses arrived at independently of those who are directly responsible for expenditures and operations. It provides data for reviewing past and for planning future budgets, revenue and expenditure programs, and for drafting needed additional legislation. The personnel of the functional units subject to postauditing should in addition look on it as a protection to them and a means of providing for official and public recognition to their honest and efficient fulfillment of the duties and responsibilities entrusted to them.

## FISCAL RESPONSIBILITY

The placement of fiscal responsibility in any political subdivision may vary from place to place. However, the principle exists and must be maintained that a public health officer must always be in the position of knowing the current status of his budget appropriation limitations.

In large cities where there tends to exist highly centralized financial operations with fiscal controls established therein and where an "executive type" rather than a "legislative type" of budget is effective, it is especially important that the health officer establish a firm fiscal basis on which he may successfully operate. A brief review of the successive steps involved in such a community that adopts this newer concept of fiscal control is presented for those who may be confronted with such an operation.

In a certain year the voters of a particular city adopted a home rule charter that had recently been authorized by the government of the state. The new charter, among other benefits, established new fiscal policies for governmental operation in the fields of budgeting, accounting practices, collection of taxes and other revenue, and the related responsibilities thereto.

The mayor of the city was made responsible primarily for the efficient fiscal operations of the various governmental functions, and through his finance director, the city's principal finance officer, was charged with the responsibility of submitting to the city council the budget requests of the various governmental units.

The city council's authority in the field of finance was restricted in the charter in favor of wider authority to be exercised by the mayor. The council retained the right to adopt the annual operating budget and the capital budget, to levy the taxes necessary for the support of the government, and to authorize debt, contingent on the approval of the voters. Under these circumstances the council was bound by the mayor's estimate of receipts and was guided in the determination of its budget appropriations by consideration of the line type budget, with detailed justifications thereof, which was submitted to the council by the mayor. This budget was presented on an "object detail class" basis. All the positions to be financed were segregated on a budget schedule, with separate schedules for personnel, contractual services, materials and supplies, equipment (detailed), and such other additional classes as the mayor recommended in his proposed annual operating budget ordinance. All budget appropriations were made in lump-sum amounts and according to the foregoing classes of expenditure for each office, department, board, or commission.

This approach to budgeting produces the executive type of budget rather than the legislative type of budget and gives the administrative officials of government more flexibility within broad limitations but does not destroy the possibility of close administrative supervision and control. Thus the responsibility for fiscal direction and control is placed more firmly on the executive rather than on the legislative branch of the government. The city council is required by law to adopt the annual operating budget ordinance for the next fiscal year at least 30 days before the commencement of that year.

On receipt of the approved budget the director of finance, with the approval of the mayor, sets up allotment accounts by departments on an expenditure class basis. Personnel appropriations may be established on a quarterly allotment pattern, and materials, supplies, and equipment on an annual basis. In the larger departments allotment accounts are set up on a departmental functional basis, with subaccount allotments for detailed object classes exceeding $20,000, for closer appropriation controls.

The multiplicity and volume of fiscal transactions handled in a centralized fiscal office of a large city necessitate the utilization of mechanized facilities. Since the director of finance is the chief fiscal officer of the city, all budget, fiscal, and accounting practices are centrally controlled in his office. There are released from the offices of the director of finance all of the official financial statements of the city. For day-to-day operations, the fiscal office of each department receives from the director of finance a daily statement that reflects the current status of each of their allotment accounts. Each transaction listed on his daily statement is documented by a copy of the voucher related thereto. These statements, however, do not include all of the encumbrances that may be involved in proposed commitments that have not reached the stage of machine recording. Therefore for this and other reasons there still remains the need of a departmental fiscal office. This need is apparent when the following are considered:

1. Most of the initial action in all fiscal transactions originates in the operating department.

2. The original departmental budgetary appropriation request is prepared in each operating department.

3. The various types of requisitions covering departmental needs are processed from each department.

4. Appropriation accounts authorized for the general fund, capital fund, and special funds must be maintained at the department level so that the health officer may direct and plan his program during the course of the year from the unencumbered balances. Therefore the departmental accounts must include those planned and proposed commitments that have not as yet currently reached the stage of machine recording.

5. Although payrolls may be prepared by mechanized methods in the finance department, the initial official time record of personnel work must originate and be prepared at the operational level.

6. Costing for evaluation of programs and activities is also essentially the responsibility of the departmental fiscal office.

In the capital fund area the principles of responsibilities are almost the same as those applicable in the general or operating fund field. However, the details of handling are somewhat different. For example, a city council may adopt each year a 6-year capital program, wherein is listed each project to be financed during these periods, showing the amount proposed to be spent for each of the 6 future years covered. The council then would also adopt a capital fund budget for the forthcoming year in which the amounts authorized to be spent therein are recorded projectwise.

In the preparation of the capital program and capital budget it is probable that the director of finance and a city planning commission, if one existed, would work jointly with the approval of the mayor to furnish the city council with a budget document that would best reflect the needs of the community with regard to the various proposed capital improvements. However, the initial budget requests would originate in the fiscal office of the operational departments.

It is evident from the foregoing that the health officer, to plan his health programs efficiently, to utilize the health dollar to the best advantage, and to remain within his budget limitations, must assure himself that he has prepared his budget properly, that its terms are applied correctly, and that shifts in programs are adjusted as the funds permit. To do this he must familiarize himself with the principles of the local fiscal requirements and must obtain the best fiscal advice and aid available.

## REFERENCES

1. Burris, J. H., and Lancaster, J. B.: Evolving concepts of governmental auditing, Footnotes: J. HEW Audit Agency, p. 16, Spring 1971.

2. White, L. D.: Introduction to the study of public administration, New York, 1955, The Macmillan Co.

3. Bahn, R.: The federal budget process, Public Health Rep. **84:**149, Feb. 1969.

4. Mitchell, W. E., and Walter, I.: State and local finance, New York, 1970, The Ronald Press Co. (see especially Chapter 18).

5. Fox, P. E., and Zwick, D. I.: Simplifying state accounting for federal health grants, Public Health Rep. **68:**1071, Nov. 1953.

6. Geiger, J.: Health officers' manual, Philadelphia, 1939, W. B. Saunders Co.

7. Draffin, E. C.: Budget presentation. In Lee, E., editor: Proceedings of the Institute on Administration in Crippled Children's Services, Berkeley, June 24-29, 1962, University of California School of Public Health.

8. Gable, W. R.: Budgeting in small communities, Mich. Munic. Rev., p. 36, Feb. 1967.

9. Klepak, D.: Performance budgeting for the health department, Public Health Rep. **71:**868, Sept. 1956.

10. Henry, M. L., and Proctor, W.: New York State's performance budget experiment, Public Admin. Rev. **20:**69, Spring 1960.

11. Michael, J. M.: Planning-programming-budgeting and health program planning. In The executive process in public health administration, Ann Arbor, 1968, University of Michigan School of Public Health.

# CHAPTER 14

# Public relations

## PURPOSES AND OBJECTIVES

Ours is a society of increasing complexity and sophistication. One of the requirements of both private and public organizations in such a society is a concern for customer or patron understanding and attitude, commonly referred to as *public relations*. The term is admittedly general and vague; it is used to describe a variety of techniques, practices, and activities, some good, some bad, designed to win the goodwill and cooperation of people individually and collectively. These activities are never an end in themselves; rather they are important merely to the extent that they enable employees to fulfill adequately their intended responsibilities to the satisfaction and understanding of all concerned.

The field of public relations is not only difficult to define but also presents a problem when one merely attempts to list or describe the various factors that contribute to it. All too often are seen instances in which executives point with pride and satisfaction to their publicity programs and refer to them as public relations programs. Although press releases, public addresses, and the like are of great importance in their place, public relations encompasses far more. It includes every conceivable factor and circumstance that may influence people's attitude toward the organization, its goals, its activities, and its personnel. Most important it includes the many seemingly incidental and casual relationships between the organization, its personnel, and those who are served. In this sense public relations may be looked on to a considerable degree as the summation of personal relations.

Another misconception with regard to the purpose of public relations activities is that they are developed for the purpose of having a reserve of support and defense when the going gets rough. Although a really good public relations program will go far in accomplishing this purpose, it is an incidental or secondary effect; the primary purpose is to make the road as smooth and effective as possible in the first place. As one writer[1] has described it: "Public relations is not an ambulance parked at the bottom of a precipice. Rather, it is a fence built at the top."

Although the public relations problem of a public health department is essentially the same as that of any other type of enterprise, certain differences in the reasons for the existence and manner of operation of the organization make good public relations peculiarly important.[2] A health department is a tax-supported public agency that belongs to the people it serves. Its existence in a democracy depends in the final analysis on their wish to maintain it. In the long run this wish can be sustained only by public understanding and satisfaction. Such reactions naturally give rise to pride of ownership, which in turn enhances cooperation and support. It might be pointed out further that modern thinking in public health is along the lines of doing things with people, not for them or to them. "With" is an interesting word which, when applied jointly to a health agency and the people it serves, implies everything that contributes to good public relations.

## GENERAL CONSIDERATIONS

Fundamental to a successful program of public relations is the desire to sell the organization and its program, not the individual. It is true that the public is interested in personalities and figureheads, but it soon tires or becomes suspicious of too frequent references to a particular public employee, including the health officer. Perhaps the most important public relations consideration for the health officer is not to regard the health program as a one-man show but to share credit as well as responsibility. When this policy is followed, the individual is automatically benefited. Thus when Enion Williams, the eminent health commissioner of Virginia, was asked to account for his long tenure of office, he replied, "I have never tried to sell the people of Virginia on the name Williams, but I have sold them on the Virginia State Department of Health."

What has been said is not meant to imply that the health officer does not have a most important personal part to play in the public relations program of his organization. After all he is the responsible leader. It is his job to ascertain that desirable relationships are formed and maintained. Beyond planning and directing the program he must cultivate certain relationships that he alone is in a position to do and is expected to carry out. He makes these contacts with other governmental officials, prominent citizens, and various important key people including representatives of the communications field in the interests of the program for which he is responsible.

This leads to a second basic consideration. Good public relations, particularly those of large organizations, seldom if ever come about spontaneously. Sometimes they may appear to, but to be effective a public relations program must be carefully and conscientiously planned and constantly watched. To do this requires initially a clearly determined overall policy of the organization and its attitude toward the public in relation to the purposes and aims of the agency. Cognizance of all potential contacts must be taken and insofar as possible arrangements made for their occurrence in the most mutually satisfactory manner. Provision must be made for employee training in good public relations, followed by checks and evaluations of the success of this aspect of the life of the agency.

With regard to the first of the two words in the term *public relations* it must be fully appreciated that there is no such thing as "one" or "the" *public*. In even the most primitive societies more than one public exists. Usually there are many, each with its particular interests, needs, and demands. The population of the typical community is subdivided into a large number of groups or publics on the basis of many characteristics, for example, religion, economic status, education, race, nationality, age, sex, and occupation, to mention only a few. The public relations program must be broken down into a similar number of subprograms. No single approach will bring success because it will touch only one or at best a few of the publics. The program must be designed as a jigsaw puzzle that eventually succeeds in reaching in one way or another all of the publics involved.

Attention should be drawn to several other general considerations. The first of these is the often overlooked fact that public relations is a two-way process. It involves a flow of information, reactions, and understanding not only from the agency to the public but also in the reverse direction. Accordingly it is important that the health agency devise and use some method of periodic determination of needs, wishes, understanding, and motivational inclinations of the public. Overlooked with equal frequency is the part played by the many informal and formal contacts between public employees and the citizenry. A health department may have the support of the press, the professions, and the business groups and may be doing a scientifically splendid job, but all this may be negated in the mind of the citizen if he is slighted, treated flippantly and rudely, or in any other way made to feel dissatisfied.

One final consideration, which is related to the next discussion, is an appreciation of the competition for the attention of the public. In addition is the often overlooked fact of extensive rivalry for attention within the health field itself.[3] In modern American society the senses of the average citizen are bombarded constantly throughout his waking hours by a barrage of publicity, propaganda, advertising, and promotional and educational forces. Some of them are subtle, whereas others resort almost to brute force. The public health worker must recognize all this as competition and must devise and employ techniques that will meet it on its own ground and obtain a fair share of public attention. In this real struggle for public attention and support the public health agency is handicapped by certain obstacles that act as deterrents to desirable public relations. Some of them relate either to the nature of the product (health) or to the means of providing for it (a public agency). Others stem from outdated, impractical, and supercilious approaches.

## OBSTACLES TO GOOD PUBLIC RELATIONS

It must be frankly recognized that people are seldom interested in public health in the general sense. Individuals are concerned with their own personal health or with that of the members of their families. By and large they are willing to pay attention to some of the larger community aspects of health only insofar as they may readily appreciate its effect on them. Even then they may weigh the possible benefits against certain other considerations such as personal freedom of action or business advantage. In other words, strange as it may seem to those imbued with the "public health spirit," public health is not necessarily a natural or spontaneous concern, interest, or wish of all people. It is in fact more than a little distressing to find that an appreciable percentage of the population is ignorant of the existence of the field and not particularly interested in enlightenment. Somewhat offsetting this is the fact that most people are to some degree hypochondriacs, including as Allen[3] admits even reporters, science writers, and editors.

Another obstacle is related to the fact that activities engaged in for the protection and promotion of health require employees with a scientific, technical, or professional background. Their training and experience usually emphasize the scientific and technical aspects of the problems and their solutions and ignores more often than not the human factors involved. Thus it is easy for public health workers to be so intent on their activities, programs, or goals that they lose sight of the personal and human aspects of the work. This professionalism may sometimes give rise to feelings of discomfort, awe, and even resentment on the part of the members of the public in their contacts with the personnel of the health department. If this occurs, it is of course a deterrent to good public relations and understanding.

Particular difficulties arise from the fact that public health programs are in large part activities of official governmental agencies and therefore subject to all of the attitudes that the public and community groups tend to have toward government. Unfortunately public employment has been held in low esteem by many in the United States, although some improvement has been noticed in recent years. All too often the public servant, professional or otherwise, has been regarded as someone incapable of successfully engaging in private business or professional practice and interested only in a political sinecure. This is due partly to the traditional American admiration of rugged individualistic business and industry and partly to occasionally unsatisfactory if not unsavory governmental operations. In addition, it must be recognized and accepted that a public agency must function much more in a case than does a private agency in which for some reason citizens tend not to feel a vested interest and demand accountability. Business and the private professions have always regarded government as a natural enemy that always seeks to control or to take over. Under these circumstances the opposition to the development and expansion of public programs is not surprising.

Related to this and accentuated by traditionally low salaries in governmental service is the frequent inferiority complex that has developed in many public employees. An unfortunate method of compensation for this is the occasional exercise of injudicious authority based on public position. This, when resorted to, only aggravates the situation.

It is easy to understand how many citizens may misinterpret planned public relations activities of public agencies as representing propaganda for the purpose of self-aggrandizement at public expense to assure reappointment or continued employment. For this and other reasons the public has been loath to provide funds for public relations purposes, thereby often making it necessary for the public agency to resort to subterfuge to accomplish this important purpose.

Finally, it should be recognized that a great many citizen contacts with the health department are unwilling contacts, whereby the individual is called on to do something not to his liking, for example, to obtain a permit. From the point of view of development of desirable public attitudes, the health department finds itself with two strikes against it from the outset. This makes it all the more necessary that the personnel of the health department take full advantage of every possible opportunity for the development and maintenance of good public relations.

## METHODS IN PUBLIC RELATIONS

Since in every community there are many publics and since societies have become so complex, it necessarily follows that there are many different approaches to the development of improved public understanding and support.

### Personal contacts

The approach by way of personal contacts is mentioned first, not only because of its importance but also because it is so often overlooked or neglected. A health department exists to serve the public, and most of its work involves contact between its staff and the individuals who comprise the public. It naturally follows that these contacts should be of a desirable nature. If a contact or association of a citizen with the personnel of the agency is unsatisfactory and leaves an unpleasant memory, the contact is a failure despite whatever service is rendered in the process. In addition to this, if the attitudes of the employees toward the public health organization, its policies, and its management are unsatisfactory, they are certain to influence the nature of the employees' contacts with the public, and this in turn will adversely affect the community's attitude toward the department.

On-the-job personal characteristics of health department employees that influence the reactions and attitudes of the public they meet may be considered under the categories of appearance, behavior, and capability.

**Appearance.** Most large private organizations have found it desirable to impose certain requirements concerning dress and other aspects of personal appearance on their employees. To do so is not without risk, since requirements of this nature, if unexplained, misunderstood, or too strict, are likely to lead to considerable intraagency friction and personnel dissatisfaction. Most employees, however, if worthy of employment in the first place, can be made to realize the purpose and desirability of their requirements.

The average person on entering a business office, especially if the office is tax supported, does not react favorably to flashy clothes or an excess of jewelry, cosmetics, or perfume. Male employees should avoid sports clothes and dazzling neckties in favor of more dignified or professional dress. Women should be similarly conservative, tending toward suits and tailored clothes. The use of cosmetics, jewelry, and perfume occupy a real place in American culture and are by no means to be denied. However, in a business environment their use should be judicious and in good taste. Under all circumstances the personnel should be neat and clean, there never being any excuse for appearance to the contrary. That this is possible is given testimony by the level of neatness and cleanliness maintained by many industrial workers and gasoline-station attendants.

No discussion of clothing can be concluded without reference to the question of uniforms. The problem arises especially in connection with one large group of employees, public health nurses. It is possible to set forth many arguments for and against the wearing of uniforms. The chief advantages relate to ease of identification and recognition of professional standing. Many believe that the public expects to find nurses in some type of uniform, lacking which they may be less acceptable. It is further considered desirable by many that a corps of readily identified uniformed workers provides visual evidence of the importance and activity of the health department. In this sense the argument rests on the promotion of public relations. Some also claim that the wearing of identical uniforms by a group of employees promotes an esprit de corps.

The opposing view points to the frequent drabness of public health nurses' uniforms. This is not necessarily a valid complaint in view of the attractive yet dignified uniforms designed for airline stewardesses and many nursing agencies. With reference to identification some call attention to the resentment felt by many citizens when their neighbors see the "city nurse" knock at the door. Added to this, they claim, is the embarrassment of both the citizen and the nurse caused by the frequent identification of a public health field visit with venereal disease or some other problem of similarly unpleasant connotation. A single conclusion does not seem possible or appropriate. Each agency must determine its own on the basis of local customs and wishes.

**Behavior.** Whereas the first impression in a personal contact is a visual one depending on appearance, the subsequent and most telling impressions are of an even more direct and personal nature. Much depends on the manner in which employees approach individual citizens or patrons in the office or in the field.

Everyone has at some time found it necessary to visit offices where, after a seemingly needless wait, he has been called on with bluntness, curtness, and occasional rudeness to state his business. In such instances the visitor is made to feel that he is an outsider, an intruder, an interruption, a nuisance to be disposed of as quickly as possible. In contrast are offices equally if not more busy where the approach is friendly, as one human being to another, where any delays are courteously and regretfully explained, and where the visitor is made to feel at home, expected, and wanted.

In their contacts with the public there are certain principles or rules that public health workers would do well to follow. The key to the situation is to look on those contacted as the real and only reason for the job and for the department. Each contact should be regarded as a contest rather than a boring routine, the goal being to win the other person over to your side, your point of view, your program. To accomplish this the public health worker must first attempt to put himself in the position of the caller, remembering that in most instances that person would much rather be doing something else. The measure of success is for the visitor to depart with no regrets. At best the circumstances of the contact will be strange to him, therefore the employee should make every effort to call forth associations that are familiar and pleasant. Explanations should be in simple terms, and strange and technical terminology should be avoided. "Vaccination," "immunization," and "shots" are examples of complicated and rather frightening words, whereas "protection" bears a connotation of something positive and desirable. A woman would much prefer to be spoken of as an "expectant mother" rather than as a "prenatal." All of us resent being referred to as cases, subjects, or numbers; we are human beings and are worthy of address as such.

Every organization of whatever size should make provision for some type of information desk. In a small organization such as the typical rural county health department this desk will not be difficult to find. In larger agencies that occupy many rooms on several floors the information desk should be placed as close to the main entrance as possible. The person in charge should be selected with care; she should appear approachable, friendly, and desirous of being of assistance to all types of persons. Her manner, although dignified, should be somewhat in-

formal, and it is perhaps preferable that she be allowed somewhat more leeway in the matter of dress than the rest of the personnel. To fulfill her purpose it is of course necessary that an individual in this position possess an encyclopedic knowledge of the organization and its program, the building in which it is housed, and also of related organizations in the community. Placed near the information desk should be an easily read and interpretable directory that indicates the location of each of the functional units in the organization and lists the names of unit directors and of any other persons frequently sought.

Next in line of travel is the office receptionist, who to a considerable degree conditions the attitude of the caller toward the organization. This position is usually filled by a woman who also serves in a secretarial capacity. She should have an air of alertness and industry backed up by competence. The position is not necessarily an easy one, since the occupant may often find herself in the middle between the person for whom she works and the visitor. By no means are all visitors important, and the receptionist has the responsibility of husbanding the limited time of the executive. On the other hand, each visitor naturally considers himself and the reason for his call of importance, otherwise he would not have taken the trouble to come to the office. The receptionist therefore must have as an outstanding qualification a sound understanding of human nature and the ability whenever necessary to turn some visitors away in such a manner as to preserve their pride and dignity and make them feel satisfied at least in some degree. Whether or not the receptionist attempts to forestall or divert the visitor, she may by her manner convey the impression that the appearance of the visitor was the most important event during the day and that any delay or refusal is extremely regretful to her, her employer, and to the organization.

When a visitor approaches, the receptionist should greet him pleasantly, arise if circumstances allow and warrant, and ask in a pleasant tone of voice, "May I help you?" When a request to see the executive is stated, the receptionist should counter with, "May I ask who is calling?" whereupon, unless impossible, she should immediately take steps to notify her superior. Should it be necessary to turn away truly important persons or individuals whom the receptionist believes her superior would want to see, she should if possible arrange or at least suggest a subsequent appointment. If the visitor is to be seen, she should usher him into the presence of the executive, announce his name, and if necessary the organization he represents. If the visitor has given her a calling card, she should place it before her superior.

An annoying problem is posed by the visitor who never knows when to leave. The time of most professional workers and executives is limited, and frequently they are tempted to terminate a call impatiently or brusquely. This is likely to be misunderstood and resented by the visitor, even though he may have inconsiderately usurped more than a fair share of time. It is possible to circumvent such occurrences either by means of a prearranged signal to the receptionist-secretary or by routine interruption on her part after a reasonable interval to remind the executive of another appointment. This allows the executive to terminate the contact regretfully and gracefully.

A common cause of ill feeling toward public officials and agencies is the manner in which visitors, clients, or patrons are frequently shunted from one place to another, no one taking the trouble to ascertain exactly what they want or assuring that they get it by the shortest possible route. This type of runaround or buck-passing has proved costly to many organizations in terms of public relations. Accordingly the person at the information desk and the receptionist and secretaries in the organization have the important responsibility of adequate referral. Moreover, whenever indicated, they should take the trouble to follow up referrals to assure the satisfaction of the caller. Usually a caller has several reasons for contacting the agency, but in each instance there is one predominant reason for the visit having been made. Under no circumstances should the visitor be allowed to depart with the feeling that absolutely nothing was done with regard to that particular reason.

Some organizations have found it possible to improve their public relations by coordinating certain services and activities and by centralizing the location of places to which the public must come. A good example of this is in connection with building permits. Ordinarily a citizen who wishes to construct or alter a building finds it necessary to make the rounds of the building department, water department, fire department, health department, and possibly others in addition to the city clerk to obtain approval of all parts of the building permit. Some communities out of consideration for the taxpayer have brought together into one office, at adjacent desks, representatives of each of the branches of government involved so that all requirements may be fulfilled in one place and in a single visit.

Many health departments have effectively built up an extensive backlog of ill feeling through their public encounters. This problem was magnified during the war years as a result of the tremendous demand for birth certificates as a prerequisite to work permits. The same applies to demands in relation to marriage and burial permits and to foreign travel. Admittedly the extent to which health department offices have been deluged with often hurried requests has not been conducive to good temper and patience. Nevertheless, by attempting to be overly efficient by the use of impersonal mass production methods, health departments have sometimes irritated large numbers of individuals. Some of the difficulty can be attributed to personnel shortages and inadequate funds.

Over and above this, however, is the ill-advised policy followed by many organizations of placing at public counters employees who do not seem to fit in anywhere else. It is strange that positions that involve the most frequent contacts with the public so often are used as reservoirs or wastebaskets for employee misfits. Examples of improper behavior at information desks and public counters are not difficult to find. I once had the misfortune of inheriting a county health department officer manager who seemed to resent the appearance of anyone and who all but physically drove out those who dared enter. She was promptly relieved of her duties. Another well-remembered instance concerns the front information desk of the health department of a large city that was staffed by two former professional employees who had become too addicted to alcohol to render professional service. In still another agency the office of statistics and records was considered more or less a place of retirement wherein the older, worn-out employees found it definitely not to their liking to have to get out of their chairs to serve applicants for copies of vital records. The organization was widely known for its outstanding achievements. Nevertheless, within its community it was evaluated by many citizens in terms of the poor, ingracious service at the counter of the office of statistics and records.

Every public agency including the health department is the recipient of many complaints.

From the point of view of public relations one of the worst things that can happen is for the public to consider that it is wasted effort to call any dissatisfaction or shortcoming to the attention of the organization. Errors of omission and commission are certain to occur to some degree, particularly in an agency that must deal with large numbers of people and problems. A forward-looking organization should welcome complaints from those whom it is supposed to serve, since this is one way to evaluate and improve the program. Furthermore, to give the citizen the feeling that his complaint or criticism was justly and fairly received, considered, and investigated is one of the best ways of making him a community salesman for the department.

Certain steps should be followed in handling complaints. The first is to assure the individual that the organization is willing and in fact anxious to hear what he has to say. Related to this is the important necessity of allowing the complainant to tell his complete story in his own words and as he sees it without excuses or alibis on the part of the listener. The next step is to check at once if possible whatever records exist that might substantiate, explain, or disprove the complaint; for example, a complaint against the health department for failure to deliver a copy of a birth certificate sometimes may be resolved by immediately checking to see if the birth was registered in the first place. After this there should be made a clear and understandable explanation of whatever contributory factors or circumstances relate to the situation and its solution. One failing of many health departments that conscientiously investigate complaints and make necessary corrections is to neglect making known what it has done, even to the complainant. People want to know what happened.

Field contacts made by representatives of the health department are subject to the same public relations influences as those that occur in the office. There should be evident a desire to help rather than to enforce or compel. The same care should be taken to make proper and effective referrals and to secure necessary follow-up. These are the things that decide the difference between cooperation and resistance or at best passive acquiescence. In addition there are certain public relations circumstances peculiar to field visits. Relatively few health departments have made any effort to give advance notice by mail or telephone of intended field visits by members of their staffs. Some may object to the procedure on the basis of cost or the possibility that some persons may attempt to forestall or avoid the contact. Against the first of these objections is the fact that notification by mail or telephone costs only a few cents, in contrast with an average cost of several dollars for a field visit.

One of the most difficult administrative problems of a health agency is the reduction of unprofitable and costly field visits caused either by the patron not being at home or having moved elsewhere. Many fruitless visits may be avoided by a program of advance notice, and a considerable saving will result. As an example, an important aspect of the disease prevention program of the Detroit Department of Health has been educational home visits of public health nurses to parents of infants between 6 months and 1 year of age. A study of a sample of 14,028 nurses' visits showed that almost 30% were wasted. In 2,568 instances, or 18.3%, the family was not at home when the nurse arrived. In 1,511 instances, or 10.8%, the nurse found that the family had moved and could not be located. The procedure was instituted of preceding the first public health nursing visit by a letter that explained the reason for the forthcoming visit and asked for confirmation of address and whether or not the child had already been immunized against certain diseases. By this means not only was the percentage of "not home" visits reduced to 8.7% but in addition 33.8% of the families who ordinarily would have been "unable to locate" were located by means of the mail-forwarding procedures of the postal department. Without presenting financial figures it is obvious that the procedure not only paid for itself but also resulted in a significant saving. In addition to the saving were the educational value of the letter and the preparation it gave for the nurse's subsequent entry into the home. In other words it was of good public relations value.

The validity of the objection to previsit contacting or notification that some people may be forewarned and thereby forestall or avoid the visit depends, of course, on the type and content of the correspondence or telephone conversation. If properly planned and conducted, it may in itself be of educational and public relations value and make the subsequent visit more acceptable and fruitful. Furthermore, it may be pointed out that citizens, particularly housewives and mothers, are frequently annoyed by nurses and other health department employees arriving when they are in the middle of their housework or caring for a child. A stated wish to avoid doing so is likely to bring about a more receptive feeling toward the health department.

Attention must be given by the health department to the frequency and multiplicity of calls. Even the most cooperative citizen becomes understandably and rightfully annoyed when health department employees arrive too often or more than one at a time. This indicates the desirability of some form of field activity coordinating device, something too frequently overlooked in the health department practice. One manner in which some form of control may be exercised is by means of a central file in which are kept all records pertaining to each person, family, household, or premise. The checking out of a folder from the file indicates that some employee is presently engaged in some activity relating to the person or household.

Whenever possible, it is desirable to follow up the field visit with some other type of contact to promote good continuing public relations. One suggestion is that each visitor, whether nurse, sanitarian, or other professional person, ask before leaving if there is anything pertaining to health or sanitation about which the householder would like further information, to be provided by a mailed brochure or a visit by some other employee of the health department.

**Capability.** A third characteristic of health department employees that influences the attitudes of the public is the extent to which they are able to demonstrate their knowledge and ability in the solution of problems with which they are faced. Little need be said with regard to this obvious requirement. Capable service breeds respect on the part of the public and their elected representatives. Continued capable professional service is the most potent safeguard against political interference. When it becomes obvious both to the public and to elected officials that here is a necessary and vital technical and professional job which requires trained and capable professional personnel, that personnel is most likely to be allowed to function effectively.

### Private life

In a certain sense public employees, particularly those in executive positions, have no private lives. Not only are they under constant scrutiny during working hours but also at all other times. Their behavior is always associated with their public positions, the citizenry always asking themselves, "Is this the kind of person I want as a health officer or public health nurse or sanitarian?" Often the public applies standards to public officials it is unwilling to apply to itself. The citizenry further tends to consider public officials and employees on call and personally accountable 24 hours of every day. "Isn't that what we taxpayers are paying them for?" This perhaps applies particularly to public health workers, since the nature of their responsibility implies a round-the-clock vigilance. With reference to personal habits and behavior, if the public employee thinks that he must drink or engage in extrafamilial activities not generally accepted by society, he owes it to the organization for which he works to avoid open scandal. As Pfiffner and Preshus[4] have stated, large numbers of influential citizens do not approve of the new freedom concerning liquor and domestic relations. On the other hand, there are ways to do things without necessarily soliciting the attention of those who disapprove. To say this is not to suggest hypocrisy and subterfuge but simply to point out that it is the better part of discretion to avoid attracting public attention in such matters.

Public employees as social human beings have many off-the-job contacts with fellow citizens. These may occur in the home neighborhood, churches, clubs, lodges, and many other occasions for social intercourse. In all such circumstances the health department worker should speak and behave in terms of the best possible representation of himself, his family, and his organization. In addition to strictly social contacts an important phase of off-the-job public relations is the participation of the health department worker in various civic and professional group activities. The health officer had best be an active member of the local and state medical societies. Similarly the other professional personnel should be active in their respective professional societies. Of a somewhat similar nature is the participation of public health personnel in chambers of commerce, councils of social agencies, service clubs, and the like.

The individual employee must always realize that others may evaluate his organization through him. In relation to this subject it is inadvisable for a public health worker to develop a reputation as a perennial joiner, handshaker, or backslapper. Membership in organizations should be judiciously and carefully decided. More than one prominent public servant has been embarrassed by association with politically or socially unsavory organizations. In most communities there exist one or two outstanding groups or organizations that are the most influential and professionally valuable. They do not always appear to be so on the surface. In one city it may be a women's club, in another an athletic club, and in a third it may be a voluntary tuberculosis and health association around which cluster the most prominent and influential citizens. The health officer and his co-workers would do well to evaluate the organizations in their community and ascertain if possible health department representation in each of the most significant groups.

Before leaving the subject of behavior in private life some comment should be made concerning gifts or gratuities. A large segment of the public takes it for granted that public service is characterized by a strong inclination toward graft and corruption. Almost every health department employee in a position of any degree of authority is certain at one time or another to become aware of this. Restaurant owners will suggest free meals, and gifts of liquor, cigars, and other things will be offered. Such forms of apparent friendliness always carry some implication of future reciprocity. It is doubtful that any citizen likes a public servant so much that he will freely press him with gifts. Once an employee falls into this trap, it is most difficult to escape. Few such gifts are worth the psychologic quandary that usually results. The best and only policy for the public health or other public worker to follow is consistent refusal accompanied by a pleasant explanation that the gift is not expected by the worker or allowed by the position.

**Professional contacts**

**Telephone etiquette.** Each day about 300 million telephone conversations are held in the United States. Most of these are in relation to business and public affairs. The possibility that both friends and enemies may be made over the telephone is often overlooked, many people apparently believing that the absence of physical and visual contact allows a certain amount of leeway in behavior. It is an interesting psychologic fact that everyone engaged in a telephone conversation consciously or subconsciously visualizes the person with whom he is speaking. Employees therefore should approach telephone contacts in the same manner as all other types of contact. The rule suggested by telephone companies themselves is to "phone as you would be phoned to." The goal should be to make these contacts brief, friendly, and fruitful. Persons calling the organization should never be left holding a silent phone for any length of time. If a protracted delay is anticipated, the caller should be so notified and asked if he wishes to be called back later. Particularly annoying is the practice of having phone connections completed by one's secretary, who must then ask the person called to hold the line while the one placing the call is located. In other words, if you place a call, be immediately available when the connection is made.

In any type of contact the first words are of great importance in conditioning the tone of the entire relationship. This is particularly true of telephone contacts, since the relationship is entirely auditory. When a call is received, the person called should identify the organization and perhaps himself in a pleasant and friendly tone of voice: "Jones County Health Department, Mr. Smith speaking." Or if a receptionist or information clerk answers, "Jones County Health Department, may I help you?" If the person placing the call neglects to state his name, it is proper to ask, "May I ask who is calling?" rather than "Who are you?" or "What do you want?" No offense will be taken at the former statement, whereas the latter tends to make the backs of most people stiffen.

If the department is large enough to justify a private switchboard, the operators should be chosen with great care as in the case of information desk attendants. They must be quick and accurate, with a pleasant and even disposition, and have a complete knowledge of the organization and its personnel. All of these characteristics are necessary. I recall a delightful woman who operated the switchboard of a large health department with the greatest efficiency. She was always cheerful and had an uncanny knowledge of where everyone was and what they were doing. Her attitude had much to do with the development of public goodwill for the department.

If an employee or a division is called by mistake, the courteous and wise thing to do is to assist the caller in making contact with the right person or the one who can best help him. Thus: "That problem is handled by the nursing division. If you wish, I will have your call transferred." If it is uncertain which unit or agency is indicated, the employee, in the interests of good public relations, should say: "I am sorry, but that is not handled by this division. I'll be happy to try to find out whom you should speak with and ask him to call you."

Courtesy demands that the person placing a call identify himself as soon as a connection is made. This should be immediately followed by a statement of the reason for the call, for example, "This is Dr. James of the Jones County Health Department. May I speak with Mr. Smith?" The business at hand should then be discussed as briefly as possible, giving the other person a chance to express his opinion, and then the call should be terminated.

**Correspondence.** A significant proportion of the contacts of an organization occurs by means of correspondence. It is often overlooked that a piece of written or printed material may be as personal as an expression on a face or an inflection in a voice. Since friends and enemies may be made by a piece of paper, it is advisable that special attention be given to this important form of social and business intercourse. It is desirable therefore that a health department establish a favorable organizational tone in its written contacts with the public rather than to leave the matter entirely to chance. There are several ways in which this may be accomplished. The organization should have a written standard practice with regard to incoming and outgoing correspondence with which all employees should become familiar. It should give consideration to matters of routing and handling of mail, restrictions concerning who in the organization should write what letters, priorities in answering, and even matters of phraseology. An important phase of correspondence control is to include instructions relating to it in preservice and in-service training programs.

Insofar as possible letters should be personalized, since the average recipient enjoys seeing his name in print. Certain words should be avoided as much as possible. Among these are "I," "we," "order," "must," and similar words implying egocentricity, compulsion, or command. By like token, "you," "your convenience," "your cooperation," and similar words and phrases should be stressed. The use of standardized, impersonal, printed form letters should be avoided. When there is indication for their use, for example, when large numbers of persons must be contacted for the same reason, it is still possible to personalize the written contact. This may be accomplished by means of electric typewriters that operate automatically in a manner similar to a player piano. A master roll or tape is made that provides for the automatic typing of the routine parts of the letter. The machine stops automatically when certain personal items in the letter are reached so that names, birthdates, "he" or "she," "him" or "her" may be typed by hand or by means of a coordinated punched card. Thus it is possible to write a letter that is both standardized and personalized. Studies have indicated a significantly greater response to this type of written approach, which although slightly higher in cost per letter, is well worth the difference in terms of results.

## Employee training

It has been indicated that good public relations do not just happen. They result only from a planned program of employee training and example. It does little good for a few at the top to formulate techniques and programs to promote good feeling on the part of the public if the rank and file of the employees of the organization are not involved. If they are not provided with opportunity to develop feelings of pride and loyalty toward the organization, if they are kept in the dark with regard to the program and its progress, if they are not taken into at least the general confidence of the organization concerning plans and aims for the future, and if they are not impressed with and shown the importance of each of their contacts with the public, the organization cannot hope to achieve an atmosphere, employee borne, that speaks for good public relations.

Some industrial concerns have found it much to their advantage to pursue a consistent employee training program for public relations. One of the most outstanding of these is the program of the Bell Telephone Company, which is well worth a few sentences of description. Before they report for work all persons employed receive a manual by mail entitled *You are the Company.*[5] On reporting for work the new employee is assigned to a school for an induction course that has three phases. First, the employee is told about the electrical and communications industry as a whole. Then he is told about the company for which he is going to work. Finally, he is told about the department in which he is going to work and the job he is going to do and its relation to the company, the industry, and society. After this he begins training to enable him to master all the technical details of his specific work. Finally, he is rated periodically by his instructors and office managers at the end of the first, third, sixth, and twelfth month. It is of interest that one phase of the customer interview rating procedure used by Bell Telephone Company is controlled by the employee himself. He records transactions and listens to the playback, comparing them with standard records. He may stop or start or discard records, depending only on his wish. After he has listened to a recorded transaction he is allowed to dispose of the record.

In the health field the American Medical Association has produced and distributed an excellent and readable booklet as a public relations guide for medical assistants.[6]

Programs and techniques such as these are well worth trial and development by public health agencies. Certainly every health department employee should be made to believe that he is taking part in much more than a means to a personal livelihood. If he believes this, and it can result only from planning and encouragement from the top of the organization, his contacts with the public are certain to be more satisfactory.

**Quarters and equipment**

As the appearance of the health department employees is important, so too is the appearance of their quarters and equipment. One of the most unfortunate characteristics of official health agencies is that they are so often forced to be satisfied with physical facilities left over after the needs and wishes of the other branches of government have been satisfied. For many years the physical appearance of many health departments was the antithesis of what they attempted to preach and, even more serious, of what they demanded of others. Under the circumstances there is little wonder that many people do not take too seriously the proposals of health departments. To require that others be what one is not oneself is hardly conducive to good public relations.

Fortunately the situation has been undergoing considerable improvement. Many local health departments have moved into quarters similar to those occupied by business organizations. An increasing number are housed in buildings designed especially as health centers. This trend has been significantly aided by the Hill-Burton Act and more recently the Hill-Harris Act, which provide matching federal funds for this purpose. In addition to

going far to provide health departments with community dignity and respect, these trends have the added value of removing the public health agency from physical connection and therefore association with the centers of partisan politics and all they represent in the public's mind.

A few specific details are worthy of mention in connection with the reactions of the public. Health in the public's mind is intimately associated with cleanliness. This being the case, the premises of the health department, of all agencies, should be clean and bright. Soap and paint alone considerably improve even the oldest quarters. If there is any question, attention is directed to the remarkable change that has taken place in the appearance of gasoline stations, earth-moving equipment, heavy-duty trucks, and the like during the past 15 years. If they can look neat, so too can a health department. If at all possible, dark woodwork and dark heavy furnishings should be avoided. The present trend in office architecture is away from a multitude of stuffy, poorly lighted cubicles toward the open-office type of layout. An increasing number of private agencies even place important executives in large open areas, set apart perhaps by a railing. It is thought that this general plan is conducive both to better personnel morale and efficiency and to better public relations, since the visitor receives a strong impression of serious business activity.

As few movable items as possible should be kept on the top of desks. In fact it is stated with good reason that only papers and other items in immediate use should be visible at any given time. In this regard a modern filing system contributes importantly to the general air of neatness and lack of confusion as well as to efficiency. It should always be remembered, however, that files are business tools and not completely enclosed wastebaskets simply for the purpose of getting things out of sight.

## AVENUES OF PUBLICITY

In any society in which they are available the formal channels of community communication play a highly important role in public relations. Predominant among these communication channels are the press, radio, and television.

**The press**

One of the most important phases of public relations concerns how to obtain and retain the cooperation of those who command the channels to community public opinion. Outstanding among these are the representatives of the press. There are in the United States over 2,000 daily and 10,000 weekly newspapers that blanket the population. Rare indeed are individuals who do not have some contact with the product of the press. An ever-present problem facing the health officer is how to reconcile his interests and those of the newspaper published in his jurisdiction. As one authority[7] has pictured it, the ideal situation would be one in which the press and the institutions in the community would have similar noble interests and in which the press could fulfill all the varying demands of all the community's institutions. No such situation exists, however, because there are no perfect newspapers with perfect publishers, editors, and reporters, and there are no perfect directors of community institutions. It is from these imperfections and also from healthy, honest differences of opinion regarding the nature of community institutions and their proper place that problems in press relations arise. It must be realized that publishing a newspaper is a big business and that each paper has a policy regarding what it considers to be news and what it will publish. That policy, although colored somewhat by altruism, idealism, and civic interest, in most instances is determined primarily by what the publisher thinks the public wants to read, which will therefore sell more newspapers and thereby attract more advertising. The average newspaper will be inclined to print material relating to health and to the health department only if it believes that it is in and of the public interest.

It must also be remembered that the press is traditionally a critic of government and its agencies. Fortunately in most instances this critical attitude is potential, since the press generally offers strong support to what it considers a good government or a good health department. Nevertheless, because it regards a government, a public health department, or any other public agency as potentially inadequate and their personnel as potentially self-seeking, the press is constantly alert, acting as the guardian of the public interest.

Each newspaper has it own style that has been developed over a period of time. It has been developed for the purpose of reader appeal. To accomplish its purpose the newspaper must write in a manner simple and interesting enough to appeal to the largest possible number of the people. This means that technical and scientific information must be translated into simple language than can be understood by the average or subaverage person. General, tedious, verbose statements must give way to sharp, precise, concise, and specific information readily applicable to the reader. It is true that sometimes emphases are changed and important points missed, but by and large the press has proved itself amazingly competent in getting rather complex ideas across to the average citizen.

A particular newspaper style is not something that the health department employee can expect to master overnight.

Because of this and in the interests of good press relations, it is best that the public health worker respect the newspaperman as a specialist in his field. Therefore it is worth while to consider the following suggestions from an experienced newspaperman to public officials.[8] These suggestions resulted from years of practical experience and contact with public agencies.

1. If I were a city official, I would have a clearly defined and systematic policy in all press relations. I would either supervise execution of such policies myself or have a responsible person, preferably with a knowledge of news and reporting techniques, do so under my direction. I would not deny reporters access to department heads but I would consult with the latter from time to time on matters of policy in regard to their own press relations.

2. I would, after this policy is clearly understood, arrange conferences with the publishers and city editors of each of the local newspapers. I would ask their advice on how to clear the news for their convenience, and how to make that news accurately reflect the best values in public administration. I would discuss the result of these conferences with the reporter on my beat and get his reaction to them. He is my daily contact; I would never make him feel I was "going over his head."

3. I would arrange a convenient, regular "press conference" time to see all newspapermen, although I would never deny any one of them admittance at any time.

4. I would develop my own "nose for news." If I found it necessary to make off-the-record statements, I would be sure the reporter understood at the outset that I was talking off-the-record. I would be free and helpful to reporters in their news-gathering jobs and answer all questions I thought fair and proper. If I could not answer a question, I would, if possible, explain why. If a reporter were after a story which would be detrimental to good government if announced prematurely, I would tell him all the facts on that story, appealing to his sense of fair play in holding it. However, I would promise his paper an equal "news break" when that story was ready.

5. I would see that news breaks were distributed as evenly as possible between the morning and evening papers. If I talked to competitive reporters individually I would be careful to give each exactly the same story.

6. I would not exaggerate the occasional petty criticisms that newspapers print so long as my general press relations were good.

7. If a "news leak" occurred and the report, because of inadequate information, was misinterpreted, I would call in newsmen and explain the proper interpretation to them.

8. I would ask editors to give me a fair chance to answer critical "letters-to-the-editor" in the same column printing such letters.

9. I would insist that all municipal and departmental reports designed for public reading be written in terms understandable to the layman, with the qualities of clarity, simplicity, and directness, and with a format that would make people, including newspapermen, want to read them.

10. On major public reports I would make the matter available to reporters from time to time before the report itself is actually published, if that is possible. These releases would be carefully timed. I would point out to the reporter the significance of more complicated passages in these reports and interpret them so he could write accurate and intelligent stories. I would also point out to him the infinite possibilities in various departments for news features and special Sunday articles. I would help him to get pictures for such articles.

11. I would prepare releases or formal written statements only on those stories of important policy where misconceptions or misquotes might result. Newspapers generally prefer to do their own local stories in their own way, and if I have the right to contact with them I can explain any story clearly.

12. I would look upon newspaper people as intelligent men engaged in a reputable work, and I would instruct all department heads and employees to treat them with respect and courtesy.

13. Finally, I would make the newspaper an effective instrument in accounting to the public for my stewardship, and I would keep in mind the significant motto of a great newspaper chain: "Give light and the people will find their way."

Several additional hints may be made with regard to relationships with the press. Occasionally public health workers, particularly some health officers, have a tendency to irritate if not insult reporters and editors by adopting a superior professional air. Overly impressed by their own apparent importance, their attitude is one of suspicious condescension. Much more is to be gained by accepting the newspaperman as an equal and to actively seek his friendship, trust, and respect. As pointed out by Allen,[3] most people involved in the communications media appreciate and welcome the gesture if made in good faith and usually respond in kind. The public health director can often profit from the advice and criticism of the reporters assigned to his beat. They and their editors can often give invaluable advice regarding public feeling, anticipated reactions, and timing of reports and announcements. It is much better to follow their opinions in these matters than to demand arbitrarily that a certain item appear on the front page of this evening's paper.

Articles should emphasize problems, programs, and the organization, not the individual. Both the press and the public soon tire of the health worker who appears to want his name in every issue of every paper. Share the credit; stress the organization. In submitting copy the customs and requirements of the trade should be followed. Material should be typed double-spaced on one side of the paper only, with extra space at the top of the first page for placement of a headline. Let the reporter reword, revise, and cut the material and write his own headline. These are his professional prerogatives that allow for individuality and pride in his work. The best safeguard against errors in reporting and headlining is to state and emphasize clearly the basic idea to be communicated. Advance copies of announcements, speeches, or articles are always appreciated by busy reporters and editors. They should not be expected, however, to use all material submitted. After all the newspaper is theirs, and so should be the choice of material.

Persons writing copy should guard against verbosity. They each tend to think that what interests them must naturally interest everyone and that every word they take the trouble to write is worth everyone's time. Newspaper writing and for that matter newspaper reading are specialized forms of writing and reading. News items must be presented "in a nutshell," since that is the form in which the newspaper reader wants them. Feature articles are seldom read in toto. Brevity and conciseness therefore are the characteristics to be sought. A page and a half, double-spaced, is a moderately long story; two typewritten pages are too long for most purposes; three and a half pages make a whole column and except in most unusual circumstances are an imposition on any editor.

Care must be given to impartiality in the handing out of newsworthy stories. Papers and editors are in competition with each other and naturally resent signs of favoritism. One of the first things a public health worker should do on beginning work in a new community is to make a complete list of all papers published in the area. Those most likely to be overlooked are the county papers in contrast with those published in the county seat, weeklies as against dailies, and foreign-language papers. The latter are of particular importance in many metropolitan cities that contain large numbers of non-English–speaking residents.

A final suggestion to be made in the interest of improved press and therefore public relations is that consideration occasionally be given to inviting reporters and editors to "come and see." If an opportunity is provided for them to visit the various activities of the health department and to take part in field trips and other in-service training activities, benefits will be reflected in better appreciation and reporting.

**Audiovisual methods**

No one medium of publicity can be used to the exclusion of all others. Whereas the press is unquestionably of great importance, it is often credited with more power and influence by the general public and many organizations than most editors and reporters would privately give it. As some newspapermen have pointed out, if the press does appear to have more power and influence than any other community institution, it is probably because the other channels of publicity and public education have been neglected. One probable reason for this neglect is that these other approaches are not as easy to use as is the press. They are more expensive, require more specialized skills and equipment within the health department, and are more time consuming because they require planning, rehearsing, or construction. Yet it must be realized that the press is applicable only to certain problems and even then only serves one phase of the total publicity. Of course, the same is true of all avenues of approach to the public. Thus an important program may be announced through the press, on the radio, on television, on posters, or in meetings. The actual launching of the program may be accomplished by exhibits, leaflets, demonstrations, and personal visits. Finally, there must be publicity follow-up, presenting the progress and results of the program.

Among the audiovisual approaches to the public, radio and television are perhaps the most important. Most stations have some responsibility for public welfare and improvement. To meet this responsibility they follow the policy of setting aside a portion of their air time for public service programs, among which may be some dealing with public health and the health department. There are certain reservations with regard to the value of such programs. In the first place the time periods that radio and television stations donate are most likely to have low listener ratings. This is understandable, since after all the stations are in a costly business and naturally reserve their most valuable time for the profitable commercially sponsored programs, particularly broadcasts over nationwide hookups. Another handicap is that the writing and presentation of satisfactory programs is a highly technical and fairly expensive job and not one for amateurs. There is a tendency on the part of many professional people, including those engaged in public health work, to think that everyone is ready and willing to listen to them. They overlook the fact that radio and television developed primarily as entertainment media and that the busy housewife or the tired workingman is not particularly interested in avidly following the serious opinions of a public health worker presented more often than not as a monotonous monologue. To insist and persist in the presentation of such performances is poor public relations, to say the least. The average member of the listening public, if he happens to hear the program at all, is most likely to turn the program off. Even that involves interruption and physical effort which the average listener may resent.

Despite this, radio and television may occupy real places in the educational and public relations programs of the health department. To do so, careful planning and judicious use are required. The fact that it is primarily a means of entertainment may be used to advantage. Many people simply turn a good program on and leave it on, tolerating short commercial or spot announcements with the knowledge that in a few minutes another entertaining program will be forthcoming. It is suggested therefore that more consideration be given to the use of spot announcements by health departments.

Beyond these short, attention-getting auditory contacts that are essentially of a sensitizing nature, health departments may find value in certain types of longer programs of 15 or 30 minutes' duration. They should not, however, take the form of talks or addresses. Instead the patterns long since proved of value in other fields should be adapted. Certain types of audiences are attracted by quiz programs, others by round-table or town-hall types of discussion. For many listeners the drama has great appeal. In any case the total program should be planned and written by professional producers and writers and if possible presented by professional actors. The period of the novelty of television is past. The role it will play eventually in social and cultural life is not yet fully determined. Already, however, it has brought about real changes, some desirable and others undesirable, in family life. Indications are that it will become a significant means of public education as well as entertainment. In fact it may eventually replace in large measure not only radio and motion pictures but also to some degree the newspapers. Many health departments in urban centers are using it as an effective means of health education of the public.

Other media of public relations and educational value are exhibits, public talks, and such miscellaneous approaches as billboards, filmstrips, streetcar and bus advertisements, throwaways, "comic" books, and paid advertising. Each of these may be made to serve particular purposes and to reach certain groups. No one of them is an end in itself but must be a part of and tied in with a larger overall program. If poorly done, they do much more harm than good and should therefore be carefully planned and evaluated.

Many public health officials attach considerable importance to their annual reports as implements for the development and maintenance of good public relations. Annual reports may be made to serve this useful purpose, but there is cause for serious doubt that they actually do in most instances. It is the uncomfortable truth that from the viewpoints of both content and format, most health departments' annual reports make extremely poor reading. Financed usually by inadequate funds, they are often poorly printed on cheap paper and consist largely of a series of disconnected reports from each of the functional units of the organization. They are illustrated merely by uninteresting columns of statistics plus perhaps the photographs of the members of the board.

An interesting and pertinent analysis of municipal public reports has been presented by the editors of *Public Management*.[9] Their criticisms, which deserve serious consideration by public health workers, may be summarized as follows:

1. Complete failure to make any kind of report
2. Extensive use of uninterpreted statistics
3. Use of graphs and statistics that may be falsely interpreted
4. Use of superfluous statistics unrelated to any purpose or accomplishment
5. Poor makeup, arrangement, paper, type, and printing, and poor or no illustrations
6. Lengthy financial statements of interest only to a few individuals
7. Disconnected combining of a collection of unrelated divisional or departmental reports rather than the synthesis of one general overall report

The distribution of annual reports presents a problem in itself. The typical situation is one in which a few thousand are printed and copies sent to the members of the board of health, city councilmen or county supervisors, prominent citizens, representatives of voluntary health and social agencies, and fellow public health workers elsewhere in the country. In many instances a sizable proportion of the edition rests in a storeroom to await some future housecleaning. The point of significance is that rarely is a copy seen by the average citizen. This gives rise to the question whether or not the annual report should be regarded at all as an education tool or a public relations technique. There appears to be a growing opinion in public health circles that the essential purposes and objectives of an annual report should be redefined. This opinion is given substance by the trend toward fulfilling legal requirements by submitting typewritten or mimeographed descriptive and statistical reports to city or county officials, conserving other efforts and funds for attractive picture-magazine types of publications designed specifically for wide public appeal and distribution.

## COMMUNITY GROUPS

Most citizens of civilized society live two lives—one as individuals, the other as members of groups. Aristotle had this in mind when he observed that the man who can live without society is either a beast or a god. Furthermore, even among primitive people a single group seldom if ever satisfies. Thus there may be found the family group, the clan or tribal group, the secret male societies, the religious groups, to mention only a few. This is the basis for the statement that there is no such thing as one public but that every community consists of many publics, each with its own characteristics. These community groups or publics manifest themselves in most instances in some form of organization. Advantage may be and should be taken by public health officials of the existence of these organizations, since they serve the triple functions of channels, audiences, and sounding boards. It therefore is important for those in responsible public health positions to establish and maintain close and friendly relationships with those in command of these valuable channels. Such a relationship is dependent on three things: mutual interest, mutual understanding, and mutual respect.

It should be realized that public health agencies do not operate in a vacuum. Problems of public health are related to many other community problems. In other words many other individuals in the community have public health as a subsidiary professional or occupational interest. The personnel of official public health agencies therefore should be constantly on the lookout for other community programs, agencies, organizations, or groups to which public health interest can be related. There should be a deliberate effort to make public health problems their problems.

Although no single approach is universally applicable, there are a few planned or formal steps that may be taken to achieve greater success. It is suggested that there be compiled a list of all groups or organizations known to exist in the community. This list in many cases will be lengthy and may include some listings that will never be of value. Nevertheless, it is well to have the information ready at hand in case it is needed. A few of the many categories of groups and organizations under which listings should be made are political, religious, racial, nationality, educational, professional, occupational, social, financial, and fraternal.

There are certain characteristics of organized community groups that must be kept in mind. Each is usually built around some special interests. Therefore if the list that is suggested takes the form of a private file, notations may well be made of any pertinent items of information relating to leadership, influence, age and social representation, chief and subsidiary interests, prejudices, and the like. This specialization referred to influences the fraction of the population that is attracted to membership in each organization; yet membership frequently overlaps several groups. Thus the same indi-

viduals may be found in the Eagles fraternal society who are also members of various labor unions. The Parents and Teachers Association may often have many members in common with the League of Women Voters and the Association of University Women. Because of this, if a group cannot be reached through one organization, they may often be approached through one or two others. Significantly, members of city councils, state legislatures, or county boards may frequently be contacted under desirable circumstances through service clubs and other community organizations.

It should also be realized that the majority of service, social, and business clubs and organizations represent the more favored in the community. As a result, they may be excellent for prestige and influencing public opinion but poor for obtaining direct results. This brings up the most difficult aspect of the problem. Despite what was said concerning man's need for society, it is a curious fact that a large proportion of the population of any community does not appear to belong to any organized community group. Several studies have been made of the subject. One of the most complete was conducted in Springfield, Mass., in the mid-1940s. It was found that in that community almost two thirds of the population appeared on the surface to belong to no organized group, including churches and labor groups. It is certain that the proportion is subject to considerable variation, and it is probable that two thirds is unusually high. Nevertheless, it is of significance that those in the community who are in greatest need are generally those not included in an organized group. In other words the people who do not come to meetings or participate are the very ones who need the help.

In planning a program or activity the public health worker should be systematic in his analysis of the community groups and organizations that may be involved. It is suggested that the following lists be made:

1. A list of the problems of the community and of the health department
2. A list of each group of the population affected by each problem
3. A list of all individuals, groups, agencies, and organizations that also may be concerned with or interested in each problem and that therefore may be considered a potential source of help
4. From the foregoing, a list of methods or channels of attack

A program for the control of venereal diseases may serve as an example. The first three lists might appear in summary somewhat as follows:

*Problems of the community and the health department*

| | |
|---|---|
| Incidence | Rehabilitation |
| Case finding | Education |
| Control of infectious individuals | Etc. |
| Treatment | |

*Groups affected*

| | |
|---|---|
| Young adults | Infants |
| Low-income groups | Prostitutes |
| Newlyweds | Etc. |

*Groups, individuals, agencies, and organizations concerned*

| | |
|---|---|
| Health department | Industry |
| Private physicians | Family and other social |
| Private laboratories | service agencies |
| Hospitals | Welfare agencies |
| Pharmacists | Recreation agencies |
| Police | Housing agencies |
| Schools | Etc. |
| Churches | |

In view of the foregoing, it is possible to classify community groups and organizations according to their representation and potential use. The following is one such suggested classification that may be of value in planning and conducting the public relations and education programs of health departments.

I. Top level (for prestige, political, professional, and financial support)

  Governmental officials—elected and employed

  Medical and other professions

  Business and industry

  Influential citizens

II. Middle level (for influencing opinions of large key citizen groups)

  P.T.A.

  A.A.U.W.

  Labor unions

  Grange, etc.

III. Lower level (for neighborhood or individual contacts)

  Local churches

  Athletic clubs

  Fraternal organizations

  Veterans organizations

  Block clubs

  "Grass roots" clubs, etc.

IV. Schools (too often overlooked as important to public relations program)

Several of the categories are worthy of special

mention. The health officer has an important public relations job with regard to elected governmental officers and to his fellow public officials. Above all he must impress the elected representatives of the people with his practicality. To do this he must have some understanding of the total problem of civic government and management with which these representatives are faced. This may be exemplified in a negative sense by occasional county health officers who have read in a book that a health department budget should be of a certain magnitude. Lacking an appreciation of the limited tax resources of county governments and of the existence of outside potential sources of funds, they may make a request to their county supervisors for a local budgetary appropriation equivalent to most of the county income. From then on the members of the county government will look on the health officer as ignorant of the facts of life.

In Chapter 34 the relationship between the medical profession and the health department with regard to medical care is discussed. It may be well to point out here that the achievement and maintenance of good relationships with this particularly important group depends on observance of several considerations. Private physicians and the professions and institutions related to them have the same ultimate objective as public health agencies—that of raising the level of health of the people. Often attention must be called to this fact. Few things will contribute as much to obtaining the support of the medical profession as competent performance on the part of the health officer and his staff. In the past health departments have not always enjoyed good standing with the medical profession because members of their staffs have not been competently trained. This situation is undergoing rapid change. It is important that the health officer keep the medical group informed with regard to new programs that the health department is planning or is ready to inaugurate. If a physician in practice hears for the first time from some other source that the health department is going to do something, he will probably react critically. If, on the other hand, he and his fellow practitioners have been taken into the confidence of the health officer, if his advice and opinions have been solicited, and best of all if he has been involved in the planning, he will most likely be cooperative.

As mentioned earlier, the health officer

should preferably be a member of the local medical society and if possible an active member of its public health committee. He should serve as secretary or some other officer of the organization. Adequate medical representation on boards of health and advisory committees is naturally important. Wherever possible and convenient, meetings of the medical society should be held occasionally in the health department quarters. If the department sponsors clinics, an attempt should be made to have the medical work performed by private physicians on a part-time or hourly fee basis. In that way, especially if the work is rotated among all the practitioners, they will become more familiar with the purposes and programs of the health department and will feel a personal interest and involvement in it. Finally, when the health officer and his department receive credit or praise, for example, in the form of an award for service, the praise and credit should be freely shared with the medical profession and any other groups in the community that may have played a contributing role.

Before leaving the subject of public relations, reference should be made to public opinion polls. Frequently it is desirable to determine the attitude of the public toward particular problems and activities. This is almost a virgin field of public relations activity as far as public health agencies are concerned and one that should bear many fruits if properly utilized. It would seem possible for health departments through the efforts of their staffs to develop modest but effective sampling systems for this purpose. In addition to aiding in the planning of programs in a manner to which the public is receptive, the technique would undoubtedly cause many citizens to believe that the health department is truly concerned with their opinions and interests.

There is an aspect of positive publicity and public relations that is readily at hand yet usually overlooked—the employees of the public health agency itself. If each employee is kept currently informed about problems, programs, activities, and goals and is actively encouraged to serve as a purveyor of information, a highly significant proportion of the public may be reached both directly and indirectly. Consider, for example, a city of 1 million persons. Its public health department may have a total of 400 employees. It is certainly not unreasonable to expect that each one has a circle of relatives and close friends totaling an average

of about 25 persons. For the entire group this means about 10,000 persons, or 1% of the population, within easy potential reach. A rather good lawn would result from such a seeding! This emphasizes again the intimate interrelationship of the various aspects of public health administration, in this case the relationship between personnel development and public relations.

## SUMMARY

Tiboni[10] presented the public relations challenge to public health in clear and succinct terms. He pointed out that the real purpose of good public relations is the development of fruitful mutual understanding and cooperation between the public health program and the community it serves, whether local, state, or national. All public health workers are engaged in public relations every day for themselves, their profession, and their organization. He perceptively asked, however, "The question is only whether we are creating a good impression by conscious design or a poor one by default." The question then forces the issue of the importance, indeed the necessity, to plan a public relations approach carefully, deliberately, and consistently as follows:

*For internal public relations planning and development:*

1. Plan and develop good public relations as a fundamental and ongoing part of the total organizational program.

2. Assign a suitable key member of the top executive's staff the responsibility to develop and coordinate the program.

3. Define and analyze with him the various publics to be reached and why.

4. Establish clearly defined policies and procedures for public relations activities.

5. Ensure that the public relations coordinator involves all appropriate staff in planning the details of the program and that he keeps you fully informed of progress and important developments.

6. Review the objectives and content of the program with your staff so that they will understand it and be fully aware of your interest in it.

7. Implement your program plan with imagination and enthusiasm.

8. Recognize staff accomplishments in public relations as significant contributions to the facilitation and success of program administration.

9. Review progress and renew your mani-

festation of interest to your staff at suitably frequent intervals.

*For external public relations activities:*

1. Establish contact with the news media in your community. Try to cultivate a personal relationship with representatives who have or may develop an interest in your programs. Within limits of agency policy and ethical conduct be frank and direct in sharing and obtaining information. Provide information on all worth-while activities to them, either informally or by formal release, depending on the situation. Whenever appropriate, stress the technical requirements of the job at hand and the professional competence of the staff needed to complete it.

2. Create and be alert to opportunities to interpret, publicize, or promote your program and its importance to the community. Use such well-known devices as speaking to community groups, spot radio and television announcements, discussion programs, and newspaper feature stories, as well as novel approaches you may develop.

3. Train all members of your staff to be ambassadors of your organization. Be sure that they understand the objectives, procedures, program, and significance of your organization. Help them to develop the right attitudes and the skills to communicate. Emphasize that to many people in the community *they are the organization*, even if they are only a voice on the telephone. Help them to understand that they are regarded in this light even in their private contacts.

4. Establish advisory committees on general program and special subjects. Give these groups a chance to express their views, not merely to react to your proposals. You need to be as interested in what they feed back to you as in what you convey to them. Remember that development of understanding is a two-way street.

5. Participate in the work of community organizations. Be of assistance to other agencies whenever possible. They will increase their understanding and respect for your organization as you work with them and assist them.

6. Maintain a sensitive ear to community opinion and reaction to your program and the areas in which it operates. Recognize these attitudes in formulating your plans.

7. Remember that a job promptly, courteously, and effectively done is the best public relations activity ever known.

### REFERENCES

1. Harral, S.: Winning community confidence through public relations, Education **61:**168, Nov. 1940.
2. Public relations for the health department. In Currents in public health, Columbus, May 1964, Ross Laboratories.
3. Allen, J. F.: How to sell your program. In Lee, E., editor: Proceedings of the Institute on Administration in Crippled Children's Services, Berkeley, June 24-29, 1963, University of California School of Public Health.
4. Pfiffner, J. McD., and Preshus, R.: Public administration, New York, 1967, The Ronald Press Co.
5. You are the company, Bell Telephone Co.
6. Winning ways with patients, Chicago, 1966, American Medical Association.
7. Maurer, W. H.: Public relations and the press. Talk presented at an in-service course on public relations, School of Public Health, University of Michigan, Oct. 8, 1945.
8. Hazelrigg, H.: A newspaper man looks at city hall, Public Management **20:**67, March 1938.
9. Editorial: Seven more sins, Public Management **20:**33, Feb. 1938.
10. Tiboni, E. A.: What you can do to improve public relations for public health, Amer. J. Public Health **54:**2083, Dec. 1964.

# PART FIVE

# Patterns of health organization

One of the almost unique characteristics of man is the instinctive tendency to draw together for the accomplishment of a common goal. To get things done requires organization as well as planning and resources. This applies especially to ventures that require the efforts of many and diverse types of people working for the benefit of the whole. On the other hand, man tends to be torn between this tendency toward organization and an inclination to function as an entirely free and independent individual. Even with the decision to organize, his views are dichotomous in the sense of agreeing that some things are best done by officially sanctioned organizations of government but others had best be kept apart from officialdom. Hence in the United States and many other countries there have occurred parallel developments of official health organizations and of voluntary or nonofficial health agencies. They can and too often function apart, but where they have worked in tandem, the whole usually turns out to be greater than the sum of the parts.

*We trained hard, but every time we formed up teams we would be reorganized. I was to learn later in life that we tend to meet any new situation by reorganization: and what a wonderful method it can be for creating the illusion of progress while producing confusion, inefficiency and demoralization.*

PETRONIUS
*The Satyricon*

CHAPTER 15

# Official health agencies

## ACTION THROUGH DIVERSITY

It is probably an understatement to say that official public health programs in the United States are organized along complex lines. That this should be found in a nation with a reputation for organizational ability is frequently puzzling, not only to visitors from other countries but also to citizens of this country whose activities and occupations bring them only occasionally into personal contact with public health agencies. This complexity of organization is attributable chiefly to the form and structure of government as it was established in the nation, and it shows the influence of democratic and more or less decentralized development. One of the clearest overall pictures was that devised by Mountin and Flook to illustrate their concise *Guide to Health Organization in the United States.*[1]

Generally speaking, official public health activities may be considered on four levels: local, state, national, and international. The first is often subdivided into municipal programs and those of rural areas, although increasingly, core cities and the areas surrounding them are merging their health resources and providing common services under a united administration. As with government as a whole, whereas each political level has its own public health structure, no one of them is by any means completely independent of the others. To the contrary and increasingly, there is a melding of local public health functions and responsibilities with those of the state and, in turn, of state functions and responsibilities with those of the federal govern-

ment. This interrelationship is implied in Fig. 15-1, which depicts the levels of governmental health activity.

## LOCAL HEALTH ORGANIZATION

On the lowest or local level, where in the final analysis most service to the public is actually rendered, there are several agencies with varying degrees of official concern for the public health. It is here that direct person-to-person contact is made between the public and their locally employed public health personnel. Although the most personal of all health services are rendered by private practitioners of medicine, dentistry, and nursing, their place in the picture will not be presented at this point other than to include them in the diagrams. Similarly the part played by the voluntary agencies is included diagrammatically here and discussed in Chapter 16. Local health departments therefore are designed to render on-the-spot, direct service to the people of a local governmental jurisdiction. The units of local governments may be municipalities, towns, townships, counties, or combinations of them. Organizations concerned with the health of towns and cities were established relatively early in United States history. In an attempt to serve the more rural areas townships or civil districts have been used extensively in the past. With the development of good roads and rapid transportation, however, this makeshift arrangement has been undergoing a process of abandonment in favor of the establishment of countywide health departments. Of additional significance, as has

**Fig. 15-1.** Levels of health organization. The complete health structure. (From Mountin, J. W., and Flook, E.: Guide to health organization in the United States, Public Health Service pub. no. 196, Washington, D. C., 1953.)

been mentioned, is the recent trend toward the formation of joint city-county health departments and even multicounty arrangements.

The establishment of public health organizations on the basis of these larger units of local government or combinations of them has been necessitated by a consideration of the number of people and the size of area adequate to raise enough public tax funds to support at least a minimum staff of qualified public health workers. In most instances it is recommended that an area should contain at least 50,000 people before it considers the establishment of a health unit of its own. Exceptions exist, of course, depending essentially on wealth, density, health problems, and geography. As of 1966, there were in the United States 1,712 full-time official local health agencies of one type or another that served 2,437 counties and 362 cities, covering areas with a combined population of more than 186 million people, or 95.4% of the population. Areas not reported as served by local health agencies included about 9 million people, or 4.6% of the nation's population.[2] Since then, although exact information is not available, it is known that additional areas have been included in county or district health units to bring the population served even closer to 100%.

The characteristics of the counties that have no organized health services other than what may be obtained from the state are generally as follows:

1. They are located in 27 states, primarily in the western Great Plains and Rocky Mountain areas.

2. They have small total populations and are sparsely inhabited.

3. The median age of their population is relatively high.

4. Generally they have lost population in recent years.

5. A high proportion of the population is employed in agriculture and relatively few in manufacturing.

6. They have a significantly smaller percentage of nonwhite inhabitants than the country as a whole.

7. They have a relatively high family income and educational level.

8. They have a higher percentage of occupant-owned dwellings than the rest of the country.

To reconsider areas with organized full-time health services the pattern throughout the nation is by no means uniform. Much variation may be observed with regard to numbers and qualifications of personnel, types of programs, and financing. Personnel and finances, hence programs, are especially thin in areas where local health services are provided by state district health units.

As a consequence of these inadequacies and inequities and because of the general broadening scope of the field of public health, the 1940s saw the development of a forceful movement to achieve complete coverage of the nation with adequate and practical full-time local health units. It was keynoted by the widely quoted Emerson report, *Local Health Units for the Nation*,[3] and promoted by a series of national, regional, and state conferences. The movement culminated in attempts to obtain legislation to provide federal subsidization of local health units through state health departments. Emerson and his committee suggested as a goal the establishment of a total of 1,197 units to include 318 single-county units, 821 multi-county units, 36 county-district units, 22 city units and 1 unit of 3 cities. The populations of these units would have ranged at the time from 10,200 to 7.5 million, with an average of 110,000.

Despite these extensive efforts, only a few additional full-time local health units were created. In 1947 there were 1,284 units covering 1,874 counties, and by 1960 they had increased to only 1,557 units covering 2,425 counties. This, in conjunction with a recognition of the nature of the uncovered areas just presented, led to a reexamination of the bases on which full-time local health units should be established—or might conceivably not be practical or needed. In reflecting on the saturation point that seemed to have been reached in the establishment of such units, Haldeman[4] stated:

This may stem from the many changes in health problems which have occurred over the years. It may be that new and additional resources such as voluntary health agencies, industrial health programs, insurance schemes and other prepayment plans are now providing, more acceptably, some services which in the past were supplied by the health department. Or perhaps the greater interest of private physicians in preventive medicine coupled with better methods of communication and transportation and increased public enlightenment regarding the individual's own responsibility for his personal health have reduced the need for organized health departments.

Another not necessarily conflicting viewpoint might hold that the plateau in organizational development of local health agencies is temporary and a reflection of the transition from a period of public attitude and professional programming based essentially on communicability to one based essentially on the complexities of the control of chronic disease and the provision of comprehensive medical care. The ultimate effect of the many medical care programs begun in the second half of the 1960s and the early 1970s will be interesting to watch.

The usual pattern of organizational interrelationships involved in the provision of health services on the local level is shown in Fig. 15-2. Necessarily a health department on the local or any other level cannot be expected to include within its organization personnel and facilities for the solution of every phase of the public health problems of the community. This was the essential theme of the National Commission on Community Health Services, which produced several concise and provocative reports

**Fig. 15-2.** Levels of health organization. The ground floor of the health structure—local official and voluntary agencies and private practitioners. (From Mountin, J. W., and Flook, E.: Guide to health organization in the United States, Public Health Service pub. no. 196, Washington, D. C., 1953.)

in the late 1960s,[5,6] that in the years ahead each community must make maximum collaborative use of all of its health resources regardless of formal organizational or other distinctions. Many other persons and agencies play important roles. In rural areas county farm agents and home demonstration agents are active in nutrition and health education. The department of public works has a most important responsibility for sanitary waste disposal. Departments of education, welfare, police, and others all contribute in some degree to the community health program. Nevertheless, the local health department should be the focal point, the catalyst, and the leader in activities in this field.

On three occasions, 1940, 1950, and 1963, the American Public Health Association has issued official policy statements concerned with services and responsibilities of local health departments.[7] It emphasizes that the fundamental responsibility of a local health department is (1) to determine the health status and health needs of the people within its jurisdiction, (2) to determine the extent to which these needs are being met by effective measures currently available, and (3) to take steps to see that the unmet needs are satisfied. It also places emphasis on the role of the local health department in social planning, particularly in the areas of medical care, regional planning of health services, effective use of natural resources, and efficient delivery of traditional services. With reference to specific functions of local health departments those listed in the 1950 policy statement were considered still valid in 1963, and they still are today, recognizing the need, however, to be constantly alert to new emerging problems. The following therefore may be regarded as appropriate basic functions of a local health department:

I.  Recording and analysis of health data
    A.  Recording and analysis of reports of births, deaths, marriages, divorces, and notifiable diseases
    B.  Maintenance of registers of individuals known to have certain specific long-term diseases and impairments
    C.  Conduct of special surveys to determine the prevalence and resultant disability from various diseases
    D.  Collection and interpretation of morbidity data from such sources as clinics, hospitals, organized nursing services, prepayment plans, industry, and workmen's compensation and disability insurance programs
    E.  Maintenance of continuing records on the number and qualifications of all types of health personnel, the quantitative and qualitative resources of available facilities, and the types and extent of health services provided through various voluntary and public programs
    F.  Periodic evaluation of community health needs and services

II.  Health education and information
    A.  Stimulation of the public to recognize health problems that exist, to study the resources available for meeting the problems, and to develop and put into action programs designed to solve them
    B.  Cooperation with and assistance of official and voluntary organizations such as departments of education and civic, youth, and other community groups in the development of their health programs
    C.  Provision of individual instruction by public health nurses and other personnel, as in the case of families in which communicable disease has occurred, of mothers attending well-baby conferences, or of diabetic and other patients who are taught to follow the regimen prescribed by the family physician
    D.  Organization of lectures, classes, and courses, such as parents' classes, courses for food-handlers, classes for diabetics, and lectures to community groups
    E.  Use of mass educational and informational media such as newspapers, magazines, pamphlets, movies, radio, and television
    F.  Development of a well-rounded program of professional education, designed to assist the local health professions to maintain and improve the quality of service

III.  Supervision and regulation
    A.  Protection of food, water, and milk supplies
    B.  Control of nuisances, sanitary disposal of wastes, and control of water and air pollution
    C.  Prevention of occupational diseases and accidents
    D.  Control of human and animal sources of infection
    E.  Regulation of housing
    F.  Inspection of hospitals, nursing homes, and other health facilities by means of
        1.  Public education and individual instruction
        2.  Issuance of regulations
        3.  Laboratory control
        4.  Inspection and licensure
        5.  Revocation of permits and, as a last resort, court action

IV.  Provision of environmental health services (as necessary)
    A.  Construction of pit privies

B. Drainage and larvicidal treatment of mosquito-breeding areas and residual spraying of homes for insect control

C. Rat proofing of buildings and other rodent and insect control measures

V. Administration of personal health services

A. Immunization against infectious diseases and other preventive measures such as the application of fluoride to children's teeth

B. Advisory health maintenance service, as in child health conferences, prenatal clinics, parents' classes, and public health nursing visits

C. Case-finding surveys of the general population, such as chest x-ray surveys, serologic tests for syphilis, cancer detection programs, and school health examination (adult health inventories and "multiphasic" surveys for the detection of various groups of diseases may also be included)

D. Provision of diagnostic aids to physicians, such as laboratory services and crippled children's, cancer, cardiac, and other diagnostic and consultation clinics

E. Provision of diagnostic and treatment services for specific diseases such as syphilis, tuberculosis, dental defects in children and expectant mothers, and orthopedic, cardiac, and other crippling impairments in children

VI. Operation of health facilities

A. Operation of health centers and clinics

B. Operation of general or special hospitals (as necessary)

VII. Coordination of activities and resources

A. Provision of effective leadership in meeting community health needs

B. Encouragement of coordination of various official and voluntary agencies to avoid duplication and overlapping and to assure efficient and economical administration

C. Participation on interdepartmental or regional boards dealing with public water supplies, sewage and refuse disposal, control of atmospheric pollution, housing, city planning, hospital planning, zoning regulation, development of recreational areas, and other public programs that have significant implications for community health

To carry out its mandate the official public health agency in rural or small urban situations requires only a relatively simple type of organizational structure. Legal responsibility for the public's health is commonly placed in a local board of health, the members of which are appointed by the locally elected officials, that is, in cities by mayors and in counties by boards of supervisors or their equivalent. The board of health usually appoints and employs a county health officer, frequently subject to approval by the state health department. Increasingly, state health departments have been establishing standards and qualifications that must be met by those appointed to local public health positions. This particular type of state supervision has met with relatively little local resistance, since in most instances local units of government have found it necessary to turn to the state health department for assistance in finding capable candidates for the position. Although assistant medical personnel are occasionally found in county health departments, the nationwide shortage of personnel and the general inadequacy of local funds have served to preclude the employment of more than one physician in a great many county health departments.

The employment of all other personnel is customarily a prerogative of the local health officer but subject to civil service regulations if they exist. This, of course, is proper. Depending on the size and nature of the jurisdiction, the health officer's staff usually consists of one or several workers in environmental health, public health nursing, and office management as well as a health educator and a laboratory worker. If possible, sometimes, nutritionists, public health dentists, and representatives of other professions are employed even in small local agencies, again depending on local needs, wishes, and resources. The workers in environmental health may consist of combinations of engineers, professionally trained sanitarians, or sanitary inspectors trained on the job. The preferred situation for most county health departments would probably be a sanitary engineer in addition to an adequate number of professionally trained sanitarians. Usually, approximately one half the funds and one half the positions of the local health department are devoted to public health nursing. This means that, of the various professions, nursing will be most represented. Even the smallest local health unit will or should have several nurses on its staff. This being the case, whereas an actual division of public health nursing may not exist structurally, one of the nurses, selected on the basis of training, experience, and personality, should be appointed as supervising nurse. Where several office workers are employed, one should be designated to serve as office manager and to supervise the work of the others. In this way responsibilities are much more likely to be clear cut and understood by those concerned. All members of the staff, as indicated in Fig. 10-2, should be ultimately responsible to the county health officer, who in turn is responsible to the board.

Current basic standards suggest the employment of the following types and numbers of professional personnel to provide the *minimum* desirable services to a community:

Medical personnel—1 per 50,000 population (the best qualified to serve as health officer, the others preferably to direct the school health program, maternal and child health program, and epidemiology program)

Environmental health personnel—1 per 15,000 population (one preferably an engineer)

Staff nursing personnel—1 per 5,000 population (1 per 2,500 population if home bedside nursing is included)

Supervisory nursing personnel—1 per 6 to 8 staff nurses

Office personnel—1 per 15,000 population

Other specialized personnel—as problems demand and funds make possible

When funds and candidates are not available to make possible the employment of other types of personnel that may be needed or when employment of full-time employees is not practical, as is sometimes the case in staffing clinics, the gap may be filled by the part-time employment of private practitioners or the use of services of district or state agencies. Wherever possible, however, the employment of full-time personnel is recommended. Obviously it is desirable that at least the health officer and the supervisory staff have had specialized training in public health.

In the larger local units of government, particularly municipalities or combinations of them with their surrounding county areas, more extensive personnel and organization obviously are required. In general the distribution of types of personnel per unit of population is similar to that followed in the smaller areas, with various numbers of different types of specialists added to meet the problems and demands inherent in the particular situation. The increased total number of employees naturally leads to the formation of a more formalized organizational structure with the bringing together of similar and related functions into divisions and bureaus. The general pattern still holds with the same basic principles of organization followed. Although there is no standard organizational structure, certain functional divisions are nevertheless almost universally encountered. Thus there usually exist divisions of vital statistics and records; sanitation, sanitary engineering, or environmental health; maternal and child health; public health nursing, either as an entity or integrated into the activities of several of the other divisions; laboratory service; epidemiologic service or communicable disease control; and health education. Increasingly one also finds a division of adult health, chronic disease and medical care. Each category large enough to comprise a unit should have its director and possibly subdirectors. The direct professional service activities of those in the top administrative positions become greatly minimized, giving way to functions of a managerial and supervisory nature. An example of a more extensive agency is presented in Fig. 10-9.

## STATE HEALTH ORGANIZATION

Still more varied is the pattern of public health organization on the state level. In each instance more than one agency has responsibility for activities in this field. A study[8] made by the Public Health Service in 1950 indicated a total of 60 different types of state agencies that contributed in some way to state health programs. The diversity of these agencies may be seen from the following consolidated tabulation:

Department of health

Department of welfare, social security, emergency relief, general assistance, etc.

Department of agriculture

Department of labor, labor and industry, labor and immigration, etc.

Department of education, public instruction, etc.

Special boards, commissions, or independent offices established specifically for the activity indicated (tuberculosis board or commission, cancer commission, workmen's compensation commission or bureau, industrial accident board, dairy and food commission, hotel commission, livestock sanitary board, water resources board, commission for the blind, crippled children's commission, mental disease commission or department, state toxicologist, state veterinarian, etc.)

Board of control of affairs, department of state institutions, etc.

Independent state hospital, independent state laboratory

Department of conservation

State university or college

Department of mines and minerals

Department of engineering, department of public utilities

State experiment station

Independent licensing and examining boards

Department of motor vehicles, department of public safety

Department of civil service and registration, department of registration and education

Other departments or offices of state government

The variety of state agencies participating in health activities is not measured alone by the aggregate count. Dispersion of health responsibility is also extreme and varied when viewed within individual states. The number of agencies performing health activities in a single state ranges from 10 to 32. . . . The variation among states in assignment of responsibility for health functions is due in great measure to two main factors: Complexity of state governmental organization and extent of health services provided by the state. The former is probably the more important in determining the total number of agencies. . . .

Numerous agencies are often responsible for a single activity within a state. As many as 13 separate agencies are engaged in accident prevention work in one state, while a total of 12 participate in some form of health education in another. Other programs in which 7 or more individual agencies participate in at least one of the States are mental hygiene,

crippled children's services, prevention and treatment of blindness, licensure for health reasons, medical care, vocational rehabilitation (restorative measures), maternal and child health, hygiene of housing, and school health services. With this multiplicity of agencies concerned with a single health program within a state, it is easy to imagine some of the difficulties encountered in developing uniform standards of performance and achieving common goals.

As indicated by a more recent analysis by the Association of State and Territorial Health Officers,[9] this complex and diffuse situation on the state level has not clarified appreciably since the earlier survey was conducted. In fact some additional agencies and offices have been added by many states. Among these are departments of human or social resources, environmental protection agencies, comprehensive health planning agencies, and a variety of others. However, in every state without exception one agency is invested with primary legal responsibility for the public health program. Usually this is a state department of public health, although in some instances public health may be a division in a larger department

**Fig. 15-3.** Levels of health organization. The second floor of the health structure—state official and voluntary agencies and professional societies. (From Mountin, J. W., and Flook, E.: Guide to health organization in the United States, Public Health Service pub. no. 196, Washington, D. C., 1953.)

of health and welfare of human resources or of social services. However, as on the local level, the state health department should provide the leadership on its governmental level in public health matters, all other agencies acting in this field as collaborating or auxiliary agencies. This relationship of a state department of public health with other agencies on its level has been illustrated by Mountin and Flook (Fig. 15-3).

In all except a few states the direct personal service functions of state health departments are decidedly few and limited essentially to the provision of traveling specialized personnel and mobile equipment to sparsely populated local areas unable to afford them. Many state health departments, for example, staff, equip, and maintain mobile chest x-ray units, dental clinics, immunization clinics, and facilities for the examination and treatment of the venereal diseases. In recent years an increasing number of states have developed and used mobile chronic disease multiphasic screening units and mobile equipment for health education, health career promotion, and nutrition services. In general the functions of a state health department are the following[10]:

1. To represent the public health interests and goals of the state to the elected governing body of the state
2. To promulgate and enforce public health rules and regulations applicable throughout the state
3. To determine state public health policy and to provide a state-wide coordinated public health program with clear objectives for the guidance of local health departments
4. To promote the establishment of full-time local health units
5. To develop an appropriate plan for the coordination of local health services with related hospital and medical programs which may be developed on a regional basis
6. To provide financial assistance to supplement the resources of local health departments
7. To make consultation and other special services available
8. To assist localities to set up demonstrations on a temporary basis
9. To establish minimum and stimulate optimum standards of performance
10. To develop a recruitment and training program for local health department personnel
11. To delegate certain legal responsibilities of the state health agency, insofar as feasible and practical, to well-organized and adequately staffed local health departments
12. To carry on all relationships with local citizens and groups through the medium of or in cooperation with the local health departments
13. To carry on a statewide program of health education
14. To evaluate continually or periodically existing state and local programs

From this list it is possible to summarize state health department functions into the several basic categories of statewide planning, intergovernmental relations, intrastate agency relations, and a certain statewide policy determination, standard setting, and regulatory functions. But above all else the chief reason for a state health department is the extent to which it stimulates and assists local departments to do a satisfactory job.

This is reflected in an analysis of the structure of health services in the states,[11] which indicates that most activities are distributed under five most common major units of organization: administration, preventive medicine, environmental health, local health services, and laboratories. In performing the details of work within each of these the several states engage in a wide variety of activities (Table 15-1). It should be noted that different terms are frequently used for activities that represent or include the same or similar activities. Thus whereas only one state lists grant-in-aid administration as an activity per se, this function is performed elsewhere in the organization as part of local health administration (4 states) and local health services (42 states).

Although this list of particular functions of state health agencies appears long, diffuse, and inadequate, the basic activities and the extent of involvement by various agencies were brought out by the recent analysis of the Association of State and Territorial Health Officers' Health Program Reporting System Project.[9] Their findings are summarized in Table 15-2.

In attempting to carry out the many activities listed, each of the 50 states has developed its own unique pattern. Some have constructed strongly centralized organizations, in contrast with others with activities decentralized insofar as possible. As discussed and illustrated in Chapter 10, the subdivisions or functional units within the structure of state health departments vary extensively both in number and in manner of emphasis and arrangement. No two state patterns are identical, but similarities are to be noted. Thus an analysis by the Association of Management in Public Health indicated that

**Table 15-1.** Frequency of activities in 50 state health departments*

| Activity | Frequency | Activity | Frequency |
|---|---|---|---|
| 1. Abattoirs | 1 | 53. Local health services | 42 |
| 2. Accident prevention | 8 | 54. Machine tabulation | 2 |
| 3. Administrative services | 9 | 55. Masseur license | 1 |
| 4. Adult health | 3 | 56. Maternal and child health | 50 |
| 5. Air pollution | 10 | 57. Meat and poultry inspection | 1 |
| 6. Alcoholism | 9 | 58. Medical and/or hospital care | 5 |
| 7. Bacteriology | 15 | 59. Mental care | 1 |
| 8. Barbers and beauticians | 6 | 60. Mental health | 27 |
| 9. Bedding and upholstery | 6 | 61. Mental retardation program | 4 |
| 10. Biologics | 6 | 62. Merit system—local | 1 |
| 11. Blood bank | 1 | 63. Merit system—state agency | 3 |
| 12. Branch laboratories | 10 | 64. Milk sanitation | 14 |
| 13. Building maintenance | 1 | 65. Narcotics control | 2 |
| 14. Camp sanitation | 2 | 66. Nursing | 50 |
| 15. Cancer control | 31 | 67. Nursing homes | 6 |
| 16. Canning and bottling plants | 1 | 68. Nutrition | 29 |
| 17. Central files | 1 | 69. Oil field pollution | 1 |
| 18. Chest x-ray survey | 3 | 70. Orthopedic program | 1 |
| 19. Child guidance | 2 | 71. Payroll | 1 |
| 20. Chronic diseases control | 30 | 72. Pedodontics | 1 |
| 21. Civil defense | 7 | 73. Personnel | 34 |
| 22. Communicable diseases | 45 | 74. Plumbing | 6 |
| 23. Crime detection laboratory | 1 | 75. Pneumotherapy stations | 1 |
| 24. Crippled children's services | 26 | 76. Poison information | 2 |
| 25. Dairy products | 2 | 77. Polio control | 1 |
| 26. Dental health | 46 | 78. Professional registration and license | 3 |
| 27. Diabetes control | 1 | 79. Program planning, development, and evaluation | 7 |
| 28. Diagnostic services | 4 | | |
| 29. Engineering | 43 | 80. Property control | 3 |
| 30. Environmental health | 50 | 81. Public relations | 1 |
| 31. Epidemiology | 11 | 82. Publications | 4 |
| 32. Examining boards | 2 | 83. Rabies control | 1 |
| 33. Film library | 1 | 84. Radiologic health | 11 |
| 34. Finance, fiscal, accounting, etc. | 13 | 85. Regional offices | 18 |
| 35. Food and drug control | 24 | 86. Research | 5 |
| 36. Funeral director licensure | 1 | 87. Rheumatic fever | 2 |
| 37. Geriatrics | 3 | 88. Sanitarian local services | 1 |
| 38. General sanitation | 19 | 89. School health services | 11 |
| 39. Grants-in-aid administration | 1 | 90. Shellfish sanitation | 5 |
| 40. Health education | 50 | 91. Social services | 6 |
| 41. Hearing and vision | 4 | 92. Staff health services | 1 |
| 42. Heart disease control | 25 | 93. Statistical services | 6 |
| 43. Hospital survey, planning, and construction licensure | 42 | 94. Training | 8 |
| | | 95. Tuberculosis control | 43 |
| 44. Hospitals and sanatoria administration | 16 | 96. Typhus control | 1 |
| 45. Hotel sanitation | 3 | 97. Vector control | 12 |
| 46. Housing | 1 | 98. Venereal disease control | 30 |
| 47. Industrial health | 36 | 99. Veterinary medicine | 13 |
| 48. Institutional sanitation | 1 | 100. Vital statistics | 49 |
| 49. Laboratories | 47 | 101. Water and sewage | 23 |
| 50. Legal services | 4 | 102. Water pollution | 19 |
| 51. Library | 4 | 103. Well drilling | 1 |
| 52. Local health administration | 4 | | |

*Included are all activities on the 50 organizational charts phrased to have a fairly clear meaning. About 40 other activities are not included because of varying degrees of ambiguity or lack of definition. None thus deleted occurred in more than 10% of the 50 charts reviewed.

**Table 15-2.** Extent of responsibility of state and territorial health departments for basic health functions, United States, 1971

| Functions | Number of programs | Involvement (%) | | | | | | |
|---|---|---|---|---|---|---|---|---|
| | | State health department only | Local health department only | State and local health departments jointly | State and local health departments and another agency | Independent agency (major state health department support) | Independent agency (minor state health department support) | Independent agency (no state health department support) |
| Preventive and personal health services | 1151 | 36 | 3 | 35 | 16 | 5 | 4 | 1 |
| Mental health care | 116 | 44 | 1 | 36 | 5 | 9 | 5 | ½ |
| Environmental control | 552 | 40 | 2 | 43 | 10 | 1 | 2 | 2 |
| Consumer protection | 192 | 50 | 1 | 38 | 9 | — | 1 | 1 |
| Certification, standard setting, and licensure | 414 | 80 | 1 | 9 | 8 | 1 | 1 | — |
| Health resource development | 367 | 70 | 1 | 7 | 16 | 2 | 3 | 1 |
| Professional services | 607 | 71 | 2 | 14 | 10 | 1 | 2 | ½ |
| Health management services | 340 | 86 | 1 | 4 | 4 | 1 | 2 | 2 |

in two thirds of the instances the state health commissioner had a span of control of 7 divisions or bureaus comprising: (1) administration (including finance, personnel, hospital administration, vital statistics, and health education), (2) local health services (usually including public health nursing), (3) preventive medicine (usually including chronic diseases and adult health and sometimes mental health), (4) maternal and child health (usually including nutrition and crippled children's services), (5) dental health, (6) environmental health (including industrial hygiene and sanitary engineering), and (7) laboratories.

In summary, the trend has been for state health departments to restrict direct services as much as possible, to limit the number of major organizational units to about a half dozen to make possible an effective executive span of control, and to decentralize activities, particularly in larger states.

## FEDERAL HEALTH ORGANIZATION

### General

The most complex organizational picture of public health in the United States is found on the federal level. The history and development of some of the federal public health agencies have been discussed in Chapter 2. The purpose at this point is merely to describe briefly the more important of them and to bring out their interrelationships. Until recently, in place of a federal department of health there existed an illogical maze of miscellaneous departments, bureaus, offices, agencies, commissions, services, and authorities, each responsible for one or several aspects of the federal government's concern with health. This situation came about through a pyramiding of special legislation, often originating from executive requests, bureaucratic expansion, or the pressure of special interest groups.

Once an agency is formed or designated to deal with a particular interest, that interest and the independence of the agency involved are jealously guarded. An extreme result of such a procedure is well illustrated by the fact that the responsibility for the health of the inhabitants of the Pribilof Islands was for long vested in the Fish and Wildlife Service of the Department of the Interior. Recent years have seen repeated and accelerating attempts to consolidate this perplexing and mushrooming group of federal agencies. At best, however, consolidation of governmental affairs is a slow process.

Secretary
Undersecretary

Assistant Secretary for Health

Office of Education

Social Security Administration

Social and Rehabilitation Service

Assistant Secretary for Administration
Assistant Secretary Comptroller
General Counsel
Assistant Secretary for Legislation
Assistant Secretary for Planning and Evaluation
Assistant Secretary for Community and Field Services
Assistant Secretary for Education
Office of Public Information

Executive Secretariat

Public Affairs

General function offices

Special function offices
Professional standards review
International health
Population affairs
Nursing home affairs

Public Health Service

Food and Drug Administration
Foods
Product safety
Drugs
Biologics
Veterinary medicine
Radiological health
National center for toxicological research

Center for Disease Control
Epidemiology
Laboratories
State services
Smallpox eradication program
Training program
Tropical disease program
National clearinghouse for smoking and health
National Institute for occupational safety and health

National Institutes of Health
Aging
Cancer
Eye
Heart and lung
Allergy and infectious diseases
Arthritis, metabolism and digestive diseases
Child health and human development
Dental research
Environmental health sciences
General medical sciences
Neurological diseases and stroke
National library of medicine
National clinical center
Division of biological standards
Division of computer research and technology
Fogarty International Center

Health Resources Administration
National center for health statistics
National center for health services research and development
Bureau of health resources development
Medicine
Nursing
Associated health professions
Comprehensive facilities utilization
Health resource planning
Regional medical programs

Health Services Administration
Community health services
Indian health service
Bureau of medical services
Bureau of quality assurance

Alcoholism, Drug Abuse and Mental Health Administration
Alcoholism control
Drug abuse control
Mental health

**Fig. 15-4.** Organization of the Department of Health, Education, and Welfare.

In the health and social services field, progress was gradually made, resulting first in the formation of the Federal Security Agency in 1939 and eventually in the establishment on April 11, 1953, of a Department of Health, Education, and Welfare.

The many federal agencies that developed over the years with responsibility for one or more aspects of public health fell into four primary categories. The first was more or less concerned with broad general interests. The only example has been the Public Health Service. The second category was concerned with the welfare of special groups in the population. Examples were the Children's Bureau, the Women's Bureau, the Administration on Aging, the Farmer's Home Administration, the Agricultural Extension Service, the Bureau of Indian Affairs, the Medical Divisions of the Army and the Navy, and the Veterans Administration. The third category included agencies concerned with special problems or programs, such as the Office of Education, the Social and Rehabilitation Service, the Food and Drug Administration, the Federal Trade Commission, the Bureau of Labor Standards, the Bureau of Labor Statistics, many bureaus within the Department of Agriculture (animal industry, entomology and plant quarantine, dairy industry, production and marketing, human nutrition and home economics, etc.), the Bureau of Mines, the Maritime Commission, and the Tennessee Valley Authority. The Social Security Administration and the Bureau of Employees' Compensation may also be included in this category in the sense that they provide medical care to special groups. The fourth category may be considered to handle the international health interests of the government of the United States. The functions of these agencies have varied from direct personal service to regulation, consultation, demonstration, research, education, and financial grants-in-aid.

As stated, the most important of the federal agencies dealing with public health matters were brought together in 1953 to form the Department of Health, Education, and Welfare. This agency was created with the purpose of grouping under one administration those agencies of the government whose major functions are to promote social and economic security, educational opportunity, and the health of the citizens of the nation.

During recent years, many of the scattered health-related functions of the national government have been transferred to the Department of Health, Education, and Welfare. Among these have been the Children's Bureau (now the Maternal and Child Health Service), the Administration on Aging, the health and medical functions of the Bureau of Indian Affairs, the Food and Drug Administration, and the Social and Rehabilitation Service. These program incorporations plus a great many new responsibilities that have resulted from recent legislative actions have made it necessary for the Department of Health, Education, and Welfare, and especially its health component to go through a difficult period of repeated searches or trials in an attempt to develop an effective and efficient organizational structure.

The frequency and complexity of these efforts have been well described by Sims,[12] using as a basis for analysis the unit entitled HSMHA (Health Services and Mental Health Administration), which functioned between April 1968 and mid-1973 as the arm of the Public Health Service responsible essentially for operational programs in contrast with the large research programs of the National Institutes of Health and the regulatory functions of the Food and Drug Administration. As Sims describes, the Public Health Service functioned during the 23 years between 1944 and 1967 with four basic units: (1) the Office of the Surgeon General, which dealt with overall management and international affairs; (2) the Bureau of State Services, which was involved with advice, consultation, and subsidization of various state programs; (3) the Bureau of Medical Services, which was responsible for all direct health care functions such as the Public Health Service clinics and hospitals, the health care programs for the Coast Guard, Amerindians, federal prisoners and others, as well as operation of St. Elizabeth's Hospital and Freedmen's Hospital in the District of Columbia; and (4) the National Institutes of Health. As indicated, this arrangement worked well for 23 years, but in the years since 1967, as a result of transfers, new programs, and new administrations, there have occurred about a dozen reorganizations of greater or lesser magnitude.

One of the most significant changes was the establishment in 1967 of a cabinet-level post in the form of an Assistant Secretary for Health. This office assumed the direct managerial and supervisory functions of the Surgeon General, who was designated as Chief Deputy to the Assistant Secretary. It should be noted that the Office of Surgeon General and the organization, the Public Health Service under which all functions are included, have a long legislative standing.

## Public Health Service

From the broad overall point of view of public health the principal organization included in the Department of Health, Education, and Welfare is the United States Public Health Service. Most of the functions of the Public Health Service take the form of research, demonstrations, interstate and international quarantine, advice on technical matters, and loan of officers to state and local health departments and other federal agencies with particular health interests. Probably its most significant contribution is made through financial grants-in-aid to state and territorial health agencies for the expansion and improvement of their programs and those of the local jurisdictions they include. The functions of the service may be summarized as follows:

1. Study of the causes and means of propagation and spread of the diseases of mankind and development of methods of prevention and control.

In this work the Public Health Service maintains several research laboratories, chief among which are those of the National Institutes of Health in Bethesda, Md., and the Center for Disease Control in Atlanta. In addition to investigations carried on at the Institutes and their field stations, financial assistance is given through research grants to universities, laboratories, and other public and private institutions for research projects on recommendation of Public Health Service advisory councils. Funds are also available for research fellowships, both in the Institutes and in various educational institutions.

2. Maritime quarantine and inspection of passengers and crews of vessels and airplanes arriving from foreign ports for protection of the country from the importation of quarantinable diseases from other countries.

Immigrants are examined for detection and isolation of persons suffering from mandatorily excludable disease. Medical inspection of aliens is performed in collaboration with the Immigration and Naturalization Service of the Department of Justice.

3. Interstate quarantine for prevention of the spread of diseases from state to state.

The Public Health Service prescribes conditions under which persons and things may move in interstate commerce from the standpoints of health and public safety. It assists states in controlling epidemics and may, on request, take complete charge of serious outbreaks. Regulation of conditions existing within the boundaries of a particular state is a duty that remains under state jurisdiction.

4. Dissemination of public health information, including collection and publication of reports of disease prevalence in the United States and foreign countries, and other pertinent information regarding conservation of the public health.

5. Assistance, through grants to states, counties, cities, and health districts, in establishing and maintaining public health services—including industrial hygiene, mental hygiene, and cancer control—and special programs for the control of the venereal diseases and tuberculosis.

Grants made under this authority represent the actual transfer of funds from federal to state treasuries for employment and training of personnel for state and local health work, purchase of supplies and equipment, provision of appropriate facilities for care and treatment of designated illnesses, and payment of general operating expenses. Services include the loan of personnel for temporary duty and the provision of consultation and advice to state and local health departments. Assistance is also furnished to states in the development of hospitalization plans and improvement of hospital and allied health facilities.

6. Supervisory control and licensure of the manufacturers of biologic products—vaccines, serums, toxins, antitoxins, and similar preparations—used in the prevention and treatment of diseases.

This control has been established to ensure safe and standard products.

7. Study of mental diseases, alcoholism, and drug addiction, and certification of legitimate needs for narcotic drugs.

8. Provision of hospitalization, general medical and dental care, and preventive health services for American merchant seamen, members of the United States Coast Guard and the Coast and Geodetic Survey, and for other legal beneficiaries of the Public Health Service.

The service also provides medical care and public health services to Indian wards of the government and Alaskan Eskimos.

9. Operation of special hospitals—the National Leprosarium and a hospital specifically for the care of mental patients and persons addicted to the use of narcotics.

10. Cooperation with other federal agencies in discharging their various health functions through assignment of personnel for assistance.

11. Collaboration with and participation in the functioning of international health organizations.

In carrying out this service particular attention is given to the direction of programs for the exchange of international health and related personnel.

12. Collection and publication of data on vital statistics, which are basic materials for public health programs and give valuable information concerning public health trends.

Through measurement of death rates from different causes the progress of health programs directed toward reduction of particular diseases or conditions can be evaluated.

At present (1974) the Public Health Service is directed by the Assistant Secretary for Health and is organized into 6 functional units: (1) the Center for Disease Control, (2) the Food and Drug Administration, (3) the Health Resources Administration, (4) the Health Services Administration, (5) the National Institutes of Health, and (6) the Alcohol, Drug Abuse and Mental Health Administration (Fig. 15-4). In addition, the Office of the Assistant Secretary has several staff offices directly related to it. These are divided as follows: (1) general functional offices (administrative management, policy development and planning, program operations, and regional operations) and (2) special functional offices (executive secretariat, public affairs, professional standards review, international health, population affairs, and nursing home affairs).

It should be noted that with the establishment of the Environmental Protection Agency at the end of 1970, most of the environmental health activities and responsibilities of the Public Health Service were transferred to it. In addition, toward the goal of getting out of direct personal services, the Freedmen's Hospital was transferred to Howard University, St. Elizabeth's Hospital to the District of Columbia, and some of the Public Health Service hospitals to the jurisdictions in which they are located. For decentralization of services and more effective assistance to States, 10 regional offices are maintained in Boston, New York, Philadelphia, Atlanta, Chicago, Kansas City, Dallas, Denver, San Francisco, and Seattle. In addition to a National Advisory Health Council, a number of special advisory councils and committees composed of nongovernmental experts are available to many of the institutes and programs. Each year the Assistant Secretary for Health (formerly the Surgeon General) meets at an annual conference with the state and territorial health officers and with certain other special groups.

In mid-March 1973 the Office of the Assistant Secretary of Health was reorganized to include five deputy assistant secretaries for program operations, for policy development, for medical and scientific affairs, for administration and management, and for population affairs. There also continue under the Assistant Secretary for Health the Office of Nursing Home Affairs, the Office of International Health, the Office of Professional Standards and Review Organizations, and the Special Assistant for Drug Abuse Prevention. In May 1973 it was decided to subdivide The Health Services and Mental Health Administration. The National Institute of Mental Health was joined with the alcoholism and drug abuse programs. The result is a Public Health Service with six functional clusters, or operational units, each reporting to the Assistant Secretary for Health.

1. The Health Services Administration, concerned with health service grants and direct health care delivery systems
2. The Health Resources Administration, containing the health service data gathering health surveillance, health service research and development, and manpower education
3. The Center for Disease Control, including the National Institute for Occupational Safety and Health and the remaining functions of the Bureau of Community Environmental Management
4. The National Institutes of Health, responsible for intramural and extramural biomedical research
5. The Food and Drug Administration, the department's major consumer protection agency
6. The Alcohol, Drug Abuse and Mental Health Administration.

It is considered that this new organizational configuration will provide a more reasonably manageable spectrum of functional units of organization and coordination of effort than has been true in the past two decades.

## Children's Bureau

Over many years, next in importance to the Public Health Service has been the Children's Bureau. Originally it was located in the Department of Health, Education, and Welfare. As a result of subsequent program and organizational changes it is now the Bureau of Community Health Services of the Health Service Administration. From a functional viewpoint the separate existence of the Children's Bureau has always appeared somewhat illogical. Its justification has been linked to the two arguments that the needs of children must be considered as a whole and that they form a population group unable to organize and to speak for themselves. A chief function of the bureau was to enable each state to extend and improve the health services for mothers and children. This has been accomplished through assistance to states in the support of prenatal, postnatal, and well-child clinics, of demonstrations of delivery and other services, and of public health nursing services for maternal and child health supervision. The bureau played an important role in the promotion and development of divisions of maternal and child health in all of the state health departments. It has also sponsored cooperative federal and state programs of services for crippled children. The programs of the Children's Bureau were carried on in a manner similar to that of the former Bureau of State Services of the Public Health Service, primarily through grants-in-aid to the states and through consultative services.

During World War II the bureau served as the administrative agency for the Emergency Maternity and Infant Care Program for the wives and infants of servicemen. By early 1949, when that program was terminated, about 1.5 million expectant mothers and about 670,000 infants had been provided with care by private physicians of their choice, paid through the program. As discussed elsewhere, this program not only represented a nationwide experiment in medical care but also provided invaluable experience in medical care administration for many public health workers. The Maternal and Child Health Amendments of 1963 made it possible for the Children's Bureau to provide grants to state and local health agencies for comprehensive maternity care of high-risk mothers. With the passage of the Social Security Amendments of 1965 the Children's Bureau received the responsibility for the administration of Section 532 of Title V, Part 4, which provides for the development of high-quality comprehensive health services to children and youth.

By collecting and distributing information the Children's Bureau, now the Maternal and Child Health Program maintains a clearinghouse on research in progress in the total field of child life, both inside and outside the federal government. It conducts surveys and studies on the nature and extent of child health problems and analyzes and reports statistics on maternal and child health and crippled children's services provided under grant-in-aid programs. It provides federal financial aid for specialized training projects in services to children, to students and workers in child health, and to teaching institutions.

Individually or as a team of specialists in maternal and child health, consultants visit state health and crippled children's agencies to advise on the operation of state programs, standards of service, and ways of extending and improving health services to mothers and children. In carrying out its responsibilities the Maternal and Child Health Program cooperates with official and nonofficial national organizations and institutions; it stimulates interest, participation, and cooperation on the part of educational, social, and welfare agencies for the coordination of resources and services; and it participates in a broad program of international cooperation.

## Food and Drug Administration

The Food and Drug Administration, a part of the Public Health Service reporting directly to the Assistant Secretary for Health in the Department of Health, Education, and Welfare, is chiefly concerned with the quality of foods and drugs. Its efforts are directed toward the promotion of purity, standard potency, and accurate labeling of substances within its jurisdiction, which include food, pharmaceuticals and drugs, cosmetics, tea, certain milk products, and poisons. Most of the consumer protection responsibilities of the federal government are vested in this increasingly important agency.

## Other federal agencies

The Office of Education of the Department of Health, Education, and Welfare is engaged in several activities related to health. It promotes programs of health education and school health and safety, engages in investigations relating to medical examination of school children and their teachers, promotes school lunch programs, and administers a grant-in-aid program for vocational education in health.

Outside the Department of Health, Education, and Welfare are several branches of the Department of Agriculture that engage in programs concerned with health. The Bureau of Animal Industry inquires into the cause, prevention, and treatment of diseases of domestic animals, which naturally have an influence on many phases of human health. Federal meat inspection services are administered by the Production and Marketing Administration, which also administers the Insecticide Act. The labor branch of this office finances medical care and health services for migrant farm workers. The Bureau of Dairy Industry is active in investigations and education relating to the sanitary production and handling of milk. The Bureau of Entomology and Plant Quarantine, although primarily concerned with the protection of crops from parasitic insects, necessarily contributes much knowledge and service to the control of insects affecting man. Active in research and service relating to foods, nutrition, and dietary habits is the Bureau of Human Nutrition and Home Economics, which with the agricultural extension service in cooperation with state land grant colleges has accomplished much in the improvement of rural health and nutrition. Of importance and interest in assistance for medical and dental care is the Farmer's Home Administration within the Department of Agriculture. Its beneficiaries are chiefly low-income farm groups. Needed medical and dental care is made available through provision of supervised credit and loans.

In the Department of the Interior are several agencies with specialized interests in public health problems. The Bureau of Mines conducts an important health, sanitation, and safety program in relation to the mining and quarrying industry. In company with the Fish and Wildlife Service it is concerned with certain phases of the problem of stream pollution. The latter agency also contributes to health protection by promoting rodent control programs. Originally the Department of the Interior through its Office of Indian Affairs had responsibility for the operation of hospitals and programs for the general improvement of health and sanitation on Indian Reservations. In 1953 this responsibility was transferred to the Public Health Service.

## Federal agencies in international health affairs

Originally the interests of the United States Government in international health affairs were limited to measures designed to prevent the introduction of certain diseases. Developments in world history, economics, and methods of transportation, however, have made it necessary to adopt a broader viewpoint and to assume responsibilities of great significance to international public health. These newer responsibilities are of two types: first, participation in development of public health programs in other specific nations and, second, participation as one of a number of partners in the promotion of worldwide health. The most important federal agencies involved in these activities are the Office of International Health of the Public Health Service and the Agency for International Development of the Department of State.

The Office of International Health of the Public Health Service was established to coordinate and give general direction to all service activities in the international health field; to maintain liaison with agencies in this field; to represent the service in international health conferences; to direct a program on international exchange of health personnel and educational material; to draft sanitary conventions and regulations and reports required by international agreements; to collect and distribute data relating to foreign medical and health institutions; to supervise special health missions to foreign countries; to advise the Department of State regarding development of plans, programs, and policies for consideration by the World Health Organization; and to advise the offices of the Secretary of Health, Education, and Welfare, and Surgeon General on International health matters. In relation to the foregoing the United States Government has representation in the World Health Organization, the Pan American Health Organization, and the Anglo-American Caribbean Commission.

The bilateral international health activities of the United States Government are centered in the Agency for International Development of the Department of State. In the planning, staffing, and conduct of its health programs it relates not only to the Office of International Health of the Public Health Service but also to other significant parts of the United States Government, to bilateral health assistance programs of other nations, and any other official or nonofficial organizations concerned with health assistance to developing nations. Much of its work is carried out through cooperative arrangements with state health departments, universities, schools of public health, and schools of medicine and professional associations or organizations.

## REFERENCES

1. Mountin, J. W., and Flook, E.: Guide to health organization in the United States, Public Health Service pub. no. 196, Washington, D. C., 1953 (subsequent changes made).
2. Organization and staffing for local health services, Public Health Service pub. no. 682, Washington, D. C., 1966.
3. American Public Health Association: Local health units for the nation, Report of Sub-Committee on Administration Practice, New York, 1945, Commonwealth Fund.
4. Haldeman, J. C.: Unpublished talk, Annual Meeting of National Advisory Committee on Local Health Departments, Washington, D. C., March 18, 1958.
5. Health is a community affair, National Commission on Community Health Services, Cambridge, 1966, Harvard University Press.
6. Health Administration and organization in the decade ahead, National Commission on Community Health Services, Cambridge, 1967, Harvard University Press.

7. The local health department—services and responsibilities. An official statement of the American Public Health Association, adopted Nov. 10, 1963.

8. Distribution of health services in the structure of state government, 1950, pub. no. 184, Part 1, Public Health Service Washington, D. C., 1952.

9. Association of State and Territorial Health Officers: 1972 inventory: Health programs in the states and territories, Washington, D. C., 1973, The Association.

10. The state public health agency. An official statement of the American Public Health Association, Amer. J. Public Health **55:**2011, Dec. 1965.

11. Shubick, H. J., and Wright, E. O.: Composite study of fifty health department organizational charts representing forty-nine states and the District of Columbia, unpublished report, 1961.

12. Sims, L. B.: Organizational history of HSMHA, Health Services Rep. **88:**117, Feb. 1973.

*Defer not charities till death;
for certainly, if a man weigh it rightly,
he that doth so is rather liberal
of another man's than of his own.*

FRANCES BACON
*Of Riches*

CHAPTER 16

# Voluntary health agencies

## DEVELOPMENT OF THE MOVEMENT

Voluntary health agencies are organizations supported by private or nontax funds and directed by privately employed individuals, the educational and experiential backgrounds of whom range widely. They have no legal powers. Although by no means unique to the United States, they are especially numerous here. This may be due in part to certain characteristics of American historic and social development: goodwill, friendliness, sympathy for the fellow who is down, an urge to improve the human condition, a penchant for carrying out studies and reforms, and a tendency to form and join organizations of all sorts for many purposes. It might be said that one aspect of the democratic philosophy as developed in America was a widespread concern for the welfare of one's neighbor or fellowman on the basis that "United we stand, divided we fall," whether one thinks of the frontier or of the depression of the 1930s, "we are all in this together!" Regrettably a change seems underway. Cunninggim[1] describes it realistically: Today's donor, he says, is often suspect whether he be a private individual, foundation, corporation or church. Earning, saving, and giving were once regarded as desirable, commendable and positive attributes in the United States. But today, he notes, negative attitudes toward giving are manifested by such questions as, "What is the donor trying to buy or hide?" in the belief that crossing the palm with silver is a time-honored way to reduce the heat or to gain advantage. As a result, the potential donor increasingly wonders why he should bother to donate at all.

The voluntary health movement began with the Anti-Tuberculosis Society of Philadelphia in 1892. Its development epitomizes the voluntary health movement as a whole. Encouraged by the formation of the local Philadelphia society, a group of unusually intelligent and enthusiastic private citizens banded together in 1904 to organize the National Association for the Study and Prevention of Tuberculosis. The membership of the group is worthy of special mention. It included Trudeau as president, William Osler, Bowditch, Bates, Janeway, Welch, Billings, Victor Vaughan, and other outstanding individuals. Among the six lay members of the board were Homer Folks, Samuel Gompers, and Edward T. Devine, who were most prominent in the development of social welfare in the United States. At that time tuberculosis caused 10% of all deaths and was the leading cause of destitution and orphanhood. From the beginning it was agreed that eventually the control of tuberculosis should be a function of government, since voluntary funds could never hope to meet the total bill. It was recognized, however, that government action in a democracy does not necessarily precede or preclude public opinion and that both the public and the government needed to be educated. This the association believed it could do, and it proceeded with the eventual organization of 50 state associations and approximately 3,000 local affiliates.

At first the financing of the National Association for the Study and Prevention of Tuberculosis posed a difficult problem. It was temporarily solved by the Russell Sage Foundation, which assumed the responsibility for the 10 years

**309**

from 1907 to 1917. Meanwhile the Tuberculosis Christmas Seal idea had been developed in Denmark. This was considered an especially desirable fund-raising technique, since it gave individual citizens a personal interest in the fight against tuberculosis. The idea was quickly adopted in the United States, and by 1914 it provided the bulk of the funds not only of the national but also of the state and local associations. As an indication of its wide appeal, about $35 million to $40 million are raised each year by the sale of Christmas Seals. The usual pattern of distribution of proceeds for most publicly supported voluntary health agencies was set from the beginning by the national association, which decided to assign most of the funds raised (95%) to the state and local associations while the national agency retained only 5%.

## NUMBER AND TYPE

Since the establishment of the Anti-Tuberculosis Society of Philadelphia in 1892, a confusing number of separate categorical voluntary health or disease related agencies (approximately 100,000) have been formed. They draw their support from literally millions of persons and serve millions of others in various ways. These agencies have been both effective and ineffective, efficient and inefficient, blessed and belittled, well and ill managed, intelligent and unreasonable, cooperative and uncooperative. These are only a few of the possible and inevitable outcomes of rapid development of a large number of independent undertakings. They have, however, one characteristic in common—they seldom die. Hochbaum[2] has summarized the all too typical sequence as follows: "In a young organization, almost all its activities are geared to deal with the very objectives and purposes for which it was created—nothing matters as much as its self-avowed mission. Later, however, increasingly strong concerns develop to maintain and strengthen the organization for its own sake, to expand its activities, to stake out a scope of goals and activities, and to protect this domain against intrusion by other agencies."

In addition to paid employees voluntary health agencies involve the time and often the money of at least 500,000 rather exceptional men and women who serve on boards or committees, as well as the time and effort of over 1 million other voluntary workers. According to the American Association of Fund-Raising Council, private philanthropy accounted for $1.4 billion in health expenditures for the year 1964-1965. These figures exclude the American Red Cross, the large philanthropic foundations, industrial health services, and a large number of agencies that only incidentally furnish health services. The American Red Cross is in a class by itself; it had a peacetime membership of about 5 million people, which increased during World War II to 36 million people. There are now about 4,000 chapters and 6,000 branches. During the 3½ years from the Pearl Harbor bombing to May 1945, contributions amounting to $654 million were raised. The American Red Cross is the only voluntary agency with quasi-official status; the President of the United States serves as its president, and the organization is regarded in effect as the official disaster relief agency of the nation.

As early as the close of World War I concern had developed about the growing number of fund-raising agencies. In 1918 the National Information Bureau that had been established laid down the following eight precepts to guide philanthropic agencies that might wish approval by that agency. So well were they stated that they have remained unchanged and useful ever since[3]:

1. Board—An active and responsible governing body (must maintain direction of the agency), serving without compensation, holding regular meetings, and with effective administrative control.
2. Purpose—A legitimate purpose with no avoidable duplication of the work of other sound organizations.
3. Program—Reasonable efficiency in program management, and reasonable adequacy of resources, both material and personnel.
4. Cooperation—Evidence of consultation and cooperation with established agencies in the same or related fields.
5. Ethical promotion—Ethical methods of publicity, promotion and solicitation of funds.
6. Fund-raising practice—In fund-raising:
   a. No payment of commissions for fund-raising.
   b. No mailing of unordered tickets or merchandise with a request for money in return.
   c. No general telephone solicitation of the public.
7. Audit—Annual audit, prepared by an independent certified public accountant or trust company, showing all income and disbursements, in reasonable detail. New organizations should provide a certified public accountant's statement that a proper financial system has been installed.
8. Budget—Detailed annual budget, translating program plans into financial terms.

Voluntary agencies concerned with health fall into several categories. Most important is a large group of agencies supported by citizen contributions and donations. These are divisible into the following four types, which demonstrate a remarkable degree of specialization:

1. Agencies that are concerned with specific diseases, for example, the American Cancer Society, the National Tuberculosis and Respiratory Disease Association, the National Foundation (poliomyelitis and birth defects), the American Social Hygiene Association (venereal diseases, narcotics, and alcoholism), and the American Diabetic Society
2. Agencies that are concerned with certain organs or structures of the body, for example, the National Society for the Prevention of Blindness, the American Society for the Hard of Hearing, the National Society for Crippled Children, and the American Heart Association
3. Agencies that are concerned with the health and welfare of special groups in society, for example, the American Child Health Association (now extinct), the Maternity Center Association, and the American Negro Health Association (now the National Health Association)
4. Agencies that are concerned with particular phases of health and welfare, for example, the National Safety Council and the Planned Parenthood Federation of America

The second large group of voluntary agencies engaged in health work is composed of foundations established and financed by private philanthropy.[4] Prominent among them are the Rockefeller Foundation, the W. K. Kellogg Foundation, the Carnegie Foundation, the Commonwealth Fund, the Johnson Foundation, the Milbank Memorial Fund, the Mott Foundation, the Rosenwald Fund, and the Markle Foundation. Organizations of this type have functioned in a variety of ways, particularly by promoting and subsidizing local health departments, especially those in rural areas, and by supporting basic research as well as public and professional education.

The third main group of voluntary health agencies is made up of professional associations such as the American Public Health Association, the American Medical Association, the National League for Nursing, and their state and local affiliates. In addition to providing a meeting ground for professional workers in their respective fields these associations do much to establish and improve standards and qualifications,

encourage research, further health education, and promote programs.

Integrating agencies such as health councils and community chests and councils constitute what may be considered a fourth group. There are now more than 1,000 of these multiple interest organizations. They are found on local, state, and national levels; their purpose is the coordination of the activities of the many specialized voluntary agencies.

A fifth group of nonofficial agencies that may be considered to have some interest in the public health consists of an increasing number of commercial organizations that have found it worth while for one reason or another to participate in the promotion of sanitary and health habits and programs. Predominant among these are several of the large insurance companies that have carried out extensive and effective educational programs and demonstrations. Some activities have also been engaged in by industries concerned with the manufacture and sale of soap, sugar, milk, meat, eating and drinking utensils, and other products. Generally speaking, this latter group must be treated cautiously, since their programs are based primarily on a desire for increased profits and improved public relations.

## FUNCTIONS AND ACTIVITIES

The Gunn and Platt study and analysis[5] of voluntary health agencies listed eight basic functions of voluntary health agencies. These may be described briefly as follows.

**Pioneering.** Pioneering involves exploring or surveying for needs not being served and for new methods of dealing with needs already recognized.

**Demonstration.** Voluntary health agencies have rendered particularly significant service by carrying out or subsidizing experimental projects designed to demonstrate practical methods for improvement of public health and for the wider application of proved methods by official and other agencies. Projects have ranged from the demonstration of the value of full-time local health departments, to home delivery service, visiting nursing service, nutrition programs, and business and record procedures.

**Education.** Education is probably the single most important function of voluntary health agencies. In fact it might be said that all other functions have education as their goal. Although activities in this field have been designed primarily for the public, many of the agencies have made provisions for or have engaged in all types of professional training by means of fellowships, in-service training courses, and the maintenance or subsidizations of field training areas.

**Supplementation of official activities.** With no legislative restrictions to encumber them the voluntary health agencies have frequently found themselves in a position to augment the activities of official health departments. Often official health agencies have been unable to enter new fields of service and action because of political restrictions or public reservation. In such instances the voluntary agencies have rendered yeoman service by stepping in to fill the gap between currently accepted practice and more advanced scientific knowledge. Usually when this is done, the custom has been to provide the new service for a limited period of time, at the end of which the official agency is expected to carry on.

**Guarding citizen interest in health.** Voluntary health agencies, because of their nature, representation, and support, have often been in a position to guard the public interest not only by promoting the official health program but also by defending it against political and other interference. By like token they have sometimes found it necessary to subject official health agencies, programs, and officials to study and criticism. This has occasionally given rise to ill feeling, and some health officials have looked on voluntary agencies as presumptuous and interfering. Health departments, however, being official, tax-supported agencies, should expect to be subject to scrutiny and if necessary criticism by the citizenry and the various groups that represent them. It has been exceedingly rare that such criticism has not been to the ultimate good not only of the community but of the official health agency itself. More than one unqualified, politically sponsored individual has been barred from health officership, and more than one qualified health officer has been supported in his program and maintained in his position by vigorous public support stemming from the voluntary health agencies.

**Promotion of health legislation.** In every state and community there is a constant stream of proposed legislation of concern to the public health. It is, of course, a responsibility of the health officer to provide leadership in the support or condemnation of each one. In many instances his voice alone is of little avail and attracts scant attention from the legislative body.

A great source of strength in this regard is the group of cooperative voluntary health agencies that are active and influential in his community. With a prime interest in health matters and representing large numbers of voting citizens, their opinions carry much weight. In addition these agencies have played an active part in the initial formulation and promotion of desirable health legislation.

**Group planning and coordination.** Group planning and coordination have been particular concerns of health federations and councils and of health divisions of councils of social agencies. With the development of many voluntary agencies in a community and their potential or actual overlapping and conflict, there has resulted a great need for action in this field. Related to this is the need for increased coordination between the programs of the voluntary agencies and those of the official agencies in the community.

**Development of well-balanced community health programs.** The development of well-balanced community health programs is really not a function in itself, but rather the total cumulative result of the successful accomplishment of the several foregoing purposes and functions. By protecting and promoting the official health department, by increasing the health consciousness of the community and by providing funds and facilities where gaps exist, the voluntary health agency may make the difference between a mediocre community health program and one that is truly effective.

## PUBLICLY SUPPORTED AGENCIES

Important to the understanding and evaluation of voluntary health agencies is the manner in which they are financed. The professional associations are supported by membership dues, whereas the health activities of commercial agencies are usually financed by budgetary items designated for education or public relations. The philanthropic foundations, of course, owe their existence essentially to large bequests from wealthy individuals. This source of funds, however, is significantly decreasing in importance with the breaking up of large personal fortunes. The most important group to be discussed is that made up of agencies supported by relatively small contributions or donations from large numbers of individuals. Several techniques have been developed by these organizations, each tending to be jealously guarded by whatever agency first devised and used them.

Some of these techniques have been spectacularly successful, depending in many instances on emotional rather than intellectual appeal, carefully developed and conducted by promotional agencies that specialize in the business of fund raising.

The first and still one of the most successful methods is the Tuberculosis Christmas Seal, previously referred to. As promoted for years, their cost of only a penny each appeared to be insignificant to most economic or social groups, and whereas most sales are in the form of several sheets of 100 each, it is not unusual to find children in poor districts purchasing at least one or a few separate stamps. Although to some this may be a point of criticism, the fact that it is done represents at least a certain amount of educational impact on all classes of society, thereby making the fight against tuberculosis truly a people's fight. An important additional incentive has been the identification of the Tuberculosis Christmas Seal with Christmas greeting cards. This campaign has been so successful that several other agencies have adopted the technique, for example, the Easter Seal, inaugurated in 1934 by the National Society for Crippled Children.

Another effective technique was developed by the National Foundation for Infantile Paralysis. Associated with the name of a great national leader, Franklin Delano Roosevelt, who was himself stricken with that disease, there developed a custom of annual drives involving careful planning, organization, and promotional activities. A gala ball to raise funds was held in the nation's capital and was attended by many dignitaries. Similar events were held in cities, towns, and even small villages throughout the nation. Concurrently the public was deluged on the streets, in their homes, and in places of amusement such as theaters with requests for contributions to the March of Dimes. These techniques have been amazingly fruitful and have brought in large sums of money. In 1958 this organization changed its name to the National Foundation and expanded its scope of interest to include arthritis, birth defects, and disorders of the central nervous system.

Other methods used to raise money are dues for nominal membership, the sale of educational literature, fees for services, personal solicitations, and direct mail appeal. Another innovation is the radio or television quiz program, which has greatly benefited several voluntary health agencies. Certain of the techniques have caused considerable public resentment, particularly when pressure or embarrassment potentially enters into the appeal. Examples of this nature are the passage of contribution boxes in a lighted theater and the use of neighbors for personal door-to-door solicitation.

Recent years have seen an increasing trend toward joint fund-raising efforts. This is epitomized by the United Fund approach, which once each year by major community effort raises funds for a large number of member organizations, the local, state, and national offices of which receive appropriate amounts. At present there are about 1,500 United Fund agencies and about the same number of Community Chests. The latter, unlike the United Fund agencies, primarily collect money only for local agencies. Also, United Fund agencies are increasingly allocating a certain proportion of the funds they raise to the United Health Foundations, Inc., which in turn supports a broad range of research and demonstration projects at universities, health departments, and other agencies. Unfortunately not only have some agencies refused to affiliate with the United Fund but also inevitably several new voluntary agencies appear which add their separate appeals to that of the Community Chest or United Fund and thereby again create confusion. Recognition must also be given to the natural wish of many people to contribute to one or a few causes in which they are personally interested rather than to what may appear as a large, vague, and indefinite fund. This problem came to a head toward the end of the 1950s, when a number of the large national foundations, notably those concerned with cancer, poliomyelitis, tuberculosis, and crippled children, forbade their local units to participate in United Fund campaigns or Community Chests. As stated by Ray R. Eppert, Vice President of United Community Funds and Councils: "These agencies who seem determined to wage a trade war for the contributors' dollars have thrown down the gauntlet to federation." He grimly warned them to "Change their policies" or "suffer the consequences."[6] That this warning may not be inevitably idle is indicated by a growing tide of questioning and criticism in the public press and professional journals.[7,8]

An important consideration in connection with the fund-raising activities of voluntary health agencies is the cost of the fund-raising campaign itself. An analysis of 7 national organizations in 1945 showed a variation of from

6 cents to about 38 cents per $1 collected.[5] An analysis of the annual report of one agency led to the conclusion that 68% of the income was spent for agency office maintenance and fund raising. This, however, was somewhat extreme. The average cost of raising a "voluntary" dollar at that time was reported as 5.9 cents by Community Chests and Councils, Inc.

In the 1956-1957 fiscal year the New York State Department of Social Welfare[9] reviewed the approximately 3,200 organizations that solicited public contributions for health, welfare, and educational purposes in that state. In that year they received a total of $324 million, of which about 13% was devoted to fund-raising costs. "Patriotic" and fraternal organizations raised $9 million, of which more than $5 million, or 57%, went for fund raising! When salaries, overhead, and other operating costs are added, sometimes there is little left for "charity." Fund raising *can* be profitable. Examples of extremes, however, should not be construed as condemning the many good organizations. A more recent study by Hamlin[10] brought out a discouraging lack of improvement. While 10 of the large national agencies claimed a cost of from 7 cents to 15 cents for each $1 raised, an auditor found the figures to vary from 12.5 cents to 36.2 cents. Some of these high costs, however, were claimed to be due to inclusion of some educational costs in the fund-raising costs.

One of the strongest recommendations of both the National Health Council study by Gunn and Platt and of the Rockefeller Foundation study by Hamlin has been for the establishment of a uniform accounting system and a standard chart of accounts. He also emphasized "It does not take over 100,000 voluntary agencies . . . to provide health and welfare services in the United States. A better job could be done by a smaller number and a greater joint effort. Furthermore, it would then be simpler to provide for the new agencies which will be needed from time to time." There has been little evidence over the years to indicate any great interest in this on the part of the individual voluntary health agencies. Hamlin found the situation so confused and discouraging that he even urged the President of the United States to establish a permanent national commission on voluntary health and welfare agencies.

## PHILANTHROPIC FOUNDATIONS

Philanthropic foundations have certain advantages over the voluntary agencies that depend on public donations. They can be more flexible and adaptive in their interests and activities, they are not directly accountable to the public, and importantly they do not depend on repetitive and wasteful fund-raising activities. There are about 25,000 private foundations in the United States with assets of about $27 billion. Only 33 of them, however, have assets of $100 million or more. Currently grants to a total of almost $2 billion are made annually, half of the amount by the 100 largest foundations. Considerable variation is observed. Thus in 1969 the Commonwealth Fund and the Danforth Foundation with combined assets of $315 million paid out $22 million—a substantial ratio. In contrast, the Kresge, Lilly, and Pew Foundations, with combined assets of $1.75 *billion,* paid out less than $22 million. There is a reason, of course. Many foundations merely spend what their investments earn each year without regard to capital gains. The Tax Reform Act of 1969 put an end to this, and by 1975 the foundations must spend the equivalent of 6% of their total assets each year. About a third of the foundation grants are devoted to various aspects of health and welfare, usually for innovative purposes. Significantly, most of the large foundations now tend to emphasize studies and demonstrations of broad social consequence rather than large expensive bioscientific laboratory research.[11] It should be noted that some of the smaller foundations have little if any active programs, and several have been established for personal or familial tax-benefit purposes.

By contrast the large foundations (and many not so large) have enviable records of efficient and beneficial philanthropic management. The essential purpose and function of a philanthropic foundation have been well described in a report of the Rockefeller Foundation[12] as ". . . to encourage and stimulate human progress. The accomplishment of this aim depends upon the intelligent distribution of its funds. Even in its institutional form, giving is highly personal, involving as it does the welfare of men, individually and collectively. Philanthropy is a complex process that is both an art and a science, and it must by necessity be creative." Cunninggim[1] indicates that on balance, "Tangibly and intangibly, foundations have done much of which they have cause to be proud," pointing to their wide involvement in all parts of the nation and throughout the world on matters of great social concern and urgency. He concludes that at worst, some foundations may have been indiscreet or naive, but not wicked. The remarkable fact about the philanthropic foundations is that their work in the public interest has in general produced benefits out of all proportion to the expenditures involved.

## DESIRABLE AND UNDESIRABLE CHARACTERISTICS

From the foregoing it is apparent that voluntary health agencies have both desirable and undesirable features. On the favorable side is the fact that these agencies have developed as a result of spontaneous reaction on the part of groups of citizens. Their leadership usually consists of devoted, personally disinterested, intelligent, nonpartisan individuals. Generally the agencies have been established to meet a real and commonly felt need. Without question, public health in America could never have reached its present high level in the absence of the voluntary health agencies. They are unrestricted by statutory or program limitations or by partisan politics. Because they are so relatively unhampered, they can adapt their programs rather readily to changing needs and conditions, thereby often shortening the lag between the acquisition of new scientific knowledge and its application. Much that has been accomplished in improved professional education, standardization of techniques and procedures, and research can be placed to their credit.

On the other hand, voluntary health agencies have certain undesirable features or disadvantages. Several official health departments have been placed in the position of having to conduct poorly balanced programs because of pressure from voluntary agencies. This may come about in two ways: A voluntary agency may exert pressure on the health department to overemphasize its particular interest or, contrariwise, some voluntary agencies have caused health departments to underemphasize certain programs because the voluntary agencies have wanted to monopolize activities in those fields. Such tactics may jeopardize appropriations for official health agencies. Similarly, despite the avowed purpose of leading the way until an activity is officially adopted, many voluntary agencies are reluctant to surrender any parts of their programs. In fact, it is rare to find a voluntary agency closing up shop as did the American Child Health Association, when it had accomplished its purpose.

With the multiplicity of existing organizations, overlapping of function and high administrative costs are certain to result. Reference has been made to the growing confusion of the public. This results from overlapping functions as well as from multiplicity of appeals. Thus one still finds many communities in which several groups of nurses operate out of an equal number of agencies, visiting homes and working in clinics. Certain of the voluntary agencies do not accede to the policy of affiliating or even coordinating their activities with each other, much less with those of local official health organizations.

Finally, and one of the most serious objections, the public tends to contribute on an emotional basis and to the organization that makes the loudest and most prolonged appeal and then believes that it has done its part toward the support of the entire public health program. An interesting example is that in recent years the agencies concerned with tuberculosis and poliomyelitis have each raised about the same amount annually, despite the fact that there are many more cases and deaths from tuberculosis each year than there are cases and deaths from poliomyelitis.

## CURRENT TRENDS AND THE FUTURE

About a third of a century ago Marquette[13] called attention to three major developments that he considered were certain to have an important effect on the future of voluntary health agencies. First was the trend toward the allotment of federal funds under the Social Security Act to the Public Health Service and other agencies for the categorical approach to important health problems such as venereal disease, tuberculosis, cancer, mental health, heart disease, and dental health. These allotments of federal funds intended for state and local as well as for national use were already making it possible for official health agencies to enter into territory previously occupied almost exclusively by the private health agency. The second development, which grew largely out of the National Health Conferences, was the increased appropriation of tax monies for hospital and medical services. Related to this was the support, albeit often reluctant, by the American Medical Association of moves for more government participation in public health, health education, mental health, the care of the mentally ill, the support of tuberculosis hospitals, facilities for convalescent care and rehabilitation, group hospitalization, and cash indemnity against sickness. A third development of great impact was the economic depression of the 1930s, followed by a trend toward higher taxes. Working together, these two factors served to eliminate some large fortunes and to reduce somewhat the inclination of many people to contribute to what they increasingly considered to be governmental responsibilities.

In light of what has occurred since, Marquette's observations appear to have been generally accurate. Previously the respective traditional roles of governmental and voluntary health agencies were more clearly defined. Education, experimentation, demonstration, and the provision of direct personal services were regarded as the strengths and proper domain of voluntary agencies. The expansion of governmental services has brought about a shift in the traditional roles. Whereas the fundamental distinction between the freedom of the voluntary agency and the statutory requirements imposed on governmental agencies remain, that distinction is becoming increasingly hazy. Community sanctions tend increasingly to limit the freedom of action of voluntary agencies, while a plethora of special grants now provide governmental agencies with greater program flexibility. As a result, today there are many areas in which both types of agencies are in a position to render essentially the same types of services for the same kinds of individuals.[14] Related to such factors as the nation's economic growth, the population increase, the changes in age distribution, and the remarkable mobility and urbanization of American society, several other developments have contributed to the shift from voluntarism to official agency action. Among these are (1) the spectacular advances in medical science, (2) a growing demand by the public for health services now possible as a result of these advances, (3) an affluent society that can and is increasingly willing to support these services through taxes, (4) a considerable improvement in the educational level of most citizenry, and (5) the development of a national social philosophy that regards health as a fundamental human right to be guaranteed by the government.

The voluntary health agencies are now faced with the problem of what to do about these trends. Some have already accepted the policy that when a tax-supported agency develops to the point where it can take over the work, the private agency should either leave the field or cease its operation entirely. To decide logically on a sound future course it has been recognized as desirable that these agencies subject themselves and their communities to careful scrutiny to reevaluate problems that do or may exist and

their relationship to them. Reevaluation is further indicated for bringing up to date the position occupied by the voluntary agency in the community and its relation to all other official and nonofficial organizations. Accordingly, recent years have seen the establishment of appraisal or evaluation committees in an increasing number of voluntary health agencies. The United Fund and Community Chests and Councils, Inc., have played an important role in the encouragement of this procedure. In speaking of agency appraisal the National Health Council suggests that the following be set up by the board of each voluntary health agency[5]:

. . . machinery for the periodical appraisal of the agency, at intervals of perhaps five years, by qualified experts with wide knowledge of the field of activity as well as of agency and community organization. This is particularly needed in the swiftly changing trends that are ahead. Valuable as is self-analysis, the outside and objective approach reduces the likelihood that smugness or self-satisfaction will establish itself. Such an appraisal should consider (a) adequacy and effectiveness of program; (b) financial status and future; (c) cooperative relationships; (d) adequacy of staff and executive direction; and (e) future opportunities and functions. Properly planned and carried out with the full cooperation of board and staff, such an appraisal will be worth more than it costs. Funds should be set aside and gradually accumulated for such an accounting and future planning. No agency would think of omitting its yearly financial audit merely to save the cost. It is even more important to have an audit of the organization itself made at intervals in order to determine how wisely it expends its money.

In addition to the evaluations sponsored by voluntary agencies themselves the past 15 years has seen the development of communitywide surveys performed by outside experts. Many of these have been sponsored by Community Chests and Councils, Inc., financial support coming from any one of several sources: the local community fund, the council of social agencies, private subsidies, or the local government itself. With the passage of the Comprehensive Health Planning and Public Health Services Amendments of 1966 Act (often referred to as the Partnership for Health Act) it is anticipated that an even more searching evaluation of voluntary and official health programs will take place. Certainly this would be fundamental to any comprehensive health planning.

Reference has been made to the National Health Council. In a sense its organization represents an attempt to adapt voluntary health agencies to the changing times. At the time of its organization in 1920 it was hailed as one of the most important steps taken in the field of public health up to that time. Its avowed goals included consolidation of funds and facilities, increased efficiency of action through joint planning, housing, and programming, and the provision of services and conferences conducive to evaluation. Its program has not been as successful as had been originally hoped because of, among other reasons, resistance on the part of many agencies to the idea of unification for fear of loss of agency integrity.

Several other steps worthy of mention have been taken to keep voluntary health agencies up to date and to increase their community value. Until relatively recently many agencies have been directed by interested lay persons. At first they served without pay, but that policy was soon recognized as being administratively unsound. Accompanying the increased employment of full-time agency directors has been a recognition of the need for some type of training. As a result, in-service training courses and other types of programs designed to fill the need have been established and conducted. Recognition of the need for training has grown to the point where at the present time not only are curricula presented (usually during the summer months) for executives of voluntary health agencies but also educational qualifications for this type of personnel have been developed by the Committee on Professional Education of the American Public Health Association.[15]

That voluntary health agencies should find themselves in the position of having to give way here and tighten up there is neither surprising nor undesirable, or do these trends necessarily indicate their approaching demise. As aptly stated by Marquette[13]:

There is really no occasion for leaders outside the tax supported health field to have any concern as to the continued importance of their work. It is rather a matter of elasticity and adjustment. Everybody in the public health field knows that so much remains to be done and that we fall so far short of using effectively the instruments that medical science has placed at our disposal for combating disease, that the combined public and volunteer health forces will be needed for years to come. It must all be properly integrated and the private agency must see the changing picture and be ready to modify its role.

However, as the Hamlin report[10] stated: "If the unstinting philanthropic spirit of the American people is to be translated into the greatest public good and their confidence in the agencies maintained, the structure and objectives of voluntary agencies should be reviewed and modernized." The study committee believed that five major steps were available to voluntary agencies.

1. Stronger voluntary agency leadership
2. Higher standards for local affiliates
3. Increased participation in organized planning
4. Better reporting of programs and accomplishments
5. Greater emphasis on research and the application of new knowledge

In the interest of objectivity it must be observed that the need for increased attention to each of these five items applies equally to official health agencies. Furthermore, if voluntary and official health agencies not only both did these things but did them in concert, the health of the public would be the better for it. Both are needed. As far as the voluntary and philanthropic health agencies are concerned, many have commented that the importance to the imaginative and perhaps unorthodox investigator of another door to knock on besides that of the government for necessary assistance should not be underestimated. Viewing this from another vantage point, Mackintosh[16] has noted: "In the United Kingdom, as people stand and watch the vast changes in health and social work that have characterized the middle of the twentieth century, especially toward the 'Welfare State,' they sometimes wonder whether there is still a place for voluntary action. Excess of officialdom carries its own hazards, notably in the suppression of the individual and his independence."

## REFERENCES

1. Cunninggim, M.: Private money and public service, New York, 1972, McGraw-Hill Book Co.
2. Hochbaum, G. M.: Health agencies and the Tower of Babel, Public Health Rep. **80:**331, April 1965.
3. Lear, J.: The business of giving, Saturday Rev. vol. 63, Dec. 2, 1961.
4. The Foundation Directory, ed. 4, New York, 1971, Columbia University Press.
5. Gunn, S. M., and Platt, P. S.: Voluntary health agencies: an interpretative study, New York, 1945, The Ronald Press Co.
6. United funds battle health agencies which aim to go it alone, Wall Street J. **38:**1, July 18, 1958.
7. Editorial: The giver's dilemma, Amer. J. Public Health **46:**1336, Oct. 1956.
8. Carter, R.: The gentle legions, Garden City, N. Y., 1961, Doubleday & Co., Inc.

9. Report of the charities registration bureau, Albany, 1958, New York State Department of Social Welfare.

10. Hamlin, R. H.: Voluntary health and welfare agencies in the United States, New York, 1961, Schoolmaster's Press.

11. Nielsen, W.: The big foundations, New York, 1972, Columbia University Press.

12. Shaplen, R.: Toward the well-being of mankind: fifty years of the Rockefeller Foundation, Garden City, N. Y., 1964, Doubleday & Co., Inc.

13. Marquette, B.: Is the private health agency on the way out? Amer. J. Public Health **29:**46, Jan. 1939.

14. Levine, S., White, P. E., and Paul, B. D.: Community interorganizational problems in providing medical care and social services, Amer. J. Public Health **53:**1183, Aug. 1963.

15. Committee on Professional Education of the American Public Health Association: Educational qualifications of executives of voluntary health agencies, Amer. J. Public Health **35:**499, May 1945.

16. Mackintosh, J. M.: Voluntary action in the British health services. In Galdston, I., editor: Voluntary action and the state, New York, 1961, International Universities Press.

# PART SIX

# The substance of public health— developmental

In building a public health program, as with so many other things, the best place to start is at the beginning. Life is a continuous spiral with a myriad of interlocking biologic, environmental, and circumstantial factors blending to determine genesis. That event in turn brings to bear a new panoply of factors over which the life that has been brought about has absolutely no control—the characteristics of the bearing mother, her socioeconomic circumstances in the broadest connotations, her habits, mental condition, and state of nutrition. And then when the cord is cut, the still helpless and dependent creature has need for physical and mental care and comfort through a long period of maturation, learning, and development. Childhood can and should be a time of joy and happiness, but biologically it, too, is a time of preparation for the hopefully fruitful years of adulthood. It is to the areas of concern toward this end that the following four chapters are devoted—maternal and child health, school health, nutrition, and dental health.

*The utmost reverence is due a child.*

JUVENAL

CHAPTER 17

# Maternal and child health*

## A CRITICAL PERIOD

The field of public health is concerned with the well being of all people, regardless of age, sex, race, or other characteristics. Traditionally, however, there have been two groups to whom particular attention has been given: pregnant women and young children, particularly infants. There are sound reasons for this. Special attention to a pregnant woman brings double health benefits: first, to her as an adult member of society and, second, to the product of her pregnancy. Other reasons are that pregnancy is a period of particular physical stress during which the woman, who ordinarily may have no difficulties, may possibly face unusual risk. Undesirable influences during the prenatal period may affect and even jeopardize the subsequent state of health of both the mother and the expected infant. Short of fatalities, these effects may result in health and economic disadvantages for the woman and child and even for the rest of the family if the mother's health is permanently impaired.

Remarkable progress has been made in many parts of the world in the saving of lives of expectant mothers and their infants. In the United States during the 55 years after World War I, maternal mortality declined about 95% and infant mortality about 90%. This may be attributed to many factors, of which public health progress is only one. Hospital and medical standards have improved, as have the national state of nutrition and the general standard of living.

Many new preventive and therapeutic agents have been introduced. Furthermore, whereas maternal and child health activities are usually given specific emphasis by public health organizations, almost every aspect of the public health program has had a direct or indirect effect on the health and welfare of expectant mothers and particularly of infants and young children. In areas undeveloped in a sanitary sense, the institution of an effective program of environmental sanitation involving the purification of water, the sanitation of milk and food, and the promotion of satisfactory facilities for the disposal of human wastes will show its first effects in a reduction in infant morbidity and mortality. Vital statistics are involved in the maternal and child health program in various ways, especially by pinpointing specific problem areas. The public health laboratory is an essential tool, particularly in prenatal management where tests must be performed to indicate the presence of venereal diseases, the Rh reaction, eclamptic tendencies, diabetes, tuberculosis, and other ailments that considerably increase the risk incurred by pregnancy and to determine appropriate medical management that must be followed. Throughout the entire antenatal, natal, and postnatal period there must be woven a strong thread of health education. The expectant mother must be constantly guarded against communicable diseases, particularly those of a viral, streptococcal, and influenzal nature, and early attempts must be made to protect the newborn child against gonorrheal ophthalmia, smallpox, whooping cough, diphtheria, measles,

---

*For a useful bibliography, see Schmidt and Valadian.[1]

and other communicable infections. It is obvious therefore that the maternal and child health program cannot be considered by itself.

## BACKGROUND OF MATERNAL AND CHILD HEALTH PROGRAMS

In the United States, programs for the promotion of maternal and child health originated with the establishment of a children's hospital in Philadelphia in 1855. Two years later the Nursery and Child's Hospital began in New York City. Little direct relationship to the health aspects of mothers and children occurred in the United States during the remainder of the nineteenth century. However, several indirectly beneficial activities occurred in relation to more humane treatment of children, especially orphans, and the inception of general public health and sanitation measures. A development of both immediate and long-range significance was the opening of the first milk station in 1893 in New York City. The original purpose of this and similar stations that subsequently were established was to combat the tremendous incidence of summer diarrhea in infants and children of the underprivileged by providing them with safe milk during the summer heat. In fact, the nature of this beginning had much to do with the ultimate development of municipal and state regulation of milk supplies. Observance of the benefits that resulted from this meager start led to the establishment of numerous infant welfare societies designed to bring medical and nursing knowledge and care to those in need. In 1908 the New York City Association for Improving the Condition of the Poor, in conjunction with the New York Outdoor Clinic, began to provide prenatal care for expectant mothers in the lower income groups. Simultaneously a Bureau of Child Hygiene was established in the New York City Health Department. These two moves were subsequently duplicated by many other communities throughout the nation. In 1909 a conference on the prevention of infant mortality was held by the American Academy of Medicine. This was followed the same year by the first White House Conference on Children and Youth called by President Theodore Roosevelt. Its purpose was "to discuss what might be done at the federal level to stimulate and help finance state and local health and social welfare programs for children." It resulted in several legislative proposals, one of which was signed into law in 1912 by President Taft to establish the Children's Bureau. Its initial charge was limited—essentially to conduct studies and report—but on this modest base astute leadership was able over the years to develop a broad program of far-reaching significance and effect.[2]

Another development of significance at about that same time was the formation of the American Association for the Study and Prevention of Infant Mortality. This group was composed of pediatricians, infant welfare nurses (who in a sense were the precursors of the present-day public health nurses) social workers, public health officials, and other interested persons, all of whom provided leadership in the rapidly expanding movement to protect the lives and health of mothers and children. This organization was the beginning of what in 1923 became the American Child Health Association, which provided most effective leadership until the time of its disbandment in 1935. The growing and widespread interest in the problem commanded national attention that resulted first in the passage of the Sheppard-Towner Act.[3] This provided the beginning of a federal grant-in-aid program to encourage and enable states to develop programs in maternal and infant care. The act functioned only from 1922 to 1929, but its goals and principles were subsequently influential in the broad national consideration of maternal and child health problems in the Social Security Act, which was approved in August 1935. These basic legislative acts, which provided initial leadership and funds, have had a significant and lasting effect on the development of maternal and child health programs in state health departments and in local areas throughout the nation.

Another occurrence of greater significance than was recognized by many at the time was the establishment during World War II of the Emergency Maternity and Infant Care Program. Designed to provide qualified obstetric care for the pregnant wives of servicemen as well as medical care for their children, it was conceived and administered by the Children's Bureau. This national program, by virtue of the necessity to establish basic standards for personnel, facilities, services, and fees in all areas that benefited from the subsidies, had perhaps a greater effect on the quality and quantity of care rendered to expectant mothers and their infants than any other factor up to that time. Furthermore, as observed by Eliot,[4] the longtime and notable director of the Children's Bureau, "The EMIC Program was the most extensive single public medical program ever undertaken in this country." As such, it provided many federal, state, and local health personnel with an opportunity to obtain experience in the administration of a medical care program, which proved to be of value to many subsequently.

The 1960s witnessed the passage of some of the most significant federal and state legislation pertaining to health in the nation's entire history.[5] The Vaccination Assistance Act was passed in 1962. It made available almost $26 million to state and local health departments to conduct intensified immunization programs, especially among preschool children, against diphtheria, whooping cough, tetanus, and poliomyelitis. The act was extended in 1965 for another 3-year period, and measles was added to the list of diseases to be attacked. It also included measures designed to establish effective ongoing immunization programs.

In 1963, recognizing that about 3% of babies born are mentally retarded and that much of this problem is attributable to inadequate maternal and infant care, Congress passed the Maternal and Child Health and Mental Retardation Planning Amendments. This made possible the start of a 5-year, $265 million program to improve maternal and child health services, especially for high-risk prospective mothers who have or are likely to have conditions hazardous to themselves or to their infants during pregnancy. Particular emphasis was placed on those who otherwise would not receive care because of low income or for other reasons beyond their control. The act also provided grants to states to plan comprehensive programs to combat mental retardation.

For health, 1965 was a banner year. The nation through its Congress and the President entered into an unprecedented assault on its health problems.[6] More progressive health legislation was passed during that year than at any time previously. One indication was that in the following year, 1966, the federal government expended through the Department of Health, Education, and Welfare about $3.1 billion for health purposes—a 50% increase in only 3 years.[7] The single most significant measure passed was the Social Security Amendments Act of 1965 (P.L. 89-97). It included several provisions designed to enhance the health and well-being of mothers and children. Not only did it extend the Maternity and Infancy Program that resulted from the 1963 legislation, but it

also enabled state and local health departments to develop comprehensive health service programs, medical, dental and psychologic, for preschool and schoolchildren. Under the amendments the federal government was empowered to provide up to 75% of the costs of projects to screen, diagnose, and treat children in low-income families as well as to carry out broad intensified child health promotive and protective activities in communities as a whole. Funds for the program began with $15 million in 1966 and increased to $50 million by 1970. The 1965 Social Security Amendments also extended and improved services to crippled children through case finding, diagnosis, and hospitalization with medical, surgical, and outpatient care. Provision was included for the training of more people to work with crippled children. Mention should also be made of legislation (P.L. 88-164, Title III, and P.L. 89-105) that provided support for research and demonstration projects relating to the education and training of youths handicapped by mental, physical, hearing, visual, or other defects.

Another event of considerable potential significance to maternal and child health was the passage of the Economic Opportunity Act of 1964 (P.L. 88-452). Through the provision relating to the Head Start Program medical and dental examinations and in some cases treatment and nutritional services were provided to economically disadvantaged preschool children. Through its Community Action Program provisions, numerous communities added significantly to their services to children of the poor, including in several instances the development of comprehensive medical or health centers. Similar programs resulted from the Appalachia Regional Development Act (P.L. 89-4).

One other legislative action destined to have far-reaching implications for maternal and child health and all other health activities was the passage of the Comprehensive Health Planning and Public Health Service Amendments Act of 1966 (P.L. 89-749), commonly known as the "Partnership for Health." This provides grants to states to finance comprehensive planning to identify public health needs and to establish priorities for health services. The act also provides block grants in place of categorical grants to states to assist in the establishment and maintenance of comprehensive public health services, some of which may, of course, relate to or affect maternal and child health. This is discussed further in Chapter 12.

**Table 17-1.** Maternal mortality, United States, 1930 and 1968

| Year | Total (per 10,000 live births) | White (per 10,000 live births) | Other (per 10,000 live births) |
|------|-------------------------------|-------------------------------|-------------------------------|
| 1930 | 67.3 | 60.9 | 117.4 |
| 1968 | 2.4 | 1.7 | 6.4 |
| Percent of decrease | 96.4 | 97.9 | 94.6 |

**Table 17-2.** Births by race, location, and type of attendant, United States, 1943 and 1968

| Place, race, and year | | | Location | | Attendant | |
|---|---|---|---|---|---|---|
| | | | Hospital (%) | Elsewhere (%) | Physician (%) | Other (%) |
| United States: | Total | 1968 | 98.5 | 1.5 | 98.9 | 1.1 |
| | White | 1943 | 77.2 | 22.8 | 97.8 | 2.2 |
| | | 1968 | 99.4 | 0.6 | 99.7 | 0.3 |
| | Black | 1943 | 31.5 | 68.5 | 55.9 | 44.1 |
| | | 1968 | 94.0 | 6.0 | 95.0 | 5.0 |

## STATEMENT OF THE PROBLEM

Despite the significant advances in the past few decades, there still is much room for improvement in maternal and child health.

### Maternal mortality

By 1971 maternal mortality in the United States had declined to an all-time low of 2 per 10,000 live births. Nevertheless, the unfinished business in maternal health becomes apparent even when the currently decreasing rates are compared with those of many economically less favored nations and especially when the rates are broken down geographically, economically, and by age, race, and other factors. During 1968, for example, although the number of all maternal deaths per 10,000 live births was 2.4 and the rate for white women was 1.7, the risk for women of other races was 6.4 (Table 17-1). However, the proportionate decrease over the previous quarter century has been about the same for women of all races in the United States.

These differences in the rates of maternal deaths by race and economics are reflected partially in the variations among the states. Generally speaking, a line drawn along the thirty-seventh degree latitude, across the northern boundaries of North Carolina, Tennessee, Arkansas, Oklahoma, New Mexico, and Arizona divides the nation into a southern area with a generally high maternal mortality and a northern area of generally low to average rates. This is epitomized by the lowest rate in Minnesota and the highest rate in Mississippi.

There is no reason to believe that true racial or geographic differences should naturally exist. Analyses of economic status, standard of living, and availability and utilization of medical, nursing, and hospital facilities bring out striking parallels with the distribution of maternal mortality rates. If for purposes of comparison one goes back to 1943, a year for which much detailed data is readily available, in all of the southern tier of states referred to, fewer than 60% of births occurred in hospitals, the figure in the case of Mississippi having been as low as 26.6%. Similarly in each of these states many women were delivered by persons other than trained physicians. The extremes were Mississippi again with 42.8% and South Carolina with 36.3%. When this is correlated with race, it is found that the majority of nonhospitalized and nonmedically attended deliveries in these states were those of black women. The overall figures for the nation in 1943 show that 97.8% of white women were delivered by physicians, 77.2% of them in hospitals, whereas 55.9% of black women were delivered by physicians, with only 31.5% of them in hospitals (Table 17-2). In Mississippi more than 80% of black women in labor had no medical attendant at all in 1943.

Since 1943, the circumstances of childbirth have improved considerably everywhere in the nation, especially for those in the poorer areas and for nonwhite women. Thus in 1968 in Mississippi, although still with the poorest record, about 90% of its women gave birth in hospitals. This represents a remarkable im-

**Table 17-3.** Maternal mortality by age and race, United States, 1952-1953 and 1962-1963*

| Age period (years) | Deaths per 10,000 live births | | | | Percent decline 1962-1963 since 1952-1953 | |
|---|---|---|---|---|---|---|
| | White | | Nonwhite | | | |
| | 1952-1953 | 1962-1963 | 1952-1953 | 1962-1963 | White | Nonwhite |
| All ages | 4.6 | 2.4 | 17.7 | 9.6 | 48 | 46 |
| Under 20 | 3.4 | 1.2 | 12.0 | 5.0 | 65 | 58 |
| 20-24 | 2.6 | 1.3 | 10.6 | 5.2 | 50 | 51 |
| 25-29 | 3.4 | 1.9 | 13.8 | 8.5 | 44 | 38 |
| 30-34 | 5.7 | 3.7 | 28.5 | 15.9 | 35 | 44 |
| 35-39 | 11.0 | 6.0 | 41.6 | 25.2 | 45 | 39 |
| 40-44 | 18.6 | 9.5 | 53.7 | 35.0 | 49 | 35 |

*From Statistical bulletin, Metropolitan Life Insurance Co., June 1965.

provement in less than three decades. Similarly the proportion of women in that state who were delivered by other than physicians was more than halved.

Overall in the nation, by 1968, not only did almost all white births (99.4%) occur in hospitals but even more significantly the proportion of black births in hospitals rose from 31.5% in 1943 to 94.0% in 1968 and medically attended black births rose from 55.9% to 95.0%. In North Dakota and the New England States all but a rare occasional birth are medically attended and take place under hospital conditions.

Maternal mortality varies significantly with age. As illustrated in Table 17-3, it is lowest in all races in women under 20 years of age, after which it increases almost geometrically with each successive age span. Of considerable current importance is the fact that the rate of decline also varies with age. Among both white and nonwhite women the greatest gains have been made in the younger age groups. The discrepancy is most noticeable, however, with nonwhite women, among whom the rate of improvement in maternal mortality slows up significantly after 35 years of age.

With respect to time of occurrence most maternal deaths take place during or soon after delivery or abortion. Thus a study in 1943, when the overall rate was 24.5 maternal deaths per 10,000 live births and figures were large enough for valid analysis, showed that 65% occurred during or soon after delivery, 16% during or soon after abortion, 14% before delivery, and 4% related to ectopic pregnancies. About 90% of maternal deaths at that time were attributable to three categories of cause: infections, 36%; toxemias, 27%; and hemorrhage, trauma, and shock, 28%. Since that time, great

gains have been made against all of these risks of maternal death before and during delivery. Table 17-4 presents the details of the comparison of the major causes of maternal deaths in 1952-1953 with 10 years later, 1962-1963.

The decline in deaths from infection is undoubtedly associated with the advances in chemotherapy, particularly in the development of antibiotics, the increased use of blood transfusions and plasma, the trend away from operative interference, and improved hospital standards. More frequent and better prenatal care with particular emphasis on diet and again the avoidance of operative delivery have undoubtedly played important roles in the great reduction of the death rate from toxemias of pregnancy. Significant inroads have been made against hemorrhage, trauma, and shock as causes of maternal mortality as a result of improved obstetric management, fewer operative deliveries, and the more common use of transfusions of blood, blood plasma, and related products. Unquestionably, considerable further success is possible against deaths related to childbearing, especially in view of existing knowledge, obstetric techniques, and the existing remarkable pharmaceutic armamentarium. Faults of human motivation and behavior remain the single greatest deterrent.

**Abortion**

This important and controversial subject was discussed briefly in Chapter 4. It is to be noted in Table 17-4 that deaths from abortion remained about as important as previously. The major proportion of such deaths were caused by illegal abortions induced either by unqualified individuals or by women themselves, usually under extremely unsatisfactory and unsanitary conditions. This resulted in

**Table 17-4.** Major cause of maternal mortality by race, United States, 1952-1953 and 1962-1963*

| Cause of death | Deaths per 10,000 live births | | | | Percent decline 1962-1963 since 1952-1953 | |
| --- | --- | --- | --- | --- | --- | --- |
| | White | | Nonwhite | | | |
| | 1952-1953 | 1962-1963 | 1952-1953 | 1962-1963 | White | Nonwhite |
| All causes | 4.6 | 2.4 | 17.7 | 9.6 | 48 | 46 |
| Toxemias | 1.4 | 0.4 | 6.5 | 1.9 | 71 | 71 |
| Hemorrhage | 0.9 | 0.4 | 2.8 | 1.7 | 56 | 39 |
| Abortion | 0.5 | 0.5 | 2.4 | 2.0 | — | 17 |
| Sepsis | 0.5 | 0.3 | 1.6 | 1.0 | 40 | 37 |
| Ectopic pregnancy | 0.2 | 0.1 | 1.7 | 0.9 | 50 | 47 |
| Other complications | 1.0 | 0.7 | 2.7 | 2.1 | 30 | 22 |

*From Statistical bulletin, Metropolitan Life Insurance Co., June 1965.

its recognition as an important social and public health problem[8-10] and the development of attacks against this needless killer of pregnant women. During the 1960s and early 1970s, an increasing number of nations liberalized their laws with regard to medically induced abortion.[11,12] This plus intrinsic social concerns led several states in the United States to undertake revision of their laws to allow induced abortion under medically acceptable circumstances and, of course, dependent on the decision of the woman involved and the advice of her physician.[13] In recognition of a trend the Public Health Service in 1968 established an Abortion Surveillance Program in cooperation with state and local departments, which were encouraged and assisted to develop abortion reporting systems. The purpose was to be able to observe and study changes in fertility, as well as maternal morbidity and mortality.[14]

Meanwhile many professional and other organizations passed strong resolutions endorsing the trend. This long-overdue movement culminated in a landmark decision by the United States Supreme Court in January 1973.[15] The court did not remove restrictions entirely. For the first 3 months of pregnancy, it said, the decision rests with the woman and her physician—a "right of privacy" in which the state cannot interfere. For the next 6 months, states if they wish, may "regulate the abortion procedures in ways reasonably related to maternal health" such as licensing and regulating the persons and facilities involved. For the last 10 weeks of pregnancy, when the fetus "has the capability of meaningful life outside the mother's womb, states may prohibit abortion except as it may be indicated to preserve the life or health of the mother." The Supreme Court stressed that the ruling does not give a woman the right to abortion on demand, nor can a physician (or presumably a hospital) be required to perform an abortion. Situations in which an induced abortion is considered especially justified include rape, incest, risk to the mental or physical health of the mother, eugenics, and exposure to viruses or drugs that might cause malformations. With the development of methods of obtaining and examining amniotic fluids for indications of genetic defects, an additional and most important indication for induced abortion is added.[16]

Already reports have appeared from various countries to indicate that the risk from induced abortion under proper circumstances, and especially during the first trimester of pregnancy, is extremely low. Thus the World Health Organization reports that in more than 2.5 million medically supervised abortions in Hungary, Czechoslovakia, and Slovenia between 1957 and 1967, only 73 women died. This is a mortality rate of 3 per 100,000 abortions compared with an average maternal mortality rate, excluding abortion, of about 20 per 100,000 pregnancies in developed countries.[17] The first year of experience in South Australia produced no deaths from supervised induced abortion.[18] In New York City, where legal abortions have been performed since 1970, it has been estimated that about 4% of women of reproductive age had medically induced abortions each year since, resulting not only in fewer maternal deaths but also "a sharp decline in the birth rate and an even greater decline reversing a long term trend in illegitimacy."[19]

In the course of these developments, and especially in view of the Supreme Court decision, recommended guidelines for abortion services have been issued, both by the American Public Health Association[20] and the American College of Obstetricians and Gynecologists.[21] Methodologies for organizations to follow in planning abortion services have also been developed.[22]

**Infant mortality**

As would be expected, the factors involved in the problem of infant mortality and the improvements that have been made closely parallel those described for the mothers of the infants. Although there is cause for satisfaction in the reduction in infant mortality, much remains to be accomplished. The situation has been depicted most vividly by comparison with war losses. "From Pearl Harbor to V-J Day 281,000 Americans were killed in action. During the same period 430,000 babies died in the United States before they were a year old—three babies dead for every 2 soldiers."[23] The nation still suffers a loss of about 55,000 infants each year. In 1973 this resulted in an infant mortality rate of 17.6 per 1,000 live births. Between 1915 and 1949 infant mortality dropped dramatically from 100 to 28 per 1,000 live births. Then the rate of decrease slowed noticeably, and between 1960 and 1965 infant mortality dropped only 5%. During the following 9 years from 1965 to 1973, however, the decrease was 30%.

It has been distressing to many in the United States to note lower infant mortality rates in several other nations.[24,25] More disturbing has been repeated use of crude comparative data collected in different ways and times and for dissimilar population groups to "prove" various professional or social theses or to obtain political advantage. Such comparisons are rife with errors, should be made with great caution, and should be viewed with great skepticism.

Although infant mortality has been steadily decreasing, as in the case of maternal mortality, internal disparities are to be noted: In 1971, for example, the death rate for white infants was 16.8, whereas for other races it was 30.2 per 1,000 live births. The rate of decline during the 1960s, however, was 23.1% for white infants but 29.2% for other racial groups. It is noteworthy that the rate of improvement in the infant mortality has not paralleled the improvement in maternal mortality. Thus between 1960 and 1970 maternal mortality decreased 36% and 41% among white and nonwhite women, respectively; during the same period, infant mortality declined 23% and 29% among white and

nonwhite infants, respectively. The geographic variation in infant mortality is approximately the counterpart of that observed with maternal deaths. The southern tier of economically disadvantaged people poses the greatest problem. However, recent reductions in infant mortality have been notably greater in the southern states. Again, as in the case of adult women, there is no evidence that the nonwhite infant is intrinsically less viable than infants born to white mothers. The same factors of lower standard of living, poor nutrition, and unavailability of professional services and hospital facilities plays a predominant role.

In an evaluation of the problem, in order to formulate a sound program for control, a knowledge of the circumstances and causes of infant deaths is fundamental. A curve of infant deaths or death rates by age in hours, days, weeks, or months is characteristically a survivorship type of curve asymptotic to both axes. It begins extremely high for the first few minutes, hours, and days of life and decreases sharply by the end of the first week. In 1968, for example, almost three fourths of infant deaths occurred during the first month of life and about 44% during the first day. The majority of neonatal deaths are due to prenatal or natal conditions or events, as shown in Table 17-5. Prematurity is by far the most important factor. The risk of death during the first month of life is almost thirty times as great for a prematurely born infant (2,500 grams or less) than for those who are of normal term (more than 2,500 grams). The problem of the premature and underweight in-

**Table 17-5.** Neonatal deaths by cause, United States, 1969

| Cause | Number of deaths |
|---|---|
| Respiratory distress, asphyxia, and other anoxias | 14,437 |
| Immaturity, unqualified | 8,890 |
| Complications of labor and childbirth | 8,683 |
| Congenital anomalies | 7,813 |
| Hyaline membrane disease | 4,778 |
| Influenza and pneumonia | 1,813 |
| Birth injury—cause not stated | 1,666 |
| Infectious and parasitic conditions | 846 |
| Accidents | 228 |
| Meningitis | 194 |
| All other causes | 6,737 |
| Total | 56,085 |

fant therefore is of predominant and increasing concern. Interestingly there is excellent evidence that nonwhite premature and underweight infants have a significantly better survival rate than do white infants of the same condition.[26] Recent studies have indicated higher neonatal death rates when mothers are under 17 or over 36 years, short in stature, underweight, and malnourished. Smoking by the mother has been found to have a surprisingly high effect, possibly as high as a 30% increase in the neonatal death rate.[27,28]

Deaths of premature infants have been reduced significantly during the past quarter century, particularly as a result of improved facilities and personnel for their prompt and adequate care. Pneumonia of the newborn used to be a much more important cause of neonatal death but has been reduced by improved nursery management and the use of antibiotics. Some inroads have been made in recent years not only against birth injuries but even against congenital malformations by means of more stringent control of environmental hazards and by examinations of amniotic fluid early in pregnancy followed by careful medically performed abortion if a malformed fetus is discovered. Survival of the first few days or weeks of life does not mean that the health and life of the infant are no longer subject to risk. There are still many threats to his well-being, and there are necessary steps that must be taken to circumvent them. A list of the leading causes of infant deaths contains several factors that surprise many (Table 17-6).

**Table 17-6.** Twelve leading causes of infant death, United States, 1969

| Rank | Cause | Number of deaths |
|---|---|---|
| 1 | Respiratory distress, asphyxia, and other anoxias | 14,508 |
| 2 | Congenital anomalies | 11,309 |
| 3 | Immaturity, unqualified | 8,946 |
| 4 | Complications of labor and childbirth | 8,706 |
| 5 | Influenza and pneumonia | 7,141 |
| 6 | Hyaline membrane disease | 4,807 |
| 7 | Accidents | 2,425 |
| 8 | Infectious and parasitic conditions | 2,287 |
| 9 | Birth injury—cause not stated | 1,691 |
| 10 | Bronchitis and bronchiolitis | 571 |
| 11 | Meningitis | 551 |
| 12 | Homicide | 151 |

Until only a few years ago infections and infectious diseases predominated. Now they are of secondary importance, with the exceptions of pneumonia and influenza, and gastroenteritis. Even these have been greatly reduced in recent years—the first by better nutrition and antibiotics and the second by improved sanitation, nursery techniques, and chemotherapy. Nevertheless, the large proportion of infant deaths attributable to a variety of respiratory ailments is notable. Numerous recent studies tend to implicate the improper or excessive use of various drugs, pharmaceuticals, and anesthetics, including some used in obstetric practice as a cause of or contributor to respiratory distress in the newborn. The significant numbers of infant deaths from accidents and homicides should also be noted. Actually, accidents represent the second leading cause of infant deaths after the first month of life is passed. With regard to homicides attention is called to the discussion of the "battered child syndrome" in Chapter 27. These are all problems that merit careful attention by all health workers. Also interesting and surprising is the occurrence of heart disease and malignancies as a cause of some infant deaths. Some success through early diagnosis and surgery is beginning to be achieved against congenital heart defects.

The infant requires a spectrum of precautions and services to get through his hazardous first year: Adequate and sanitary feeding, protection against infections and accidents, supervision preferably by a family pediatrician, home follow-up if necessary by a public health nurse, prompt correction of any defects that may exist, early diagnosis and treatment of any illnesses that may occur, and the provision of a satisfactory emotional environment. Failure to provide these needs invites more serious difficulties later in life.

### The preschool child

There are in the United States approximately 18 million children between the ages of 1 and 5 years, customarily referred to as the preschool period. When a child passes his first birthday, he enters a phase of development that is most favorable from the standpoint of the risks of mortality. At the present time the risk of death between the first and the fifth birthday is only about 1 per 1,000 preschool children. This was not always the case. At the beginning of the century the death rate of this age group was about 20 per 1,000. The preschool period benefited most from many of the greatest triumphs of

**Table 17-7.** Ten leading causes of death for children 1 to 4 years of age, United States, death registration area, 1900 and 1967

| 1900 | Rates per 100,000 population | 1967 | Rates per 100,000 population |
|---|---|---|---|
| Influenza and pneumonia | 386.6 | Accidents | 32.4 |
| Diarrhea and enteritis | 303.0 | Congenital malformations | 9.7 |
| Diphtheria | 271.0 | Influenza and pneumonia | 9.2 |
| Tuberculosis (all forms) | 101.8 | Malignant neoplasms | 8.2 |
| Measles | 87.6 | Meningitis (except meningococcal and tuberculous) | 2.0 |
| Accidents (nonmotor vehicle) | 75.3 | Gastritis, enteritis, and colitis | 1.9 |
| Scarlet fever | 64.1 | Bronchitis | 1.4 |
| Whooping cough | 60.0 | Meningococcal infections | 1.2 |
| Dysentery | 29.4 | Homicide | 1.1 |
| Nephritis | 19.5 | Diseases of heart | 1.1 |

**Table 17-8.** Acute conditions, restricted activity days, and bed disability days by age, United States, 1971*

| Age (years) | Acute conditions per 100 persons per year | Restricted activity days per 100 persons per year | Bed disability days per 100 persons per year |
|---|---|---|---|
| Under 6 years | 373 | 1165 | 494 |
| 6-16 | 296 | 903 | 433 |
| 17-44 | 206 | 823 | 366 |
| 45+ | 123 | 840 | 340 |
| All ages | 219 | 882 | 387 |

*U. S. Public Health Service: Current estimates from the health interview survey, U. S.—1971, DHEW 1971, DHEW pub. no. (HSM) 73—1505, Rockville, Md., 1973.

preventive medicine and public health. The dramatic decreases in deaths, illnesses, and disabilities in this group may be credited chiefly to the successful treatment and, what is of greater importance, to the prevention of the so-called acute communicable diseases of childhood. This is emphasized by a comparison of the leading causes of death in this age group for 1900 as against 1967 (Table 17-7). In the earlier year, 1900, the preschool death rate from influenza and pneumonia was about 387 per 100,000 as compared with a rate of about 10 per 100,000 in 1967. At the beginning of the century diarrhea, enteritis, and dysentery were important causes of death, accounting for a combined death rate of about 330 per 100,000, compared with about 2 preschool deaths per 100,000 population in 1967. The decrease in deaths from diphtheria, measles, scarlet fever, and whooping cough have been equally dramatic. Whereas deaths from motor vehicle accidents in this age

group have necessarily gone up since 1900, it is interesting that accidents from other causes have decreased significantly. In fact, the 1900 rate was more than twice the current rate.

Of greater significance than the forces of mortality in the preschool ages is the fact that although deaths are infrequent, morbidity is high. Thus the National Health Survey indicates an annual frequency rate of acute conditions during the first 6 years of life of 373 per 100 children. Similarly, restricted activity days and bed disability days are high during this period of life. Fortunately, as indicated in Table 17-8, not only is the recovery rate for preschool children high but the duration of their illnesses is brief.

The preschool years represent a period of significant nutritional and emotional change for the child as well as of increased effective contacts for the acquirement of communicable diseases and involvement in accidents. From the point of view of the public health approach therefore this stage of life is now one to which more attention must be given, not so much for the prevention of death as for the prevention of physical and mental illnesses and trauma that may handicap the future lives of those concerned. Since the individual in this age span is undergoing extremely rapid growth and development, what may often appear at the moment to be inconsequential influences of a nutritional, emotional, dental, or physical nature may have an ultimate cumulative effect far out of proportion to their initial appearance. The need therefore is for programs designed to minimize the daily impact of influences of this nature, programs for nutritional improvement, accident prevention, and continuous health and dental supervision, including techniques for the prevention of dental caries such as topical application of sodium fluoride. Mental illness is one of the greatest causes of disability in the adult population at the present time. It is during the preschool period that the seeds of much of this are sown. There is an important need, therefore, for the application of sound mental health principles and for the more widespread establishment and use of mental health and child guidance services.

## APPROACH TO THE PROBLEM

Since so many factors can affect the well-being of mothers and children, programs related to them must be multifaceted and involve the hopefully coordinated efforts of many disciplines, organizations, and agencies. For children, of course, well-informed and concerned parents necessarily must provide the keystone for the arch of proper child care and development. There are many important and sometimes critical roles for the health department.

### General

To meet adequately the many problems in maternal, infant, and child health the official health agency of a community should carry out a well-conceived and coordinated series of activities, each of which looks forward to the subsequent periods of life. Personal and community services and education are involved. As has been implied, however, the health department cannot function alone. In fact no other part of the health department program requires the cooperation of so many people and agencies in the community. In the final analysis, except in economically disadvantaged areas, most of

the direct medical and dental service to mothers, infants, and children will be rendered by private physicians and dentists. Similarly the health department can probably never substitute for the health teaching of children in the home and in the classroom under the guidance of intelligent parents and professionally trained teachers. No other phase of the public health program requires so many cooperative contacts with nonofficial nursing agencies and with the many social agencies that usually exist in the community. Within the health department itself the cooperation of all the staff is necessary. Everyone in the organization, including the vital statistics and environmental staffs as well as nurses, contributes to the protection and improvement of the health and welfare of these unusually vulnerable population groups.

Beyond this the active cooperation and assistance of many lay persons and community groups must be obtained. Few aspects of the public health program can capture the active interest of the public, and especially the news media, as much as the maternal and child health program. In addition to using lay advice and support by means of advisory committees, maternal health councils, or similar techniques, many health departments have found it possible to improve and expand their service programs considerably by using volunteer workers both in clinics and in the field.

One further general consideration deals with the necessity to conduct continuous research and surveys to keep the total health program in tune or in balance with maternal and child health needs. This involves attack from several angles. In areas with good reporting, morbidity and mortality data provide the most obvious source of guidance. Much useful data is available in many nations. In the United States the Bureau of the Census and the National Center for Health Statistics and the Division of Maternal and Child Health of the Public Health Service are especially good sources of data. In addition, the state and community agencies can provide regionally and locally pertinent information.

Generally speaking, the statistical needs for maternal and child health programs can be divided into two categories: vital statistical data and supplemental statistical information that is usually necessary for the proper interpretation of the vital statistics. The following vital statistics relating to maternity and infancy are usually available for any state, county, or large city and are a part of the basic information in planning any health service for mothers and infants:

1. Live births and stillbirths (number and rate)
   a. Urban, rural
   b. Resident and nonresident
   c. In hospitals, in homes
   d. Attended by physician, not attended by physician
   e. Legitimate or illegitimate
   f. Race
2. Maternal deaths (number and rate)
   a. Urban, rural
   b. Resident and nonresident
   c. In hospitals, in homes
   d. Attended by physician, not attended by physician
   e. Causes of death
3. Neonatal deaths (infant deaths under 1 month of age) (number and rate)
   a. Urban, rural
   b. Resident and nonresident
   c. In hospitals, in homes
   d. Attended by physician, not attended by physician
   e. Race
   f. Causes of death
   g. Age at time of death

This list must be supplemented by information relating to available medical and nursing and hospital resources, the occupations of women in the childbearing ages, educational, cultural, and many other socioeconomic factors. In addition, data must be sought with regard to the quality of health care available and the complications of pregnancy and infancy that occur in the geographic area under consideration. There should also be conducted and available to the health agency periodic analyses of hospital and medical records. This is best done by an acceptable and unbiased peer review procedure.

## MATERNAL HEALTH PROGRAM

The natal process naturally divides itself into several discrete physiologic phases, each of which presents certain problems and needs, and for many of which state and local health departments have developed programs and services.[29,30]

### Preconceptional period

Contrary to the understanding of many individuals, an adequate maternal health program should begin long before the child is conceived and even before the expectant mother reaches physiologic maturity and marriage. The preconceptional aspects of the program involves a threefold approach of education, medical service, and eugenics. Much education that may have a direct and significant influence on future parenthood can be accomplished with the high school and even grade school girl and boy. Scientifically correct and socially acceptable facts may be presented to school children relating to many phases of social hygiene, including the anatomy and physiology of reproduction, the dangers of venereal diseases and abortion, the importance of medical supervision during pregnancy and infancy, and the responsibilities of parenthood. In secondary or high schools it is appropriate to include information on and discussion of the reasons for and methods of contraception and family planning. The staffs of health departments should cooperate actively with school and other groups engaged in such educational programs.

The health department is the chief agency for the promotion, implementation, and enforcement of legislation dealing with premarital and prenatal examination requirements, of which serologic tests for syphilis and pulmonary x-ray examination should be only a part.

The eugenic approach to maternity health may be manifest by any one or a combination of three activities. The first of these is education, the basic principles of eugenics being an important and necessary part of any teaching program of sex education, social hygiene, or preparation for parenthood. Second, an increasing number of health departments sponsor programs on family planning often in cooperation with the Planned Parenthood Federation. These programs may provide contraceptive information and material and sometimes operate clinics for the remedying of sterility. In addition, it is now possible to visualize health agencies offering directly or by referral amniocentesis service for the early diagnosis of genetically damaged fetuses so that appropriate medically induced abortions may be performed promptly. Programs and services such as those described may be implemented in several ways: through supplementary service in maternal health clinics, through specifically established planned parenthood clinics, through the activities of the public health nurse in the home, or by means of referral to private physicians. A third manner in which the health department may be concerned with eugenics is where, as in some communities and states, commissions exist to pass on the desirability of sterilization of certain defective individuals. In several such instances the health officer is made a member of the commission. The fourth activity, and one that will probably grow in importance, is to serve in company with other professional and community groups in the establishment and enforcement of standards and qualifications in relation to legal induced abortion facilities and personnel. Coupled with this, and in a way related back to the first activity, education, is the role of consultant advisor and referer for those who wish or would benefit by such assistance.[31]

**Antepartum period**

The antepartum period of pregnancy is most important. The objective is to get expectant mothers under early and continuous supervision of a qualified medical advisor. This objective should be supplemented by related activities including antepartum public health nursing service and instruction in the home; the provision of auxiliary facilities such as consultants, laboratory service, and nutritional aid; and an organized approach to special problems such as illegitimate pregnancy, abortion, care for women engaged in industry during pregnancy, and such technical problems as the management of Rh incompatibility.

So that as many expectant mothers as possible receive prenatal medical and nursing supervision it is necessary to set up some form of administrative procedure to locate them as early in their pregnancies as possible. The need for and manner of doing this varies from one community to another, depending on many social factors. The health department has at its disposal several sources of information. Knowledge of pregnancies may come to the health department staff through their personal observations during their daily rounds, by statements or suggestions from neighbors of expectant mothers, and from previous patients. Some health departments have found it worth while to maintain continuous contact with business establishments that sell layettes and other baby equipment. A highly desirable goal is for the private physicians practicing in the area to notify the health department of each new obstetric case. Part of the problem is already solved in that the patient is already under medical supervision. However, even here the health department may render service through public health nursing supervision and education wherever the medical attendant wishes and with follow-up of women who miss appointments.

Antenatal medical supervision may be rendered in one of three ways: by general practitioners, by obstetricians, or in prenatal clinics operated by the health department or other agencies. Considering the country as a whole, the first of these provides the largest part of the care, and the last provides the least care. Great social and geographic variations exist. The majority of obstetric specialists practice in the large cities. Prenatal clinics are found serving primarily the lower economic groups in large urban centers and certain rural areas, particularly in the southern states. Most of the prenatal medical care rendered in rural areas is provided by general practitioners of medicine. It should be remembered, however, as previously pointed out, that although almost all white women have some medical supervision during their pregnancies, about 5% of black expectant mothers receive none.

One of the most significant developments in recent years toward the solution of these and related problems in the United States has been a changing attitude toward the use of professionally trained nurse midwives.[32] An increasing number of medical and allied health training centers are now adding this valuable health resource to society's cadre of health workers. For example, in 1970, there were 12 schools for midwives and 4 more in planning stages. Several midwives are now in group practice with obstetricians. Demands for midwives' services have sharply increased in the last few years, especially from obstetricians, and it has been predicted that a larger percentage of hospital births will be attended by nurse-midwives because of the physician shortage. A few health departments that serve areas with significant numbers of home confinements conduct programs designed for the improvement of this type of service. Some of the activities in this regard are the provision of sterilized obstetric packs and layettes, the preparation of the expectant mother for delivery in her home, and the provision of obstetric nursing assistance to the general practitioners who officiate at the deliveries. The purpose of the latter activity is threefold: service to the patient and the physician, education of the patient, and in some instances education of the physician.

**Intrapartum period**

Although the actual delivery of a pregnant woman would appear to be the concern of the woman, her husband, and her accoucheur, there are many places where the health department may enter into the intrapartum period. It has been pointed out in Chapter 9 that many health departments, primarily on the state level, have legal responsibility for the licensure, inspection, and regulation of maternity hospitals and nurseries. In many places public health agencies maintain active programs for the purpose of assuring hospitalization of selected obstetric cases and emergencies. Where midwives exist, states and communities have the legal responsibility for their regulation and control. Ordinarily this is accomplished by licensure, supervision, provision of some training, and examination.

Throughout the entire maternal health program, and particularly in its intrapartum phase, the role of the public health agency is preferably to support, assist, and promote the use of private physicians to supplant them. Additional ways in which assistance is rendered are by provision of materials for ophthalmia prophylaxis, umbilical packages, birth registration materials, and in some instances loan of equipment for blood typing, transfusion, and other emergencies. Many health departments have been active in the development of standards for obstetric consultation and in some instances in the provision of the consultants themselves by direct employment or subsidization.

A procedure of far-reaching consequence that has been promoted by many health departments in conjunction with their related medical societies is the formal review of all maternal deaths by a maternal and child health committee of the medical society. In many such instances the physician who attended the deceased mother must appear before the committee, outline his management of the case, and attempt to explain the reasons for its unfavorable outcome. This represents in effect a review of the attendant's work by a jury of his peers, and where forthrightly carried out, it has undoubtedly encouraged more careful supervision and obstetric management of women in labor.

### Postpartum period

As in the antepartum program, the first essential in the postpartum program is case finding. The location of women who have recently delivered is accomplished with relative ease. Where an efficient birth registration program is in effect, birth records provide a fruitful source of data. In addition to this is the arrangement achieved in some localities whereby hospitals routinely and promptly notify the health department of all deliveries that have occurred within their confines. In many instances the health department is notified when the patient is about to return home. Early notification is

most desirable, since it enables the public health nursing staff to make primary contact while the patient is still in the hospital in order to facilitate her hospital discharge and reentrance into the home and to prepare her home to receive her. Unfortunately a great many postpartum public health nursing visits are first made after the mother and her new infant have been home for some weeks. By then much of the potential value is lost. It is when the woman first returns to the confusing cares of her home, with the added burden of a new infant, that she really needs and appreciates help. This is especially true if the mother is socioeconomically disadvantaged. The value of meeting the mother and infant practically at the doorstep has been demonstrated by several health agencies, and the secret of its accomplishment is one of interagency cooperation and administrative timing. The problem of contacting women and infants after delivery has been greatly complicated during recent years by the frequency of change of address and by the fact that many women come into cities for hospital delivery as a convenience but return to small communities or rural areas after discharge from the hospital. These factors have also caused much difficulty in the handling of premature and ill infants, especially those who are illegitimate.

The health department's postpartum program has two purposes: to provide whatever public health nursing service and education to the mother is indicated in each case and to accomplish a smooth and automatic carry-over to the infant health program. The nurse should instruct the mother in proper postpartum care, infant care, the advantages and hygiene of breast feeding, and the preparation of infant formulas. She should make certain that the birth of the infant has been registered and that the mother and infant are both under medical supervision. She should maintain a watchful eye for the development of postpartum complications in the mother and of illness in the infant. Referrals should be made to appropriate agencies wherever medical, economic, or social problems are found to exist. Finally, the groundwork should be laid for the pediatric supervision of the infant, including all indicated protective treatments from either private physicians or health and well-baby conferences and clinics.

### THE INFANT AND PRESCHOOL PROGRAM[30,33-35]

With regard to the neonatal program, early case finding is again a prerequisite and may be accomplished by means of (1) routine check of birth certificates, (2) notification from the accoucheur, the hospital, or the family itself, and (3) from the records of prenatal clinic attendance. Neonatal cases should be classified into priority groups, with premature infants at the top of the list, followed by those known to have been born with physical defects, and those who have become ill or injured during or after birth. Many health departments maintain several portable warm beds that may be loaned to parents of premature babies who have worked out arrangements, sometimes with other agencies, for example, fire or police departments, for resuscitation services and for emergency transfer to hospitals. A number of communities provide electrically heated beds for prematures that may be fitted into taxicabs or helicopters for the emergency transportation of premature infants. A few local health departments, usually in company with other community agencies, have become involved in the provision of breast milk to infants who are premature and suffering from certain illnesses.

For the usual infant and preschool child the health department's aim is one of supervision and education. As much as possible this aim is effected by reliance on the many persons and agencies that exist as resources in the community. The most obvious and important of these are the private practitioner of medicine, the pediatrician, and the general practitioner. A large proportion of all well-child care is rendered by general practitioners. This occurs despite the fact that general practitioners tend to give less attention to health supervision as against therapy. Of general practitioner's visits to children (29% of his total practice), less than one in three visits are for health supervision. Thus whereas pediatricians see an average of 9 children a day for health supervision, the general practitioner averages 1.3. Nevertheless it is the general practitioners who provide most of the health supervision for the nation's children, since they outnumber pediatricians about 20 to 1. Only about 1.5% of the total medical services to children is rendered in community health clinics. In view of these proportions it is all the more important for the health department to solicit the active and interested cooperation of the local medical society. One of the most effective steps in this regard is the promotion of an active participation in a medical society committee on maternal and child health by the health officer.

Within the health department the larger proportion of the visits and services of the public health nursing staff should be devoted to the infant and preschool program. The services are essentially educational in nature, the teaching being done wherever possible by demonstration. One of the primary objectives of the public health nurse in her visit to the home of an infant or preschool child is to assure continuous well-baby medical supervision, preferably by the family physician or pediatrician, and failing that, in a well-baby conference conducted by the health department. Public health nursing visits on behalf of infants and preschool children should be made according to a set schedule that should be elastic enough, however, to allow for additional visits for special cases and emergencies. Generally speaking, at least two visits should be made during the first month of the infant's life. The first visit, as stated before, should be made within the first 48 hours after return to the home from the hospital or within the first 24 hours after delivery in the home. A third visit should be made as the child approaches 6 months of age, followed by another between the ninth and twelfth months. One of the primary purposes of the 6-month and 9-month visits is the promotion of the protective treatment of the baby against whooping cough, diphtheria, tetanus, measles, and poliomyelitis. Chapter 39, which deals with vital statistics, includes a description of the manner in which this part of the program may be integrated with some other activities of the health department to achieve ultimately the desired result of a high level of community protection.

Despite the emphasis of the foregoing on the well child, the infant and preschool program of the health department must take special cognizance of the sick and handicapped child population,[36,37] seeking them out and referring them to the proper community or state facilities and agencies. It should be pointed out that in one half of the states, services for crippled children are under the jurisdiction of the state health department. In the remaining states these services are usually found in departments of welfare; in 6 states there are separate crippled children's commissions, in 4 states the program is conducted by the department of education, in 2 by a branch of the state university, and in 1 state by a board of control. Rehabilitation is discussed in detail in Chapter 35.

Other activities that are gradually receiving increasing attention in infant and preschool health programs include the promotion of dental health, nutrition, and mental health. These subjects are discussed in detail in Chapters 20, 19, and 23, respectively.

## REFERENCES

1. Schmidt, W. M., and Valadian, I.: A bookshelf on maternal and child health, Amer. J. Public Health **54:**551, April 1964.
2. Eliot, M. M.: The 50th anniversary of the maternal and child health section, Amer. J. Public Health **62:**1018, July 1972.
3. Schlesinger, E. R.: The Sheppard-Towner era: a prototype case study in federal-state relationships, Amer. J. Public Health **57:**1034, June 1967.
4. Eliot, M. M.: The Children's Bureau: fifty years of public responsibility for action in behalf of children, Amer. J. Public Health, **52:**576, April 1962.
5. U. S. Department of Health, Education, and Welfare: HEW catalogue of assistance, DHEW pub. no. (OS)73-44, Washington, D. C., 1972, Government Printing Office.
6. Forgotson, E. H.: 1965: The turning point in health law—1966: reflections, Amer. J. Public Health **57:**934, June 1967.
7. U. S. Public Health Service: A report to the people on health, Washington, D. C., 1967 (unnumbered publication).
8. Calderone, M. S.: Illegal abortion as a public health problem, **50:**948, July 1960.
9. Beck, M. B., Newman, S. H., and Lewit, S.: Abortion: a national public and mental health problem—past, present, and proposed research, Amer. J. Public Health **59:**2131, Dec. 1969.
10. David, H. P.: Abortion: public health concerns and needed psychosocial research, Amer. J. Public Health **61:**510, March 1971.
11. Roemer, R.: Abortion law: the approaches of different nations, Amer. J. Public Health **57:**1906, Nov. 1967.
12. Scientific group on spontaneous and induced abortion, WHO Tech. Rep. Ser. no. 461, Geneva, 1970, World Health Organization.
13. Gold, E. M.: Abortion—1970, Amer. J. Public Health **61:**487, March 1971.
14. Smith, J. C., and Bourne, J. P.: Abortion surveillance program of the Center for Disease Control, Amer. J. Public Health **88:**255, March 1973.
15. Rowe v. Wade 41 USLW 4213, 1973; Doe v. Bolton 41 USLW 4233, 1973.
16. Harris, M., editor: Early diagnosis of human genetic defects; proceedings of a symposium, HEW pub. no. (NIH)72-25, Bethesda, 1972, National Institutes of Health.
17. Spontaneous and induced abortion, WHO Chron. **25:**104, March 1971.
18. News item: No deaths from abortion in year of South Australia's law, Hosp. Tribune **7:**2, March 26, 1973.
19. Pakter, J., O'Hare, D., Nelson, B. A., and Svigir, M.: Two years experience in New York City with the liberalized abortion law—progress and problems, Amer. J. Public Health **63:**524, June 1973.
20. Recommended program guide for abortion services, Amer. J. Public Health **62:**1669, Dec. 1972.
21. Guidelines on abortion, Chicago, Feb. 1973, American College of Obstetricians and Gynecologists.
22. Williams, S. J.: A methodology for the planning of therapeutic abortion services, Health Services Rep. **87:**983, Dec. 1972.
23. Committee for the Study of Child Health Services, The American Academy of Pediatrics: Child health services and pediatric education, New York, 1949, Commonwealth Fund.
24. U. S. Public Health Service: International comparison of perinatal and infant mortality, PHS pub. no. 1000, ser. 3, no. 6, Washington, D. C., 1967.
25. Chase, H. C.: The position of the United States in international comparisons of health status, Amer. J. Public Health **62:**581, April 1972.
26. Erhardt, C. L., et al.: Influence of weight and gestation on perinatal and neonatal mortality by ethnic group, Amer. J. Public Health **54:**1841, Nov. 1964.
27. Haworth, J. C.: Cigarette smoking during pregnancy and the effect upon the fetus, Canad. J. Public Health **64**(supp.):S20-4, March 1973.
28. Williams, H. S., and Meyer, M. B.: Cigarette smoking, infant birth weight, and perinatal mortality rates, Amer. J. Obstet. Gynec. **116:**890, July 15, 1973.
29. U. S. Public Health Service: Maternal and child health service programs—administering agencies and legislative base, DHEW pub. no. (HSM) 72-5000, Rockville, Md., 1972.
30. Lesser, A. J.: Promoting the health of mothers and children, DHEW pub. no. (HSM) 73-5002, Rockville, Md., 1972.
31. Harting, D., and Hunter, H. J.: Abortion techniques and services: a review and critique, Amer. J. Public Health **61:**2085, Oct. 1971.
32. Levy, B. S., Wilkinson, F. S., and Marine, W. M.: Reducing neonatal mortality with nurse midwives, Amer. J. Obstet. Gynec. **109:**50, Jan. 1, 1971.
33. U. S. Public Health Service: Infant care, DHEW pub. no. (OCD)72-29, Rockville, Md., 1971.
34. Standards of child health care, Evanston, 1967, The American Academy of Pediatrics.
35. U. S. Public Health Service: The children and youth projects, DHEW pub. no. (HSM) 72-5006, Rockville, Md., 1972.
36. U. S. Public Health Service: Illness among children, PHS pub. no. 2074, Rockville, Md., 1970.
37. U. S. Public Health Service: Children and youth, selected health characteristics, U. S. 1958 and 1968, PHS pub. no. 1000, ser. 10, no. 62, Rockville, Md., 1971.

*The excesses of our youth are drafts upon
our old age, payable with interest
about thirty years after date.*

C. C. COLTON

# CHAPTER 18

# School health

## THE SCHOOLCHILD

After the preschool period the child enters a world that involves more extensive contacts, a wider geographic range, an increasing number of personal and social conflicts, and many varied learning experiences. There are at the present time over 63 million children in the age group between 5 and 20 years, of whom 52.5 million are between 5 and 17 years of age. The majority are enrolled in schools, over 27 million in elementary and about 20 million in secondary schools. In addition, some in the lowest age are in kindergarten, and many in the highest 2 or 3 years are enrolled in colleges, universities, or technical schools.[1]

The situation with regard to mortality and morbidity among schoolchildren is similar to that of preschoolchildren. Again the death rates are low, having dropped from about 4 per 1,000 in 1900 to less than 1 per 1,000 at the present time. This reduction is largely attributable to success in prevention and treatment of acute communicable diseases of childhood (Table 18-1). In addition, the lowering of the threat of tuberculosis is noteworthy. At the beginning of this century over 36 schoolchildren per 100,000 died each year from this single cause. At the present time it is relatively inconsequential as a cause of death in this age group. Of further interest is the reduction in the number of deaths of school-age children from diseases of the heart to approximately one tenth what they were in 1900.[2]

As in the case of the preschool child, schoolchildren represent a group that, although subject to low death rates, experiences at the same time a high incidence of illness. To illustrate this the number of acute conditions per year per 100 individuals in each age group is presented in Table 18-2.

As a result, here again mortality data provide a poor measure of health problems and progress. Thus although the death rate in this age group from heart disease, essentially rheumatic, was

**Table 18-1.** Leading causes of death for children 5 to 14 years of age, United States, death registration area, 1900 and 1967[2]

| 1900 | Rates per 100,000 population | 1967 | Rates per 100,000 population |
|---|---|---|---|
| Diphtheria | 69.7 | Accidents | 19.3 |
| Accidents, nonmotor vehicle | 38.3 | Malignant neoplasms | 6.6 |
| Pneumonia and influenza | 38.2 | Congenital malformations | 2.4 |
| Tuberculosis | 36.2 | Influenza and pneumonia | 1.7 |
| Diseases of the heart | 23.3 | Cardiovascular and renal disease | 1.1 |

**Table 18-2.** Incidence of acute conditions by age, United States, July 1967-June 1968[3]

| Age group | Acute conditions in thousands |
|-----------|------------------------------|
| Birth-4 | 63,128 |
| 5-14 | 99,673 |
| 15-24 | 62,107 |
| 25+ | 143,448 |

only 0.8 per 100,000 in 1967, it has been estimated that almost 1% of the school population suffers from this disease, the crippling and life-shortening effects of which are delayed until later in life. Similarly, despite the great reduction in the tuberculosis death rate in this age period, it is probably here that a significant amount of the remaining new infection with the tubercle bacillus takes place. Throughout this period of life the stresses of rapid growth remain evident and are emphasized both from a physical and mental standpoint by the sexual maturation of the individual in the later school years.

Two circumstances are of considerable importance to the community health program as far as the older schoolchild is concerned: The first is that throughout this period the individual is preparing himself for living by learning. In addition, the often overlooked fact is that the older schoolchild of today is the parent and citizen-voter of tomorrow. Both of these factors have a direct bearing on the support and success of the public health program in any community. In other words this receptive impressionable period should be the most fruitful for the dissemination of health knowledge and for the establishment of understanding and support of community health measures.

## SCHOOL AND COMMUNITY HEALTH

Between the fifth or sixth year and early adulthood children spend a large part of approximately one half the year in a school environment. During this important formative period, the essential influences for physical and mental health and for education are shared by the home, the community, and the school. If the schools are to meet their responsibilities, it is necessary to formulate and to put into effect sound policies and programs for health protection and promotion during the hours of school experience.

The school is of particular importance for

several reasons: In addition to its potential importance with regard to health instruction and the development of desirable habits it represents a gathering place for a population group that is particularly susceptible to many communicable diseases and accidents. School health, therefore, must be thought of as one part of the total community health pattern, concentrating its efforts on the individual during a specific period of his existence. School health is actually the common concern of the school, the parent, and the community at all levels of government. The success and effectiveness of the program depends in large measure on the common understanding on the part of each group and each individual involved as to (1) the precise scope of its sphere of action, (2) its role in the total community health picture, and (3) the need for consistent cooperation in its implementation. In other words at its best it must be a concerted attempt to put into practice for the school-age child the thought embraced in the Children's Charter: "Every child has the right to be well-born and to attain the best possible quality of health of which it is capable."[4] All community health personnel need to pool their efforts to realize this obviously desirable goal to the greatest degree possible.

## THE SCHOOL HEALTH PROGRAM

Because of the various influences and inter-relationships as well as the dynamic nature of children and the health problems they may potentially develop, a program must be developed that focuses on circumstances that may affect the health and well-being of the schoolchild, that may derive from school personnel, and that may have their origin within the school and reach out to affect the home and the community or vice versa. With this purpose in mind the school health program has been defined as "the school procedures that contribute to the understanding, maintenance, and improvement of the health of pupils and school personnel, including health services, health education and healthful school living."[5] In other words the concern here is with (1) the school environment, (2) the protection and promotion of health, including the handling of special problems of certain children, and (3) health instruction. With this triad in mind the basic components of the school health program and the activities involved in each of them are presented in Table 18-3. Of necessity there is a certain amount of overlapping and interrelationship among these. This is desirable,

**Table 18-3.** Components of the school health program*

| School environment | Health protection and promotion | Health instruction |
|---|---|---|
| Maintenance of a safe sanitary plant | Health appraisal | Planned, direct health teaching |
| Buildings | Periodic medical examination | Indirect health education |
| Grounds, playfields | Screening examinations | Assembly programs |
| Gymnasiums, swimming pools | Dental examination | Exhibits, etc. |
| Health service unit | Special examinations | Incidental health education |
| Seating, lighting, ventilation, heating, sanitation, drinking fountains | Referrals | Integrated health education |
| | Athletes | Correlated health education |
| | Follow-up procedures | Health units in other subject courses |
| Safety and accident prevention | Referrals | |
| Protective equipment | Correction of remediable defects | In-service health education |
| Fire drills | Care of exceptional children | School personnel |
| General safety | Prevention and control of disease | Planning sessions |
| Civilian defense and disaster | Planned emergency care | Workshops |
| Safety patrols, traffic safety | Illness | Conferences |
| Transportation | Injury | Courses |
| Driver education | Health counseling | Parent education |
| Administrator-teacher-pupil relationships | Health of school personnel | Preparation of health curriculum guides |
| | Cooperation with community agencies | Utilization of resources |
| Recreation program | Official | Teaching aids |
| School luncheon | Voluntary | Textbooks, supplementary books, periodicals |
| Custodial care | Civic | |
| Healthful school day | Parent | Community personnel |
| Length | Program coordination | Community facilities |
| Class size | | Museums |
| Routine | | Libraries |
| Grading and marking procedures | | Health centers |
| Promotions | | Cooperation with community health education efforts |
| Classroom procedures | | Official agencies |
| | | Voluntary agencies |

*Modified from Hanlon, J. J., and McHose, E.: Design for health—the teacher, the school, and the community, ed. 2, Philadelphia, 1971, Lea & Febiger.

since each part of the program should be designed and used as much as possible to augment other parts. Thus certain aspects of the school environment or health appraisal activities should provide valuable firsthand health instructional material.

## THE SCHOOL ENVIRONMENT

In relation to schools the term *environment* should be interpreted in its broadest sense. It should take cognizance not only of the immediate school premises but also of its surroundings and not only of its sanitation but also of its location and safety. In other words it should include consideration of every potential physical, mental, and moral hazard with which the child may come in contact in connection with his school experience. As stated by the National Committee on School Health Policies,[7] "The author-

ity which requires pupils to attend school implies the responsibility to provide an environment as evocative as possible of growth, learning and health."

A discussion of the details of each of the many factors involved in the school environment is considered beyond the province of this book. Attention should be directed, however, to the general factors that call for supervision by public health and other authorities. Of primary importance is the location of the school. It should be chosen with a view to accessibility, salubrity, and adequacy. Proper choice of location will preclude the development of many sanitary problems. Attention should be given to drainage, shade and sunlight, freedom from industrial wastes, excessive noise, and excessive traffic. Provision should be made for adequate recreational space and for the possibility of future expansion. Although the actual choice of location will not be a responsibility of the public health department, it should offer its consultative services to whatever agencies are involved.

The health department should play a role in the assurance of the proper construction and maintenance of the school. Conformance with accepted sanitary and safety standards should be assured by frequent inspection by representatives of the public health agency and by consultation with the school authorities. Consideration must be given to ventilation, lighting, heating, and acoustics; to adequacy and location of stairways and exits; to construction materials and methods from the viewpoints of sanitation and safety; and to the adequacy and design of toilet and handwashing facilities. Because of the numbers and characteristics of those involved, the water supplies and sewage disposal facilities serving schools are considered of a public nature. Even if they are part of larger municipal systems, facilities of this type merit particular scrutiny and supervision. In rural and developing suburban areas the provision and maintenance of satisfactory water and sewage disposal facilities is particularly troublesome and requires especially persistent supervision by the health department.

Many schools, even in rural areas, provide lunchrooms and cafeterias that often have rather extensive facilities for the preparation and serving of foods. Such facilities should be under the constant surveillance of the sanitation staff of the health department to prevent their becoming a threat rather than a benefit to the children who use them. In addition, as discussed in the chapters on health education and nutrition, the staff of the public health agency should work closely with school authorities and staff to make school meals and lunchroom sanitation a practical firsthand learning experience.

Schools that contain gymnasiums, play areas, and swimming pools place an added supervisory responsibility on the health department. Standards of construction and maintenance should be established by the health agency and enforced in cooperation with the school authorities. This becomes particularly important in view of the laudable trend toward making such facilities available to the entire community rather than to restrict their use to schoolchildren during school hours. Related to these facilities and to the school as a whole should be adequately equipped and adequately staffed health service rooms for the provision of first aid. This

will be mentioned further in relation to health protection and promotion.

The most ideally located and constructed school can rapidly deteriorate and become a sanitary menace unless provision is made for its proper maintenance. As implied earlier, many aspects of the physical school plant must be subject to frequent inspection. In addition, the health department staff, as a matter of policy, should annually conduct a complete and detailed survey of the sanitary conditions and facilities of each school, public or private, within its jurisdiction. Often this is best done during the summer months when some of the other community problems slacken and during which time whatever repairs as may be indicated may be made before the reopening of the schools in the fall. Written reports with recommendations for improvements should be submitted to the school principal and the superintendent of schools. Shortcomings should be discussed with them and all assistance possible given to remedy whatever defects are found. Subsequently follow-up inspections should be made to assure the correction of any undesirable conditions.

## HEALTH PROTECTION AND PROMOTION

Present-day thinking indicates a social responsibility to prepare schoolchildren physically and psychologically as well as intellectually for adulthood. For many individuals this means graduating them in better physical condition than when they entered school. To accomplish this purpose it is necessary to establish base lines by means of physical examination. At one time it was the custom to attempt to examine every schoolchild every year. Eventually this was realized to be inefficient and pointless. This procedure had two undesirable features: So many children had to be examined each year that they usually received what amounted to a cursory scanning rather than ever getting a truly complete physical examination. Furthermore, so much attention was given to getting the children examined that it either became an end in itself or else left no time for the follow-up necessary to secure the correction of defects.[8,9]

Accordingly a more reasonable approach has been developed and is followed by progressive communities. Currently accepted standards[7] state that children should be examined only three or four times during their entire school experience, for example, at entrance to grade school, the fourth grade, junior high school, and senior high school. Preferably a parent should be present at the examination of elementary school children for purposes of explanation and education. The examinations must be carefully conducted and complete examinations, regardless of the circumstances under which they are performed. By reducing the total amount of time spent on examinations more funds and personnel time and energy are left available for securing the correction of defects.

The arrangements whereby schoolchildren are examined varies. In some communities salaried school physicians do the work, whereas in others private physicians are employed on an hourly or daily basis. There may still occasionally be seen in large schools the grossly unsatisfactory system whereby one physician examines all throats, another all ears, another all chests, and so on without consideration of the total child.

Some communities follow the interesting policy of restricting the school medical work, particularly in relation to periodic examinations, to the younger and newer men just entering practice in the community. This is based on the philosophy that everyone concerned benefits. The school and health departments get the examinations accomplished; the new physicians not yet completely established benefit from the part-time salaries and from the experience and family contacts; and the children are given more thorough examinations because the younger physicians usually relate better to children and devote relatively more time to the examination, whereas older practitioners are spared the necessity of using their time in routine examinations in which they often are not too interested. Finally, a learning situation is provided in which hopefully the younger physicians experience a satisfactory and helpful relationship with the health department that should bear sound fruits in terms of future professional relations.

Probably the most desirable system in the long run is one in which the health department and the schools educate and prompt parents to the maximum extent possible to take their schoolchildren to their family physician, if they have one, for periodic physical examinations and other protective and promotive services as well as for their illnesses. Furthermore, when the schoolchild becomes accustomed to going to his own physician for such services, the likelihood of his continuing to consult a physician after his school years is considerably greater than if he had come to expect such services

from a full-time school physician. Interesting and important variations exist as to the extent that this is possible.[10]

An important administrative technique that is of value as an adjunct to the periodic physical examination is the screening of pupils by their classroom teachers. The health department may cooperate by providing in-service training for teachers to acquaint them with the signs and symptoms of illness, particularly the communicable diseases. Without attempting to make diagnosticians out of them or to overburden them the teachers are encouraged to survey their pupils briefly each morning, referring any pupils with suspicious indications to the medical personnel available to the school. Comparative tests have demonstrated the ability of teachers to pick out sick or ailing children without reference to the exact cause.

The discovery of physical and mental defects or illnesses in schoolchildren in itself is of relatively little value. In fact, whatever value it has is contingent on what is done with the information obtained. This means a successful follow-up program from the school and health department to the home, to the private physician or dentist, or to the social agency, whichever is needed for correction of the condition.

Another phase of the school health protection and promotion program deals with the control of communicable diseases. Of primary importance is the degree to which the parents of the community bring their children to school already protected against acute communicable diseases such as diphtheria, smallpox, whooping cough, measles, and poliomyelitis. Some school systems attempt to secure these protections by mandate. When this approach is followed, some parents tend to delay immunizations until the time of school entrance, which is too late for epidemiologic value. On the other hand, a high degree of community and school protection may be obtained by educational methods, and it is foolish for a health department to make lasting enemies for its general program by stubbornly and needlessly insisting, on the basis of law or regulation, on the immunization of every last child. Too often some health or school officials have been so concerned with the achievement of high paper scores and ratings that they have overlooked much harm of a public relations nature that has been done in the process.

The screening of pupils by teachers has been discussed in relation to the periodic physical examination. When conducted routinely each morning, this becomes of some added value in the school's communicable disease control program and as an educational device. Children with suspicious signs and symptoms should be excluded from class and referred to the school medical service or to their private physician. It is desirable that there exist a policy of prompt notification of the health department. Similarly a release should be obtained from the health department or private physician before the child is readmitted to his classroom.

A question that inevitably arises in every community is whether or not schools should be in session during epidemic periods of communicable disease. In general the public tends to want the schools closed. However, when this is done, greater and more intimate contact between children usually follows, since they tend to play in their neighborhoods and circulate among crowds rather than remain at home. Therefore in communities with well-organized and efficient public health and school health services epidemics can best be controlled if the schools remain open and engage the children in controlled activities under intelligent and watchful surveillance.

In discussing the subject the National Committee on School Health policies suggested that the decision regarding the closing of schools when epidemics occur or threaten may be decided locally by answering the following two questions: (1) Are nurses and medical staffs so adequate and the teaching staff so alert that the inspection, observation, and supervision of students will keep sick students out of school? (2) If schools are closed, will students be kept at home and away from other students so that the closing of schools will not increase opportunities for contact with possible sources of infection?

As a general policy, when the first question can be answered affirmatively or when the second question is answered negatively, schools should be kept open in the face of an epidemic. This is most often the case in large public schools and in thickly settled communities. Schools should be closed when the first question is answered negatively or the second question affirmatively. In smaller communities with scattered homes, where chances for personal contact are limited, this is frequently the situation. In rural communities where pupils are transported in buses and close contact is unavoidable, it also may be advisable at times to close the schools.

## SPECIAL PROBLEMS

Of particular concern to the school health program are measures designed to meet the special needs of certain handicapped children. It is estimated that about 1.1 million children under the age of 15 years have one or more chronic disabilities that limit activities. This represents 1.8% of all those in that age group; of these, 0.9% are limited but not in a major activity, 0.7% are limited in amount or kind of major activity, whereas 0.2% are unable to carry on a major activity. Among the disabilities or impairments in children under 15 years of age are included visual defects (5.5 per 1,000), hearing defects (7.8 per 1,000), speech defects (9.1 per 1,000), and orthopedic defects (21.0 per 1,000).[3] In addition, of course, are children with other types of physical and mental defects. Most of these children are educable, and for the majority educational services can be met in conjunction with special care necessitated by physical or mental handicaps. Many localities follow a policy of complete segregation of these children, if not in special institutions, at least in separate classes for the blind, hard of hearing, crippled, pretubercular, or those with cardiac ailments and epileptic tendencies. Although such classes undoubtedly make possible much specialized care, they have the undesirable result of making the handicapped child feel still more apart and different from other children. This is not conducive to good mental health and development or to complete rehabilitation. Most authorities consider that the best policy is to allow the handicapped to intermingle with other children in the same general classrooms and to provide special classes or rest periods if needed for them, depending on their handicap. It is believed that this policy has a beneficial effect on both the handicapped children and their more fortunate classmates and results in all children considering each other as at least basically the same.

Programs of this nature may be criticized as being impractical, time consuming, and expensive. In many instances specially trained teachers are indicated. However, in terms of the most desirable end result such programs must be considered worth while. In any case time and money must be spent for the education and care of handicapped children, and some specialized personnel will have to be employed. By careful curriculum and administrative planning and by using the specialized personnel partly as consultants and in-service trainers for the general teaching staff, possibly more can be accomplished than by any other approach to the problem.

## HEALTH INSTRUCTION

Schools are primarily places where children go to learn for living. Most people consider health important for successful living. It logically follows therefore that schoolchildren should have presented to them in an understandable and interesting manner a considerable amount of information dealing with the present and future health of themselves and their community. Customarily "health teaching" is a requisite in most school curricula. However, in a great many instances the job is poorly done. Too often "health classes" turn out to be physical training periods. With equal frequency the material is presented by unqualified and sometimes disinterested persons. On about the same level are the situations where didactically unsuited members of the health department staff or private physicians are asked to give "health talks" to the students. All of these are poor substitutes for what is really needed. Empathy with students is a highly important ingredient for success in this field.

Teaching is a profession in itself. Everyone is not fitted by temperament and training to teach. Certain skills, aptitudes, and training are necessary to accomplish a satisfactory result. Therefore, inasmuch as possible, the teaching of health as well as of arithmetic and geography should be left to the trained classroom teacher who is already well acquainted with the pupils. The health department can be of greatest assistance to her by offering advice, consultative service, in-service training, and teaching materials and by aiding her in planning her health teaching program. This can best be done by a health educator or health counselor who may meet with the teachers collectively and individually to discuss goals and problems. Ever-enlarging sources of visual aids are becoming available, and the health department, as one of its justifiable activities, should make them accessible to the schools of the community.

Wherever possible, health teaching should be related to other subjects or to other school activities. Civics, geography, and many other subjects offer opportunities for the incidental inclusion of health information. As already mentioned, if a school lunch program exists, much education in food sanitation and nutrition may be associated with it. Many local health departments and school authorities have developed programs of field trips and special health study projects designed to demonstrate to schoolchildren community activities that have an influence on the health and well-being of themselves and their families. When properly planned and carried out, these study programs can have a considerable educational impact. A few health departments have progressed further to the point of allowing high school students to take turns working at simple jobs in the health department offices or even clinics as volunteers or at a nominal temporary salary. This is a doubly worthwhile venture by virtue of its educational effect and because it is also a form of vocational guidance. To be of value, however, a judicious choice of jobs and constant supervision are necessary. Since, if properly planned and conducted, it represents a learning process under supervision, the granting of academic credit for the time spent is considered justified.

## RESPONSIBILITY FOR THE SCHOOL HEALTH PROGRAM

A long-standing problem in public health administration but one that has been satisfactorily solved in many progressive communities is concerned with which agency in the community should be responsible for the school health program. Children are an important part of the total community. They can affect the health of the community, and the community in turn can affect them. It would appear obvious that to attempt to operate the school health program apart from the general community health program is inefficient, costly, and administratively unsound. An important factor is that in many communities, school systems were established earlier than public health agencies. In the absence of the latter it was natural and commendable for departments of education to attempt to provide for the health problems of the schoolchild. However, the widespread development of sound community health programs tends to negate these excuses. In general there is a much greater tendency for education authorities to provide the service in metropolitan areas and for health agencies to be responsible in isolated counties.

The advantages of operating the school health program as part of the community health program are many. More facilities, people, and sources of information are thereby readily available. Activities are more logical and fall more readily into their relative positions in the total picture of health. As just one example, consider the problem of securing the correction of physical defects. This is accomplished most effectively by qualified, generalized public health nurses who, rather than limit their interests and activities narrowly to the school situation, secure the correction of defects in schoolchildren as part of their general, family, and community public health nursing program. Such an approach cannot fail to broaden the understanding and increase the capability and efficiency of the nurse, and what is said for her holds true for the other participants in the school health program. If adequate control and supervision of the school environment are outside the field of training of the medical, physical training, or custodial staffs of the schools, the well-organized local health department will have available the services and knowledge of a qualified engineer and sanitarian to perform this important function. The efficient health department will also have up-to-the-minute reports of illness in the community and can often prevent the infected child from reaching school in the first place. Furthermore, since the community health program operates the year around, the problem of lack of professional functions and activities during the summer months is obviated.

On the other hand, there are certain activities that are rightfully considered within the jurisdiction of the schools. The most important of these is the actual teaching of health, to which reference has already been made. This is best accomplished by the professionally trained classroom teacher who should feel free to call on the official and nonofficial health agencies for assistance in planning and presentation. Many of the larger schools and departments of education employ a health coordinator to expedite these interagency relations and generally to plan and integrate the health instruction program. Beyond this all schools should have some system for providing first aid or emergency medical care or consultation. Many larger school systems employ full-time school physicians for this purpose, whereas others rely on one or several practicing physicians who agree to be on call as a public service or at a nominal fee. Even when the official health agency has general responsibility for the school health program, the employment of a school health nurse by a large school or by a department of education is not unusual. In such instances her function, although subject to variation, generally includes

responsibility for the first-aid or health room, care of minor injuries, referral to private physicians or school physicians, and consultant services to the teachers, the principal or superintendent, and the public health agency.

Although it may often appear theoretically better to center responsibility for the school health program in one or the other agency, in most instances many nontheoretical factors such as community tradition, relative acceptabilities of the respective agencies, funds and other resources available, and yes, politics too. It is realistic to recognize that different patterns do exist, that they often have good bases, that they will continue to exist for a long time, and that the advantages of each type of administration need not necessarily be lost because of the existence of the other.

## SCHOOL HEALTH COUNCILS

In dealing with most health problems of schoolchildren no single person or agency can bring about a complete solution. Fortunately interest in the health and well-being of schoolchildren is widespread. The primary responsibility, of course, rests with parents. In addition to them society as a whole and particularly private physicians, dentists, nurses, official and nonofficial health, social, and welfare agencies, and professional societies all have a rightful concern and responsibility. Here, therefore, intelligent and cooperative planning and teamwork are what spell success. Only thus can balanced and effective programs of school health education, protection, and promotion be developed. School health policies must be formulated therefore in a manner that makes the maximum use of the resources of the community. This is best accomplished by means of school health councils. Every school and school system should have a health council or committee with representation from all groups concerned in school health. At the top level in the community, where general cooperative community relationships and policies are best developed, membership should include such persons as the superintendent of schools, the local health officer, the president of the Parents and Teachers Association, a representative of the medical and dental societies, and whatever other individuals may be in key positions with relation to the health and well-being of the schoolchild. The relationship of the central school health council to each of the individual school health councils or committees is best determined by experience in each community. In general it has been recommended that the central council guide and give leadership but leave each individual school health council with considerable authority.[7]

The health council or committee of each school need not follow any particular pattern. In a one-room rural school it might consist only of the teacher, an interested parent, and a public health nurse. In larger schools the numbers of those who may play an active role are many and varied and depend on local circumstances. The essentials are that they be representative of all in the community who are concerned and may be helpful and that they provide a simple, democratic, and orderly means of determining and implementing wise school health policies.

## REFERENCES

1. Statistical abstract of the United States, Washington, D. C., 1971, Government Printing Office.
2. U. S. Public Health Service: Facts of life and death, PHS pub. no. 600, Rockville, Md., 1970.
3. U. S. Public Health Service: Children and youth: selected health characteristics, United States 1958 and 1968, PHS pub. no. 1000, ser. 10, no. 62, Rockville, Md., 1971.
4. The White House Conference, New York, 1931, The Century Co.
5. Report of the Committee on Terminology in School Health Education, J. Amer. Ass. Health, Phys. Educ. Recr. **22:**14, Sept. 1951.
6. Hanlon, J. J., and McHose, E.: Design for health —the teacher, the school and the community, ed. 2, Philadelphia, 1971, Lea & Febiger.
7. Suggested school health policies, ed. 4, Washington, D. C., 1966, National Education Association and American Medical Association.
8. Editorial: The annual school health examination —an archaic anomaly, Amer. J. Public Health **41:**448, April 1951.
9. Yankauer, A., et al.: A study of periodic school medical examinations, Amer. J. Public Health **45:**71, Jan. 1955; **46:**1553, Dec. 1956; **47:**1421, Nov. 1957; **51:**1532, Oct. 1961.
10. Cauffman, J. G., Petersen, E. L., and Emrick, J. A.: Medical care of school children: factors influencing outcome of referral from a school health program, Amer. J. Public Health **57:**60, Jan. 1967.

*A hungry man is not a free man.*

ADLAI STEVENSON

CHAPTER 19

# Nutrition*

## FOOD AND THE HEALTH OF NATIONS

In a dissertation written in 1851 on *Food and the Development of Man*,[2] Ule stated as follows:

Of all the influences which determine the life of the individual, and on which his weal and woe depend, undoubtedly the nature of his food is one of the weightiest. Every one has for himself experienced how not only the strength of his muscles, but also the course of his thought and his whole mental tone, is affected by the nature of his food. . . . The foods we use must contain the indispensable elements of nutrition in due proportion; our food must be mixed, varied, and alternating. And what is here said with regard to individuals, holds good also for nations. The foodstuffs of an energetic population are up to the standard only when they are multifariously blended, and when there is a due proportion of substances belonging to the three groups mentioned above. [The three groups the author mentioned were blood-formers or albuminates, heat-producers or respiratory foods rich in carbon, and the nutritive salts.] Now, this relation between the nutrition and the physical and the mental development of people must be apparent in the history of their civilization. When the food is insufficient, fluctuating between want and excess, uniform and undiversified, the capacity of the people for work must be inferior; their bodily strength and their mental culture must be of a low grade.

The importance of nutrition on a national scale was probably fully realized for the first time in the United States as a result of the White House Conference on Child Health called in 1930 by President Hoover. Although not at first anticipated, nutrition loomed as a factor of

predominant concern, not only because of its specific importance but especially because of its relationship to so many other circumstances related to the well-being of children. Shortly thereafter, the League of Nations began what was called a world food movement in an attempt to remedy the dire nutritional difficulties of so much of the world population that resulted from the economic depression. It emphasized the importance of adequate diets to health and suggested that agriculture, by supplying the necessary foods to the world, could overcome the depression not only for itself but for the many industries related to it. Under the League's auspices many studies of the relation of nutrition to the health of various groups were carried out. Two specific results were the formulation of the first table of optimum dietary standards and the organization of national nutrition committees in about 20 countries. Boudreau[3] states, "It was the belief of many that had this movement been started early enough the train of events leading to the Second World War might have been halted." Few things cause discontent as much as hunger, especially in the midst of plenty.

Most of the fruits of war are bitter, but some of its better fruits will be considered. Much has been written about the use of food as a weapon. The idea is not new. Captains of war recognized early the relationship between food and conquest. All would-be conquerors, from Caesar to Napoleon and Hitler, had as one of their fundamental military precepts that an army travels on its stomach and saw to it that their soldiers received the best food available. The use of siege as a means of subjugation

---

*For a useful bibliography, see Brennan.[1]

**344**

is so old as to be obscure in its origin. The cutting off of the supply of food was, of course, its chief purpose. The technique is continued in modern time in the form of embargoes, blockades, and mine fields. Once conquest was effected, the importance of food did not diminish; if anything, it increased. The Roman soldier has been described as entering conquered lands carrying a sack of flour on the point of his lance. To keep the conquered peoples contented their Roman rulers gave them bread and circuses. In this connection it is interesting to note the position of bakers in the Roman state. During the Roman Empire bakers were considered as persons important to the welfare of the nation and were made civil servants, licensed and paid by a department of food supply. It might be asked why a state such as Rome, which was anything but socialistic, followed such a nutritional policy. Undoubtedly it was because in the period of the Roman Imperium bread had become a political factor of enormous importance. A sufficient supply of bread meant social peace; lack of it implied hunger and bloody revolution.

During World War II food was used as a weapon as usual but this time as a defensive weapon as well as for offense. The story of the stupendous efforts of the allied nations to produce not only more food than ever but also food of a better quality in the face of many difficulties is well known. Less well realized, however, is the effect of this effort on the general health and well-being of the countries involved. Taken as a whole, it is justifiable to state that not only did the millions of young men and women of the allied nations who were in uniform get better meals than they otherwise would have obtained but also civilians benefited enormously both in terms of education and the substitution of nutritionally more desirable foods for some that were scarce and less beneficial. The effects of this were to be far reaching and long lasting.[4]

Boudreau, who was then Executive Director of the Milbank Memorial Fund, and Wilder,[5] his co-chairman on the Food and Nutrition Board of the National Research Council, gave some indications of these effects:

It is perhaps too early to appraise the contribution of workers in nutrition to the winning of this war, but some credit undoubtedly is due them for the fact that the country has come out of the war with unusually good health reports. Infant mortality has continued its decline despite the war, and in contrast to the usual experience in war. Deaths from tuberculosis have not increased as they always did

before in war; indeed a new all-time low record has been obtained. The figures for maternal mortality are better than they were before the war, and the same is true for virtually all death rates which reflect in any way the influence of diet on the public health. We might be less assured of the contribution of nutrition to these better records were it not that in Great Britain the fall in these rates has been even more pronounced, and over there all environmental factors except nutrition were worsened by the war.

The situation in Great Britain was summarized by Magee,[6] Consultant in Nutrition to the British Ministry of Health:

The war-time food policy was the first large-scale application of the science of nutrition to the population of the United Kingdom. . . . A diet more than ever before in conformity with physiological requirements became available to everyone, irrespective of income.

The other environmental factors which might influence the public health had, on the whole, deteriorated under the stress of war. The public health, far from deteriorating, was maintained and even in many respects improved. The rates of infantile, neonatal mortality, and the still-birth rate reached the lowest levels ever. The incidence of anemia declined, the growth-rate and the condition of the teeth of school children were improved, and the general state of nutrition of the population as a whole was up to or above prewar standards. We are therefore entitled to conclude that the new knowledge of nutrition can be applied to communities with the expectation that concrete benefit to their state of well-being will result.

This was supported by Jameson,[7] who served as Chief Medical Officer to the Ministry of Health of England and Wales during and after the war. He stated:

This can't be just an accident. All that's been done to safeguard mothers and children must have had some effect—such things as the national milk scheme, vitamin supplements for mothers and children, the great extension of schemes for school meals and milk in schools. There are doubtless other factors—full employment and higher purchasing power in many families, especially in the old depressed areas; as well as the careful planning from a nutritional point of view of the restricted amount of food available for the nation.

His conclusion was that "nutrition is the very essence and basis of national health."

## NUTRITION IN THE WORLD COMMUNITY

A measure of the importance of food to people other than its value in times of strife is the proportion of the productive resources that is devoted to providing it. The figure is always considerable, varying from about 37% of the total productive resources in the United States to about 90% in China. It depends on many factors such as wealth, social constitution, the nature of the soil, the national economy, industrialization, scientific development, and transportation. Of great importance are habits, customs, and education. "Food does more than satisfy hunger and provide pleasure, it also helps man to reach his genetic potential. The health and well-being of the people of the world now and in the future depend upon how efficiently man develops, protects, and uses his food supply. Unfortunately the gap between the world's population and its food supply is widening; therefore *every* person now alive has a responsibility to make good use of today's food supply to prevent further widening of this gap."[8]

Jelliffe[9] has defined malnutrition as a pathologic state caused by a relative or absolute deficiency or excess of one or more essential nutriments, the clinical results being detectable by physical examination or biochemical, anthropometric, or physiologic tests. Four types of malnutrition are distinguishable[10]:

1. *Undernutrition,* which results from consumption of an inadequate quantity of food over an extended period of time. Marasmus and inanition are synonymous with severe undernutrition. Starvation implies the almost total elimination of food. Such conditions as illnesses of various sorts, malabsorption syndromes, age, and continued use of antibiotics may all contribute to deficiencies of particular nutrients.

2. *Specific deficiency,* which results from the relative or absolute lack of a specific nutrient. With the exception of ascorbic acid and vitamin D deficiency in infants, specific deficiency conditions are uncommon in human malnutrition.

3. *Overnutrition,* which results from the ingestion of excess food over an extended period of time.

4. *Imbalance,* which results from a disproportion among essential nutrients, with or without the absolute deficiency of a particular nutrient required in a theoretically balanced diet.

It is difficult to determine the number of people in the world who are malnourished. The Third World Health Survey by the Food and Agriculture Organization concluded in 1963 that in the less developed countries at least 20% of the population was undernourished (insufficient calories) and about 60% had diets of inadequate nutritional quality. Overall it estimated that up to one half of the world's population (1 to 1.5 billion people) suffer from undernutrition or malnutrition or both.[11,12]

The most vulnerable group is young children. The World Health Organization estimates that about 100 million children under 5 years of age in developing countries are moderately or severely malnourished. Their malnourished state, complicated by disease, often leads to premature death. Relatively minor infections like measles, whooping cough, or chickenpox often become fatal. Studies by the Pan American Health Organization show that in the Americas malnutrition is directly or indirectly responsible for the deaths of children under 5 years of age in 53% of cases, and the situation in Asia is even more severe.[13] In addition to increased susceptibility to illness and death, malnutrition has long been recognized to have a significant and long-lasting adverse effect on intellectual development and social behavior.[14,15] It is now well demonstrated and accepted that only a well-nourished and healthy population can learn readily and have high productivity. In an excellent review by Birch[16] of many studies on this subject in many parts of the world, it is important to note his closing comment:

Malnutrition never occurs alone, it occurs in conjunction with low income, poor housing, family disorganization, a climate of apathy, ignorance and despair. The simple act of improving the nutritional status of children and their families will not and cannot of itself fully solve the problem of intellectual deficit and school failure. No single improvement in conditions will have this result. What must be recognized rather is that within our overall effort to improve the condition of disadvantaged children, nutritional considerations must occupy a prominent place, and together with improvements in all other factors of life, including relevant and directed education, contribute to the improved intellectual growth and school achievement of disadvantaged children.

Protein deficiency is one of the most severe forms of malnourishment in terms of its consequences. Since animal protein is the most expensive food, the extent of its availability and consumption is essentially a function of the economy of a family or nation. Whereas the proportion of animal products—milk, meat, eggs, and fish—in the North American diet reaches the exceptionally high figure of 40% and in the British diet nearly 30%, the figure for Latin America is only 17%, for Africa 11%, for the Near East 9% and for the Far East 5%.[17] Approximately 350 million children, or 70% of the world's population under 6 years of age, are estimated to be stunted by protein deficiency.[18] This condition is known by various names around the world in places where diets are habitually poor; in South America it is called *culebrilla*, in Africa, *kwashiorkor*. It is characterized by retarded growth and development, apathy, gastrointestinal irritability, a reddish golden appearance of the skin and hair, edema which produces a swollen abdomen, and fatty infiltration of the liver. Untreated, the mortality is high. The United Nations, recognizing protein deficiency as a major world public health problem, has charged three of its related specialized agencies—Food and Agriculture Organization, World Health Organization, and UNICEF—to collaborate in a search for a solution.

In view of the great advances in the science of nutrition it is paradoxical that so much malnutrition still exists. It must be realized, however, that there is always a great lag between research and interpretation to the masses. In the field of nutrition there is not only a lag in interpretation but also in human acceptance. Food has been said to represent the crossroads of emotion, religion, tradition, and habit—and food habits usually are changed extremely slowly. In addition to ignorance, prejudice, and poverty, however, agricultural practices and economic policies also play their part in the total picture of malnutrition. World leaders are beginning to realize that people are rationed by economic status and agricultural practices as well as by an understanding of their needs. Food intakes often reflect external circumstances rather than the fundamental needs, and some of these external circumstances are man made and can be man controlled.

## WORLD EFFORTS TOWARD IMPROVED NUTRITION

Significant steps have been taken to avoid a repetition of the failure to control some of the man-made external circumstances, which so disastrously followed World War I. During 1943 at the United Nations Conference on Food and Agriculture, in Hot Springs, Va., 44 nations agreed to work together to secure a lasting peace through freedom from want. In the records of this conference[19] the bearing of nutrition on human health was summarized as follows:

1. The kind of diet which man requires for health has been established.
2. Investigations in many parts of the world have shown that the diets consumed by the greater part of mankind are nutritionally unsatisfactory.
3. Diets which do not conform with the principles of satisfactory nutrition lead to impaired physical development, ill health and untimely death.
4. Through diet a new level of health can be attained, enabling mankind to develop inherited capacities to the fullest extent.

In planning the United Nations organization one of the earliest considerations was the establishment of the Food and Agriculture Organization (FAO) as one of the specialized agencies of the United Nations. The meeting of the Preparatory Commission held in Washington from October 28, 1946, to January 24, 1947, was attended by representatives of 17 nations: Australia, Belgium, Brazil, Canada, China, Cuba, Czechoslovakia, Denmark, Egypt, France, India, Netherlands, Philippine Republic, Poland, United Kingdom, and the United States of America, with Thailand present in discussions concerning rice. Russia and Argentina were invited to send representatives; the latter sent observers. Other international organizations represented included the International Bank for Reconstruction and Development, the International Labor Office, the International Monetary Fund, the United Nations Economic and Social Council, and the World Health Organization.

The following challenges were recognized:
1. How to expand the total food production of the world
2. How to increase buying power so that people who are now poor and underfed can buy the additional foods they need to maintain health
3. How to improve distribution among nations so that farm prices will be stable and so that starvation and surpluses will not exist side by side

The organization considered that primary responsibility rested with national governments and that the functions of the international organizations might consist of research, supplying information and consultation, encouraging cooperation, and assistance in making farming more efficient with the result that many farm workers in the less developed nations might transfer to small industries. It also hoped to play a role in the stabilization of agricultural prices as a step toward reaching a balance between food production and consumption. A conference such as this could not have been held even 25 years earlier because the relation of nutrition to the health, peace, and happiness of the world had not yet been recognized. The Food and Agriculture Organization, headquartered in Rome, has a membership of 131 nations (1974). Representatives of these governments meet annually to review the world situation in food and agriculture, forestry and fishery, to discuss common problems, and to agree on common action. Representatives of 18 governments comprise a smaller council and act between the annual sessions on the decisions made by the Conference.

What can be expected for the future of these international efforts? The potentials were well expressed by Orr,[20] a former Director General of the Food and Agricultural Organization:

I feel confident that both the highly industrialized countries and the underdeveloped countries will realize that cooperation in making this new machinery work is in their own interests . . . and that they will cooperate wholeheartedly. . . . In that case, we can look ahead to a happier future in which there will be food for the people, prosperity for agriculture, and an expansion of world trade, all of which are absolutely essential for a permanent peace.

In an effort to support the United Nations FAO program the United States passed P.L. 480. The following summarizes some of the main points of this law,[21] which was effective between 1954 and 1962:

TITLE I: Millions of tons of food have been shipped to foreign ports, paid for in local currencies and then the currencies made available to the recipient nation as aid in local developmental projects.

TITLE II: Some 60 countries received food grants until 1962 valued at about $800 million. These were government-to-government grants. Foods were made available through the Food and Agriculture Organization of the U.N.

TITLE III: Foods were made available to needy countries through the intermediary of UNICEF and non-profit voluntary relief agencies such as CARE and religious groups. Most foods under this title have been used for child feeding.

TITLE IV: Includes a barter program under which, by 1962, about $1.5 billion of supplies had been exported.

TITLE V: Provides foods on long-term dollar credit.

In 1962 the Food and Agriculture Organization and the United Nations created a World Food Program. It had two advantages: (1) Its multilateral sponsorship precluded any accusation of political or economic intent. (2) Nations other than the United States could contribute surplus supplies and personnel to it.

It began with a budget of $95 million for 3 years, by which time its need and value were so well proved that it was extended. Contributions to date add up to over $1 billion in commodities and services. About 50 nations, both poor and affluent, have participated in support that has made possible more than 525 projects in about 87 countries.[22] Meanwhile, the United States augmented its efforts with the Food for Peace Program, which had three general goals: (1) obtainment of higher protein foods for distribution, (2) enrichment and fortification of available foods, (3) formulated food development. A formulated food is a single food that can serve either as a beverage or a gruel, or perhaps be added to bread—a food that includes all nutrients a child requires.

A highly significant event during this period was the development of grain hybrids that produce greatly increased yields. Their use has spread rapidly throughout the world, initiating what has been referred to as the "green revolution." The importance of this development and its application brought Borlaug the Nobel Peace prize.

In 1966 the President of the United States appointed a panel of technical experts to study world food problems. After a year of study it expressed the view that hunger and malnutrition are not primary diseases of the last half of the twentieth century. Rather, along with the so-called population explosion, "They are symptoms of a deeper malady—lagging economic development of the countries of Latin America, Asia and Africa in which nearly two-thirds of the people of the earth now live." The panel's deliberations led to four basic conclusions:

1. The scale, severity, and duration of the world food problem are so great that a massive, long-range, innovative effort unprecedented in human history will be required to master it.

2. The solution of the problem that will exist after about 1985 demands that programs of population control be initiated now. For the immediate future the food supply is critical.

3. Food supply is directly related to agricultural development, and in turn agricultural development and overall economic development are critically interdependent in the hungry countries.

4. A strategy for attacking the world food problem will, of necessity, encompass the entire

foreign economic assistance effort of the United States in concert with other developed countries, voluntary institutions, and international organizations.[23]

The overall current situation has been summed up by Goldsmith[24] as follows:

The promises of the green revolution, the potentials of family-planning programs and the possibilities of economic development in the underdeveloped countries through international cooperation are great, and give us hope that famine can be averted. However, there is no room for complacence. Our accomplishments are meager in the face of a tremendous task. We have just started a long, difficult, and grueling race. If all of us, governments, industries, national and international organizations and individual citizens appreciate the scope of the problem and work together, it should be possible to improve nutrition, produce more food and limit population growth, thus winning the race against starvation.

## THE DETERMINANTS OF DIET

Given all cooperation among agencies, countries, and individual scientists, many practical problems remain to be solved by education, by agricultural and industrial production, by better food sanitation procedures, and by proper food storage.[25] One of the most difficult problems relates to the eating customs and habits to which a people are accustomed. Reeducation in this regard usually is difficult. Even to list the factors that decide the nature of the diet of an individual or of a community or nation is a formidable task. They may, however, be placed within a relatively few categories. Adapting from Margaret Mead,[26] they might be said to depend on six types of influences: (1) physiologic needs, (2) social organization, (3) advances in food technology, (4) economic resources and cost, (5) attributes of food, and (6) psychologic attitudes. To these may be added nutrition education, the availability of fuel and water with which to prepare food, and the all-important parental responsibility and maternal efficiency. Merrill[27] has compressed these by indicating that those concerned with public health must remain cognizant of the factors that influence food intakes. He grouped them into four headings: geographic factors, biotic factors, economic factors, and cultural factors. "Men eat," he says, "not only what the soil and the climate allow them to eat, not only what the saleability and desirability of the products they grow allow them to purchase from their neighbors, but essentially they eat what they saw their parents and grandparents eat before them."

Physiologic needs are affected by at least two types of desires: the wish to avoid the discomfort of hunger and the desire for health and vigor. For most people the former is probably the factor of predominant concern. The extent to which the feeling of hunger is produced varies to a considerable degree with the energy expenditure, which in turn is influenced by hundreds of diverse factors such as the extent of industrial and agricultural mechanization, indoor and outdoor temperatures, recreation, and methods of earning a living.

With regard to the physical attributes of foods and psychologic attitudes toward them it is obvious that different foods have different characteristics which may tend to make them pleasant or unpleasant, desirable or undesirable, practical or impractical to the individual. Among these are flavor, odor, texture, color, form, temperature, nutritive value, cleanliness, and perishability. It is a rare person indeed who can honestly deny having some food biases or idiosyncrasies. This, of course, is closely interrelated to the question of psychologic attitudes toward food. Some foods are shunned for fear that they might be fattening, poor chemical mixers, or other real or imagined physiologic reasons. Some foods are identified with low social or economic status (e.g., corned beef and cabbage); others are identified with affluence (e.g., lobster). Certain foods are symbols of hospitality, for example, wines and in some groups, ice cream. Of common knowledge is the relationship between certain foods and religion. It is not without significance that every known religion has rules relating to some foods.

Because of some and in spite of other factors that influence dietary habits and customs, some remarkable changes have taken place in the types and amounts of foods consumed by the American public during the past half century and particularly during the war years. The most outstanding changes have been steady increases in the consumption of dairy products, citrus fruits and juices, and leafy, green, and yellow vegetables. Steady downward trends have occurred in the consumption of potatoes, grain products, and some fruits.

Some changes in food consumption have naturally had an effect on the intake of the various specific nutrients. Surprisingly, the number of calories has remained more or less constant, except for a short drop during and after World War I and during 1935, a year of both economic depression and drought. Although the use of potatoes and cereals has declined, the increase in use of fats, oils, and sugar has made up the otherwise lost calories. Per capita intake of protein decreased steadily from 1909 to 1933. It increased sharply in 1934 because the drought in that year necessitated slaughtering of many animals for lack of pasture and feed. As a result, the amount of protein available in 1935 was the lowest for the entire period from 1909 to 1945. Since then, the figure has increased until now it is equal to the 1909 figure. The recent increase, however, is due in part to increased consumption of milk and eggs and the return to normal of the use of meat, poultry, and fish.

The greatly increased use of dairy products has resulted in considerable increases in calcium and riboflavin. The bread and flour enrichment program also contributed to the riboflavin increase, as it did to the increase in thiamin, niacin, and iron. The latter decreased temporarily when the consumption of meats and grain products declined. With increases in meat consumption and when the enrichment program went into effect, an increase of 15% in the amount of thiamin, niacin, and iron resulted. With the greatly increased use of leafy, green, and yellow vegetables considerable increase in the amount of vitamin A available has occurred. A similar change in the amount of ascorbic acid has resulted from the increased consumption of tomatoes and citrus fruits.

Taken as a whole, although the situation preceding World War II tended to be somewhat unfavorable, the changes in the food habits of the American public since then are encouraging, with significant increases in most of the essential nutrients coupled with a continuing awareness of "excess baggage," partly based on increased appreciation of the relationship between obesity and cardiac ailments. Nevertheless, the two most significant nutritional problems in the United States at this time are iron deficiency[28][31] and obesity.[32][33] Both problems have commanded ever-increasing attention in recent years because of awareness of their long-term consequences.

## RECOMMENDED DIETARY INTAKE

In 1968 the Food and Nutrition Board of the National Research Council issued its seventh revised edition of *Recommended Daily Dietary Allowances*.[34] Because of decreasing physical activity and a corresponding tendency to overweight on the part of many Americans, the

**Table 19-1.** Recommended daily dietary levels for the reference man and woman*

| Nutrient | Man | Woman |
|---|---|---|
| kcal. | 2,800 | 2,000 |
| Protein (gm.) | 65 | 55 |
| Vitamin A (I.U.) | 5,000 | 5,000 |
| Vitamin D (I.U.) | — | — |
| Vitamin E (I.U.) | 30 | 25 |
| Ascorbic acid (mg.) | 60 | 55 |
| Folacin (mg.) | 0.4 | 0.4 |
| Niacin (mg. equiv.) | 18 | 13 |
| Riboflavin (mg.) | 1.7 | 1.5 |
| Thiamin (mg.) | 1.4 | 1.0 |
| Vitamin $B_6$ (mg.) | 2.0 | 2.0 |
| Vitamin $B_{12}$ ($\mu$g.) | 5 | 5 |
| Calcium (g.) | 0.8 | 0.8 |
| Phosphorus (g.) | 0.8 | 0.8 |
| Iodine ($\mu$g.) | 140 | 100 |
| Iron (mg.) | 10 | 18 |
| Magnesium (mg.) | 350 | 300 |

This table refers only to the needs of the "reference man" (22 years old, 154 pounds, and moderately active) and the "reference woman" (22 years old, 128 pounds, and moderately active).
* From National Research Council, Washington, D. C., 1968.

recommended daily calorie allowance for adults was lowered about 3% to 5%. Other changes from the previous (1964) recommendations included an increase in thiamin for both sexes, a decrease in protein in both sexes, a decrease in ascorbic acid for men, an increase of riboflavin for women, and a 20% increase in iron for women. It considered that women of childbearing age require more iron than an otherwise adequate diet would provide but suggested that it was impractical to depend on ordinary food and that iron supplementation was necessary. Supplementation of water with fluoride where deficient is supported for the effect on teeth and to some extent on bones. The report provides recommended allowances for 24 age categories. For convenience and example the recommendations for a "reference man and woman" are presented in Table 19-1.

## PUBLIC HEALTH NUTRITION IN THE UNITED STATES

King[35] has provided a good brief review of nutritional developments in the United States during the 50 years that followed World War I. It was during this period that so much fundamental research was conducted and nutrition became well established as a medical and social specialty. He pointed out, however, that "the horizon is still crowded with questions and challenges that we are obliged to meet."

Recent changes in social organization in the United States have had far-reaching effects on national food habits. It is conceivable that the process of "Americanization," involving the intermarriage of many nationalities results in considerable interchange of dietary customs, ideas, and habits. Increased travel enables individuals to experience many new types of foods and methods of food preparation. Of course, the one social change that has had the most far-reaching effect has been the shift of American culture from an agrarian way of life to an industrialized, urban existence. This has resulted in a considerable shift away not only from the production of food at home but also from eating at home. The development of school lunches, the workingman's lunch box, tremendous expansion and use of restaurants, cafés, drugstore lunch counters, and drive-ins have become part of the American way of life. Eating at home often tends to promote a habitual and limited choice of food, whereas eating in groups outside causes a trend toward greater variety, interest, and choice. However, it must be remembered that steam tables often provide food of impaired vitamin content.

Many of the food problems caused by urbanization have eventually been met to an amazing degree by developments in the field of food technology that have played a dominant role in recent changes in food habits. Thousands of refrigerator cars, possibly one of American civilization's most significant inventions, move along railroads. Good highways have made possible the use of extensive fleets of food trucks and milk tank cars. Canning, dehydration, and quick freezing have produced great changes in dietary lives. Now only the smallest communities lack frozen food lockers and supermarkets. These and many other developments have made commonplace types of foods that only a short time ago were seasonable, rare, expensive, or exotic. Today's citizen of Middletown may have milk from Illinois, cereal from the Dakotas, oranges from Florida, beef from Texas, avocados from California, pineapples from Hawaii, celery from Michigan, and eggs from New Jersey.

Of course, the mere desire for food and its availability do not necessarily ensure procurement. After all, food is a commodity and can be had only for a price. It follows therefore that those who are economically disadvantaged cannot afford any but the simplest and least expensive food habits. Furthermore, they cannot afford the auxiliary factors that influence dietary development such as education, travel, and the like. As a result, large numbers of low-income population in the United States suffer from marginal or frank deficiency diseases, often in the face of food surplus. For the rural family in these circumstances much good has been done by the Agricultural Extension Service in promoting vegetable gardens in addition to cash crops, home canning, and other methods of food preservation, the construction of food cellars, and instruction in soil care and crop planning.

For urban populations with low incomes the problem has been more difficult. The school lunch program represented in its inception an attempt to supplement the diets of children of this group of the population. Subsequently it became a means of providing a noon lunch for all children who could not conveniently return home at midday. Since 1946, the school lunch program has grown considerably, and by 1973 it served 26 million school children at a cost of $1.3 billion. "Attesting to the value and potential of school feeding, the 89th Congress passed the Child Nutrition Act of 1966, authorizing a School Breakfast Program together with a Special Milk Program."[36]

Although the school lunch program has generally been considered a joint enterprise of federal, state, and local authorities, it is of critical importance that the principal, teachers, parents, and school lunch managers be interested in and understand the program. This has been part of the reason for the formation of the American Food Service Association, which now has more than 50,000 members. On the federal level, information regarding the establishment and management of the program and the use of surplus foods has been available through the United States Department of Agriculture. On the state level, inquiry can be made through the state health department and through the state department of education. On the local level, health departments and school authorities can provide information necessary to the establishment and management of a school lunch program. However, the mere serving of food is not enough; the art of incorporating nutrition education into the entire curriculum so that the feeding experience is really a learning laboratory is essential if the aim of developing good food habits in children is to be achieved.[37] Todhunter[38] has aptly described some goals that must be attained if the school lunch is to contribute to the lifetime nutritional well-being of the child:

1. Educators and school administrators must understand the importance of nutrition for school children and recognize the value of the school lunch in nutrition education.
2. The school lunch must be a part of the total school program. Teachers need to have training which will provide sufficient background in nutrition to be able to give children adequate guidance in food selection and the development of desirable food habits.
3. The school lunch program must be managed by trained lunch managers, assisted by employees who have been given adequate training for their specific jobs.
4. The school lunch must be eaten by "trained" children—that is, children who are learning about foods in relation to nutrition and health as a laboratory for educational experiences.
5. The school lunch program must run on a nonprofit basis, financed in the same way that other school services are financed. The sale of nonessential foods and beverages at lunch times or at any other period of the school day should not be permitted.
6. There must be further research and study of the nutritional needs of children, of ways of developing new food habits, and of how to teach nutrition to boys and girls so that they will put into practice what they are taught.
7. Nutritionists, dietitians, public health workers, and health educators must be alert to the significance of the school lunch as a contribution to the nutritional well-being of the child and must direct their efforts to the fulfillment of such a program as has been described.

Nutrition education can and should be an integral part of the total school curriculum and be carefully planned as such. It should develop and adapt, beginning with kindergarten and progressing through secondary school and college. As Sinacore and Harrison[39] propose, it should be regarded as an important part of the conceptualization of health and health education and be constructed upon ten basic concepts:

1. Nutrition is the use of food by the body.
2. Adequate nutrition is essential for physical health and for realization of growth potential.
3. The body needs nutrients rather than specific foods; there are many combinations of foods which can provide an adequate diet.
4. All people need the same nutrients, but quantitative requirements are unique for each individual at any given stage in his life.
5. Many factors determine what foods people eat.
6. Food is important to people because it fulfills

social, psychological, and emotional needs as well as physical ones.
7. An individual's nutritional status is determined by an interaction of his nutrient intake with heredity, disease, and environment.
8. Food is the most sensible source of nutrients for people under most circumstances.
9. The responsibility for nutritional health rests with the individual, the family, and the community.
10. Nutritional challenges change as our society changes and as knowledge accumulates.

Interesting and sound information can be incorporated into many parts of the total educational experience. This can be accomplished best by collaboration between nutritionists (school or health department), curriculum committees, and individual teachers.[40] History, for example, can be used to emphasize the important and sometimes critical role that food or the lack of it has played in the major development and tragedies of the world. Many factors such as religion, emotions, agricultural practice, and income must be considered in the study of racial and individual food habits. Food habits are slowly developed. Once formed, they are even more slowly changed. Nutrition education and the true appreciation of the part that food plays in the attainment of total health are slowly acquired but should be presented. Consequently, nutrition education and application should not be limited to one class, one semester, or one year if its true value is to be translated into healthier, happier children and adults.

The extensive urbanization of the United States and the diminished ability of the small farmer to make a profitable living has had an adverse affect on many families, as pointed out by Schorr.[41]

In 1963, of the 69 million children in the United States who lived in families, 15.6 million were poor. Depending upon one's definition of poverty, the number of poor children can be enlarged or diminished. It may be well, therefore, to be explicit about what the figure means. The portion of income that a family uses for food may be regarded as a rough indicator of its prosperity. That is, as total income goes up, a smaller and smaller percentage is devoted to food. The poorest families spend a third or more of their income on food; other families generally spend a smaller proportion. The point at which total income is less than three times the cost of the basic nutritional requirements of a family (of specific size and ages) may be viewed as the brink of poverty. Basic requirements are determined here—some will think too stringently by the economy food plan developed by the Department of Agriculture. The economy food plan is for "temporary or emergency use when funds are low." In the long run it cannot provide an adequate diet. It is by this standard that almost one fourth of the children in the United States are counted as poor.

During the years of the economic depression of the early 1930s, the federal government, to combat a general inability to obtain sufficient food, established the Federal Surplus Relief Corporation, later reorganized as the Federal Surplus Commodities Corporation, which, working with other agencies, provided food for school lunches and other programs. In 1939 an unprecedented program was begun by the Department of Agriculture to supply low-income families and those on relief with foods at public expense. One of the interesting aspects of this program was that the foods, which consisted of surpluses, were distributed not by a governmental agency but by independent grocers. Known as the Food Stamp Plan, a form of scrip was printed and distributed to low-income and relief families who could use it at markets of their choice. The grocer could subsequently turn in his accumulated stamps to the federal agency for reimbursement. The Federal Surplus Commodities Corporation actually served as a food-purchasing agent, bidding for surplus foods and then arranging for distribution and packaging. Throughout, however, supplies flowed through the regular channels of trade. The plan as a whole was successful in that it satisfied private enterprise and at the same time allowed the recipient of the food to enjoy more nearly the status of the independent purchaser. The magnitude of the initial program was $235 million made available by Congress for the use of agricultural surpluses in 1940 and 1941. Considerable nutritional and dietary education resulted from the plan, and unquestionably it had a significant effect on the eating habits of a large faction of the nation's population.

Based largely on the success of the surplus food program, in 1961 Congress enacted a 3-year pilot program to improve the nutritional status of low-income families by the provision of food stamps. Eight economically depressed areas were selected for study. After 3 years the families who participated showed better diets than similar families who had not participated. "Findings showed food stamp families made significant increases in the value of food purchased with more than 80 percent of this increase accounted for by animal products— meat, poultry, fish, milk and eggs—and by fresh fruits and vegetables."[42] As a result, the program was expanded in 1964 and now includes many areas in about half of the states. In 1972 about $43 billion in food stamps and food certificates were distributed to needy families and individuals affected by national disasters.

## RELATION OF NUTRITION TO SELECTED HEALTH PROBLEMS

**Pregnancy.** In perhaps no phase of the public health program is nutrition more important than in maternal and infant health activities. Although the relationship of the nutrition of the expectant mother to the nutrition and health of her fetus seems self-evident, it is only recently that sound, scientific proof has been forthcoming. Studies in many clinics and laboratories in this and many other countries all lead to the same conclusion: Mothers who are well nourished protect their health and the health of their babies; mothers who are not well nourished jeopardize their own physical well-being and give birth to infants not adequately equipped to withstand the trauma of extrauterine life. In addition, miscarriages, stillbirths, and premature or underweight infants are more likely to occur in poorly nourished mothers. Reports further indicate that although both the fetus and the mother may be affected by the mother's poor nutritional status, the fetus tends to suffer the most. It is also recognized that only to a limited extent is the fetus a parasite and that the extent is limited apparently by the mother's nutritional state. If the findings reported in several studies applied to all women in the United States, as they well may, better nutrition of all pregnant American women would result in more than 1 million American babies each year beginning their lives at a higher level of health and with fewer subsequent illnesses.

Many questions remain inadequately answered. For example, does maternal malnutrition play a role in the development of congenital anomalies? Can a woman poorly nourished all of her life compensate for long-term malnutrition by consuming adequate food during the period of pregnancy? What are the added risks for the woman who at conception is malnourished? Despite the fact that research groups have not yet been able to unravel many of the unknowns in this important aspect of preventive medicine, there exists adequate knowledge of the relation of nutrition to the health of both the mother and the baby to justify use of all resources at hand to encourage the best state of nutrition possible in all pregnant women. Furthermore, good nutrition throughout the entire prior life-span, as well as during the period of pregnancy, is essential if optimal nutrition is desired in the offspring. Nutritional status, good or bad, cannot be turned on and off like a faucet. Adequate nutrition during the pregnancy must be based on adequate nutrition before pregnancy.

How then should the pregnant woman's diet be managed? Circumstances place the responsibility fundamentally on the woman and the medical attendant to whom she goes for care. Her diet should be neither ignored nor considered merely in terms of a table of standards. Each woman is an individual and should be treated as such, and the physician who fails to study his pregnant patient's dietary problems as carefully as he checks her blood pressure is clearly negligent. Public health nurses and nutritionists can assist the physician or midwife by interpreting the nutritional needs of pregnancy and lactation to women individually or in mother's classes.[43] There is much misinformation about proper nutrition during pregnancy and during the period of lactation. The average pregnant woman in the United States obtains enough vitamins from her ordinary diet. On the other hand, there is no evidence that extra vitamins are harmful with the exception of vitamins A and D. Additional iron (30 to 60 mg. daily) and folic acid (200 to 400 $\mu$g. daily) are needed both during and after pregnancy, whether or not the infant is breast-fed. Ordinarily supplementary calcium is unnecessary, and prenatal fluoride does not reduce the future incidence of dental caries in the child. The pregnant woman requires additional calories, and restriction of caloric or salt intake as well as the routine use of diuretics can be dangerous. The average woman gains 22 to 25 pounds during the course of her pregnancy, and moderate weight gain apparently has no particular physiologic importance. Excessive weight gain, however, should be avoided because of the problem of future obesity and its complications.[44]

**Infancy.** Once the woman has been delivered of her infant, he has certain nutritional requirements and dietary problems peculiar to his early age. Many factors are involved, including the infant's lack of teeth, limited digestive powers, spectacular rate of growth, and need to acquire a taste for foods of a variety of flavors and textures. The mother also has nutritional needs peculiar to her own recovery from the physiologic strain of pregnancy and to the production of adequate breast milk for the feeding of her infant. The advantages of breast-feeding are many and will not be recounted here, except to make passing reference to one that is related to mental health. Suffice it to say that food habits, good or bad, are established extremely early; the security, comfort, and ideal food that breast-feeding affords start the infant out with mealtime being a psychologically as well as physiologically satisfying experience.

Federal agencies are cognizant of the problems of the medical and nutritional needs of the prenatal population, and in 1964, under the guidance of the Children's Bureau, funds were made available to local and state groups for comprehensive maternity and infant care projects.[45] By 1973 Maternity and Infant Care projects in many parts of the nation had provided much needed services, including nutritional services, to more than 1 million poor expectant mothers.[46]

**School nutrition.** The school health program is perhaps the activity to which nutrition is next most closely allied. The relationship is threefold: (1) the assurance of a satisfactory midday meal while the child is away from home, (2) the imparting of sound nutritional information, and (3) growing out of proper integration of the first two, the development of desirable nutritional habits.

Nutrition education should be a basic part of school studies for all socioeconomic groups, from kindergarten through the primary, secondary, and college levels. Major obstacles to the inclusion of more nutrition education in school curricula appear to be a combination of a lack of understanding of educational concepts on the part of nutrition specialists and a lack of workable information about nutrition on the part of the teachers. In the past, teachers' colleges have not provided their students with an adequate background in health, and nutrition has been particularly neglected. Consequently graduate in-service nutrition education is now being provided in many states. The training is offered by one or several agencies or institutions that employ personnel who are experienced in both the field of education and the field of nutrition. Included are county, city, and state health departments; colleges and universities, particularly those engaged in training home economics teachers; the American National Red Cross; and government agencies such as the Agricultural Extension Service.

Graded programs in nutrition education are now receiving increased attention, and both commercial and academic groups as well as official agencies have developed and made available helpful guides planned on graded levels. The use of tools appropriate to the age and interest of all grade levels is an absolute necessity in this field, as in all health fields. In the primary grades the emphasis is best placed on food itself, that is, how it grows, how it tastes, and so on. In the upper elementary grades simplified technical information should be presented, such as the need of particular foods for growth. In secondary schools a more scientific approach will hold the student's interest, provided his earlier nutrition education has given him the information necessary for this more mature approach.

As has been mentioned, nutrition education that can accompany a well-managed school lunch program holds great potentialities—potentialities that unfortunately are often ignored. Schools that feed but do not teach fall short of one of the aims of providing a lunch at school. Through the school lunch, children have an opportunity to become acquainted with foods not familiar to them and simultaneously to learn good patterns of eating by practicing them throughout their school years, at least at the noon meal. The school lunch program should, of course, be a part of the broad health program for all children in a school.

**Handicapped children.** Children with special health problems, such as physical, mental, or economic handicaps, also need the personal services of a nutritionist. The feeding of premature infants is the responsibility of the physician and mother, but a nutritionist can aid them. The preschool child needs an adequate diet to develop his full potential. As President Lyndon Johnson[47] pointed out in 1967, the Head Start Program "has dramatically exposed the nutritional needs of poverty's children. More than 1.5 million preschoolers are not getting the nourishing food vital to strong and healthy bodies." The President also proposed child and parent centers that would meet a wide spectrum of the following needs: (1) health and welfare services, (2) nutritious meals for needy preschoolers, (3) counseling for parents in prenatal and infant care and instruction in household management, accident prevention, and nutrition, (4) day care for children under 3 years old, and (5) a training base for specialists in child development.

Mentally handicapped children are increasing in number and require special help in meeting their dietary needs. "Nutritional factors may be

directly involved in retardation in conditions due to inborn errors of metabolism, such as phenylketonuria and galactosemia. Mental retardation may result if these conditions are not detected early and accompanying medical and specific dietary treatment provided."[48] The 1963 Maternal and Child Health and Mental Retardation Planning Amendments increased the crippled children's services "so that care may be provided to children handicapped by any form of disability or long-term illness."[49]

Welfare departments and juvenile courts, migrant workers programs, and child care facilities all can use consultant services of the nutritionist or dietician. The nutritionist must be perceptive to programs that can incorporate her services and must be flexible enough to meet the variety of needs in children and youth programs to which she can offer valuable consultative service.

**The aging population.** Inadequate nutrition is one of the greatest concerns in an aging and an aged population. In many respects the former group is of more importance than the latter because there are many more people growing old than there are those already infirm by virtue of age. Far more can be accomplished for those who are still in the aging process than for those already advanced in years. Furthermore, the circumstances of middle life determine in large part whether the subsequent advanced years will be healthy or infirm. If life is worth prolonging, it is worth nurturing in a healthy condition rather than in a state of chronic illness, senility, and dependency. Man's most productive years should be during the fifth and sixth decades, yet it is here that incapacitating chronic illness strikes so often. Arteriosclerosis, hypertension, arthritis, diabetes mellitus, degenerative conditions of the kidneys and liver, cancer, and various other disorders increasingly are becoming dominant challenges to the public health and medical professions. These are all conditions of as yet somewhat uncertain etiology. However, it is known that the way of life has much to do with the development of all of them, and considerable research indicates a frequent direct or indirect relationship with nutrition.

Certain facts about the older population should be borne in mind. In general, they tend toward a more sedentary type of existence involving less physical activity. A larger percentage of their time is spent indoors where the temperature is warm. The period of tissue and organ development is largely past, and certain changes in food habits have been enforced by virtue of impaired dental function, elimination difficulties, various physiologic changes, boredom, or economic limitations.

One of the most common effects of changes in food habits is the acquisition of excess weight. A relationship between obesity and shortened life expectancy has been clearly demonstrated. From middle age onward there is almost a direct line relationship—the age-specific death rates are increased roughly 10% for each 10 pounds of excess weight. Thus an excess of 25 pounds will lessen life expectancy by 25%. The exact reasons for this are not entirely clear because the premature deaths are not all just due to cardiac failure from carrying an overload. For example, the incidence of diabetes mellitus is two and one half times as great and of cardiovascular. and renal disease, one and one half times as great in the obese as in those of average weight.[50,51] Sebrell[52] has pointed out the following:

. . . As we pass through the middle years, the percentage of body fat usually rises, though the overall weight may remain the same. Thus, among groups of standard weight, fat may comprise only 10 per cent of the body weight in younger men, as compared with 21 per cent in older ones. The prevalence of obesity increases to about age 40 for men and 50 for women, and declines after age 60. This decline is due not only to loss of fat, but also to the loss of fat people.

The fact that obesity is correlated with aging and chronic disease does not in itself imply a causal relation. Unknown etiological factors may be common to these conditions. In various studies, however, caloric restriction has prevented cancer in mice, prolonged greatly the life of rats, and reduced the signs of diabetes in humans. Moreover, striking decreases in the incidence and severity of diabetes and hypertension accompanied undernutrition and loss of weight in certain European countries during both World Wars.

In the final analysis all obesity results from overeating in relation to one's physiologic and environmental requirements. The second of these factors has tended to be overlooked, indicating the importance of obtaining assistance from workers in several other fields in the development and conduct of obesity control programs. Sometimes excessive eating may be an expression of disturbed emotional balance—as Waife[53] has said, a substitute for some lack in the pattern of living, as the vicarious satisfaction for emotional starvation. The possible psychologic roots of excessive eating are many. "Pau-

city of companionship, love, and affection, dearth of opportunities for expression of personality, meager sources of pleasure, and sensuous gratification are some of the factors. Fear of economic insecurity, frustration from undesired social position, shame for inadequate capabilities, and shyness are often compensated by overeating." The discovery and solution of these causative problems may be more successful if the services of psychiatrists, psychologists, and social anthropologists are involved in certain phases of the public health nutritional activities.

With one out of every three Americans who are 20% overweight,[54] a variety of formula foods, fad diets, and medications have become a psychologic crutch. Apparently the overweight person would rather not revert to a proper and adequate diet. Diet was originally a Greek word meaning "way of life," and control of weight is a lifelong series of habits that must be cultivated.

In contrast with obesity in the middle and advanced years is the problem of underweight and excessive leanness due to caloric restriction. The reasons may be impaired dental function, allergic difficulties, economics, disinterest in eating because of living alone, or as in many instances of overeating, for emotional reasons such as anorexia nervosa. Significant underweight may lower resistance to tuberculosis and various other infections, and it may also cause serious disability from ocular, vasomotor, endocrine, and skeletal changes. In addition, there is the risk of mild to fullblown avitaminoses, particularly pellagra, beriberi, and scurvy. These in turn may aggravate further the underlying causes by brining about additional oral or psychic conditions.[55]

Although all concerned agree that much is still to be learned about the relationships between nutrition, chronic diseases, and the aging process, there is ample justification, if not urgency, for public health agencies to use in their planning and to disseminate among the public the considerable knowledge that is available, and also to stimulate motivational research. In addition, there is a need, as Keys[56] suggests, to protect the public from nutritional nostrums: "Part of the problem of providing nutritional help for older persons consists in countering the claims of the food faddists, the purveyors of special nostrums offered for nutritional purposes, and the writers who find a ready sale for books and articles promising miracles from peculiar diets. The older person who observes deteriorative changes in himself is especially vulnerable; the greater the loss of the sense of well-being, the stronger is the urge to believe any promise of help."

Interest of Congress in the nutritional aspects of aging is reflected in the Medicare amendments to the Social Security Act. Written into the Conditions of Participation for Extended Care Facilities are requirements for the dietary supervision and adequacy of meals. The Home Health Care section has given the professional worker an obvious responsibility for all of the acute and chronic nutritional implications of the aged. Another important step has been the inclusion in the Older American's Act of a program to provide one hot meal each day to the elderly poor. It became operational during 1972, and during its first year served 212,000 people daily. Legislative extension in 1974 allowed for an approximate doubling during the following 2 years in the number of persons benefited.

In the field of oral hygiene and public health dentistry good nutrition practices play a very important role. Conversely, there is much that the dental worker can do to promote healthier food habits.[57] It begins with the diet of the expectant mother and continues with the nature of the feedings and the subsequent more substantial diet of the infant. Also the relationship between dietary inadequacies and the development of pathologic conditions of the gingivae may be emphasized. As Massler[58] has stated, "The physical character of the food is not a nutritional factor but it is an important dietary consideration. The natural cleansing action of the food is an important adjunct to good oral hygiene. The detergent action of the food must supplement the toothbrush in preventing the accumulation of food debris, with subsequent caries and local gingivitis. Since relatively few individuals use the toothbrush correctly or effectively, the physical character of the food is an important consideration in planning a well-balanced diet."

A further consideration of consequence is the effect that a diet high in carbohydrates, especially free sugars, has on the growth of lactobacilli and *Streptococcus mutans* in dental plaques with resultant carious breakdown of the enamel and other tooth substance.[59,60] Certainly here is a fruitful area in the realm of public health nutrition for the partial solution of a large and difficult problem. Some aspects of this are discussed in more detail in Chapter 20.

## THE PLACE OF NUTRITION IN THE PUBLIC HEALTH PROGRAM

Nutrition should be considered an important activity of a health department because good nutrition is a prerequisite of good health and because good health is necessary for the full realization of useful, enjoyable lives. When public health workers speak of good health and nutrition, they should not mean just adequate health and nutrition but rather those qualities plus a reserve; in other words, health and nutrition might be thought of in three gradations; negative, borderline (or just adequate), and positive. It is for the latter that those in the public health field must strive. Unfortunately, as Christakis of the Mount Sinai School of Medicine has indicated, some health workers have presumed, perhaps more on hope than on fact, that nutrition has little contemporary relevancy, since classic nutritional deficiency states are so seldom seen in the United States. Although it is true that frank pellagra, rickets, and scurvy are now rare in this country, other significant nutritional problems still exist.

From what point of view should a department of public health be concerned with nutrition? It should not be in terms of dispensing foods or nutritive concentrates to the undernourished and needy because that constitutes a part of public welfare. Neither in most circumstances should it be in terms of diagnosing and treating individuals. Rather, as with all other problems, the health department's approach to nutrition should be all-embracing, viewing the people as a whole and not as individuals. This applies to both investigative and remedial activities.

Because of fiscal inadequacies and especially because of insufficient numbers of adequately trained personnel, relatively few local health departments, except those in large urban centers, have distinct programs of public health nutrition. This is good reason to provide nutritional expertise at least on a regional or state level. Many states have nutrition committees that serve as nuclei around which to build the program. Many related agencies, such as the Agricultural Extension Service, are organized on the state level. Many of the problems are state wide rather than local. Finally the type of program visualized should involve local contacts by accepted local public health personnel rather than by the nutrition staff whose function would be most efficient and fruitful in an advisory and consultative capacity. Because of this, it appears practical in most circumstances to limit attention essentially to specialized programs carried out on the state level, which after all exist in large part to assist and support the efforts of local health personnel.

The first states to employ nutritionists were Massachusetts and New York in 1917, and they have maintained continuous service ever since. At first their activities were merely those of specialized educators working essentially with the schools. Gradually they expanded their interests to include work with tuberculosis clinics, community education, and staff education. Largely as a result of federal funds made available under the Maternity and Infancy Act (Sheppard-Towner Act), Illinois, Michigan, Mississippi, and Connecticut began nutrition services. Because the Children's Bureau was the source of funds, these activities were all placed in the respective state divisions of maternal and child health. In 1929 the law was repealed, and despite the economic depression, only Connecticut, Massachusetts, and New York continued the activities. In 1935 the passage of the Social Security Act enabled the Children's Bureau, and through it the states, to pick up where they had left off. Soon afterward, World War II, with its attendant food shortages and rationing plus the disturbing results of military draft tests, made the public and health officials more nutrition conscious than ever before in history. As a result, by 1948, 50 out of 53 state and territorial official health agencies were budgeting funds for the employment of 170 nutritionists. At first most of the nutrition services were financed by outside funds. Thus in 1945 and 1946, 63% came from the Children's Bureau, 9% from the Public Health Service, and only 28% from the states.[61] Since then, state and local health departments have increasingly assumed responsibility for these activities.

## ORGANIZATION AND FUNCTIONS OF STATE NUTRITION PROGRAMS

Up to the present there has been much difference of opinion concerning the manner in which a nutrition program should fit into the structure of a state health department. In some states it has been organized as a separate division or as a staff agency directly responsible to the commissioner. In others it has been placed in divisions of medical services, public health nursing, and local health services. Most commonly it has been allocated to the bureau or division of maternal and child health. Un-

doubtedly this has come about as a result of the noteworthy pioneering of the Children's Bureau, and a suggestion for a different arrangement should not be construed as an attempt to detract from the credit due its far-sighted leadership. To the contrary, it is believed that public health activity in the field of nutrition is of such importance as to justify its inclusion as a more fundamental activity of wider scope rather than to risk the possibility of its benefits becoming limited to one or two groups in society, in this case children and expectant mothers.

Whereas each state or locality must of necessity organize its program in terms of its peculiar problems, facilities, and organizational history, it is believed that the most logical place for the nutrition program in most instances is in a division of local health services. The outstanding function of a state health department in nutrition, as in most other fields, is to provide leadership, guidance, consultation, and advice to those who work on the local level where the public is ultimately found. The tested pattern is the channeling of services of the state specialists through a division of local health services. This administrative technique has proved itself to make for economy, efficiency, and coordination from the viewpoints of both the state and local staffs.

The nutrition program should be under the direction of an individual who is immediately responsible to the director of local health services. The ideal qualifications of the director of nutrition should include a medical education with special clinical experience in nutritional diseases, a basic background in biochemistry, and training and experience in public health. The obvious difficulty in obtaining such a person can be solved to some extent by careful choice of a balanced staff who will carry out the detailed specialized activities of the program under his or her direction. The most important qualifications are the medical and public health backgrounds which will enable the director of nutrition to give the necessary medical guidance and to integrate the program into the other activities of the health department. The program should be so organized as to carry out a double purpose: first, because of the ever-present need and the unusual present demand for education and promotion in the field of nutrition, a service program should be organized; second, since it behooves all progressive health departments to assume some responsibility for evaluation and the advancement of knowledge, especially as it relates to potential public health practice, a research program is advisable.

## LOCAL NUTRITION PROGRAMS

To carry out any corrective and promotive program on a sound basis it is desirable, if possible, to determine at the outset the type and extent of existing problems and to furnish a base line from which to appraise any changes that might result from subsequent activities on the one hand or economic and biologic influences on the other. It is necessary therefore that everything possibly related to the state of nutrition of the people in the area be carefully considered and studied. The nutrition staff should accumulate and appraise data about groups of individuals or districts of the jurisdiction that might be of value in the service program. This involves (1) a study of the material and economic resources of the community, that is, types and amounts of foods produced, exported, retained, imported, (2) a study of food production potentialities, (3) a study of food preparation customs, (4) a study of actual food consumption patterns, and (5) a study of the nutritional status of the population, including an appraisal of the incidence, distribution, and types of deficiency diseases. Jelliffe[9] has developed a useful checklist for the World Health Organization to be used for the assessment of community or national nutritional status (Table 19-2).

Depending on the amount of funds and personnel available, assessment activities or nutritional evaluations may vary considerably from a mere study of reports of illness and death to the carrying out of extensive surveys on representative groups of the population. Survey methods have been applied to the field of nutrition to good avail to evaluate existing nutritional conditions of populations. A common procedure followed has been a threefold approach, using clinical examinations and histories, dietary analyses and/or food inventories, and various laboratory tests. Admittedly all of these procedures are subject to considerable variation and error because of the influence of the personal factor in clinical examinations and the listing of food intake, the difficulty of measuring food accurately, the variables introduced by various types of cooking, and the fact that many of the laboratory tests are still in the developmental stage. Nevertheless, by recognizing these drawbacks and by reasonable applications

of the results, the survey method can be useful in indicating outstanding problems in any given area. These procedures are admittedly too costly for most local health departments. However, in some areas they have been carried on as a cooperative enterprise of the health department and the departments of home economics, biochemistry and medical centers.

It was previously stated that a health department's service activities in nutrition should not be of the nature of dispensing public welfare. If not, then what remedial measures can be taken? They can take the form of ever-increasing education by showing the people what is wrong, by teaching them why it is wrong, and finally by assisting them in their efforts to find ways and resources to overcome the problems. This sometimes involves the breakdown of almost traditionally faulty diet habits and the translation of scientific diet analysis and planning into readily understandable and usable layman's terms. As one writer aptly put it, the facts of good nutrition must be made part of the local folklore.

A change in the mores of a people, especially as related to such a self-preserving function as nourishment, is usually accomplished slowly and with considerable difficulty. In the process one must deal with deeply ingrained ethnic, regional, and familial customs, as well as prejudices, prides, jealousies, and even superstitions and fears. To tell individuals and communities what is wrong and what remedies are needed is not enough. The more subtle but more fruitful approach is one that maneuvers community thought into the position of itself recognizing the needs and the remedies at hand.

How may this be done? In most communities in the United States there already exist many agencies and individuals not only interested in but actually already engaged in the promotion of better nutrition. State and local departments of education, welfare, and health; home demonstration and county farm agents; state agricultural extension services; the federal Departments of Agriculture and Labor; the American National Red Cross; home economics teachers; community garden, canning, and lunchroom projects; and many more are already in the front lines of activity. Working separately, there results not only some duplication of effort but also failure to recognize the existence of some problems that are perhaps of too great a magnitude for any single agency but not for the concerted effort of a combination. The development of intelligent cooperation and initiative among all these groups through health department leadership, then, is one function of a public health nutrition service. In other words, much of the function of the health department is that of a coordinator and catalyst for existing community resources.

Beyond this, consultative service should be offered by well-qualified nutritionists to the various persons and agencies mentioned, the end in view being to demonstrate how nutrition education can be injected into daily routine without adding appreciably to the daily burden.

These phases of the work should be under the immediate supervision of a well-trained and experienced nutritionist with a knowledge of the area and its governmental and voluntary agencies. Working under her direction should be several regional consulting nutritionists and possibly one or more institutional nutritionists with a special background in institutional dietetics. The area, such as a state, should be divided into regions roughly comparable in size, number of counties, population, inclusion of large cities, industries, etc. It is suggested that at first activities be restricted to counties or

**Table 19-2.** Assessment of nutritional status*

| Sources of information | Nature of information obtained | Nutritional implications |
|---|---|---|
| 1. Agricultural data<br>Food balance sheets | Gross estimates of agricultural production<br>Agricultural methods<br>Soil fertility<br>Predominance of cash crops<br>Overproduction of staples<br>Food imports and exports | Approximate availability of food supplies to a population |
| 2. Socioeconomic data<br>Information on marketing, distribu-tion, and storage | Purchasing power<br>Distribution and storage of foodstuffs | Unequal distribution of available foods between the socioeconomic groups in the community and within the family |
| 3. Food consumption patterns<br>Cultural-anthropo-logic data | Lack of knowledge, erroneous beliefs and prejudices, indifference | |
| 4. Dietary surveys | Food consumption<br>Distribution within the family | Low, excessive, or unbalanced nutrient intake |
| 5. Special studies on foods | Biologic values of diets<br>Presence of interfering factors (e.g., goitrogens)<br>Effects of food processing | Special problems related to nutrient utilization |
| 6. Vital and health statistics | Morbidity and mortality data | Extent of risk to community<br>Identification of high-risk groups |
| 7. Anthropometric studies | Physical development | Effect of nutrition on physical development |
| 8. Clinical nutritional surveys | Physical signs | Deviation from health due to malnutrition |
| 9. Biochemical studies | Levels of nutrients, metabolites, and other components of body tissues and fluids | Nutrient supplies in the body<br>Impairment of biochemical function |
| 10. Additional medical information | Prevalent disease patterns, including infections and infestations | Interrelationships of state of nutrition and disease |

*Modified from Jelliffe, D. B.: The assessment of the nutritional status of the community, WHO Monogr. Ser. no. 53, Geneva, 1966, World Health Organization.

communities with full-time public health services, since their existence will facilitate public acquaintance and acceptance of the work of the nutritionist. The length of time to be spent in each local area, the frequency of visits, and the particular type of activity and approach should be worked out on the basis of cumulative experience in the locality by the regional nutritionist herself. In some places frequent visits of short duration or irregular visits of several weeks' duration may be more successful than regularly scheduled routine visits of 1 week.

At all times the nutritionist should keep in mind the actual and potential contributions that local home economists, teachers, home demonstration agents, and many others can make, and she should plan accordingly to promote the use of their services whenever possible. She should remember that efforts on her part to render direct service to the public will reach only a few and that her real contribution is to promote the use of local talent and facilities for nutritional betterment by timely suggestions, correlation, and cooperation.

The rapid expansion of nutrition services in both public and private health agencies in recent years has lead the Food and Nutrition Section of the American Public Health Association to formulate the following statement of functions of a nutrition service to be adapted to the local conditions in an area.[62]

1. To determine the nature and magnitude of nutrition needs and to establish long-range objectives and short-term program goals.

2. To work toward the integration and coordination of nutrition service with all other appropriate services within the health agency.

3. To keep own agency informed and to work with other official agencies and organizations engaged in food and nutrition programs in a coordinated approach to the improvement of the population's nutrition status.

4. To provide a nutrition education program, including inservice education. Such a program should lead to the establishment, improvement (when indicated), and maintenance of sound eating habits throughout life, and should thereby foster the promotion of nutritional health and prevention of disease.

5. To provide consultation services on nutrition problems, on developments in nutrition research, and on the administration of nutrition aspects of programs within the agency, to professional personnel—such as physicians, nurses, and dietitians—and to groups, organizations, and other agencies.

6. To emphasize nutrition services for persons most susceptible to nutritional difficulties, for example, expectant and nursing mothers, infants and children, adolescents, the aged, those with chronic illness or physical handicap, and those with limited food budgets or restricted sources of food. The persons responsible for nutrition of such groups should be given practical instructions on the planning and value of an adequate diet, how to use available foods, and how to make prescribed dietary modifications.

7. To promote programs for adequate nutrition and food service and the provisions of suitable physical facilities by offering consultation, technical assistance, and training programs to management and food service personnel in institutions of all kinds, such as hospitals, penal institutions, sanatoriums, nursing homes, homes for the aged, industrial establishments, child care institutions and day care centers, and schools and colleges. This should make the administrative and food service personnel aware of the nutritional needs of the people they serve, and better able to meet those needs.

8. To develop, evaluate, and promote the use of nutrition education materials.

9. To participate in (or conduct) studies and investigations on the relationship of dietary factors to health and to disease.

10. To provide direct nutrition services where indicated.

11. To evaluate continually the effectiveness of the public health nutrition programs.

12. To record, report, or summarize progress and activities at regular intervals.

With the rapid expansion of the services of the public health nutritionist, there is a critical need to evaluate the services they render and determine what services could be delegated to other personnel. The 6 or 7 years of training required is barely enough to provide all the many experiences needed to face the complex nutrition problems in urban and rural society in an age of advancing technology. The University of California has developed a 5-year program that produces graduates with a master's degree, ADA internship, and some experience in public health. Various countries have developed other approaches suitable to their situations. Japan, for example, meets its personnel needs by graduating 2-year nutrition technologists. Just as the hospital dietician has promoted the use of food service supervisors, so must the public health nutritionist look for ways of extending her services through lesser trained workers. The underdeveloped nations have selected village workers, trained them for 1 year, and returned them to their homes to teach health and nutrition to their peers. Might not this principle be used to teach women in the ghetto areas of American cities, to saturate the neighborhoods with adequate nutrition information on food buying and budgeting, and to provide enough sound nutrition information so that people would not become vulnerable to fallacious practices and beliefs?

## LEGISLATION FOR ENRICHMENT OF FOODS

One other activity in the field of nutrition that should be mentioned concerns a more centralized and forceful kind of activity. This is the possibility of a community or of a state attacking nutritional problems at their source, that is, the place of production or distribution of a product. Perhaps the earliest example of this was the addition of iodine in the form of sodium or potassium iodide to public water supplies, chocolate, and more practically, to table salt.

During periods of war, animal foods become scarce because animals are expensive to feed and to produce; cereal products are consumed in greater quantities because they are the least expensive to produce in terms of acreage, man-hours, and cost. Consequently it was apparent to the Food and Nutrition Board of the National Research Council during the World War II period that cereals as a major part of the nation's diet must offer adequate nutrients.

On January 18, 1943, a government order known as War Food Order No. 1 went into effect. This order required that all white bread be enriched to meet the requirements of the order in thiamin, niacin, riboflavin, and iron. It remained in effect until October 18, 1946. By extending the practice of enrichment to low-priced bread, this program brought its benefits to low-income groups where the need was greatest. Since the War Food Order was an emergency measure and in peacetime inapplicable to interstate situations, an increasing number of states have passed legislation for the continuance of a policy of enrichment of all white flour and bread within their borders. By now, well over half of the states have adopted flour and bread enrichment legislation.

Because corn is a staple food in the southern states and substantially replaces white flour products, the Food and Nutrition Board recommends the enrichment of all corn products to the level of federal standards in areas where the consumption of corn is substantial. In some areas of the South the enrichment of corn products has met with remarkable success. For example, during a period of about 15 months, the Alabama Extension Service persuaded over 450 corn mills representing about 90% of the state's milling industry to begin voluntary enrichment of corn meal. South Carolina inaugurated its program in 1943, and the program has been continuously successful. In March 1949 the South Carolina legislature strengthened the program by amending the state's degerminated corn products enrichment law, making it mandatory to enrich all types of cornmeal and grits sold for human consumption. Several other states have since followed this example. In some areas the corn enrichment program has been delayed principally because of the nature of the corn milling industry; some products are degerminated, whereas others are not, and a large proportion of both kinds is marketed through small mills.

The repeal by some states of legislation that imposes class or restrictive taxation on margarine and the enactment of laws providing for its enrichment by the addition of 15,000 units of vitamin A per pound are further examples of centralized approach to the problem of ensuring adequate food, especially to low-income groups. A particularly important step forward was made on March 16, 1950, when the United States Congress enacted P.L. 459, which repealed the federal tax on margarine.

## REFERENCES

1. Brennan, R. E.: A bookshelf on foods and nutrition, Amer. J. Public Health **58:**621, April 1968.
2. Ule, O.: Food and the development of man (translated from the German by J. Fitzgerald, from Die Natur, 1851), Pop. Sci. Month. **5:**591, 1874.
3. Boudreau, F. G.: Nutrition in war and peace, Milbank Mem. Fund Quart. **25:**232, July 1947.
4. King, C. G., and Salthe, O.: Developments in the science of nutrition during World War II, Amer. J. Public Health **36:**879, Aug. 1946.
5. Boudréau, F. G., and Wilder, R. M.: The Food and Nutrition Board of the National Research Council: a review of its accomplishments and a forecast of its future, Fed. Proc. **5:**267, June 1946.
6. Magee, H. E.: Application of nutrition to public health, some lessons from the war, Brit. Med. J. **1:**475, March 1946.
7. Jameson, W.: The place of nutrition in a public health program, Amer. J. Public Health **37:**1371, Nov. 1947.
8. White, P. L.: Let's talk about food, Chicago, 1967, American Medical Association.
9. Jelliffe, D. B.: The assessment of the nutritional status of the community, WHO Monogr. Ser. no. 53, Geneva, 1966, World Health Organization.
10. LeRiche, W. H., and Milner, J.: Epidemiology as medical ecology, Harlow, Essex, 1971, Longman Group, Ltd.

11. Third World Food Survey, FFHC Basic Study no. 11, Rome, 1963, Food and Agriculture Organization.

12. Scrimshaw, N. S.: Food and health, contrasts deepen, Technol. Rev. (M.I.T.) **68:**20, Nov. 1965.

13. Malnourished children, Hosp. Tribune **7:**20, March 19, 1973.

14. Scrimshaw, N. S., and Gordon, J. E., editors: Malnutrition, learning and behavior, Cambridge, 1968, Massachusetts Institute of Technology.

15. Latham, M. C., and Cobos, F.: The effects of malnutrition on intellectual development and learning, Amer. J. Public Health **61:**1307, July 1971.

16. Birch, H. G.: Malnutrition, learning and intelligence, Amer. J. Public Health **62:**773, June 1972.

17. Wolstenholm, G., and O'Connor, M., editors: Health of mankind, Boston, 1967, Little, Brown & Co.

18. Randal, J.: Hunger: Does it cause brain damage? Think, p. 3, Nov.-Dec. 1966.

19. Consumption levels and requirements, United Nations Conference on Food and Agriculture, Final Act and Section Reports, Appendix 1, Report of Section 1., 1943.

20. Orr, J. B.: Nutrition and human welfare, Nutr. Abstr. Rev. **11:**3, July 1941.

21. Van Veen, A. G.: U. S. food production and world food needs, J. Amer. Dent. Ass. **48**(6): 473, June 1966.

22. Dustin, J. P.: World food program: the first ten years, World Health, p. 3, Jan. 1973.

23. President's Science Advisory Commission: The World food problem. Report of panel on the world food supply, Washington, D. C., 1967, Government Printing Office.

24. Goldsmith, G. A.: Where are we in the race against starvation, Amer. J. Public Health **61:** 1478, Aug. 1971.

25. King, C. G.: Trends in international nutrition programs, J. Amer. Dent. Ass. **48**(4):267, April 1966.

26. Mead, M.: The factor of food habits, Ann. Amer. Acad. Polit. Soc. Sci. **225:**136, Jan. 1943.

27. Merrill, M. H.: Meeting the challenges of the coming decades—the role of medicine in nutrition. Talk given at the Western Hemisphere Nutrition Conference, Chicago, Nov. 1965.

28. Filer, L. J.: The USA today—is it free of public health nutrition problems? Amer. J. Public Health **59:**327, Feb. 1969.

29. A.M.A. Council on Foods and Nutrition: Iron deficiency in the United States, J.A.M.A. **203:**119, Feb. 5, 1968.

30. Beal, V. A., and Meyers, A. J.: Iron nutriture from infancy to adolescence, Amer. J. Public Health **60:**666, April 1970.

31. White, H. S.: Iron deficiency in young women, Amer. J. Public Health **60:**659, April 1970.

32. Nordsiek, F. W.: An epidemiological approach to obesity, Amer. J. Public Health **54:**1689, Oct. 1964.

33. Mann, G. V.: Obesity, the nutritional spook, Amer. J. Public Health **61:**1491, Aug. 1971.

34. Food and Nutrition Board: Recommended daily dietary allowances, pub. no. 1694, Washington, D. C., 1968, National Academy of Science–National Research Council.

35. King, C. G.: Fifty years of experience in nutrition and a look to the future, Amer. J. Public Health **58:**2015, Nov. 1968.

36. Leverton, R.: Food and nutrition news, National Livestock and Meat Board, vol. 38, no. 6, March 1967.

37. Todhunter, E. N.: School feeding from a nutritionist's point of view, Amer. J. Public Health **60:**2302, Dec. 1970.

38. Todhunter, E. N.: Child feeding problems and the school lunch program, J. Amer. Diet. Ass. **24:**422, May 1948.

39. Sinacore, J. S., and Harrison, G.: The place of nutrition in the health education curriculum, Amer. J. Public Health **61:**2282, Nov. 1971.

40. Semrow, E. H.: Programming nutrition education, Sch. Lunch J., p. 28, Nov. 1962.

41. Schorr, A. L.: Poor kids, New York, 1966, Basic Books, Inc.

42. Currents in public health, Ross Laboratories, vol. 5, no. 2, Feb. 1965.

43. Lowenberg, M.: Coordinating maternity care: the role of nutrition, Amer. J. Public Health **41:**13, Nov. 1951.

44. Pitkin, R. M., et al.: Maternal nutrition, a selective review of clinical topics, Obstet. Gynec. **40:**773, Dec. 1972.

45. Hill, M., editor: Nutrition program news, U.S. D.A., May-June 1967, U. S. Department of Agriculture.

46. U. S. Public Health Service: Promoting the health of mothers and children, DHEW pub. no. (HSM) 73-5002, Rockville, Md., 1972.

47. Johnson, L. B.: The White House message on America's children and youth, Washington, D. C., Feb. 8, 1967.

48. Shoun, F. N.: An overview of nutrition programs for children in the United States. The nutritionist in health and welfare programs for children, Pittsburgh, 1962, University of Pittsburgh Press.

49. Egan, M. C.: Opportunities for nutritionists and dietitians in rehabilitation programs, J. Amer. Dent. Ass. **49**(4):295, Oct. 1966.

50. Vilter, R. W., and Thompson, C.: Nutrition and the control of chronic disease, Public Health Rep. **66:**632, May 1951.

51. McCay, C.: Effect of restricted feeding upon aging and chronic disease in rats and dogs, Amer. J. Public Health **37:**521, May 1947.

52. Sebrell, W. H.: Potentialities in chronic disease, Public Health Rep. **68:**737, Aug. 1953.

53. Waife, S.: The pathogenesis of obesity, Amer. Pract. **2:**47, Sept. 1947.

54. The National Observer, Jan. 13, 1964.
55. Editorial: Nutrition and vital resistance, Amer. J. Public Health **37:**915, July 1947.
56. Keys, A.: Nutrition for the later years of life, Public Health Rep. **37:**484, May 1952.
57. Davis, W.: What can the dental health worker teach regarding nutrition and diet? Amer. J. Public Health **31:**715, July 1941.
58. Massler, M.: Nutrition and the oral tissues, Amer. J. Public Health **35:**926, Sept. 1945.
59. Jay, P.: The role of sugar in the etiology of dental caries, J. Amer. Dent. Ass. **27:**393, March 1940.
60. Hoerman, K. C., et al.: The association of *Streptococcus mutans* with early carious lesions in human teeth, J. Amer. Dent. Ass. **85:**1349, 1972.
61. Report to Food and Nutrition Board, National Research Council, nutrition programs in state health departments, Public Health Rep. **65:**417, March 1950.
62. Educational qualifications of nutritionists in health agencies, Amer. J. Public Health **52**(1): 116, Jan. 1962.

*There was never yet philosopher
that could endure the toothache patiently.*

SHAKESPEARE
*Much Ado About Nothing, v.1*

CHAPTER 20

# Public health dentistry[*]

## MAGNITUDE OF THE PROBLEM

Studies of incidence and prevalence of dental ailments carried on during recent decades have placed problems of dental health clearly in a position of major importance with regard to national health needs. Fortunately the same interval has seen the dramatic development of the field of preventive dentistry and of public health dentistry—something which at the beginning of that period could not have been forecast. To put what has occurred in perspective, in 1938 two of the major contributors[3] to the progress that has since been made stated:

Inasmuch as the etiology of dental caries is unknown, prevention of the disease causing these defects is still in the experimental stage. It is generally acknowledged, however, that the treatment of early carious lesions by the proper placement of chemically and physically stable filling materials will largely prevent carious teeth from terminating in tooth loss, or tooth mortality. A primary purpose of dental health programs becomes, therefore, the promulgation of procedures whereby the early detection and treatment of carious teeth is accomplished, and tooth mortality thereby prevented.

When this statement was made, people were certainly aware of their teeth and the ailments to which they were subject. The general attitude, however, was one of fatalism and complacent acceptance of the fact that teeth were a necessary evil and that one necessarily had

to expect increasing difficulties with them as one became older. Fortunately, however, and despite obvious difficulties of prime magnitude, that situation did not continue to hold true so that it was possible for Knutson[4] to state before the American Public Health Association in 1953, "I look back over the past ten years and conclude that more has been accomplished during the decade than during the previous fifty years."

Three factors in particular contributed to the tremendous change in outlook that occurred during this period. First was the generally progressive attitude of the dental profession in the United States. This was exemplified by its many inquiries into ways of preventing dental ailments and methods of providing dental care of good quality to large numbers of the people. Second was the tremendous impact that resulted from the military drafting of a fourth of American dentists during World War II and particularly the shocking results of the physical examinations of inductees. One of the most startling findings was that of the first 2 million men examined for service in the armed forces, more were rejected because of dental defects than for any other physical reason. In fact, about 1 out of every 12 men examined was rejected on this basis.[5] Even now the United States Army finds that every 100 inductees require 600 fillings, 112 extractions, 40 bridges, 21 crowns, 18 partial dentures, and 1 full denture.[6] The third contributing factor in the progress of recent years is to be found in the brilliant researches and studies that have been made by various investigators and particularly

---

[*] For excellent bibliographies, see "Toward a Sociology of Dentistry"[1] and "A Book Shelf on Dental Public Health."[2]

by dental officers of the Public Health Service, the Eastman and Forsyth Dental Institutes, several of the schools of dentistry, and some community dental health programs. It has been estimated that dental research has expanded 1,000 times since the late 1940s. These inquiries into the incidence and prevalence of dental disease, dental physiology and pathology, the relationship of various dietary factors and particularly sugars, and the studies of the relationship of fluorides to mottled enamel and the prevention of caries are already considered epidemiologic classics.[7,8]

To appreciate the magnitude of the problem that confronts the dental profession and especially those in public health dentistry, one must consider the incidence and prevalence of dental disease and the backlog and maintenance needs for many types of dental services including diagnosis, prophylaxis, fillings, extractions, treatment of soft tissue diseases, prosthetics, orthodontics, and special services such as oral surgery, correction of congenital oral deformities, and radiation therapy. Overlying all of these, of course, is the constant need for dental health education.

Many studies have demonstrated that almost everyone in the nation has some type of dental health problem. Dental caries affects 98% of the population and is the most prevalent affliction of children. By the time the average child reaches school age he has 3 decayed teeth, and by age 15 years he has 11 decayed teeth. Each year the United States spends $2 billion just to treat caries in the 40% of the population that seeks care. If all caries incurred each year were treated, the annual cost would be about $10 billion. Americans have an estimated total of 700 million unfilled caries. Ten percent of children under 5 years have 8 or more cavities. Approximately 24 million American children 6 to 11 years of age have an estimated DMF index of 1.4, consisting of 0.5 decayed, 0.1 missing, and 0.8 filled permanent teeth per child.[9] About 10% of children 15 to 19 years of age have 10 or more cavities. At least 1 in 4 persons 18 years of age or more has lost all his permanent teeth. This is true of 1% of those 18 to 24 years, 25% of those 45 to 54 years, and 60% of those 65 to 74 years of age.[10,11] Twenty percent of school-age children have need of orthodontic treatment,[12] whereas 1 child in 800 is born with a cleft lip or palate.[13] By middle age almost 75% of the adult population is estimated to have or to have had periodontal

disease, 48% without pockets and 24% with pockets of infection. This is true of almost all persons who reach the age of 65 years.[14,15]

This leads to a consideration of the size and distribution of the personnel available to serve the dental needs of the nation. In mid-1969 there were 115,610 dentists in the United States. This represents a decline from 50 nonfederal dentists per 100,000 civilians in 1950 to 46.6 in 1969, despite the fact that graduates increased by 44% during the period—from 2,565 in 1950 to 3,700 in 1969. Twelve new dental schools were established since 1950, making a total of 53 for the nation.[16]

An additional factor to consider in relation to the adequacy of dental resources is that due to improved average economic status and more extensive health education activities on the part of dentists and health agencies, a much larger proportion of the population now seeks care. Thus in 1950 about 20% to 25% of the population visited a dentist during the year, whereas at the present time about 45% does so. It is notable, however, that more than 30 million Americans have never visited a dentist. As might be expected, urban dwellers obtain dental care more frequently and readily than do rural dwellers. The ratio of male to female dental visits is almost 1 to 1.3.[17]

Also unfortunate is the fact that dentists are not distributed evenly in relation to population and need. Low ratios of dentists to population are found particularly in the South, in rural counties, and in low-income areas. In 1968 there were 239 counties in the United States that lacked dentists. One state had almost five times as many persons per dentist as the state that was at the other extreme.[18]

Trained dental hygienists and dental assistants have more than proved their worth in recent years. Confronted with personnel shortages during World War II, studies made by Klein[19] indicated that many service hours can be gained and many more patients served through the expansion of operating equipment and the use of dental assistants. He found that the added availability of a dental hygienist or a dental assistant increased the patient load capacity per dentist 33%. If a second chair were added in addition to the assistant, the patient load capacity increased 62%. More recent studies by Soricelli and other investigators have substantiated this, especially in relation to the care of children.[20,21] In terms of his observations Knutson said[4]:

An extra dividend of this study was data and experience on the effective utilization of dental assistants. It was found that a dentist can double his out-put with the help of one fulltime and one halftime assistant. In addition, the dentist who uses assistants effectively can give better service at less cost and with less fatigue. The study showed too that once the children are on a maintenance level, one dentist with the help of trained chairside assistants can render service to approximately 1,300 children annually.

Despite the proved value of dental hygienists and dental assistants, their numbers and centers in which to train them are very inadequate. In 1970 there were about 16,000 registered dental hygienists active in the United States. This is only 16 per 100 practicing dentists. Jensen[22] deplores the negative, self-defeating attitude of many dentists and of many schools of dentistry and dental associations. He exclaims that it is their responsibility to educate practicing dentists not only to the necessity of maximizing their efficiency but to the many advantages, increased challenges, and personal satisfaction of delivering oral health care as leader of the dental team. Dentists, he claims, must be made to realize that dentistry has a responsibility to all of the public.

The average length of the dental hygienist's career is estimated to be about 7 years after graduation. About one fifth return after an interval as a homemaker. The number of schools of dental hygiene has increased rapidly in recent years from 37 in 1960 to 100 in 1970. As a result, students have increased by 50%. About 2,500 were graduated in 1970. All states now have laws for licensing dental hygienists. With their value proved so conclusively, it would seem reasonable to anticipate much greater expansion of the field of dental hygiene. In addition to increasing numbers of dental hygienists there has developed a large number, now estimated at 95,000, of dental assistants with varying amounts of short-term training usually superimposed on a high school education. The number of training institutions has grown from 26 in 1960 with 658 graduates to 154 in 1970 with 3,075 annual graduates.[16] Properly qualified individuals are certified by the American Dental Assistants Association.

There is now underway a movement to go beyond the usual dental assistant and to train what are being called dental technotherapists who can perform certain minor intraoral procedures that until now have been done by dentists.[23] A key problem is restrictive legislation,[22] and at present only a few states have allowed expansion of the functions of dental hygienists regardless of additional training. Meanwhile, dental therapy assistants are being employed by the Indian Health Service and the armed forces.[24] Obviously the nature and quality of work of such paraprofessionals must be competently supervised, but those who have them so far have not found this to be a problem.[25]

Thirty years ago, McCall[26] visualized the dentist in the future as a highly trained expert director of a cooperative team that would include a dental hygienist who would place amalgam and other plastic fillings for children, a dental technologist who would take impressions or insert and adjust dentures, and a dental assistant. The dentist himself would be free to devote himself to diagnosis, prescriptions for preventive dentistry, operative periodontic and orthodontic treatment, crown and bridge work, and direction of auxiliary personnel. Actually this has come about in the more advanced dental clinics and private practices.

A few words should be said about cost. Despite the inadequacies of dental facilities and personnel, the American public spends about one tenth of its health dollar or $2 billion per year for this purpose. In addition, the Veterans Administration pays about $70 million per year more to private dentists for veterans' service-connected dental benefits as well as providing dental care at veterans' hospitals and clinics. If nothing were possible to decrease the incidence of dental disease, it could be estimated that about $10 billion a year would be necessary to serve the dental needs of the American population adequately. One other facet of the cost picture should be mentioned. Insurance statistics have shown that "employees with poor mouth conditions have a greater incidence of illness resulting in absence from work than those with good mouth conditions. Current surveys corroborate this statement, revealing an average of four and one-half days per employee per year lost from work because of toothache or some dental ailment. An industrial manager should have to consider only such figures to see that a dental care program can save the plant money by reducing absentees."[27]

## FACTORS INVOLVED IN CARIES

Before considering some of the remarkable developments that have led to the possibility of practical and fruitful public health dental programs, it may be of value to explore briefly some of the many factors that have been considered to have a relationship to the development of dental caries. Dental caries and the consequences thereof constitute by far the major proportion of the total dental problem. It has been defined as follows[28]:

Dental caries is a disease of the calcified tissues of the teeth. It is caused by acids resulting from the action of microorganisms on carbohydrates, is characterized by a decalcification of the inorganic portion, and is accompanied or followed by a disintegration of the organic substance of the tooth.

Innumerable factors have been related at one time or another to the development or lack of development of dental caries. Some of those particularly considered have been pregnancy, chronic debilitating diseases (e.g., diabetes and tuberculosis), endocrinopathies, radiation, psychic trauma, nutritional deficiencies, inadequate dental exercise, inadequate dental cleansing, enzymes, bacteria of various species, and inherited or acquired immunity or susceptibility.

One of the commonest ideas is that the general state of health and nutrition has a close relationship with the presence or absence of dental caries. It is now known that once the teeth have erupted, their enamel is thenceforth unaffected by increased intake of calcium, phosphorus, or any of the vitamins. Similarly it has been shown that except in the most extreme instances calcium is not withdrawn from the formed teeth. This disproves one of the oldest and still extremely common folk ideas of a tooth loss for every baby. As far as can be determined the state of health and nutrition of a mother during pregnancy and lactation have little or no relationship to the subsequent possible development of dental caries in her child. As Florio[29] has stated: "Any woman should have regular dental supervision. It is highly questionable whether there is any particular virtue in having a dental examination and corrections made during pregnancy, unless it is simply easier to impress the mother at such times." He continues, "There are excellent reasons for vitamin and mineral supplement for the mother, but the soundness of the baby's teeth is not one of them." Not only does general health and nutritional status have no significant bearing on the amount of caries but there is also some evidence that malnourished people tend to have a decreased incidence of dental caries, apparently as a result of the change in composition, quantity, viscosity, and bacterial or antibacterial nature of the saliva.

Disturbances of various endocrine glands have been claimed from time to time to have an effect on the development of dental caries. The reasoning has been based on the role that some endocrine substances play in determining the structure and configuration of the dental arch, in their effect on the composition of the saliva, and possibly in relation to the development of resistance or susceptibility to caries. There has been no acceptable substantiation of such claims, and it is generally considered that no relationship exists between endocrine disturbances and the amount of caries. Much attention has been given to the possibility of inherited susceptibility or immunity to dental caries. The subject has been approached by (1) animal breeding studies, (2) human family studies, and (3) twin studies. By selective breeding, caries-resistant and caries-susceptible strains of hamsters and rats have been developed. Family studies in the United States and Sweden indicate less caries in the children of caries-free parents. Twin studies show less intrapair difference in the incidence of caries than among children selected at random.[30] Many investigators, including Klein, Jay, and Bunting, have reported the existence of families that appear to experience few or no caries. Bacterial and serologic analyses in some of these instances have shown that the lactobacillus was absent from the mouths and digestive tracts of such individuals and that the blood agglutination titer to lactobacilli was high. Despite these various studies, the general belief is that inherited or acquired susceptibility or immunity to dental caries, if a reality, plays a minor role in the total caries picture and that further investigation is indicated.

Significant racial differences appear to exist. Klein and Palmer[31] found the average numbers of decayed, missing, or filled teeth per person of both sexes at 15 years of age to be 6.6 for Hagerstown Whites, 6.5 for San Francisco Whites, 4.1 for Hagerstown Blacks, 3.1 for Indian children of all tribes studied, and only 1.1 for Navajo Indian children. In other words, at the age of 15 years white children were found to have about 1.5 times more decayed, missing, and filled permanent teeth than Black children and more than twice the number discovered in Indian children. With regard to the latter, however, it should be noted that the rate for Indian children of the Northwest was higher than for the white children studied and that the Navajo children lived in a high fluoride area.

Perhaps as a result of highly successful commercial salesmanship, it is widely accepted that various oral hygienic practices will reduce the probability of development of dental caries. Included in this category is the use of the toothbrush, dentifrices, miscellaneous mouthwashes, lozenges, medicated chewing gum, and professional dental prophylaxis. The conclusion of the American Dental Association has been that, except for certain dentifrices containing stannous fluoride, whereas these agents and procedures are worth while from the standpoint of general oral hygiene, cosmetic effect, and the stimulation of healthier gingival tissues, no evidence exists to indicate that their use bears a relationship to the suppression of caries. Of particular interest is the conclusion that even professional dental prophylaxis cannot remove all bacterial plaques from the surfaces of the teeth, especially in the pits, fissures, and contact points, and that even when they were removed they tended to re-form in a matter of days. Plaque does appear to play a significant predisposing role both in the development of caries and periodontal disease. Plaque is a soft, adherent, mucinous substance composed of bacteria, epithelial cells, leukocytes, and debris. It may become calcified by salts in the saliva precipitating. Acid-producing bacteria in the plaque erode the tooth substance causing caries, whereas calcified salts at the gingival line may irritate the soft tissues causing gingivitis, which may result in periodontal disease. Unfortunately there is no statistical evidence up to now showing that prophylaxis three or even more times a year will reduce the dental caries attack rate.[32]

Considerable research has been carried on to determine a relationship between various microorganisms and the development of dental caries. Most attention has been given to the streptococci, proteolytic bacteria, and acidogenic bacteria. These researches, especially those relating to the lactobacilli, have brought investigators much closer to the goal of understanding the mechanism of dental caries development and of devising practical preventive measures. By now it may be considered to have been conclusively demonstrated that a relationship between the formation of dental caries and the number of lactobacilli in the mouth exists. The careful studies of Jay, Bunting, and their associates, in particular, appear to have settled this question as well as the question of the correlative part that is played by a high intake of carbohydrates, especially free sugars.[33-36]

That the situation is perhaps more complicated, however, is evidenced by studies of groups fed different types of carbohydrate and carriers of free sugars. For example, those fed free sugars in the form of toffee developed significantly more caries than those who were fed chocolate, which was less adherent and was swallowed more quickly.[37] Among the bacteria, *Streptococcus mutans* has been receiving increased attention as an important cause of caries.[38] The report by a group of dental scientists that all decay-causing bacteria they have studied so far are infected with a provirus has been unexpected. A provirus is the reproductive nucleic acid portion of a virus without a protein coating. Eight strains of *S. mutans* and *S. salivarius* were treated with ultraviolet light and other agents that caused the bacterial walls to break down, releasing what appeared to be viruses with hexagonal heads and long tails. Some of the bacteria that behaved this way were found in carious teeth and produced decay in animal teeth. Strains of bacteria with no demonstrable provirus did not cause decay.[39] The potential of this observation and subsequent research tempts conjecture concerning the possibility of eventual artificial immunization against caries.

Because of the long-standing unsolved nature of the problem, much more now appears to be known of the nature and cause of caries than is realized by the public in general. Before proceeding to a consideration of some of the other developments of recent decades that have brought dental research to the point where a practical preventive dental program is possible, it is worth noting that Easlick's[40] summary of what is known about the etiology of dental caries is still valid:

Somewhat over-simplified perhaps, but nevertheless quite readily understandable, the factors may be outlined which are essential for dental caries. In the first place, the patient must be susceptible to dental caries; very few people are immune. In the second place, the patient must have teeth and the hard tissues of his teeth must be soluble in weak organic acids. In the third place, acidogenic (acid-forming) bacteria, certainly, and apparently aciduric (acid-tolerating) organisms must be present and active in large numbers in the patient's mouth. In the fourth place, the food, the substrate on which aciduric bacteria live, must be made available frequently in the patient's mouth; in other words, the host must ingest fermentable carbohydrate and usually in the form of sugar. In the fifth place, certain specialized "promoters" of chemical activity, the necessary enzymes, must be present in the patient's mouth or must not be inhibited when manufactured by resident bacteria, because at least 13 chemical reactions are required to degrade a fermentable sugar to lactic acid. Finally, in the sixth place, the organic acids, once produced, must be protected from the neutralizing effect of the patient's saliva in order that they may react with the mineral surface of a tooth. A tough, adherent film, the bacterial plaque, therefore, appears essential to the caries process.

These six essential factors, (1) susceptible patient, (2) acid-soluble tooth structure, (3) aciduric organisms, (4) carbohydrate substrate, (5) bacterial enzyme system, and (6) bacterial plaque, deserve careful consideration. They serve as research guideposts since interference with any of these factors, or any combination of them, presents possibilities for prevention or for the reduction of the patient's dental caries.

At the annual meeting of the American Public Health Association in 1953, Knutson[4] reviewed the events of the preceding decade that presaged a new era in dental health:

At the beginning of the decade we did not have a single practical method for preventing dental caries on a public health basis. To be sure, we had an abundance of evidence of high correlation between the consumption of refined sugars and the prevalence of dental caries. However, the practicability of a preventive program based on reduced sugar consumption had not been demonstrated. Our dental programs were confined largely to the early detection of new carious lesions and the prompt filling of carious teeth.

Detailed knowledge of the characteristics of the disease suggested programs designed to care for the dental needs of children on an incremental basis rather than those which were attempting to deal with the consequences of postponed care. Such dental care programs would minimize needs arising from neglect and would avoid the totally unmanageable problem posed by the accumulation of dental defects over many years. This practical approach to the dental care problem is as sound today as it was then. However, the need for emphasizing care rather than prevention made those early years in dental public health trying, indeed. Because they provided direct dental care, it was difficult to win acceptance of those programs. Public health administrators and dentists were overwhelmed by the size of the problem and the projected costs of a program designed to meet it.

No wonder those of us who lived through the days of the early, limited substance programs appreciate present caries preventive measures which can be applied so effectively and economically on a public health basis.

From the vantage point of 1974, four advances merit special mention: (1) the development of a practical method of assessing and stating the dental health status or problem of an individual group, (2) the application of fluorides directly to the teeth or indirectly through public water supplies, (3) the development of public health dentistry as a specialty, and (4) the beginning of an attack on the economic deterrents to good general dental health.

## MEASUREMENT OF DENTAL NEEDS

One of the most important developments of recent decades was the devisement of a practical definitive means of evaluation of dental needs and problems. To study the prevalence of caries in the children of various Indian tribes, Klein and Palmer were faced with the necessity of finding some means of defining the overall condition of the teeth of an individual and of large groups. Collins,[41] in compiling data to depict the physical state of school children in 1931, presented the condition of their teeth in terms of the numbers per child that were carious, extracted, and filled. Several years later Messner and associates[42] presented similar data on dental needs and treatment but in terms of the amounts in each category per 100 children specific for age groupings. Klein and Palmer[43] then combined these ideas and developed the D.M.F. (decayed or missing or filled) concept by means of which they were able to define and statistically handle the prevalence of caries, defining prevalence rate as the number of children per 100 children examined who have one or more teeth decayed or missing or filled. They explained:

The term "decayed or missing or filled," which is abbreviated throughout this report as D.M.F., means, with respect to a child, that the mouth contains one or more actively decayed, one or more filled, or one or more missing permanent teeth. It follows that a child having one or more teeth affected in any or all these classes has a D.M.F. or carious mouth. It follows also, that a count of the number of teeth decayed, plus the number filled, plus the number missing, gives a count of the total number of teeth affected by caries which in this report is synonymous with the D.M.F. count.

Simple as this concept may appear to us now, its development was a necessity to the advancement of the epidemiology of dental disease. Subsequently Klein, Palmer, and others devised variations in the method of use of the D.M.F. count. Thus the percentage of people with one or more D.M.F. represents the prevalence of caries experience in a group. The number of D.M.F. teeth per person represents the caries tendency of a group of people. The number of D.M.F. tooth surfaces per person represents the total caries tendency. The differences in the numbers of D.M.F. teeth between one point in time and another represents the incidence of caries. By means of these factors it has been possible to depict by use of graphs not only incidence and prevalence but also expectancy curves.[31]

Several other indices should be mentioned. One is the "debris index," which measures the amount of plaque formation; similar is the "calculus index." The "oral hygiene index" is a combination of the debris and the calculus indices. Several indices have been proposed to measure the extent of periodontal disease. For a different purpose a "malocclusion index" has been developed. Each of these is a valuable descriptive, programming, and evaluative tool.

## FLUORIDATION

By far the most dramatic and significant development in dental health has been the discovery of the relationship of fluorides to dental caries. Teeth blackened by minerals or, more correctly, hypoplastic teeth, which in areas of high fluoride concentration develop posteruptively a characteristic brown stain, were first described two thirds of a century ago by Eager,[44] who studied the condition in a localized area of Italy. Not long afterward, in 1916, Black and McKay[45] presented the first of an outstanding series of reports on what was called "mottled enamel" in children in certain areas of Colorado. Repeated searches for the cause of mottled enamel culminated in the report by Smith, Lantz, and Smith[46] in 1931, which definitely implicated a relatively high amount of fluorides in the soil and water. Up to this time and for several years thereafter mottled enamel was looked on exclusively as a pathologic condition and fluorine as its undesirable causative agent.

During the 1930s, however, some investigators not only in the United States but also in Argentina, China, Japan, and South Africa began to notice and question a possible relationship between high fluorine content of soil and water and mottled enamel on the one hand and apparent resistence to caries on the other. Fosdick and Hansen,[47] in their 1936 report on dental changes in Pueblo Indian children, commented, "It is interesting to speculate on the possible relationship of fluorides in fermentation and the reduced susceptibility of mottled enamel to decay." In early 1937 Arnim, Aberle, and Pitney[48] reported on unusual complete freedom from caries in 1,605 permanent incisors of 204

Indian children examined in New Mexico and Arizona. The water used by the tribes contained more than 1 part per million of fluoride. Meanwhile, Armstrong and Brekhus[49] reported a fluorine content of 0.0111% in the enamel of noncarious teeth of individuals from high fluoride areas compared with 0.0069% in carious enamel.

In connection with their 1937 report on dental caries in American Indian children, Klein and Palmer[43] raised the question of the possible beneficial effect of a certain amount of fluoride in the drinking water. They noticed that children of certain tribes in the southwestern part of the United States had much lower caries attack rates than those living elsewhere. They noted that the section involved had been found to be an endemic fluorosis area. They suggested the following:

This fact may have important implications, and would seem to justify some discussion. Fluorides are well known as enzyme inhibitors, and it may be suggested that perhaps a measure of the responsibility for low caries attack rates in the southwestern area may be the result of the drinking of fluoride water. Such water may provide an enzyme inhibitor which will operate to limit the chemical degradation of tooth-impacted carbohydrates to organic acids, so reducing the production of local acidity about the teeth, and so limiting an important vector in caries initiation.

There followed a large series of investigations by many scientists who compared the fluoride content of the enamel of teeth from different areas and of carious as against noncarious teeth, animal feeding experiments, and many comparative community studies. All substantiated the thesis that whereas an excessive amount of fluoride in water would produce mottled enamel, a certain amount, as low as 1 part per million of fluoride in water consumed during the period of tooth calcification, resulted in a significantly lower incidence of dental caries.

Of significance, especially in view of some antifluoridation arguments, is the recent discovery that rather than harming the skeletal structure and general physiology, sodium fluoride does just the opposite. In one study, for example, only 3% of females aged 55 to 64 years in high fluoride towns had signs of osteoporosis as compared with almost 21% in low fluoride areas. The study also showed less evidence of hardening of the arteries.[50] These observations have since been duplicated by a number of other investigators. Among such studies is a comparison of the incidences of fractured hips, long bones, and wrists; osteoporosis; collapsed vertebrae; and calcification of the aorta in low fluoride Kingston, N. Y., as opposed to fluoridated Newburg, N. Y.[51]

Because of the lack of knowledge at the time with regard to toxicity and costs, the first step to be taken for the practical use of the new knowledge was to apply fluorides directly to the teeth. This procedure was reported independently in 1942 by Bibby[52] and Cheyne.[53] Bibby painted the permanent teeth of children every 4 months with a solution containing 1,000 parts per million sodium fluoride. Cheyne used a solution half that strength of potassium fluoride but at 3-month intervals. Both reported a 50% reduction in caries as compared with the respective control groups. The success of these studies, which were widely publicized, led to a $1 million nationwide demonstration program sponsored by the Public Health Service for the purpose of bringing about widespread knowledge and use of the technique.[54] Another event of this period to which attention should be called was the establishment of the National Institute of Dental Research in 1948 by the Public Health Service. The establishment of this institute in itself may be considered one of the outstanding developments of recent years. Not only did it represent formal recognition by the Congress of the importance of dental health problems, but it provided funds and facilities for research, research grants, and fellowship programs.

Meanwhile studies underway demonstrated that fluorides in the concentrations being considered were nontoxic.[55-59] The Kettering Laboratory and the Institute of Industrial Health listed over 8,500 carefully analyzed and accepted scientific reports on the subject. The result was summarized by Kehoe,[60] the director of the institute: "The question of public safety of fluoridation is nonexistent from the standpoint of medical science." At the same time sanitary engineers and waterworks chemists and operators developed policies, procedures, and mechanisms for maintaining within extremely narrow limits the fluoride levels in water.[61-63] With public sanction a number of carefully controlled community studies were initiated in which fluorides were added to the public water supplies. The results of these studies indicated conclusively that the addition of fluorides up to a concentration of about 1 part per million of the drinking water supply resulted in up to two-thirds reduction in the incidence of dental caries in children who consumed it from birth.[64] If they began to drink it when they were 5 or 6 years of age, the reduction was still 22%.[65] Even those who at 16 years of age had received fluorides for only 6½ years experienced a reduction in expected caries of 18.1%.[66]

The acceptance of the fluoridation of public water supplies as an exceptionally safe, effective, and inexpensive procedure was for long disappointingly slow. However, by 1970 over 80 million people in 4,834 communities in the United States received water with the fluoride concentration adjusted to optimal levels.[67] An additional 8.4 million people in 2,624 communities were protected by naturally occurring fluoride in their water supplies.[68] The combination represented 56% of the national population. It is interesting to note that every state now has some communities with fluoridated water, and 8 states have passed statewide fluoridation laws (March 1973). Among the large cities, New York, Chicago, Philadelphia, Detroit, Baltimore, Cleveland, Washington, D. C., Minneapolis-St. Paul, St. Louis, Milwaukee, and San Francisco are now included. In fact 56% of the communities with populations over 50,000 are included.

Ireland, after much study and debate, now requires by its Health Act of 1960 the fluoridation of all public water supplies. Many other nations have enacted permissive legislation, and no government has prohibited the procedure. Thirty three nations in 1969 reported some fluoridation to the World Health Organization. Every reputable professional, civic, and governmental organization or agency endorses it. After several years of discussion and debate the World Health Organization, at its twenty-second annual assembly in July 1969, passed a resolution concerning both the effectiveness and safety of fluoridation of water supplies as a proved method of limiting the amount of dental caries.[69]

Despite this, progress has been much slower than would have been expected. This has been essentially because of the successful tactics of a relatively small group of obstructionists—the antifluoridationists. The characteristics, motivations, and methods of these people have interest and meaning for public health workers far beyond the subject of fluoridation. They are the same type and often the same individuals who tend to oppose many progressive and liberal advances, be they immunization procedures, pasteurization of milk, civil rights, or international technical assistance. Their personal motivations vary from sincere convictions based on misunderstanding, religious tenets, or deepseated cultural factors to what can only be described as fanaticism. Some find the role of professional "anti" economically rewarding. Former Vice President Hubert Humphrey mentions this in his book, *Cause is Mankind.*[70] He describes the extreme right wing of American politics as composed of a small minority of fanatics who are "against civil rights, against the United Nations, against Social Security, against fluoridation of water, against disarmament" and basically "against people." They have been well analyzed by Hoffer[71] as including certain of the socioeconomically underprivileged, the misfits, the lonely, the innately self-centered and selfish, the bored, the self-accused sinners, and various other groups. He also describes their techniques and unifying forces as including hatred, demagoguery, persuasion and coercion, suspicion, quoting out of context, and guilt by association.[72] As Paul[73] has pointed out, the arguments of antifluoridationists fall basically into three categories: its benefits are uncertain, it may be injurious, and it violates individual rights. In addition, some object on the basis of added public cost.[74]

The first two arguments have already been commented on. With reference to economics a simple calculation to compare the per capita, per family, or community cost of fluoridation with the tremendous expenditures required to repair carious teeth makes the argument absurd. An exact picture has been developed, comparing the costs of dental care for children in nonfluoridated Kingston, N. Y., with those in fluoridated Newburgh, N. Y.[75] The mean cost per child for initial dental care in Kingston was $27.61 as opposed to $11.92 for Newburgh. The mean cost of incremental dental care per child was $11.51 in Kingston compared with $6.17 in Newburgh.

Perhaps more serious is the charge that fluoridation constitutes enforced medication, violates individual rights, and is illegal.[76-78] Fortunately this charge no longer is valid. The right of communities to adjust the amount of fluoride in their public water supplies as a dental disease preventative has been upheld by courts all the way up to the United States Supreme Court, which has refused review of several appeals on the basis that no federal constitu-

tional question was involved. It is of further significance that in 1966 the Michigan branch of the American Civil Liberties Union considered the issue and concluded that there was no basis on which to consider a violation of personal or civil liberties. One of the problems that has confronted many communities and their health agencies is that antifluoridationists increasingly succeed in placing the issue on the ballot. It has long since been demonstrated that one can obtain sufficient signatures to get almost any referendum before the people and by adroit choice of words so confuse the voters that either they do not vote or vote contrary to their wishes. The question naturally arises whether this type of issue, which is in the interests of the general public health, should ever be the subject of a public referendum. As stated by Rhyne[79] at the 1966 National Dental Health Assembly, "I think that on the local level the proponents of fluoridation too frequently go through a referendum without raising the question of whether or not this is a proper issue for submission to the people. . . . I recommend that you think more in terms of presenting this issue to the courts. I think you will find that the courts will hold there is no right to a referendum on a health issue such as this."

## PUBLIC HEALTH DENTISTRY
## A SPECIALTY

Another significant development during the past 25 years should be mentioned. Because of the growing public and professional awareness of the importance of the problems of dental health and because of the remarkable strides that were taken in rapid succession and that provided several practical measures that could be taken for the solution of those problems, the specialty of public health dentistry was firmly established. Early in the period a Dental Health Section of the American Public Health Association was established, which by 1945 had defined the field of public health dentistry and had established educational qualifications of public health dentists, since revised.[80] About the same time the American Association of Public Health Dentists came into being, along with a Dental Health Section of the American Dental Association. Annual professional and official conferences of those most directly concerned with programs of dental health were instituted with the establishment of the Conference of State Dental Directors with the Surgeon General of the Public Health Service and the Chief of the Children's Bureau, on the one hand, and Council on Dental Health of the American Dental Association, on the other. The specialty was formally recognized in 1952 through the establishment of the American Board of Dental Public Health, which is sponsored jointly by the American Association of Public Health Dentists and the Dental Health Section of the American Public Health Association.

## PREPAID DENTAL CARE

To plan and provide for adequate dental care of adults is more costly and complex than to do so for children. The oral ills of adults are more varied and often require more meticulous and time-consuming work than do those of children. Dental care for adults involves the prevention and treatment of (1) diseases of the teeth, (2) periodontoclasia, (3) anomalies, (4) cysts, (5) malignant and precancerous lesions, (6) oral manifestations of systemic disturbances, and (7) traumatic injuries and the preservation or restoration of mouth function. None of these can be handled on other than an individualized basis. Furthermore, the increasing number and proportion of older people and the increasing hazards of facial injuries because of automobile and other accidents mitigate against an early lessening of the group needs for some of these services. Even a significant decrease in the total amount of dental caries, which would make available a larger proportion of a dentist's time for the care of these adult ailments, will not change their magnitude or cost.

It is obvious by now that adherence to the "fee for service" payment mechanism cannot begin to solve the basic problem. The ultimate provision of reasonably adequate dental care for adults will depend on the development of practical, widely acceptable, and available prepayment dental maintenance programs. The first such plan in the United States actually began in 1867, and by 1900 four others had been established.[81] For the next half century, progress was slow. Since 1950, some notable developments have occurred. Group practice clinics that employed their own dental staffs began and have been multiplying. One of the oldest, largest, and most successful has been the Naismith group, which for almost a quarter century has been practicing in the San Francisco Bay area.[82,83] This, however, is a closed panel system that serves essentially higher educational and income government workers. Dental service corporations have been formed my many local and state dental societies or by groups of dentists by means of which contracting groups receive treatment in the private offices of participating dentists.[84] A highly comprehensive plan is that of the California Dental Service, a nonprofit corporation sponsored by the California Dental Association. About 90% of dentists in active practice in the state are members, and the plan covers well over 1 million of the state's 20 million people. Increasingly school districts are adopting the plan as a supplement to teachers' salaries.[85] By 1968, 36 private insurance companies had extended medical prepayment plans to include dental care, essentially accidental injury to teeth and major dental surgery. However, it is doubtful that private insurance will ever play a significant role.[86] In addition, several labor unions, beginning with the St. Louis Labor Health Institute in 1945, have sponsored prepaid dental plans with some success.[87] Since then, several labor unions, notably the International Longshoremen's and Warehousemen's Union,[88] have made some dental care benefits one of their bargaining priorities. Of particular interest is the prepaid dental insurance package in the 1974 contract agreement between the United Steelworkers of America and the major steel companies.[89] The program, which takes effect on August 1, 1975, will be paid for by the employer and will cover 100% of preventive services for children under 19 and half the cost of orthodontics for children. Benefits for retired and active union members also are expanded.

Since 1942, the American Dental Association has sponsored numerous studies of prepayment mechanisms. Its original plan[90] proposed to provide family dental service to low-income groups and involved the payment by the subscriber of $1 each month for himself plus an additional $1 monthly for his first dependent and 50 cents a month more for additional dependents. Thus the total fee for a subscriber with two or more dependents amounted to $2.50 a month. Certain services, such as orthodontics and the construction of crowns, bridges, and dentures, were not included. It must be remembered that the suggested fees applied to the year 1944.

With all of this apparent activity it is regrettable to note that by 1968, only 1.7 million Americans, or less than 2%, were involved in any type of prepaid dental health care program. It is notable that a major proportion of those covered are in California, a state which has long been a leader in this field. No single approach yet tried appears to be without drawbacks. Fisher[91] has reviewed the three most common payment formulas as follows:

1. The *fee per service* mechanism rewards productivity and penalizes patient dropout and extensive follow-up; emphasizes high-fee services; erodes quality by stress on quantity; and de-emphasizes time-consuming services such as children's dentistry.

2. The *fee per visit* mechanism rewards inefficiency and unproductiveness, multiple short visits, and minor restorative services; encourages manipulation to achieve multiple-visit records by a single patient in a single day; and de-emphasizes laboratory-related and long-visit rehabilitative services.

3. The *capitation* device rewards prevention and patient turnover by either completion or dropout; encourages minimums of treatment; emphasizes inexpensive (again nonrehabilitative) services and quantitative efficiency; encourages neglect of certain needs; and encourages more extensive services to the cooperative and token care to the uncooperative.

At this point in time further experimentation and demonstration are indicated and urgent. As Fisher emphasizes, "Dentistry's concern with costs cannot be limited to promoting usual and customary fees."

In 1953 the House Delegates of the American Dental Association adopted a set of principles in relation to prepaid dental health plans. These were revised most recently in 1973. Among the more significant points covered are the following:

Carriers should develop plans in conjunction with dental societies.

Plans should permit participation by all licensed dentists.

Patients should be free to choose dentists.

Dentists should be free to refuse patients.

Plans should allow maximum and efficient use of dental personnel and facilities.

Professional standards and treatment plans should be controlled by dentists.

Third parties should make full use of peer review mechanisms in fee disputes.

Administrative policies should be flexible and allow experimentation with various methods of payment.

The earlier insistence on direct payment to the dentist has been deleted. However, the revision states that "The usual, customary and reasonable fee reimbursement method is preferred but various methods may be allowed. A capitation reimbursement system should not be imposed."

Premiums should be based on accurate current data on fees in the area to be served and should be developed with the advice and assistance of the dental society and adjusted when necessary.

Plans should include preventive as well as treatment activities.

Programs should provide dental health education for all participants.

With specific reference to capitation as a method of prepayment of dental care, Schoen[92] points out that a capitation rate for a population has to be based on its need for dental resources and the cost of supplying them. Factors requiring consideration are the amount of dentists' and hygienists' time required, which is affected by the need for initial care, as opposed to maintenance care, stability of the population, utilization of services, family size, age of eligible persons, fluoridation, and socioeconomic variables. Provider time and cost are also affected by the type, quantity, and use of facilities and auxiliary personnel. He has devised a method that takes account of these various cost factors and provides a realistic basis for arriving at a capitation rate per person or family for a given population. The method is applicable to populations with differing dental requirements and financial capabilities, since the pertinent formulas and priorities include numerous variations. For example, to lower the capitation rate, members of families may be phased into treatment. Also, surcharges or copayments can be placed on patients for all services or only for specific ones. He considers that if this method is used to provide care under a rational system of priorities, capitation group practice of dentistry can achieve results not obtainable under the fee-for-service solo practice system. He also believes that in prepaid group practice there are incentives for using expanded-duty auxiliaries, containing costs, and improving the level of dental health of the eligible population through both treatment and prevention.

Prepayment for dental services is now at about the same point that medical and hospital prepayment was in the mid-1940s. The extent and rate at which it will develop further will depend on many factors, not the least of which is much better public understanding of the problem and a wish and willingness to solve it. Germane to the latter is the enormous backlog of existing dental defects that would have to be corrected at a great cost to achieve a position where continuity of maintenance services would become possible. Add to this the real shortage of dentists and dental auxiliaries, restrictive laws relating to the latter, and continuing reservations by the majority of practicing dentists concerning compensation by other than the guild-type fee-for-service. In view of these limitations, rapid and extensive change in the near future does not seem probable, although the widespread formation of Health Maintenance Organizations and certainly the passage of National Health Insurance legislation would be certain to have a significant effect.

## PUBLIC HEALTH DENTAL PROGRAMS

In summing up the situation as it existed in 1954, Knutson[4] stated:

The nature of accomplishments during the past 10 years made this a decade of beginning in the field of dental public health. Water fluoridation, topical fluorides, oral cancer detection and control programs, the team approach to the diagnosis and treatment of cleft lip and cleft palate cases, orthodontic care programs, utilization of chairside assistants, the National Institute of Dental Research, approaches to the epidemiology of dento-facial deformities and periodontal diseases, and principles of prepayment for dental care services—all these are no better than well begun and several are in the budding stage. The objectives of all and the merits of most of them have been firmly established . . .

In view of this, it can readily be understood that present-day public health agencies and the relatively few but well-qualified public health dentists on their staffs are in a different situation from that which existed a few years ago, when all they could do was try to devise ways and means of reducing by dental therapy the discouraging flood of accumulating dental needs. By now a practical approach has been unfolded, with some clearly defined and proved preventive measures that, if properly applied, hold promise of reducing the needs for caries correction to a point at which they may be handled reasonably adequately along with the prosthetic, orthodontic, and dental surgical needs of the community.

Although recognizing that most preventive and promotive dental health activities must be aimed primarily at the child population, they should also be adapted to the total population as follows: Using all modern knowledge available, dentistry and society could (1) prevent and control most dental caries; (2) prevent or control soft tissue inflammation and disease of the supporting tissues of the teeth; (3) with specialist cooperation, correct maloccluding teeth and prevent a relatively small number of the gross tooth irregularities that may interfere with mastication, with the health of the supporting tissues, and with the emotional stability of the individual; (4) with specialist cooperation, can treat the problems arising from anomalies of the oral cavity, for example, the cleft palate, congenitally missing teeth, supernumerary teeth, hypoplastic teeth, and other developmental dental abnormalities; (5) can treat and restore teeth involved in accidents; (6) can detect oral cancer in the early stages; and (7) can prevent and eliminate oral infection that may contribute to body disease.

In reflecting on how society's existing considerable knowledge may be applied to the successful accomplishment of these goals, the following areas of activity should seem to be indicated: (1) planning and evaluation, (2) prevention of dental caries, (3) remedial treatment of caries, (4) remedial treatment of other dental and oral defects, (5) public dental health education, (6) professional and paraprofessional development, (7) development of public and private methods to overcome economic deterrents to obtaining dental health services, and (8) research and development of improved methods of prevention, treatment, and public education.

Except for large municipalities, state health departments are the chief governmental agencies that provide dental health services. They operate principally, however, through local health departments that work in cooperation with the dental profession, the schools, and other local organizations. Although the state and local health agencies and their public health dentists are often in the position of having to spearhead community activities in this field, the establishment of policies and the development of programs should always be carried out in conjunction with members of the dental societies and for certain components of the program with school health committees, departments of education, and other key groups. A close relationship with the dental profession and schools is particularly important, since their understanding, cooperation, and support are fundamental to a successful dental program.

On the basis of experience acquired in the successful development of a dental health program in Oak Ridge, Tenn., Stroud and Brumback[93] have set down certain guideposts to planning that because of their practicality and good sense are repeated here in part:

1. The first step should be a survey of local needs in order to determine the nature and extent of the problem.

2. A list of resources already available to aid in meeting the needs should be prepared. This should include practicing dentists, official and nonofficial agencies, civic organizations, parent-teacher associations, and their attitudes.

3. Resources outside the community should be called on early in planning. The state public health department can help in many ways. The United States Public Health Service has many aids available for use. (To these may be added the state dental society and the American Dental Association.)

4. Local practicing dentists should be active members of the planning group from the start. A committee of dentists should advise the group throughout the inauguration and operation of the program.

5. In planning, representatives of all local organizations having an interest in health should be invited. Their advice can help to avoid many pitfalls, and their active interest is essential to a really successful program.

6. If the program operates under the auspices of a lay group as in Oak Ridge, the active administration and supervision should be provided by the local public health department. If funds are to be administered by the lay governing council, this council should be incorporated. Officers responsible for such funds should be bonded, and the budget should include an amount to pay for a periodic audit of accounts.

7. Before a program begins operation, policies and procedures should be agreed on. Personnel policies should be established before employing anyone.

8. In program planning, every opportunity for education should be considered. As many community residents as possible should be encouraged to participate in the organization and operation. In Oak Ridge, several hundred people have taken part in the planning or operation up to the present time. They are members of various community official agencies, private practitioners of dentistry and medicine, housewives, members of clubs and voluntary organizations, scientific workers, teachers, students, businessmen, and private citizens not falling into any of the preceding categories. Each has made a valuable contribution to the program and all have learned something about dental health.

Soricelli[94] also emphasizes the importance of building evaluative procedures into any planned program. Since caries constitutes the bulk of the dental problem and since the chief goal to be attained is a reduction in the amount of dental caries, the prevalence of that condition in the population to be served should be determined. Since the D.M.F. count of adults is closely correlated with that of children, an initial survey of a sample of the child population alone may

serve the purpose. This is based on the observation that a functional relationship exists between the proportion of children having at least one D.M.F. permanent tooth and the average number of D.M.F. permanent teeth per child,

Since it has been clearly shown that proper fluoridation of water supplies will decrease dental caries prevalence up to 65%, it is obvious that the primary goal of a public health dental program should be the acceptance and development of this procedure. To accomplish this several steps should be suggested. Probably the first thing that should be done is to obtain a positive statement of policy on fluoridation by the state dental society and the state health agency. After this it will probably be advisable to promote the establishment of a state fluoridation committee to work with the state public health dentists and the state dental society. Such a group may be of considerable value in providing information and data on fluoridation to the general public and the press, to local dental societies, and to state and local nonprofessional organizations and officials. It may also assist by drawing up a sample fluoridation ordinance in conformance with state legislation and by collecting information on costs. On the local level the local dental society might preferably provide the leadership in organizing a local committee and should play an active role in the planning and establishment of the local program.

Despite its greater cost and more difficult method of use, topical application of fluoride to the teeth of children has a place in many if not all public health dental programs. This is especially true in rural areas or where there is shortsighted but effective opposition to fluoridation of public water supplies. Thus as has been pointed out previously, opposition, procrastination, and scattered populations account for the fact that by 1970 only 88 million people in 7,458 communities had the benefit of fluoridated water. Incidentally it should be noted that now more than two thirds of the population of the United States lives under urban circumstances.

Another reason for retaining the topical fluoride procedure is that since water fluoridation is most effective during the years of enamel calcification, it is advisable that children, whose teeth were already calcified when fluoridation is begun, have topical fluoride applications. Subsequently, as the benefits of fluoridated water become effective, topical fluoride applications may be discontinued gradually beginning with the younger age groups. The extent to which the topical procedure is carried out in the offices of private practicing dentists on the one hand, or through public facilities on the other, will depend entirely on the local situation.

Wertheimer[95] has described some of the difficulties encountered by the program in Michigan, which was one of the first to be established. Of particular interest was the partial solution of the difficult personnel problem by means of summer employment of junior dental students. With proper preparation and demonstration as well as discussions on the place of dentistry in public health, public relations, the group method approach, and the care of equipment, students were found to do a creditable job. Incidentally this approach has reduced the cost of topical fluoride application per child by about 50%. Wertheimer also points out that this approach gives the following additional benefits to the dental students: (1) experience in group method of topical fluoride application, (2) development of skill in handling children, (3) learning about dental conditions of children in communities in contrast to select groups usually seen in dental schools, (4) orientation in public health and the concept that dental disease is a public health problem, and (5) opportunity to observe community action as an approach to the solution of the problems.

Horowitz[96] has demonstrated the practicality of fluoridation of a school's water system in the absence of general fluoridation. To duplicate the optimum fluoride intake the school water received 4.5 times the usual dosage. An overall reduction in tooth decay of 40% was achieved with no signs of dental fluorosis.

It must be recognized that fluoridation of water and topical application of fluorides do not bring about complete caries control and do not eliminate the need for other dental health measures. A certain amount of caries will always develop; hence there probably always will be a need for some remedial treatment of caries. For this and other reasons an essential part of the public health dental program should be the promotion of regular dental supervision as an essential part of individual hygienic living. With a major proportion of caries subject to prevention, it may be possible to repair the backlog of caries on an incremental basis. Even in the face of vast accumulated dental needs it has been found practical and fruitful in several places to restrict caries corrective programs

to children in a restricted age span. For example, some programs that began by caring for children from 5 to 10 years of age have found it possible during the second year of the program to add the new crop of 5-year-old children and, in addition, to continue with the 11-year-old children who were in the original group the year before. As each year goes by, new 5-year-olds have been added, and all children previously cared for were continued.

The part of a community dental health program that relates to the remedial treatment of dental and other oral defects, including orthodontics, prosthetics, and dental surgery for congenital defects, would seem to rest largely in the hands of private practicing dentists aided to whatever degree may be possible by the services, facilities, and contributions of public clinics for indigent or low-income groups, philanthropic agencies, and prepayment dental care plans. The scant attention sometimes given to these conditions is in no way indicative of their relative importance. Indeed, as Gruebbel[97] visualized in the late 1940s,

Orthodontic services . . . may some day prove to be high on the list of essential services. The health professions are finding increasing evidence of the value of orthodontic care to the physical and mental well-being and social adjustment of children and youth. It has been estimated that there are approximately 40 million children under the age of 16 years in the United States, of whom 7 to 8 million need major orthodontic care, and of whom less than 4 out of every 100 who need it are actually receiving treatment.

At the present time increasing numbers of underprivileged children with such oral and dental defects that would ordinarily be uncorrected are being cared for by the health components of some of the Economic Opportunity Programs, the Maternal and Child Health Programs, or by the Comprehensive Health Care section of Title V of the 1965 Amendments to the Social Security Law (P.L. 89-97).

Underlying all the other activities should be a carefully planned dental health education program so varied as to reach all segments of the public, with particular emphasis on "sensitive" groups. For many years those who attend prenatal, well-baby, and other public health clinics have been exposed to dental health educational procedures. It is puzzling, however, to understand why so few hospital waiting rooms and private physicians' offices do anything to encourage their clients to seek dental supervision. In consideration of the numbers of persons involved and the receptive circumstances in which they find themselves this is suggested as a channel of public education worthy of much more intensive exploration and use.

An extremely important area for dental health education is in relation to the school health program. Those responsible for the community dental health program should work particularly closely with the board of education, classroom teachers, and physical education personnel, assisting them in the preparation of sound and practical information in the field, screening of classroom teaching aids, and obtaining material for them from the various dental and public health associations.[98]

On the state level public health dentists should work closely and in a similar manner with state departments of education, dental schools, and teachers' colleges. Another area worthy of particular attention is that concerned with the school lunch program. The public health dental personnel in collaboration with teachers of nutrition and home economics and with the school lunchroom managers should attempt to bring about a change in lunch and snack habits, particularly with regard to the intake of carbohydrates. With this in mind a great many school systems have discouraged the use and even availability of candy and soft drinks in their lunchrooms and elsewhere on school premises. Whereas it is fully recognized that school children may obtain these products elsewhere, it is at least a partial step in the right direction to bring about a change in the habit pattern at mealtime.

A final and basic part of the community dental health program should be concerned with the improvement of professional standards and practices. This is particularly appropriate at this time, when one considers the many recent developments that have come about since the graduation of many of those now practicing dentistry. Still another reason is the increasing awareness of the relationship of various fields in medicine, economics, and sociology to the modern practice of dentistry. Several states have found it highly worth while to sponsor postgraduate seminars on subjects related to modern dental practice. Such activities go far in strengthening the local dental society, raising the standards of local practice, and assuring the cooperation and active participation of the dentists of the community. In connection with seminars and postgraduate

training it is suggested that the subject matter not be restricted to dentistry or even public health dentistry but include also appropriate aspects of mental health, economics, newer techniques for the diagnosis and treatment of cancer, and other similar subjects.

A previous section of this chapter briefly discussed the need for the usefulness of dental hygienists and dental assistants. It was pointed out at that time that only a minor percent of practicing dentists are making use of this valuable potential source of assistance. The promotion of the use of dental hygienists, assistants, and technotherapists is certainly a worthwhile and legitimate aspect of the community dental health program, since its success would provide a greater total amount of dentists' time available to the community.

An easily overlooked area of action in a program such as that under consideration is related to the solution of the ever-present problem of personnel shortages. Those responsible for the program should consider activities in the nature of career guidance to high school and college students as an important responsibility.

## REFERENCES

1. Toward a sociology of dentistry, Milbank Mem. Fund Quart. vol. 49, no. 3, 1971.
2. A book shelf on dental public health, Amer. J. Public Health **56:**467, April 1966.
3. Knutson, J., and Klein, H.: Tooth mortality in elementary school children, Public Health Rep. **53:**1021, June 1938.
4. Knutson, J.: Dental public health accomplishments and predictions, Amer. J. Public Health **44:**331, March 1954.
5. Causes of rejection and incidence of defects, Med. Stat. Bull. **2:**1, Aug. 1943.
6. Ten year program of research and development, Bethesda, Md., 1970, National Institute of Dental Research.
7. Federal Security Agency, U. S. Public Health Service: The epidemiology of dental disease. Collection of papers of Henry Klein and others, 1937-47, Washington, D. C., 1948.
8. Law, F. E.: Highlights of research in dental public health, 1956-1960, Amer. J. Public Health **51:**825, June 1961.
9. U. S. Public Health Service: Decayed, missing and filled teeth among children, DHEW pub. no. (HSM) 72-1003, Rockville, Md., 1971.
10. American Council on Education: Commission on the Survey of Dentistry in the United States, Washington, D. C., 1961, The Council.
11. U. S. Public Health Service: Selected dental findings in adults: by age, race and sex, PHS pub. no. 1000, ser. 11, no. 7, Rockville, Md. 1965.

12. Starnbach, H. K.: Orthodontia needed by 1 in 5 children, Pediat. News **7:**2, Feb. 1973.

13. Grace, L.: Study on incidence of cleft palate, J. Dent. Res. **22:**495, Dec. 1943.

14. U. S. Public Health Service: Periodontal disease among children, DHEW pub. no. (HSM) 72-1060, Rockville, Md., 1972.

15. U. S. Public Health Service: Periodontal disease in adults, DHEW pub. no. (HSM) 72-1078, Rockville, Md., 1965.

16. U. S. Public Health Service: Health resources statistics, PHS pub. no. 1509, Rockville, Md., 1971.

17. U. S. Public Health Service: Dental visits, volume and interval since last visit, U. S., 1969, DHEW Pub. no. (HSM) 73-1502, Rockville, Md., 1972.

18. U. S. Public Health Service: Health manpower, PHS pub. no. 2044, Rockville, Md., 1971.

19. Klein, H.: Civilian dentistry in wartime, J. Amer. Dent. Ass. **31:**648, May 1944.

20. Soricelli, D. A.: Implementation of the delivery of dental services by auxiliaries—the Philadelphia experience, Amer. J. Public Health **62:**1077, Aug. 1972.

21. Myers, S. E.: Operating dental auxiliaries, WHO Chron. **26:**511, Nov. 1972.

22. Jensen, J. R.: Dental manpower and the responsibilities of the dental schools, Amer. J. Public Health **61:**1565, Aug. 1971.

23. Della Pella, N., Soricelli, D. A., and Bronstein, E.: Training technotherapists for use in an urban dental care program, Health Services Rep. **88:**181, Feb. 1973.

24. Heid, T. H.: Dental therapy assistant: effect on team productivity, Health Care Research Division Rep. no. 7, Ft. Sam Houston, 1973, Brooke Army Medical Center.

25. Soricelli, D. A.: Controlling quality in the delivery of dental care, Amer. J. Public Health **61:**2046, Oct. 1971.

26. McCall, J. O.: Dental practice and dental education in the future, J. Amer. Dent. Ass. **31:**16, Jan. 1944.

27. Aston, E. R.: Responsibility of the American Association of Industrial Dentists, Public Health Rep. **67:**694, July 1952.

28. Easlick, K. A.: Dental caries, mechanism and present control techniques, St. Louis, 1948, The C.V. Mosby Co.

29. Florio, L.: In Leavell, H. R., et al.: Textbook of preventive medicine, New York, 1953, McGraw-Hill Book Co.

30. Finn, S. B.: Clinical pedodontics, Philadelphia, 1968, W. B. Saunders Co.

31. Klein, H., and Palmer, C.: On the epidemiology of dental caries, University of Pennsylvania Bicentennial Conference, Philadelphia, 1941, University of Pennsylvania Press.

32. Volker, J. F.: Dental science. In Contributions of the biological sciences to human welfare, Proceedings of the Federation of American Societies for Experimental Biology, vol. 31, Part 2, Bethesda, Md., Nov.-Dec. 1972, The Federation.

33. Jay, P.: *Bacillus acidophilus* and dental caries, J. Amer. Dent. Ass. **16:**230, Feb. 1929.

34. Jay, P.: The problem of dental caries with relation to bacteria and diet, J. Pediat. **8:**725, 1936.

35. Bunting, R. W., and Palmerlee, F.: The role of *Bacillus acidophilus* in dental caries, J. Amer. Dent. Ass. **12:**381, April 1925.

36. Jay, P.: The role of sugar in the etiology of caries, J. Amer. Dent. Ass. **27:**393, March 1940.

37. Gustafsson, B. E., et al.: The effect of different levels of carbohydrate intake on caries activity in 436 individuals observed for five years, Acta Odont. Scand. **11:**232, 1954.

38. Hoerman, K. C., et al.: The association of *Streptococcus mutans* with early carious lesions in human teeth, J. Amer. Dent. Ass. **85:**1349, Dec. 1972.

39. Greer, S. B., et al.: Report on viruses and tooth decay, Research News no. 96, Bethesda, Md., June 1972, National Institute of Dental Research.

40. Easlick, K. A.: The caries problem of the school child, Amer. J. Public Health **39:**984, Aug. 1949.

41. Collins, S.: The health of the school child, a study of sickness, physical defects and mortality, Public Health Service bull. no. 200, Washington, D. C., Aug. 1931.

42. Messner, C. T., Gafafer, W. M., Cady, F. C., and Dean H. T.: Dental survey of school children, ages 6-14 years, made in 1933-34 in 26 states, Public Health Service bull. no. 226, Washington, D. C., May 1936.

43. Klein, H., and Palmer, C.: Dental caries in American Indian children, Public Health Service bull. no. 239, Washington, D. C., Dec. 1937.

44. Eager, J.: Chiaie teeth, Public Health Rep. **16:**2576, 1901.

45. Black, G. V., and McKay, F. S.: Mottled teeth: an endemic developmental imperfection of the enamel of the teeth heretofore unknown in the literature of dentistry, Dent. Cosmos **58:**129, 1916.

46. Smith, M. C., Lantz, E., and Smith, H. B.: The cause of mottled enamel, Science **74:**244, 1931.

47. Fosdick, L., and Hansen, H.: Theoretical considerations of carbohydrate degradation in relation to dental caries, J. Amer. Dent. Ass. **23:**406, March 1936.

48. Arnim, S., Aberle, S., and Pitney, E.: A study of dental changes in a group of Pueblo Indian children, J. Amer. Dent. Ass. **24:**478, March 1937.

49. Armstrong, W., and Brekhus, P.: Chemical constitution of enamel and dentin, J. Biol. Chem. **120:**677, Sept. 1937.

50. Bernstein, D. S., et al.: The prevalence of osteoporosis in high and low fluoride areas in North Dakota, J.A.M.A. **198:**499, Oct. 1966.

51. Korns, R. F.: Relationship of water fluoridation to bone density in two New York towns, Public Health Rep. **84:**815, Sept. 1969.

52. Bibby, B. G.: Preliminary report on the use of sodium fluoride applications in caries prophylaxis, J. Dent. Res. **21:**314, 1942.

53. Cheyne, V. D.: Human dental caries and topically applied fluorine: a preliminary report, J. Amer. Dent. Ass. **29:**804, 1942.

54. Knutson, J. W.: The nationwide topical fluoride demonstration program, J. Amer. Dent. Ass. **39:**438, 1949.

55. Cox, G. J., and Hodge, H. C.: The toxicity of fluorides in relation to their use in dentistry, J. Amer. Dent. Ass. **40:**440, April 1950.

56. Heyroth, F.: Toxiocological evidence for the safety of the fluoridation of public water supplies, Amer. J. Public Health **42:**1568, Dec. 1952.

57. Hagan, T. L., Pasternack, M., and Scholz, G. C.: Waterborne fluorides and mortality, Public Health Rep. **69:**450, May 1954.

58. Geever, E. F., Leone, N. C., Geiser, P., and Lieberman, J. E.: Pathological studies in man after prolonged ingestion of fluoride in drinking water, Public Health Rep. **73:**721, Aug. 1958.

59. Hodge, H. C.: Safety factors in water fluoridation based on the toxicology of fluorides, Proc. Nutr. Soc. **22:**111, 1963.

60. Campbell, I. R., editor: The role of fluoride in public health, a selected bibliography, Cincinnati, 1963, Kettering Laboratory, University of Cincinnati.

61. Tentative standard specifications for sodium fluoride, J. Amer. Waterworks Ass. **42:**899, Sept. 1950.

62. Bull, F. A., Hardgrove, T. A., and Frisch, J. G.: Methods and costs of water fluoridation, J. Amer. Dent. Ass. **42:**29, Jan. 1951.

63. Maier, F. J.: Engineering problems in water fluoridation, Amer. J. Public Health **42:**249, March, 1952.

64. Ast, D. B.: Effectiveness of water fluoridation, J. Amer. Dent. Ass. **65:**581, Nov. 1962.

65. Horowitz, H. S., Law, F. E., and Pritzker, T.: Effect of school water fluoridation on dental caries, Public Health Rep. **80:**381, May 1965.

66. Hutton, W. L., Linscott, B. W., and Williams, D. B.: The Brantford fluorine experiment, Canad. J. Public Health **42:**81, Jan. 1951.

67. Fluoridation census, 1969, Bethesda, 1970, National Institutes of Health.

68. Natural fluoride content of community water supplies, 1969, Bethesda, 1970, National Institutes of Health.

69. Fluoridation and dental health, Resolution, World Health Assembly, Boston, July 23, 1969.

70. Humphrey, H. H.: Cause is mankind, New York, 1964, Fredricka Praeger, Inc.

71. Hoffer, E.: The true believer, New York, 1958, Mentor Press.

72. Comments on the opponents of fluoridation, J. Amer. Dent. Ass. **71:**1156, Nov. 1965.

73. Paul, B. D.: Fluoridation and the social scientist, J. Soc. Issues **17**(4):1, Oct. 1961.

74. Fluoridation facts—answers to criticisms of fluoridation, pub. G 21, Chicago, 1965, American Dental Association.

75. Ast, D. B., et al.: Time and cost factors to provide regular periodic dental care for children in a fluoridated and nonfluoridated area, Amer. J. Public Health **57:**1635, Sept. 1967.

76. Roemer, R.: Water fluoridation: public health responsibility and the democratic process, Amer. J. Public Health **55:**1337, Sept. 1965.

77. Legal note—dental health and fluoridation, Public Health Rep. **77:**639, July 1962.

78. Tobey, J. A.: Water fluoridation and civil rights, Public Health News, New Jersey Department of Health **43:**121, April 1962.

79. Rhyne, C. S.: Fluoridation and the law, Public Health Service pub. no. 1552, Washington, D. C., 1966.

80. Educational qualifications of public health dentists (revised), Amer. J. Public Health **42:**188, Feb. 1952.

81. Penchansky, R., and Safford, B. M.: Prepayment for dental care: need and effect, Public Health Rep. **81:**541, June 1966.

82. Smith, A., Mitchell, G., and Lucas, G.: An experiment in dental prepayment: the Naismith dental plan, PHS pub. no. 970, Washington, D. C., 1962.

83. Naismith, R.: Group practice and prepayment, talk presented before 23rd National Dental Health Conference, Chicago, 1973, American Dental Association.

84. U. S. Public Health Service: The dental service corporation—organization and development, PHS pub. no. 1274, Washington, D. C., 1965.

85. U. S. Public Health Service: Digest of prepaid dental care plans, 1963, PHS pub. no. 585, Washington, D. C., 1964.

86. Follmann, J. F.: The role of private insurance. In a symposium on the group purchase of dental care, Amer. J. Public Health **50:**28, Jan. 1960.

87. McNeel, J. O.: Dental program of the St. Louis Labor Health Institute, Amer. J. Public Health **44:**878, July 1954.

88. U. S. Public Health Service: Report on the dental program of the ILWUPMA, PHS pub. no. 894, Washington, D. C., 1962.

89. News item, Amer. Med. News, April 29, 1974.

90. American Dental Association: Proposed plan for prepayment of dental insurance, Chicago, 1944, The Association.

91. Fisher, M. A.: New directions for dentistry, Amer. J. Public Health **60:**848, May 1970.

92. Schoen, M. H.: Methodology of capitation payment to group dental practice and effects of such payment on care, Health Services Rep. **89:**16, Jan.-Feb. 1974.

93. Stroud, H., and Brumback, C.: A dental health program for your community, Amer. J. Public Health **40:**1426, Nov. 1950.

94. Soricelli, D. A.: Comprehensive dental care in a

metropolitan community (Philadelphia). Paper presented at American Dental Association Conference, Las Vegas, Nov. 7, 1970.

95. Wertheimer, F.: Michigan summer topical fluoride program, Amer. J. Public Health **44:** 484, April 1954.

96. Horowitz, H. S.: Fluoridating school's water supply protects against decay, Research News no. 96, Bethesda, Md., June 1972, National Institute of Dental Research.

97. Gruebbel, A. O.: Standards of dental care for different age groups, Amer. J. Public Health **39:**981, Aug. 1949.

98. American Dental Association: A dental program for schools, Chicago, 1963, The Association.

# PART SEVEN

# The substance of public health— disease control

Certainly all agree that one of the most fundamental reasons for the existence of health programs relates to disease control. Immediately the two words give rise to questions. Which diseases? How control? Until a few years ago it was rare to find public health agencies concerned with any but communicable diseases, and many of them could be controlled and a few have been almost eradicated. But what of noncommunicable ailments—metabolic diseases, degenerative conditions, accidents, and the like. It was convenient for many to allocate them either to the realm of therapeutic medicine or to acts of God. Their inevitability was accepted as a fact of life —or death. The emphasis was all on repair or amelioration with little thought to the possibility that some might actually be prevented.

Probably the discoveries of insulin and thyroid were significant turning points, along with the development of some safety measures in industry. Then with the explosion in biologic science that occurred especially since World War II, more eyes and more minds were turned to more noncommunicable diseases that might be, and increasingly could be, at least controlled if not prevented or eliminated. Etymologic evidence of this expanded viewpoint may be seen in the adroit change in name of the Public Health Service's Communicable Disease Center to the Center for Disease Control. Similar evidence has taken the form of increased attention to the possibilities of applying through public programs the findings by the National Institutes of Health and the many other scientific and clinical research centers. It is to these two companion fields, communicable diseases and metabolic and degenerative diseases, that Chapters 21 and 22 are devoted.

*In quenching the flames at one point,
the good work is begun but not ended.
Can infectious disease of all kinds
never be quenched?*

WILLIAM FARR
(1875)

CHAPTER 21

# Communicable diseases

## BACKGROUND

Since there are many excellent texts on the clinical and bacteriologic aspects of the various communicable diseases,[1,2] the purpose of this chapter is essentially to present certain broad aspects of the subject, particularly those concerned with administrative control measures. Great reductions have been achieved in the incidence of many communicable and infectious diseases in all parts of the world.[3-6] Table 21-1 illustrates, for example, the dramatic extent of the decline in death rates from several once common diseases in the United States. For all practical purposes they appear to have been eliminated.

As recently as the mid-1940s about 80 countries reported smallpox, and a majority of the world's population lived in smallpox-endemic areas. By the end of 1971 the disease was confined mainly to 4 endemic countries—Ethiopia,

**Table 21-1.** Decline in deaths from selected communicable diseases, United States, 1900 to 1971

| Causes of death | Deaths per 100,000 population per year | |
| --- | --- | --- |
| | 1900-1904 | 1971 |
| Diphtheria | 32.7 | 0.0 |
| Pertussis | 10.7 | 0.0 |
| Measles | 10.0 | 0.0 |
| Typhoid fever | 26.7 | 0.0 |
| Diarrhea and enteritis | 115.3 | 1.1 |
| Syphilis | 12.9 | 0.2 |
| Tuberculosis | 184.7 | 2.1 |

India, Pakistan, and Sudan. Residual foci of the disease elsewhere are limited in extent and are regarded as susceptible to prompt eradication.[7] So successful has been the attack on smallpox that by the end of 1972 vaccination requirements for travel among all European countries and the United States were dropped, and worldwide eradication is predicted by about 1980 if not sooner. Also by the end of 1971 the United States Public Health Service recommended the discontinuance of routine smallpox vaccination in the country. The recommendation was based on the current greater danger from vaccination itself than from risk of the disease. Thus during the preceding year there had been 7 deaths and 572 complications in relation to more than 14 million smallpox vaccinations. It would take six importations of the disease each year to result in the same death rate, and experience in recent years has been less than 1 case per year actually imported to the United States. It was recommended that public health efforts be devoted to assuring adequate immunization of all personnel in health services and of all travelers to and from continents where smallpox had not yet been eradicated.[8]

Malaria provides another good example. Only 20 years ago it was estimated that of 2,500 million people then on the earth, more than 250 million, or one tenth, had experienced clinical attacks of malaria each year, and about 2.5 million died from the disease annually. Currently deaths from malaria throughout the world are estimated at about 350,000 per year. By the end of 1971, of the estimated 1,844 million people living in the originally malarious areas of the world, 1,372 million (74%) were in areas where malaria had been eradicated or where eradication programs were in progress. Of the 472 million people living in areas without eradication programs, 36 million were partially protected by malaria control measures, while governments were attempting to ensure antimalarial drugs for an additional 161 million people.

Numerous other examples of success could be presented (see Chapter 8). More appropriate for the present purpose, however, is to indicate some important reservations that must be constantly kept in mind. It is a false hope that man will ever be free from the threat of bacterial or viral infections—new or old. Jekel[9] presents the case very well:

Most infectious agents have existed for a long time. They are a tougher and more resilient foe than many realize. As far as is known, every pathogenic organism that has ever been identified is still active somewhere in the world; very few organisms have been eliminated from so much as a single continent and now a number of factors are emerging in our changing world that are detrimental to efforts to control infectious disease. If we are to cope with these factors we must identify them and establish their relationship to communicable disease today. Some of the critical factors are: the population explosion, contemporary urbanization, increasing mobility, declining levels of acquired immunity, increasing resistance to antibiotics and insecticides, new epidemiologic circumstances, decreasing diagnostic acuity for infectious disease, infections in wild animal populations, and man's most regrettable contribution—lack of concern.

He concludes that the communicable diseases require a long-term commitment to their surveillance and control, which is based more on their potential danger than on their actual incidence or prevalence at any given point in time. The relevance of this is indicated in a recent statement by the chief of the Immunization Branch of the Center for Disease Control, who in mid-1971 warned,[10] "Measles is out of control, diphtheria is at its highest incidence in 8 years, and poverty areas of some of our major cities as well as certain rural areas are ripe for a polio epidemic. Overall the picture of immunization practice in the United States in 1971 is far from bright. The time for us to be complacent about these diseases has run out."

Increasingly reports are seen of the development of resistance to insecticides, especially where large amounts are used for agricultural purposes; the malaria eradication program, despite its spectacular progress during the past two

decades, appears to be slowing down, and the number of reported cases in the United States has risen from 62 in 1960 to 3,997 in 1970. It is true that the majority of the latter occurred among military personnel. Nonetheless, 125 were civilians and at least a dozen were known to have acquired the infection in the United States. As most public health workers are well aware, the saying "out of sight out of mind" applies to protection against communicable diseases as well as to many other things, and experience shows that the absence of disease leads to a neglect of immunization.

Evidence of the folly of complacency is found in the fact that the communicable diseases still represent the major cause of illness and death in much of the world. The extent of their real and present danger is indicated in Table 21-2, compiled by Le Riche,[11] who also estimates annual world incidences of 2 million cases of typhoid, 50 million cases of dysentery, and 750 million cases of gastrointestinal infections, not including diarrhea of the newborn.

**Table 21-2.** Deaths from communicable diseases, estimated world totals, 1963*

| Cause of death | Number of deaths in thousands |
|---|---|
| 1. Pneumonia | 5,701 |
| 2. Gastritis, duodenitis, enteritis, and colitis, except diarrhea of the newborn | 3,094 |
| 3. Tuberculosis of respiratory system | 2,839 |
| 4. All other diseases classified as infective and parasitic | 1,347 |
| 5. Infections of the newborn | 1,131 |
| 6. Bronchitis | 1,085 |
| 7. Measles | 508 |
| 8. Malaria | 326 |
| 9. Influenza | 313 |
| 10. Dysentery, all forms | 202 |
| 11. Smallpox | 172 |
| 12. Diphtheria | 127 |
| 13. Whooping cough | 112 |
| 14. Typhoid fever | 98 |
| 15. Syphilis and its sequelae | 68 |
| 16. Acute poliomyelitis | 35 |
| 17. Meningococcal infections | 31 |
| 18. Cholera | 12 |
| 19. Typhus | 7 |
| 20. Scarlet fever and streptococcal sore throat | 6 |

*From Le Riche, W. H.: In Wolstenholme, G., and O'Connor, M., editors: Health of mankind, London, 1967, J. & A. Churchill, Ltd.

## BIOLOGIC SIGNIFICANCE OF INFECTION

At first glance it may seem extraneous to discuss the essential meaning of infection. However, although human beings may be members of advanced societies, they are nevertheless influenced to a surprising degree by many elemental emotions and superstitions. Man may strive to convince himself and others that he is different from the other creatures of the earth. Insofar as possible people consciously or subconsciously attempt to avoid recognition of the fact that they share with all living things certain fundamental needs, desires, and drives, that is, the need for food and shelter, the desire for personal survival, and the drive for perpetuation of their species.

Any approach to the communicable diseases and their control should be based on a frank recognition and understanding of these ecologic facts. It must be realized that the microorganisms that cause disease in man have no innate malevolence toward him, but in their own struggle for survival and perpetuation have found in his body merely a convenient stepping-stone and have adapted their biologic life cycle accordingly. By like token it may be said that man himself, probably more than any other species, in his struggle for survival has contrived to take advantage of many other living creatures, from the myriad microorganisms that exist in his intestinal tract and assist his digestive process to the fish, fowl, and cattle that give him sustenance and the beasts that bear his burdens.

By far the most desirable situation for a microorganism is one in which it lives in nonfatal harmony with the other creatures upon or within which it exists. For a microorganism to so evolve that its multiplication results in the demise of its host represents perhaps the ultimate in biologic failure; by killing its host, it kills itself.[12] The anthrax bacillus, for example, depending on multiplication in the bloodstream of its human host, completely defeats its purpose when it kills its host and thereby traps itself within the dead body, whence only with great difficulty it can be transmitted to others. If for the purpose of discussion one was to assume the tuberculosis organism to be endowed with some form of intelligence, it might be said that the more astute of its kind would be content with producing only moderate degrees of tuberculosis. By allowing its host to continue unsuspectingly his customary life, the organism assures itself not only of continued existence but also of ample opportunity for further transfer and perpetuation. In a biologic sense the more virulent and more toxic strains that kill and do so quickly also represent impatient and overambitious biologic failures.

## GENERAL REQUISITES FOR MICROORGANIC SURVIVAL

In order for a microorganism that has involved itself in a biologic relationship with man to survive successfully a certain chain of circumstances must be followed (Fig. 21-1). As long as a parasitic microorganism is entirely confined within its definitive host, it cannot present an immediate threat to other potential hosts. Many examples may be cited. Except for certain stages of the disease it causes, the spirochete of syphilis is completely contained within the body of its host, who although actually infected, cannot transmit the disease. Similarly in the field of protozoology the malarial parasite, except for relatively short intervals is nontransmissible.

The necessity for the parasite to leave the host implies a mode of exit. This is not as simple as it sounds, since each parasitic microorganism has adaptively restricted itself to a few paths and often one particular path. Thus the parasite of malaria is restricted to egress through the skin of its host and even then only at certain phases of its life cycle. The spirochete of syphilis, because of overspecialization that has resulted in great frailty, must rely essentially on exit through the sexual organs of humans, which in the process of their use provide the spirochete with the maximum protection against its most lethal natural hazard, that is, drying. A great many parasitic species have so adapted themselves that the nose and throat offer the most expeditious exit. Still others rely essentially on the discharges of the gastrointestinal tract. If in some way the typhoid bacillus were suddenly to decide on the skin or genitalia as a means of exit, it would in all probability cease to be a threat to man. All external parts of the human body, including of course the openings of the respiratory, genitourinary, and gastrointestinal tracts, serve as sites of exit for various microorganisms that affect man. Obviously the more limited the means of egress the greater is the opportunity for successful control, at least in a theoretic sense.

The picture becomes greatly complicated, however, by certain other biologic and cultural aspects of human existence. Thus although for all practical purposes the spirochete of syphilis

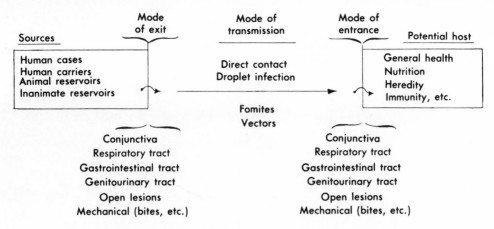

**Fig. 21-1.** Sequence of events in transmission of diseases.

has restricted itself to a single mode of exit, successful control or elimination of the disease is more easily proposed than accomplished. In theory syphilis could be completely eradicated by prohibiting all human sexual intercourse. Such a prohibition, however, even if tolerated, would in turn eliminate man himself. This being impractical, it therefore becomes necessary to find some other approach to the problem. Theoretically typhoid fever and many related diseases could be eradicated by complete control over the defecatory functions and habits of man. This function, however, is essential to continued human existence, and the regulation of it is no mean task considering its involvement in various superstitions, social attitudes, and agricultural economies. Therefore it must always be borne in mind that the theoretically ideal or obvious approach to the control of a communicable disease is not necessarily practical or successful. As a result, the indirect attack is often the most fruitful. Furthermore in many instances the greatest handicaps to control are factors relating to man himself rather than to the pathogen.

On gaining exit the parasitic organism must find some means of transportation to the new potential host. Here again, depending on the biologic characteristics of the particular pathogenic organism, the method of transfer is limited. Some organisms, for example, the syphilis spirochete, require direct and intimate conditions of transfer. Certain others, of which those causing malaria and yellow fever are examples, must rely for transfer not only on another living thing such as a mosquito but even only on certain species of that insect. Many organisms, however, have made themselves more adaptable and have allowed for relatively prolonged exis-

tence outside the human host and for transfer in any one of a number of ways. The typhoid bacillus can be cited as an example.

Even when the proximity of a potential host is gained, successful transfer of infection does not necessarily follow. The pathogen must now find a biologically suitable mode of entrance. The limitations surrounding this requirement are similar to those that relate to the mode of exit. To be successful the choice must conform with the adaptive processes through which the organisms, both parasite and man, have gone. Generally speaking, but by no means exclusively, the mode of entrance is the same as the mode of exit, that is, the diphtheria organism leaves and enters through the nasopharynx, the tuberculosis organism through the respiratory tract, the typhoid organism through the gastrointestinal tract, and the malarial organism through the pierced skin.

Finally, several factors come into play in deciding whether or not the parasite that has gained entrance will survive and thrive. Among the most important of these are the general state of health and nutrition of the host, the presence or absence of immune bodies, and the virulence and toxicity of the parasite. Because of the future need of the parasite to continue still further beyond the present host, consideration must be given to some other characteristics of the host. For example, the typhoid organism is most successful if it achieves infection of a food-handler or of someone who is indiscriminate in his defecatory habits. Its chances of future success are considerably limited when it finds itself within a business or professional person who works and lives according to a social pattern that provides obstacles to further transfer. Gono-

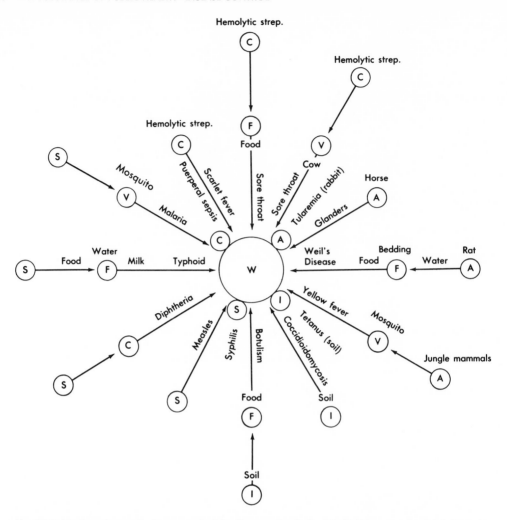

**Fig. 21-2.** Modes of spread of communicable disease. Symbols: *W*, Well human; *S*, sick infected human; *C*, well infected human (carrier); *F*, inanimate transmitter (fomite); *V*, animate transmitter (vector); *A*, animate reservoir; *I*, inanimate reservoir.

coccal infection of the eyes of a newborn child does not nearly parallel the degree of success from the point of view of the gonococcus that is represented in the infection of a prostitute. In the first instance the organism has been sidetracked. Likewise infection of an individual about to move to a mosquito-free area is longrange wasted effort on the part of the malarial organism.

Each step mentioned represents a necessary link in the chain of disease perpetuation. Each also presents a point at which control measures may be applied. The chain is only as strong as its weakest link, and the successful severance of any one link will go far in controlling and in some instances completely eradicating particular diseases.

This concept may be approached in still another way. In Fig. 21-2 the well person, represented by [W], is the center of potential attack by many types of organisms in many different ways. He finds in his environment several factors that threaten him: [S] clinically ill and infected humans; [C] apparently well but infected human carriers; [F] inanimate transmitters of disease (fomites); [V] animate transmitters (vectors); [A] animate nonhuman reservoirs of disease in the form of lower animals; and [I] inanimate reservoirs of disease, for example, soil.

The well person may receive infection by means of many combinations of these factors, depending on his biologically adapted habits and activities, those of other humans, and those of vectors, animal reservoirs, and the pathogens. In certain instances, as in the case of the venereal diseases, direct and intimate contact must take place between the well and the infected human. This is indicated diagrammatically as [S] [W]. In certain other instances the well person may be infected across a certain distance by droplets from an infected human in a nonintimate relationship, [S] ——→ [W]. Measles and smallpox present examples of this. With some diseases an apparently healthy human carrier may be interposed, as in the circumstance of a clinically ill diphtheria patient passing the organism to another human who remains apparently well but in turn transmits the organism to another well person who then becomes clinically ill, [S] ——→ [C] ——→ [W]. The intervening factor in some diseases, for example, typhoid, may take the form of inanimate transmitters, often referred to as fomites. Thus the typhoid patient or carrier may transmit the disease indirectly to a well person by means of food, milk, or water, [S] ——→ [F] ——→ [W]. With diseases such as malaria and the rickettsial diseases the intervening factor may take the form of a mosquito, tick, louse, or other biting insect. The pattern here is [S] —— [V] ——→ [W]. Healthy individuals may sometimes be infected as a result of intimate contact with healthy carriers, [C] [W]. An example of this is found in the transfer of hemolytic streptococci from the hands of an accoucheur to the tissues of a woman in labor, thereby resulting in puerperal sepsis. Certain pathogenic organisms may be transferred over a distance from healthy human carriers to the well person, [C] —— [W]. Here again may be mentioned hemolytic streptococci, now causing scarlet fever in the recipient. Furthermore, many organisms, of which the hemolytic streptococcus is again an example, may be transferred first from a carrier to an inanimate fomite such as food, thence to the new human host according to the pattern [C] ——→ [F] ——→ [W]; if the organism is the hemolytic streptococcus, it may perhaps result in a case of septic sore throat. On the other hand, the healthy human carrier may infect an animate transmitter such as a cow, which develops mastitis and thereby infects its milk, causing septic sore throat in a new human host; the resulting pattern is [C] ——→ [V] ——→ [F] ——→ [W].

Animate but nonhuman reservoirs of disease may threaten the well person in several ways similar to the foregoing. Again instances exist in which intimate contact is necessary between the animate reservoir and the potential human host. Thus the handling of the carcass of an infected rabbit may result in the transfer of tularemia to man, [A] [W]. Bites from rabid animals and bites resulting in rat-bite fever are further examples in this category. Some animal diseases, for example, glanders in horses, may be transmitted over a distance in a manner similar to measles, with the pattern [A] ——→ [W]. Other animal diseases may be passed on to human hosts by means of inanimate intermediaries, or fomites, [A] ——→ [F] ——→ [W]. Here might be mentioned the contamination by rats of bedding or food from which the human host becomes infected with the leptospira causing infectious jaundice. Some diseases that primarily affect lower animals but with which humans may be infected may require an intermediate vector, usually in the form of a biting insect. An important example is jungle yellow fever, transferred by mosquitoes from small jungle mammals to man. Here the pattern is [A] ——→ [V] ——→ [W]. Finally, even man's inanimate environment may be a source of infection, either by direct contact as in the case of tetanus acquired from the soil, [I] [W], or over a distance as may possibly be the case in transmission of coccidioidomycosis [I] ——→ [W].

The foregoing scheme by no means presents an all-inclusive picture. Some diseases of man, particularly those caused by protozoa and helminthes, involve far more complicated patterns of transmission. The large fish tapeworm *Diphyllobothrium latum,* for example, infects man according to the following scheme:

dog      water    crustacean    fish      human
[A] ——→ [I] ——→ [A] ——→ [A] ——→ [W]

Of a similar magnitude is the pattern of schistosome infection:

sick
human      water    snail    water    human
[S] ——→ [I] ——→ [A] ——→ [I] ——→ [W]

A still more complicated cycle is that of the sheep liver fluke:

grasses and
sheep  water  snail  water  vegetables  sheep
[A] ——→ [I] ——→ [A] ——→ [I] ——→ [F] ——→ [A]

human

[W]

For purposes of further discussion, however, it is probably best to ignore these more complicated methods of infection and to limit consideration to the simple circumstances shown in Fig. 21-2. It is observed that the ultimate sources of infection in the diagram occur at the periphery and that, if it is found possible to place a block between any given peripheral source and the central potential host, infection cannot take place. Considering the problem from the standpoint of total diseases, it might be said that the central potential host would be completely safeguarded from all diseases if a cordon could be thrown around him at any point between him and all of the various peripheral sources of infection. Careful consideration of the diagram indicates the possibility of a series of concentric cordons, the most central of which would bar all infections and the more peripheral affecting the more complicated types of infection patterns.

Theoretically speaking, the more links there are in a chain of infection the more difficult it is for the organism to survive. Each link presents another place where something may go wrong. From the point of view of humanly conceived control measures each additional link provides another point of attack where obstacles to disease transmission may be interposed. Because of this, syphilis, with the simple [S] [W] pattern involving only the spirochete and man, is proportionately more difficult to control than malaria. In the latter instance control measures may be applied singly or jointly to any of a number of factors: the plasmodium (by treating or isolating infected persons), the adult mosquito, breeding places, the mosquito larvae, or the potential hosts.

By the same token it is equally true that the greater the number of ways an organism may be transmitted the greater are its chances of survival. When a pathogenic organism is restricted completely to one particular path, for example, the malarial parasite, the problem of control, once the basic facts about the disease are discovered, is theoretically simplified. Contrast with this the hemolytic streptococcus, which as shown in Fig. 21-2, may be transmitted by direct or indirect contact with either a sick infected human or a carrier or through a wide variety of fomites and vectors acting as intermediaries. An organism that could so adapt itself as to be transmissible by any or all of the paths indicated would present a dire threat indeed. Probably the best example of this is the

*Pasteurella pestis,* which can spread by intimate contact, by droplet infection, by innumerable fomites, and by several animal vectors. It is not without significance that this particular organism came closer to eradicating the human species than any other known factor in its history.

In view of the foregoing the details of the control of specific communicable diseases must take into consideration the biologic characteristics of the pathogenic organism, of the potential host, and of any vectors or animal reservoirs that might be involved. To acquire essential knowledge concerning the disease and to apply that knowledge effectively attention must be given both to the adaptive habits of the organisms and to the social and cultural habits of the hosts.

## GENERAL PRINCIPLES OF THE CONTROL OF COMMUNICABLE DISEASES

Control measures may be aimed at any factor or at any link involved in the chain of transmission, that is, the organism, its present host, its vectors, its reservoirs, or the potential host himself. Following is a general classification of these measures.

### Prevention of spread

**Measures aimed at the organism.** The ultimate point of attack here is the pathogenic organism itself. Since the goal is the destruction of the living cause of disease, any measures that could be devised to strike directly at it would be of great value. This is unfortunately difficult, since pathogenic organisms by their very nature seldom exist in the free state. It is interesting that some of the earliest attempts by primitive people to combat communicable diseases were along these lines, taking the form of the generation of noise and smoke, the latter subsequently dignified by the term *fumigation*. These methods were intended originally to drive away the evil gods of disease and were later continued against miasms. Although current scientific knowledge makes their use ridiculous, it may be pointed out that as recently as the beginning of the twentieth century pitch barrels were burned and cannons were fired in New Orleans as a means of combating yellow fever. Man's ties with the past are further demonstrated by the continued sale of materials for fumigation and the wearing of asafetida bags in some areas of the world. A somewhat direct approach of attacking the organism is found in the treatment of persons who are infected. The community as well as the personal benefit that results from so doing has justified even in the minds of those with narrow horizons the treatment under public health auspices of individuals infected with syphilis, tuberculosis, and certain other diseases.

**Measures aimed at sources of infection.** Sources of infection may be eradicated, their communicability may be reduced, or they may be rendered noninfectious by treatment.

*Eradication of sources.* When the source of infection is a known accessible animal reservoir, its elimination provides an effective means of eradication of the disease. Many instances of this method of attack in modern public health practice may be mentioned. Bovine tuberculosis has been almost eradicated in the United States by the destruction of infected cattle. However, this would be extremely difficult or impossible in a Hindu society for cultural reasons. Psittacosis may be eradicated by the elimination of infected parrots and other psittacine birds. Plague, typhus fever, leptospirosis, anthrax, tularemia, and several other diseases may be controlled by a similar attack against their animal reservoirs. Theoretically this approach could be applied effectively to diseases peculiar to man by the eradication of persons found to be infected. In a sense this was done at least partially during medieval times with regard to lepers, the deliberate neglect of whom was tantamount to elimination. A more conscious and direct use of this method was made occasionally in recent times by the leaders of the Nazi regime. A more humane and scientific adaptation of the method is seen in the surgical removal of a chronically infected part of the human body. Thus cholecystectomy has been used in an attempt to cure chronic typhoid carriers, and tonsillectomies have frequently been performed on chronic carriers of diphtheria and streptococci. Even these techniques, however, have become less justified with the introduction of antibiotics.

*Reduction of communicability of sources of infection.* The eradication of the sources of infections is often unnecessary for the control of the infections they contain. When dealing with diseases in human beings, the most practical primary point of attack sometimes takes the form of reducing the communicability of those infected. This may be accomplished by a combination of two control measures: (1) limitation of their movement and (2) treatment of their infection. Limitation of human activity

for public health purposes takes the form of isolation of those known to be infected and quarantine of those known or suspected to have been exposed to the risk of infection. Customarily the free movement of known infected individuals is restricted until clinical observation and/or laboratory tests indicate the absence of infectiousness. Quarantine for a disease generally has been extended over a time interval equal to the usual maximum incubation period of the disease.

These techniques, although of long historic standing, have never been too popular. First, it is human to resist and to circumvent restriction of personal action. Second, the measures are usually economically costly both to those restricted and to those enforcing the restriction. Beyond these objections are some more scientific reasons for their limited value. There are many unreported, hidden, or undetected cases of most if not all communicable diseases. The ineffectiveness of isolation and quarantine for the control of measles is evidence of this. Of even greater significance is the large number of apparently healthy carriers of some diseases who effectively spread pathogenic organisms. For this reason isolation of a diagnosed case of poliomyelitis and its contacts is futile. Furthermore, the majority of acute communicable diseases are most infectious during their early stages before diagnosis is made or confirmed. Nevertheless, when rigidly applied under certain circumstances and to certain diseases such as smallpox and bubonic plague, isolation and quarantine may constitute effective means of control. At the present time there are only six human diseases on the international list of quarantinable diseases: cholera, plague, smallpox, yellow fever, louse-borne typhus, and louse-borne relapsing fever. Under special circumstances, quarantine of animals may be a valuable control measure. An interesting example of this is found in the rabies control program of England.

To be segregated and subsequently rendered noncommunicable, diseased individuals first must be discovered. Fundamental to this is a system for the reporting of cases of communicable diseases both by physicians in the area and by health authorities in other localities to which infected individuals may emigrate. Other sources of information are hospital records, requests for biologics, death certificates, and burial permits. The value of a report of a case of communicable disease is not in the counting of a "vital fact" or merely in the control of the patient but in the lead it gives in finding sources and contacts. This implies engaging in what some have termed *shoeleather epidemiology.* A routine procedure must operate to determine and locate for subsequent examination members of a group in which active infection of either recent or earlier origin is most likely to exist.

Human sources of infection may also be discovered by means of various screening and diagnostic procedures, for example, tuberculin tests and chest x-ray examinations for tuberculosis, stool examinations for typhoid fever and other intestinal infections, nose and throat cultures for diphtheria, and vaginal and urethral smears for gonorrhea. Such tests are most useful when applied on a selective basis at certain times to certain groups of high average incidence and risk of infection.

*Treatment of sources of infection.* Merely to find a source of infection is of little value. Prompt treatment is indicated to render the patient noninfectious as well as to cure him. Thus treatment of individuals with communicable diseases is primarily for the protection of contacts and of the community and secondarily for the benefit of the patient. This has served in the past as justification for the establishment of publicly supported communicable disease treatment clinics and hospitals. In a few instances complete treatment or cure of the patient is unnecessary to eliminate the threat to those about him. The syphilitic person, for example, may be rendered noninfectious by prompt administration of therapeutic agents. Similarly many tuberculosis patients may be made noninfectious by partial lung collapse or by drug therapy. It is important under such circumstances, however, that treatment be continued to ultimate success because the patient may relapse to a communicable stage. Furthermore, one must be concerned not only with the control of a disease from the standpoint of spread but also in terms of eliminating it as a cause of disability and premature death. In this sense public health is considered increasingly as a summation of personal health.

**Measures aimed at transmitters of disease.** Many communicable diseases require some kind of transmitting agent either in the form of an inanimate fomite or of a living vector. Not infrequently the most fruitful attack is one that is aimed at these transmitting agents. In fact some of the most spectacular examples of successful control have depended on this approach. Truly remarkable results have followed programs of water purification, sanitary excreta disposal, food and dairy sanitation, and pasteurization. Success in these instances is greatly enhanced by the ability to apply effective control measures at central focal points such as water-treatment plants, pasteurization plants, canneries, bakeries, etc. It is worthy of particular mention that the healthfulness of American urbanized society and its economy depends in no small measure on the penchant for convenient processed foods, the sanitary quality of which is controlled with relative ease.

Almost equally spectacular results are possible and in some instances have been achieved by the control or elimination of animate vectors of disease. Here the public health worker has the advantage of finding a chain of events with numerous links, each of which is subject to attack. For example, the control of mosquito-borne disease may be achieved in several ways: The adult mosquito may be destroyed by chemical or other means. Its breeding places may be eliminated by filling or impounding or made unsuitable by spraying with oils and other larvicides. The mosquito's effective biting contact may be eliminated by the use of screens, nets, mosquito bars, and repellents. Finally, persons with malaria may be isolated from the mosquito, and healthy potential hosts may avoid the consequence of actual mosquito bites by routine chemoprophylaxis. Similar measures aimed at other vectors may take the form of delousing, cattle dipping, ship fumigation, rat proofing, proper garbage disposal, and the destruction of rats and biting flies. Measures relating to inanimate transmitters include the cooking of pork, the boiling of water or milk, the disinfection of typhoid stools, the burning of tuberculous sputum, and the ultraviolet disinfection of air.

## Increasing the resistance of potential hosts

**Maintenance of general health and nutrition.** Although each communicable disease is attributable to a specific infectious agent, certain factors enter into the decision of whether or not the organism can thrive and cause disease once it gains entrance to the body of a potential host. The inverse relationship between general health and nutrition, on the one hand, and susceptibility to many infectious agents, on the other, is well established. Examples of this are found in connection with pneumonia, tuberculosis, some streptococcal diseases, and even some intestinal infections. A rather striking example is hookworm infection, in which spontaneous elimination of adult worms has been achieved merely by improving the diet of the host.

**Production of passive immunity.** If available, passive immunization is important when recent exposure of persons susceptible to diseases with short incubation periods is known to have occurred. Measures of this nature are exemplified by diphtheria and tetanus antitoxins. Still others are convalescent sera for the prevention of scarlet fever, measles, pertussis, chickenpox, mumps, and some other diseases. Certain precautions must be observed in using passively immunizing products. Applicable to all of them is the need for prompt administration of large enough doses. In the case of antitoxin, particular care must be taken to avoid serum reactions by obtaining careful therapeutic histories and by testing for sensitivity to horse serum.

**Production of active immunity.** Where available and popularly accepted, active immunization against communicable diseases may offer an ideal control measure. If applicable, this approach has produced spectacular successes comparable to those effected by sanitary engineering procedures. The widespread use of such simple measures as smallpox vaccination and diphtheria immunization has eradicated the threat of these two diseases in the United States and many other countries. Active immunization of a practical nature is also available against several other infectious diseases, including tetanus, pertussis, poliomyelitis, measles, rubella, mumps, influenza, cholera, typhoid fever, yellow fever, and spotted fever. Of more limited value and applicability are active immunizing measures against scarlet fever, meningococcic meningitis, and pneumococcal pneumonia.

Although there is no universally followed schedule of immunizations, Table 21-3 presents what is practical for most situations.

**Prevention of complications.** A procedure similar to active immunization is the deliberate exposure of susceptible persons to measles, followed in 5 or 6 days by the administration of immune serum in an amount not sufficient to prevent the disease completely but enough to modify its clinical severity. In this way the patient obtains a lasting immunity by undergoing a controlled, greatly attenuated attack of the disease. The recent availability of an effective antimeasles vaccine, however, makes this procedure unnecessary. For a somewhat

*Text continued on p. 401.*

**Table 21-3.** Immunization schedule

| Age | Immunization |
|---|---|
| PRIMARY IMMUNIZATIONS | |
| 2 months | |
| 3 months | Diphtheria, pertussis, and tetanus, combined 0.5 ml. each time |
| 4 months | |
| 5 months | Smallpox vaccine (if epidemiologically indicated) |
| 6 months | |
| 7 months | Salk or Sabin polio vaccine, 1 ml. each time |
| 14 months | |
| 21 months | |
| 1 year | Live measles virus vaccine (if Edmonston strain used, administer measles immune globulin also) |
| 1 year to puberty | Live rubella virus vaccine* (not before first birthday) |
| BOOSTER DOSES | |
| 18 months | Diphtheria, pertussis, tetanus, 0.5 ml. |
| 5 years | Diphtheria, pertussis, tetanus, 0.5 ml. |
| | Salk or Sabin vaccine |
| | Smallpox vaccine (if epidemiologically indicated) |
| 7 years | Diphtheria and tetanus, 0.25 ml. |
| 10 years and each | Smallpox vaccine (if epidemiologically indicated) |
| 5 years after | Salk or Sabin vaccine |
| OTHER IMMUNIZATIONS | |
| Appropriate immunizations if possible exposure to yellow fever, typhoid fever, cholera, plague, or rickettsial fever is anticipated | |

*Live rubella virus vaccine should not be given to known or possibly pregnant women—if women considered, lack of pregnancy must be assured for the following 2 months.

**Table 21-4.** Case, contact, and disinfection control of reportable infectious diseases*

| Disease and incubation period | Isolation (cases) | Quarantine (contacts or premises) | Environmental control (disinfection) |
|---|---|---|---|
| Amebiasis (dysentery, amebic) (a few days-several weeks) | None; exclude patient from food handling | None | *Concurrent:* sanitary disposal of feces; handwashing after defecation<br>*Terminal:* cleaning |
| Anthrax (within 7 days, usually 2-5 days) | Until lesions are healed; inhalation type—strict isolation | None | *Concurrent:* of discharges from lesions and soiled articles; spore sterilization requires steam under pressure, prolonged heat above 284° F., or burning<br>*Terminal:* thorough cleaning |
| Brucellosis (usually 6-21 days; sometimes longer) | None | None | *Concurrent:* of purulent discharges<br>*Terminal:* none |
| Cat-scratch fever (2-18 days; average 7-14 days) | None | None | *Concurrent:* of discharges from lesions<br>*Terminal:* none |
| Chancroid (1-3 days) | Exclusion from sexual contact with others until lesions are healed | None | *Concurrent:* personal hygienic measures<br>*Terminal:* none |
| Chickenpox (12-21 days) | None; exclusion from school for 1 week after eruption first appears; avoidance of contact with susceptibles | Susceptible child contacts may be excluded from school from twelfth to twenty-first day after exposure; none | *Concurrent:* of articles soiled by discharges from nose and throat<br>*Terminal:* none |
| Cholera (1-5 days; in common-source outbreaks, 2-3 days) | Unnecessary if attendants maintain high levels of cleanliness; patient should be treated in hospital | Surveillance of contacts for 5 days from last exposure and longer if feces contain cholera vibrios | *Concurrent:* of feces and vomitus and of articles used by patient; disinfection of hands each time after handling articles contaminated by fees<br>*Terminal:* cleaning |
| Coccidioidomycosis (1-3 weeks) | None | None | *Concurrent:* of discharges and soiled articles<br>*Terminal:* thorough cleaning |
| Conjunctivitis (see Keratoconjunctivitis; see Ophthalmia neonatorum) | | | |
| Cryptococcosis (unknown) | None | None | *Concurrent:* of discharges and contaminated dressings<br>*Terminal:* cleaning |
| Cytomegalovirus infection (little information available; several weeks after transfusion of blood containing agent) | None | None | *Concurrent:* of discharges from hospitalized patients and soiled articles<br>*Terminal:* none |

| Disease and incubation period | Isolation | Quarantine | Concurrent and terminal disinfection |
|---|---|---|---|
| Diarrhea of newborn, epidemic (variable; 1½-6 days; average 2-4 days) | Immediate removal of infected infant to isolation room; suspects should be held in separate quarters | Of nursery; no admission of newborn to affected nursery | *Concurrent:* of all discharges and soiled articles<br>*Terminal:* thorough cleaning of nursery and equipment |
| Diphtheria (1-10 days; average 2-5 days) | Until afebrile 24 hours and thereafter until two consecutive negative cultures from nose and throat have been obtained not less than 24 hours apart and reported from a registered laboratory | Wage earners may be permitted to enter and leave premises if they have no contact with the patient, with children, or with food for public consumption; all intimate contacts until nose and throat cultures negative | *Concurrent:* of discharges and articles soiled therewith<br>*Terminal:* cleaning and airing of sickroom |
| Dysentery, bacillary (see Shigellosis)<br>Encephalitis (4-21 days) | None | None | *Concurrent:* of discharges from nose and throat and articles soiled therewith<br>*Terminal:* none |
| Enteroviruses (see Poliomyelitis)<br>Food poisoning (1-36 hours after ingestion of food) (*Salmonella,* staphylococcal, *C. botulinum*) | None; for food infections— exclusion of infected persons from food handling and from care of young children | None; food infections—family contacts should not be employed as food handlers during contact and only after repeated negative feces cultures obtained | *Concurrent:* of feces and articles soiled therewith; with adequate sewage treatment, sewer disposal satisfactory<br>*Terminal:* cleaning |
| Gonorrhea (2-5 days in males; as long as 21 days) | None; antibiotics in adequate dosage; genitourinary lesions— no sexual contact; conjunctival lesions—exclusion from school or contact with children | None | *Concurrent:* disposal of discharges from lesions and articles soiled therewith<br>*Terminal:* none |
| Granuloma inguinale (variable; probably 8 days to 12 weeks) | Exclusion from sexual contact until lesions healed | None | *Concurrent:* disposal of discharges from lesions and articles soiled therewith<br>*Terminal:* none |
| Hepatitis, viral (variable; Virus IH, 2-6 weeks) | During first 2 weeks of illness; 1 week after onset of jaundice | None | *Concurrent:* sanitary disposal of feces and urine<br>*Terminal:* none |
| Hepatitis, serum (Virus SH, 1½-6 months) | (Same as viral hepatitis) | None | *Concurrent:* of equipment contaminated with blood<br>*Terminal:* none |
| Herpes simplex (2-12 days; average 6 days) | None | None | *Concurrent:* none<br>*Terminal:* none |

*From Top, F. H., and Wehrle, P. H., editors: Communicable and infectious diseases, ed. 7, St. Louis, 1972, The C. V. Mosby Co.

*Continued.*

**Table 21-4.** Case, contact, and disinfection control of reportable infectious diseases—cont'd

| Disease and incubation period | Isolation (cases) | Quarantine (contacts or premises) | Environmental control (disinfection) |
|---|---|---|---|
| Histoplasmosis (unknown; in epidemics, 5-18 days) | None | None | *Concurrent:* of discharges from skin lesions; sputum, and soiled articles<br>*Terminal:* thorough cleaning |
| Hookworm disease (ancylostomiasis) (unknown) | None | None | *Concurrent:* of feces and articles soiled therewith<br>*Terminal:* none |
| Impetigo (1-5 days) | Of infected infants; of children, exclusion from school | Of exposed infants; of children, none | *Concurrent:* careful disposal of dressings or moist discharges; sterilization of towels and underclothing before laundering<br>*Terminal:* thorough cleaning of hairbrushes, combs, and other toilet articles |
| Influenza (1-3 days) | Until recovery | None | *Concurrent:* of discharges from nose and throat<br>*Terminal:* none |
| Keratoconjunctivitis, epidemic (uncertain; probably 7-10 days) | None; hygienic measures important | None | *Concurrent:* of conjunctival and nasal discharges and articles soiled therewith<br>*Terminal:* none |
| Larva migrans, visceral (probably weeks to months) | None | None | *Concurrent:* none<br>*Terminal:* none |
| Leprosy (months to several years) | In treatment center for initiation of treatment | None | *Concurrent:* of nasal discharges from lesions and articles soiled therewith<br>*Terminal:* thorough cleaning of living premises |
| Leptospirosis (4-19 days; usually 10 days) | None | None | *Concurrent:* none<br>*Terminal:* none |
| Lymphocytic choriomeningitis (indefinite; meningitic probably 8-21 days) | None | None | *Concurrent:* of discharges of nose and throat<br>*Terminal:* none |
| Lymphogranuloma venereum (variable; 7-12 days usual for primary lesion) | Exclusion from sexual contact while lesions are open | None | *Concurrent:* of discharges from lesions and articles soiled therewith<br>*Terminal:* none |
| Malaria (10-28 days; average 12 days for *P. falciparum*, 14 days for *P. vivax* and *P. ovale*, and 30 days for *P. malariae*) | None; protect from bite of mosquitoes | None | *Concurrent:* a single concurrent residual spraying where potential vectors are active<br>*Terminal:* none |

| Disease (incubation period) | Isolation | Quarantine and control of contacts | Disinfection |
|---|---|---|---|
| Measles (8-12 days; average 10 days) | For 7 days from appearance of rash | Quarantine impractical; in face of outbreak in large communities in sparsely settled rural areas, exclusion of exposed susceptible school children and teachers from school and all public gatherings until 14 days from last exposure may be justifiable | *Concurrent:* of articles soiled with secretion of nose and throat<br>*Terminal:* thorough cleaning |
| Meningococcal meningitis (2-10 days; average 4 days) | Until 24 hours after initial of chemotherapy | None; surveillance profitable | *Concurrent:* of discharges from nose and throat of articles soiled therewith<br>*Terminal:* thorough cleaning |
| Mononucleosis, infectious (variable; 30-50 days for young adults; average 6 weeks) | None | None | *Concurrent:* of articles soiled by nose and throat discharges<br>*Terminal:* none |
| Mumps (14-21 days; average 18 days) | Until swelling has subsided; not less then 9 days from onset of swelling | None | *Concurrent:* of mouth discharges and articles soiled therewith<br>*Terminal:* none |
| Ophthalmia neonatorum (1-3 days) | For first 24 hours after administration of antibiotic | None | *Concurrent:* of conjunctival discharges and articles soiled therewith<br>*Terminal:* none |
| Paratyphoid fever (1-10 days; longer for paratyphoid A than B or C) | Until recovered and until three consecutive negative stool cultures obtained at weekly intervals | None; family contacts should not act as food handlers | *Concurrent:* of feces and urine and articles soiled by them; with modern sewage plants, feces and urine can be disposed of directly into sewer without preliminary disinfection<br>*Terminal:* thorough cleaning |
| Pertussis (7-10 days; rarely longer) | For minimum of three weeks; patients should be allowed access to open air on premises, weather permitting | Of nonimmune children until patient released from isolation | *Concurrent:* of discharges from nose and throat and articles soiled therewith<br>*Terminal:* thorough cleaning |
| Plague (2-6 days in bubonic type; 2-3 days in pneumonic type; may be shorter, rarely longer) | Rid patient, clothing, and baggage of fleas; hospitalize if practical; ordinary hospital precautions for bubonic type; strict isolation with precautions against airborne spread with primary pneumonic plague | Contacts: bubonic plague—disinfestation with insecticide powder and surveillance for 6 days; pneumonic plague—dust with insecticide, institute chemoprophylaxis, and maintain surveillance for 6 days | *Concurrent:* of sputum and purulent discharges and articles soiled therewith and with urine and feces of patients<br>*Terminal:* bodies of patients dying of plague should be handled with strict aseptic precautions |

*Continued.*

**Table 21-4.** Case, contact, and disinfection control of reportable infectious diseases—cont'd

| Disease and incubation period | Isolation (cases) | Quarantine (contacts or premises) | Environmental control (disinfection) |
| --- | --- | --- | --- |
| Pneumonia, mycoplasmal (20-35 days; range, 11-35 days) | None | None | *Concurrent:* of discharges from nose and throat. *Terminal:* thorough cleaning and airing |
| Pneumonia, pneumococcal (less then 24 hours to 2-3 days; not well determined) | Desirable | None | *Concurrent:* of discharges from nose and throat. *Terminal:* thorough cleaning |
| Poliomyelitis (limits, 3-35 days; average, 7-14 days) | For 7 days from onset and for the duration of fever, if longer | Of doubtful value; restricting the movement of intimate contacts for 7-21 days may be desirable under certain circumstances | *Concurrent:* of discharges from nose and throat and articles soiled therewith. *Terminal:* none |
| Psittacosis (4-15 days; often 10 days) | Of patient during the acute and febrile stages | None; of premises if infected birds in home | *Concurrent:* of all discharges; infected or suspect birds must be removed and destroyed. *Terminal:* thorough wet cleaning |
| Q fever (commonly 2-3 weeks) | None | None | *Concurrent:* of sputum and blood and articles freshly soiled therewith. *Terminal:* none |
| Rabies (variable; 2-8 weeks or longer) | With warning to attendants concerning danger of inoculation of virus from saliva | None | *Concurrent:* of saliva and all articles soiled therewith. *Terminal:* thorough wet cleaning |
| Rickettsialpox (probably 10-24 days) | None | None | *Concurrent:* none. *Terminal:* none |
| Rocky Mt. spotted fever (3-14 days; average 2-5 days) | None | None | *Concurrent:* all ticks on patient should be destroyed. *Terminal:* none |
| Rubella (14-21 days; average 17 days) | Of no practical value unless for 5 days after onset when contact to patient is a woman in early months of pregnancy | None | *Concurrent:* none. *Terminal:* none |
| Salmonella enteritis (6 hours to several days) (see also Paratyphoid fever and Typhoid fever) | Exclusion of infected persons from food handling; patient care of young children and the elderly until cultures of feces are free of *Salmonella* for 3 successive days | None | *Concurrent:* of feces and articles soiled therewith. *Terminal:* thorough cleaning |
| Scabies (indeterminate) | Exclude infected children from school and public gatherings until adequately treated | None | *Concurrent:* of personal underclothing and linen. *Terminal:* desirable |

| Disease (incubation period) | Isolation | Quarantine/Contacts | Concurrent and terminal disinfection |
|---|---|---|---|
| Shigellosis (1-7 days; usually under 4 days) | None; exclude patient from food handling | None; family contacts should not be employed as food handlers during contact and only after repeated negative feces cultures obtained | *Concurrent:* of feces and soiled articles; with adequate sewage treatment, sewer disposal satisfactory. *Terminal:* cleaning |
| Smallpox (8-17 days; average 10-12 days) | Until skin clear of crusts | For 21 days from last exposure unless successfully vaccinated | *Concurrent:* oral and nasal discharges should be burned; all articles should be steam sterilized or boiled. *Terminal:* thorough washing of sickroom and furniture; sterilize bedclothing and mattress |
| Staphylococcal infections, general (variable; newborn 3-10 days); pyodermas (to 10 days) | All known or suspect cases, immediately | None; surveillance of all suspect or exposed persons, including the newborn | *Concurrent:* collect and burn dressings; autoclave towels, linens, and bedclothing before laundering. *Terminal:* thorough washing with hexachlorophene detergent of all nonexpendable articles in cubicle or unit; boil basins and instruments and autoclave mattresses |
| Streptococcal infections (erysipelas, scarlet fever, septic sore throat) (12 hours to 3-4 days; rarely longer) | Until recovery; scarlet fever—on the basis of recovery or not less than 7 days from onset; may be removed after 24 hours of adequate treatment with penicillin, provided therapy is continued for 7-10 days | None | *Concurrent:* of nose and throat discharges and all articles soiled therewith. *Terminal:* thorough cleaning of all contaminated articles and scrubbing of all horizontal surfaces |
| Syphilis (variable; 10-90 days; average 3 weeks) | Unnecessary 24 hours after adequate treatment; no sexual contact, particularly with untreated partners | None | *Concurrent:* of discharges and all articles soiled therewith. *Terminal:* none |
| Tetanus (3-10 days [average 6 and possibly 1-50] for neonatal tetanus; median, U.S., 6.2-7.6 days and 90% less than 14 days) | None | None | *Concurrent:* none. *Terminal:* none |
| Trachoma (variable; experimentally, 5-14 days) | Exlude from school and public gatherings until recovery | None | *Concurrent:* of eye discharges and articles soiled therewith. *Terminal:* none |
| Trichinosis (2-28 days; variable) | None | None | *Concurrent:* none. *Terminal:* none |

*Continued.*

**Table 21-4.** Case, contact, and disinfection control of reportable infectious diseases—cont'd

| Disease and incubation period | Isolation (cases) | Quarantine (contacts or premises) | Environmental control (disinfection) |
|---|---|---|---|
| Tuberculosis (variable; 2-10 weeks or longer) | In hospital or sanatorium desirable; necessary for uncooperative patients | None | *Concurrent:* of sputum and articles and eating utensils; patient should cover mouth when speaking or when care given. *Terminal:* thorough wet cleaning of walls and floors |
| Tularemia (2-7 days; average 3½ days) | None | None | *Concurrent:* of discharges from ulcer, lymph nodes, eye. *Terminal:* none |
| Typhoid fever (5-14 days; range, 1-3 weeks) | Until 3 successive negative fecal cultures obtained at 1-week intervals | None; family contacts must not be employed as food handlers until repeated negative feces and urine cultures obtained | *Concurrent:* of feces and urine and articles soiled by them; with modern sewage plants, feces and urine can be disposed of directly into sewer without preliminary disinfection. *Terminal:* thorough cleaning |
| Typhus fever, classically louse-borne (6-15 days; average 10-12 days) | In a vermin-free room; not required after proper delousing of patient, clothing, living quarters, and household contacts | Exposed lousy susceptibles should be quarantined for 15 days; may be released after application of insecticides with residual effect | *Concurrent:* appropriate insecticide powders to clothing and bedding of patients and contacts; treatment of hair for louse nits with tested chemical agents. *Terminal:* if death occurs before delousing, thorough application of insecticide to body and clothing |
| Typhus fever, murine, flea-borne (6-15 days; average 12 days) | None | None | *Concurrent:* none. *Terminal:* none |
| Typhus fever, scrub (6-21 days; average 10-12 days) | None | None | *Concurrent:* none. *Terminal:* none |
| Vincent's infection (variable) | Exclusion from school | None | *Concurrent:* of mouth discharges. *Terminal;* none |
| Whooping cough (see Pertussis) | | | |

different reason some advocate the deliberate exposure of female children to rubella (German measles) to preclude subsequent acquisition of the disease during the first trimester of pregnancy, when certain malformations of the fetus may result. Here again the recent development of an effective vaccine has replaced this approach.

Every communicable disease program must provide for the eventuality of dealing with cases or outbreaks of communicable diseases, which occur despite preventive measures. Many large cities have met this problem by maintaining communicable disease hospitals wherein adequate isolation and treatment are possible. Smaller jurisdictions usually have not found this to be economically feasible and have provided treatment under the necessary isolation precautions either in a small general hospital or in the home of the patient. The dramatic decline in acute communicable diseases, the availability of antibiotics, and the perfection of isolation techniques have made special isolation hospitals superfluous even in large communities. For reference convenience Table 21-4 from Top and Wehrle[1] is included to provide certain basic control information for the various communicable and infectious diseases.

## ADMINISTRATIVE AIDS IN COMMUNICABLE DISEASE CONTROL

As with all other activities in public health work, certain administrative or management aids are necessary for the control of communicable diseases.

### Legislation

A large part of public health law in the United States is concerned with the control of communicable diseases. The most important basis on which rests the enactment and enforcement of public health law is the police power, which is considered in more detail in Chapter 9. It will suffice here to remind the reader of the folly, even in a democracy, of allowing individuals complete freedom of action. In fact individual freedom, in order truly to exist, must be limited to the right to engage in all activities except those that may be detrimental to the common welfare. An individual infected with a disease transmissible to others must necessarily forfeit some of his personal freedom for the common good. It is the exercise of the police power over these restricted freedoms that endows the health officer with actually greater potential legal power than anyone else in so-

ciety. Only the health authority may summarily enter premises without a search warrant or deprive an individual of his personal freedom without a trial or even a subpoena. The necessity and legality for such action has fortunately been well established in the courts.

To make possible the administrative control of communicable diseases, the states and their communities have found it necessary to enact many types of legislation. The ultimate responsibility for the promulgation and enforcement of communicable disease laws, rules, and regulations rests with the state. All state and territorial health departments have this responsibility. In some states, however, power of enforcement is either not included in the regulatory authority or is limited to situations in which local action is inadequate. With regard to diseases of animals that are transmissible to man, the responsibility is shared with the department of agriculture or special commissions in about one half of the states. Other components of state government that are occasionally involved in communicable disease control include departments of welfare, social security, public assistance, education, and in two instances the state university. Where responsibility is thus divided, it is done in consideration for the particular portions of the general health program for which the respective departments are responsible.[13]

The problem of communicable disease is ever changing because of ecologic factors and the application of newly acquired knowledge. It is important therefore that states revise their communicable disease codes periodically. In analyzing the undesirable features of communicable disease legislation, Emerson[14] pointed to six characteristics in particular:

1. Lack of notification of some diseases for which modern standards of health service appear to demand notification
2. Placarding premises where cases of various communicable diseases are reported, under circumstances that make observance of isolation or quarantine neither likely nor helpful in preventing secondary or subsequent related cases in the home of the index case or elsewhere
3. Failure to verify the diagnosis of certain important diseases by an expert clinician, by laboratory test or by both
4. Requiring isolation periods for infected persons and quarantine periods for exposed susceptibles which are significantly inconsistent with the known periods of communicability and incubation of the particular disease
5. Failing to provide for a consecutive sanitary

**Table 21-5.** Diseases usually considered reportable in the United States*

| | |
|---|---|
| Anthrax | Poliomyelitis |
| Aseptic meningitis | Psittacosis |
| Brucellosis | Rabies, in man or animals |
| Chancroid (soft chancre) | Relapsing fever |
| Cholera | Rickettsial fevers |
| † Conjunctivitis, acute infectious, in newborn infants, not including trachoma | † Ringworm of the scalp or body |
| | † Salmonellosis |
| †Dengue | † Scabies |
| † Diarrhea of the newborn, epidemic | Smallpox (variola) |
| Diphtheria | † Staphylococcal infection |
| Dysentery, bacillary (shigellosis) | Impetigo |
| Encephalitis, arthropod-borne | Pemphigus |
| Food poisoning (bacterial intoxications) | Surgical and nursery outbreaks |
| Staphylomycosis | Streptococcal infection, respiratory |
| Botulism | Scarlet fever |
| Glanders | Streptococcal sore throat, streptococcal |
| Gonorrhea | nasopharyngitis, streptococcal tonsillitis, |
| Hepatitis, serum or acute infectious | septic sore throat |
| † Influenza | Streptococcal infection other than respiratory |
| † Keratoconjunctivitis, infectious | Erysipelas |
| Leprosy | Puerperal infection (puerperal septicemia) |
| Leptospirosis | Syphilis |
| Malaria | Tetanus |
| Measles (rubeola) | Trachoma |
| Meningococcic meningitis (cerebrospinal meningitis) and meningococcemia | Trichinosis |
| | Tuberculosis, pulmonary |
| † Mononucleosis, infectious | Tuberculosis other than pulmonary |
| Paratyphoid fever | Tularemia |
| Pertussis (whopping cough) | Typhoid fever |
| Plague | Typhus fever |
| † Pneumococcal pneumonia | Yellow fever |

* Modified from The control of communicable diseases in man, ed. 11, New York, 1970, American Public Health Association.
† Epidemics only.

**Table 21-6.** Diseases not ordinarily considered reportable in the United States

| | |
|---|---|
| Actinomycosis | Hookworm disease (ancylostomiasis) |
| Amebiasis | Lymphogranuloma venereum (inguinale) and climatic bubo |
| Ascariasis | |
| Blastomycosis | Mumps (infectious parotitis) |
| Chickenpox | Pediculosis |
| Choriomeningitis | Pneumonia, bacterial, other than pneumococcal |
| Coccidioidomycosis (coccidioidal granuloma, valley fever) | Primary atypical pneumonia |
| | Rheumatic fever (acute rheumatic fever, acute rheumatism) |
| Common cold | |
| Filariasis (mumu) | Rubella |
| Granuloma inguinale | Schistosomiasis (bilharziasis) |
| Helminthiasis | Vulvovaginitis in children |
| Histoplasmosis | Yaws (frambesia) |

supervision of carriers from the time of the clinical course of the disease, or the first discovery of a carrier state, until it can be shown that these persons are no longer spreaders of infection

6. Use of fumigants for terminal disinfection in some diseases

## Reporting[15]

The most basic communicable disease legislation relates to reporting to the official health agency of all cases of certain diseases listed in a communicable disease code. This information is necessary to any subsequent steps the health authorities may take to control those diseases. It is the starting point for the application of isolation and quarantine measures and for all routine epidemiologic investigations. Although states vary somewhat in the particular diseases for which they require reports, the accompanying list (Table 21-5) is more or less typical.[16]

In addition to those listed in Table 21-5, there are several other communicable diseases the reporting of which is not frequently required. Obligatory reporting of these diseases (Table 21-6) is not ordinarily considered justified by the benefits that may accrue from whatever steps the health authority may be in a position to take.

At the present time many states also include certain noncommunicable diseases in their lists of reportable conditions. Occupational diseases constitute the bulk of these, although some of the southeastern states particularly include some of the avitaminoses, especially pellagra.

On the local level it is usually required that diseased individuals and carriers or suspected carriers of communicable diseases be reported to the local health officer, who acts as the agent of the state. In cities and countries without local health departments it is generally required that reports be made directly to the state health department. Although "immediate" notification is ordinarily specified, in most cases this is interpreted to mean within 24 hours following diagnosis. Although in most instances it is the private physician who is in the position of having to make a report, several other persons or institutions are usually specified in the laws, rules, and regulations as also having this responsibility. Generally included are physicians; dentists; directors of registered laboratories; veterinarians; parents and guardians; superintendents, principals, and teachers of all schools; nurses engaged in private duty and school, public health, or industrial work; pharmacists;

keepers of hotels, lodging houses, motels, and trailer parks; superintendents of public or private hospitals, nursing homes, clinics, dispensaries, asylums, or jails; owners or managers of dairy farms or any place where dairy products are handled or offered for sale; and licensed embalmers when the death certificate certifies that the primary or contributory cause of death was one of the reportable diseases.

Reporting is effected locally in either one or a combination of two ways. Some jurisdictions require written reports on all reportable diseases; many others, however, make the much more reasonable compromise of accepting telephoned reports on all diseases and requiring written confirmation for only a few of the more serious diseases such as smallpox or typhoid fever. Written reports are usually in the form of printed postal cards that provide space for entry of the patient's name, address, age, color, sex, and disease, and the name and address of the person reporting.

Various techniques have been tried in an attempt to minimize the "bookkeeping" burden of reporting while still making available prompt and accurate information on the occurrence of communicable disease. One interesting method has been to pay a sample of medical practitioners as consultants, emphasizing rapidity of both reporting and feedback to physicians in general. Interestingly, although it reduced the responsibility of most other physicians, the total number of cases of the more common communicable diseases reported actually increased. This system could not, however, relieve physicians in general from their responsibility to report the more serious diseases.[17] The internationally quarantinable diseases must be reported immediately by telephone and/or telegraph.

Since the collection of data on the incidence of communicable diseases is a function of all state health departments, the regulations of every state provide for the transmission of information from the local health authorities or, in their absence, from physicians directly. About two thirds of the states collect weekly reports and only one third require daily reports. Occasionally states pay fees for reports of communicable diseases. In most instances this is in lieu of salary to part-time officials acting in the absence of a full-time health officer.

Despite the fact that failure to report a case of communicable disease usually implies liability to prosecution, it is common knowledge that reporting is far from complete. A health officer would be utterly lacking in wisdom if he were to attempt to obtain reports, particularly from private physicians, only on the strength of his legal prerogatives. A legal point and a demonstration of authority might be gained only at the expense of having made one or several lasting antagonists who henceforth might avoid cooperation with the general public health program.

Persistent tact, educational efforts, and good professional relationships are the keynotes to success. Certain generalizations may be arrived at in this regard. The more serious a disease the more faithfully it is likely to be reported. Thus physicians seldom fail to report cases of smallpox; on the other hand, they might pay little attention to a requirement to report mumps. Furthermore, it is not surprising that many physicians are negligent in reporting diseases if past experience indicates that little official action results. It is recommended therefore that requirements for reporting be limited to diseases that present a real social threat and about which some fruitful, official steps may be taken or assistance might be given to the physician. Sometimes a public health agency requests information concerning minor diseases or those about which at present it can do little. In such instances it is advisable that the true reasons be presented frankly to those from whom the reports are requested rather than simply to notify them that as of a certain date a certain disease must be reported. The one approach invites cooperation based on understanding, whereas the other suggests bureaucratic dictation.

The hesitancy of many physicians to report the names of patients suffering from certain socially stigmatized diseases such as syphilis is understandable. In many areas a practical compromise has been reached. In the long run, of course, public and professional education is the path to follow toward the attainment of a more mature attitude toward these and other diseases. Meanwhile it is possible to arrange for reports to list numbers rather than names, with the provision that an infectious patient who has become negligent in his treatment be subsequently reported to the health authorities by name and address in order that field follow-up may be carried out.

### Isolation and quarantine

For many years legal authority was freely invoked to isolate diagnosed patients and to quarantine individuals who have had contact with any one of the many communicable diseases. Careful studies during the 1930s, however, by several investigators, particularly Chapin[18] in Providence, Holst[19] in Norway, and Gordon and Badger[20] in Detroit, brought out the limitations of these methods. The trend has been toward shortening, individualizing, or in many cases eliminating the periods of restriction, using severity of infection, complications, age, and occupation of the patient as a guide, combined with competent hygienic nursing technique. The decrease in the extent to which these restrictive measures are used has resulted not only in improved public relations but also in considerable financial savings, both to private citizens and to publicly supported hospitals and health departments.

Historically isolation and quarantine have been associated with placarding, a procedure that has also for all practical purposes become obsolete. The case against placarding was so well stated in *The Control of Communicable Diseases in Man*[16] by the American Public Health Association that it is included here as follows:

Placarding—This official procedure under local or State authority consists of posting a warning notice upon the door or entrance to living quarters of persons isolated because of communicable disease. The object of such placarding is primarily to keep unauthorized persons from entering upon the premises during the period of communicability of the isolated patient. Such placarding may incidentally protect the patient against additional or secondary infection which may be carried to him by visitors. Its use may have some educational value.

Placarding, however, does not aid significantly the efforts of a health department to control the acute communicable diseases ordinarily spread directly from person to person in the United States (chicken pox, mumps, pertussis, measles, diphtheria, scarlet fever, anterior poliomyelitis, meningococcus meningitis, pneumonia, tuberculosis, gonorrhea, syphilis) and consequently is not recommended for these diseases.

Placarding has definite disadvantages: it is difficult to enforce, it may be a deterrent to reporting, it is costly in transportation. The most serious objection is the loss of time of public health nurses and other public health department employees that should be devoted to practical instruction in the observance of isolation and concurrent disinfection at the bedside of patients suffering from the more serious of the communicable diseases.

The current policies of the health department of a large city illustrate the trend toward more reasonable control of communicable disease patients and contacts. The requirements are summarized as follows:

*Quarantine of contacts*

Chickenpox–none

* Diphtheria—pending negative nose and throat cultures
* Poliomyelitis—none
* Scarlet fever—none

Measles—none

Pertussis—nonimmune children excluded from school and public gatherings for 14 days after last exposure

Smallpox—16 days after last exposure unless successfully vaccinated

Typhoid and paratyphoid—none; familial contacts should not act as food-handlers

*Isolation of infected individuals*

Until recovery—erysipelas, influenza, leprosy, meningococcus, meningitis, mumps, ophthalmia neonatorum (from other infants only), septic sore throat, typhus fever

For specific periods

Chickenpox—until skin entirely clear

Smallpox—until skin clear of crusts

Diphtheria—until two successive negative nose and throat cultures 24 hours apart, otherwise 14 days

Measles—7 days from rash minimum

Pertussis—3 weeks minimum

Poliomyelitis—7 days minimum from onset

Psittacosis—during acute clinical stage

Scarlet fever—7 days minimum in uncomplicated cases, otherwise until recovery

Typhoid and paratyphoid—until three consecutive negative stool cultures at least 24 hours apart

Excluded from school, public gatherings, or work until recovery—impetigo, epidemic keratoconjunctivitis, scabies, trachoma

Excluded from intimate contact—chancroid, gonorrhea, syphilis, granuloma inguinale, lymphogranuloma venereum

Not required but desirable—common cold, amebic dysentery, bacillary dysentery, pneumococcal pneumonia, primary atypical pneumonia, tuberculosis (preferably in hospital or sanatorium)

Separation from women in early pregnancy—rubella

## Compulsory immunization

An important type of communicable disease legislation until the recent past dealt with im-

---

* Wage earners are permitted to enter and leave premises provided they have no contact with the patient, with children, or with food intended for public consumption.

munization requirements. With the development of protective measures against specific major communicable diseases, it is natural that many persons in positions of authority have attempted to enforce their use by all people. Most notable in this regard has been smallpox, a sufficiently serious disease for which a spectacularly easy, safe, and powerful preventive is available. Many countries have seen fit to require vaccination against smallpox by law. The pattern in the United States varies. In the face of repeated epidemics, by 1915, 15 states and territories* and the District of Columbia had laws that required vaccination as a prerequisite to school attendance. Twenty-one others† had laws or regulations that enabled local jurisdictions to enact compulsory vaccination regulations or to require vaccination under certain conditions, for example, threatened epidemics, exposure to patients, or the existence of a case in a school or in the community. In striking contrast were several states that had certain statutory prohibitions concerning vaccination (Table 21-7).[21] Many of these regulations have been changing.

Without question, where smallpox has occurred to a significant extent, compulsory vaccination brings about results, as illustrated in Fig. 21-3. The map shows that from 1936 to 1945 the incidence of smallpox was significantly lower in the states that had compulsory vaccination laws and higher in the states where compulsion was prohibited. Since that time, the incidence of smallpox has undergone a great reduction throughout the nation. In the process those states that were negligent and those that opposed forthright action undoubtedly rode on the successes of the states and areas that undertook forceful epidemiologic action. As mentioned at the beginning of this chapter, the Public Health service now recommends not only no compulsory smallpox vaccination but the cessation of its routine use.

Compulsory immunization laws have occasionally been used in the past in relation to several other diseases.[22] A few states and a num-

---

* Arkansas, Kentucky, Maryland, Massachusetts, New Hampshire, New Mexico, New York, Pennsylvania, Rhode Island, South Carolina, Virginia, West Virginia, Hawaii, Puerto Rico, and the Virgin Islands.

† Alabama, Arizona, Colorado, Connecticut, Georgia, Iowa, Kansas, Louisiana, Maine, Michigan, Minnesota, Mississippi, Montana, New Jersey, North Carolina, Ohio, Oregon, Tennessee, Wisconsin, Wyoming, and Alaska.

**Table 21-7.** Statutory prohibitions relative to vaccination*

| State | Action prohibited or made unlawful |
|---|---|
| Arizona | Subjection of minor child to compulsory vaccination without parent's or guardian's consent |
| California | Adoption by school or local health authorities of any rule or regulation concerning vaccination |
| Minnesota | Rule of state board of health or of any public board or officer compelling vaccination of child or excluding, except during smallpox epidemics and when approved by local board of education, child from public schools because unvaccinated |
| North Dakota | Requirement of any form of vaccination or inoculation as a condition precedent to admission to any public or private school or college of any person or for exercise of any right performance of any duty or enjoyment of any privilege by any person |
| South Dakota | For any board, physician, or person to compel another by use of physical force, to submit to operation of vaccination with smallpox or other virus |
| Utah | For any board of health, board of education, or any other public board to compel by resolution, order, or proceedings of any kind the vaccination of any person of any age or to make vaccination a condition precedent to attendance to any public or private school, either as pupil or teacher |
| Washington | Requirement of child to submit to vaccination against parent's or guardian's will |

*Modified from Fowler, W.: Principal provisions of smallpox vaccination laws and regulations in the United States, Public Health Rep. **56:**188, Jan. 31, 1941.

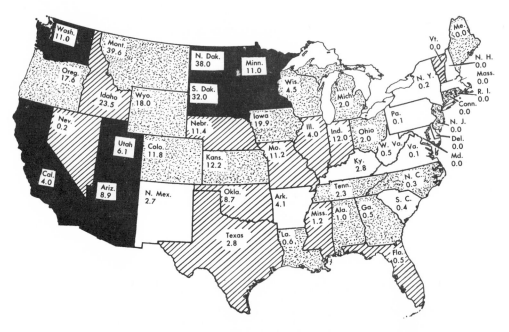

**Fig. 21-3.** Vaccination legislation and average annual smallpox incidence per 100,000 population, by states, 1936-1945. *White,* vaccination required for school; *stippled,* local option in face of threat; *diagonal lines,* no vaccination laws; *solid,* compulsory vaccination prohibited.

ber of local communities have required immunization against diphtheria as a condition for admission to school. The inaptness of this is to be found in the study of the age distribution of diphtheria patients and deaths. Where laws of this nature exist, there is a known tendency on the part of parents to defer obtaining the protection until their children are ready to enter school. This practice overlooks the fact that the greatest threat from the disease is during the preschool period from the first to the sixth birthday.

At one time Arkansas, Mississippi, and New Mexico required immunization against typhoid fever for family contacts and known carriers, all food-handlers, and all susceptibles. Whereas the development of immunity in such persons may have decreased somewhat their chances of developing clinical typhoid fever, it in no way assured their being noninfectious to others. Furthermore, in view of certain questions concerning the efficacy of typhoid vaccination and the current availability of several antibiotics that have considerable effect on typhoid and related organisms, the continuation of compulsory immunization in such circumstances became inappropriate. More appropriately certain countries require vaccination against yellow fever, and many nations insist on valid evidence of vaccination against yellow fever, typhus fever, and plague as a condition of entry from areas affected by these diseases.

Related to the attempts to control communicable diseases in man is the legislative requirement in some jurisdictions that all dogs be actively immunized against rabies. Strangely, this useful and justified measure to protect dogs as well as humans sometimes calls forth greater public indignation and vituperation than do attempts to obtain immunization of children against various preventable diseases.

**Compulsory examination**

Another area in which legislative control of communicable diseases has been attempted involves the compulsory examination of certain people under certain circumstances. At the present time most states have laws that require examination of all applicants for marriage licenses.[23] Unfortunately the premarital examination too often consists merely of the performance of a serologic test for syphilis, despite the decline in that disease concurrent with a considerable increase in gonorrhea and to a lesser extent several other sexually related conditions.

Based on the same general philosophy as premarital examinations, legislation requiring prenatal examinations has been enacted by many states. Again the chief target is syphilis. At the present time all but a few states have enacted such laws. Prenatal health examination laws are confined to blood serologic tests for syphilis, with the responsibility placed on the attendant of the pregnant woman. Exceptions to this are Georgia and North Carolina, where the pregnant woman also has the responsibility to request a test. One of the obvious difficulties is the time factor. Most state laws specify a serologic test during or within 15 days of the first examination. This of course is of limited value if the first visit is shortly before delivery.

The remaining states' laws tend to be even more general.[23]

As a result of dramatic changes in the incidence, treatment, and control of the venereal diseases after the widespread use (and abuse) of antibiotics, the legal requirement of premarital and prenatal examination for these diseases became subject to question. Condit and Brewer,[24] for example, pointed out that between 1949 and 1951 the 511,160 premarital examinations in California discovered only 1,079 cases of syphilis, of which only 162 were in the primary and secondary states, at a cost of $2,741 per new case found. Only 4.3% of all primary and secondary cases were discovered by this means. Hedrick and Silverman[25] compared the experiences of the states that require premarital examinations with those that do not. They found that during the decade from 1945 to 1956 both groups enjoyed a dramatic 97% decline in infant deaths from syphilis and a 93% decline in primary and secondary syphilitic morbidity. They concluded that since premarital blood tests had little influence on syphilitic mortality and morbidity and were in addition extremely expensive to carry out, compulsory laws were no longer justified. However, there has been a resurgence of syphilis in recent years, partly because of changes in sexual mores and partly because of the appearance of more resistant strains of the spirochete. Thus an analysis of reports from 26 states in 1964 and 1965 indicated that about 1 out of every 85 prospective brides or grooms was suspected as having syphilis. Similarly almost 1% of all pregnant women examined was suspected as having the disease.[26] In view of this and the previously mentioned "epidemic" of gonorrhea, the continuance of premarital and prenatal testing appears wise.

A wide variety of laws and regulations exist in the United States that require compulsory examination of various types of workers and groups in society. The most common and significant of these are persons known to have contact with individuals having communicable diseases. It is also common practice to require a medical examination, especially for tuberculosis, as a condition for employment as a schoolteacher. It is not unusual, however, to find that no further periodic examinations are required subsequent to actual employment.

Food-handlers have been singled out as a key group for which preemployment and periodic examinations and laboratory tests are required.

It is unfortunate that more often than not the chief if not exclusive concern for the requirement of food-handler examination is a search for syphilis. Obviously this ignores the fact that it is highly unlikely that a food-handler will transmit the spirochete of syphilis while engaged in activities customarily related to food-handling. To examine these individuals for signs and symptoms of tuberculosis, the typhoid fever carrier state, and a few other pertinent conditions may well be warranted, but the singling out of this occupational group with particular regard to the venereal diseases, however, does not appear to be justified.

Some states have enacted regulations that require the preemployment and periodic examination of workers in certain of the heavy industries, particularly those in which risk of silicosis or radium poisoning is known to exist. A few communities have adopted the policy of routinely examining all persons arrested for certain offenses, particularly prostitution, narcotic and drug charges, or alcoholism because those involved are considered to constitute key epidemiologic groups.

**Compulsory treatment**

The police power is sometimes resorted to in requiring treatment and if necessary enforced hospitalization of recalcitrant individuals infected with certain communicable diseases. Every large health department has found it necessary to resort to this undesirable and unpopular procedure occasionally with regard to cases of smallpox, typhoid fever, the venereal diseases, and tuberculosis.[27] In a sense, to do so represents an admission of failure on the part of the educational and public health agencies of the community. However, a certain few adamantly unreasonable and uncooperative persons always exist and if necessary must be controlled by law.

**Regulation of vehicles of disease transmission**

Of tremendous public health importance are the regulations dealing with the many vehicles of disease transmission. There exists a formidable array of laws, regulations, and codes, unfortunately sometimes contradictory, concerned with the production, treatment, and distribution of milk, milk products, food, water, and drugs. Other factors that might be included deal with plumbing, sewage disposal, stream pollution, air pollution, and the care and transportation of the bodies of persons who have died from communicable diseases. No reasonable person would contest the wisdom of providing legislative regulation of these factors. The criticisms that may be raised against such laws, however, are based on the wide variability of their provisions and their not infrequent contradictions and anachronisms.

Some mention should be made of the wisdom of placing too much reliance on legislative action in the accomplishment of public health goals. It must always be remembered that it is natural for a free people to resent laws and restrictions and occasionally to regard them as challenges that provide an incentive for the popular game of circumvention. It should be realized further that the enactment of law in no sense constitutes an accomplished end. Ill-conceived and poorly administered laws almost inevitably lead to undesirable and costly court actions that often end in dismissal for lack of evidence or the levying of a relatively small fine. Generally speaking, publicity attending such cases is not particularly desirable and often tends to crystallize hitherto unorganized opposition to the general public health program.

Whereas it is always desirable to have a practical, scientifically correct, complete body of public health laws to fall back on whenever necessary, it is equally wise to avoid insofar as possible the exercise of those laws. On the other hand, there is little sense in the enactment of laws and regulations in the absence of intent or inability to enforce them whenever truly necessary. For the greatest ultimate success, reliance should be placed on intelligent cooperation by the public. This means that in the final analysis an effective program of community health education is the most fruitful approach to communicable disease control as it is to other public health problems. To tell an individual that he must not do a certain thing does nothing to make him a better person or citizen; this merely calls forth either dumb, unthinking acquiescence or sullen resentment. To educate him in an intelligent, cooperative manner, with regard to the undesirability of following a certain line of action, offers much more chance of success, which when it occurs, instills the idea not only in the individual but also in those about him and those who follow.

## MATERIAL AIDS IN COMMUNICABLE DISEASE CONTROL

The provision or use of certain material aids has become standard practice in official public health agencies. Of primary importance among these are standardized forms furnished to private physicians on which they must report births, deaths, cases of communicable diseases, certain prophylactic treatments, and other significant information. The keynote for administrative success in designing such forms is simplicity and brevity. To require extensive written reports from busy medical practitioners, particularly if they have to pay the postage, is to invite failure. Such reports should be looked on by public health agencies only as points of departure and should therefore be restricted to a minimum of requested information, for example, identification and location of an individual affected, the condition with which he is affected, and possibly a few other items of basic information, depending on the disease, service, and other circumstances. Prestamped or the more economical prepaid reply cards should be made freely available to all practicing physicians, along with simple instructions concerning their legal responsibilities. This is particularly important when physicians first enter practice in the locality and whenever responsibilities undergo a change.

An important adjunct to communicable disease control is the furnishing of biologic and certain other diagnostic, prophylactic, and therapeutic material and diagnostic laboratory service to physicians on request and preferably free of charge. In addition the laboratory serves a basic function in the sanitary control of foods, milk, and many environmental factors that may influence the public health. This phase of the public health program is specifically considered in a subsequent chapter.

### Consultation service

Consultation service in the diagnosis or control of communicable disease represents another type of material assistance frequently offered by public health agencies. All state health departments at the present time provide this service to local health departments, which in turn include it as a primary part of their service to local practicing physicians for two reasons: (1) the health department is responsible for the control of communicable diseases and (2) the health officer or his assistants usually see more cases of communicable diseases than does the average physician. Therefore they tend to have a more extensive diagnostic background in this field on which to draw.

### Graphic aids

Several material aids and techniques have been found useful for the efficient administra-

tive control of communicable diseases. Generally speaking, they fall into the two categories of graphic aids and registers. Probably the most common graphic aid is the spot map, which indicates the geographic location of each case. One of the simplest and most instructive ways of depicting multiple occurrences of communicable illnesses is to mark them on some form of time scale.[28] Thus graphs showing the incidence of disease by day, week, month, or year are frequently found useful. Various types of time and place charting are discussed and illustrated by MacMahon, Pugh, and Ipsen.[29] With certain diseases, particularly measles, incidence charts that include 5-year or 7-year moving medians for epidemic and nonepidemic years have been found to be particularly useful in estimating disease expectancy (Fig. 21-4). Every health jurisdiction and the statistical data relating to it should be fractionated to some degree to make more evident the predominant trends and problems. For this purpose health departments have relied particularly on census tracts, voting areas, or sanitary districts for which basic population data may be conveniently available. A particularly interesting and useful adaptation of this is found in the so-called epidemiologic master chart, described and illustrated in Chapter 39 on vital statistics. Tools such as these enable the public health worker to maintain a continuous and adequate grasp of the total disease situation and the factors relating to it.

### Registers

The maintenance of case registers has proved to be of incalculable value in the operation of adequate programs for the control of many diseases. Most commonly used in connection with tuberculosis, registers have also been developed by some health departments for venereal diseases, some of the more important acute communicable diseases and their carriers, and occasionally for cancer, rheumatic fever, and other chronic diseases. To be of value the register should readily indicate by some combination of filing and tickler system the location of the patient or carrier, the stage of his condition, and the date of next indicated treatment or follow-up procedure.

### ADMINISTRATIVE PROGRAMMING IN COMMUNICABLE DISEASE CONTROL

The official program for the control of communicable diseases should be based on all the known epidemiologic facts and should be care-

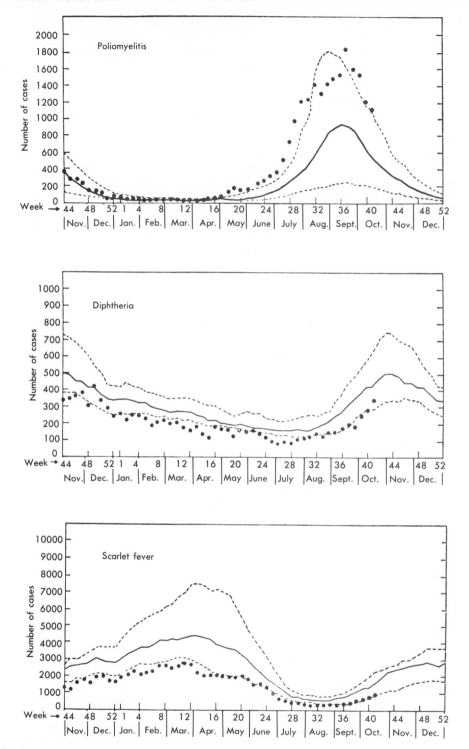

**Fig. 21-4.** Communicable disease charts. All reporting states, November 1947 through October 16, 1948. Upper and lower broken lines represent the highest and lowest figures recorded for the corresponding weeks in the 7 preceding years. Solid line is the median figure for the 7 preceding years. All three lines have been smoothed by a 3-week moving average. Dots represent numbers of cases reported for the weeks of 1948.

fully and logically planned and balanced rather than allowed to pursue a hit-or-miss policy. The total program may be divided into routine control measures and those activities necessitated by emergency or epidemic situations. Much of the program may be routinized to a greater or lesser degree. To do so successfully it is necessary for the public health agency to obtain satisfactory answers to the following series of questions about each disease with which it is concerned:

1. What groups of the population are most likely to have or to acquire the infection?
2. Which of these groups is in the best position to expose others?
3. Where are they most conveniently and efficiently found?
4. What possible groups are most likely to be exposed?
5. When, where, how, and why are they subject to exposure?
6. What practical and economical control procedures and facilities are available?
7. What practical and economical control procedures and facilities are acceptable to the people involved?

For practical purposes the factor of timing is of paramount importance. Communicable diseases may be subdivided into those that vary in incidence by season and those that occur constantly, or endemically, throughout the year. Under usual circumstances a certain relatively constant incidence of new cases of tuberculosis and the venereal diseases may be expected. Programs aimed at combating them must therefore involve a constant hammering at the factors involved in their spread. Contrasted with these

are the so-called acute communicable diseases of childhood that are subject to considerable seasonal and in some instances annual fluctuation. A very simplified picture is presented in Fig. 21-5, which indicates the general seasonal prevalence of several of these diseases as they have occurred in North America in the past. The incidences of most of the diseases generally increased during the spring months of the year. Pertussis tended to lag a month or two behind the main group, whereas poliomyelitis was usually most prevalent in the fall and diphtheria occurred mostly in the winter months.

Although it is desirable that children receive immunizing protection against various diseases routinely as they reach certain ages, it is obvious that any special immunization program that may be considered necessary should precede the period of expected high incidence. Accordingly it would be more practical for health departments in the Northern Hemisphere to engage in a special pertussis immunization program during February and March rather than to wait until August or September when the seasonal threat of that disease has passed. Similarly, antimeasles immunization is most practically provided during the late winter rather than in the summer or fall. In places where the disease might occur, the promotion of a postgraduate institute in the management of poliomyelitis patients would probably be of greatest value in the late summer months rather than at any other time of the year.

Control programs should be similarly keyed with regard to age, since particular diseases tend to affect certain age groups more than others (Fig. 21-6). A pertussis immunization program for entering school children would be

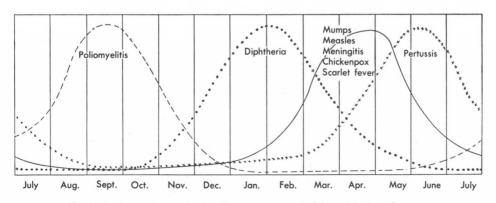

**Fig. 21-5.** Seasonal prevalence of acute communicable respiratory diseases.

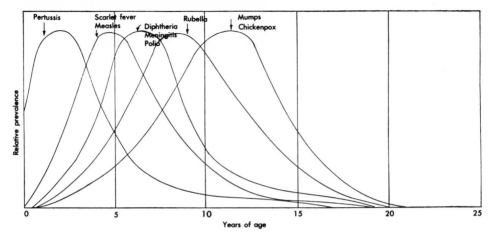

**Fig. 21-6.** Relative prevalence by age of acute communicable respiratory diseases.

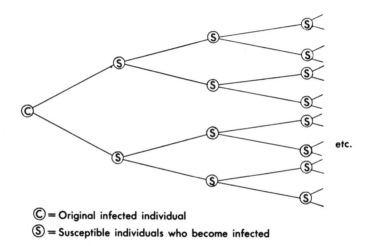

ⓒ = Original infected individual
Ⓢ = Susceptible individuals who become infected

**Fig. 21-7.** Geometrically progressive transfer of infection in absence of immunization.

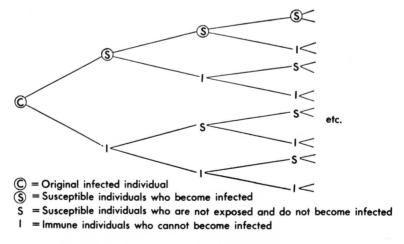

ⓒ  = Original infected individual
Ⓢ  = Susceptible individuals who become infected
S  = Susceptible individuals who are not exposed and do not become infected
I  = Immune individuals who cannot become infected

**Fig. 21-8.** Linear transfer of infection with 50% immunization.

of little avail, since the period of greatest risk is during the first 2 years of life. Emphasis therefore should be placed on the immunization against this disease during infancy. For similar reasons the diphtheria preventing program should stress immunization between the ninth and fifteenth months of life. The importance of this was clearly established many years ago by Godfrey,[30] who demonstrated that immunization of as high as 65% of entering schoolchildren against diphtheria was relatively ineffective in the community control of the disease, whereas immunization of as few as 35% of early preschool children would effectively prevent the disease from ever reaching epidemic proportions.

In this connection it is of interest to point out the statistical explanation for the lack of necessity, from a community's standpoint, of protecting every member of the community or even every susceptible member of the community. For the purpose of explanation it might be assumed that a given individual has an average epidemiologically effective rate of contact of two during the period he is infectious. That is, the average infectious person, while he is still able to circulate, may have contacts of an intimate enough nature to fulfill the biologic conditions necessary for the transmission of his infection to two susceptible persons. This of course varies with disease, location, culture, and many other factors. In a totally unprotected community therefore the original patient would give rise to two new patients, who in turn would produce a total of four, each of whom would infect two others to produce a total of eight persons. The picture therefore is one of geometric progression: 1-2-4-8-16-32-64-128, etc. (Fig. 21-7). If, on the other hand, merely one half of the susceptible individuals in the community are protected against the particular disease, the average rate of effective contact of patients with susceptible persons is reduced 50%. Each case therefore, on the basis of probability, will now give rise to only one new case, and everything but the main trunk of the tree of infection will have been pruned. The picture of transmission now becomes 1-1-1-1-1 (Fig. 21-8). Although by chance an occasional case may give rise to two or more new cases, the chances are equally great that at some point the existing case will not have effective contact, and the chain of infection may die out completely.

The modern approach to tuberculosis provides an excellent illustration of administrative programming in the routine control and eradication of a communicable disease. Some years ago the notable epidemiologist Frost[31] stated the epidemiologic prognosis for this disease as follows:

We need not assume that tuberculosis is permanently and ineradicably engrafted upon our civilization. On the contrary, the evidence indicates that in this country the balance is already against the survival of the tubercle bacillus; and we may reasonably expect that the disease will eventually be eradicated. It is necessary only that the rate of transmission be held permanently below the level at which a given number of infection spreading cases succeed in establishing an equivalent number to carry on the succession. If, in successive periods of time, the number of infectious hosts is continuously reduced, the end result of this diminishing ratio, if continued long enough, must be extermination of the tubercle bacillus.

However, there are many signs of impatience. A realization has come about that although the biologic tide has turned in our favor, it is needlessly expensive and wasteful to be satisfied with the present rate of decline in the tuberculosis incidence and death rate. The question arises of how to accomplish the reduction and hopefully eventual eradication most effectively and efficiently. Early case finding is obviously the key. By finding those who are already infected as early as possible, not only is it less expensive to restore them to health, but the length of time during which they may infect others is significantly shortened. With the development of new and relatively inexpensive diagnostic tools such as the photofluorograph, the examination of large groups of people has become a practical technique. In addition there are now available drugs for more effective treatment and prophylaxis. It must be remembered that tuberculosis still requires a major part of state and local health expenditures. The economic savings alone, were the process of eradication adequately pursued, obviously would be enormous.

Tuberculosis is known to be a socially selective disease. The health department must therefore familiarize itself with the extent and location of tuberculosis in its community. This involves a careful and fractionated analysis of all statistical and other sources of information, for example, reports of cases, deaths, hospital admissions, etc. To know that a community's tuberculosis death rate is 5 per 100,000 is not sufficient. Careful consideration must be given to the size and location of population groups

**Table 21-8.** Summary of gastrointestinal diseases

| | Typhoid fever | Paratyphoid fever | Bacillary dysentery | Amebic dysentery | Cholera | Brucellosis | Hookworm |
|---|---|---|---|---|---|---|---|
| Cause | Salmonella typhosa | Salmonella (several species) | Shigella (several species) | Entamoeba histolytica | Vibrio comma | Brucella (several species) | Necator americanus |
| Incubation period | 3-38 days, usually 7-14 days | 3-15 days, usually 4-10 days | 2-7 days | 2 days-several months, usually 3-4 weeks | 1-5 days | 6-30 days | None in true sense |
| Prevalence | Worldwide, warm seasons especially; affects mostly males and young adults | | Tropics and subtropics, especially warm season; affects all ages and sexes | | India and China | Mediterranean, U.S., Canada, Scandinavia; warm season | Limited to warm, moist, sandy soil; affects white children especially |
| Period of communicability | Prodromes, illness, and convalescence until stools negative | | | | | 20-300 days | While infected |
| Source | Feces and urine of cases and carriers | | | | Exception: Brucellosis; milk, tissues, blood, and discharges of infected cows, swine, goats | | |
| Spread | Infected water, food, fomites, flies, direct contacts | | | | Exception: Brucellosis; milk and contact with tissues and discharges | | |
| | | | | | Hookworm; contaminated soil (neither man to man) | | |
| Susceptibility | General susceptibility, decreasing with age | | | | Exception: Brucellosis; most persons have some natural immunity | | |
| Immunity | | | | | | | |
| Passive | None | | | | | | |
| Active | One attack gives long-lasting immunity to typhoid; relative immunity in paratyphoid and bacillary dysentery; short immunity with vaccines in typhoid and paratyphoid (about 2 years) and cholera (about 1 year) | | | | | | |
| Control measures | 1. Early diagnosis and reporting of cases and carriers; | | | | 4. Quarantine—cholera only (5 days) | 10. Milk sanitation | |
| | 2. Isolation in all but hookworm, amebic dysentery, and brucellosis | | | | 5. Immunization (q.v.) | 11. Shellfish sanitation | |
| | 3. Disinfection—concurrent—terminal in all but hookworm and brucellosis | | | | 6. Source finding—cases and carriers, important in all | 12. Prevention of fly breeding | |
| | | | | | 7. Water sanitation | 13. Carrier control | |
| | | | | | 8. Excreta sanitation | 14. Education of patients and carriers | |
| | | | | | 9. Food sanitation | | |

**Table 21-9.** Summary of acute respiratory diseases

| | Diphtheria | Scarlet fever | Pertussis | Measles | Smallpox | Chickenpox | Mumps | Meningitis | Poliomyelitis |
|---|---|---|---|---|---|---|---|---|---|
| Cause | Corynebacterium diphtheriae | Hemolytic streptococci | Haemophilus pertussis | Filtrable virus | Filtrable virus | Filtrable virus | Filtrable virus | Neisseria meningitidis | Filtrable virus |
| Incubation period | 2-7 days | 2-7 days | 7-16 days | 8-12 days | 8-16 days | 14-21 days | 14-21 days | 2-10 days | 7-14 days |
| Period of communicability | Variable; usually under 2 weeks, seldom over 4 weeks | Variable; usually 3 weeks from onset until no discharges | Catarrhal stage (7-14 days) and 3 weeks of whoop | Catarrhal stage (4 days) and 5 days of rash | Catarrhal stage (2-4 days) to disappearance of lesions | Catarrhal stage (0-2 days) and during 6-10 days of lesions | Unknown; assumed while glands enlarged | From onset until 2 weeks after recovery | Unknown; assumed incubation period and first week of disease |

Prevalence: Worldwide, but especially temperate zone—winter and spring except pertussis (spring), poliomyelitis (late summer), and diphtheria (fall and winter); affects children most; incidence usually less and older age group affected more in rural than urban communities

Source: Discharges from nose and throat of cases—occasionally other lesions in diphtheria, scarlet fever, and smallpox; carriers in diphtheria, scarlet fever, meningitis, and poliomyelitis

Spread: I° cases, II° fomites; occasionally milk in diphtheria and scarlet fever (explosive epidemics); carriers in diphtheria, scarlet fever, meningitis, and poliomyelitis

Susceptibility: Everyone after 6 months of age not having active or acquired immunity. Exceptions: scarlet fever varies geographically; smallpox and pertussis susceptible from birth; some immunity probably acquired without disease by age and contact in all but smallpox and measles

Immunity
Passive: Convalescent serum and gamma globulin give some protection for several weeks in all but smallpox; whole adult blood in pertussis, measles, mumps; placental extract in measles; artificial immunity in smallpox, diphtheria, pertussis, poliomyelitis, rubella, rubeola, and mumps

Active: An attack gives long-lasting immunity; artificial immunity in smallpox, diphtheria, pertussis, poliomyelitis, rubella, rubeola, and mumps

Control measures:
1. Early diagnosis and reporting (laboratory in Diph., Pert., Mening., Polio)
2. Isolation: Diph., SF, Pert., SP; of little value in the rest
3. Disinfection
   Concurrent
   Terminal
4. Quarantine like isolation
5. Immunization, q.v.
6. Source finding—Diph. and SF (cases, carriers, milk); SP (cases); of little value in the rest
7. Pasteurization of milk, especially in diphtheria and pertussis
8. Prevention of overcrowding, especially in meningitis
9. Education

in which the disease is likely to exist to an undue degree because of genetic, biologic, economic, or occupational influences. These are the groups among whom mass case-finding techniques should be particularly stressed. Among the more important are (1) persons with suspicious pulmonary symptoms, (2) contacts to known cases of tuberculosis, (3) members of certain racial and nationality groups (e.g., blacks, Esquimoux, Amerinds, Scotch, Irish, Poles), (4) workers exposed to silica dust, (5) general clinic and hospital patients, (6) adolescents and young adults, (7) pregnant women, and (8) attendants of tuberculous patients. Several other groups should receive special attention by virtue of their occupational opportunity to infect others. Outstanding among these are schoolteachers and food-handlers.

Many of the groups mentioned are most conveniently and effectively reached for diagnostic purposes through certain channels. Thus it is more efficient and fruitful to arrange for the mass examination of industrial workers at their place of work, schoolteachers and adolescents at their schools, and pregnant women and clinic and hospital patients at the time of their admission to service. Suspected cases and contacts of known cases require routine persistent field contacts by public health nurses.

Although it is true that each of the communicable diseases is a biologic entity, certain similarities make it practical to group them into several categories for administrative and control purposes. Since control measures depend essentially on modes of spread, this factor is also the most convenient for grouping diseases. Thus, although strictly speaking hookworm infection is not a gastrointestinal disease, the nature of the factors involved in its transmission justifies including it for administrative control purposes in that group of diseases.

The point of practical significance, of course, is that by grouping diseases in this manner many control measures may be applied to group rather than to a single disease. This is illustrated by Tables 21-8 and 21-9, which summarize in a general manner the essential epidemiologic facts concerning acute respiratory diseases and gastrointestinal diseases. Similar groupings may be made for insect-borne diseases, chronic respiratory diseases, and genitoinfectious or venereal diseases. This concept has been reflected organizationally in the frequent establishment in health departments of states and large cities of categorical divisions or bureaus for venereal disease control, tuberculosis control, and sometimes others. Present trends, however, are toward consolidation of all units into one major administrative division of communicable disease control or epidemiology, perhaps with bureaus for various subcategories, depending on the relative magnitudes of problems. This trend is further manifest by the increasing number of organizations with a division of medical services, a bureau of which relates to disease control in general. This in turn may be further subdivided.

In addition to the more prosaic activities of the routine program of communicable disease control, public health organizations must be ever alert to the potentiality of circumstances that may be considered of an emergency or epidemic nature. The health department should be so organized that "without slipping a gear" it can marshal its resources and those of related agencies. An example of how this may be done is shown in the "responsibility schedule" on p. 417. This represents one page of a complete responsibility breakdown of all the components of the program of a large urban health department. It has been found useful to list points in the agency's effort in this form and to indicate exactly what part of the health agency is responsible for which activities, under what circumstances, and at what time.

Much has been said and written about the definition of the word *epidemic*. This is like arguing over the number of angels on the head of a pin. From a practical standpoint one might consider epidemic to refer to any disease (or indeed injury) situation that calls for unusual or strenuous epidemiologic control measures. The staff of a modern health department should become as concerned over a report of a single case of smallpox or an increase in drug abuse as it does with an outbreak of poliomyelitis or typhoid fever involving a score of persons. All such situations are unusual, present a serious threat to the community, and call for immediate action. Accordingly a strong case could be made for avoiding the use of the word *epidemic* and substituting the term *public health emergency*.

On being confronted with evidence that indicates a possible emergency the public health official or epidemiologist must take a series of logical steps. Most obvious, although sometimes overlooked, he must first ascertain the true existence of an emergency. This involves careful consultation with those making the reports, followed by confirmatory diagnosis in which the

## RESPONSIBILITIES IN ACUTE COMMUNICABLE DISEASE CONTROL
### Division with primary responsibility: Epidemiology

**SCOPE AND PURPOSE**

To control the incidence and transmission of acute communicable diseases.

**COMPONENT PHASES**

1. Acute infectious diseases
2. Parasitic infections
3. Food-borne outbreaks
4. Epidemic outbreaks of communicable diseases
5. Tropical and exotic infectious diseases

### Typical activities

**PRIMARY DIVISION**

1. Furnishing consultation services to physicians requesting diagnostic help
2. Epidemiologic investigation and surveillance of diseases—medical
3. Food-borne disease investigation and control
4. Direction and control of follow-up procedures for the control of carriers
5. Validation of foreign travel immunization certificates
6. Professional direction of clinic for diagnosis and treatment of parasitic diseases
7. Detection and surveillance—with epidemiologic services in occurrences of unusual, tropical and exotic diseases
8. Direction of epidemiologic investigation and control of epidemic outbreaks of communicable diseases
9. Analysis of statistical reports
10. Research into cause and control of communicable disease

**PARTICIPATING DIVISION**

**Public health nursing**

1. Nursing services in clinics
2. Public health nursing services in the home for
   a. Nursing care when ordered
   b. Instruction and counseling for family health
   c. Referral to appropriate community agencies when indicated
   d. Epidemiologic investigation and follow-up in selected cases
   e. Consultation to other health and welfare agencies
   f. Interpretation of health department policies to families and social agencies

**Laboratory**

1. Providing laboratory tests to aid diagnosis and/or treatment including, but not limited to, the following:
   a. Enteric diseases
   b. Diseases of nose and throat
   c. Food poisoning outbreaks
   d. Hospital staphylococcal diseases

**Environmental health**

1. Food-borne disease investigation

**Health education**

1. Preparation and distribution of educational audiovisual materials
2. Preparation of educational-professional news releases
3. Promoting speaking engagements

health official or epidemiologist himself takes an active part. Diseases are poorly diagnosed or understood from behind a health department desk. The determination of the etiology of the disease is of obvious importance in deciding on subsequent steps to take. Diagnostic assurance makes it possible to avoid some missteps and wasted effort and to decide what laboratory or other aids will be of assistance.

Once the nature of the condition is determined, the next step is to establish the fact of undue prevalence and incidence. False diagnoses because of either hysteria or faulty clinical judgment must be eliminated. By like token missed cases must be found. These may be attributable again to faulty diagnosis or to unrecognized or undiagnosed cases. Occasionally cases are missed, not because of lack of diagnosis but because they are deliberately concealed for misguided personal, social, or economic reasons. More than one vacation resort area, for example, has attempted to quash knowledge of the presence of disease. The occurrence of typhoid fever in several places in the past has been ignored because of false pride in some new sanitary installation. These possibilities for missed cases therefore make it necessary for the investigator to decide whether there is undue prevalence of recent origin or whether cases have been occurring for a considerable period of time and are just now being recognized. It is a common experience, for example, for the first one or two definitely diagnosed cases of poliomyelitis in a community to make the public and the private physicians particularly alert to the possibility of that disease in former as well as new patients.

Once the disease is diagnosed and a distinct departure from normal prevalence has been noted, the next step in many situations is to contact all persons involved, the public in general, and practicing physicians in particular to apprise them of the situation in a nonemotional manner and to solicit their assistance in whatever matter is indicated. This may take the form of public education to boil water or to avoid crowds, or of professional education in special diagnostic methods and techniques or in reporting.

Known patients should now be studied in relation to certain pertinent factors, including time, place, events, groups of the population affected, sex, race, age, and occupation. Each of the patients or at least a representative sample of them, depending on the disease and the size of the outbreak, should be visited. A standardized epidemiologic case card should be filled out for each patient. This has a twofold purpose: (1) to find the source and (2) to find contacts who may become future patients or in whom the development of the disease may be prevented. Out of a careful analysis of the epidemiologic case cards it is hoped that some common denominator may be discovered—a particular milk supply, social event, form of personal behavior, and so on. If such a factor can be brought to light, it can then be made the subject of intense laboratory or other study to confirm the suspicion of its causal nature, and appropriate steps can be taken to prevent a recurrence of the emergency.

Anyone who has been engaged in such activities will agree that the foregoing paragraphs read much too easily. The investigation of a communicable disease emergency is no mean task. It involves intelligence, intuition, patience, and persistence. It is seldom a venture one can undertake alone. Reliable medical cooperation, laboratory assistance, and many other things are necessary for its successful completion. When truly complete, however, an epidemiologic investigation is a work of art.

**REFERENCES**

1. Top, F. H., and Wehrle, P. H., editors: Communicable and infectious diseases, ed. 7, St. Louis, 1972, The C.V. Mosby Co.
2. Baer, J. G., et al.: Pathogenic organisms and infectious diseases, Basle, 1971, Ciba-Geigy.
3. Stolnitz, G. J.: A century of international mortality trends, Pop. Studies **9:**24, July 1955.
4. Hinman, E. H.: Current status of eradication of infectious diseases, Trans. Stud. Coll. Physicians Phila. **30:**133, Jan. 1963.
5. Gregg, M. B.: Communicable disease trends in the United States, Amer. J. Nurs. **68:**88, Jan. 1968.
6. Communicable diseases in 1971, WHO Chron. **26:**6, June 1972.
7. World Health Organization: Second report of Expert Committee on Smallpox Eradication, WHO Techn. Rep. Ser. no. 493, Geneva, 1972.
8. U. S. Public Health Service: Routine smallpox vaccination unneeded, Hosp. Tribune, **5:**11, Nov. 15, 1971.
9. Jekel, J. F.: Communicable disease control and public policy in the 1970's—hot war, cold war, or peaceful coexistence, Amer. J. Public Health **62:** 1578, Dec. 1972.
10. Polio, diphtheria, measles: immunization lag is feared, Hosp. Tribune, **5:**4, April 19, 1971.
11. Le Riche, W. H.: World incidence and prevalence of the major communicable diseases. In Wolstenholme, G., and O'Connor, M., editors: Health of mankind, London, 1967, J. & A. Churchill, Ltd.
12. Flennes, R.: Man, nature and disease, New York, 1965, Signet Books, New American Library.
13. 1972 Inventory, health programs in the states and territories, Washington, D. C., 1973, Association of State and Territorial Health Officers.
14. Emerson, H.: Uniformity to control of communicable diseases, Amer. J. Public Health **32:**133, Feb. 1942.
15. Manual of procedures for national morbidity reporting and surveillance of communicable diseases, Atlanta, 1968, National Communicable Disease Center.
16. The control of communicable diseases in man, ed. 11, Washington, D. C., 1970, American Public Health Association.
17. Schaffner, W., et al.: Innovative communicable disease reporting, HSMHA Health Rep. **86:**431, May 1971.
18. Chapin, C. V.: Papers of Charles V. Chapin, M.D., New York, 1934, Commonwealth Fund.
19. Holst, P. M.: Concerning isolation in contagious disease, T. Norsk. Laegeforen. Nov. 9, 1933.

20. Gordon, J. E., and Badger, G. F.: The isolation time of scarlet fever, Amer. J. Public Health **24:** 438, May 1934.

21. Fowler, W.: Principle provisions of smallpox vaccination laws and regulations in the United States, Public Health Rep. **56:**188, Jan. 31, 1941.

22. Jackson, C. L.: State laws on compulsory immunization in the United States, Public Health Rep. **84:**787, Sept. 1969.

23. Today's VD control program, New York, 1966, American Social Hygiene Association.

24. Condit, P. K., and Brewer, A. F.: Premarital examination laws—are they worthwhile? Amer. J. Public Health **43:**880, July 1952.

25. Hedrick, A. W., and Silverman, C.: Should the premarital blood test be compulsory? Amer. J. Public Health **48:**125, Feb. 1958.

26. Resurgence of venereal disease, Bull. N. Y. Acad. Med. **40:**802, July 1964; **41:**820, July 1965.

27. Kupka, E., and King, M.: Enforced legal isolation of tuberculosis patients, Public Health Rep. **69:** 351, April 1954.

28. Paul, J. R.: Clinical epidemiology, Chicago, 1966, University of Chicago Press.

29. MacMahon, B., Pugh, T. F., and Ipsen, J.: Epidemiological methods, Boston, 1960, Little, Brown & Co.

30. Godfrey, E. S.: A study in the epidemiology of diphtheria in relation to the active immunization of certain age groups, Amer. J. Public Health **22:** 237, Feb. 1932.

31. Frost, W. H.: How much control of tuberculosis? Amer. J. Public Health **27:**759, Aug. 1937.

*Is it with us as clearly shown*
*By slant and twist, which way*
*The wind hath blown?*

ADELAIDE CRAPSEY
*On seeing weather-beaten trees*

CHAPTER 22

# Metabolic and degenerative diseases[*]

## EMERGENCE OF THE PROBLEM

The form and substance of the practice of both medicine and public health have been undergoing considerable change during recent years. Not the least of the reasons for this is the spectacular shift that has occurred in the relative age distribution of the population. This shift may be attributed to three factors: (1) the decrease in immigration, (2) a decrease in the birthrate, and (3) an increase in the life expectancy and an accompanying rise in the average age at death. Of the three, the last has been of greatest significance and has been largely the result of prior activities in preventive medicine and public health. Up to the present time these activities have been designed of convenience or necessity to benefit primarily infants and children, with relatively little attention paid to those in the older age groups. That this has been true is not so surprising. In one sense it has been a case of first things first. In another sense it is characteristic of a growing nation that major attention be focused on the younger age groups so necessary for the development of that kind of nation.

However, the population has matured as far as its age distribution is concerned in the United States. The extent to which this is true is shown in Fig. 22-1, which indicates the shift that has

---

[*]For an excellent and convenient guide, see *Control of Chronic Diseases in Man.*[1]

taken place in the age distribution of the population since the middle of the last century and the distribution anticipated by the end of the twentieth century. It will be noted that in 1860 only 13% of the population was 45 years of age or over, in contrast with an expected proportion of 40% by the year 2000. Similarly in 1860, 51% of the population was under 20 years of age, in contrast with an anticipated 25% by the end of the twentieth century. Considering a shorter and more recent interval, in 1900 only 2.5 million persons or 4.1% of the population of the United States were in the age group over 65 years. Currently about 10% of the population is over 65 years, and one third of them are 75 years or older. If present growth and rates of natality and mortality continue, in 50 years the population of the United States will be 300 million, with 48 million persons over 65 years and about 16 million over 75 years of age.

"In a society which is now having great difficulty in providing adequate income, housing, social services and health care for its 20 million older persons, the next few decades should provide a considerable test of our social ingenuity and our commitment to social justice."[2] Changes in the need and demand for certain types of public health and medical care have resulted. With the increased control of acute communicable diseases the number of beds needed for patients being treated for these diseases has necessarily decreased. At the same time the need and demand for facilities for the care of chronic dis-

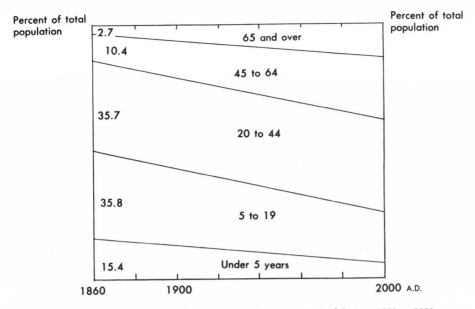

**Fig. 22-1.** Change in age distribution of the population in United States, 1860 to 2000 A.D.

eases and the aged have increased. By like token private physicians and public health workers must expect to devote more and more attention to problems of a geriatric and gerontologic nature.

This points to one of the most distressing aspects of the growing problem. Elwood[3] has pointed out that the elderly resemble minority groups when viewed not only in terms of socio-economic criteria but also inclination to care for them by those on whom they must depend. He cites several studies to illustrate this. Surveys of medical students place care of the chronically ill and the elderly at the bottom of the list of interests. An important reason for this is the nature of their training. Greatest attention is focused on medical and surgical treatment, preferably dramatic, of acute conditions. To the contrary, a review of the 99 medical schools existing in 1970 showed that 51 of them made no mention of the subject of aging, geriatrics, or gerontology in the school history, curricula deliberations, course outlines, staff structure, research, or otherwise. It is no wonder that so few medical graduates enter this field or even devote reasonable attention to it in their practices. Neither are schools of public health free of censure. Again, curricula analyses and faculty staffing are disappointing. One indication of disinterest is provided by the number of doctoral dissertations on aging, which numbered 667, or 0.25% of the total in all scholarly fields. In the

biologic, medical, psychologic, and social science fields the proportion was only 0.5%. The health sciences were credited with a mere 29 dissertations on problems of aging in 35 years! As for the discipline of psychology, Elwood observed that "It is likely that more dissertations on child development are produced in a single year than have been produced on aging for that entire period."

Another indication of the history of disinterest in and neglect of this important and growing problem is the recency of social and professional efforts. This is illustrated by the following chronology of events in gerontology in the United States.[2]

| | |
|---|---|
| Club for Research on Aging | 1940 |
| Gerontological Society formed | |
| *Journal of Gerontology* started | 1945 |
| Social Science Research Council Report: | |
|   *Research on Social Adjustment in Old Age* | |
| First International Gerontological | 1948 |
|   Congress—Belgium | |
| Private foundation support of research in | 1950 |
|   gerontology: Carnegie, Rockefeller | |
| Second International Gerontological | 1951 |
|   Congress—St. Louis | |
| Beginning of major government support of | |
|   research in gerontology | |
|   NIH: Intramural and Extramural | 1955 |
| *Gerontologist* started—reports on | 1960 |
|   applied social gerontology | |
| Handbooks on research in social gerontology: | |
|   Birren, Tibbitts, Burgess | |

Fifth International Gerontological Congress—
San Francisco

First White House Conference on Aging 1961
U. S. Senate Special Committee on Aging
established

Ford Foundation support of research on aging
Medicare

Older Americans Act of 1965. Established 1965
Administration on Aging

NICHD Grants to universities for research and
training in area of adult development and
aging

Russell Sage Report on *Aging and Society* 1968

Administration on Aging grants for research 1968
and development in applied gerontology

Eighth International Gerontological 1969
Congress—Washington

President's Task Force on Aging 1970

Second White House Conference on Aging 1971

Ninth International Gerontological 1972
Congress—Kiev

National Institute on Aging established 1974

Although chronic and metabolic diseases are not restricted to older age groups, it is that period of life in which they most commonly occur or become evident and cause disability and ultimate death. As a result of the population changes that have occurred, many more persons are now surviving to ages that are characterized by a high incidence of cardiovascular and renal diseases, cancer, diabetes mellitus, arthritis, rheumatism, gout, and the mental and physiologic changes associated with the climacteric. That this has occurred is emphasized by a comparison of the leading causes of death in the United States in 1900 and in 1970 (Table 22-1).

The overall picture may be summarized by stating that whereas at the beginning of the century 61% of deaths were caused by infectious and parasitic diseases and only 28% by chronic and metabolic diseases, the situation is now reversed, with over 80% of deaths caused by chronic and metabolic diseases and only 1% by infectious or parasitic diseases.

**EXTENT OF THE PROBLEM**

It is difficult to determine accurately how many persons are affected at a particular time by the various chronic noncommunicable diseases. The insidious nature of most of these conditions results in delayed diagnosis, which not infrequently is made first at the time of death.

However, interviews by the National Health Survey of a representative sample of families throughout the United States during the year ending June 30, 1966, indicated that approximately 49% of the population have one or more chronic conditions. Of these, almost one quarter were limited in the amount or type of their activity, and over 2% were unable to carry on their customary major activity. Thus it may be stated that more than 11% of the noninstitutionalized population has some degree of long-term limitation of activity because of chronic illness or impairment. The amount varies from 1.9% among individuals under 17 years of age to 45.1% among those 65 years and older (Table 22-2).[4]

Beyond this, as might be expected, the fre-

**Table 22-1.** Twelve leading causes of death, United States, 1900 and 1970

| 1900 | | 1970 | |
|---|---|---|---|
| *Cause* | *Death rate per 100,000 population* | *Cause* | *Death rate per 100,000 population* |
| Influenza and pneumonia | 202.2 | Diseases of heart | 360.3 |
| Tuberculosis | 194.4 | Malignant neoplasms | 162.0 |
| Diarrhea and enteritis | 139.9 | Cerebral hemorrhage | 101.7 |
| Diseases of heart | 137.4 | Accidents | 54.2 |
| Cerebral hemorrhage | 106.9 | Influenza and pneumonia | 30.5 |
| Nephritis | 88.7 | Diseases of early infancy | 20.9 |
| Accidents | 72.3 | Diabetes mellitus | 18.5 |
| Cancer | 64.0 | Arteriosclerosis | 15.9 |
| Diseases of early infancy | 62.6 | Cirrhosis of liver | 15.8 |
| Diphtheria | 40.3 | Bronchitis, emphysema, asthma | 14.9 |
| Simple meningitis | 33.8 | Suicide | 11.1 |
| Typhoid and paratyphoid | 31.3 | Congenital malformations | 8.1 |
| All causes | 1719.1 | All causes | 940.4 |

quency with which more than one chronic disabling condition exists increases with age. This is shown in Table 22-3.[5] Among individuals 15 years of age or younger only 3.3% had more than one chronic condition. By contrast, 51% of persons 65 years of age or over had more than one chronic condition.

Only about 30% of those in the higher age group suffer 1 or more days per year from respiratory conditions. This is actually less than the incidence in the population as a whole. Eighty-five percent, however, have a chronic or metabolic disease; about 20% are ill from a digestive condition; 32% suffer from arthritis or rheumatism; 3% suffer from a chronic skin condition; 2% suffer from a nervous disease; and more than 8% are incapacitated for a day or more because of accidental injuries. In addition, there is a considerable frequency of foot ailments and visual defects that limit ambula-

tion and promote accidents, many hearing defects, and many dental problems that affect mastication and therefore diet and nutrition.

The prevalence of specific chronic diseases or impairments in the older component of the population is shown in Table 22-4.[6] It is well to note that impairment of locomotion and limitation of relationship with the surrounding world (visual and hearing defects) are major handicaps which tend to be underrated by many, including health workers. Casual inquiry indicates that limitation of locomotion and of communication rank high among older people as most annoying and worrisome handicaps. This appears to hold true even when individuals are aware that they also have some more serious chronic condition. Apparently many people learn to live with the knowledge of the latter, whereas the less serious handicaps of locomotion and communication are constant limitations

**Table 22-2.** Limitation of activity due to chronic conditions, percent of population by age, United States, July 1965 to June 1966*

| Age in years | All persons | Persons with no chronic conditions | Persons with 1 + chronic conditions | | | | |
|---|---|---|---|---|---|---|---|
| | | | Total | With no limitation of activity | With limitation, but not in major activity | With limitation in amount or kind of major activity | Unable to carry on major activity |
| All ages | 100.0 | 50.9 | 49.1 | 37.9 | 2.8 | 6.3 | 2.1 |
| Under 17 | 100.0 | 77.6 | 22.4 | 20.5 | 1.0 | 0.7 | 0.2 |
| 17-44 | 100.0 | 46.1 | 53.9 | 46.6 | 2.6 | 4.1 | 0.6 |
| 45-64 | 100.0 | 29.4 | 70.6 | 51.7 | 5.0 | 11.1 | 2.8 |
| 65+ | 100.0 | 14.8 | 85.2 | 40.1 | 6.2 | 25.4 | 13.5 |

*From U. S. Public Health Service: Limitation of activity and mobility due to chronic conditions, PHS pub. no. 1000, ser. 10, no. 45, Rockville, Md., 1968.

**Table 22-3.** Number of chronic conditions, percent of population by age, United States, July 1957 to June 1958*

| Age in years | Number of chronic conditions (%) | | | | |
|---|---|---|---|---|---|
| | Total | None | One | Two | Three or more |
| All ages | 100.0 | 58.6 | 23.0 | 10.0 | 8.4 |
| Under 15 | 100.0 | 82.5 | 14.2 | 2.6 | 0.7 |
| 15-44 | 100.0 | 57.7 | 26.0 | 10.2 | 6.1 |
| 45-64 | 100.0 | 39.4 | 28.8 | 16.6 | 15.2 |
| 65+ | 100.0 | 21.9 | 26.6 | 20.5 | 31.0 |

*From U. S. Public Health Service: Health statistics, limitation of activity and mobility, PHS bull. no. 584-B-11, Washington, D. C., July 1958.

**Table 22-4.** Percentage prevalence of chronic diseases and impairments, disabling and nondisabling, 65 years and older*

| Condition | Male | Female |
|---|---|---|
| Heart conditions | 70.1 | 58.5 |
| High blood pressure | 29.9 | 23.2 |
| Arthritis and rheumatism | 33.7 | 31.0 |
| Digestive conditions | 22.7 | 19.1 |
| Vascular lesions of central nervous system | 71.3 | 69.6 |
| Visual impairments | 32.7 | 31.2 |
| Hearing impairments | 6.2 | 5.6 |
| Orthopedic impairments (excluding paralysis or absence) | 35.3 | 32.7 |

*From U. S. Public Health Service: Age patterns in medical care, illness and disability, U. S. July 1963-June 1965, PHS pub. no. 1000, ser. 10, no. 32, Rockville, Md., 1966.

to daily living. With reference to the various chronic illnesses and impairments it is important to note the consistent increases in the older age groups and the higher prevalence in most age groups for women in contrast with men. This is surprising, considering the significantly greater expectation of life for women. It could, of course, indicate a greater tendency on the part of women to be seen by diagnosticians.

With reference to mental disorders in the elderly, interest has been similarly scant and delayed—not that society has been unaware of the problem, however. Thus a study of people over 65 years of age showed 33% of men and 42% of women in need of psychiatric or social help. The highest rate of mental illness in terms of age exists in this age group. They make up almost 30% of first admissions to mental hospitals, yet they constitute only 2% of the psychiatric outpatient department population. It is also noteworthy that suicide is a significant cause of death in older age groups, especially among men. In a sample of 278 persons in nursing homes and homes for the aged in Ottawa, Goldstein[7] found the following psychiatric conditions.

| | |
|---|---|
| Chronic brain syndrome | 136 |
| Neurotic depression | 83 |
| Psychotic depression | 5 |
| Manic-depressive, depressed | 3 |
| Manic-depressive, manic | 2 |
| Paranoid state | 12 |
| Late paraphrenia | 7 |
| Chronic schizophrenia | 3 |
| Anxiety state | 11 |
| Personality disorder | 12 |
| Alcoholism | 2 |
| Mental retardation | 1 |
| Drug addiction | 1 |
| Total | 278 |

## CHRONIC DISEASES INCREASING

There is no denying that many more people suffer from chronic diseases now than formerly. An important question, however, is whether the increase is real or apparent, absolute or relative. The use of crude morbidity and death rates in the evaluation of health problems is fraught with considerable danger. Unfortunately, because of the ease and convenience of their calculation and use, most of the information that is available to and discussed by the health professions as well as the public is of this nature. Since the older age groups in the population that are most likely to develop chronic ailments have increased, it would appear only natural that the crude morbidity and death rates from these causes should have increased. Thus the crude death rate for diseases of the heart increased from 137.4 per 100,000 in 1900 to 360.3 per 100,000 in 1970, and the rate from cancer during the same period increased from 64.0 to 162.0. These represent increases of about two and a half times for both diseases during the intervening 70 years. Quite a different picture is obtained, however, by a more careful analysis by means of age specific standardization of rates. In brief this procedure consists of the calculation of a series of death rates, one for each age group of the population, instead of a single crude rate for the entire population. These age specific death rates are then applied to the present population as it would appear if distributed by age in a manner similar to some standard or previous population such as that of 1900. Thus, as an example, when this procedure was applied to industrial policyholders of the Metropolitan Life Insurance Co., it brought out the surprising fact that during the third of a century between 1911 and 1945, the death rate standardized for color, age, and sex decreased 29% for diseases of the heart, arteries, and kidneys and increased only 8% for cancer. The observation was made that the slight increase recorded for cancer was rather less than might be expected from improvements in diagnosis.[8]

On the other hand, it has been pointed out that the population is not now aging as rapidly as before World War II and that the increase in chronic diseases cannot be linked as closely to increased age of the population as previously assumed.[9] Granted that older populations have more chronic diseases than do others, careful analysis indicates that there are not really enough of them proportionately to alone account for the difference.

## AGING AS OPPOSED TO SENESCENCE

Information such as presented here is not meant to imply an inevitability of chronic illness and disability in the adult and aging population. Aging is not necessarily synonymous with chronic illness or senescence. This has been pointed out by many writers. Widmer,[10] having studied 100 persons past 90 years of age, summarized his conclusions in this forceful sentence: "The old people of sixty are all ill, the centenarians are healthy." He described his patients as taut, lean, and dry. None of them was invalid or bedridden, and all were rather young in appearance.

Rejoicing is heard on all sides for the consistent lengthening of the life-span that has been the privileged experience of recent generations. For many it would appear to represent a matter of scorekeeping in a contest with fate. If the increasing numbers of persons achieving advanced ages did so by being physically and mentally fit, there would be real reason to rejoice. The cruel fact remains that despite any mathematic readjustments that may be made, increasing numbers of individuals, not rates, are growing not only old but sick and senile as well. As Piersol[11] has opined, "Longevity marred by an accompaniment of a disabling disease and suffering has little to commend it; it is a distinct liability rather than an asset." He therefore considers that the most important responsibility of medicine and public health is prevention or delay of the development of the degenerative diseases so that the potentialities of elderly persons may be more widely developed and utilized.

But there is an even deeper aspect of this problem. For those who have passed middle age there is little reason to rejoice in the average increased longevity not only because of their accumulating or developing chronic and metabolic ailments but also because they actually are not beneficiaries of the increased average life-span. For all practical purposes in terms of years of life remaining once an individual passes his forty-fifth birthday, he is essentially no better

**Table 22-5.** Average years of life remaining at specific ages, United States, 1900 and 1970*

| Age in years | Average years of life remaining | | Increase in years |
|---|---|---|---|
| | *1900* | *1970* | |
| Birth | 49.2 | 71.1 | 21.9 |
| 1 | 55.2 | 71.5 | 16.3 |
| 5 | 55.0 | 67.7 | 12.7 |
| 25 | 39.1 | 48.6 | 9.5 |
| 65 | 11.9 | 15.2 | 3.3 |

*Modified from U. S. Department of Health, Education, and Welfare: Toward a social report, Washington, D. C., 1969, Government Printing Office.

off than was his great grandfather. This is brought out by Table 22-5,[12] which presents life expectancies at various ages in 1970 compared with those at the beginning of the twentieth century.

These figures illustrate vividly that the much vaunted lengthening of the life-span is the result largely of preventive measures of which infants and young children have been the chief beneficiaries. The figures also point an unequivocally accusing finger at critical health issues and population groups who have been subject either to inadequate attention or frank neglect. Here is one of many answers to those who may believe that there is not much challenge left in public health.

## SOLUTION OF THE PROBLEM

Much attention is currently being given to steps that may be taken by the individual, the medical profession, and society in general to meet successfully the problems posed by the aging of the population and the accompanying increase in chronic diseases. The voluntary health agencies provided the first and continuing organized attack in the form of associations concerned with heart disease, cancer, arthritis, diabetes, and other chronic ailments.

A quarter of a century ago a document entitled "Planning for the Chronically Ill," issued jointly by the American Medical Association, the American Public Health Association, the American Hospital Association, and the American Public Welfare Association,[13] contained this significant statement, "The basic approach to chronic disease must be preventive. Otherwise the problems created by chronic diseases will grow larger with time, and the hope of any substantial decline in their incidence and severity will be postponed for many years." How literally this statement has been lived up to in the ensuing years might be debatable. The ultimate hope must of course be for prevention. With reference to chronic diseases, prevention may be regarded in several ways. In general there are two kinds of prevention: (1) the total community approach as represented by the attack against certain public health problems and (2) the more individualized approach represented by the personal service rendered in the offices of private physicians or in a variety of public or private clinical settings. The total community approach is inapplicable to most problems of chronic disease and preventive geriatrics. The threats to the well-being of the older segments of the population or to any who may be subject to chronic illness cannot be avoided by the turning of a valve or the mass injection of an antigen. Necessarily, therefore, the predominant role must be played by physicians, assisted by a variety of other professionals and technologists, as well as by the increasing types of sophisticated devices for rapid and multiple screening and diagnostic tests. Geriatrics undoubtedly will pattern much of its thinking and development after the concepts and experiences of pediatrics. As a matter of fact, paradoxical as it may appear, pediatricians probably have been more conscious of the factors involved in aging than any other physicians.

The immediate problems that must be faced, however, are somewhat different. As pointed out by Stieglitz[14] in his discussion of the social urgency of research in aging, "Whereas the commoner diseases in youth have acute and florid onsets, obvious symptoms, and, being of infective origin, tend to be self-limited and self immunizing, the disorders frequent in later years are characterized by insidious and asymptomatic onsets, slowly progressive course and endogenous, or at least nonspecific, etiology." Fundamental as it is to the solution of the problem of adult health and chronic diseases, the personal approach of the private physician is not without its limitations and handicaps. Not the least of these are the expense and inadequacy of facilities for adequate early diagnosis and treatment. The inequalities in the distribution of members of the healing professions and of auxiliary aids such as hospitals is the subject of discussion in Chapter 34, which deals with medical and hospital care. Also discussed is the inability of a large proportion of the population to meet the mounting costs of

medical care. The average elderly person can usually afford the fee for the first physician seen but in many instances finds it difficult to meet the costs of consulting physicians, diagnostic aids, hospitalization, and surgery. This problem was pointed up by former President Johnson in a message to Congress: "One third of the aged who are forced to ask for old age assistance do so because of ill health, and one third of our public assistance funds going to older people is spent for medical care."

Although the cost of health care has been rising for everyone, it affects the elderly doubly or triply. They have only about half the income of those under 65 years of age, but even with Medicare and Medicaid they pay more than twice as much for health services—if they get them. They are twice as likely as a young person to have one or more chronic diseases, and much of the care needed is of a prolonged and expensive type.[15] Added to this is the extra effort and cost involved in the process of physically obtaining the care. "The elderly," as James[16] states, "have been pushed out of the mainstream of life ahead of their time." The percentage of older people in the labor force has declined by half since 1940. This necessarily makes more difficult the maintenance of proper health and nutrition and encourages a delay in proper early diagnosis. A few figures emphasize the economic plight of many in the older age groups, hence their inability to assure themselves of adequate nutrition, housing, and health care.[17]

In 1969 the median income of an aged family was 48% of that of families headed by younger persons.

One out of 4 of the older people lived in poverty (as compared with 1 out of 9 of the younger people).

More than one half of all older families had annual incomes below $4,800; one fifth had less than $2,500.

More than one half of all older single persons living alone or away from relatives had less than $2,000; one third had less than $1,500.

Prevention may be regarded in still another way. It includes measures that avert the occurrence of disease in the first instance and measures that halt or retard the progression of disease, which has been allowed to occur, into disability or death. These are referred to as primary and secondary prevention, respectively. Whereas some might deny the possibility of prevention of chronic diseases, it is nevertheless possible to a significant although indirect extent.

In fact even 20 years ago the Commission on Chronic Illness, which functioned between 1950 and 1956, listed more than 50 chronic diseases against which preventive action is possible.[18] The present potential is even greater in view of the many biomedical and biophysical advances of the past few decades. The successful approach of the prevention and treatment of the communicable diseases of early life precludes the development of much tissue damage and foci of infection that, if permitted to occur, would be manifested later on as syphilitic or rheumatic hearts, nephritis, arthritis, or other chronic conditions. Careful obstetric management with the avoidance of cervical tears and the proper repair of those that occur is certain to prevent many future cervical carcinomas. The increasing precautions taken by industry for the protection of its workers not only prevent many disabling injuries but for some processes also remove potential hazards that might lead to bronchitis, silicosis, occupational cancers, and other chronic diseases. Breslow[19] and others have emphasized that better nutrition is a major immediate goal in the primary prevention of chronic disease. He pointed, on the one hand, to the common protein, vitamin C, and mineral deficiencies in the diets of many elderly persons and, on the other hand, to overweight as an increasingly important national health problem of the middle aged. The latter has been shown to account for a significant proportion of the unnecessary mortality from cardiovascular disease, diabetes, and other chronic diseases. These are only a few of the direct preventive measures that may be taken against chronic illness.[1]

Beyond this are the potential fruits of current biochemical and physiologic research that may inhibit some of the degenerative processes that tend to occur with increased age. For example, Comfort[20] lists several substances that might modify the rate of aging. They include antioxidants that could scavenge the free radicals and prevent molecular decompensation; certain chemicals that have been shown to protect against the effects of background or other types of radiation; protein synthesis inhibitors; lysosome stabilizers that can prevent the escape of vital enzymes; immunosuppressants that may be used to suppress the autoimmune response; and chemical agents that could be used to impede cross-linking. Furthermore, the potential of hormonal agents, including anabolics, somatotrophins, prednisolone, and 17-keto-steroids, as well as antimetabolic drugs, remains to be explored. Moreover, reduction in calorie intake and lowered environmental temperature are known to retard the process of aging in experimental animals. Theoretically, Comfort says, prolonging the more productive years of human life rather than just extending life is a distinct possibility. The possibility, he adds, is an extraordinarily tantalizing one.

Secondary prevention, that is, prevention of the progression of diseases which have already begun, is now possible with an increasing frequency. The keynote here, of course, is early diagnosis. This may be achieved in several ways. One is by intelligent and consistent self-observation and examination based on sound personal health education. Self-palpation of the breasts, alertness to abnormal discharges, and other signs and symptoms are examples. Participation in screening programs and periodic complete medical examinations are other ways. Of great importance is the role of the personal physician, who should not be satisfied with treatment alone, much less treatment of only one complaint, but who should approach each patient as a total person with pathologic potentials as well as pathologic actualities. A serious handicap, of course, is the insidious nature of the development of most chronic illnesses. Their onsets tend to be asymptomatic, and they often progress slowly with little or no pain or discomfort in the earlier stages. This encourages the person afflicted, even when he suspects the condition, to delay in seeking medical advice and care. One of the most fundamental handicaps therefore is the difficulty of getting persons to protect themselves, to obtain periodic medical examinations, and if necessary, to obtain early and adequate treatment. Steiglitz[14] has aptly stated, "The privilege of longevity carries with it the obligation of personal effort toward health maintenance." This in consideration of the inherent frailties of human nature is the source of much of the problem. Several psychologic blocks must be counteracted. The individual must overcome a considerable amount of inertia and do something that is not of immediate or apparent benefit, much less pleasure. For many, a truly complete and adequate physical examination represents a decidedly unpleasant and embarrassing experience. Furthermore, it not infrequently requires time off from gainful work. Fear of a positive diagnosis serves as a deterrent for some, and other rebel at the thought of potential restrictions on their personal habits and pleasures. The only weapon available against these deterrents is increased and persistent education. The ultimate goal should be the establishment of periodic medical examinations as part of the accepted process of living.

One effect of these psychologic and cultural blocks may well be the fact that the outlook for the reduction of deaths from chronic diseases in the United States and probably elsewhere is more favorable for females than for males. This has been pointed to by Bright[9] not only on the basis of the slight advantage that women have over men with respect to cardiovascular and renal diseases but also the trend of a declining cancer death rate among females, whereas the rate for males has been moving upward. These differences are observed in both the white and nonwhite races.

## ROLE OF THE HEALTH DEPARTMENT

For a long period chronic diseases and adult health were not regarded by many as a concern of official public health agencies. Fortunately this attitude has undergone considerable change. Interestingly it is often overlooked that the more commonly accepted public health activities may play an extremely important although indirect part in the eventual alleviation and prevention of many of the disease problems of advanced years. As pointed out previously, the reduction in morbidity from acute communicable diseases not only is important in the prevention of early death but also in the avoidance of infectious foci and structural changes that may give rise to chronic ailments that may impair or limit one's life. Maternal health not only eases the burdens and immediate risks of motherhood but prevents the development of complications that formerly invalided many women in later life. Most of the benefits of services to children, such as well-child conferences and clinics, school health programs, and medical examinations for the correction of defects, are reaped in later life. Recognition should be given to the delayed benefits of the present extensive use of antibiotics, ataraxics, antihypertensives, and other drugs as well as to recent nutritional improvements.

Good nutrition of the expectant mother and the child is said to contribute more than anything to physiologic and mental health in later life. Davis,[21] for example, believes that "The involutional, biochemical processes which lead to senescence may be influenced by all factors that in any way modify cellular metabolism." He lists the following factors as important in determining the onset and relative severity of these changes: (1) heredity, (2) health and nutrition of the parents at conception, (3) health and nutrition of the mother during pregnancy and lactation, (4) any illnesses that the individual may have had at any time in his life, (5) quantity and quality of the nutrition at all periods of life and its relation to the individual needs, (6) environment of the individual during his past life, his occupation, habits, and manner of living, and (7) any gases, dust, or chemical compounds to which the individual has been exposed and any drugs used at one time or another.

Official public health agencies should not be expected to assume the entire burden of the attack against the diseases of middle and older ages. As already indicated, the predominant role must be played by practitioners of medicine, and the place of the voluntary health and social agencies must likewise become increasingly important. The necessary combination to meet the need is a three-cornered partnership made up of the medical profession, the social agencies, and the public health agencies working together toward the amelioration and solution of the problem. Such a partnership would not be new, having operated successfully for many years in other fields such as maternal and child health, tuberculosis, and venereal disease control. With the precedent well established it is logical to visualize, for example, the establishment of screening and diagnostic centers and home care programs financed wholly or in part by public funds, staffed by private physicians and consultants on any of the acceptable bases of payment, with the educational and promotional work carried on by the public and voluntary health agencies, and the necessary social service work performed by the appropriate agencies which exist for that purpose. The impetus and leadership, however, may well be furnished by the official public health agency, which may serve to stimulate, correlate, and integrate the contributions and activities of all concerned.[22]

## DEVELOPMENT OF PUBLIC PROGRAMS

Chronic disease programs are being established at an increasing rate. Up to this time, however, the major focus of attention has been on cancer. This was the first of the chronic diseases to receive recognition in the official public health program. In this country Massachusetts merits priority for the provision in 1919 of funds for the establishment in its state health department of a program for the study of the prevalence, prevention, and control of cancer. As far as can be ascertained, Detroit was the first city to explore the problem after a specific appropriation in 1928 to the health department for this purpose. The objectives of the program were as follows: first, to get the factual information, that is, the statistical background with regard to cancer in the community; second, to encourage physicians to diagnose and to treat cancer through the various channels of undergraduate and postgraduate medical education; third, to institute a service for early detection and the encouragement of treatment; fourth, to institute a follow-up system for cases that received surgical, radium, or x-ray treatment; and fifth, to educate the public in simple terms and with frank statements with regard to the existing knowledge concerning the early treatment of cancer.

Slow to develop, by 1950 every state had established a cancer program. Some services are provided by all 50 state health departments. State cancer commissions, university medical centers, departments of welfare, and a variety of other agencies participate. Many of the statewide cancer programs are carried on with the assistance of the state chapters of the American Cancer Society, and state medical societies.[23] In most states the general goals set forth by the National Advisory Cancer Council are more or less adequately approached. These include (1) statistical research to determine the nature and extent of the cancer problem of the state and to evaluate the results of activities; (2) educational activities for the public and all professional groups concerned in the detection, diagnosis, and treatment of cancer; (3) activities to provide adequate detection, diagnostic, and treatment facilities and services accessible to persons of all economic groups in all sections of the state, including facilities for care of the terminal case either at home or in an institution.

Progress has been much slower in relation to the other diseases and health problems of later life. A few states are beginning to turn their attention to some of the broader aspects of the situation. Here again Massachusetts has long been the leader, with Connecticut and New York not far behind. Already many public health programs include, in addition to the cytologic smear for detection of cancer, the clinitron for diabetes screening, the tonometer for early glaucoma detection, and screening tests for various other chronic conditions. Significant also is the trend toward expanding programs for diagnosing tuberculosis into programs for diagnosing all chest disease, placing greater emphasis on cardiac conditions, pulmonary carcinoma, and silicosis. The goal of such programs is the earliest possible diagnosis with referral to physicians and hospitals for prompt treatment.

Unfortunately, although a large number of local health departments now provide many *services* in relation to various chronic illnesses, few can be said to have yet developed what might genuinely be considered chronic disease *programs,* and surprisingly few have organizational units specifically concerned with chronic diseases. This situation may well stem from the categorical approach forced on state and local health agencies by the various special legislative actions of Congress that have provided funds for the development and conduct of chronic disease services in a piecemeal and generally uncoordinated manner. This has been partially offset by the Comprehensive Health Planning and Public Health Services Amendments Act of 1965 (P.L. 89-749), which provides block grants to states (and local agencies) in place of categorical grants for the purpose of broader based program planning. It is hoped that the recent trend toward intergovernmental revenue sharing will also have some effect.

## CONTENT OF A CHRONIC DISEASE PROGRAM

Knott[24] has indicated five processes by which a community may establish and pursue a chronic disease program: (1) health maintenance, (2) prevention of disease or injury, (3) detection and treatment of illness in its earliest possible state when cure is often feasible, (4) limitation of disability to preserve the maximum normal function, and (5) restoration of the capacity for the highest level of independent activity of which the patient is capable. In other words, he emphasizes the critical need to regard chronic disease control in a broad comprehensive sense. For example or comparison he indicates that probably the nearest that public health and society have approached this goal is in the care of the individual during infancy and childhood. "Here," according to Knott, "to a greater extent than in any other stage of life, we more nearly practice—laymen and professional—the concept of total health care." Furthermore, "Examples of such health care during adult life are unfortunately few and far between. And even these seldom cover the entire life span of those individuals who are served." The development of a truly comprehensive and adequate program of chronic disease control requires extremely careful planning as a joint enterprise by a variety of disciplines. In this regard attention is directed to an excellent planning guide for the development of community chronic disease programs recently produced by the Public Health Service.[25]

A complete program for chronic diseases should be based on both primary and secondary preventive concepts and should include the following activities: (1) research, (2) case finding, (3) hospitalization and treatment, (4) follow-up, (5) rehabilitation, (6) education, and (7) custodial care.

### Research

At the present time continued and expanding research is still a fundamental necessity. In addition to the obvious need for the study of the causes, diagnosis, and treatment of chronic diseases, research activities should include statistical studies of prevalence, incidence, and mortality in the various component groups of the population and administrative studies for the development of satisfactory and efficient methods of implementing a community program. The source of the greatest impetus in this regard is the National Institutes of Health. In 1972 the very names of and appropriations to some of the institutes give testimony to this: National Institute of Cancer ($337.5 million), of Heart and Lung ($232.1 million), of Arthritis and Metabolic Diseases ($153.2 million), and of Neurological Diseases and Stroke ($116.6 million). In addition, all of the other institutes have direct or indirect involvement with other chronic diseases. This does not preclude, however, an important role for state and local official and voluntary health agencies in research and demonstration.

### Case finding

Early diagnosis is a primary step in controlling any chronic disease regardless of whether it is communicable. For some diseases diagnosis is relatively simple and inexpensive, whereas for many others it is difficult, time consuming, and produces an economic burden of considerable magnitude. Several approaches are possible to overcome this aspect of the problem. Private physicians and hospitals might be called on to render an increased amount of free or reduced-fee medical care. This, however, would be impractical and unfair to the medical profession and institutions as well as undesirable for the public. One compromise that has been arrived at and that has met with reasonable success is to provide periodic screening examinations of limited scope in the offices of private physicians with the patient paying the fee customarily charged for a general examination. If possible, medically indigent patients may be examined free, or an agreement may be reached whereby the physician is paid out of public funds.

Up to the present this approach has been more or less limited to examination for signs of cancer. Studies have shown, for example, that more than 60% of cancer cases involve five readily accessible sites: the skin, lips, breasts, cervix, and rectum. These sites can be easily examined by any well-trained physician in his office without recourse to unusual equipment or procedures. The examination is so relatively simple, brief, and inexpensive that both the patient and the physician can afford its repetition every 6 to 12 months. The only potential danger of this approach is that the patient, on receiving a negative report from this limited examination, may believe that he is free of all types of cancer and of all disease. It is of great importance therefore that these limitations be stressed to the public whenever such a program is put into effect.

Another approach has been the use of specialized cancer detection centers. Generally these have not been economical and efficient, and if the idea were extended to the establishment of similar special facilities for other chronic diseases, the cost would be prohibitive, and the program might well be inefficient and ineffective in view of the total need. The approach therefore should be more general and concerned with broad aspects of the chronic disease diagnostic problem. Multiphasic screening programs have been developed as one attempt to meet the need. In these a variety of tests may be performed quickly and efficiently for large numbers of people. Carefully designed and conducted multiphasic screening tests would appear to provide the answer. At best they should be available on a continuous rather than on a one-shot basis.[26] Attention is also called to the use of the concept of prospective medicine, discussed briefly in Chapter 1, as a method of meeting the need.

## Hospitalization and treatment

The majority of patients who are diagnosed as having a chronic disease are hospitalized for at least a period of several days or weeks for a complete decision as to diagnosis, therapy, and prognosis to be made. In addition, many hospital beds are needed for long-term care so that certain patients may receive the surgical, medical, and nursing treatment necessary to return them eventually to normal or near-normal existence. Here the problems of availability of sufficient hospital beds and the ability to pay for them appear. Private or public prepayment hospitalization insurance plans provide some solution to the problem of payment. Medicare and Medicaid, made possible by the Social Security Amendments of 1965 and as extended by the Social Security Amendments of 1972 (Title II, P.L. 92-603),[27] have had a significant impact on the payment aspect of the problem. The inevitable enactment of comprehensive national health care legislation will, of course, go much further in providing an adequate solution. There appears to be unanimous agreement concerning the need for large numbers of additional publicly supported hospital beds for chronic diseases. Some of these undoubtedly will have to be provided by additional appropriation and construction, such as are provided for by the Hill-Burton hospital survey and construction program.

The need for more beds for patients suffering from chronic diseases provides one answer, however, to a problem with which public health administrators have already begun to be concerned, that is, the most efficient use of hospital beds formerly needed for acute communicable diseases and tuberculosis in the face of declining incidences and shortened hospital stays. It would appear logical that many of these beds might eventually be made available for the care of patients with chronic noncommunicable diseases. It is interesting that the first public hospital established for the care of cancer patients many years ago in Pondville, Mass., was a reconverted tuberculosis sanatorium.

## Follow-up

The active follow-up of posthospitalized patients is an important and expanding part of the chronic disease program. Often the chronically ill and aged patient is happier and mentally better off in his own home with familiar surroundings and proximity of those he loves. It has been estimated that about 70% of such patients could be cared for satisfactorily in their own homes if adequate auxiliary services, such as visiting nurse, home health aid, and housekeeper services,[28] were available and if the other members of the family were given some training. It is here that the public health nurse especially can make a significant contribution to the program for the care and education of the chronically ill and aged.[29,30] The needs and wishes have already been made evident by the public in terms of demands for this type of service. This constitutes a strong argument in favor of the more widespread and more effective joining of the forces of the official public health nursing services and the bedside nursing programs of the visiting nursing societies. An important result has been the passage of the Older Americans Act of 1965 and its subsequent amendments. This has made it possible for every state to have an agency to aid the elderly and has provided funds for community projects, nutrition programs with hot meals, some housing improvements, and transportation for the elderly.

An early demonstration of the value of home nursing service in relation to chronic illness was provided by the home nursing service for policyholders of the Metropolitan Life Insurance Co. In 1925 nearly 50% of requests for service related to acute and communicable conditions, most of which occur in early life, and only about 5% for chronic diseases. Only 20 years later in 1945 the figures were reversed to 14% and 28%, respectively.[31] In addition to rendering direct services in the home the visiting nurse may be of assistance in returning the posthospitalized patient to the care of a private physician, providing him with information helpful in the handling of the case and assisting the patient in putting the physician's suggestions into effect. Patients may also be aided in the use of outpatient clinics and departments of general hospitals by patients residing in their own homes.

For those who no longer require the extensive medical services of a hospital but who are not yet ready to function on an independent basis, the convalescent home provides an important bridge. Here, as is the case with nursing homes subsequently mentioned, the health department has an important role in establishing and enforcing standards and qualifications with reference to personnel, type and quality of care, food quality and service, and general sanitation and safety. Many health departments have the responsibility of licensing these institutions.

## Rehabilitation

A program of rehabilitation for chronically ill and disabled patients should be carried on concurrently with other activities. The need for this is indicated from two points of view. The most obvious is assistance to enable patients to become partially self-supporting or at least to take care of their own personal needs and to be less of a burden to their relatives and friends. Many patients may be returned to their previous occupations, although often on a reduced work-time schedule. Others may be guided into new endeavors more suitable to their present capabilities.

Too frequently overlooked is the need for rehabilitation in the mental health sense. Not uncommon is the woman who, having undergone a breast amputation or a hysterectomy, is returned to her home and family with no psychiatric preparation and who spends the remaining years of her life feeling incomplete, half a woman, and perhaps unwanted. The same applies, although in a somewhat different sense, to the man who is summarily directed to give up his daily work, his sports, and his other activities that made life worth living because of a stroke or a cardiac ailment. The tremendous need for activity in this area represents as yet a vast virgin territory and provides an area of great potential service by public health nurses and medical and social service advisors.

## Education

The need for public education with regard to the chronic illnesses of later life is very great. On first consideration it appears incomprehensible that large numbers of the population of the United States are so utterly lacking in knowledge and have so many misconceptions and superstitions regarding chronic ailments. Related to this is the substantial number of people who allow themselves to fall prey to all sorts of quacks and charlatans when afflicted with a chronic disease. However, when the fundamental forces that motivate human thought and behavior are considered, the result is not so surprising. Up to the present this challenge has been met almost singlehandedly by the various voluntary agencies, and as a result it is they who deserve the major credit for the contemporary interest and progress that is taking place in this field. In the final analysis it may well be that increased public education in these matters would represent the single most important service that may be rendered by public health agencies in company with the schools.

## Nursing homes and custodial care

The final phase of any program designed to serve those who suffer from chronic diseases is the provision of custodial care. In a sense the extent of the need for this type of care is the best measure of the degree of defeat or failure of the total program. A certain number of patients require custodial care of long duration because of indigency and lack of family or because of progressive incurability and incapacitation due to their illness or age. What is needed here is not so much medical and hospital treatment as mothering, the alleviation of pain and discomfort during the remaining period of life, and psychosocial support for a death as comfortable and dignified as possible. This last is extremely important, and regrettably health professionals or institutions give it little attention.[32,33] At present relatively few facilities for this type of care are maintained at public expense. Dependence must be placed also on facilities established and operated by religious and fraternal organizations or conducted as proprietary, profit-making institutions—some excellent but others abominable. The regulation and supervision of custodial care institutions are certainly a proper and necessary public health function. As strongly stated by Kosberg,[34] "The aged in institutions are perhaps the most powerless, voiceless, invisible, and uncared for groups in this country. The conditions under which they live in these facilities are for the most part dehumanizing and tend to make them more lonely and dependent. Nowhere is the plight of the institutionalized elderly more evident than in nursing homes." To this Nader[35] has added, "The few homes that are humane, competent, and mindful of their residents' need for activity and meaning in their day, highlight the staggering gap between what an affluent society should attain, and what is too frequently the reality for most nursing homes." On the basis of eligibility to receive federal funds for payment of care rendered under the provisions of the Medicaid legislation, and in response to strong pressures from the 1971 White House Conference on the Aging, the United States Department of Health, Education, and Welfare has undertaken an extensive and vigorous program to train inspectors to inspect and to certify nursing homes.[36] During the first 11 months of the program (up to July 1972), 579 or 1 in 12 of the 7,000 nursing homes that had been qualified for Medicaid payments had dropped out or had been decertified. Although

2,860 patients were moved to certified homes, almost 16,000 patients had to be left in or moved to homes that were reclassified as "intermediate care facilities" for which regulations were subsequently developed. The department has also taken steps to ensure that those who need "skilled care" are in skilled-care facilities.[37]

## ROLE OF INDUSTRY

Industrial establishments are key spots of great potential advantage to any program of adult health and chronic disease service and control. They may be regarded as places where, because large numbers of adults are concentrated, they may be conveniently and efficiently reached and served in the same way that schools represent focal points for much of the public health programs designed for children. This is particularly significant when it is realized that chronic illnesses are particularly prevalent among wage earners in the lower and middle income groups (Table 22-6).[38]

Progressive industrial concerns now realize that the promotion of the health and education of workers represents a sound investment. There are many ways in which industry may play an important role. An increasing number of businesses and industries are establishing policies that require preemployment and periodic medical examinations of workers. Considering the many persons involved, this serves as a fruitful means of diagnosing chronic ill-

nesses in their early stages and makes a large part of the population aware of the need for constant self-surveillance. Many industries conduct praiseworthy programs of health education for their workers. Reference has already been made to the potential preventive value of the removal of industrial hazards. Hospital and medical care insurance is frequently an employment benefit and one increasingly demanded in union contract negotiations. Rehabilitation programs work to the advantage of business and industry. World War II brought about a belated realization that there exists in the population a large pool of industrial manpower in the form of persons only partially handicapped by chronic disease and disabilities. In the face of serious shortages of manpower the contributions of such persons to the national war effort was by no means insignificant and has been said by some to have turned the scale on the production front. As a result many industries have continued their wartime policy of job placement of partially handicapped workers on the basis of aptitude tests and a careful study of their physical capabilities. This is the best possible type of rehabilitation, physical, mental, moral, and economic, and it should be done by more employers.

An important contribution that may be made by industry is the development of more reasonable and individualized retirement procedures. The picture is an all too familiar one of an individual's having to accept retirement at a

**Table 22-6.** Work-loss days from selected chronic conditions by family income, United States, July 1959 to June 1960*

| Selected chronic conditions | Work-loss days (in thousands) | | Work-loss days per 1,000 employed persons per year | |
|---|---|---|---|---|
| | Family income | | | |
| | Under $4,000 | Over $4,000 | Under $4,000 | Over $4,000 |
| Heart conditions | 6,247 | 7,821 | 318.4 | 184.8 |
| High blood pressure | 3,905 | 3,423 | 199.0 | 80.9 |
| Varicose veins | 950 | 1,023 | 48.4 | 24.2 |
| Hemorrhoids | 2,092 | 3,355 | 106.6 | 79.3 |
| Chronic bronchitis | 1,732 | 1,609 | 88.3 | 38.0 |
| Peptic ulcer | 4,759 | 4,412 | 242.5 | 104.3 |
| Skin conditions | 1,275 | 1,997 | 65.0 | 47.2 |
| Diabetes | 1,153 | 1,026 | 58.8 | 24.2 |
| Fracture and dislocated residuals | 1,739 | 1,419 | 88.6 | 33.5 |
| Arthritis and rheumatism | 9,014 | 2,220 | 459.4 | 52.5 |
| Other diseases of muscles and joints | 5,360 | 2,441 | 273.2 | 57.7 |

*From U. S. Public Health Service: Health statistics, currently employed persons, illness and work-loss days, PHS bull. no. 584-C7, Washington, D. C., April 1962.

certain age on the basis of chronology rather physiology, with the result that the enforced idleness and apparent lack of purpose limit the remaining years of life. Actually human beings are much less similar at the age of 65 years than they are at birth. Productive potentials are subject to great individual variation until the end of life. Most people are not promoted to positions of great responsibility and opportunity until about the age of 50 years. This being true, it is important to find means to help older individuals keep physically and mentally fit and then to allow them to use their fitness and ability. It would appear therefore to be highly inefficient as well as illogical and cruel to attempt to place all persons in exactly the same retirement mold.

## RECENT EVENTS ON THE NATIONAL LEVEL

Uncoordinated as the total picture has been up to the present, it now appears to be coming into focus. Not many years ago chronic illness and problems of adult health were subjects that tended to be underemphasized in public health and in other circles. The situation has rapidly changed during recent years, with the role of leadership being assumed more and more by agencies on the national level, perhaps more notably epitomized by the National Institutes of Health and the various chronic disease program units of the Public Health Service. One may also point to several important national meetings and conferences since the 1947 National Conferences for Planning for the Chronically Ill, which involved the American Hospital Association, the American Medical Association, the American Public Welfare Association and the American Public Health Association.[13] There has been a National Health Forum on Chronic Disease in 1956[39] and the work of the Commission on Chronic Illness, a national voluntary group that carried out studies in the United States between 1945 and 1956 and produced useful volumes on various aspects of the problem based on its extensive deliberations. On the federal level there have been held two White House Conferences on the Aging, one in 1961[41] and another in 1971.[42]

Finally, attention must be directed to the flood of recent national legislative proposals that relate to a long list of chronic ailments and disabilities including cancer, heart disease, arthritis and rheumatism, mental diseases, dental diseases, addictions, multiple sclerosis,

cerebral palsy, birth defects, epilepsy, poliomyelitis, blindness, leprosy, and venereal diseases. Many of those have been enacted into law and have resulted in the establishment of several National Institutes of Health, previously mentioned, as well as in the promotion of many state and local chronic disease activities by means of grants-in-aid and consultation. Several recent acts of Congress deserve particular mention as major steps toward the more effective solution of the chronic disease problem.

One is the so-called Partnership for Health or more correctly the Comprehensive Health Planning and Public Health Services Amendments Act (P.L. 89-749), subsequently amended. Whereas this law applies far beyond chronic disease considerations, as indicated earlier, it should greatly assist and encourage state and local health agencies to develop broadly gauged and properly balanced chronic disease control programs. In addition, because of the provisions that require the establishment of state and local or regional planning agencies and advisory committees with representation from official and nonofficial agencies as well as representatives of the public, voluntary health agencies and official health departments should be expected to work more closely and effectively together than previously. The Social Security Amendments of 1965 and 1972 (P.L. 89-97) have also been referred to. This significant breakthrough assures payment for needed medical, hospital, and related services not only for the older component of the population by means of Medicare or Title XVIII but also for many young as well as older persons financially incapable of meeting medical expenses through Medicaid, Title XIX, or Grants to the States for Medical Assistance Programs. Obviously these provisions should encourage and make possible earlier diagnosis and secondary preventive treatment of many cases of chronic illness.

Another national legislative act of great and specific consequence for chronic disease control was the Heart Disease, Cancer, and Stroke Amendments Act (P.L. 89-239). This act grew out of the report of the President's Commission on Heart Disease, Cancer, and Stroke,[43] which recommended a series of regional medical complexes that would bring quality care directly to the patient with relation to these three diseases, which account for 7 out of every 10 deaths in the United States. However, the law as passed provided for regional cooperative arrangements among medical schools, research institutes, hospitals, and other health institutions to make available to their patients the latest advances and treatment of heart disease, cancer, stroke, and such related diseases as kidney disorders and diabetes. The law also provided for continuing education of physicians in these fields. This program was discontinued in 1973. At the same time, however, greatly accentuated programs were established with the specific targets of cancer and hypertension.

In May 1974 the Congress took the significant step of establishing a National Institute on Aging within the U. S. Public Health Service. It is charged with the responsibility to conduct and to support biomedical, social, and behavioral research and training relating to the aging process and diseases and special needs of the elderly. In view of the effects and influence of other components of the National Institutes of Health, this could hold great promise for the increasing proportion of our older more chronically ill citizens.

These steps, momentous as they are, cannot be regarded as solving the problem completely. Further action can certainly be contemplated in these and related fields. Although the control of chronic diseases still appears difficult, the situation is probably no different from that presented by communicable diseases a half century ago. That problem has been largely conquered. In the light of recent trends workers in public health may well look forward to similar results in the field of chronic diseases with the ever-increasing knowledge provided by persistent research and the cooperation of the medical, public health, and social professions.

As implied in the course of this discussion, the equal or greater challenge is the personal humane aspects of the problem. If these cannot be solved satisfactorily, all scientific and professional advances will be to no avail. This has been expressed in a challenging manner by Townsend,[44] whose comments referring to Britain are equally applicable to America.

At a time when we stand perhaps on the threshold of a new era in social policy we are in danger of being stigmatized by future generations as grudging, indifferent and parsimonious to those among us who are unable because of chronic illness, disability, poverty, loss of family or inadequacy of housing, to stand up to the rigours of a competitive society. We look back with horror at some of the cruelties perpetuated in the 1860s, just as our descendants, a hundred years hence, will look back with horror at some of the cruelties we perpetrate today. Possibly

the ultimate test of the quality of a free, democratic and prosperous society is to be found in the standards of freedom, democracy, and prosperity enjoyed by its weakest members.

## REFERENCES

1. Blum, H. K., and Keranen, G. M.: Control of chronic diseases in man, Washington, D. C., 1966, American Public Health Association.
2. The future of aging and the aged, Atlanta, 1971, Southern Newspaper Publishers Association Foundation.
3. Elwood, T. W.: Old age and the quality of life, Health Services Rep. **87:**919, Dec. 1972.
4. U. S. Public Health Service: Limitation of activity and mobility due to chronic conditions, PHS pub. no. 1000, ser. 10, no. 45, Rockville, Md., 1968.
5. U. S. Public Health Service: Health statistics, limitation of activity and mobility, PHS bull. no. 584-B-11, Washington, D. C., July 1958.
6. U. S. Public Health Service: Age patterns in medical care, illness and disability, U. S., July 1963-June 1965, PHS pub. no. 1000, ser. 10, no. 32, Rockville, Md., 1966.
7. Goldstein, S.: Community psychiatry and the elderly, Canad. Med. Ass. J. **108:**579, March 3, 1973.
8. Statistical bulletin, Metropolitan Life Insurance Co. **27:**11, Nov. 1946.
9. Bright, M.: In Lilienfeld, A. M., and Gifford, A. J., editors: Chronic diseases and public health, Baltimore, 1966, The Johns Hopkins Press.
10. Widmer, C.: Die Neunzigjaehrigen, München, Med. Wschr. **76:**840, 1929.
11. Piersol, G. M.: Medical considerations of some geriatric problems, Arch. Ophthal. (Chicago) **29:** 27, Jan. 1943.
12. U. S. Department of Health, Education and Welfare: Toward a social report, Washington, D. C., Government Printing Office.
13. Planning for the chronically ill; joint statement of recommendations by the American Hospital Association, American Medical Association, American Public Health Association, and American Public Welfare Association, Amer. J. Public Health **37:**1256, Oct. 1947.
14. Stieglitz, E. J.: The social urgency of research in aging. In Cowdry, E. V., editor: Problems of aging, Baltimore, 1942, The Williams & Wilkins Co.
15. U. S. Public Health Service: Health in the later years, DHEW pub. no. (HSM) 72-1207, Rockville, Md., 1971.
16. James, G.: Poverty as an obstacle to health progress in our cities, Amer. J. Public Health **55:**1757, Nov. 1965.
17. Social Security Administration: Resources of people 65 or over, SS pub. no. 1-71, Washington, D. C., 1971.

18. Prevention of chronic illness. In Report of the Commission on Chronic Illness, Boston, 1957, Harvard University Press.

19. Breslow, L.: Prevention of chronic illness, Amer. J. Public Health **46:**1540, Dec. 1965.

20. Comfort, A.: Basic research in gerontology, Gerontologia **16:**48, Jan. 1970.

21. Davis, N. S.: Factors which may influence senescence, Ann. Intern. Med. **18:**81, Jan. 1943.

22. Ames, W. R., and Longood, R. J.: Home care of the sick—Monroe County acts, New York Health News, p. 4, March 1962.

23. 1972 Inventory, health programs in the states and territories, Washington, D. C., 1973, Association of State and Territorial Health Officers.

24. Knott, L. W.: Components of a chronic disease program, Amer. J. Public Health **52:**2080, Dec. 1962.

25. U. S. Public Health Service: Development of community programs for the chronically ill, Washington, D. C., 1967, Government Printing Office.

26. Getting, V. A.: Multiple screening: organizing a program in chronic disease control, Continued education Ser. no. 88, Ann Arbor, 1960, University of Michigan Press.

27. A guide to provisions related to Medicare, Medicaid, and maternal and child health—enacted as Title II of Public Law 92-603, the Social Security Amendments of 1972, Chicago, 1972, American Medical Association.

28. Ryder, C. F., et al.: Home health services—past, present, future, Amer. J. Public Health **59:**1720, Sept. 1969.

29. Drenckhahn, V. V.: Educational role of the nurse in chronic disease control, Public Health Rep. **80:**1103, Dec. 1965.

30. Morris, R., and Harris, E.: Home health services in Massachusetts, 1971: their role in the care of the long-term sick, Amer. J. Public Health **62:**1088, Aug. 1972.

31. Dublin, L. I.: Problems of an aging population setting the stage, Amer. J. Public Health **37:**155, Feb. 1947.

32. Barnard, C. N.: A good death, Family Health **5:**40, April 1973.

33. Pickering, G.: Medicine and society—past, present and future Brit. Med. J. **1:**191, Jan. 23, 1971.

34. Kosberg, J. J.: The nursing home: a social work paradox, Social Work **18:**104, March 1973.

35. Nader, R.: In Townsend, C.: Old age: the last segregation, New York, 1971, Grossman Publishers, Inc.

36. Doten, D.: Nursing home surveyors HSMHA Health Rep. **87:**114, Feb. 1972.

37. Pressure on nursing homes, Mod. Med. **40:**16, Aug. 7, 1972.

38. U. S. Public Health Service: Health statistics, currently employed persons, illness and work-loss days, PHS bull. no. 584-Cy, Washington, D. C., April 1962.

39. National Health Forum on Chronic Disease, Public Health Rep. **71:**675, July 1956.

40. Commission on Chronic Illness: I. Chronic illness in the United States; II. Care of the longterm patient; III. Chronic illness in a large city, Cambridge, 1957, Harvard University Press.

41. White House Conference on Aging, Washington, D. C., 1961, U. S. Department of Health, Education, and Welfare.

42. White House Conference on Aging, Washington, D. C., 1971, U. S. Department of Health, Education, and Welfare.

43. Report of the President's Commission on Heart Disease, Cancer, and Stroke: a national program to conquer heart disease, cancer, and stroke, Washington, D. C., 1964, Government Printing Office.

44. Townsend, P.: The last refuge, London, 1964, Routledge & Kegan Paul, Ltd.

# PART EIGHT

# The substance of public health— mental and behavioral

Despite Juvenal's well-known and widely quoted aphorism, *Mens sana in corpore sano,*[1] far too many people, including a substantial proportion of health workers, tend to think of health and illness only in relation to the physical body. This is thrice in error! It errs first in that it ignores the complex of mental and behavioral disorders that afflict a large proportion of mankind, second in that it ignores the various mental and behavioral conditions that may have their genesis in physical illnesses, and third in that it ignores the fact that few, if any, physical illnesses or injuries are without a mental or behavioral component or consequence.

Much of the problem relates to difficulty of definition. The case has been stated particularly well by Lipscomb[2]: "The attempts to study mental illness, delinquency, alcoholism and drug use have demanded that epidemiologists ruefully accept that they can no longer classify the occurrences of these events by single precise labels—'the alcoholic,' 'the addict,' 'the delinquent.' They have had to consider the events under study—drinking, drug use, delinquent behavior—in the ecological content in which an indexed individual lives, a context which inevitably changes over time as the person himself changes."

This is especially evident among those who find themselves, by no personal choice, in socioeconomically disadvantaged circumstances, epitomized by the slum or ghetto, that constitute a complex morass of human problems. The choices open to such a marginal person in his attempt to cope with the intolerable externalities that confront him have been summarized as follows[3]:

1. He may adopt a delinquent or criminal pattern.
2. He may become a drug addict and consequently a criminal.
3. He may passively accept his lot in life or divorce himself from it as the latent schizophrenics do.
4. He may reject the Horatio Alger myth that appears as the primary ingredient which predisposes him to the above solutions, and he may instead struggle for change in the external intolerable conditions. In so doing, the individual would change himself and the whole world around him.

It is essentially within this conceptual framework that the next group of chapters are presented.

## REFERENCES

1. Juvenal: Satires X.
2. Lipscomb, W. R.: An epidemiology of drug use-abuse, Amer. J. Public Health **61:**1794, Sept. 1971.
3. Abrams, A., Gagnon, J. H., and Levin, J. J.: Psychosocial aspects of addiction, Amer. J. Public Health **58:**2142, Nov. 1968.

**437**

*If a patient is poor he is committed to a
public hospital as "psychotic"; if he can
afford the luxury of a private sanitarium,
he is put there with the diagnosis of "neurasthenia";
if he is wealthy enough to be isolated in his own
home under constant watch of nurses and physicians
he is simply an indisposed "eccentric."*

PIERRE MARIE FELIX JANET
(1859-1947)

*La Force et la Faiblesse
psychologiques*

CHAPTER 23

# Mental illness

## THE PROBLEM WITHIN

The subjects of mental and emotional health and illness constitute one of the frontiers of public health that has been the subject of considerable exploration and activity during recent decades.[1] As a result of increasing attention from both the public and the professional press, there has developed an acute awareness of the relationship between mental illness of various types and degrees of severity and crime, violence, juvenile delinquency, prostitution, alcoholism, addictions, accidents, suicides, familial discord, occupational inadequacies, and a host of other social and physical phenomena. These are now recognized as components of what the Committee on Mental Health of the American Public Health Association has referred to as the "Social Breakdown Syndrome."[2] Similarly the public as well as the medical and health professions have become conscious of the increasing mental stresses of urban and especially of industrialized life.[3,4] Furthermore, the large number of individuals in need of professional and institutional care and the great cost of providing it have become matters of common knowledge and concern.

As with many other social problems, preliminary study and experimentation in this field derived chiefly from the interest of a few individuals and private or voluntary groups or agencies. Until relatively recent historic time, mentally ill persons were incarcerated without treatment in filthy jails and other institutions, often in company with criminals and diseased persons; they were exhibited as curiosities or sources of amusement; and they were restrained for long periods of time in chains and straightjackets, cruelly beaten, and rendered stuporous by drugs. Some were even burned at the stake on the assumption that they were witches or possessed by evil spirits. Their greatest and most courageous champion was Philippe Pinel in France, who in the 1790s agitated for reforms for their more humane treatment. His efforts to remove their chains, to have them considered victims of illness, and to transfer them from prisons to hospitals were pursued in the face of strenuous opposition and ridicule not only from the public but also from his fellow physicians. About 50 years later a similar movement got under way in the United States largely because of Dorothea Dix. During the late nineteenth century, the foundations of the related fields of psychology and psychiatry were laid, leading to consideration of possible preventive and promotive approaches to the problem that eventually crystallized in the form of the mental health movement.

The mental health movement may be said to have begun in 1908 with the publication of Clifford W. Beers' book *A Mind That Found Itself.*[5] It presented in dramatic and effective manner his experiences as a patient in several institutions for the mentally ill. The narrative ended with a plea for drastic reform and public education in mental health. Prompt encouragement and support enabled Beers to establish the first organization of its type, the Connecticut Society for Mental Hygiene. Its purpose was to combat the widespread ignorance about mental illnesses and their causes. One year later, in 1909, the National Committee for Mental Hygiene was organized. Rapid growth occurred during the ensuing two decades, as evidenced by the organization of 19 state mental hygiene societies as well as societies in 16 different nations. In 1922 the International Congress for Mental Hygiene came into being, and in 1930 it called the first International Mental Hygiene Congress in Washington, D. C.

Meanwhile a few local and state governmental units including some health departments began to introduce activities in the field of mental health. Usually they were exploratory and experimental and often were integrated with some other activities of the agency rather than identified separately. As future developments illustrated, this was a fortuitous necessity. A great stimulus came in 1946, when the National Mental Health Act (P.L. 487) was passed by Congress. It authorized $7.5 million for the construction and equipment of hospital and research facilities by the Public Health Service as a center for research and training in mental problems. Ten million dollars were provided for grants to states to expand their facilities, and an additional $1 million for demonstrations and the employment of personnel. In 1948 these responsibilities were reorganized to form the National Institute of Mental Health. By this means the act has made possible much of the expansion of thought and action that since has occurred at all levels of government in the United States and to which subsequent reference will be made.[6,7]

## NATURE AND EXTENT OF PROBLEM

In terms of both incidence and prevalence, on the one hand, and of social and economic consequences, on the other, mental illness is one of the most compelling public health problems. So widely do problems of this nature pervade all aspects of community health that Jensen,[8] a sociologist, has claimed: "If it isn't mental health, it isn't public health." Indeed, it is difficult to think of any aspect of public health work that does not have a mental or psychologic component. Mental illness, like cancer, is not a clear discrete entity. Rather it is a mixture of a variety of conditions that limit or destroy the individual's effectiveness. By now much mental illness has been clarified and classified on an organic basis. Much of what remains, including the large area of schizophrenia, is still obscure.[9] Accelerated research, however, is shedding

more light on these dark areas. Evidence has been accumulating to indicate that somatic and psychic functions are so closely related that they operate in health and illness as parts of an entity.[10] As a result, the integration of psychiatry with general medicine is considered to be the most significant trend in modern psychiatry. This is evidenced by psychiatrists' increasingly moving out of their hospitals, clinics, and consulting rooms into close relationships with other physicians and groups in the community. Similarly more work is being done in the form of family and group dynamics.

Each year in the United States over 1 million persons, including 4,000 children and youths, are treated in mental hospitals. Although only about 2% of all hospital admissions are for psychiatric disorders, about one half of the hospital beds in the nation are occupied by mentally ill patients. In addition, 1.5 million adults and children visit outpatient clinics and private physicians for psychiatric diagnosis and treatment each year. It has been estimated that about one half of all children and adults who consult private physicians for any reason have some kind of emotional disorder. Similarly it is estimated that of the 20 million patients who go to general hospitals for physical ailments each year, about 6 million have illnesses caused by emotional disturbances. There is evidence that at any given time about 1 out of every 10 persons in the country has some form of mental or emotional disorder that needs treatment. Among the many factors that contribute to the increase in mental patients are increased stresses of urbanization and industrialization, extended longevity, increased population, improved and more acceptable diagnosis, and increased facilities for diagnosis and care.

Among patients hospitalized for mental illnesses, schizophrenia is the most common condition, accounting for 45.6% of the total. The following comprises the frequency of other important conditions: mental diseases of the senium, 12.2%; manic depression, 7.6%; syphilitic psychosis, 6.7%; and psychosis with mental deficiency, 6%. Alcoholic and involutional psychoses each accounts for about 3% of those hospitalized.

The incidence of mental illness depends on many factors. Type of condition in relation to age is especially important. Most mental illnesses have their origins in early childhood but do not become manifest until the developmental or productive years of life. Despite this, schizophrenia is being diagnosed in children with increasing frequency. In general, however, when measured in terms of age at first hospitalization for mental illness, about one half are between 35 and 64 years, about one fourth are between 15 and 34 years, and about one fourth are over 65 years, whereas only slightly more than 1% are under 15 years of age. It is interesting that one of the reasons Gibson[4] gives for the increased need for psychiatric help is increased longevity. As he says, one's tendency to psychiatric breakdown increases with age, depression being more common in the middle aged and elderly and pathologic intellectual deterioration occurring most often in the older age groups. Also, as Silverman[11] describes, personal and nutritional neglect as well as more dramatic phenomena such as suicide are common manifestations of depression in the elderly.

As to type of illness, mental deficiency, epilepsy, personality disorders, and schizophrenia usually appear early in life; alcoholic and manic-depressive psychoses are centered in the middle productive years of life; whereas involutional and senile psychoses occur during the later years. Mental illness seems to be more frequent among women than among men. About 50% more women than men enter hospitals because of schizophrenia and manic-depression. The incidence of psychoneuroses appears to be about twice as common in women as in men, whereas involutional psychoses are three times as high. On the other hand, personality disorders are twice as frequent and alcoholic psychoses are about four or five times as frequent in men as in women. There is no significant difference between the sexes in the incidence of mental deficiency or of senile psychoses.

These differences by type and age are especially significant in relation to the chances for recovery and play a determining role in the enormous hospital bed requirements and treatment costs for mental illness. This is summarized in Table 23-1, which presents various mental conditions in the order of their general ultimate importance, considering numbers of persons affected, duration of illness, length of hospitalization necessary, and chances of recovery.

Some interesting socioeconomic variations may be noted in the incidence of mental illness. Thus neuroses are twice as common as the more severe psychoses among the wealthy, professional, and top managerial groups; the opposite is true among semiskilled and unskilled laborers. Another way of looking at this is that neuroses are twice as common in the higher than in the lower socioeconomic groups, whereas severe psychoses occur about twice as frequently in the lower than in the higher socioeconomic groups of the population. Part of these discrepancies may result from a greater awareness of and economic ability to seek medical attention for neuroses by the more educated and affluent. Similarly many in the lower socioeconomic group may not consider neurosis as an illness

**Table 23-1.** Hospitalization for mental illness by age, sex, and chance of recovery

| Condition | Usual age at first admission | First admissions (%) | | | Hospitalized mental patients (%) | Chances of recovery |
|---|---|---|---|---|---|---|
| | | Men | Women | Both | | |
| Schizophrenia | 16-35 | 18.6 | 26.8 | 22.6 | 45.6 | Poor after age 50; long hospitalization |
| Manic-depressive psychosis | 35-50 | 3.1 | 5.3 | 4.2 | 7.6 | Poor; long hospitalization |
| Psychosis with mental deficiency | 15-44 | 2.7 | 1.8 | 2.3 | 6.0 | Poor; long hospitalization |
| Alcoholic psychosis | 25-54 | 21.8 | 5.2 | 13.7 | 3.0 | Fair; short hospitalization |
| Involutional psychosis | 48-58 | 3.0 | 8.3 | 5.6 | 3.0 | Poor; die soon; short hospitalization |
| Senile psychosis | 60+ | 21.1 | 20.5 | 20.8 | 12.2 | Poor; die soon; short hospitalization |
| Personality disorders (nonalcoholic) | 15-34 | 7.2 | 3.9 | 5.6 | 4.0 | Fair; short hospitalization |
| Psychoneurotic | 25-44 | 6.3 | 12.4 | 9.3 | 6.0 | Fair; short hospitalization |
| Other disorders, each of low incidence | All ages | 16.2 | 15.8 | 15.9 | 12.6 | Generally poor; long hospitalization |

in relation to the pressures from many other problems.[12,13] On the other hand, some of the causes of the more severe psychoses are more prevalent in the environments and family milieus of the socioeconomically deprived. Gibson[4] notes that the higher one is on the socioeconomic scale the less the chance will be of developing a psychologic illness, except manic-depressive psychosis.

At present the most dramatic and effective role is being played by pharmacologic research.[14,15] The discovery of the ataraxics or tranquilizers has revolutionized both inpatient and outpatient care. Many who previously would have been institutionalized now are not because the length of institutional stay has been shortened significantly. Indeed the very atmosphere of mental institutions has changed dramatically. The year 1955 was the turning point. In that year the number of patients discharged from institutions increased sharply and the number of persons institutionalized declined. Further evidence of the effect is that in 1964, although there were 300,000 admissions to state and county mental hospitals, the largest number in history, the number of resident patients on any one day dropped below 500,000 for the first time in 15 years. By 1971 the average daily census had dropped almost to 300,000 patients. The economic saving to society inherent in this decline of hospitalized patients hence tax funds required for hospitalization is tremendous.

The limitations of data restricted to hospitalization are obvious. Many individuals receive some psychiatric guidance through public and private medical facilities other than hospitals, but the amount is unknown. Many more are in need of varying degrees of assistance for relatively minor personality adjustment and psychiatric problems but never receive it. In many ways the latter represents perhaps the greatest social and economic aspect of the total problem. It has been estimated that the overall annual cost of mental illness in the United States is about $21 billion, of which about 43% is borne by those other than the mentally ill or their families. The average annual cost is about $5,400 per patient. Almost $2 billion of the total represents the cost of care and maintenance in public mental hospitals. The cost to the Veterans Administration is $1.25 billion per year. Then there is the cost of care rendered in community mental health centers and by private psychiatrists. The value of the extensive

mental health counseling by other private physicians, public health nurses, family counselors, social workers, clergymen, and others is, of course, unknown.[16]

The possibility of insuring against the costs of mental illness naturally arises. Although several health insurance organizations and plans that operate their own facilities have psychiatrists on their staffs and some provide mental health clinics, only rarely do they include the costs of psychiatric treatment among their benefits. The few that have attempted to do so have encountered substantial difficulties. Among these, Reed[17] has listed high costs in a setting where all types of health insurance plans are finding their costs expanding; the indeterminateness of these costs, particularly when care over a long period in a hospital or physician's office is required; the question of how mental hospitals in this country should be financed and of demarcation of the respective roles of patient, private insurance, and government in financing mental hospital care; and a rather complete lack of information as to what the utilization of psychiatric services would be if they were available on an insured basis. Nevertheless, forward movement has been under way. An increasing number of state Blue Cross and Blue Shield plans have included provision for payment of certain psychiatric services. The 1967 amendments to the Social Security Act expanded significantly the benefits under Medicare and Medicaid for the mentally ill.[18] Beyond this the movement toward the development of comprehensive health maintenance organization implies an increase in community mental health resources. Meanwhile, following a contract negotiated in 1964 between the United Auto Workers and the automobile and agricultural implement industries under which about 2.5 million workers and their families will receive coverage for psychiatric care, plans have been made for a study of the effect on the provision and ability of community mental health services.[19]

## DEFINITION AND GOAL OF MENTAL HEALTH

Mental health represents a broad field and one that is difficult to define. Potentially there are few if any areas of public health with which it is unrelated and to which it cannot make a real contribution. The increased provision of facilities and the improvement of techniques for treatment of the mentally ill are not, of course, the complete or ultimate goals. Rather, the primary concerns include improved and increased detection of psychiatric and prepsychiatric conditions that may result in personal and social handicaps, the study of their causes, and the initiation of efforts to eliminate as far as possible the factors that bring them about. Thus the goal may be considered a more satisfying and effective life, free of adverse mental deterrents for more people or, to state it even more simply, the development of emotionally mature people.

Lemkau,[20] in his excellent discussion of the field of mental health, outlined its goals and indicated that desirable program content should be two dimensional. He points out that the vertical or categorical dimension, consisting of early diagnosis and treatment of existing mental ills, as in the case of tuberculosis control, meets several needs: (1) the prevention of the development of more serious and handicapping illness, (2) the removal of sources of stress from family and social environments, and (3) the making available of the services of specialist personnel to the broader horizontal aims of the mental health program. The horizontal goals of mental health he visualizes in terms of the work of every member of the health agency being influenced by mental health principles. Some of the many ways be which this may be accomplished follows.

## MENTAL HEALTH PROGRAMS

Because of the relative newness of the field of mental health as a broadly applied social responsibility and the amount of exploration occurring, it is not possible to state clearly what a mental health program should include or who is or should be administering it. However, a consideration of some of the activities that already have been attempted is of some interest.

The National Mental Health Act passed in 1946 provided federal grants-in-aid to states for research, training, and assistance in the establishment and development of community mental health programs, particularly for the prevention and early treatment of mental and emotional disorders. A particularly noteworthy result of the act was the establishment several years later of the National Institute of Mental Health. This institute has provided national leadership of high quality. Already significant progress may be noted in having made state public health personnel aware of mental health and in integrating it into various parts of their programs and activities. Within 4 years after the passage of the act specifically identified bu-

reaus, divisions, or sections for mental health were founded in 28 state public health agencies, and in several others a consultant in mental health served on the staff, usually of the bureau or division of preventive medical services. At the present time the functions of these mental health units variously include the maintenance of lists or rosters of mental health facilities; the gathering of reports or data on mental health needs and problems; the development of and assistance to state and local, lay and professional educational programs; the direct operation of mental health clinics, inpatient facilities, and day-care centers; the promulgation of rules and regulations relating to mental health and the administration of certain aspects of some of them; financial assistance to local agencies; promotional, supervisory, and consultative services to local official and voluntary agencies; and special surveys and research. In mid-1963 another milestone occurred in the fight against mental illness in the United States in the form of P.L. 88-164, the Mental Retardation Facilities and Community Mental Health Centers Construction Act. Its purpose was to assist all levels of government to deal more vigorously with the problems of mental illness and mental retardation. In addition to providing more funds for research it also authorized grants to states for the construction of additional community mental health centers, the extension of community mental health preventive and promotive programs, and the initial staffing of these facilities and programs.[21] The purpose of the act was extended and strengthened in 1965 by an amendment (P.L. 89-105), which provided additional support for community-based programs for the care of the mentally ill and encouraged general hospitals to become major community psychiatric resources.

However, as DuVal and Venable[22] have indicated, the greatest hindrances to the development of truly efficient and effective community mental health services have been the lack of coordination and cooperation among the agencies on the several levels of government, on the one hand, and between public or community health advocates and mental health advocates, on the other. With reference to the former, significant progress has been achieved in recent years, and more is anticipated. Thus the states have been provided with federal stimulus and assistance to enact legislation for the establishment of community mental health services boards and the provision to them of state matching funds for the extension and coordination of mental health activities. Improvement of the second hindrance, however, is still subject to question. It is true that throughout its history the field of public health generally gave less than adequate attention and leadership to various aspects of mental health and related fields. This, plus the fact that psychiatry had developed along a mind-body distinction and a one-to-one concept, led the American Psychiatric Association in the early 1960s to adopt an official position that community mental health services as they developed should function through separate departments of mental health. As a consequence, there has developed a situation in which, whereas mental health services are carried on in all states and territories, responsibility is divided among departments of public health, mental health, and welfare, or institutions, as well as in some instances special boards or commissions. Understandably this resulted in considerable anguish among many public health workers, inefficiency from the viewpoint of responsible governmental managers, and confusion for the public. In most circumstances, adoption of reasonable methods of coordination and cooperation have appeared unreasonably difficult to achieve.

It is interesting to note that by 1967 the Conference on Education in Psychiatry of the American Psychiatric Association regarded the mind-body distinction and the one-to-one approach anachronistic and strongly endorsed training and practice to be comprehensive in the total-person sense and in the form of group and community action. Meanwhile, as DuVal and Venable[22] note, both public health and mental health are in active ferment: "In some states each . . . appears to be moving in a different path and often in a different direction, as both search for new methods of approaching the same problems." Still holding the beliefs that the mind and body are irrevocably related parts of the whole and that "in union there is strength," they urge the development, not of a single organizational model, but of a variety of bilaterally endorsed and supported accommodations based on the customs, mores, relationships, responsibilities, and authorities of the different governmental jurisdictions. This seems reasonable and must come about. It must be realized by all that solutions to the exceedingly complex problems of mental health, especially as they impinge on or are effected by physical health, society, and the environment, cannot be found within any single group or profession. This has been emphasized by Felix and Kramer[23]: "Because of the complexity of the problem, effective research on the community aspects of mental illness must be interdisciplinary, combining the skills and knowledge of the psychiatrist, psychologist, social scientist, public health physician and nurse, psychiatric social worker, epidemiologist, and statistician." This was also clearly indicated in the report of the National Health Assembly,[24] which stated: "Clergymen, teachers, lawyers, social workers, nurses, recreation and group workers, law enforcement officers, public health personnel, representatives of management and labor, and many others, are constantly presented with opportunities for recognizing emotional problems." A most important omission by each of these listings, and perhaps the key group toward which the efforts of all of the others should be primarily aimed, are parents—both actual and prospective. These important concepts have been clearly illustrated by Blain and Robinson,[25] as shown in Fig. 23-1.

As of 1968, more than 2,280 psychiatric outpatient clinics were reported to be in operation in the United States in contrast with fewer than 500 in 1947. They served an estimated 1.5 million persons during the year.[16] To be considered adequate for reporting purposes, it is necessary that a center be staffed at least by a psychiatrist, a clinical psychologist, and a psychiatric social worker. The clinics are located in all states and territories with the exception of Nevada. However, more than half of the clinics are in the northeastern states, which have only one quarter of the total population. State governments operate 41% of the clinics, and another 23% receive some state aid; 5% are operated by the Veterans Administration.

As has been implied, the relationship between the staff of the mental health center or program and the personnel of the official public health agency sometimes presents an administrative problem. It involves especially the relationship between the psychiatric social workers and the public health nursing staff. The obvious goal is for the public health nurses and the psychiatric social worker to look on each other as sources of referral and as a resource for consultation, advice, and in-service education. This can best be accomplished through joint planning, joint conferences, and joint in-service training. Perhaps the key consideration to be kept in mind

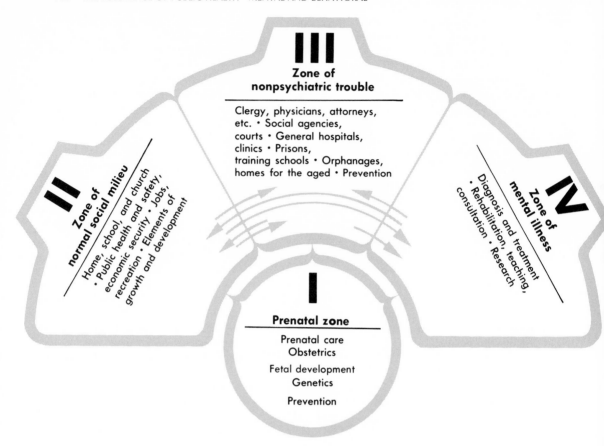

**Fig. 23-1.** Population and service zones in relation to mental health and illness. (Modified from Blain, D., and Robinson, R. L.: New York J. Med., Jan. 15, 1957.)

by the nursing staff is that social work, especially as it relates to the mentally disturbed, is a specialized field. In turn the limited numbers of psychiatrically trained social workers must recognize that they are physically incapable of making all the contacts and of meeting all the needs and that public health nurses have wide and well-established contacts and entrée throughout the community. Beyond this, all concerned, including the health officer and the director of the mental health center, should bear in mind that the promotion and maintenance of smooth and fruitful interpersonnel and interprofessional relationships is in itself a manifestation of sound mental health and in turn is a prerequisite to the planning, development, and implementation of an effective community mental health program.[26]

### ROLE OF THE HEALTH DEPARTMENT

At an Institute on Mental Health in Public Health held in the University of California at Berkeley in 1948[27] it was agreed that one of the most important problems for health departments at that time was to clarify their responsibilities in their communities with respect to mental health in order that citizens and other agencies might know what to expect. It was thought that unless effective organization took place among the various agencies concerned with the problem and unless each understood its specific role and the roles of the others, confusion would result. Unhappily a large proportion of health departments have yet to clarify their positions and roles, and confusion still exists. This has also been indicated in the report of the Joint Commission on Mental Illness and Health[28] not only with reference to public health but also in relation to most other types of agencies.

Aronson[29] has proposed that the health officer, in attempting to face the challenge of the mental health problem, should turn to well-established patterns used so successfully in the control of communicable disease. First, he looks for broad, well-documented epidemiologic patterns. Second he searches for elements in existing programs that most nearly meet the needs of those patterns. Finally, he explores ways to use existing personnel in the new areas of activity. He emphasizes the opportunity for the health officer "to act as a catalyst—to be the voice of the community, in calling for the co-ordination of the variety of services and efforts being made by a number of agencies, in pointing out imbalance and gaps in available services, and in securing the widest community support for a broad spectrum of mental health services consistent with recognized scientific evidence and readily available to all who need them."

Others[30,31] have suggested health department activities to orient and train its own staff and personnel of other community agencies in mental health and illness, to provide diagnostic and referral services as well as community follow-up after discharge of patients from psychiatric hospitals, to operate community mental health clinics and day-care centers for mentally retarded children, to cooperate with industrial mental health programs, and to educate the public in mental health. In addition, attention is directed to the important psychologic and psychiatric implications of children institutionalized for any reason: geriatric problems, alcoholism, suicide, marital and other family discord, crime and delinquency, and accident proneness. Some of these are discussed elsewhere in this book. To assist the public health agency in defining and developing its role the American Public Health Association has developed a useful handbook on mental disorders and their control.[32] In addition, attention is directed to a highly provocative series of presentations on the potentials for mental health involvement by the various components of traditional health agencies.[33]

## FUTURE OF COMMUNITY MENTAL HEALTH

With the ever-increasing complexity of American society, the accelerating pace of living, and the concentrations of people, it would appear that mental and emotional problems would tend to increase in the years ahead. Offsetting this to a significant extent is the increase in understanding of human behavior and the continuing advances in psychopharmacology. For the immediate future certainly more community-based facilities are needed. In 1964 Felix[34] envisioned

them as multiservice centers designed to provide preventive services, early diagnosis, and treatment of mental illness on both an inpatient and outpatient basis, and to serve as a locus for the aftercare of discharged hospital patients. He itemized the spectrum of services to include the following:

A general diagnostic and evaluation service (precare)
An acute inpatient service and an outpatient service
A day-care service and a night-care service
An emergency service available around the clock
Rehabilitation services
Consultation services
Public information and education services
Supervision of foster homes
Research and training

By means of these he believed true continuity of mental and emotional care would become possible to the enormous advantage of the patient and of the community of which he is a member. Fortunately it is now possible to point to many such comprehensive community mental health facilities that have developed during the ensuing decade.[35,36] Thus aid for stressful mental problems is being brought ever closer to the people and the sources of their problems. The importance of the establishment and operation of 24-hour emergency mental health facilities deserves particular emphasis.[37] Although it appears in Felix's list, actually it relates to many of the other needs in the list. Furthermore, its importance to problems discussed in the next four chapters is self-evident.

Dreizel,[38] in his perceptive work on the social organization of health, states:

The creation of mental hospitals was a great achievement for the nineteenth century. For the first time mentally disturbed persons were ascribed the role of the sick and treated accordingly. However, these hospitals, in which most psychotics are still kept, are . . . "total hospitals" with an internal power structure and the norms of a community of prisoners. Though once a humane alternative to almshouses and jails, they serve today as asylums for the socially unwanted, radically isolating the patient from his family, neighborhood, and work. They thus more often than not function as a self-fulfilling prophecy, producing in the patient the illness that originally served as a pretext to run him in, rather than providing help for his life problems.

Among the rewards of biochemical and surgical approaches to mental illness and the development of community mental health centers during recent years has been the opportunity for increasing numbers of patients to avoid or escape from the confines of the artificial and generally unhelpful closed institutional environments of the not-so-distant past back to the more normal environment whence they came and wherein may be some true hope and opportunity of social reentry. It is good to read of the announcement by Great Britain at the Fifth World Congress on Psychiatry held in Mexico City in 1971 that it plans to close all its mental hospitals within the next 15 years. Let us hope that all nations may look forward to a similar eventuality.

## REFERENCES

1. Sanders, D. S.: A bookshelf on mental health, Amer. J. Public Health **55:**502, April 1965.
2. Gruenberg, E. M., et al.: Social breakdown syndrome: environmental and host factors associated with chronicity, Amer. J. Public Health **62:**91, Jan. 1972.
3. Society, stress and disease, Report of symposia, WHO Chron. **25:**168, April 1971.
4. Gibson, A. C.: Stress disorders of modern life, Roy. Soc. Health J. **91:**172, April 1971.
5. Beers, C. W.: A mind that found itself, New York, 1948, Doubleday & Co., Inc.
6. U. S. Public Health Service: The national mental health program and the states, PHS pub. no. 629, Washington, D. C., 1959.
7. National Institute of Mental Health: The National Institute of Mental Health, NIMH pub. no. 5027, Rockville, Md., 1970.
8. Jensen, H. E.: Mental health: a local public health responsibility, Ment. Hyg. **37:**530, Oct. 1953.
9. Causes of mental disorders: a review of epidemiological knowledge, Proceedings of a symposium, New York, 1961, Milbank Memorial Fund.
10. Lapouse, R.: Problems in studying the prevalence of psychiatric disorder, Amer. J. Public Health **57:**947, June 1967.
11. Silverman, C.: The epidemiology of depression, Baltimore, 1968, The Johns Hopkins Press.
12. Halpert, H. P.: Surveys of public opinions and attitudes about mental illness, Public Health Rep. **80:**589, July 1965.
13. King, S. H.: Perceptions of illness and medical practice, New York, 1962, Russell Sage Foundation.
14. Drugs for the troubled mind, **5:**2, Med. World News, March 13, 1964.
15. Kline, N. S., Kris, E. B., Ayd, F. J., and Cameron, W. R.: Symposium on psychopharmacology and community mental health services, Amer. J. Public Health vol. 52 (supp.), Sept. 1962.
16. What are the facts about mental illness in the United States? New York, 1971, National Health Education Commission.
17. Reed, L. S.: Health insurance coverage for mental illness, Public Health Rep. **73:**185, Feb. 1958.
18. National Institute of Mental Health: Mental health benefits of Medicare and Medicaid, PHS pub. no. 1505, Rockville, Md., 1969.
19. Editorial: Insurance coverage for psychiatric care, Public Health Rep. **80:**1118, Dec. 1965.
20. Lemkau, P. V.: Mental hygiene and public health, New York, 1955, McGraw-Hill Book Co.
21. Felix, R. H.: The national mental health program, Amer. J. Public Health **54:**1804, Nov. 1964.
22. DuVal, A. M., and Venable, J. H.: Mental health and public health—organization of state services, Amer. J. Public Health **57:**878, May 1967.
23. Felix, R. H., and Kramer, M.: Research in epidemiology of mental illness, Public Health Rep. **67:**160, Feb. 1952.
24. America's health—a report to the nation by the National Health Assembly, New York, 1948, Harper & Row, Publishers.
25. Blain, D., and Robinson, R. L.: Personnel shortages in psychiatric services, a shift of emphasis, New York J. Med. **57:**257, Jan. 15, 1957.
26. Coleman, J.: Relations between mental health and public health, Amer. J. Public Health **46:**805, July 1956.
27. Ginsberg, E. L.: Public health is people, New York, 1950, Commonwealth Fund.
28. Action for mental health, Report of Joint Committee on Mental Illness and Health, New York, 1961, Basic Books, Inc.
29. Aronson, J. B.: Mental health and the local health department, Amer. J. Public Health **51:**89, Jan. 1961.
30. Sparer, P. J.: Mental hygiene in a modern health department program, Amer. J. Public Health **51:**892, June 1961.
31. Turner, W. E., Smith, D. C., and Medley, P.: Integration of mental health into public health programs—advantages and disadvantages, Amer. J. Public Health **57:**1322, Aug. 1967.
32. Mental disorders: a guide to control methods, New York, 1962, American Public Health Association.
33. Goldston, S. E., editor: Mental health considerations in public health: a guide for training and practice, PHS pub. no. 1898, Rockville, Md., 1969, National Institute of Mental Health.
34. Felix, R. H.: A model for comprehensive mental health centers, Amer. J. Public Health **54:**1964, Dec. 1964.
35. National Institute of Mental Health: The comprehensive community mental health center, PHS pub. no. 2136, Rockville, Md., 1970.
36. Feldman, S., and Goldstein, H. H.: Community mental health centers in the United States: an overview, Int. J. Nurs. Stud. **8:**247, Aug. 1971.
37. Resnik, H. L. P., and Ruben, H. L., editors: Emergency psychiatric care, Bowie, Md., 1974, Charles Press Publishers.
38. Dreizel, H. P.: The social organization of health, New York, 1971, The Macmillan Co.

*To be, or not to be:–that is the question:–*
*Whether 'tis nobler in the mind to suffer*
*The slings and arrows of outrageous fortune,*
*Or to take arms against a sea of troubles,*
*And by opposing end them?*

HAMLET (III. I)

CHAPTER 24

# Suicide*

## HOW GREAT THE PROBLEM

Hamlet's question is one that many people ask themselves at some time or another and it is a question to which many respond by some form of self-destructive act. Unquestionably suicide is the most frequently concealed of the major causes of disability and death. Furthermore, as Schneidman[4] emphasizes, "Suicide is the first leading cause of *unnecessary* and *stigmatizing* deaths." Each year more than 22,000 suicides are reported in the United States.[5] This is equivalent to the deaths from all of the infectious and parasitic diseases including among others tuberculosis, influenza, meningitis, and the enteritides. However, various authorities consider the true incidence to be two or three times the reported number.[6] This places its toll at more than that attributed to vehicular accidents or possibly 2.5% of all deaths. World wide, the World Health Organization estimates that each year more than 500,000 successful suicides occur. This is the equivalent of the entire population of Richmond, Nashville, or Salt Lake City. In addition, it is estimated that there are about ten times as many attempts as there are successful suicides—the equivalent of the populations of Pittsburgh or Seattle for the United States, or in relation to the world-wide figures the combination of Los Angeles and Philadelphia, or of Vienna, Paris, and Copenhagen, or of Rio de Janeiro and Montevideo.

---

*For a comprehensive review of the literature, see Farberow.[1] For excellent current overviews of all aspects of the subject, see Resnik and Hathorne[2] and Schneidman and co-authors.[3]

Official international death rates for suicides vary from 2 to 25 per 100,000 population. The highest rates for both sexes are reported from Germany (Democratic Republic), Hungary, Austria, Finland, Switzerland, Japan, and Denmark. The lowest rates are in Italy, Spain, Ireland, the nonwhite population of the United States, Columbia, and Costa Rica.[7] However, such data must be regarded with considerable scepticism, since they are significantly affected by customs and mores, the quality and quantity of medical care, the frequency and accuracy of autopsies, official vital statistical procedures, and many other factors. For example, as McCulloch and Philip[8] point out, even in Great Britain where public records are accurate, Northern Ireland has a rate of one half that of England, with Scotland and Wales between the two. As they indicate, it is probably not coincidental that the attitude of the law to suicidal acts over the years has tended to be punitive in Northern Ireland in contrast to indifference in England and Scotland. Whatever the reservations, the fact is that suicide now ranks as the third leading cause of death among persons 15 to 45 years of age in the 8 leading industrialized countries of the world.

## SUICIDE OR ACCIDENT?

A comparison has been made between suicidal and vehicular accident deaths. In this regard McCulloch and Philip[8] have stated:

. . . suicidal behavior, especially completed suicide, tends to be ignored as a public health or social action problem by all but a few bodies. It seems anomalous

447

that death by suicide should be so treated, while road fatalities, which account for approximately the same number of deaths per year, are combated by publicity campaigns and legislation which attempt to change people's attitudes and behavior. It is strange that road deaths, where the human factor looms no larger than it does in suicide and where in some cases there are suicidal connotations, strike people as being untimely and avoidable while these sentiments are felt less often about suicide and other forms of disease.

The question of the use of the automobile as a suicidal agent is therefore important.[9] A relationship has been suspected for some years, but only relatively recently has it been subjected to study by means of the technique of "psychological autopsy."[10-12] This involves reconstruction of the life-style and personality of the deceased and a careful inquiry into recent events and behavior. Interviews are conducted with his spouse, mature children, parents, physicians, employers, friends, and others who knew him well to determine on a probability basis whether the deceased died accidentally or intentionally. Using this method, in combination with site and vehicle inspections and toxicologic analyses, several studies in American cities indicate that perhaps 15% of fatal automobile crashes are conscious, goal-directed suicides. On these and similar bases it has been estimated that as many as 8,000 of the 55,000 deaths from motor vehicular accidents each year in the United States should be more properly attributed to suicide.

There appear to be some interesting similarities and differences between *true* suicides and *true* accidents. For example, it has been noted that in about one half of both fatal accidents and suicides the subjects had been drinking alcohol prior to their deaths and that drinking had been used frequently as a method of response to problems in their lives. One difference is that those who die by accident do not appear to have encountered any clear psychologically traumatic situation just before the fatal event. This is in contrast with suicides who have suffered recent losses (death, money, affluence, status) and who tend to be more closely integrated and involved with others. However, it is interesting that true accident victims, more often than not, are involved in potential or recent moves to situations of greater responsibility. They also tend to be hypersensitive to criticism, relatively exhibitionistic, and poorly integrated with others.[13]

The foregoing begs the question of definition or determination of suicide. This is not always simple. Frequently it can be established fairly easily that an injury or poisoning was deliberately self-inflicted. Whether or not actual death was the intended goal, however, is less easy to determine. Often the act is essentially a reaction to a crisis of despair or despondency and represents a dramatic appeal for help, an attempt to attract attention, a means of spiting others, or submitting one's self to trial by ordeal. It should be recognized that many individuals engage in various forms of the last few of these, subconsciously if not consciously, while driving, engaging in certain sports, or in choosing certain occupations. Then there is the dilemma that results from an individual *not* doing something necessary to the protection or preservation of life—not taking insulin or not wearing automobile seat belts. Certainly some deaths attributed to diabetes and certain cardiac and other ailments are actually willful suicides carried out by the simple expedient of inaction, the intent of which is unprovable. To place the problem in a rational context Shneidman[14] pointed out that whereas deaths from a bullet, a vehicle, a poison, or an infection may be classified as a homicide, an accident, a suicide, or a disease, as far as the individual affected is concerned they are all simply threats to life or means to death.

## EPIDEMIOLOGY OF SUICIDE

Despite the difficulties indicated in the introduction, much is known about the epidemiology of suicide. An interesting observation is that *actual* suicide presents a different age pattern from *attempted* suicide. The incidence of suicide increases with age, climbing from a rate of 0.3 per 100,000 among those 5 to 14 years of age to more than 24 per 100,000 in persons over 75 years. For both sexes the mode is in the late forties. Suicidal attempts, on the other hand, are most common in young people, being highest in the late teens and early twenties. Contrary to common belief, Litman,[15] Co-director of the Los Angeles Suicide Prevention Center, in discussing the approximately 100,000 self-poisonings each year in the United States involving children between the ages of 6 and 17 years, estimated that on the basis of his studies not only were 75% intentional but more than 25% were attempted suicides. This coincides with the findings of a similar study[16] of 1,103 poisoned patients, aged 6 to 18 years, admitted to the emergency departments of a group of midwestern hospitals. The conclusion was that self-poisoning in that age group is rarely accidental. Boys predominated in the 6- to 10-year-old group, but after 11 years of age girls showed an abrupt increase in self-poisoning. However, a significant relative increase was observed among boys 17 to 18 years old, entirely independent of drug use. The investigators noted that the histories of children and youths involved in self-poisoning, suicidal attempts, and suicide seemed to be patterned into what they called "the five Ps"—privation (either poverty or privilege), parents, peers, punctured romance, and pregnancy. The importance of pregnancy among certain groups as a factor in teen-age suicidal attempts has been emphasized by several investigators.[17] In the United States it is commonly estimated that about 1 out of every 1,000 teen-agers attempts suicide.[18] Some investigators, such as Jacobziner[19] and Ross[20] however, believe suicidal attempts by young people to be much more common, perhaps in the ratio of 1 out of every 100 individuals. In their detailed studies in Edinburgh, McCulloch and Philip[8] note that currently 1 teen-ager in every 250 deliberately poisons or injures himself, a rate almost double that of the mid-1960s! An adequate explanation is yet to be found.

Especially tragic is the incidence of suicide among college students for whom it is considered, on the basis of numerous studies, the second leading cause of death (after accidents) and a 50% greater risk than among nonstudents of the same ages.[21] Enigmatically it is noted that texts on "college health" rarely give more than a few paragraphs' attention if any to this important problem. In recognition of the problem, however, colleges increasingly are establishing "hot lines" so that troubled or suicidal students can call for help or advice. Fox[22] makes the cogent observation that ". . . the student who takes his life represents the tip of an iceberg of youthful distress. The more we can learn of it, the better we can understand the mass with emotional problems falling short of fatality. Furthermore, any measures designed to prevent suicide must serve also to relieve distress at other levels." Ross and others have pointed to the collegiate atmosphere of intense competition, rapid social mobility, and expectations greater than can be realized by many students. Drugs, incidentally, have been found to play little if any role in the picture. There

have been some indications that students who achieve high or even highest scholastic grades are more likely to attempt suicide, perhaps because they often place greater demands on themselves than do their professors, schools, or parents. Although depression is the most frequently noted precursor, Ayd[23] points out that suicide in the young is usually an impetuous act which occurs soon after a real or imagined wrong or failure and at a time when the young person has been manifesting personality and behavioral changes. "Thus," he concludes, "prior to age 30 it is the tense, confused, and deluded schizophrenic and not the depressed person who commits suicide, whereas after age 30 it is primarily the depressed manic-depressives, including the involutional melancholics, and the chronic alcoholics who take their own lives." The distinctions become greater in the advanced years of life. In his studies of the psychodynamics of suicide among almost 7,000 elderly patients, Seidel[24] found the following factors significant: an increasing failure of psychophysical capacity, affective changes associated with aging, poor integration, a tendency toward hypochondria and paranoia, a feeling of rapid passage of time and the nearness of death, the loss of influences that give life a meaning and value, and restricted social existence.

Suicide is observed three times as frequently among males as among females, although more women appear to attempt suicide than do men. In recent years the gap has been narrowing with a rise in female attempts. Possibly this is one of several prices to be paid by women for their increased emancipation, or liberation and the resultant changing role of women in society. A similar increase is being noted with regard to hypertension, coronary heart disease, cancer of the lung related to smoking, and other stress-related conditions. Among the races, suicide is four times as common among whites as among blacks, although some investigators have noted more attempts among blacks. It should also be noted that suicide rates for blacks have begun to move upward in recent years. The phenomenon is highest among Orientals. This appears to be essentially culture linked. If age, sex, and race are considered together, some interesting contrasts are seen. Among white males in the United States suicide death rates increase consistently with each age group from 9.3 per 100,000 males between 15 and 24 years to 65.1 per 100,000 in those 85 years and older. Among white females, rates peak at 12.5 per 100,000 among those 45 to 54 years, then decrease. The rate for nonwhite males peaks at 16.2 per 100,000 between ages 25 to 34 years, then levels off. For nonwhite females the peak is also between 25 to 34 years, but much lower, 4.7 per 100,000, and declines from there.

There are significant variations depending on marital status.[25] Below the age of 35 years single women are more a suicidal risk than are single men, but after 35 years this is reversed. Although married women tend to have higher rates than single women of comparable age, this is not true of men. Under 35 years of age both single and married men have comparable rates, but among those over 35 years the suicide rate for single men is double that of those who are married. Contrary to what is often assumed, rates for those widowed are low, but among those who are divorced or separated the rates are extremely high. This difference may be related to some of the personality and behavioral characteristics involved in many divorces or separations.

Successful suicides are more common among the more affluent and better educated than among the economically and educationally poor. With reference to occupation, laborers, miners, teachers, and clergymen have low suicide rates in contrast with high rates among entertainers, artists, businessmen, the military, and professionals, especially dentists, lawyers, and physicians. It is interesting that rates among the military are highest during peacetime, but rates for the military and most other groups drop sharply when a nation is confronted with a military emergency. Among the professions those in medicine and especially psychiatrists and psychoanalysts have the highest rate. Indeed, the annual suicide rate among physicians in the United States is at least 33 per 100,000, three times the national average, and among psychiatrists and psychoanalysts the rate is an astounding 70 per 100,000 per year. Among the conjectured reasons for high rates among physicians and psychiatrists are the tendency to suppressed and introspective personalities, confrontation and preoccupation with morbid situations, ready availability of drugs and poisons, and limitation of family and social life.[26] In their studies in Edinburgh, Sainsbury and Barraclough[27] discovered an interesting contrast with reference to attempted suicides. One tenth of attempted suicides occurred among families of professionals and middle management personnel, one tenth occurred among families of skilled occupations, two tenths occurred among families of skilled workers, and four tenths occurred among families of unskilled workers. They recognize, however, that more affluent individuals are more likely to be quietly treated in their own homes or even hospitals than are the less affluent. Based on this and other observations they conclude that social class is largely irrelevant and that potential or actual suicides resemble each other more than nonsuicidal persons of their own social class.

## ENVIRONMENT AND SUICIDE

Many aspects of the environment appear to influence suicidal tendencies. The further west one goes in the United States the higher become the rates. The meaning of this is not clear. Suicide rates are also higher in the temperate than in the colder or warmer climates. They also rise with altitude. An interesting study in Philadelphia showed a rise whenever the barometer dropped. Contrary to what many would expect, the phenomenon is more common in the United States during the months of May and June and on clear sunny days. A similar contradiction is its more frequent occurrence early in the week, on a Monday or Tuesday morning soon after arising, rather than at the end of a possibly long and arduous week. Interestingly, in Edinburgh, April and November account for one fourth of all suicides, and weekends and holidays have particularly high rates with midweek the lowest. Obviously a knowledge of local time-occurrence relationships is important for effective program planning so that suicide peak hours, days, and seasons will be related to ready availability of staff resources.

Suicide rates are higher in central cities than in suburbs, which in turn are more threatened than rural areas or small towns, where it is less difficult to be unknown. Suicide is more common among immigrants than among the native born. Religion plays an important role; rates are highest among those who follow Oriental religions, next highest among Protestants and Reformed Jews, low among Roman Catholics, and very low among Orthodox Jews.

An aspect of the environment that calls for detailed study is the effect of mass communications media on suicide. Although it did not address itself specifically to suicide, the Surgeon General's Scientific Advisory Committee on Television and Social Behavior[28] did find evidence of some relationship between violent types of television programs and aggressiveness in children. More directly to the point are studies that indicate that news media may stimulate destructive action in young people by vivid and detailed portrayal and sometimes even glorification of various forms of destructive behavior. This certainly appeared to play some role in the epidemic of campus violence during the late 1960s. If this can be true of externalized violence, why not internalized violence? It appears significant that during the 268-day "news blackout" in Detroit between November 1967 and August 1968, the suicide rate in both sexes and all age groups dropped significantly.[29]

## METHODS

A wide variety of methods are used by individuals intent on terminating their existence. Women tend to use nonviolent or nondisfiguring methods, apparently maintaining some concern about their appearance even after death. An analysis[30] of the methods used by over 20,000 Americans who committed suicide in 1964 is shown in Table 24-1.

Incidentally, some question may be raised concerning the validity of the data for hanging and strangulation as well as for some of the other methods listed because of erotic implications in some instances.[31,32]

During recent decades, and especially in the United States, a significant shift in method has been noted. Although firearms and explosives still rank far above other methods (58%) and hanging and strangulation is still second, poisonings especially with drugs and pharmaceuticals have become more common. Thus between 1950 and 1964 the use of drugs rose from 5% to 12.4% and of gas, including automotive fumes,

**Table 24-1.** Methods used in successful suicides, United States, 1964

| Method | Percentage |
|---|---|
| Firearms and explosives | 47.2 |
| Hanging and strangulation | 14.7 |
| Analgesics and soporifics | 12.4 |
| Gases | 11.5 |
| Other solid and liquid substances | 3.6 |
| Jumping from high places | 3.6 |
| Submersion (drowning) | 2.6 |
| Piercing instruments | 1.8 |
| Other and unspecified means | 2.6 |
| Total | 100.0 |

from 6% to 11.5%. Barbiturates now account for 75% of drug-related suicides.

## SUICIDE AND THE LAW

The attitude of the law toward suicide, as Silving[33] well summarizes, depends on the prevailing ethics in a particular place at a particular time. As she indicates, whereas most monotheistic religions prohibit suicide, they are sometimes inconsistent. For example, Buddhism forbids the killing of any form of life yet recognizes suicide as a religious practice under certain circumstances. Similarly there may be social approval of suicide on the basis of national honor or security. Generally, throughout history governments and their laws have frowned on suicide. According to Blackstone, the great English legal commentator, in ancient Athens attempted suicide was punished by cutting off the hand that committed the forbidden deed. Another approach was described by Plutarch in relation to an epidemic of suicides among women in Milesia, who for certain reasons preferred death to matrimony. The epidemic was brought to a stop by a decree that the bodies of those who committed suicide would be displayed naked in the public marketplace. Although it is unknown whether suicide was punishable under Roman law, an attempted suicide to evade trial for a crime was punished. Early Christians venerated martyrs who invited death, but the church prohibited suicide in A.D. 452, following the edict 250 years later with the punishment of excommunication.

English common law, which provided the basis of law in the United States, was itself based on Roman law and church or canon law. Suicide in England originally fell under the jurisdiction of the ecclesiastic courts, which condemned it. In A.D. 673 it became part of English law, which made suicide subject to severe civil penalties including forfeiture of land and goods. For more than 1,000 years it was a felony, and at one time the punishment was ignominious burial in the highway without religious rites and with a stake driven through the body. The last crossroads burial of a suicide occurred in 1882, in London's Grosvenor Place. Meanwhile the law had been amended to allow burial in church grounds, although unconsecrated and only between the hours of 9 P.M. and midnight! Blackstone himself regarded suicide as among the worst crimes, considering it a double offense—spiritual by invading the prerogatives of the Almighty, and temporal against the King by depriving him of a subject. Suicide is still considered a felony under English law, and one who aids and abets a suicide is a principal in the second degree to the crime of murder. Before 1916, imprisonment was normal punishment, but now the individual may be institutionalized, placed under guardianship, or still sent to prison.[34] When canon law spoke against suicide, both France and Italy made it a crime. However, when the French criminal code was written in 1810, it ignored suicide, and other countries of Europe followed suit, and it has not been punishable as a crime in continental Europe since the last half of the nineteenth century.

Although as Curran[35] says, the harshness of English law toward suicide was never applied in America, "The current law in the 50 states is in hopeless confusion with some states still 'punishing' suicide as a crime; some 'punishing' attempted suicide, with or without punishing the 'crime' itself; and some, with or without either of these, punishing a person who aids another in committing suicide. There is no pattern or purpose to the law which is at all discernible from a reading of the law and the last few law review commentaries published in recent years."

Diggory,[36] in discussing some of the attitudes and laws concerning suicide in various cultures and religious groups, emphasizes the importance of the professional worker consciously putting aside his own value system, be it religious, philosophic, or scientific, when he works with a suicidal person. He complains that an integrated value system involved in dealing with suicidal people has not been given the careful thought that is necessary if people are to develop functional concepts that are meaningful, both to the person who is contemplating or has attempted suicide and to those close to him. Such a value system, to the maximum degree possible, should be objective, empiric, and functionally oriented. He concludes with the provocative question, "Do we value life in the sense of continued individual development of skill, knowledge, affiliations and achievements; or do we value it as a prolongation of vegetable metabolism?" In any case to regard suicide or its attempt as self-murder is a curt way of justifying an indictment and trial of an unfortunate person who has succumbed to the stresses and exigencies of his life. His act is neither sinful nor a crime. He is a distressed sufferer from a severe emotional disorder and

if a survivor, should be placed under expert medical and social care and not imprisoned. The implications of this go far beyond suicide and involve attitudes toward contraception, the limitation of treatment of those in extremis, and euthanasia.

## SUICIDE AND THE PHYSICIAN

There has been a tendency even among members of the medical and health professions to regard suicide fatalistically, either as if it was none of their concern or as if nothing could be done about it. By now, even the inadequate efforts that have been made to attack the problem provide sufficient evidence that suicides can be prevented. Several facts are known to justify some measure of optimism. Among them are the following: Potential suicides do not act impulsively; the majority of them talk about it or give other clues to their thoughts or intentions frequently for a long period of time.[37] Thus in a highly detailed study of a significant number of successful suicides Robins and associates[38] observe, "One of the most striking findings of this study was the high frequency with which these persons communicated their suicidal ideas, by specific statements concerning their preoccupation with death and the desire to die, and by making unsuccessful suicide attempts. The statements were made to family, friends, job associates, and many others." In another recent study[39] an even higher proportion, 70%, were found to have communicated their suicidal ideas to several persons, often a physician.

How fortunate medical practitioners would feel if 70% of potential tubercular or coronary patients could give them prior warning, and what rigorous action the practitioners would undoubtedly take. Regretfully that does not apply to warnings about impending suicide. Kobler and Stotland[40] view ". . . verbal and other communications of suicidal attempts, as efforts, however misdirected, to solve problems of living, as frantic pleas for help and hope from other people; help in solving the problem and hope that they can be solved. Whether the individual then actually commits suicide seems to depend to a large part on the nature of the responses by other people to his pleas." Havens[41] also considers suicidal efforts to spring from despair and helplessness. Illustrations of the extent to which these cries for help offer a challenge to the medical profession are frequent.[42] In one study in New Hampshire nearly 50% of individuals who committed suicide consulted a physician a short while before for a wide range of illnesses considered as masks for underlying depressions or anxieties. In a San Francisco study 1 out of every 6 suicide victims was known to have seen a physician during the preceding week, and more than 2 out of 5 persons within the preceding 6 months. Schneidman and Dizmang[43] of the Center For Studies of Suicide Prevention of the National Institute of Mental Health insist, "A well-trained and skillful physician should be as able to identify a potentially suicidal patient on a routine examination as he can detect an early heart murmur or slightly enlarged spleen." Similarly they indicate that a past suicidal attempt or history of suicide in a family ". . . must be looked at just as carefully as a history of familial diabetes or previous history of glucose in the urine."

In other words, failure by physicians to prevent suicide is due not so much to ignorance of the causes as to failure to recognize the signs and symptoms of impending suicide among those in their practices. Beyond this many physicians are hesitant to report a death officially as a suicide. This is especially true if they have known the patient and his family. Furthermore, the fact that some life insurance policies refuse payment in the case of suicide not only causes many persons to mask the act but also leads some physicians to mask the diagnosis.

## MOTIVATION IN SUICIDE

What then are the causes of suicide? The actual phenomenon appears to result from the interplay between (1) factors inherent in the patient and (2) factors in the environment. Of the two, the first is without question the most critical. Numerous studies indicate that the most significant characteristic of those who attempt suicide is a state of frank psychosis. For example, Robins and associates[38] observe that 98% of the suicides they studied had been clinically ill and 94% of them psychiatrically ill. Of the group, 68% had been suffering from one of two diseases: manic-depressive depression or chronic alcoholism. None of the individuals in the study had an uncomplicated neurosis (anxiety reaction, conversion reaction, or obsessive compulsive reaction). It is of interest that 73% of the manic-depressives and 40% of the alcoholics had been under medical or psychiatric care for illnesses associated with their suicide during the year preceding their death.

To approach this question from a different direction, as evidence of the significance of mental aberration among would-be suicides are the following observations: Suicide is the most common cause of death among those known to be mentally ill. The method chosen for the actual suicide is often irrational; individuals have been observed to hang themselves out of a high window instead of jumping. Related to this is the tendency to irrational response. Thus although the suicidal person cannot be handled adequately by reasoning or logic, he may be influenced often by suggestion: "Come in from that window ledge or I'll close the window!" or "Come aboard this boat or you'll catch a cold!" In such instances a favorable response of course is merely temporary and unrelated to the heart of the problem. Another significant observation is that rarely is insufferable pain a factor in suicides. Much more often it is an obsessive hypochondriac concentration on a trivial ailment, which of course is not the fundamental cause of the problem. Not infrequently the depression that precedes an actual suicide is out of proportion to the cause of the depression. This provides the rationale for the prompt institution of antidepressant drugs or even electroshock therapy in some cases of emphatically threatened or attempted suicides.[44]

For another view of the relationship between suicide and mental illness, although as indicated some investigators point to high incidences of psychiatric disturbances among attempted suicides, this has not been subscribed to by some others.[45] As Kessel[46] says, ". . . distress drives people to self poisoning acts, and distress is not the exclusive province of the mentally ill." Similarly there is no justification for assuming, as some investigators seem to do, the existence of a specifically suicide-prone personality per se. Such would be in distinction for acquired behaviorisms or exposure to undesirable environmental and social conditions.

The result of the combination of psychiatric, environmental, social, and acquired behavioral forces is illustrated by a study[8] of 50 men and 50 women after recovery from suicidal attempts. Almost 50% of each group were rated as character disordered. Forty percent showed other signs of psychiatric disturbance, one half of these had personality disturbances, and the remainder were of uncertain pathology. The remaining 12% showed no signs of psychiatric pathology. As would be expected, a higher proportion of psychiatrically disturbed individuals are found among suicide repeaters.

Many investigators have noted a close association between alcoholism and drug addiction, on the one hand, and attempted suicide, on the other. It is especially significant that whereas only an estimated one fifth of those involved in first attempts are alcoholics or problem drinkers, almost one half of repeaters may be so classified. This points to a group at much greater than average risk that merits special community or public health attention. Essentially the same is true of those involved in drug abuse or addiction. Thus the suicide rate for "mainlining" narcotic addicts is fifty times greater than that for nonaddicts. It is important to realize, however, the complexity of these situations in that alcoholics, addicts, and attempted suicide victims all tend to share many or most of the various precipitating or contributing factors such as inadequacy, escapism, loneliness, dejection, and the like.

A fascinating sidelight of some studies of the behavior of dolphins is the discovery that these perceptive, affectionate, and intelligent mammals seem deliberately to commit suicide not only if they are sick or injured but also out of frustration and boredom. This perhaps provides further commentary on one of the consequences of a well-developed forebrain!

One of the greatest problems in the field of suicidology, as indeed it is in the mental health field as a whole, is the wish or tendency to oversimplify. Life—and death—are exceedingly complex phenomena. There is no easy answer or explanation for either. And when death comes by one's own hand, the complexities are multiplied. As Stengel[47], Professor of Psychiatry at the University of Sheffield, sees it,

Human behavior usually has multiple motivations, not all of them obvious and some antagonistic to each other. People, according to some psychiatrists, either want to die or to live. That most people who commit suicidal acts want to do both at the same time, and that these suicidal acts may also serve as punishment for others, seems difficult to grasp. Yet there is ample evidence that this commonly happens. . . . Why should we expect those people who commit suicidal acts to behave as if they knew exactly what they wanted and to act accordingly? Only rarely is human behavior governed by one tendency only. The outcome of most human actions, especially of most irrational actions such as suicidal acts, depends on the quantitative relationship of conflicting tendencies and on many other factors, some of them unpredictable.

Prominent among factors associated with suicidal attempts may be listed broken homes or frequent household moves during childhood, marital disharmony, emotional immaturity, cruelty to children, and jealousy bordering on the pathologic. Not infrequently these factors are coexistent, as indicated in Table 24-2.

Loneliness has been noted as highly significant. Indeed it has been claimed that of all factors associated with suicide, isolation and loneliness may be the potentially most lethal. This would seem to justify special community effort toward identification of such persons and provision of easy and multiple channels of social communication and involvement for them. Organized "befriending" or "buddy" systems have been effective in this regard.[48] In the adult male an important factor is anxiety related to inability to obtain and retain employment or advancement. This is worthy of particular concern at this time in view of the current rapid changes in science and technology, fears of automation, and the decreasing time-

**Table 24-2.** Rates of occurrence of certain social variables in attempted suicides, Edinburgh*

| Variable | Rate per 1,000 for attempted suicides | Rate per 1,000 for Edinburgh |
|---|---|---|
| Overcrowding | 294.7 | 93.0 |
| Rented accommodation | 389.5 | 193.6 |
| Divorce | 73.7 | 9.7 |
| Separation | 94.7 | 25.3 |
| Persistent truancy | 684.2 | 2.1 |
| Court prosecutions | 410.5 | 39.6 |
| Children in care | 200.0 | 3.4 |
| Referrals for child cruelty | 105.3 | 6.6 |
| Repeated attempted suicide | 442.1 | 0.5 |

*From McCulloch, J. W., and Philip, A. E.: Suicidal behavior, Oxford, 1972, Pergamon Press, Ltd.

value of specialized training and education. Concern applies especially to middle-aged men who, coincident with real or feared decline in economic values, begin to observe the independence of their children and the waning of their own physical and sexual strength. It is suspected that the much vaunted shorter work week may exacerbate these problems. Some studies have indicated that about one third of men who attempt suicide have frequent or prolonged periods of unemployment unrelated to work capability or availability. To emphasize this further, unemployment has been noted as a precipitating factor in one third of male suicidal attempts and as a contributing factor in one half of male and one fourth of female suicidal attempts. In terms of elicited precipitating factors it stands fourth, after financial difficulties, alcoholism, and marital discord, and often all four factors combine to form a vicious chicken-and-egg cycle.

All these points were well summarized by Cautela,[49] who indicated that in essence three factors were determinants in suicidal attempts: (1) aversion stimuli, such as acute pain or rejection, (2) absence of adequate reinforcement, and (3) escape conditioning as a learned response. He added that it was noteworthy that all three factors tend to be present in the elderly male. Not only do more elderly men take their own lives compared with younger men and with women of all ages but the gap between attempts and completions narrows alarmingly. As some investigators have pointed out, "Suicidal old men seldom miss!" One is reminded of the comment by Weisman[50] that one of the aspects of terminal behavior is an attempt to create a distance between oneself and a noxious situation, and as he notes, the suicide, if successful, achieves this in a most complete way.

## DIAGNOSIS OF IMPENDING SUICIDE

In most instances the presuicidal state is temporary. If the condition is recognized and the patient is protected from himself through this critical period, he stands a good chance of being saved. This also provides time for appropriate treatment.

How may the potential suicide be diagnosed? Shneidman[51] states that the suicide syndrome is a constellation of symptoms and lists these under the headings of depressed, disoriented, defiant, and dependent-dissatisfied. The preceding discussion gives some indication of the types of signs and symptoms that should be watched for. As for the type of person to watch, the potentiality of suicide should be kept in mind with reference to (1) all depressed persons, (2) all manic-depressive patients, (3) especially all those who have previously attempted suicide —no matter how long ago, (4) those who often speak of suicide with apparent seriousness, and (5) those who have suddenly lost interest in previously important and valued things and events.

A question commonly asked is, "What about those who *think* of suicide?" This in itself would not appear to be dangerous. Several studies indicate that suicide is considered by the majority of individuals at one time or another. Fortunately, however, only a minor proportion of them act on the idea and, as indicated previously, because of deep inherent psychologic problems. A number of warning signals are worthy of attention. Among these are evidence of depression, especially with manifestations of guilt, tension, or agitation; insomnia, especially if great concern is expressed about it; severe hypochondriasis; expressions of fear of losing self-control; frequent discussion about and apparent preoccupation with the idea of suicide or death; and, of course, previous attempts. The depths of depression may be judged by an otherwise inexplicable loss of weight, appetite, and sexual desire; a slowing and blurring of speech and action; an unusual hesitancy or unwillingness to meet people; an attitude of hopelessness, often indicated by a drawn and wrinkled facial expression and dullness of the eyes; chronic low back pain that does not respond to appropriate medical treatment; chronic recurring headaches with elusive etiology; vague and frequent gastrointestinal complaints; and interestingly, as Ross[52] has observed, not only peculiar vague sensations and a bad taste in the mouth but actual dental pain and discomfort. Ross gives a good general word picture of such people: "One's first observation may be of a pale faced sallow person sitting huddled in a waiting room chair evidencing little or no spontaneous activity. Further inspection may reveal evidence of weight and sleep loss, perhaps accentuated facial wrinkles and eyelid folds, and lacklustre hair. There may be careless or unkempt grooming." He also calls attention to the manner in which such individuals present complaints to physicians or others. For example, the highly anxious patient may tell his story rapidly and without interruption or be preoccupied with minutiae. "Immobility of facial expression and body," he says, "can communicate underlined discouragement," and notes that "it is remarkable how often the patient presents the notion that things are different for him: his world, his life, his bodily function, his outlook and his habits."

## HANDLING THE IMPENDING SUICIDE

The question arises concerning how best to handle the individual with apparent or frank suicidal intent. If he can be contacted, every effort should be made to continue conversational contact, while eliciting as much meaningful information as possible and alerting appropriate sources of assistance.[53] He should be encouraged by "gatekeepers"[54] (spouse, friends, neighbors, clergyman, policeman, bartenders, employer, etc.) to be examined by a physician. The physician in turn should give the patient an opportunity to talk out his troubles and problems, great or small, real or imagined, in his own way. The reality of the intent or attempt to commit suicide should be accepted and discussed forthrightly and the patient encouraged to discuss his thoughts, problems, reactions, and motivations. A complete medical examination should be done, of course, since it has been found that a large number of would-be suicides have physical as well as mental complaints and that these are not infrequently interrelated. This also provides the patient and the physician with a specific physical focus of attention and goal. Those who are mildly troubled should be given helpful suggestions. Single and lonely persons should be encouraged to participate in group and religious activities. On the other hand, agitated and depressed patients and those who have previously attempted suicide may be given antidepressant medications and should be referred promptly to a psychiatrist rather than rely, as so often is the case, on the police or prison or on the county or municipal general hospitals.[55,56]

To the contrary, it is the consensus that such individuals should be immediately referred by physicians for hospitalization in a closed psychiatric ward.[38] This provides the best opportunity for further clinical and psychiatric study, psychotherapy, and whatever drugs or shock therapy might be indicated. After the acute episode is past and the patient is considered eligible for discharge from the psychiatric institution, careful provision should be made for follow-up in the community by a competently staffed community mental health facility.

## SUICIDE PREVENTION PROGRAMS

Recent years have seen a gradually growing interest in the problem of suicide and its prevention. First various essentially nonprofessional volunteer groups, then social workers, psychiatrists, public safety officers, and the courts, the medical and public health professions, and then the public in general became interested and willing to discuss and act on the problem. The trend bears out Dublin's[57] point that although by no means are all the questions answered, the practicality of developing effective programs already has been well demonstrated in many communities and nations. Suicide is now recognized as a problem of great significance that lends itself to intelligent public health control efforts. It is surprising for many to learn that the first effort goes back almost three quarters of a century to the Anti-suicide Bureau of the Salvation Army.[58] This was established in London in 1905 and in purpose and method bore many similarities to the programs of today. The work of the Samaritans[59] in England also merits special mention in view of its length of service and its pioneering of blending the forces of theology, medicine, psychiatry, and social work. Similar organizations are to be found in Vienna, Berlin, Milan, and other European cities. Most notable in the United States for its leadership has been the Los Angeles Suicide Prevention Center.[60] In an address to state and territorial mental health authorities in 1966 Shneidman[61] predicted, "Now at the end of 1966, we stand on the threshold of an efflorescence and burgeoning of suicide prevention activities." He illustrated this by the fact that whereas in 1958 only two states had programs, by the time of his address 15 states were included. Within the half year after, 4 more states were added, and in the interval since, great progress has been made toward the goal of all 50 states. Similar growth has occurred on the local level, and by now there are more than 200 suicide prevention programs in cities throughout the nation. Obviously many more are needed. These centers are conducted by a variety of agencies including hospitals, medical centers, mental health facilities, official and voluntary social service agencies, religious organizations, and some health departments. They operate under a variety of names, often chosen for easy identification and an implication of empathy—Hotline, Life Line, We Care, Help, Call for Help, Rescue, Crisis Service, Crisis Intervention, and many others. It is regrettable that many are little more than telephone answering and referral services, which accomplish little but delay. This viewpoint is subscribed to by Kiev[62] of Cornell University Medical Center, who stated that current programs that rely on receiving calls and referring have shown no evidence of reducing the suicide rate. He noted that whereas suicides are most common among men, most patients in psychiatric clinics and office practices are women. Because of this, he urged that active links be established with industry, schools, prisons, alcohol rehabilitation facilities, and similar institutions. Welu[63] has voiced similar concerns and recommendations warning as follows:

> . . . we have artificially severed the phenomenon of suicide from the habitat in which it exists. Thus our suicide prevention efforts have been quite parochial. We have disassociated suicide prevention from the bigger arena of suicidogenic constituents, namely, society's rejection of the aged, retirement, social readjustment, social isolation, society's growing disregard for life, and other factors or elements existing and/or exhibited in a society which may have a causal relationship to suicide or be a condition which predisposes the individual to begin travelling on the suicidal continuum.

He proposes that suicide prevention programs should be based on the concept of a suicidogenic continuum that depicts movement, not necessarily causality, and includes suicidogenic constituents, a prodromal phase and a terminal phase. These views are subscribed to and have been presented in depth by many of the current leaders in suicidology.[64]

On these premises a suicide prevention program may be visualized as follows:

A. *Primary prevention.* This should be aimed, as Stengel views it, to eliminate or reduce all factors that tend to increase the incidence of suicidal acts and to strengthen all those that tend to reduce it. This is recognized as going far beyond suicide and involves a ". . . drastic reorientation of society to the social needs of its members."
   1. Preservation of the family
   2. Active membership in a religious community or some other social group
   3. Fight against alcoholism and drugs
   4. Improved mental and physical health
   5. Improved medical services
   6. Employment for all to the extent of their ability
   7. Improved medical and social care for the elderly

B. *Secondary prevention.* This should be aimed, as Welu views it, in terms of the public health model, at early discovery, diagnosis, and prompt treatment to prevent progression and hopefully repetition.
   1. An active outreach program to contact the older population who exhibit prodromal clues
   2. Identification of the suicide-attempt population and initiation of follow-up treatment and continuity of care after discharge
   3. Education of professionals and the public concerning prodromal clues and emergency and antisuicidal resources
   4. Improvement of treatment facilities to assure prompt, correct, and adequate response to suicidal attempts
   5. Mobilization of the entire community to recognize the magnitude of the problem and their role in its solution
   6. Provision of a 24-hour crisis intervention service including efficient coordination of all pertinent resources
   7. Development of a continuous research effort in all aspects of the problem and its solution

There are many sources of input for a suicide prevention program of this nature. Earlier, for example, the term gatekeeper was used to describe the types of individuals who are in a position to observe and to be alert to the potential suicide and who might refer him to adequate sources of assistance. In addition, there might be listed the major roles possible by private physicians, outpatient clinics and hospitals, mental health programs, poison control centers, accident prevention programs, agencies that deal with juvenile delinquency, alcoholism, and narcotic addiction programs, and many other agencies and groups in the community. Generally speaking, on the basis of preventive philosophy, if suicide is essentially a psychiatric problem, it necessarily follows that the earlier the age at which emotional or mental problems might be identified the closer one comes to the inception of the motivating factors for suicide. Because of this, particular emphasis should be placed on the care and training of young children.

Based on their various studies of suicide and in line with what has been presented here, Tuckman and associates[65,66] suggest the following as the basis for a community suicide prevention program.

1. Evaluation and referral services for persons showing suicidal thinking and behavior
2. Consultation services for physicians, social agencies, and the community at large with respect to potential suicides
3. Community education, including the preparation of suitable educational materials with emphasis on diagnosis, prevention, and treatment, and the introduction of material on suicide in the medical school curriculum
4. Development of follow-up procedures for attempted suicides with special emphasis on children and young adults
5. Casefinding to obtain a more accurate estimate of suicidal behavior in the community as well as to gather systematically life experience, personality structure, and environmental stresses

To these should be added the need for a type of 24-hour service to which the individual under stress could resort. This is perhaps best illustrated by the Nightwatch part of the Los Angeles program[67] or by the program of the Samaritans in England. Callers receive immediate sympathetic consideration with evaluation of the emergency, appropriate counseling, and referral. If indicated, appropriate individuals and teams may be sent to the caller on an emergency basis. Response to this service has been great, and its success and usefulness have been obvious.

## NATIONAL CENTER FOR STUDIES OF SUICIDE PREVENTION

An event of great significance in the movement to understand and do more about the problem of suicide was the establishment in 1966 of the Center for Studies of Suicide Prevention in the National Institute of Mental Health. Shneidman,[4] who organized it, considers it to have five basic functions:

1. To serve as the focal point within the Institute to coordinate and direct activities throughout the nation in support of research, pilot studies, training, information, and consultation aimed at furthering basic knowledge about suicide, and improving techniques for helping the suicidal individual
2. To compile and disseminate information and training material designed to assist mental health personnel, clergy, police, educators, and others in obtaining a better understanding of suicidal actions and learning to utilize research findings
3. To assist in developing and experimenting with the variety of regional and local programs and organizational models to coordinate emergency services and techniques of prevention, case finding, treatment, training and research

4. To maintain liaison with studies and programs on suicide prevention undertaken by other agencies, both national and international
5. To promote and maintain the application of research findings by state and local mental health agencies

More specifically, Shneidman lists ten aspects of a comprehensive national suicide-prevention program to include the following:

1. A program of support of suicide-prevention activities in many communities throughout the nation
2. A special program for the "gatekeepers" of suicide prevention
3. A carefully prepared program in massive public education
4. A special program for followup of suicide attempts
5. An active NIMH program of research and training grants
6. A redefinition and refinement of statistics on suicide
7. The development of a cadre of trained, dedicated professionals
8. Governmentwide liaison and national use of a broad spectrum of professional personnel
9. A special followup program for the survivor-victims of individuals who have committed suicide
10. A rigorous program for the evaluation of the effectiveness of suicide-prevention activities

This ten-point program for suicide prevention is indicated as a mutual enterprise, which to be successful will require the active interest, support, and activities of many groups, individuals, and professions in communities throughout the country. Particularly important to this is the development of a group of individuals whom Shneidman has labeled as "suicidologists," who will focus on the problem as their chief interest. In this regard it is significant that in 1967 the first students of this new profession began a year's fellowship study at the Henry Phipps Psychiatric Clinic of Johns Hopkins University under a grant from the National Institute of Mental Health. Fellowships are offered to qualified members of a variety of disciplines including psychiatry, psychology, social work, anthropology, sociology, public health education, and psychiatric nursing. Also in mid-1967 the Center for Studies of Suicide Prevention inaugurated its *Bulletin of Suicidology*.

In view of the accelerating interest in the subject of suicide and the recent actions that have been taken there is now good reason to anticipate that at last a forthright and intelligent attack will be launched against this major cause of disability and death.

## REFERENCES

1. Farberow, N. L.: Bibliography on suicide and suicide prevention, 1897-1970, DHEW pub. no. (HSM)72-9080, Rockville, Md., 1972, National Institute of Mental Health.
2. Resnik, H. L. P., and Hathorne, B. C., editors: Suicide prevention in the '70s, DHEW pub. no. (HSM) 72-9054, Rockville, Md., 1973, National Institute of Mental Health.
3. Shneidman, E. S., Farberow, N. L., and Litman, R. E.: The psychology of suicide, New York, 1970, Science House, Inc.
4. Shneidman, E. S.: The N.I.M.H. center for studies of suicide prevention, Bull. Suicidol., p. 2, July 1967.
5. U. S. Bureau of Census: Statistical abstracts of the United States, ed. 92, Washington, D. C., 1971, Government Printing Office.
6. Shneidman, E. S.: Some current developments in suicide prevention, Bull. Suicidol., p. 31, Dec. 1967.
7. Mortality from suicide, WHO Chron. **16:**15, Jan. 1962.
8. McCulloch, J. W., and Philip, A. E.: Suicidal behavior, Oxford, 1972, Pergamon Press, Ltd.
9. Litman, R. E., and Tabachnick, N.: Fatal one-car accidents, Psychoanal. Quart. **36:**248, April 1967.
10. Curphey, T.: The role of the social scientist in the medico-legal certification of death from suicide. In Farberow, N., and Shneidman, E., editors: The cry for help, New York, 1961, McGraw-Hill Book Co.
11. Weisman, A. D., The psychological autopsy and the potential suicide, Bull. Suicidol., p. 15, Dec. 1967.
12. Weisman, A. D., and Kastenbaum, R.: The psychological autopsy: a study of the terminal phase of life, New York, 1968, Columbia University Press.
13. Tabachnick, N., Litman, R. E., Osman, M., et al.: Comparative psychiatric study of accidental and suicidal death, Arch. Gen. Psychiat. **14:**60, Jan. 1966.
14. Shneidman, E. S.: Suicide, sleep and death, J. Consult. Psychol. **28:**95, Feb. 1964.
15. Litman, R. E.: Presuicidal states in adolescents, Amer. J. Orthopsychiat. **39:**315, 1969.
16. McIntyre, M. S., and Angle, C. R.: Is the poisoning accidental, Clin. Pediat. **10:**414, Oct. 1971.
17. Gabrielson, I. W., Klerman, L. V., Currie, J. B., et al.: Suicide attempts in a population pregnant as teen-agers, Amer. J. Public Health **60:**2289, Dec. 1970.
18. Faigel, H. C.: Suicide among young persons, Clin. Pediat. **5:**187, Jan. 1966.
19. Jacobziner, H.: Attempted suicides in adolescence, J.A.M.A. **191:**7, Jan. 1965.
20. Ross, M.: Suicide among college students, Amer. J. Psychiat. **126:**220, Aug. 1969.
21. Peck, M. L., and Schrut, A.: Suicidal behavior among college students, HSMHA Health Rep. **86:**149, Feb. 1971.
22. Fox, R.: Suicide among students and its prevention, Roy. Soc. Health J. **91:**181, July-Aug. 1971.
23. Ayd, F. J.: Psycho-drugs as suicide inhibitors, U. S. Med. **4:**19, Feb. 1, 1968.
24. Seidel, K.: The independent internal dynamics of suicide in the aged, Bibl. Psychiat. Neurol. **142:**42, Jan. 1969.
25. Paffenbarger, R. S., and Asnes, D. P.: Precursors of suicide in early and middle life, Amer. J. Public Health **56:**1026, July 1966.
26. Anonymous: High rate of suicide among physicians, Med. World News, **4:**5, July 3, 1964.
27. Sainsbury, P., and Barraclough, B.: Differences between suicide rates, Nature **220:**1252, 1968.
28. Surgeon General's Scientific Advisory Committee on Television and Social Behavior: The impact of televised violence, DHEW pub. no. (HSM) 72-9090, Rockville, Md., 1972, National Institute of Mental Health.
29. Anonymous: Suicide and the press, Lancet **7623:** 731, 1969.
30. Felix, R. H.: Suicide, a neglected problem, Amer. J. Public Health **55:**16, Jan. 1965.
31. Resnik, H. L. P.: Eroticized repetitive hangings: a form of self destructive behavior, Amer. J. Psychother. **26:**4, Jan. 1972.
32. Litman, R. E.: Eroticism, aggression and suicides in depressions. In Masserman, J. H., editor: Science and psychoanalysis, New York, 1970, Grune & Stratton, Inc., vol. 17.
33. Silving, H.: Suicide and law. In Shneidman, E. S., and Faberow, N. L., editors: Clues to suicide, New York, 1957, McGraw-Hill Book Co.
34. St. John-Stevas, N.: Life, death and the law, Bloomington, 1961, Indiana University Press.
35. Curran, W. J.: Suicide: civil right or punishable crime?, Amer. J. Public Health **60:**163, Jan. 1970.
36. Diggory, J. C.: Suicide and value. In Resnik, H. L. P., editor: Suicidal behaviors: diagnosis and management, Boston, 1968, Little, Brown & Co.
37. Bell, J. N.: Lifeline for would-be suicides, Today's Health **45:**31, June 1967.
38. Robins, E., Murphy, G. E., Wilkinson, R. H., Gassner, S., and Kayes, J.: Some clinical considerations in the prevention of suicide based on a study of 134 successful suicides, Amer. J. Public Health **49:**888, July 1959.
39. Lewis, J. M.: The family doctor and the suicidal crisis, Texas Med. **64:**52, Jan. 1968.
40. Kobler, A. L., and Stotland, E.: The end of hope: a social-clinical study of suicide, Glencoe, Ill., 1964, The Free Press.
41. Havens, L. I.: Recognition of suicidal risks

through the psychological examination, New Eng. J. Med. **276**(4):210, Jan. 26, 1967.

42. Anonymous: M.D.'s held able to prevent suicides, Med. World News **8**:24, Jan. 2, 1967.

43. Shneidman, E. S., and Dizmang, L. H.: In Discussion on suicide, M.D. **11**:93, Sept. 1967.

44. Ayd, F. J.: Suicide: a hazard in depression, J. Neuropsychiat. **2**:S52, Feb. 1961.

45. World Health Organization: Prevention of suicide, Public Health Paper no. 35, Geneva, 1968.

46. Kessel, N.: Self poisoning, Brit. Med. J. **5473:** 1265, 1965; **5474**:1336, 1965.

47. Stengel, E.: The complexity of motivations to suicide attempts, Bull. Suicidol., p. 35, Dec. 1967.

48. Resnik, H. L. P., and Cantor, J. M.: Suicide and aging, J. Amer. Geriat. Soc. **18**:152, Feb. 1970.

49. Cautela, J.: Proceedings of the Annual Meeting of American Psychology Association, Washington, 1970.

50. Weisman, A. D.: Suicide, an attempt to reach for normality, U. S. Med. **7**:23, Jan. 1, 1971.

51. Shneidman, E. S.: Preventing suicide, Amer. J. Nurs. **65**:111, May 1965.

52. Ross, M.: The presuicidal patient: recognition and management, Southern Med. J. **60**:1094, 1967.

53. Danto, B. L.: Assessment of the suicidal person in the telephone interview, Bull. Suicidol., p. 48, Fall, 1971.

54. Snyder, J. A.: The use of gatekeepers in crisis management, Bull. Suicidol., p. 39, Fall, 1971.

55. Litman, R. E.: Emergency response to potential suicide, J. Mich. Med. Soc. **62**:68, Jan. 1963.

56. Litman, R. E.: Acutely suicidal patients; management in general medical practice, Calif. Med. **104**:168, March 1966.

57. Dublin, L. I.: Suicide: a public health problem, Amer. J. Public Health **55**:12, Jan. 1965.

58. Levine, M., and Kay, P.: The Salvation Army's Anti-Suicide Bureau, London—1905, Bull. Suicidol., p. 57, Fall, 1971.

59. Varah, C., editor: The Samaritans, New York, 1965, The Macmillan Co.

60. Shneidman, E. S., and Farberow, N. L.: The Los Angeles suicide prevention center: a demonstration of public health feasibilities, Amer. J. Public Health **55**:21, Jan. 1965.

61. Shneidman, E. S.: State programs in suicide prevention, Address presented to the Surgeon General's conference with state and territorial mental health authorities, Washington, D. C., Dec. 6, 1966, National Institute of Mental Health.

62. Kiev, A.: United program urged to lower suicide rate, U. S. Med. **7**:8, April 1, 1971.

63. Welu, T. C.: Broadening the focus of suicide prevention activities utilizing the public health model, Amer. J. Public Health **62**:1625, Dec. 1972.

64. Beck, A. T., Resnik, H. L. P., and Lettieri, D. J., editors: The prediction of suicide, Bowie, Md., 1974, Charles Press Publishers.

65. Tuckman, J., Youngman, W. F., and Bleiberg, B. M.: Attempted suicides by adults, Public Health Rep. **77**:605, July 1962.

66. Tuckman, J., and Cannon, H. E.: Attempted suicide in adolescents, Amer. J. Psychiat. **119**:228, Sept. 1962.

67. Litman, R. E., Farberow, N. L., Shneidman, E. S., Heilig, S. M., and Kramer, J. A.: Suicide prevention telephone service, J.A.M.A. **192**:107, April 5, 1965.

*Every inordinate cup is unblessed
and the ingredient is a devil.*

OTHELLO (II. 3)

CHAPTER 25

# Alcoholism*

## FRIEND OR FOE

In addition to the more evident communicable and organic disorders to which man is subject and which in many instances he may share with other creatures, another group of conditions exist that are peculiarly his own invention. These are behavioral disorders that involve the unreasoned, compulsive consumption of certain chemical substances, some natural and some manmade, to his ultimate physical, psychic, and social detriment. It is interesting that all of these substances have numerous beneficial uses and effects when used properly and judiciously and generally adversely affect only a minor proportion of those who are exposed to their use. Most prominent among these agents is alcohol, a substance of ancient development and widespread consumption. Alcohol has played a fascinating role in the history of mankind.[5] The production of alcoholic beverages appears to have been one of man's earliest discoveries.

Undoubtedly early it was recognized that among those who consumed it were some who developed an uncontrollable necessity for continued use, regardless of the consequences. Thus the drunkard is mentioned in the Old Testament. Through time, society typically frowned on the undesirable results of the abuse of alcohol but was at a loss to understand them. Generally they were attributed to innate depravity, some hereditary weakness, or the loss

of the soul. Such attitudes have continued down to the present time. Only recently have more enlightened attitudes developed, based on clearer understanding of the function of the mind, its relationship to the body, and the effects of pressures of society.

Alcohol is used in many different situations, that is, in religious ceremonies, as a food, as a relaxant, as a customary base for many social affairs; by many different kinds of people, that is, men and women, young and old, well-adjusted and emotionally disturbed; with many different results, that is, an improved appetite, a warm glow of well-being and conviviality, a blackout, or personality deterioration.

Alcohol has a long history of use in medicine and at one time was one of the most commonly prescribed drugs and the most commonly used anesthetics. Although some of the supposed health values ascribed to it have been disproved, certain others have been scientifically confirmed. For example, certain alcoholic beverages are now used in the diets of diabetic patients, since alcohol, unlike sugar, does not require insulin for metabolism. It is also used as an aid in the treatment of arthritis, certain digestive diseases, hypertension and coronary disease, and as a tranquilizer or sedative for convalescent and geriatric patients.[6]

More often than not its use and its effects are regarded in terms of a gradient, with all persons being distributed along a scale of consumption with a concurrent scale of response. Thus ordinarily the less the intake is the less will be the response, and the more the intake

---

*For excellent overviews of the subject, see references 1 to 4.

is the greater will be the response, its consequences, and the probability of becoming an alcoholic. Unfortunately the situation is not as simple as this. There are some individuals who may actually consume, even on a relatively consistent basis, a considerable amount of alcohol yet never become alcoholics. Conversely there are those whose intake may be significantly less or occasional, yet they may be obvious problem drinkers. The reason for drinking and for continuing to drink has much to do with the making of an alcoholic. Similarly the attitude toward other aspects of life and the world has much to do with deciding whether or not a person is an alcoholic. Still another deciding factor is the relative ease or difficulty of reduction or elimination of the consumption of alcohol.

## DEFINITION

The foregoing points up the factors that make alcoholism difficult to define. Nevertheless, the more the problem is studied the more apparent it becomes that certain types of persons, especially under certain circumstances, do tend to become alcoholics, whereas others do not. The alcoholic has been defined by some as an individual under emotional pressure who drinks to get away from the way he feels but eventually is drinking because of his drinking. This is a practical definition in that it stresses the initial psychosocial trigger followed by the eventual psychophysiologic entanglement.

From an epidemiologic viewpoint alcoholism may be defined as an acquired chronic progressive disease of adult life involving the compulsive intake of excessive amounts of alcohol and leading in its more advanced stages to certain psychologic, social, and physical deteriorating sequelae. It affects predominantly males to the ratio of about 6 to 1, that is, adults between 35 and 55 years of age in the most productive period of life to an extent of 85% of cases. This problem is particularly common in certain occupations, such as those involving non-routine, pressure, decision making, and transiency, is significantly greater in urban areas, and is more frequently found in certain nationalities, especially Scandinavian, Nordic, Celtic, and Polish, in contrast to its infrequency among Italians, Greeks, and Jews.

## EXTENT OF PROBLEM

The determination of the true magnitude of the problem is also difficult because so many cases never come to definitive social or medical attention and because of the number of individuals at any time who are on the borderline between problem drinking and chronic alcoholism. In 1952, the Yale Committee on the Study of Alcoholism[7] on the basis of surveys estimated that there were about 70 million drinkers of alcoholic beverages in the United States. Of these, only an estimated 4.5 million were considered to be problem drinkers, 1 million of them chronic alcoholics. This was a prevalence, however, of 2.4% of the total population or almost 7% of those who drink. Furthermore, since 6 out of 7 were adult males, this means an estimated prevalence of problem drinking in the male population 20 years of age and over of about 7.5%! These proportionate figures still hold 20 years later. To complicate the picture further alcoholism is not a disease primarily of the ignorant or of unskilled labor. To the contrary, about 80% of alcoholics are regularly employed up to the point of disability, and three fourths of them belong to the executive class in large and small businesses, professional men, salesmen, and skilled laborers.[8]

Some further insight is provided from studies by Cisin and Cahalan,[9,10] who distinguished between the characteristics of those who drink at least once a year and those who fall into the category of "heavy drinkers." Their findings are summarized in Table 25-1.

As they note, their survey produced some unexpected findings and confirmed others:

1. It showed that drinking is (at least statistically) normal behavior, and that both abstinence and heavy drinking are statistically atypical.
2. Whether a person drinks at all is primarily related to sociological and cultural variables rather than to psychological variables. This is obvious from the great difference in the proportion of drinkers by sex, age, social status, region, urbanization and religion.
3. However, certain personality measures helped to account for some of the "heavy" drinking—particularly alienation from society, neurotic tendencies, and psychological involvement with alcohol or "escape" drinking.
4. There appears to be a high turnover in the drinker or nondrinker status of many individuals, in addition to the general tendency for older persons to drop out of the drinking and heavy-drinking classes.

The implications of this with regard to social, economic, and professional productivity and morale are obvious. The reality of the problem becomes evident from several business and industrial surveys[11] which indicate that the

**Table 25-1.** Comparison of groups most likely to be drinkers and heavier drinking groups*

| Groups in total population with highest rates of drinking at least once a year (total sample, 68%) | Among those who drink, groups with highest rates of "heavy drinking" † (total among drinkers, 18%) |
|---|---|
| Men 30-34, 88%; women 35-39, 73% | Men 40-49, 40% |
| Men of highest social status, 88% | Men of lowest social status, 33% |
| Professional people, 81%; semiprofessional or technical, 78%; sales workers, 79%; managers or officials, 75% | Operatives, 24%; service workers, 23% |
| College graduates, 82% | Men who completed high school but not college, 32% |
| Single men, 83% | Single men, 26%; divorced or separated men, 21% |
| Residents of suburban cities of 50,000 to 1 million, 87% | Residents of central cities over 50,000, 22% |
| Those whose fathers were foreign-born, 80%; especially of Italian origin, 92% | Those whose fathers were Latin-American/Caribbean, 30%; Italian, 22%; British, 21% (Irish, when adjusted for age levels, 33%) |
| Jews, 92%; Episcopalians, 91% | Protestants of no established denomination, 29%; Catholics, 23%; those without affiliation, 25% |

*Data from the National survey, conducted 1964-1965 by the Social Research Group, a national probability sample of 2,746 persons.
†For definitions of "heavy drinkers," see Cahalan, D., Cisin, I. H., and Crossley, D.: American drinking practices, Monogr. no. 6, New Brunswick, 1969, Rutgers Center of Alcohol Studies. Most "heavy drinkers" drank nearly every day with 5 or more drinks per occasion at least once in a while, or about once weekly with usually 5 or more drinks per occasion.

average company can expect about 3% of all its employees to be alcoholics in need of special attention. Little wonder that alcoholism is now included among the seven categories of diseases that cause outstanding numbers of deaths and disabilities and that represent major unsolved public health problems. The others are cardiovascular disease, mental illness, crippling and handicapping conditions, cancer, dental disease, and diabetes. It should be noted incidentally that all of these, including alcoholism, are conditions about which something is known and about which something can be done.

## COST OF ALCOHOLISM

Although it is obviously impossible to determine, the cost of alcoholism to society must be great. Many different factors contribute to the cost, which The National Institute on Alcohol Abuse and Alcoholism estimates at $15 billion annually in the United States. Absenteeism, high spoilage rates, decreased productivity while on the job because of lowered ability and apparently avoidance of work situations involving hazard or ones that are likely to indicate the worker's condition, personnel turnover, and lowered morale of the alcoholic and those working with him account for some of these costs.

Added to them is the expense to society of many facilities for grappling with various aspects of the problem, for example, police, courts, jails, religious organizations, hospitals and medical care, various social and charitable agencies, departments of welfare, domestic relations organizations, visiting nurse agencies, and industrial personnel guidance offices. Less tangible is the ultimate cost of the frequently disastrous effects on other members of the family and circle of friends, for example, on children at school and on other adults at work in the home or at the alcoholic's place of employment. Still another social loss due to alcoholism is the amount of crime and prostitution that is related to it as either or both cause and effect. The amount is indeterminate but on the basis of observations by many would appear to be significant.

The relationship of accidents to alcoholism is interesting.[12] Surveys carried out by the Yale University School of Alcohol Studies in 1943[13] indicated that the estimated 1.37 million alcoholics employed in industry accounted for 1,500 fatal accidents at work and 2,850 fatal accidents at home, in public places, and in traffic, or a total of 4,350 fatalities. This was a fatal accident rate of 321 per 100,000 men or more than twice that of nonalcoholic workers in the same occupations. More recent analyses,[14] however, indicate that whereas alcoholics lose more work time than nonalcoholics, they do not appear to suffer a higher rate of occupational accidents. This substantiates earlier studies by Trice,[15] who hypothesized that the alcoholic while actually on the job tends to be over-cautious, concentrates more on what he is doing in a deliberate attempt to avoid accidents, is subject to fewer of other types of distractions, develops a well-planned work routine, is sometimes "covered up" by his fellow workers, and if actually in an alcoholic or hangover state, tends to be absent rather than to risk discovery or a work accident. The only work relationships in which Trice found alcoholics to indulge their addiction and to have work-related accidents were (1) as participants in fellow-worker drinking groups after working hours and (2) on jobs that require geographic mobility, hence separation from protecting or inhibiting influences coupled with greater accessibility to alcohol.

Alcohol-related accidents away from work present a different picture from the nonmobile work situation. This is best illustrated by the relationship between automobile accidents and alcohol consumption, which has been the subject of many studies. Problem drinkers have about twice as many accidents per mile of driving as does the nondrinking population. As little as 0.03% of alcohol in the blood reduced driving skill,[16] and the probability of accidents increased consistently with an increase of alcohol in the blood. The risk at 0.1% blood alcohol has been found to be twice that at 0.05%, whereas an increase of the blood level to 0.15% multiplied the risk tenfold.[17] With this in mind the percentage of automotive accident fatalities involving persons with significant blood alcohol levels is illuminating. For instance, in Nassau County, N. Y., a series of 269 autopsies of driver fatalities showed 52% with blood alcohol levels over 0.1%. Numerous studies in many places have shown that about 50% of automobile-related fatalities involved significant blood alcohol levels in either or both drivers and pedestrians, if the latter were involved.

It is somewhat more difficult to relate alcohol with home accident fatalities. However, recalling Jellinek's findings that the total fatal accident rate in alcoholic workers was twice that of nondrinkers, coupled with Trice's findings that this was not caused by on-the-job accidents, and recognizing further that in the

United States home accidents are about twice as frequent as work accidents and at least four times as frequent as vehicular accidents,[18] it would seem reasonably certain that a close relationship exists between drinking and the probability of home accidents. To paraphrase the slogan "If you drink, don't drive," one might say, "If you drink, don't climb a ladder."

Another relationship of alcohol that merits mention is its role in suicide. It has been noted that as in the case of fatalities from vehicular accidents, about one half of successful suicide victims have been drinking immediately prior to their self-destructive act.[19] Furthermore, by means of the technique of "psychologic autopsy," an extremely high proportion of successful suicides were found to have been chronic alcoholics.[20,21]

## EFFECTS OF ALCOHOL

The Alcoholism Subcommittee of the Expert Committee on Mental Health of the World Health Organization has concluded that although alcohol must be regarded as a drug, it can be classified neither as an addiction-producing drug nor as a habit-forming drug, but that it must be placed in a category of its own, intermediate between these two groups.[22] After ingestion alcohol is rapidly absorbed directly from the stomach and upper intestine into the bloodstream. It is detectable in the blood within 5 minutes after ingestion and by this medium is distributed throughout the body. The average adult body can oxidize about 10 ml. of alcohol per hour, releasing energy and carbon dioxide and water. Any that is not oxidized is excreted in the urine and through the lungs. Thus ingestion of excessive amounts gives rise to a build-up in the bloodstream and in the tissues, awaiting either oxidation or excretion. Blood concentrations of 0.2% usually result in mild to moderate intoxication, whereas more than 0.3% causes significant effects. Blood concentrations between 0.5% and 0.8% result in death. Repeated and extensive use of alcohol tends to result in increased tolerance.

Alcohol affects all parts of the body, especially the central nervous tissue. Contrary to common belief, it acts not as a stimulant but as a depressant. In so doing it inhibits the controls of behavior in the cerebral cortex. The pulse increases and vasodilation occurs, especially in the skin, and results in decreased body temperature due to heat loss. Because of this, again contrary to common thought, the use of alcohol to warm the body is not physiologically sound. Vision and sense of balance are impaired relatively early. In more advanced states of intoxication the centers in the brain that regulate breathing, cardiac function, and body heat are depressed. As with so many things, the moderate consumption of alcohol actually appears to have little or no effect on longevity. There is good evidence, however, that heavy drinking does shorten life in various ways. Some estimates indicate that the life expectancy of alcoholics is about 10 to 12 years less than the average.[22]

Much of the ill effect of excessive consumption of alcohol is due to malnutrition. The alcoholic typically eats inadequately because of the dulling of the appetite and general disinterest in food and because calories for energy are obtained from alcohol. Since the latter are so readily available, what food is eaten often is stored unused in the body. Hence many alcoholics, especially in the earlier stages, may become overweight. Most important among the nutritional deficiencies that occur are those involving vitamin B complex. This may result in polyneuritis, so-called beer heart, with cardiac weakening and enlargement with attending edema, pellagra, and the typical skin and ocular manifestations of riboflavin deficiency. Fatty degeneration of the liver may result, probably from a combination of vitamin B deficiency and direct toxic effects of alcohol on the liver cells. Because of lowered mineral intake, anemia is frequent. Among the more dramatic effects are those relating to the psyche such as delirium tremens, Korsakoff's psychosis, and personality changes due to alcoholic degeneration of cortical tissue. In connection with the latter the advanced alcoholic tends to become socially unstable, careless about his appearance or actions, suspicious, irritable, belligerent and quick to take offense, crafty, overemotional, and frequently brutal and callous toward those around him, especially those he may love. Much of the latter, of course, is attributable to the severe guilt complex that is typically developed.[23]

## TYPES OF ALCOHOLICS

It is important to consider first of all how alcoholics differ from the much larger number of persons who drink but are not alcoholics. As Bacon[24] has indicated, there are many reasons for drinking, such as to fulfill a religious ritual, to be polite, to have a good time, to make friends, to experiment, to show off, to get warm or cool, to quench thirst, to go on a spree, or to flavor food. He states, however:

> None of these is the purpose of the alcoholic, although he might claim any or all to satisfy some questioner. The alcoholic drinks because he has to if he is to go on living. He drinks compulsively; that is, a power greater than rational planning brings him to drinking and to excessive drinking. . . . Most alcoholics hate liquor, hate drinking, hate the taste, hate the results, hate themselves for succumbing, but they can't stop. Their drinking is as compulsive as the stealing by a kleptomaniac or the continued hand washing of a person with a neurosis about cleanliness. . . . It is useful to think of their drinking behavior as a symptom of some inner maladjustment which they do not understand and cannot control. The drinking may be the outward, obvious accompaniment of this more basic hidden factor.

Many psychiatrists have pointed out that if the alcoholic did not drink, unadjusted he would consciously or subconsciously seek some other outlet for his unresolved conflicts and tensions. In addition, there is some evidence that certain physical causes for alcoholism exist. Some investigators believe that the problem drinker may have some abnormal psychologic and physiologic reaction to alcohol that others do not have.[25]

The frank alcoholic is intensely introspective and is disinterested in anything except himself and his problem. He has few if any diversional interests, such as hobbies, entertainment, or social activities. A large proportion of alcoholics are socially unattached to family or social group, which tend to be regarded as secondary to the drinking pattern and to drinking "buddies." This introspection and social isolation presents particular difficulty to persons, programs, or agencies that may try to relate meaningfully to them in order to assist them. Sometimes part of the difficulty derives from the sense of failure and guilt that the alcoholic commonly feels and that may even result in a willful rejection of attempts to help. Alcoholics may reject help on the basis that they deserve to be miserable because of their real or imagined failings and because of the compulsive drinking pattern itself, which they developed in relation to their conflicts and failings.

Generally speaking, there are two main types of problem drinkers: The first or primary type is the individual who was maladjusted to begin with, that is, before he embarked upon compulsive drinking. He was what is commonly referred to as neurotic, that is, subject to a sense of constitutional psychoneurotic inferiority. Usually his personality was developed improperly from early childhood with gradual realization of vague and constant feelings of anxiety, apprehension, inadequacy, or inferiority. Often he thinks that he is defeated before he begins and that he will be unsuccessful in school, in courtship, in work, and in society. He fears such situations and, if at all possible, wants to avoid them. Occasionally such a person finds that indulgence in alcohol brings a sense of release and gives some degree of confidence and apparent success. Perhaps more than anything it enables him to forget temporarily his own feeling of inadequacy and dissatisfaction with himself. What is more logical than to repeat the experience? The problem is compounded, however, when the effects of alcohol wear off. There are unpleasant memories or, worse, uncertainties about behavior while under the influence of alcohol, providing additional feelings of anxiety and guilt. This leads to the additional use of alcohol, often the morning after, to overcome the postalcoholic sense of guilt, and a vicious circle is established.

The second type of compulsive drinker begins as an apparently well-adjusted person. He is not neurotic; his personality has not been improperly developed; and in fact he appears to get along well in his family, in his work, and with the group. If anything, he may tend to be an extrovert. He becomes involved in situations and with groups, in connection with either or both his social or his work life, which lead to considerable drinking. He participates with enthusiasm but is not yet an alcoholic. He is in fact indulging himself without any particular feeling of compulsion. However, the continued use of more alcohol gradually lowers his senses of discrimination and responsibility. He becomes less efficient, becomes careless, and begins to put things off or to let things slide to meet the preferred social demands. Almost imperceptibly at first his relationships and behavior at home, on the job, and in society begin to deteriorate. This becomes noticeable to those around him, he becomes aware of it and because of fear or worry drinks more. Meanwhile, his family, friends, and employer, usually indulgent or tolerant at first, become impatient. There occurs a mutual loss of regard, and blunt words are exchanged. Because of arguments at home or perhaps a demotion or loss of a job, he begins to believe that everyone is down on him, and with increasing self-pity blames it all on the misunderstanding and intolerance of others or on just plain bad luck. The only thing that provides escape or supports the ego is the very thing that began the process—alcohol. Hence again a vicious circle is begun. As time goes by and the situation becomes worse, he appears on the surface more and more like the primary type of alcoholic. However, because his alcoholism is not superimposed on a basic inferiority, his chances of recovery and rehabilitation are decidedly better. Fortunately from society's viewpoint the larger proportion of alcoholics appear to fall into this category.

## WHAT CAN BE DONE

Until recently and even now in many places the approach to the alcoholic has been to tolerate him if possible; "dry him out" periodically either in jail, a public hospital, or a private sanatorium; or if he were beyond recovery, to provide him with some type of refuge in skid row or elsewhere in which he could subsist on handouts from friends, strangers, missions, or other charitable organizations during the intervals between employment at usually undesirable types of work. With the relatively recent acceptance of the condition as a disease and on the basis of an increasing amount of social, medical, and psychiatric study and research, a growing number of programs are being established with increasingly fruitful results. Much is still on the basis of trial and demonstration.

It is interesting that the real impetus arose from within the group affected. This took the form of the organization in 1935 of Alcoholics Anonymous (A.A.). It considers itself "a fellowship of men and women who share their experience, strength, and hope with each other that they may solve their common problem and help others to recover from alcoholism." It states, "The only requirement for membership is an honest desire to stop drinking"; that it is "not allied with any sect, denomination, politics, organization, or institution; does not wish to engage in any controversy, neither endorses nor opposes any causes." The primary purpose of its members "is to stay sober and to help other alcoholics to achieve sobriety." Since its foundation, A.A. has helped more than 500,000 men and women in the United States, Canada, and many other countries. These people constitute the core of the membership and the nucleus to which others in need of help may relate. There are now about 12,500 groups throughout the world: 7,821 in the United States, 1,241 in Canada, 2,136 outside of Canada and the United States, 569 in hospitals, and 677 in prisons.[26] The organization operates on a few simple but sound and effective premises. Participation must be voluntary—there can be no checking up or compulsion. An alcoholic can never indulge in controlled drinking; either his drinking will become progressively worse or he must abstain completely from alcohol and develop a new pattern of constructive living. Belief and faith in God is a fundamental source of strength in the attempt toward recovery. A recovered alcoholic can best understand the problems and motivations of the alcoholic and is therefore in the best position to be of assistance. Group meetings for group therapy and open discussion of problems are valuable in obtaining an understanding of the underlying causes of one's alcoholism. Individual anonymous assistance in the form of moral support is instantly available by visit or phone at all times. The process of trying to help other alcoholics in itself is an important aid to staying sober oneself. Members do not swear off alcohol for life or for any other period in the future—they merely concentrate on the 24 hours of today. Contributions toward recovery and rehabilitation by other groups, such as the medical profession and social agencies, are recognized, and members are referred freely as indicated.

In a similar vein have been the efforts of the Salvation Army and various "Gospel Mission" programs. Although they tend to be underrated by many, including health professionals, it must be recognized that in the face of a social and professional vacuum over many years they have provided for some basic needs: psychologic encouragement, shelter, and nutrition.

Meanwhile over several years an ever-increasing knowledge about the psychologic and physiologic causes and effects of alcoholism has been accumulated. One result has been the development of three schools of thought with regard to explaining and handling the problem: the social, the psychiatric, and the medical or physiologic schools of thought. More and more it is recognized that rather than conflicting, the three are complementary—each approach contributing to the solution of the problem. Not until recently have attempts been made to apply

knowledge as it became available. In 1944 the Laboratory of Applied Physiology at Yale University established two public clinics in Connecticut, one at New Haven and the other at Hartford, to attract and guide alcoholics and to bring to bear the various resources and approaches to their treatment. Soon after, schools of alcohol studies were established first at Yale then at Rutgers University. A journal, *The Quarterly Journal of Studies on Alcohol*, devoted exclusively to the subject was begun.[27] The success of the Yale clinics led to the establishment in 1949 of a pilot program by the Western Electric Corporation, which now estimates that about 70% of its recognized alcoholics are rehabilitated. Since 1949, the number of companies with planned programs for the recognition and treatment of alcoholics has rapidly increased. For companies without programs, assistance in the form of consultation and information has been made available through the numerous local committees of the National Council on Alcoholism.

## ALCOHOLISM PROGRAMS

Until 1945, no state had a program specifically for alcoholism. In that year, largely as a result of the success of the Yale clinics, Connecticut began the first state program under an independent commission. Since then, most states have established programs. There is no consistency with reference to their organizational location; 11 programs are in independent commissions, 15 programs are units of state health departments, 1 program is related to a welfare department, 12 programs are in state mental health agencies, and 3 programs are in departments of institutions.[28] The programs carried on are various combinations of educational, research, and treatment activities.

Until recently, federal interest in alcoholism has been minimal. In 1966, however, President Lyndon Johnson dealt with alcoholism explicitly for the first time in United States history in his health message to the Congress. New legislation was passed and a National Advisory Committee on Alcoholism appointed. In addition, a National Center for the Prevention and Control of Alcoholism (now the National Institute of Alcohol Abuse and Alcoholism) was established within the National Institute of Mental Health to provide consultation and grants for education, research, and demonstrations to states and through them to localities and institutions. One of the institute's most significant activities has been to stimulate the formation of state mental health planning agencies and community mental health boards. As a result, a significant and increasing number of competent community mental health programs with well-grounded alcoholism components have been established. These activities were strengthened further by the passage on December 31, 1970, of the Comprehensive Alcoholism Prevention Treatment and Rehabilitation Act (P.L. 91-616), which in addition to making possible more grants and contracts in this field, also created a National Advisory Council on Alcoholism.

Too often local programs have tended to be parochial and limited to treatment of cases brought to public attention. There is a trend, however, toward broadening the base of approach by utilizing more effectively and extensively resources of all pertinent fields, professions, and agencies.[29,30] Among the resources, services, and activities that should be included if possible are the following[2]:

*For alcoholics*
Information and referral
Intensive care facilities
Extended care facilities
Physicians
Outpatient clinic services
Halfway houses
Day-care facilities
Custodial care facilities
Pastoral counselors
Social agencies
Psychiatrists
Vocational rehabilitation
Industrial health services
Surveys
Case finding
Follow-up
Evaluation

*For providers of services*
Information and referral
Consultation
Coordination
Training programs
Resource materials
Evaluation and standards
Reports
Morbidity and mortality data
Demographic and social data
Follow-up

*For prevention*
Information and referral
Consultation
Resource materials
Educational activities
Surveys and reports
Teacher training programs

Social agencies
Research (especially etiologic)
Coordination

*For opinion molders*
Informational services
Surveys and reports
Coordination
Consultation
Evaluation and standards
Resource materials

The problem is so vast and complex, with multiple causes, different types of cases, and numerous agencies of potential value, that no standard program is possible or even desirable at this time.[31] Certainly, as Vogel[32] has stated:

Treatment of the alcoholic is not the sole province of the psychiatrist, internist, sociologist, minister, or any scientific or lay discipline. Recognition of this is fundamental. . . . A total push is necessary and mobilization of all methods and facilities is necessary to improve results and make help available to more alcoholics. The nonspecificity of present-day treatment should not result in therapeutic nihilism, which is often used by physicians and others as rationalization to avoid this important problem. There are definitely ways to treat the alcoholic.

An unusually well-thought out community-wide program has been developed on a systems basis by the South Central Mental Health Region of North Carolina[33] and is shown in Fig. 25-1.

Basically there is no reason why the approach to the problem of alcoholism should not follow the well-established principles of epidemiology and program planning that have been so successful in many other areas.[34] This should include the gathering of data by survey, reporting, or other means to determine the extent of the problem. The data should be analyzed to pinpoint problem areas and problem groups, existing or incipient, and to determine places and circumstances in which alcoholism is or tends to become a problem. Early case finding should be carried out by enlisting the participation of public health and visiting nurses, police, clergy, institutional staff, and many others. Since about one half of the problem drinkers are in the pre-addict stage, special effort should be made to reach them as early as possible for attempts at prevention of progression.

Another 30% of problem drinkers are in the early acute addict stage. This group probably represents the combination of the most accessible and potentially most susceptible to rehabilitation. Treatment centers, providing a

**Fig. 25-1.** Points of intervention in the public-private system for dealing with problem drinkers. (From the Regional Alcoholism Systems Project, Raleigh, N. C., 1971, South-Central Mental Health Region.)

spectrum of therapies utilizing the services of Alcoholics Anonymous, internists, psychiatrists, sociologists, and others, should be available especially for those in the early acute addict stage. Provision should be made for individual counseling, group therapy, medical treatment as required, and hospital referral if indicated. Increasing use has been made of the drug Antabuse (tetraethylthiuram disulfide), which taken orally produces no effect unless alcohol is subsequently used. In such an event acetaldehyde is formed and causes severe nausea, vomiting, increased pulse rate, and decreased blood pressure. This should be prescribed and used only under medical guidance and, if at all possible, should be combined with psychotherapy. Concurrent with the treatment, steps should be initiated for the other aspects of rehabilitation, that is, social, familial, religious, economic, and the like. In the process the patient's family, especially the spouse, should not be overlooked.[35] The occasional importance of this has been emphasized by Lewis,[36] as follows:

When the wife of an alcoholic remarries, she very often remarries an alcoholic. We often see reciprocal relationships between the alcoholic and his spouse, and as an alcoholic improves the adjustment of the spouse deteriorates. Strange as it may seem, the spouse is often ambivalent about her alcoholic husband's recovery; she frequently derives neurotic satisfaction, which may be unconscious, from his alcoholic binges. The inadequacy of her husband makes her feel needed and more adequate. . . . Wives often resent their alcoholic husband's therapists whom they see as threatening their control of their husbands. A part of this psychological mechanism between husband and wife is the nagging and the pressure which the wife puts on her alcoholic husband, making him feel more inadequate and thus less likely to stop drinking.

Many male alcoholics do tend to exhibit some degree of an Oedipus complex, and not infrequently their wives play the role of the long-suffering but protective mother figure. Literature on female alcoholics, on the other hand, indicates that they have strong emotional conflicts about their womanliness; they have been described[37] as having "a fragile sense of feminine adequacy"; and when confronted with self doubts, they turn to alcohol in an attempt to gain artificial feelings of womanliness. Steinglass and Weiner,[38] however, raise the interesting question of ". . . whether the marital structure is the result of the preexisting needs of each partner or the result of stress placed upon the marriage by the introduction of drinking behavior essentially after the fact." To the extent that this may be true the emphasis perhaps should be not so much on the alcoholic per se as on the quality and form of the marriage.

Suggestions for meeting this situation are to align oneself with the spouse's positive motivations, to urge her to join Alanon, a group of spouses of A.A. members, or if possible to get her to accept some psychiatric consultation in order that she might better understand her husband's problem and her relationship to it.

## PREVENTION

The development of most cases of alcoholism is so insidious and the causative factors so complex and often buried in the individual's past that prevention is difficult. Experience has shown that prohibition of alcoholic beverages by law is impractical. Even if it could be achieved, the maladjustments and inferiorities that give rise to alcoholism, in the presence of alcohol, would still be there. In a utopian world the elimination of these underlying factors might be anticipated, but under existing conditions this is too much to hope for.

Nevertheless, increasing attention to mental health, the greater equalization of social and economic opportunity, and more understanding parents may make some inroads. In the practical sense, however, it would appear that the best chance for prevention still lies along the path of education. This should have as its goal a willingness on the part of all to regard, discuss, study, and deal with alcoholism and its precursors frankly, dispassionately, and intelligently toward the end of combatting the development of the precursors and of seeking in the face of their existence patterns of behavior other than hiding behind the screen of an alcoholic haze. Education in the school can be important, but as Bacon[39] has stressed, ". . . only if (a) the lesson to be taught is realistic, understandable, meaningful to the student, (b) the community is largely in agreement with what is taught and (c) the teachers themselves are taught and properly equipped." It is utterly pointless and farcical for an uninformed teacher to utter prohibitory preachments to students about drinking, when they know that he, their own families and friends, and society in general partake of alcoholic beverages to some extent. Far better for an informed teacher to present the realities of living and on that basis to discuss its risks and why and how they may be avoided.

Earlier it was stated that one of the most important needs is to recognize alcoholism for what it really is—a disease. Paradoxically, this is still lacking to a considerable degree in the medical profession.[40] Surprisingly few schools of medicine teach to any consequential extent about alcoholism. The average physician and, indeed, the average public health worker still regards the alcoholic as a socially undesirable misfit who refuses to pull himself together. If physicians and public health workers cannot face the problem honestly and properly, how can anyone else? A few recent events serve to emphasize the point. Only within the past few years have some hospitals begun to take alcoholics on their general wards. Only within the past few years have hospitalization insurance organizations begun to pay for hospitalization due to alcoholism. Even yet only about one half of such organizations do so, and benefits vary widely. Indeed, it was only in the early part of 1958 that the House of Delegates of the American Medical Association unanimously passed a resolution stating that alcoholism is a disease and that it should be treated by a physician in a hospital setting when necessary.

Once having done so, the association moved rapidly. Its Committee on Alcoholism prepared a manual on alcoholism,[41] which was distributed to all physicians. It urged the development of uniform legislation dealing with alcoholism based on scientific fact. This has since been done by the National Conference of Commissioners on Uniform State Laws.[42] It is urging hospitalization insurance organizations to allow hospital benefits for alcoholism, and most important with its Committee on Professional Education it is working toward the much-needed improvement in the teaching of alcoholism as a disease in the nation's medical schools. It is encouraging to note that most schools of public health as well as many schools of nursing and social work are following suit. Obviously an enlightened and progressive viewpoint by all health-related professionals is crucial to the amelioration of this severe health and social problem.

## REFERENCES

1. Alcoholism in the United States, Ann. Amer. Acad. Polit. Soc. Sci. **315:**entire issue, Jan. 1958.
2. Cross, J. N.: Guide to the community control of alcoholism, New York, 1968, American Public Health Association.
3. National Institute of Mental Health: Alcohol and alcoholism, PHS pub. no. 1640, Washington, D. C., 1970.
4. National Institute of Mental Health: Alcohol and Health, DHEW pub. no. (HSM) 72-9099, Rockville, Md., 1972.
5. Alcohol, World Health (special issue), Jan. 1966.
6. Leake, C. D., and Silverman, M.: Alcoholic beverages in clinical medicine, Chicago, 1966, Year Book Medical Publishers, Inc.
7. Jellinek, E. M., and Keller, M.: Rates of alcoholism in the United States of America, Quart. J. Stud. Alcohol **13:**49, 1952.
8. Clark, G. A.: The doctor and the alcohol problem, Penn. Med. J. **58:**790, Aug. 1955.
9. Cisin, I. H., and Cahalan, D.: Some correlates of American drinking practices. In Mello, N. K., and Mendelsohn, J. H., editors: Recent advances in studies of alcoholism, pub. no. (HSM) 71-9045, Rockville, Md., 1971, National Institute of Mental Health.
10. Cahalan, D., Cisin, I. H., and Crossley, D.: American drinking practices, Monogr. no. 6, New Brunswick, 1969, Rutgers Center of Alcohol Studies.
11. Presnall, L. F.: Quoted in Business Week, Sept. 21, 1963.
12. U. S. Department of Health, Education, and Welfare: Alcohol and accidental injury, Conference proceedings, Washington, D. C., 1966, Government Printing Office.
13. Jellinek, E. M.: Phases in the drinking history of alcoholics, Quart. J. Stud. Alcohol **7:**1, 1946.
14. "Observer," and Maxwell, M. A.: A study of absenteeism, accidents and sickness payments in problem drinkers in one industry, Quart. J. Stud. Alcohol **20:**302, 1959.
15. Trice, H. M.: Work accidents and the problem drinker, I.L.R. Research, New York State School of Industrial and Labor Relations, Cornell University **3:**2, March 1957.
16. Loomis, T. A., and West, T. C.: The influence of alcohol on automobile driving ability, Quart. J. Stud. Alcohol **19:**30, 1958.
17. McFarland, R. A.: The role of preventive medicine in highway accidents, Amer. J. Public Health **47:**288, March 1957.
18. Accident facts, Chicago, 1970, National Safety Council.
19. Tabachnick, N., Litman, R. E., Osman, M., et al: Comparative psychiatric study of accidents and suicidal deaths, Arch. Gen. Psychiat. **14:**60, Jan. 1966.
20. Robins, C., Murphy, G. E., Wilkinson, R. H., Gassner, S., and Kayes, J.: Some clinical considerations in the prevention of suicide based on a study of 134 successful suicides, Amer. J. Public Health **49:**888, July 1959.

21. Weisman, A. D., and Kastenbaum, R.: The psychological autopsy: a study of the terminal phase of life, New York, 1968, Columbia University Press.

22. Alcohol as a drug, WHO Chron. **8:**144, April 1954.

23. Mello, N. K., and Mendelson, J. H., editors: Recent advances in studies of alcoholism: an interdisciplinary symposium, pub. no. (HSM) 71-9045, Rockville, Md., 1971, National Institute of Mental Health.

24. Bacon, S. D.: Alcoholism, nature of the problem, Federal Probation, vol. 11, no. 1, 1947.

25. Hirsh, J.: The problem drinker, New York, 1949, Duell, Sloan & Pearce, Inc.

26. World directory of Alcoholics Anonymous, Box 459G, New York, 1966, Alcoholics Anonymous, Inc.

27. McCarthy, R. G.: Public Health approach to the control of alcoholism, Amer. J. Public Health **40:**1412, Nov. 1950.

28. Membership list, North American Association of Alcoholism Programs, 323 Dupont Circle, Washington, D. C., 1967 (mimeographed).

29. Prothro, W. B.: Alcoholics can be rehabilitated, Amer. J. Public Health **51:**450, March 1961.

30. Hewlett, A. H.: State and municipal alcoholism programs and their relationship to health services, Amer. J. Public Health **57:**964, June 1967.

31. Brightman, I. J.: The future of alcoholism programs, Public Health Rep. **75:**775, Sept. 1960.

32. Vogel, S.: Psychiatric treatment of alcoholism, Ann. Amer. Acad. Pol. Soc. Sci. **315:**99, Jan. 1958.

33. Holder, H. D., and Hallan, J.: Systems approach to planning alcoholism programs in North Carolina, Amer. J. Public Health **62:**1415, Oct. 1972.

34. Cross, J. N.: Public health approach to alcoholism control, Amer. J. Public Health **57:**955, June 1967.

35. Futterman, S.: Personality trends in wives of alcoholics, J. Psychiat. Soc. Work **23:**37, 1953.

36. Lewis, J. A.: Alcoholism, Amer. J. Nurs. **56:**433, April 1956.

37. Wilsnack, S. C.: Quoted in Feelings of feminine inadequacy motivate most women who drink, U. S. Med. **8:**26, July 15, 1972.

38. Steinglass, P., and Weiner, S.: Familial interactions and determinants of drinking behavior. In Mello, N. K., and Mendelson, J. H., editors: Recent advances in studies of alcoholism, pub. no. (HSM) 71-9045, Rockville, Md., 1971, National Institute of Mental Health.

39. Bacon, S. D.: Alcoholism, its extent, therapy and prevention, Federal Probation vol. 11, no. 2, 1947.

40. Symposium article: Alcoholics face a "therapy gap," Amer. Med. News **15:**8, Feb. 7, 1972.

41. Committee on Alcoholism of Council on Mental Health: Manual on alcoholism, Chicago, 1958, American Medical Association.

42. National Institute of Mental Health: Uniform Alcoholism and Intoxication Treatment Act. In Alcohol and health, DHEW pub. no. (HSM) 72-9099, Rockville, Md., 1972.

*Not poppy, nor mandragora,*
*Nor all the drowsy syrups of the world*
*Shall ever medicine thee to that sweet sleep*
*Which thou ow'dst yesterday.*

OTHELLO
(III. 3)

CHAPTER 26

# Addictions, habituations, and drug abuse

## WHAT ARE DRUGS?

Next to alcohol in prominence and historic discovery are the narcotizing alkaloids. More recently have been added certain substances that have been developed synthetically, usually for therapeutic purposes, such as the barbiturates and related drugs, amphetamine, and to some extent, certain of the so-called tranquilizers, euphoriants, and ataraxics.[1] To these may also be added the psychedelic or psychotomimetic drugs, natural and synthesized, of which mescaline, psilocybin, and lysergic acid diethylamide (LSD-25) are the best known.

Alkaloid-bearing plants were probably discovered very early. Because of the physiologic effects they produced, they soon became important adjuncts to social intercourse, religion, and politics and have played an important part in the literature of all cultures. Through the ages there has been much speculation about them, especially about certain of the psychic effects they produce. They seemed to release the usually pent-up spirit from the tangible body and allow it to wander freely. Sometimes these substances seemed to bring about the phenomenon of second sight. Some mystical results, coupled with the unusual appearance and behavior of the person affected, inevitably led to great wonder and awe, especially on the part of primitive peoples. From the beginning therefore, although these substances appeared to be similar to other materials ingested such as food and drink, they were nevertheless considered different and special. Indeed, in many instances they were treated as sacred, to be prepared only by certain persons, and to be used only at certain times such as festivities, religious events, or in instances of individual or group catastrophe.

Here again, as in the case of chronic alcoholism, the health worker is dealing with a condition and a situation that appears on the surface to be something different from what it really is. Whereas the typical attitude toward the alcoholic is that he is a weakling, lacking in self-control and self-respect, the narcotic addict has usually been regarded as an essentially depraved person and a criminal. This has been subject to change, however, during recent years with the advent of the so-called "drug culture," characterized by peer envy, approval, and imitation. This phenomenon has affected the affluent, educated, and adult components of American and other societies as well as the young and the socioeconomically disadvantaged.

## DEFINITION

Drug addiction lends itself somewhat more easily to definition than does alcoholism because fewer people regularly use these drugs and because ordinarily they are obtained and used clandestinely. Furthermore, the addiction that results from their use is more clear cut and appears within a relatively short time. The World Health Organization's Expert Committee on Addiction-Producing Drugs[2] believes that it

**473**

is important to distinguish clearly between drug habituation and drug addiction. It defines *drug habituation* (habit) as "a condition resulting from the repeated consumption of a drug," and lists its characteristics as (1) a desire (but not a compulsion) to continue taking the drug for the sense of improved well-being it engenders, (2) little or no tendency to increase the doses, (3) some degree of psychic dependence on the effect of the drug but absence of physical dependence and hence of withdrawal or abstinence symptoms, and (4) detrimental effects, if any, primarily on the individual. The majority of affinities to synthetic drugs fall in this category.

On the other hand, the committee defines *drug addiction* as "a state of periodic or chronic intoxication produced by the repeated consumption of a drug (natural or synthetic)," and lists its characteristics as (1) an overpowering desire or need (compulsion) to continue taking the drug and to obtain it by any means, (2) a tendency to develop tolerance or decreased effect hence a tendency to increase the dose, (3) a psychic (psychologic) and usually a physical dependence on the effects of the drug, and (4) detrimental effects not only on the individual but also on society. The continued compulsive use of the narcotizing alkaloids and of certain synthetic drugs are included herein. For purposes of orientation it should be pointed out that the World Health Organization considers alcohol as intermediate between the addiction-producing and the habit-forming drugs. It points out that alcoholism and drug addiction have certain similarities but also certain important differences. Thus the severe symptoms that occur on withdrawal of alcohol can be more dangerous to the individual than those which occur when morphine, for example, is withheld. On the other hand, it takes much longer to develop tolerance to and dependence on alcohol than is the case with narcotics. Also, up to the present time, treatment of alcoholism is much more possible and successful than is treatment of narcotic addiction.[3]

## REASONS FOR DRUG USE

The use and misuse of drugs, especially alkaloids, is not new. No society is without a substitute to chew, swallow, or smoke to transform feelings about reality. Some substances have been used for many centuries without legal or social restrictions, and on several occasions international strife resulted from attempts to curtail their open sale and use. It is also interesting to note that in the past, stronger attitudes and sanctions existed against certain substances that are now accepted readily than against substances that are now considered undesirable and dangerous. Thus in the seventeenth century in various parts of Europe and western Asia the use of tobacco invited flogging, slitting of the lips, life prison sentences, and in some instances even the death penalty. Incidentally, none of these severe punishments stopped the increased use of tobacco. Even tea and coffee were regarded as evil and dangerous. Lewis,[4] Professor Emeritus of Psychiatry, University of London, described the attitude that existed in many places as recently as the beginning of this century.

The results of excessive coffee are painted in alarming colours: "The sufferer is tremulous and loses his self-command; he is subject to fits of agitation and depression. He has a haggard appearance. . . . As with other such agents, a renewed dose of the poison gives a temporary relief, but at the cost of future misery." Tea is no better: "tea has appeared to us to be especially efficient in producing nightmares with hallucinations which may be alarming in their intensity. Another peculiar quality of tea is to produce a strange and extreme degree of physical depression. An hour or two after breakfast at which tea has been taken a grievous sinking may seize upon a sufferer, so that to speak is an effort. The speech may become weak and vague. By miseries such as these, the best years of life may be spoilt."

The writers quoted were eminent in their days, one a Regius Professor at Cambridge, another a leading British pharmacologist. Their attitude toward the use of opium presents an interesting contrast, one not at all uncommon in America as well as in Britain and the European continent at that time. They wrote, "Opium is used, rightly or wrongly, in many oriental countries, not as an idle or vicious indulgence, but as a reasonable aid in the work of life. A patient of one of us took a grain of opium in a pill every morning and every evening for the last fifteen years of a long, laborious and distinguished career. A man of great force of character, concerned in affairs of weight and of national importance and of stainless character, he persisted in this habit as being one which gave him no conscious gratification or diversion, but which toned and strengthened him for his deliberations and engagements."

Somewhat similar is the age-old practice of chewing coca leaves by the Indians of the

Andes. It is estimated that 6 million, or 1 out of every 2.5, persons of all ages in that area indulge in this habit. There is some slight stimulating and sometimes a mild hallucinatory effect, but essentially the slow, sustained release of a small amount of cocaine makes possible a tolerance to a depressing existence and an ability to perform otherwise exhausting work at physiologically antagonistic altitudes and temperatures. Indeed, when its common use in the Andes became known, laudatory articles appeared in several leading medical journals both in England and America recommending its use for everything from tuberculosis to impotence.[5]

Without at all intending to minimize the great significance of the problem, it must be recognized that not all drug users are necessarily addicts any more than all people who drink alcohol are alcoholics. It is important to recognize further that there is nothing new about drug use, even common drug use. Addiction, predominantly to opiates and morphine, became prevalent among Civil War veterans who had been administered large amounts of these narcotics in relation to their severe battle wounds and amputations. In fact, morphine addiction was referred to as "the Army disease." Ironically, both cocaine and heroine, which were considered to be nonaddictive, were deliberately introduced later as substitutes for morphine.[6] It is well to realize that it was not until the second decade of this century that serious steps began to be taken against the free and common use even of narcotics. As Brotman and Freedman[7] point out, it is estimated, for example, that in 1910 in the United States narcotics, predominantly opium and cocaine, were used by 1% to 4% of the population, predominantly adult males, among whom the incidence was therefore about 10%. These materials could be openly purchased over the counter with no restrictions in grocery stores and pharmacies. It should also be remembered that into the 1920s many cough syrups, products for soothing babies, headache remedies, and "tonics" for female ailments, as well as several popular drinks contained narcotic substances, sometimes in significant amounts.

There are actually many and sometimes complex reasons for drug use and abuse. Addiction that results from medication to relieve severe pain has been mentioned. In this connection it has been pointed out that whereas the pain that led to addiction in the last century was usually physical, today it is mainly psychic. Most of today's addicted persons appear to have discovered that drugs relieve their anxieties, tensions, feelings of inadequacy, and other emotional conditions with which they cannot cope in a normal way and which they find handicapping and sometimes psychically unbearable in terms of the demands of current living circumstances.[8] Peculiarly, although it was logically anticipated that a generally improved standard of living and the reduction of poverty would eliminate escape phenomena such as drug abuse and addictions, the opposite seems to be the result. Under circumstances in which changes are rapid and the beliefs, customs, and values of yesterday are attacked and eroded, affluence allows the time and funds to support drug excesses. When a person no longer needs to work as much in order to eat and clothe himself, he easily develops problems of leisure. If he has no viable goals and no motivation or drive to create, to study, or to help others, or if he is denied the opportunity to do so, he may become bored or alienated and vulnerable to the temptation of using artificial substitutes. Some of the factors involved in the recent increase in drug use are as follows[9]:

1. The widespread belief that "medicine" can magically solve problems
2. The easy access to drugs of various sorts in an affluent society
3. Enjoyment of the euphoria or excitement induced by drugs
4. "Peer pressure" which leads an individual, especially a young one, to conform to current styles in dress, behavior, entertainment, and drugs
5. A search for sharpened perception and heightened creativity which some persons believe they obtain from mind-altering drugs
6. The use of drugs, especially marihuana, in a social context, with a role similar to that of alcohol
7. The numbers of young people who are dissatisfied or disillusioned, or who have lost faith in the prevailing social system
8. The tendency of persons with psychological problems to seek easy solutions with chemicals
9. The statements of proselytizers who proclaim the "goodness" of drugs
10. A lack of alternatives which appear meaningful to "counter culture"

## CLASSIFICATION OF DRUG ABUSERS

Yost[10] has classified drug addicts into the following three groups, to which a fourth may be added:

1. Emotionally    well-adjusted    individuals

**Table 26-1.** Characteristics of narcotics and drugs

|  | Slang names | Description |
|---|---|---|
| Alcohol (sedative) | Booze, liquor, cocktail, night-cap, moonshine, white lightning, mountain dew, firewater | Liquid, made through natural process by the fermentation of sugars and starches |
| Amphetamines, or uppers (stimulant) | Bennies, dexies, hearts, speed, pep pills, wake-ups, uppers, co-pilots, meth | Capsules or pills in a variety of shapes and colors; bitter taste, odorless |
| Barbiturates, or downers (depressant) | Peanuts, barbs, goof balls, red devils, yellow jackets, rainbows, blue devils, spacers, downs | Capsules or pills in a variety of shapes and colors; bitter taste, odorless |
| Cocaine (anesthetic) | Snow, dust, flake, stardust, girl, Corine, Cecil, C, coke | White, flaky powder, bitter, odorless; numbs lips and tongue |
| Codeine (mild depressant) | C, poppys, school boy | Liquid, ingredient in cough medicine |
| Hallucinogens (includes LSD, STP, DMT, psilocybin, etc.) | Acid, cubes, sugar, pearly gates, heavenly blue, royal blue, DOM, serenity, tranquillity, and peace | White crystalline powder or a tasteless, odorless, colorless liquid that can be placed on any type of tablet, capsule, or transporting agent |
| Heroin (analgesic-depressant; narcotic made from morphine) | Horse, H, smack, white stuff, joy powder, junk, dope, goods, hard stuff, heavy stuff | White (or possibly brown) powder, packed in paper bundles or balloons; bitter taste, vinegar-like odor |
| Marihuana (*Cannabis sativa;* hallucinogen, stimulant) | Pot, grass, weed, hashish, joint, stick, reefer, roach, Mary Jane, rope, ashes, jive, hay, loco, sweet Lucy, gaga, griefo, bhang | Greenish-brown plant material, coarsely ground, powdered leaf; weedy, burned-rope odor |
| Mescaline (hallucinogenic drug from peyote cactus) | Peyote, mescal, mesc, buttons | Powder made from cactus plant top; bitter, odorless |
| Morphine (analgesic narcotic) | Junk, morpho, morphie, Miss Emma, white stuff, hard stuff, dope, goods, stuff, Big M | Bitter white powder or tablets |
| Solvents (includes glue, paint thinner, gasoline, etc.; volatile chemicals) | Sniffing | Any volatile substance whose fumes are capable of producing an intoxicating effect, such as glue, paint thinner, gasoline, lighter fluid, air fresheners |

| Effects | How used | Medical use |
|---|---|---|
| Slurred speech, uncoordination, confusion, tremors, drowsiness, agitation, nausea, respiratory depression; continued use can damage the liver and enlarge and weaken the heart | Orally | For mild sedation and appetite stimulation |
| Excitability, rapid and unclear speech, restlessness, tremors, insomnia, sweating, dry mouth, bad breath, itchy nose, dilated pupils; continued use results in increased pulse and blood pressure, hallucinations, psychoses | Usually orally or by injection (speed) | For weight reduction, mild depression, narcolepsy |
| Similar to alcohol intoxication, drowsiness, confusion, uncoordination, tremors; continued use results in depressed pulse and blood pressure, possible convulsions | Orally or by injection | For sedation and sleep, analgesic for minor pain; sometimes used as anesthetic for minor surgery |
| Excitability, talkativeness, headache, nausea; continued use results in increased blood pressure and pulse rate, possible hallucinations and violent or dangerous behavior | Usually sniffed or injected | Has been used (very rarely now) for local anesthesia in oral-nasal surgery |
| Drowsiness, pinpoint pupils, stupor, sometimes nausea develops; continued use develops a tolerance to drug | Orally | To relieve pain, coughing |
| Trance, anxiety, confusion, tremors, euphoria, depression, dilated pupils, increased pulse rate and blood pressure; continued use may result in psychoses, possible chromosomal breakdown and organic brain damage | Orally, dissolved on sugar cubes, tablets, stamps, etc., and swallowed or licked; can be injected for faster high; DMT is often smoked in pipe or cigarette | None, LSD has been used for psychiatric experimentation |
| Relaxation, drowsiness, confusion, euphoria, slurred speech, flushing of skin or face, nausea, constricted pupils, respiratory depression; continued use results in scars or abscesses at injection points | Dissolved in water and injected, called skin popping or mainlining; sometimes sniffed | None in the United States |
| Euphoria, dizziness, excitability, hallucinations, increased appetite, dryness of mouth, increased pulse and blood pressure, nausea | Usually made into cigarettes (joints) and smoked; sometimes sniffed or swallowed (baked in cookies) | None |
| Resembles LSD effects; distortion of senses, anxiety, confusion, tremors, euphoria, depression, dilated pupils, increased pulse rate, psychoses, and possible hallucinations | Orally, powder form in capsule | None |
| Lethargy, drowsiness, confusion, euphoria, slurred speech, flushing of skin, nausea, constricted pupils, respiratory depression; continued use results in scars or abscesses at injection points | Dissolved in water and injected, or sometimes used orally | For relief of pain |
| Similar to alcohol intoxication, slurred speech, blurred vision, uncoordination; ringing in ears, nausea, and vomiting; continued use results in psychoses, hallucinations, liver and blood damage, respiratory depression | Inhaled; fumes from the glue tubes are inhaled by the user after the glue has been squirted into a sack or paper bag | None |

who take addicting drugs on medical advice for treatment of pain, sleeplessness, and the like. After protracted use they find they cannot get along without them. This type constitutes only 5 in 1,000 of those hospitalized at the Public Health Service Hospitals at Lexington, Ky., and Fort Worth, Texas.

2. Neurotics who turn to drugs because drugs make them forget their feelings of inadequacy, fear, and the like, making them feel better and more normal, either physically or mentally or both. These constitute the largest group of drug abusers.

3. Psychopaths who take drugs in a deliberate search for thrills and "kicks." This is probably the smallest group numerically.

4. Otherwise relatively normal individuals, usually adolescents, who try narcotics to maintain face with the group. This would appear to be a variable group, its numbers depending considerably on variations and fluctuations in group behavior and fads and on the extent of law enforcement and availability of supplies.

Yost applies the apt phrases of "addiction prone" to the second and third categories (neurotics and psychopaths) and "accidental addicts" to the first group. As might be expected and in line with the experience with alcohol, the first and fourth categories of addicts present the least important and least difficult part of the problem and are much more susceptible to rehabilitation because undesirable underlying personality problems are generally absent. The second and third categories, neurotics and psychopaths, present the core of the problem of addiction in terms of numbers and presence of personality insufficiencies, hence difficulty of cure.

With regard to the type of person who is likely to become an addict a study in 1951 of 260 boys and girls admitted to Bellevue Hospital in New York City is illuminating. It was concluded that there was a striking uniformity in personalities and backgrounds of the boys. The subjects were all nonaggressive and used passive techniques that gave a superficial appearance of ease and poise. Their interpersonal relationships were weak and superficial, with the notable exception of their relationships with their mothers. They had many acquaintances but few friends, but their relationships with their mothers were extremely close. Often they were their mother's favorite. Many had chosen definitely domestic types of occupations such as cooking or tailoring. On the other hand,

there appears to have developed a reversal of this essentially complacent and introverted prototype. In more recent years the usual and normal level of conflict between adolescents and adults has risen to a high pitch as standards and established social institutions have been increasingly challenged and attacked by the young. It would appear that one manifestation of this has been the use of drugs as familial and social defiance.[11]

Substantiating part of the earlier New York study is a recent analysis[12] in Portland, Ore., of an array of social factors in relation to adolescent drug use. Significant positive association was identified with regard to broken families, low income, adult crime, substandard housing, low valuation of owner-occupied dwelling, and extent of rented occupancy. Obviously most of these are interrelated as well as related to other problems or indices of low socioeconomic status. At the same time (1969) a national survey[13] of a representative sample of high school senior students indicated that they make a sharp distinction between marihuana and more serious drugs. Over two thirds of students strongly disapproved of the regular use of each of the more serious drugs, but the same proportion approved of or were neutral about the use of marihuana.

Table 26-1 presents in condensed form some of the characteristics and effects of various narcotics and drugs that are considered later in this chapter. Alcohol is included for comparison and because it is actually a drug.

## NARCOTIC ADDICTION
### Extent and cost of the problem

It is extremely difficult or impossible to determine the extent of the narcotic addiction problem.[14] Estimates of the number of addicts vary from 60,000 to 600,000 in the United States.[15] The lower figure, however, is based on those who have had encounters with law enforcement agencies,[16] and as Mattick[17] colorfully observed, "Any attempts at extrapolation from arrestees to addicts is sheer metaphysics." On the other hand, the higher figures are estimates based on usually limited or biased surveys or on amounts of narcotics known or thought to have entered the country. This, of course, ignores the facts that many individuals use narcotics only once, a few times, or sporadically, that some who use them more often are not necessarily addicted, and that some persons who may be classified as addicts may nevertheless continue as useful, productive members of society.[7]

As an example of the undependability of data in this field, whereas the Federal Bureau of Narcotics and Dangerous Drugs counts 32,000 "known" narcotic addicts in the State of New York, the New York State Narcotic Control Commission reports about 60,000 addicts, essentially the same figure given by the federal agency for the nation as a whole.[9] Furthermore, a careful survey by the New York City Addiction Service Agency concluded there were about 100,000 narcotic addicts *in New York City alone!*[18] One reasonably dependable figure is the 1,259 narcotic-related deaths that occurred in New York City during 1971. This represented an increase from 311 such deaths in 1961 and constituted the leading cause of death in persons between 15 and 35 years of age in that city. A recent report[19] of a Task Force of the Drug Abuse Council (established by the Ford, Carnegie, Commonwealth, and Kaiser Foundations in cooperation with pertinent federal and state agencies) estimates between 150,000 and 250,000 active heroin addicts in the United States, about one half of whom live in New York. From 60% to 70% are Black, Puerto Rican, or Mexican-American; about 85% are males between 15 and 35 years of age; and from 40% to 60% also use amphetamine or barbiturate regularly. Since about 95% of active narcotic addicts are currently on heroin, the 250,000 figure is probably reasonably close to the total picture at this time.

It is impossible to make even a crude guess as to what drug addiction costs society. Included should be the loss or decrease of production by those afflicted, the costs of hospitals, enforcement agencies, and prisons, losses due to crime stimulated by the search for money with which to purchase drugs, the costs of accidents and illnesses connected with their use, and the cost of the drugs themselves.

Most opium, which is the raw source of heroin, is grown in Asia and the Middle East. About 1,300 tons are sold illicitly each year, enough for 24 million doses of heroin. North America and especially the United States is the principal consumer of both the legitimate (morphine) and illegitimate (heroin) refined products. As an estimate of the amount of heroin smuggled into the United States each year, federal narcotic authorities have applied the average daily dose just to the number of known addicts and arrive at a minimum of 3,300 pounds of refined drug. An average of less than one tenth of this amount is seized annually by all enforcement agencies. Another indication of the magnitude of the problem is that in a recent typical year, United States agents working abroad seized 888 kilograms of raw opium, 128 kilograms of morphine base, and 84 kilograms of heroin destined for the United States.[20]

The Permanent Central Narcotics Board of the United Nations Economic and Social Council points out that raw opium sells for $30 to $40 per kilogram in areas where there is little control and about ten times that where there is risk of discovery. Hence the value of the illicit raw opium is between $36 and $360 million. But when processed into heroin, it brings thousands of dollars per ounce. Another way of emphasizing the profit, or markup, is that the true cost of 1 kilogram (2.2 pounds) of heroin is about the same as 1 kilogram of potatoes. When it ultimately reaches the street where it is sold, it is worth about $50,000. This, of course, is why traffic in illicit narcotics has attracted the criminal classes in various countries and why dealers in illicit drugs so frequently encourage free trials to get additional sure customers "on the hook." Once hooked, it has been estimated that the average cost of supporting the habit is from $75 to about $150 per day. One hard drug addict is worth about $5,000 per year to a "pusher." Where does the confirmed addict obtain the necessary funds, especially if his addiction affects his ability to work? Essentially the source of funds is illegal—theft, prostitution, or pandering. In Chicago alone 50% of all crime is attributed to addicts, and the Drug Abuse Council[19] estimates that heroin addicts in the United States steal from $1 to $2 billion annually.

**Effects of narcotics**

Each narcotic produces certain characteristic effects. Generally speaking they all cause general stimulation, euphoria, and contentment, with release from pain or concerns that arise from worries, neuroses, and conflicts. Various sensory manifestations occur, such as a tingling of the skin, hallucinations, and feelings of ecstasy. All these pleasures, of course, are of temporary and short duration for which the addict pays a high price in continued and progressive misery. Contrary to popular opinion, although these substances act generally as stimulants, they depress certain functions, notably the sexual drive. Continued use produces a considerable loss of appetite, resulting in weight loss and nutritional disorders; the typical addict is thin, wan, and undernourished. Severe constipation is common, as is severe itching. The addict suffers from nervousness, insomnia, and depression, and suicidal attempts are not uncommon, especially during the typical postjag depression. Because of the anxiousness of the addict to experience the drug and because dilution by those who sell it is so common, the addict frequently does not know how much he is actually taking. As a result, serious toxic reactions and even death may occur from an overdose. This is the most deadly complication of narcotic addiction.

Overdose is estimated to kill 1% of New York's addicts each year. Even when not lethal, heroin excess can cause pulmonary congestion, edema, and fibrosis. Most complications, however, are caused not by the effects of the drug but by infections introduced through a contaminated needle or solution. Prominent among these are viral hepatitis, bacterial endocarditis, pneumonia, syphilis, malaria, bacteremia, and various skin and subcutaneous infections at the site of injection. Viral hepatitis, occasionally fatal and frequently recurrent and severe, was observed in 42 out of 100 reported complications among New York addicts. Almost equally prevalent was bacterial endocarditis caused by a variety of microorganisms, the most common being *Staphylococcus aureus*. Contrary to the usual types of endocarditis, that of the heroin addict did not spare healthy valves or the tricuspid valve.[21,22] Because of lowered resistance, the addict is much more susceptible than the average person to many other infections and organic diseases. Furthermore, one effect of the drug is to dull awareness to pain, fever, and other symptoms. All told, life expectancy is greatly shortened.

The most unfortunate effect of narcotics is what they do to the morale, morals, and social behavior of those so unfortunate as to become addicted to them. The typical narcotic addict lives only for the next time he can experience the drug; nothing else really matters. As a result, to obtain the drug he will forfeit anything—job, social position, family, self-respect. He will beg, borrow, or steal to satisfy his craving, and considering the combination of lowered ability to earn and the high daily cost of the required drugs, much petty crime results. Male addicts commonly turn to picking pockets, shoplifting, burglary, dishonest gam-

bling, and pandering. Women and girls frequently become prostitutes. Very frequently the addict becomes a willing "pusher" of the drug, the riskiest link in the delivery chain, to assure his own supply. In effect, the unfortunate addict literally does not own his soul.

A particularly tragic consequence of heroin addiction has become evident within the past few years. Because of the increased prevalence of the use of this narcotic among women of childbearing age, an increasing number of infants are being affected. During the 9 years, 1960 through 1969, 384 infants were born to 382 heroin-addicted mothers in a New York hospital.[23] About one half of the infants weighed less than 2,500 grams. During the first 4 days of life, 259 of the infants had withdrawal signs, 178 of them severe enough to require treatment with chlorpromazine. Fourteen infants died during the neonatal period, 9 of them during the first 9 hours after birth. Most disturbing has been a sharp increase with more than 500 addicted infants born in New York City During 1970[24] and continuing upward in 1971.[25]

**Epidemiology**

As with infectious disease or any other human malfunction, the problem of narcotic addiction may be approached from an epidemiologic point of view. This was well illustrated by Jacobziner[26] in connection with the program in the New York City School Health Program. In reviewing it he said the following:

An epidemic of narcotic addiction must be studied in the same manner as any other outbreak of a communicable disease. The agent, host, and environment and their impact and interrelationship must be studied and investigated. In an epidemic of narcotic addiction the *agent* is perhaps of far lesser significance than the *host* and *environment*. It should be emphasized that drug addiction is not a primary disease entity, but merely symptomatic of an underlying deep-seated disturbance: narcotic addiction being only one of many forms of social maladjustment. Narcotic users are not definitely psychopathic, but in the main, products of an unhealthy and an unhappy environment. Therefore, the underlying causes and motivations must be investigated, discovered, and understood. It is not the *process of addiction* which is important to know, but what causes an adolescent to use a drug or to become socially maladjusted. . . . Two factors are needed for the production of addiction: There must be a vulnerable soil—the individual or host must suffer from a psychological or emotional disturbance—and the drug or agent must be capable of resolving the conflicts, tensions, and anxieties of the maladjusted individual.

A more recent and meticulously developed example of this approach has been presented by Hughes and associates[27] in relation to an almost classic epidemic of heroin addiction in the south side of Chicago during the late 1940s and early 1950s.

From the standpoint of general and statistical epidemiology a predilection for the younger component of the population is evident. The most susceptible age group since the end of World War II until the early 1960s was from 15 to 30 years, but the past decade has shown a downward shift to even younger ages of inception.[28] Although males outnumber females (85% to 15%), it is interesting that the predominance is not as great as among evident alcoholics. Earlier[19] it was pointed out that about one half of addicts lived in New York, and if the metropolitan New York City area is included, the proportion is even greater. In the latter area, as was indicated, 60% to 70% of narcotic addicts are black, Puerto Rican, or Mexican-American. Also earlier[12] the tendency for narcotic addiction to coincide with substandard conditions that accompany or result from a low socioeconomic status was emphasized. In this sense addiction becomes just another trap within a complex of traps.

The import of this was illustrated by an analysis of a sample of 400 individuals, in this instance in Chicago.[29] As the investigators summarized: "The potential for addiction is widely spread through the children of the migrants in the deprived areas of the city, and the ultimate use of drugs by any specific individual depends on many fortuitous circumstances. The high rates of mental disease, alcoholism and other social pathologies which are sown by thwarted desires are the harvest of the same social conditions." And to emphasize the infectiousness of these situations they point out that the addict in such an environment becomes dehumanized and brutalized and in turn dehumanizes and brutalizes others. The terrible end result is indicated by the fact that in the addict population studied the average addict between the ages of 10 and 25 years has spent 15% of his life in prison and that there was every indication that they would continue to spend about 2 months out of every year in a prison setting. They conclude that: "Once the addict enters the cyclical pattern of arrest, incarceration, release, and readdiction, the re-sultant personality makes the addict's role practically irreversible except through certain specific modes of therapeutic intervention, 'burning out' and/or active involvement in social change." It is the possibility of the alternatives to which attention is now turned.

## Approach to the problem

Initially and traditionally attempts to combat the narcotic problem in the United States have been based on legislation, prohibition, judicial action, and punishment. Simrell[6] has detailed the sequence of events well. A few highlights may be of interest. Police action goes back to 1885. In 1909 Congress passed legislation "to prohibit the importation and use of opium for other than medicinal purposes," the latter undefined, but to be regulated by the Secretary of the Treasury. An international convention was called in 1912 in the Hague that not only considered control of international commerce in opiates but also included national obligations to control domestic manufacture, traffic, and use. The Hague convention of 1912 was eventually superseded by a new convention adopted by the United Nations in 1961. The United States withheld signature until 1967, when it felt secure that certain controls stipulated in the earlier convention would not be weakened. Meanwhile the United States Congress, to implement its agreement with the Hague convention, passed the Harrison Act of 1914, administered by the Department of Justice through the chief federal policing agency for criminal narcotics activities, the Bureau of Narcotics and Dangerous Drugs. Based essentially on the taxing power, it strictly limited the importation, production, sale, and use of opiates with the specific exemption of the use of narcotic drugs by a registered physician in the course of his practice only. Since then, the Congress has taken several actions to broaden the base to include such concepts as United States international obligations and the promotion of the public health, safety, and welfare. Throughout, the fundamental administrative tool has been the exercise of criminal sanctions. In 1929, however, the Congress enacted legislation that added four important responsibilities to the Public Health Service:

1. Treatment and rehabilitation of federally convicted narcotic drug addicts
2. Prevention of federal narcotics offenses by means of treatment and rehabilitation of voluntary patients
3. Encouragement and assistance to states

and local communities to provide adequate and acceptable facilities and methods for the care of narcotic addicts

4. Research and training in the causes, diagnosis, treatment, control, and prevention of narcotic addiction

One result of this was the establishment by the Public Health Service of a specialized hospital at Lexington, Ky., in 1935 for the study, treatment, and rehabilitation of addicted prisoners, probationers, and voluntary patients in circumstances "less prison-like than most prisons and more prison-like than most hospitals."[30] In 1938 a second hospital for this purpose was established at Fort Worth, Texas, but this was recently closed. It should be noted that these activities led eventually to the passage of the National Mental Health Act on July 3, 1946, and provided the genesis of the now broad-ranging National Institute of Mental Health on April 1, 1949. The responsibilities and potentials of the institute in the field of narcotic addiction were significantly expanded by the passage of the Narcotic Addict Rehabilitation Act of 1966, which established a national policy of civil commitment for treatment and aftercare of addicts even if they are charged with or convicted of violating federal criminal laws.[31] Added to this was the Comprehensive Drug Abuse Prevention and Control Act of 1970, which provided funds for additional research into the causes and prevention of drug abuse and dependence; additional funds for treatment and rehabilitation of addicts; and strengthening of existing drug abuse law enforcement authority. It also provided for the establishment of a Commission on Marihuana and Drug Abuse to report to the President and the Congress. Subsequently, in December 1970, the Drug Abuse Education Act was added, which authorized funds for public education about the problem.

The past decade has witnessed a considerable reexamination of attitudes and methods.[32,33] Increasingly the addict is being regarded separately and differently from those who promote addiction for substantial economic profit. There has been occurring a gradual shift from a national philosophy and approach based on punitive action against addicts who had been assumed to be intrinsically evil, hence criminal, toward an acceptance of the addict as a sick victim of an unfortunate social and physiologic phenomenon. In the process more enlightened legislation has been appearing in relation to the addict concurrent with a constantly tightening of law enforcement and judicial action against those who promote narcotic traffic, who are still and must continue to be regarded as criminals.[34]

Any program designed to attack the problem of narcotic addiction must be multipronged and involve the understanding and cooperation of many disciplines, that is, religion, law and law enforcement, and education, to mention only the most obvious. The most logical first step is case finding. Police and other law-enforcement personnel are probably the primary sources of case finding; physicians, hospitals, and health centers are the secondary source. In addition, public health and visiting nurses and social workers occasionally learn of addicts from patients and clients. Regardless of the circumstances, on discovery the addict should be regarded primarily as an ill person and not as a criminal. Instead of being treated in a punitive fashion, he should be admitted promptly to a hospital or other suitable institution for evaluation and appropriate medical and psychiatric treatment. It is not possible to treat a confirmed narcotic addict as an outpatient, at least in the initial stages. If local facilities are not available or suitable, arrangements may be made for admission to the Public Health Service hospital in Lexington, Ky., which is specially equipped to handle this type of case.

As to chances of cure, studies of patients after discharge from the Lexington hospital are far from encouraging. Usual experience is that 3 out of every 4 addicts relapse at some time. Frequently the road to ultimate cure involves several relapses. A study[35] of the 43,215 patients treated at Lexington between 1935 and 1966 showed a total of 77,076 admissions. Some returned as many as six times. The overall patient readmission rate was about 38%. For white male voluntary patients under 21 years the rate was 53%. The readmission rate for those discharged as cured was 37%, whereas for those who left against medical advice before 31 days it was 40%, and for those who stayed longer it was 42%.

The high relapse rate points to the most difficult part of the problem, that is, rehabilitation and follow-up.[36] An important part of the treatment is to make the addict aware of the underlying reasons for his addiction and to help him rehabilitate himself psychologically and socially. Many investigators have emphasized the importance of qualified field personnel, public health nurses or social workers, who may obtain pertinent background information about the patient, his family, and his environment. Repeated visits to the home and neighborhood environment are suggested, not only before and after the discharge of the patient but also prior to the patient's admission for treatment. In addition to the patient, the family and the community need to be reeducated and prepared for the return of the patient. With special reference to the adolescent the importance of a good parent-child relationship is emphasized, and parents must be made to understand that a poor quality of parent-child relationship is responsible for many forms of social maladjustment. Those close to the patient should be forewarned of the possibility of a relapse and warned not to castigate the patient if this should occur but to contact appropriate professionals or institutions as soon as possible. In 1949 an organization known as Synanon, patterned after Alcoholics Anonymous, was formed. It has developed into a valuable adjunct in the rehabilitation of narcotic addicts. It has branches in several cities and is gaining experience in providing effective resources for addicts. Since then, a variety of other types of rehabilitative groups and organizations have formed throughout the country, especially in centers of high addiction prevalence. These facilities, which are called "halfway houses" and other names, play an increasingly important role in assisting in the return to community life.[36] Since a sense of inadequacy and failure often plays an important role, efforts should be made to assist the discharged patient in obtaining employment so that he may develop a feeling of fulfillment and confidence. Much remains to be done toward development of a willingness on the part of most potential employers to give the ex-patient an opportunity and to provide encouragement whenever possible.

During the past few decades, there has been much controversy about the validity of the so-called British system, wherein drug addiction is handled primarily by specially licensed members of the medical profession with controlled legal distribution of drugs to those who use them. The premise is that by removing the profit motive there is no temptation to resort to crime to obtain the drug and there is no incentive to create new addicts. In reviewing it, Kolb[37] advocates strenuous attempts to cure the addict during periods of hospitalization but believes that when after several such attempts the patient is apparently not amenable to cure but will get along well with a minimum amount of narcotic, he should be given this for the rest of his life under medical supervision. He believes, on the basis of his experience, that the majority of such addicts would work, support themselves, and create no public problem. Variations of this approach are followed in several other countries, and it has been advocated on a selective and demonstrative basis by the New York Academy of Medicine.[38]

Many investigators, however, object on the basis that the procedure removes the incentive for real cure. The Study Group on Treatment and Care of Drug Addicts,[39] called by the World Health Organization in November 1956, discouraged this approach, "While complete withdrawal of the drug of addiction might be deferred in certain circumstances, the maintenance of drug addiction is not treatment." Similar reservations were reiterated in other terms by the WHO Expert Committee on Drug Dependence in 1970.[40]

Recent experience in England indicates a significant rise in the number of known narcotic addicts from 500 in 1964 to about 1,500 in 1967. In addition, the number of drug-related complications and crimes has increased, despite the system.[40] Whether this may correctly be attributed to the system or to more complex sociologic changes is unclear. It has resulted, however, in placing the system in disfavor. As Hess[41] disclaims, "Reference is made to 'the successful British system.' But how can a program be called successful when the addicted population has doubled in the past 10 years? In addition, it has been shown that 35% of a study group in England became involved in crime within a year." Furthermore, as Larimore and Brill[42] point out, not only is the number of known narcotic addicts in England small (about 700) but about one sixth of them were physicians to begin with. In this regard it has been noted[43] that drug addiction, like alcoholism, is an occupational hazard of physicians. It is estimated that physicians make up 15% of all the drug addicts in the United States, England, Germany, Holland, and France, where data on the subject have been collected. They conclude that these factors plus a lower cultural susceptibility to drug addiction on the part of the British people account for any difference between the United States and England rather than between the American and British method of handling addicts. This is agreed to by the WHO Expert Committee on Drug Dependence,[40] which states that the "British approach" has developed in a social and medical setting that is probably unique and that it is impossible to make valid comparisons between the situations and methods in the United Kingdom and North America.

**Methadone.** The most significant event that has occurred with relation to possible eventual solution of the narcotic and especially the heroin problem was the discovery by Dole and Nyswander[44,45] in the early 1960s of the effectiveness and values of methadone hydrochloride in the treatment and rehabilitation of addicts. Methadone is a synthetic narcotic drug with many of the properties of heroin, morphine, and other opiate drugs. For example, taken either orally or intramuscularly it is a highly effective analgesic. However, there are several unique and important differences when used properly to treat chronic opiate addiction. It does not lose effectiveness when taken by mouth. Its effects are longer lasting, a single dose suppressing heroin withdrawal symptoms for 24 to 36 hours. It suppresses the action of other opiates without itself producing sedation or euphoria, hence the addict ceases to have obsessive and compulsive thoughts about or craving for opiate drugs. As a result, the individual typically renews interest in normal life and can return to school, maintain employment, and present no social problems. Although a dependence on methadone is substituted for the heroin dependence, the individual develops a tolerance to most of the effects of the drug, which incidentally is remarkably free of side effects or complications when used properly. Sensitivity to pain is normal, and there is even a normal response to intramuscular morphine if its use should be indicated for other medical reasons. Sleep, digestion, alertness, reaction time, and libido usually become normal. Infants of methadone-dependent individuals are born normal. DuPont, and Katon[46] describe it as one of the most important medical discoveries of the twentieth century and add that, "Like Fleming's discovery of penicillin and Enders' discovery of virus tissue culture techniques, the Dole-Nyswander discovery enabled physicians to deal constructively with a major health problem that was previously unsolvable."

Methadone was first used by its discoverers in 1963 in New York City. Since then, its use has increased in that area and has spread throughout the country. By mid-1972 more than 50,000 heroin addicts (an estimated one third to one fifth of the total) were receiving the drug in about 300 clinics throughout the country, most of which have long waiting lists.[47] Despite its wide acceptance and the many advantages just described, the use of methadone is not without problems. It has no usefulness against nonopiate drugs. Taken in large, uncontrolled doses it can produce undesirable reactions and even death. Because of this, early in 1973 the Food and Drug Administration placed strict limitations on the method and circumstances of its use. Methadone maintenance programs will be permitted to expand, but prescribing of the drug by physicians who are not involved in such programs must be voluntary, limited to heroin addicts who have been drug dependent for at least 2 years and who are over the age of 18 years, except in special circumstances. Only liquid methadone will be administered in the presence of an attendant, and the privilege of taking it home will be severely restricted.

Methadone programs typically are two phased. Initially there is an inpatient detoxification phase, during which the addict is detoxified from heroin and stabilized on methadone. This is followed by the outpatient maintenance phase, which involves the patient reporting to the methadone clinic to take the orally administered drug. Dole and Nyswander, on the basis of their experience, claim that 80% of new patients need not be admitted to a hospital for the first phase but can be supervised on an ambulatory basis. Furthermore, the experience of DuPont and Katon[46] at their active center in the District of Columbia leads them to believe that methadone is so effective that many patients cannot conceive of wanting heroin again. This causes them to believe that they can be detoxified, but every patient detoxified had some recurrence of drug hunger and almost all either resumed methadone treatment or returned to heroin.

This necessarily directs attention to cost. Methadone itself is inexpensive and currently costs only 25 cents for a single day's dosage. However, as Maidlow and Berman[48] point out, since the addict must be maintained on methadone for the remainder of his life, the cost for the drug alone is about $100 per year, or $5,000 over 50 years of remaining life. This, however, is the minor part of the cost, since the drug must be administered in a controlled center. Generally administrative overhead and medical personnel result in an estimated total cost of $1,000 per addict per year, or $50,000 during the life expectancy. What is gained by this? In their interesting cost-benefit analysis, Maidlow and Berman point to a twofold benefit (1) reduced thefts by addicts and (2) increased addict productivity. The value of thefts by heroin addicts has been established at about $30,000 per addict per year. Since each lives an average of 28 years as an addict, the present total value of thefts discounted at 8% is about $330,000, which, of course, is avoided with the addict on methadone. Furthermore, assuming a productive or earning life of 28 years at a constant average of $5,084 per year, again discounted at 8%, the present value of the productivity of the individual on methadone would be about $57,000. The lifetime gain therefore from a maximum lifetime expenditure of $50,000 for methadone maintenance would be about $337,000 per patient ($330,000 plus $57,000 minus $50,000).

**Preventive measures.** Currently, of course, much research is underway toward the goal of developing longer lasting and safer narcotic antagonists, implantable capsules, or effective prophylactic measures. Meanwhile in the psychologic arena a number of "self-regulating" communities have been developing, the first founded in 1958 in California. Their conceptual basis is that the use of drugs is a symptom of an underlying character disorder or emotional immaturity which requires a restructuring of the individual's character and personality. Typically new members are given the most menial or degrading tasks from which they may advance to more desirable roles and greater responsibilities. Drugs and violence are strictly forbidden, and criticisms and punishments are deliberately harsh. This is offset, however, by a unique form of group concern for the individual that is rarely if ever found on the outside. Some communities have the advantage of assistance from professionals in mental health and public health as well as various social agencies. The value of such communities is subject to question. Experience so far is that only about two thirds of those who contact them become residents and of these fewer than one half remain more than a few months.

With reference to general preventive measures, several points should be considered. First, certain legislation is necessary (1) to control strictly the importation, production, distribution, and sale of all drugs that potentially may cause addiction, (2) to provide adequate organization and financing for carrying out the foregoing and other activities, (3) to provide for severe punishment of those found guilty of the illicit importation, handling, and sale of narcotics, and (4) to allow for addicts who are apprehended to be turned over to suitable institutions for mandatory treatment without court action. More adequate educational activities are indicated to bring about better understanding and cooperation on the part of all those in society who may play a role in attacking this problem. This applies to physicians, nurses, public health workers, teachers, clergy, police, welfare workers, and many others. Most authorities, however, believe strongly that direct propaganda to young people on the subject of narcotics is not only of no value but is actually dangerous. Thus H. J. Anslinger, former United States Commissioner of Narcotics, believes that it may only serve to awaken the interest or stimulate the curiosity of potential adolescent addicts. Similarly Artis, supervisor of the Chicago office of the United States Bureau of Narcotics, has stated: "We do not recommend or promote direct education on narcotic drugs. In this conclusion, we agree with the conclusions of the 68 nations of the United Nations who passed a resolution on this subject. Narcotic education is open to controversy and great objections. We prefer to educate at the parent-teacher level." Recent experiences of several secondary schools that conducted courses on narcotics and drugs appear to substantiate these views.

Beyond the activities of adequate legislation and education it is to be anticipated that, as in the case of alcoholism, increased and improved methods in mental health and their wider availability and acceptability will play a significant part in the prevention and amelioration of the narcotic problem. Added to this are the benefits that are sure to result from constantly improving and equalizing social conditions and opportunities. These in the long run may remove many of the underlying factors that lead some to escape unpleasant realities through the insidious medium of narcotics.

Public and official awareness and concern are illustrated by the dramatic increase in facilities relating to narcotic and drug abuse. Thus a study[49] in 1962 showed that only 28 states had programs. Eight programs were operated by state health departments and most of the rest by state departments of mental health. In cities with populations over 100,000 only 4 local health departments reported programs, whereas 11 cities had programs under auspices other than the health department. Only 5 years later, in 1967, another study[50] identified 110 governmental and 55 nongovernmental programs. Only 12 states reported no program, and in the interval since, at least one half of them have instituted activities. Facilities consisted of the following types: hospital and/or clinic 120, rehabilitation and/or treatment 28, coordination and/or referral 27, information and education 27, halfway house 11, and other 19. Two thirds of the facilities sponsored by governmental agencies were in hospitals or clinics, usually under a department of public health, mental health, or public welfare. Services provided consisted of group and/or individual psychotherapy 65, medical treatment including detoxification and withdrawal 66, casework services and guidance 42, vocational and recreational therapy 38, referral 32, rehabilitation and treatment of unspecified types 21, other services 26, and no direct services 6. With reference to sponsorship of the governmental facilities or programs, 2 were federal, 82 were state, and 26 were city or county. Although two thirds of the facilities or programs were government sponsored, annual use figures indicated a total of only about 35,000 individuals served: one sixth by local governmental agencies, two sixths by state governmental agencies, and three sixths by nongovernmental agencies. In the several years since, more facilities have been established and many more addicts served as a result of the advent of methadone. Nevertheless, it is obvious that much more needs to be done and that this is still essentially a pioneering territory for health agencies.

## NONNARCOTIC DRUGS

As indicated earlier, there are a variety of substances, both natural and synthetic, which although not addictive, are included here for convenience. Among other reasons is the fact that they share certain characteristics with narcotics: they produce some unusual psychic effects; their use is not ordinarily socially acceptable in most cultures; commerce in them is ordinarily illegal and tends to attract certain socially undesirable types of individuals; and the majority of them have certain undesirable physical or mental consequences. Included are certain drugs with valuable legitimate medical uses.

Lipscomb[51] categorizes these many drugs into "ups" and "downs" (Table 26-1). The first he describes as having a centrifugal action on the human organism. Their effect is to elicit or enhance and sustain greater numbers of stimuli than the individual would ordinarily experience. Included in this group are the amphetamines, STP, LSD, marihuana, and caffeine. The second category is described as having a centripetal action on the human organism by diminishing, subduing, or reducing the number of stimuli that might be experienced. Included (in addition to alcohol and opiates) are tranquilizers and barbiturates. Increasingly in American culture these substances, rather than being used singly, are used synergistically or more commonly "in tandem." Thus Lipscomb describes the all too familiar "sine curve individual," who takes a "wake-me-up" pill in the morning (caffeine or amphetamine), a midday "soother" (perhaps a martini), an evening "turn-me-down" (highball), and a nighttime "put-me-to-sleep" (barbiturate). To dispel any idea that the common use and abuse of many of these substances is limited to some insignificant "depraved" component of the population, it is well to point out that more than 200 million prescriptions for psychoactive drugs, most of them to alleviate anxiety, frustration, agitation, boredom, and depression are filled annually in the United States, despite the common realization that they will not solve any problems. In addition, of course, is the enormous amount of caffeine-containing and alcoholic beverages that are consumed in American society. Obviously most of these materials are consumed by ordinary members of society who store much of it in overstocked "medicine" cabinets in their homes. This profligate use has significance beyond the apparent. Children learn much from the examples of their parents. Studies in Canada,[52] for example, found that marihuana and other illicit drug use was more common among students who reported their parents to be users of both alcohol and tobacco, and if their parents used tranquilizers daily, the students were twice as likely to use illicit drugs. Dumont[53] asks the pertinent question, "Shall we ever know the full costs of our mania for prescribing medicines? A world of antibiotic-resistant infections and amphetamine and barbiturate dependency, a whole generation incapable of coping with anxiety and grief, and an ambience of pill-taking that induces our children to believe that there is a chemical for everything, including a world gone mad." And to this one may add the soft piped-in music provided in some mortuaries and cemeteries! For purposes of descriptive discussion the various nonnarcotic substances will be considered in the four categories of depressants, stimulants, ataraxics, and hallucinogens.

## Depressants

Depressants include sedatives and hypnotics. Predominant in this group are the barbiturates, the most widely abused of the depressants. These substances are commonly used in medicine for their sedative or calming effect, especially in anxiety states, hyperthyroidism, and high blood pressure, as well as to allay pain and to control convulsions such as occur with epilepsy. When chronically misused, they may in some ways become more dangerous than narcotics. Physical dependence on them may develop, and tolerance is never complete. A person who is habituated to them shows evidence of slurred speech, staggering and even falling from lack of balance, quick temper, and quarrelsome disposition. Overdose produces coma, and pneumonia is not an uncommon complication. When these drugs are withheld from a habitué, the withdrawal symptoms may be as serious and dangerous as those of narcotic withdrawal. Central nervous system symptoms develop, leading possibly to epileptiform convulsions with subsequent delirium and hallucinations similar to delirium tremens. Indeed, this is becoming a serious aspect of the drug scene with increase in multiple drug use. Treatment for withdrawal from one type of drug, such as heroin, may lead to neglect of withdrawal stress from another, such as barbiturates, which may be fatal.[54]

Among persons who use these substances illicitly there is a variety of colorful names, such as goof balls, peanuts, red devils, rainbows, and blue heavens, to mention only a few. In 1973 drugstores in the United States filled 478 million prescriptions for barbiturates. In any one year enough amphetamines and barbiturates are medically prescribed to provide every man, woman, and child with a month's supply. However, a former commissioner of the Food and Drug Administration has testified that enough raw material was produced in 1962 to make over 9 billion doses of barbiturates and amphetamines combined. He estimated that at least one half ended up in the illicit market.

## Stimulants

The second group of substances are stimulants, which include drugs that directly stimulate the central nervous system, producing alertness, wakefulness, excitation, and sometimes a rise in blood pressure and respiration. The most common substances in this category are the amphetamines, which have been used for the 25 years in the treatment of a variety of mental diseases and as adjuncts in the correction of excessive weight. They appear to have a specific effect on the appetite center in the brain. They are also valuable in the treatment of narcolepsy and Parkinson's disease. Because of their unusual stimulant action, amphetamines and related compounds tend to be abused by individuals whose occupations require long periods of wakefulness or vivaciousness and by those who attempt to "burn the candle at both ends." A relatively high degree of tolerance can be developed with these substances without necessarily causing physical or psychic damage if dosage is gradually increased. In some instances, however, a true drug psychosis resembling schizophrenia may develop with delusions and hallucinations. Under ordinary misuse, however, the individual appears to be unusually excitable, talkative, and restless, with a tremor of the hands and an enlargement of the pupils, sleeplessness, and perspiration. Under certain circumstances a psychic or emotional dependence on these chemicals may develop.

As in the case of the depressants, these materials have many colloquial names, including bennies, co-pilots, peaches, cartwheels, hearts, and dexies. The economics of the illicit drug market as a whole are well illustrated by amphetamines, which can be purchased wholesale for $1 per 1,000, sold in the illegal market for $30 to $50 per 1,000, and retained to the individual for as much as 10 to 25 cents per tablet. The true medical need of oral amphetamines is not more than several hundred thousand units. However, the annual production in the United States is 8 billion doses! Effective March 1973, all the amphetamine-type drugs were banned from the open market and their medical use restricted to narcolepsy, minimal brain dysfunction in children, and short-term adjunctive management of exogenous obesity refractive to other measures.

## Ataraxics

The third category of nonnarcotic drugs that tend to be abused are the ataraxics, or tranquilizers. These materials introduced during the 1950s are in one sense a type of nervous system depressant. They have revolutionized the treatment of many psychiatric disorders and, as such, represent a major advance in pharmacology and therapy. Their use under medical direction or otherwise has become extremely commonplace and would appear to be generally lacking in toxic side effects and much less likely to produce habituation among those who use them. More than 1 million pounds are produced and over 60 million prescriptions written for them each year in the United States. The economic value of the tranquilizer market is now measured in the hundreds of millions of dollars annually.

### Hallucinogens

The fourth group of substances of a non-narcotic nature and one that has been rapidly increasing in use are the various hallucinogens.[55,56] Pharmacologically they are referred to as psychedelics or psychotomimetics. Included are lysergic acid diethylamide (LSD-25), a semi-synthetic derivative of ergonovine; the seeds of some varieties of morning glory ("Ololiuqui," *Rivea corymbosa*, and *Ipomoea violacea*), the active principle of which is closely related to LSD; mescaline, a phenethylamine present in the buttons of a small cactus ("mescal," "peyote," or *Lophophora williamsii*), which has been used by Indians in southwestern United States and Mexico in certain accepted religious rituals of the Native American Church; psilocybin, an indole found in a mushroom ("teonanacatl," *Psilocybe mexicana*); and DMT or dimethyltryptamine, a synthetic indole, also found in the seeds of a South American plant (*Piptadenia peregrina*). LSD is an extremely powerful drug, 100 times more potent than psilocybin and 7,000 more potent than mescaline. Since it has been brought under legal control, however, the relatively newer synthetic DMT with a shorter and stronger action appeared on the illicit market. An LSD "trip" or "experience" usually has a fairly gentle onset and lasts about 12 hours, whereas a DMT "trip" has a sudden "rough" onset and lasts only about 2 hours. One of the characteristics of these substances, especially the synthetics, is that eating, inhaling, or injecting only minute amounts, as little as 1/280,000 of an ounce of LSD for example, may produce severe and dramatic effects that sometimes may recur, even without taking the drug again.[57]

The illicit use of these substances, especially by certain psychosocial cults, by groups such as beatniks or hippies who attempt to withdraw from society, or by some misguided young people or older pseudosophisticates in search of a new and different "experience" or of their "identity," has been attributed to the mind-expanding effects of the drugs. It is true that many individuals may use them without serious effects and in the process experience a wide variety of stimulating and colorful hallucinations. Even in such instances the physical effects of LSD are usually disturbing. There is an increase in blood pressure and heart rate; the blood sugar level goes up; there may be nausea, chills, flushes, irregular breathing, sweating of the hands, and trembling of the extremities. Sleep is virtually impossible until at least 8 to 10 hours after the LSD episode is over. The pupils of the eyes are widely dilated so that dark glasses are often worn, even at night, for protection against the light. Beyond these more "usual" effects there is ample evidence of the development in some individuals of overwhelming fear and panic, paranoid delusions, distressing distortions of time, place, and position, and intense self-loathing. Unprovoked violence toward others, loss of sanity, and suicide are by no means rare.

As evidence of these serious manifestations, in 1966, for example, more than 100 individuals were admitted to Bellvue Hospital in New York City suffering from LSD-induced psychosis. Many other hospitals elsewhere have been confronted with similar experiences. One example of the condition of such patients is given in an analysis[58] of 70 patients (53 males and 17 females, 16 to 36 years of age) admitted to the psychiatric service of a university hospital during 7 months of a recent year. Diagnoses included psychotic disorders (19 patients), neurotic disorders (15), character disorders (13), addiction (7), adjustment reaction of adolescence, borderline, etc. (8), and multiple diagnosis (8). Over one half of the patients had taken other drugs 6 weeks and more prior to admission. The side effects presented after the use of LSD included hallucinations (2 patients), anxiety (17), depression (15), suicide attempt (5), suicidal manifestations (5), paranoia (10), and confusion (14). Some of the patients presented more than one symptom. Seventeen of the patients required more than 1 month of hospitalization.

Prolonged or rebound effects of LSD use have been mentioned. Some insight into this phenomenon is provided by a study[59] of the clinical effects of LSD in a group of schizophrenic patients in whom LSD-induced psychotic reactions persisted beyond 24 hours in 3 out of

158 experiences. The reactions responded poorly to therapy and persisted for as long as 3 months. The prolonged reactions appeared as exaggerations of the affective and emotional liability observed before the use of LSD and paralleled the instances of prolonged psychoses observed in adolescent and psychopathic individuals, where the induced state had been characterized by depressive episodes, suicidal preoccupations, delusional states, and aggressive outbursts. The hazard of LSD administration appears to be in decreasing emotional and affective controls and inducing a persistent state of altered consciousness. It is suggested that in experimental and therapeutic programs the hazards of LSD administration may be minimized by the prophylactic administration of a phenothiazine after the acute LSD syndrome has been observed.

At present there is much difference of opinion concerning possible genetic effects of hallucinogens, especially LSD. Observation of chromosomal damage was first reported in 1967 and since has been substantiated or discounted by various investigators in the United States and other countries. An especially provocative recent study[60] reported 46 persons who ingested LSD and 4 persons who were exposed to the drug in utero. Fourteen drug-free controls had a chromosomal breakage rate of 6% to 16.5%, whereas among the drug users it was 8% to 45%. In addition to observed chromosomal breakage several reports have been appearing in the United States and British medical literature indicating possible relationships between LSD use and clinical teratologic malformations. A key problem is the concurrent use of a variety of other substances as medications, as additional drugs, or as foods that could conceivably cause or contribute to the phenomenon. The problem and its potentials are so significant as to encourage careful studies that separate clearly any effect on chromosomes produced by LSD from effects that might be attributed to other substances or factors.[61]

## Marihuana

Because of the considerable attention given to it during recent years, specific mention should be made of a much milder but more widely used hallucinogen, marihuana. Marihuana is a drug found in the flowering tops and leaves of the Indian hemp plant *Cannabis sativa,* which is related to the fig, hop, and nettle. It is used commercially in making rope, textiles, and birdseed. The consumption of cannabis in one form or another—marihuana, bhang, ganja, charras, maconha, kif, or hashish—has been known for at least 5,000 years. Although it has no use in modern medicine, it was included in a Chinese medical compendium dated 2737 B.C. as a means of relieving pain during surgery. It was regarded as a useful medicinal in ayurvedic medicine of the subcontinent of Asia and in Arabic medicine. It was introduced into western medicine in 1839 by Sir William O'Shaugnessy, a British physician who had served in India. He used it to treat rheumatism, tetanus, and seizures and described its use in an apparently rabid dog, which after dozing, awoke, wagged its tail contentedly, ate greedily, and "assumed a look of utter and hopeless drunkenness," after which it was perfectly well and lively! Its use spread, and many reports were published concerned with its effectiveness in insomnia, dysmenorrhea, erysipelas, and numerous other ailments. Sir William Osler considered it the most satisfactory remedy for headaches, and in 1890 Reynolds wrote "when pure and administered carefully, it is one of the most valuable medicines we possess."[62] At that time it was also recommended as a treatment for opiate addiction. In 1941 it was removed from the *United States Pharmacopoeia* and *National Formulary*, but as recently as 1949, THC, a synthesized concentrate, was reported effective in preventing epileptic seizures, and it is being studied as an antidepressant and analgesic, as well as a remedy for sunstroke.

Marihuana was introduced to the United States as an intoxicating drug in 1920, and its use became especially well known among "jazz" musicians who attributed to it an enhanced ability to perform. In 1931 the Food and Drug Administration limited the importation of cannabis except for medicinal purposes and as birdseed. Largely to eliminate fears about its use by immigrants from Mexico, the United States Government in 1937 passed the Federal Marihuana Tax Act. This was followed by strict laws and enforcement in every state. During the 1960s, apparently spurred by the examples and statements of several well-known personalities, a sharp increase occurred in its use, especially in college and university groups. This attracted greater law enforcement efforts, and arrests on marihuana charges more than doubled. This did not, however, diminish its use and indeed may even have contributed to its increase.

It is estimated that currently in the United

States about 600,000 individuals smoke marihuana "habitually," 2.4 million socially, and 3 million occasionally. A national poll in early 1973 indicated that 12% of Americans over 18 years of age had tried it. This represented a tripling over the previous survey a mere 2½ years before. Most who had tried it, however, stated they would not use it again, even if it were legalized.[63] Its use was found to be most common in the age group 18 to 19 years and twice as common among men than among women and among those who attended college as those who did not. The percentage use by region was West, 18%; East, 12%; Midwest, 10%; and South, 7%.[64] Another recent study[65] by the Columbia University School of Public Health indicated that about 15% of America's youth between 12 and 17 years of age (boys 17% and girls 14%) had smoked marihuana. Incidentally this study brought out the close relationship between the use of marihuana and experimentation with other mood-changing drugs. Among nonusers of marihuana only 3% said they had used any of five other drugs included in the study, but among the marihuana users 91% had also tried amphetamines, 82% had taken barbiturates, 62% had tried LSD, 33% had sniffed glue, and 11% had used heroin. Such data must be interpreted with care. For one thing almost one half of the marihuana users admitted having tried three or more of the other substances. Another interesting finding was that only 6% of teen-agers from families with an annual income under $10,000 had tried marihuana in contrast to 19% of teen-agers from families with an annual income of $15,000 or more. These and other findings point to factors not intrinsic to marihuana as a basic reason for drug use. As the recent report[66] of the National Commission on Marihuana and Drug Abuse states: "Youth of today are better fed, better housed, more mobile, more affluent, more schooled and probably more bored with their lives than any generation which has preceded them."

It is interesting to read Treadway's comments when the 1937 legislation was being considered.[67] He indicated that cannabis does not produce dependence or increased tolerance as does opium addiction. He did not consider marihuana to be habit forming "in the same sense as alcohol might be with some people, or sugar or coffee." He admitted that sometimes it produced a delirium with a frenzy that might result in violence, but he added that

this is also true of alcohol. Ordinarily when smoked, the active ingredient is absorbed through the respiratory system, enters the bloodstream, and acts on the brain and nervous system. The most obvious signs and symptoms include a rapid heartbeat, lowered body temperature, and reddening of the eyes. The blood sugar level drops, the appetite especially for sweets is stimulated, and the body is dehydrated. The user may become loud and loquacious, uncoordinated, or drowsy.

The effects on the emotions and senses vary, depending on the amount of strength of the marihuana, the social setting, and the experience, previous mood and expectations of the user. Ordinarily its effects appear in about 15 minutes and may last from 2 to 4 hours. The effects may range from excitement and exhilaration to deep depression, and some users experience no change of mood. A common phenomenon is the distortion of time and distance. A moment may seem like an hour, hence musicians may think they are playing much more rapidly than they really are. Similarly objects nearby may appear distant and distorted in shape. Since decision-making ability and reaction time are affected, as is the case with alcohol, individuals should not drive while under the influence of the drug. There is no evidence that marihuana by itself as ordinarily used causes permanent effects, and acute toxic reactions are relatively rare (certainly less so than with alcohol). Intensive studies of 30 long-time Jamaican cannabis users and 31 chronic hashish users in Greece were noteworthy for the relative absence of pathology.

In consideration of its history, its widespread use, its mild reactions, and especially in relation to a long list of obviously more serious social offenses, legal sanctions in the United States in relation to marihuana have been surprisingly harsh. Under federal law to have, give, or sell marihuana in the United States is a felony, which is a serious crime. Federal and many state laws deal with the drug as severely as if it were a narcotic. The federal penalty for possessing the drug is 2 to 10 years' imprisonment plus a possible fine of up to $20,000 for the first offense, 5 to 20 years for the second offense, and 10 to 40 years for further offenses. For transfer or sale of the drug the first offense may bring a 5- to 20-year sentence and a fine of up to $20,000; two or more offenses may bring 10 to 40 years in prison. If a person over 18 years of age sells to a minor under 28 years, he is subject to a fine of up to $20,000 and/or 10 to 40 years in prison for the first offense, with no suspension of sentence, probation, or parole.

The recent report, "Marihuana and Health,"[68] issued by the National Institute of Mental Health, stated that current penalities for use and possession are much too severe and out of keeping with knowledge about its harmfulness. It is also interesting that the former Deputy Director of the Bureau of Narcotics and Dangerous Drugs of the Department of Justice recently accepted membership on the board of the National Organization for the Reform of Marihuana Laws, remarking that he had decided it was wrong to jail young people for smoking pot and that both liquor and tobacco have far more harmful effects. Numerous other professions, organizations, and individuals have been taking similar stands. During 1972, the National Commission on Marihuana and Drug Abuse[66] recommended in its report to the President that marihuana be "decriminalized." The commission suggested elimination of state and federal penalties for possession of small amounts with fines of about $100 for public use, possession of more than 1 ounce, and disorderly conduct or driving associated with marihuana intoxication. It also urged, however, that there be continued strong measures against the production, importation, or sale of marihuana. These modest yet practical recommendations, despite their coincidence with the recommendations of an international panel of experts convened by the World Health Organization[69] are yet to be accepted or acted on favorably, largely because of opposition from several officials whose reactions could readily be anticipated.

## SOLVENT INHALATION

To shift finally to a more bizarre phenomenon, brief mention should be made of the use of several other substances by children and teenagers—airplane glue, lighter fluid, gasoline, nutmeg, and ether.[70] Smelling or inhaling these substances tends to provide a momentary sense of exhilaration, euphoria, and intoxication, but all of them have serious toxic side effects. An important aspect of the use of these materials by adolescents is the fact that frequently their use is by a group. Part of the reason is apparently a shared boredom, a lack of definite goals, a revolting against adult rules, and as a manifestation of wanting to belong to a group. Not uncommonly their use begins in a gang or party setting with one of the group introducing the material or practice and the rest responding for fear of appearing to be "chicken" or cowardly. Whereas some of these practices may on the surface appear innocuous, they may lead to criminal acts. For example, although there is no dependable data concerning the number of those who use these materials in the young population, there is mounting police and court evidence of violations of the law by juveniles after having engaged in the practice. These violations extend from breaking and entering and stealing of automobiles to more serious actions. In one instance the murder and rape of two small twin sisters was committed by a 15-year-old boy who had spent the afternoon sniffing glue. As is often the case, the boy afterward remembered none of the circumstances.

The solution to these problems is not easy, and as in the case of alcoholism or narcotic addiction, it requires the interest and joint action of several concerned groups. Public education, particularly in the schools, is important. In certain circumstances legal restrictions with reference to the sale of certain materials may have some effect. Development by industry of substitutes for dangerous chemicals that are nonetheless necessary for legitimate purposes may offer some hope. In addition to this is the need for persistent and consistent surveillance of the problem by public health officials, law enforcement officials, and other groups. There is also a critical need for the apprehension and prosecution of any who are involved in the sale, dissemination, and use of these dangerous materials for improper purposes.

## FRAUDULENT MEANS OF OBTAINING DRUGS

A few words should be said concerning the methods of obtaining dangerous drugs and particularly those that require prescriptions. Certain of the narcotics are smuggled through customs checkpoints into the United States by various devious means. In addition, however, a large amount of potentially dangerous materials legally produced within the country manages to slip into illegal channels of distribution. Normally drugs move from manufacturer to wholesaler to pharmacist. At each step and point some pilferage or illegal sale may occur. The record of professionals involved in the normal channels of sale and use is excellent. Each year very few arrests are made for illegal sales by pharmacists or physicians. Thus in 1963, despite a total of 300,000 physicians and pharmacists in the country, the Food and Drug Administration recorded only 74 abuses. The three great problem areas are large-scale theft, clandestine drug manufacturers, and individuals who are adept at fraudulently obtaining drugs from physicians and pharmacists. Some concept of the magnitude of theft in transit was indicated by the previously mentioned discrepancies between the amount of barbiturates and amphetamines produced, for example, and the amount legitimately sold. The ability to synthesize certain drugs such as LSD has led to large-scale clandestine manufacture of certain of these materials. Usually the counterfeit products appear as exact duplicates of the legitimate drugs, although the product may vary significantly in potency and may be contaminated because of inadequate quality control. In the same category with the clandestine manufacturer is the repackager and the bulk peddler.

A worrisome problem to the ethical physician and pharmacist is the individual user who has become adept at fraudulently obtaining needed supplies through normal channels. A favorite method is the forging of prescription orders. This is done in a variety of ways—by altering legitimate prescriptions, by stealing prescription blanks or having prescription blanks printed illegally, by impersonating a physician either in person or by telephone, and by shopping around from one physician to another. Not infrequently such individuals watch carefully for new young physicians opening practice in the community and take advantage of a combination of the lack of experience and a desire to build up a practice. Such pseudopatients often become proficient in quoting medical journals and relating lengthy medical histories that require stimulants, barbiturates, or narcotics.

## INTERNATIONAL CONTROL

The United Nations and its specialized agencies have evidenced considerable interest and concern in relation to narcotics and drug abuse. The World Health Organization has been especially active and has supported expert committees, scientific discussions, and researches relating to various aspects of the subject. The results of some of these are included in the references for this chapter.

With specific reference to the circumstances under which control measures should be in-stituted the World Health Organization's Expert Committee on Drug Dependence has stated as follows[71]:

There are two main conditions, at least one of which must exist for a drug to be considered in need of control:

1. The drug is known to be abused other than sporadically or in a local area and the effects of its abuse extend beyond the drug taker; in addition, its mode of spread involves communication between existing and potential drug takers, and an illicit traffic in it is developing.

2. It is planned to use the drug in medicine and experimental data show that there is a significant psychic or physical dependence liability; the drug is commercially available or may become so.

If neither of these conditions is fulfilled, there is no need for an agent to come under consideration for control.

The role of the World Health Organization in this field is well described by Royall[72] who discusses the initiation of the WHO international drug monitoring program in 1962, the establishment of a center for this purpose in Alexandria, Va., in 1968, and the various pilot projects and other activities engaged in.

Meanwhile, the United Nations Economic and Social Council established a Permanent Central Narcotics Board, which in many respects has developed supranational powers in the enforcement of treaties that govern all phases of the narcotics problem. In reviewing international control activities, which actually began in 1909 with the conference in Shanghai of the International Opium Commission, the board noted that efforts had long been directed mainly toward limiting legal narcotics to medical uses, controlling crops of narcotizing plants, licensing legal producers and accounting for their output, and tracking down illegal producers and smugglers. Little attention, they observed, was devoted to the medical and particularly psychologic problems of addiction. Whereas the board recognizes that efforts to eliminate illicit supplies constitute an effective and indispensable weapon in the fight against addiction, it considers realistically that even the most perfect regimen cannot completely accomplish this and that the more rigorous the action the greater is the probability of the development of a prosperous black market in illicit drugs. Accordingly the treatment and rehabilitation of addicts, including studies of etiologic factors, and measures to meet the risk that addicts deprived of narcotic drugs by tight controls may turn to the abuse of other harmful substances have now become the principal items of deliberation and action by the board. This shift in emphasis, it believes, has been so pronounced as to justify speaking of a new chapter of international collaboration in the field of narcotic drugs.

## TOBACCO

One of the greatest events of history was the discovery of the "New World," the Western Hemisphere. It was not devoid of drawbacks. One was that literally from the beginning, the return of Columbus to Spain, two unfortunate curses were introduced into Europe and beyond—syphilis and tobacco. In addition to its use as a symbol of peace and friendship, the American Indians attributed various medicinal values to it. These were transferred to Europe, and for a period its virtues were advertised for everything from deafness to problems of the womb and, ironically, even cancer. Its popular use was greatly accelerated when Sir Walter Raleigh brought some to Queen Elizabeth. From England and Spain it spread to the Middle East, Asia, and throughout the world. As Diehl[73] comments, "Such widespread distribution and use of a plant which until the past few centuries was limited to North America is an amazing phenomenon." A measure of the magnitude of the phenomenon is provided by the fact that during the American colonial period and the early years of the American republic, it was the leading export product. Currently (crop year 1970 to 1971) 2,331 million pounds of tobacco were grown in the United States and 7,704 million pounds elsewhere in the world. The United States exports annually about 600 million pounds of tobacco leaf and about 5% of the 2,320 billion cigarettes manufactured each year. This provides about $1.2 billion to farm income and about $6.6 billion to manufacturers annually in the United States.[74] On this basis many point to tobacco as a valuable economic asset, but this conclusion would seem subject to serious question in view of the lack of physiologic benefit, the use of large amounts of land that should be used for more important and less soil-destructive purposes, plus the costs of the devastating damage done to health.

Another measure of the magnitude of the problem is the annual consumption of tobacco. The number of cigarettes consumed per person per year in the United States was 49 in 1900; 1,365 in 1930; 3,322 in 1950; and 4,000 in 1970. Actually a slight decline occurred since 1965. Thus the percentage of smokers in the adult population (17 years and older) dropped from 41.6% in 1965 to 36.7% in 1970. It was especially significant among men—from 51.0% to 43.2%, in contrast to women among whom the decline was only from 33.2% to 30.9%. Nearly 8 million people stopped smoking during the 5-year period, whereas the percent of those who never smoked did not change significantly. In the age group 17 to 24 years, however, the percent who never smoked improved from 52.4% to 55.6%.[75]

Tobacco is in a somewhat different category from the other substances discussed in this chapter. Although its use commonly leads to a genuine habituation, its undesirability is related not to any psychic or ethical changes. Rather it is because of its relationship to several chronic diseases of major significance. Prominent among these are carcinoma of the respiratory system and mouth, emphysema, hypertension, coronary heart disease, Buerger's disease, sinusitis, and peptic ulcer. There are also indications that it influences the incidence of spontaneous abortion and prematurity, both of which phenomena appear to be twice as common in habitually smoking mothers as compared with nonsmoking mothers.[76,77]

Cigarette smoking is associated with a 70% increase in the age-specific death rates of men and to a lesser extent of women. The total number of excess deaths causally related to cigarette smoking in the United States population cannot be accurately estimated. In general, the greater the number of cigarettes smoked daily the higher is the death rate. For men who smoke fewer than 10 cigarettes a day, the death rate is about 40% higher than for nonsmokers; for those who smoke 10 to 19 cigarettes a day it is about 70% higher; for those who smoke 20 to 39 cigarettes a day it is 90% higher; and for those who smoke 40 or more cigarettes a day the death rate is 120% higher than for nonsmokers. It is interesting that the ratio of death rates of smokers to nonsmokers is highest in the earlier ages (40 to 50 years) and declines with increasing age.[78]

When one considers the time lags that exist between cause and most effects attributable to tobacco smoking, the identifications represent true classics of long-term epidemiologic studies. By now the literature is so replete that it would be pointless to try to separate out a few studies for reference. This is especially true in view of a series of readily available reports and reviews with extensive bibliographies.[73,76-80] As a result of these studies, several nations have taken steps to try to decrease the use of tobacco. In the United States, in no small part because of concern crystallized by the report of the Royal College of Physicians of London,[76] the President established a Surgeon General's Advisory Committee on Smoking and Health. This committee led to the development of a National Clearinghouse on Smoking and Health within the Public Health Service, which has gathered, prepared, and disseminated data and information on the subject, carried out extensive public educational efforts in company with other interested organizations, promoted scientific and professional conferences, and was instrumental in the development and enactment of the Federal Cigarette Labeling and Advertising Act in 1965. This resulted in the requirement that all packages of cigarettes bear a warning of danger to health. In 1971 it was successful in having cigarette advertising banned from radio and television. These steps had already been taken in several countries, beginning in 1962 in Italy and New Zealand. The National Clearinghouse on Smoking and Health issues an annual compilation of antismoking legislation and programs in the nations of the world.[81] The importance of these efforts is not to be underestimated, as evidenced by a statement by the Surgeon General of the Public Health Service that "Cigarette smoking is the greatest preventable cause of illness, disability and premature death in the United States."

## REFERENCES

1. Addiction-producing drugs, WHO Chron. **11:**81, March 1957.
2. Drug addiction and drug habituation, WHO Chron. 11:165, May 1957.
3. Dependence on alcohol and other drugs, WHO Chron. **21:**219, June 1967; Glatt, M. M.: Problems common to alcoholism and drug dependence, WHO Chron. **21:**293, July 1967.
4. Drugs, World Health (special issue), April 1971.
5. Musto, D. F.: A study in cocaine, J.A.M.A. **204:** 125, April 1, 1968.
6. Simrell, E. V.: History of legal and medical roles in narcotic abuse in the U. S., Public Health Rep. **83:**587, July 1968.
7. Brotman, R., and Freedman, A.: A community mental health approach to drug addiction, (SRS) pub. no. 9005, Washington, D. C., 1970, U. S. Department of Health, Education, and Welfare.
8. U. S. Department of Health, Education, and Welfare: Narcotic drug addiction, PHS pub. no. 1021, Washington, D. C., 1963.
9. National Institute of Mental Health: A federal source book: answers to the most frequently asked questions about drug abuse, Rockville, Md., 1971.
10. Yost, O. S.: The bane of drug addiction, New York, 1954, The Macmillan Co.
11. Drugs and the adolescent, WHO Chron. **25:** 263, June 1971.
12. Johnson, K. G., et al.: Survey of adolescent drug use, Amer. J. Public Health **61:**2418, Dec. 1971; **62:**164, Feb. 1972.
13. Johnson, L.: Survey of high school drug use, Ann Arbor, 1969, University of Michigan Institute for Social Research.
14. Bullington, B., et al.: Concerning heroin use and official records, Amer. J. Public Health **59:**1887, Oct. 1969.
15. Richards, L. G., and Carroll, E. A.: Illicit drug use and addiction in the United States: a review of available statistics, Public Health Rep. **85:**1035, Dec. 1970.
16. Winick, C.: The narcotic addiction problem, New York, 1964, American Social Hygiene Association.
17. Mattick, H.: The epidemiology of drug addiction and reflections on the problem and policy in the U. S., Illinois Med. J. **130:**439, Oct. 1966.
18. Burham, D.: Census of addicts in state started, N. Y. Times, June 23, 1968.
19. Dealing with drug abuse. Report of a Task Force of the Drug Abuse Council, New York, 1972, Frederick A. Praeger, Inc.
20. The challenge of crime in a free society. A report by the President's Commission on Law Enforcement and Administration of Justice, Washington, D. C., 1967, Government Printing Office.
21. Louria, D. B., Hensle, T., and Rose, J.: The major medical complications of heroin addiction, Ann. Intern. Med. **67:**1, July 1967.
22. Cherubin, C. E.: The medical sequelae of narcotic addiction, Ann. Intern. Med. **67:**23, July 1967.
23. Zelson, C., Rubic, E., and Wasserman, E.: Neonatal narcotic addiction, Pediatrics **48:**178, Feb. 1971.
24. Drug abuse problem, M.D. **16:**85, April 1972.
25. Amer. Med. News **15:**2, Dec. 11, 1972.
26. Jacobziner, H.: Investigating narcotic addiction in school children, Amer. J. Public Health **43:** 1138, Sept. 1953.
27. Hughes, P. H., et al.: The natural history of a heroin epidemic, Amer. J. Public Health **62:**995, July 1972.
28. Poll says 6% of youths tried heroin, Washington Post, p. A1, May 10, 1972.
29. Abrams, A., Gagnon, J. H., Levin, J. J.: Psychosocial aspects of addiction, Amer, J. Public Health **58:**2142, Nov. 1968.
30. Lowry, J. V.: Hospital treatment of the narcotic addict, Federal Probation **20:**42, Dec. 1956.

31. Yolles, S. F.: Narcotic Addict Rehabilitation act of 1966: a legislative summary and background paper, Washington, D. C., H.E.W. Indicators, Feb. 1967.

32. Koran, L. M.: American responses to heroin addiction and marihuana use, In Coelho, G. U., and Rubinstein, E. A., editors: Social change and human behavior, Rockville, Md., 1972, National Institute of Mental Health.

33. Pattison, E. M., Bishop, L. A., and Linsky, A. S.: Changes in public attitudes on narcotic addiction, Amer. J. Psychiat. **125**:160, Jan. 1968.

34. Geis, G.: Not the laws business: an examination of homosexuality, abortion, prostitution, narcotics and gambling in the United States, Center for Studies of Crime and Delinquency, pub. no. (HSM) 72-9132, Rockville, Md., 1972, National Institute of Mental Health.

35. Ball, J. C., Thompson, W. O., and Allen, D. M.: Readmission rates for 43,215 narcotic drug addicts, Public Health Rep. **85**:610, July 1970.

36. Sells, S. B., editor: Rehabilitating the narcotic addict: Report of Institute of New Developments, Washington, D. C., 1967, Vocational Rehabilitation Administration, U. S. Department of Health, Education, and Welfare.

37. Kolb, L.: Narcotic addiction—an interview, Spectrum **5**:136, March 1957.

38. Drug addiction—III. A statement by the New York Academy of Medicine, Bull. N. Y. Acad. Med. **41**:825, July 1965.

39. Treatment and care of drug addicts, WHO Chron. **11**:323, Oct. 1957.

40. Prevention and treatment of drug dependence: Report of the Expert Committee on Drug Dependence, WHO Techn. Rep. Ser. no. 460, Geneva, 1970, World Health Organization.

41. Hess, C. B.: New trends in narcotic addiction control, Public Health Rep. **81**:277, March 1966.

42. Larimore, G. W., and Brill, H.: Epidemiologic factors in drug addiction in England and the United States, Public Health Rep. **77**:555, July 1962.

43. Alcoholism, addiction, suicide and physicians, Mod. Med. **41**:138, Jan. 1973.

44. Dole, V.P., and Nyswander, M.: A medical treatment of diacetylmorphine (heroin) addiction: a clinical trial, J.A.M.A. **193**:646, Aug. 23, 1965.

45. Chambers, C. D., and Brill, L., editors: Methadone: experiences and issues, New York, 1973, Behavioral Publications.

46. DuPont, R. L., and Katon, R.: Physicians and the heroin addiction epidemic, Mod. Med. **39**:123, June 1971.

47. Drug abuse problem, M. D. **16**:85, April 1972.

48. Maidlow, S. T., and Berman, H.: The economics of heroin treatment, Amer. J. Public Health **62**:1398, Oct. 1972.

49. Facilities for the treatment and rehabilitation of narcotic addicts, New York, 1962, American Social Hygiene Association (mimeographed).

50. Winick, C., and Bynder, H.: Facilities for treatment and rehabilitation of narcotic drug users and addicts, Amer. J. Public Health **57**:1025, June 1967.

51. Lipscomb, W. R.: An epidemiology of drug use-abuse, Amer. J. Public Health, **61**:1794, Sept. 1971.

52. Drugs, World Health (special issue), p. 32, April 1971.

53. Dumont, M. P.: Why the young use drugs, Mod. Med. **40**:46, Feb. 1972.

54. Abeles, H. P., Ralph, L. T., and Rosenthal, H. M.: Multiple drug addiction in New York City in a selected population group, Public Health Rep. **81**:685, Aug. 1966.

55. Cole, J. O., and Katz, M. M.: The psychotomimetic drugs—an overview, J.A.M.A. **187**(10): 182, March 7, 1964.

56. For detailed references see (a) Hallucinogens—a select bibliography (1967); (b) Adverse effects of LSD—a select bibliography (1964-1968), Bethesda, National Library of Medicine.

57. Dependence on LSD and other hallucinogenic drugs: Report of Committee on Alcoholism and Drug Dependence and the Council on Mental Health, J.A.M.A. **202**:141, Oct. 2, 1967.

58. Ungerleider, J. T., Fisher, D. D., and Fuller, M.: The dangers of LSD: analysis of seven months' experience in a university hospital's psychiatric service, J.A.M.A. **197**:389, Aug. 8, 1966.

59. Editorial: Prolonged adverse reactions to LSD, J.A.M.A. **198**:658, Nov. 7, 1966.

60. Egozcue, J., Irwin, S., and Maruffo, C.: Chromosomal damage in LSD users, J.A.M.A. **204**:122, April 15, 1968.

61. Editorial: A genetic trip, J.A.M.A. **204**:167, April 15, 1968.

62. Proliferating problem, M.D. **14**:101, Sept. 1970.

63. News item of Survey for National Commission on Marihuana and Drug Abuse, Amer. Med. News **16**:2, March 3, 1973.

64. The Gallup poll: 11% of Americans have tried marihuana, Baltimore Sun, p. A3, Mar. 26, 1972.

65. Fifteen percent of young Americans have smoked marihuana, Hosp. Tribune **7**:14, Jan. 8, 1973.

66. Marihuana: a signal for misunderstanding, First Report of the National Commission on Marihuana and Drug Abuse, Washington, D. C., 1972, Government Printing Office.

67. Fishbein, M.: Historical perspective on drug legislation, Med. World News **13**:88, May 19, 1972.

68. National Institute of Mental Health: Marihuana and health, Report to the Congress, Rockville, Md., 1971.

69. The use of cannabis: report of the WHO scientific group, WHO Techn. Rep. Ser. no. 478, Geneva, 1971, World Health Organization.

70. Mullings, E. B.: Airplane glue, Mich. Health, Sept.-Oct. 1966.

71. Criteria for determining the need for drug control: Report of the WHO Expert Committee on Drug

Dependence, Techn. Rep. Ser. no. 407, Geneva, 1969, World Health Organization.

72. Royall, B. W.: International aspects of drug monitoring: the role of the World Health Organization, WHO Chron. **25:**445, Oct. 1971.

73. Diehl, H. S.: Tobacco and your health: the smoking controversy, New York, 1969, McGraw-Hill Book Co.

74. Statistical abstract of the United States, Washington, D. C., 1971, Government Printing Office.

75. World almanac, New York, 1973, Newspaper Enterprise Association, Inc.

76. Smoking and health: summary and report on smoking in relation to cancer of the lung and other diseases, Royal College of Physicians of London, London, 1962, Sir Isaac Pitman & Sons, Ltd.

77. Smoking and health: Report of Advisory Committee to the Surgeon General, PHS pub. no. 1103, Washington, D. C., 1964.

78. The health consequences of smoking: a Public Health Service review, PHS pub. no. 1696, Washington, D. C., 1967.

79. World conference on smoking and health: summary of the proceedings, New York, 1967, American Cancer Society.

80. U. S. Public Health Service: Health consequences of smoking: Report of the Surgeon General (HSM) pub. no. 72-7514, Rockville, Md. 1972.

81. U. S. Public Health Service: Smoking and health programs around the world, Rockville, Md., annual.

*Have a heart that never hardens,*
*A temper that never tires,*
*A touch that never hurts.*

CHARLES DICKENS

CHAPTER 27

# Violence and delinquency

## A NEW LOOK AT AGGRESSION

The several chapters in this section have attempted to deal with various aspects of antisocial behavior, all with a psychiatric base—mental ill health, alcoholism, addictions, drug abuse, and suicide. Each of these at one time or another, to some degree or another, has been the subject of legal and criminal justice measures. Historically the legal profession has philosophically attributed insanity to "the guilty mind." Even now much debate takes place between those who advocate the legal or criminal justice approach to the problems under consideration and those in the health and social service professions who regard them as manifestations of "the deprived and sick mind," which either cries for help or attempts to escape from unwanted or intolerable situations, often in what may appear to be bizarre ways. Fortunately a rapprochement has been under development. Matthews,[1] a lawyer and director of the project on Mental Illness and the Criminal Law of the American Bar Foundation, has presented what is taking place and some of its rationale.

If one observes both the persons who crowd our criminal courts . . . and the population of our mental hospitals, one is struck not by the differences between the two but by the similarities. Our preoccupation with trying to separate the "mentally ill" from the "criminals" may have led us to overlook a more central reality: both mental illness and criminality are tributaries of some deeper and more mysterious channel. Certainly there are differences between "criminals" and the "mentally ill" but it seems possible that the problems of mental illness and crime frequently lend themselves to similar if not identical methods of handling. This possibility is reinforced when one reflects to what extent entry into . . . and continued presence in the criminal process may be a result of what we call the "random factor"; that is, decisions based not so much on reason and scientific differentiation as on chance circumstances, social class, available mental health resources, divisions of political authority, and education and training levels of the officials whose responsibility it is to make decisions. There is a need for individualization at every step of the criminal process in order to neutralize the random factor as much as possible. If the wide range of alternatives available for handling persons thought to be mentally ill, especially alternatives in the individual's home community, should be made available to persons involved with the criminal law, then the accident of labels, whether civil or criminal, would be reduced. A wide spectrum of diagnostic and treatment facilities should be made available to the administrators of the criminal law to assist them in the related tasks of preventing crime and dealing effectively with persons legally convicted of criminal acts. If mental health resources are available both in mental hospitals and correctional facilities, much of the sting of criminal convictions will have been removed.

Matthews concludes that an imaginative change in present competency procedures by prosecutors, judges, attorneys, and even defendants themselves would make available a new wide range of dispositional alternatives to the criminal process. Many of these alternatives, he believes, are or should be available at progressive mental health centers. But, he notes, unfortunately there is the reality of a limited

**497**

supply of mental health resources as well as an inefficient use of those which exist.

This emphasizes perhaps that neither criminal justice nor public and mental health can stand or function alone. Each to a significant degree must depend on and work with the other.[2] In terms of "health" statistics it is significant that the major risks of death for young white males in the United States are, in order, vehicular accidents, suicide, and homicide, and for young black males they are homicide, vehicular accidents, and drowning accidents. Hall,[3] as President of the American Medical Association, pondered possible methods to prevent some of this tragic violent loss—the elimination of human judgment in driving by a complex computerized highway system, the tranquilization of all young men so they will not kill themselves or each other, the fencing of all lakes and rivers. Obviously, Hall notes, none of these is practical, much less acceptable, although it should be mentioned that the second, in the form of leucotomy (brain surgery in certain cases) or chemotherapy, has been attempted on a limited selective basis in several countries.[4] General reaction to such Orwellian approaches is negative, in part because of the macabre path down which they might lead civilization. To the contrary, the only practical approach is to attempt a better understanding of the underlying causes of hostility, aggression, and violence and to seek effective methods of public motivation to avoid or neutralize the causes. It is against this background that the following discussion is presented.

## HOSTILITY

### Source of hostility

Underlying most if not all of man's antisocial behavior and of his violence toward himself or others is a deep-seated sense of hostility, which the affected individual may or may not recognize. Hostility is a unique and much misused term. In an attempt to describe it precisely Saul[5] defines it as "a motivating force—an impulse, urge, tendency, intent, motivation or reaction—toward injury or destruction of some kind or degree, toward an object which can be animate (including oneself) or inanimate, usually accompanied in humans by the feeling or emotion of anger." To elucidate he emphasizes that hostility is not merely aggression, anger, or hatred, although any or all of these may be components or manifestations of overt hostility. Aggression, which means "to move actively,"

may actually be constructive. Indeed to be progressive, to achieve, one must have some measure of aggressiveness. It does not necessarily have to be hostile or is hostility necessarily aggressive. Indeed, it may be passive. Hostility may be manifested in many ways and for many purposes, varying in intensity from a simple unnoticed glance, a fixed stare, or facial tenseness, to active vindictiveness in the form of malicious gossip, the smashing of objects, brutality toward animals or other humans, and in the extreme, murder or suicide. Mere anger should not be confused with hostility, since typically it is a transient reaction and may be, and often is, expressed toward a loved one. As such, the storm of sudden anger quickly passes away, usually leaving in its wake some measure of remorse. With hostility there is no place for remorse. It is the inherent Cain—the essential evil in people.

Some may find this an objectionable or unpleasant thought, but it must be realized that everyone, to varying degrees because of complex circumstances, is pulled by two opposing forces—strong social and self-satisfying motivations and strong asocial or antisocial motivations that may be equally or even more satisfying. An understanding of these opposing forces or motivations and the social application of that understanding offers the only ultimate hope of headway against individual or collective brutality and violence which constantly threatens man and his societies. It is significant that toward the end of his life Sigmund Freud[6] wrote "I can no longer understand how we could have overlooked the universality of non-erotic aggression and destruction and could have omitted to give it due significance in our interpretations of life." Then he added that "Those who love fairy tales do not like it when people speak of the innate tendencies of mankind toward aggression, destruction and cruelty.... The tendency toward aggression," he concludes, "is an innate, independent, instinctual disposition in man and ... it constitutes the most powerful obstacle to culture."

In his well-known studies of behavior and conditioning, Cannon[7] observed that an animal confronted with a threat, irritation, or frustration is physiologically stimulated and prepared spontaneously for either one or two maximum responses—to fight or to flee. Early in man's history in competitive biologic circumstances this was necessary for survival. It may still be observed in some primitive people. But in supposedly cooperative and civilized contemporary life this automatic physiologic response if misunderstood and uncontrolled in relation to existing stresses and problems is likely to flood the mind with unwise and unwarranted feelings of fear and hostility and result in destructive reactions against others or oneself. Unfortunately this eventuality is common, as a reading of man's history or an issue of a newspaper gives ample testimony. This tendency, this characteristic, has already been referred to as inherent or innate to man. It also appears to be unique to him. Almost all animals have some form of organization based on protective and productive aggregations—hives, flocks, herds, and the like. So does man, but with an additional significant use—purposeful aggressive attacks on and destruction of his own kind. Thus Allee[8] notes, "One species of animal may destroy another, and individuals may kill other individuals, but group struggles to the death between members of the same species, such as occur in human warfare, can hardly be found among non-human animals." To this one may add the observation that only a human could have written Thanatopsis. Only a human could have conceived and composed a Gotterdammerung. And only a human could have attempted it.

### Hostility—a disease

Because of such considerations, Saul[5] regards man's hostility as the central problem in human affairs and urges its recognition in its many forms. He provides health workers with the challenge in these terms:

Hostility is a disease to be cured and prevented like cancer, tuberculosis or smallpox, . . . its cure will result in healthier, better living—not only for society in general but for each individual in particular. . . . Hostility cannot be passed off as something we inherit and hence can do nothing about. The fact is that hostility is a disease of the personality, transmittable from person to person and group to group, and, basically, by contact from parents to children, from generation to generation. . . . Indeed if the major motivating forces in each of us could develop normally, healthily, without interference or coercion from the outside, friendly social cooperation would be the result. Only when this development is disturbed during the earliest formative years of infancy and childhood, by active mismanagement or by gross neglect (whether unconscious and well meaning or conscious and willful) does the fight-flight reaction, with its resulting hostility, flower into full strength.

To this he adds the pertinent health-related observation that through all the various forms of physical, physiologic, and psychologic reaction—withdrawal, depression, manic episodes, hysteria, phobias, compulsions, perversions, addictions, paranoias, schizophrenia, and the rest as well as the psychosomatic conditions in which emotions play a role—ulcers, hypertension, stroke, thyroid disease, and some allergies and arthritis—"however prominent the element of flight, invariably the power of the fight reaction with its rage, hate and hostility is also unmistakable." He concludes that "The elucidation of hostility in its causes, effects, transformations, connections, and the means of reducing and preventing it, could well be the great contribution of this generation of students of the human mind and human motivations."

### Extent and form of hostility

Cannon's choice between flight or fight therefore has special implications for modern man's survival. He now has available such effective weapons with which to fight. These weapons are not necessarily limited to physical form. As Saul[5] points out, fighting may now range from direct overt action to indirect hidden, subtle, and even masked forms disguised as justice, righteousness, and love. "It can be acted out within or outside the law by single persons on their own, by unorganized crowds or mobs, or by highly organized gangs or armies. It finds easy expression in crime, delinquency and warfare, the prevalence of which serves as an index of how widespread the problem is."

Obviously its true dimensions elude determination. Nevertheless some indications, with varying degrees of accuracy, are available. In the United States, for example, there occur annually an estimated 2 million crimes, and the rate is increasing about four times as rapidly as the population. Thus between 1960 and 1970 the number of murders increased 76% from 9,000 to 15,812; forcible rapes increased 121% from 16,860 to 37,273; and aggravated assaults increased 117% from 152,000 to 329,937. During 1970, in addition, there were 3.489 million arrests for nonaggravated assaults and 78,500 for offenses against family and children. These, it must be emphasized, are only those offenses actually known to the police.[9] Other manifestations of hostility are significant proportions of the 10 million persons injured and the more than 100,000 killed in "accidents." Self-directed hostility takes the lives of about 22,000 known suicides each year. Social but nonfatal indications of hostility include many of the annual 750,000 divorces, and the 1.5 million children termed delinquent by the courts. In the world arena one can point to the minimum of 25 million people killed and several times that number injured in wars of this generation alone. These figures are influenced, of course, by several variables. Included are the definition of crime; the size, nature, and vigilance of the law enforcement and judicial systems; the education, customs, and attitudes of the public; the economic and employment levels; and numerous other factors. Despite the influence of these variables, however, the actual magnitude is unquestionably great. In addition, it is interesting to contemplate the extent to which this line of reasoning may explain man's attitude toward his physical environment, which he "conquers," "subdues," "exploits," and "rapes" (note the words commonly used) in the name of productivity and development.

## CRIMINAL HOMICIDE

Every hour in the United States 15 or more people are stabbed, clubbed, or shot. A significant number of them die. During 1970, felonious murders and nonnegligent manslaughter accounted for about 16,000 deaths, or 1 every 33 minutes with a constant increase. Homicide decreased through the early 1950s, but in about 1958 it leveled off and began to increase. Between 1960 and 1970 the average annual increase was 6%, with a total increase over the decade of 76%. These, of course, are only the incidents known to the police and do not take into consideration the unknown numbers of individuals whose deaths are classified erroneously as accidents. The statistical chance of an American being murdered in any one year is about 1 in 20,000. The risk varies considerably, however, among different components of the population.

Differences among the color groups far outweigh differences by sex, with homicide rates for the nonwhite population eight to ten times greater than for the white population. When data are limited to males, the differences by color are even greater. Age adjustment further emphasizes the disparity among the color groups, especially for nonwhite males whose rates are raised about an additional one fourth. Homicide occurs most frequently in persons between the ages of 25 and 44 years, for whom the rate is twice the national average. At these ages the color difference is most pronounced, with a level ten to twelve times higher than among the nonwhite population. The male to female homicide rate is a ratio of about 3 to 1. With reference to residence, rates are higher in urban areas, especially center city circumstances, compared with rural areas. Some changes are taking place, however, in all of these dimensions. During the past decade, for example, the age-adjusted homicide rate for all ages combined increased nearly 30% among whites as compared with a 10% increase among nonwhites. The ratio of male to female homicides declined slightly, as did the average age, and the residential rates altered with an increasing number of homicides in suburbs.

It is important to distinguish murder from other homicides. The term *homicide* includes not only "murder and nonnegligent manslaughter" but also "justifiable homicide" (such as the killing of a felon by a policeman in line of duty and some other types of killing in self-defense). It also does not include legal executions. Practically speaking, homicide includes any violent death that is neither a suicide nor an accident, although as pointed out previously, some of each of these are actually conscious or subconscious homicides. *Murder,* or *criminal homicide,* is a more restricted term. Most criminologists consider a murderer as "one who kills a fellow member of his society not by accident or negligence but with purpose or to defend himself in connection with an attempt to commit another crime, such as robbery, or to shield himself from accusation by a person whom he has offended or abused."[10]

Homicides therefore may be considered to fall into three categories. The best known and the type toward which the criminal justice system, as well as the public in general, has centered their attention is planned killing that is consciously acceptable to the perpetrator at the time. Contrary to popular belief, this type of killing, criminal homicide, represents only a small fraction of the total homicides in American society. By far the most common type of homicide is a form of resolution of conflict that usually has extended over a significant period of time. In these instances, which comprise about 80% of the total, often an insignificant provocation may develop an intense emotional response leading to the homicidal act, which has not been consciously planned. The perpetrators of such acts apparently do not have the ability to satisfy their aggressions consistently and, as a result, on occasion may do so impulsively and explosively. The third type of homicide is that which was mentioned earlier as justifiable acts taken by a law enforcement officer or an individual in self-defense.

It is notable that, except for the third or noncriminal type of homicide, in about 65% of cases a relationship either by birth or choice exists between the victim and the murderer. In other words it is not the stranger who is to be feared as much as it is a person with whom one has some degree of intimacy. This has prompted Judge George Edwards of the National Commission of Reform of Federal Criminal Laws, in an address before the American Psychiatric Association in 1971, to deflate what he referred to as the "four myths about murder." They are that the average citizen is justified in living with a top priority fear of being murdered, that most murderers are premeditated killers for money, that the most likely murderer is a stranger, and that you can protect yourself from murder by keeping a pistol handy. None of these myths, he emphasized, is true. What is true about murder, as pointed out by King of the International Association of Chiefs of Police, is that it is the least suppressible of crimes—that greater police visibility and more sophisticated police techniques have little effect on homicide because it occurs most often in the privacy of the home, with an existing prior relationship between victim and killer, which means that the murder is almost always an act of blind rage, of illogical violent passion that cannot be anticipated. It has also been pointed out by Pasternack,[11] a psychiatrist and a specialist in violent behavior, that perhaps as many as 40% of murders of passion are actually victim precipitated, wherein one person taunts another beyond endurance or where a philandering husband parades his mistress in front of his wife, daring her to do anything about it. This type of situation, says Pasternack, is far from rare and when it happens, the killer as well as the killed is a victim.

Since the majority of so-called criminal homicides are committed in moments of explosive passion, it is interesting to observe the profile of the typical convicted murderer. Gillin,[10] in a study of a sample of 486 out of 1,700 prisoners, including 92 murderers, in the Wisconsin State Prison, found that those convicted for murder differed from their fellow prisoners in eight ways: (1) they left school earlier; (2) a greater proportion had full-time jobs before their fourteenth year (seven tenths contributed to the family support before the age of 14 years and nine tenths before the age of 19 years, that is,

they were from homes where children were given early economic burdens that limited education); (3) fewer remained on a job for more than a year at a time; (4) more of them (43% as opposed to 12%) believed that they were favorites of someone (mother, father, or someone else); (5) more of the married murderers and their wives lived disharmoniously than other married fellow prisoners and wives; (6) a higher percent of married murderers than of their married fellow prisoners had married women with more education than themselves; (7) they showed a greater appreciation of their mothers than did their fellow prisoners; and (8) fewer murderers were farmers, although Wisconsin is a farming state.

Seven out of 10 murderers came from families in which there were unfavorable conditions. During the typical murderer's boyhood, his mother worked outside the home about twice as often as average mothers in the nation. He was thirty four times as likely to be a black and eleven times as likely to be an Indian than a white. Also he was 1.5 times as likely to be from foreign-born parents. (Note: These figures are for Wisconsin.) The murderer stood not more than one chance in two of feeling that his parents were affectionate toward him. In at least one case in five he thought his parents were cruel, fault finding, moody, domineering, or indifferent. There was a history of family intemperance in one third of the cases and of insanity, epilepsy, mental defect, or "queerness" he knew about in his ancestry in 1 out of every 6 cases. Typically he had been sentenced for life at the age of 32 years—slightly older than for other prisoners. His education was somewhat less than that of males committed in the United States for all crimes. Seven tenths of the convicted murderers in Wisconsin were skilled or unskilled laborers. It is important to note that they did not tend to be professional criminals. Two thirds had no prior institutional experience of any type, even in an orphanage, and fewer than one half had been arrested or in court before. One third were single, one half married, one eighth divorced, and one fourteenth widowed. Of the 42 married "lifers," 18 had killed their wives. More than one fifth of those convicted had committed murder as a result of an immediate quarrel and two fifths as a result of long-standing marital difficulties or a long-term grudge. In other words the convicted murderer was essentially a criminal as a result of a momentary, passionate, hostile act. Gillin then makes the interesting observation that "Abnormal mental conditions characterize the Wisconsin lifer to a much greater degree than other people in the State or even the other inmates of the prison. In over one case in four he was committed as insane or became insane after incarceration. Moreover, there was not quite one chance in three that his intelligence quotient was over 70. Furthermore, there was more than one chance in four that he was drunk at the time he committed the crime."

## PREVENTION OF HOMICIDE

The question logically arises, "Can anything be done to reduce this needless loss of life?" For one thing those in the health professions—public health workers, private practitioners of medicine, hospital administrators, and all the rest—must recognize, as many still do not, that an individual killed with a weapon is just as dead and just as tragic as one who has succumbed to tuberculosis or cancer and that most if not all of the so-called criminal homicides are largely influenced by some aspects of mental ill health. This is not the place for a detailed discussion of the psychiatric measures, individual or collective, that are needed. There are two other aspects of prevention, however, that must be mentioned. The first is social conditioning. Banay[12] pointed out two decades ago that the American public is conditioned to murder, that it was no exaggeration to consider that except for maintaining the traditional legal penalty (in itself a form of murder) for taking another's life, "the society we live in almost reaches out to encourage murder." It is the most common topic in children's so-called "comic" books, the focal point of mystery stories that are sold by the tens of millions each year, and the stock-in-trade of television, radio, and motion picture "thrillers." Typically it receives the top headlines in American news media. The gun is probably the most common toy sold and encourages the most popular form of play, especially among boys, which takes the form of a travesty of killing. Significantly, the American Rifle Association, which staunchly opposes any limitation on the sale and ready availability of guns is one of the strongest and best supported political lobbies in Washington. It is also interesting that when an individual disagrees with someone or dislikes him, he is likely to say "Drop dead!" Banay concluded that "a psychologist studying our culture might fairly deduce that we are obsessed with the idea of

sudden, violent and retributive death." Washburn,[13] in his discussion of aggressive behavior and human evolution, goes even further. After considering development in several mammalian species he observes that "All the evidence would indicate that evolution has built into man a propensity for learning to be aggressive. Our early ancestors' way of life was not easy . . . the group was defended by the young adult male who hunted and formed the army. The order of killing was very high." It has been estimated "that in many primitive tribes about 25 percent of the males were killed off in combat. This, of course, does not mean that man must continue to be aggressive, but it does suggest the importance of institutional controls over aggression." In contradistinction Endleman,[14] in his studies of street violence and riots, believes strongly that although violence is prevalent, it is not endemic or necessarily natural to the human condition and that preconditions of violent behavior must be sought in social rather than in genetic or instinctual characteristics of man. He also points out what has increasingly been observed that violence begets violence, that is, there is a tendency to respond to violence violently and that this response leads in turn to even more conflict and violence. This viewpoint has justified the trend in recent years of many mental health workers and of law enforcement agents to encourage aggressive or violent individuals or groups to "cool it" and to use the cooling period for joint exploration of the causes of dissension and their possible solutions. This, of course, represents an extremely valid applied mental health approach.

During recent years much attention has been focused on the possible influence of television on aggressive behavior, especially in view of the pervasiveness of television in the United States. As pointed out by the Surgeon General's Scientific Advisory Committee on Television and Social Behavior,[15] 96% of American homes have one or more television sets, and the average home set is turned on for more than 6 hours per day. Most of the studies inquired into by the committee indicated positive relationships between exposure to television violence and aggressive tendencies, although most of the relationships between exposure to television violence and aggressive tendencies, although most of the relationships were of low magnitude. However, the observation raised other questions: (1) Does violence viewing lead to aggression? (2) Does aggression lead to violence viewing? (3) Are both violence viewing and aggression products of a third set of conditions? The studies tended to support the first and third of these propositions. Bandura,[16] who has studied the subject for more than a decade, makes the interesting point that an investigation of violence per se in relation to television seems less likely to yield information on the underlying process of influence than the study of the visual media with regard to its impact on learning in general. He strongly believes that the environment in which the media is viewed is extremely important. A possibly related observation[17] that has been made is that countries or cultures with high homicide rates tend to have low suicide rates and vice versa. Thus in Mexico, where 18.7 out of every 100,000 people were murdered in 1966, only 1.6 killed themselves. This is in contrast with West Germany, for example, where only 1.3 murders per 100,000 were recorded in contrast to 25 suicides per 100,000 population. The question is raised whether a country is homicidal or suicidal depending on the level of its labor force status integration, that is, the degree of certainty among individuals about what society expects of them in view of their age, sex, and other factors. In rigid societies where roles are well defined and people have little freedom of choice in directing their lives, homicide rates are high. This is in contrast to societies where people have the opportunity to choose their life style from a variety of alternatives and where suicide rates tend to be high.

There is a second and very important area for preventive action in this field. Among those with expertise in the field there is almost unanimous agreement that the most urgent need is effective gun control. Thus Burka[11] says firmly, "The single most effective step we can take is to ban hand guns and to use stringent methods to make the ban work. A hand gun is meant for police work and that is the only place it belongs —not in the hands of criminals and would-be criminals, not in the pockets of frightened citizens, and not in the home. Anyone who thinks possession of a gun protects him and his family is deluding himself." King[11] of the International Association of Chiefs of Police, who has studied the problem extensively, is equally emphatic, stating "By far the greatest number of homicides are shootings, so reduction of homicides starts with elimination of hand guns. Nobody denies that people are also murdered with every imaginable weapon besides guns—knives, fists,

rocks, clothes lines, 2 by 4s, and so on." He responds to those who scoffingly say that there is as much sense to banning hand guns as getting rid of lumber yards because some murders are committed with 2 by 4s by pointing out that "... a gun is the most lethal of weapons; it has a range far greater than an attacker's arm, and recovery from a bullet wound is much rarer than recovery from a knifing or beating." There is an obvious need to extirpate the almost juvenile avid retention by many individuals of the primitive urge to destroy other species long after the necessity to fear them or require them for sustenance. In the process all sorts of specious justifications are presented: that guns are needed not only for hunting but also "to protect one's castle," "that guns do not kill, people kill." The variety of illogical themes are many. As Pasternack[11] expresses, "We are victims of the mystique of the gun. Who in his right mind could dispute that if there were no guns in the home or in the streets there would be a dramatic reduction in killings. Murders of passion would certainly diminish greatly with no chance for the impulsive, irreversible pulling of a trigger before passion can cool; street killings would plummet if the criminal had no gun to hide behind to draw false courage."

The unfortunate fact is that the "gun lobby" is one of the largest, best financed, and most powerful in the national and state capitals. As a result, the acquisition of a gun, not merely a hunting rifle, is absurdly simple. As the late J. Edgar Hoover, while Director of the Federal Bureau of Investigation, stated, "The easy accessibility of fire arms is a significant factor in murders committed in the U. S. today." Approximately 2 million guns are sold in the United States each current year—many by mail. Far too many are purchased by the deranged, the hardened criminal, the convict, the addict, and the alcoholic. It is unreasonable to expect such individuals to be prudent in their use. Bakal[18] in his book *The Right to Bear Arms* speaks of a plague of guns that sweeps over our land and points out that since 1900, more than 750,000 American civilians have been killed by gunfire —a higher toll than all of the Americans killed in battle since the American Revolution and through the Vietnamese war. Only 7 states at present even require a permit or a license before purchase of a pistol or revolver, and as Bakal indicates, almost every place one can purchase a rifle more easily than getting a dog or cat license or even a hunting permit. The total result is an estimated 90 million guns in the hands of private individuals in the United States.

## CHILD ABUSE

A manifestation of aggression and violence of direct concern to the fields of public health, medicine, and social service is the "battered child." Children have probably been misused and abused throughout much of man's history. The inception of the Industrial Revolution accentuated the problem, as was indicated in the earlier chapter on the history of public health. Child labor laws in the United States and many other countries have gone far to eliminate this social evil.[19] However, the battered child is a much less evident and more elusive aspect of child abuse, one that has attracted increasing attention during the past several decades as a significant cause of disability and death in children.[19,20] Usually the battered child is a rejected child and not infrequently the only one of several children in a family subjected to abuse. Rejection may result from exhausting demands on the parents from too many children, from poor marital adjustment, from resentment of a marriage forced by pregnancy or other persons, or often from the fact that the parents, especially the mother herself, was rejected as a child. In such cases the parent, through identification with her child, manifests her feelings of self-deprecation and inward hostility by abuse of the child. Other causes may be mental illness in one or both parents, social and economic frustrations, unusually young and immature parents who may treat a baby like a doll or toy or may mistreat it during a tantrum to "teach the other parent a lesson," jealousy by one parent over the attention given the child by the other parent, jealousy on the part of older children in relation to a new baby in the family, or sexual aberrations on the part of one or both parents, older children, or other relatives or acquaintances.

The abuse of children may run the gamut from overprotection in the form of isolation to general neglect with poor hygiene and malnutrition, constant nagging and scolding, sexual abuse, severe and often irrational punishment, sometimes leading to death. It is these latter instances that have been given the name *battered child syndrome*. Reliable statistics are understandably difficult to obtain, but the Children's Division of the American Humane Association[21] estimates that there are about 10,000

cases a year in this country—probably a conservative estimate. The association's study revealed that more than one half of the affected children were under 4 years of age. One fourth of them died, and most of the deaths were in children less than 2 years of age. Fathers were guilty more often of child abuse than mothers but sometimes both parents actively participated. Battered children are not limited to any particular socioeconomic group, and not all abused or battered children are found among the very young. Thus a study in 1968 of 6,617 abused children showed 8.1% were under 6 months; 5.5% were between 6 months and 1 year; 10.8% were between 1 and 2 years; 9.4% were between 2 and 3 years; 19.9% were between 3 and 6 years; 15.1% were between 6 to 9 years; 12.2% were between 9 and 12 years; 10.8% were between 12 and 15 years; and 5.6% were over 15 years of age with 2.6% of age unknown. As has been indicated, however, the highest fatality rate is in the very young, commonly those under 3 years who are too young to explain their bruises, fractures, and swellings. Among older children, many are too frightened or convinced of guilt to discuss what actually transpired. It is estimated that 5% of battered children are killed outright and another 30% eventually suffer permanent injury. Furthermore, of those who are not killed outright, it is estimated that 1 out of every 2 dies after being returned to his or her parents. This point is extremely important to bear in mind. Regretfully it is estimated that very few cases of battered or abused children, perhaps as low as 1%, are brought to the attention of appropriate authorities. Since most incidents occur in the home, all but the most serious tend to go unnoticed even by neighbors. Physicians represent a critical point of first suspicion and action. However, even here reporting has tended to be minimal. A physician sometimes is so concerned with clinical signs that he literally may give no thought to their source. If he does have suspicions, they are difficult to prove, and he takes the parent's word about accidents, clumsiness, or other children. Furthermore, most people, including physicians, find it difficult to believe that any parents would injure their own children. In this regard Sanders[22] expresses the opinion that most parents have both hostile and negative attitudes as well as warm and loving feelings toward their children and that the members of the medical profession also often have ambivalent childhood memories which makes them reluctant to deal with parents of battered children. In addition, some may fear becoming involved in time-consuming legal processes. These reactions, Sanders points out, overlook the possibility that, although few abusive parents are actually psychotic, most are immature, impulsive, and suspicious and although frightened by the medical and legal professions, they recognize that something is wrong and want help themselves.

In 1963 the Children's Bureau and the American Humane Association developed a model law[23] to provide for mandatory reporting of suspicious cases of child abuse by physicians while protecting them against criminal or civil liability. Reporting would lead to investigation and if suspicions were confirmed, appropriate steps would be taken to protect the child and rehabilitate the family if possible. Meanwhile the Committee on the Infant and Preschool Child of the American Academy of Pediatrics made the following recommendations[24]:

1. Physicians should be required to report suspected cases of child abuse immediately to the agency legally charged with the responsibility of investigating child abuse—preferably the county or state department of welfare or health or their local representatives, or to the nearest law enforcement agency.

2. The agency should have ample personnel and resources to take action immediately upon receipt of the report.

3. Reported cases should be investigated promptly and appropriate service provided for the child and family.

4. The child should be protected by the agency either by continued hospitalization, supervision in home, or removal from home through family or juvenile court action when indicated.

5. The agency should keep a central register of all such cases. Provision should be made for the removal of case records from the register when it is found that abuse did not, in fact, occur.

6. The reporting physician or hospital should be granted immunity from suit.

By now all 50 states have enacted laws based on either or a combination of the proposed model law or the American Academy of Pediatrics recommendations. These laws and increased professional publicity concerning the problem have led to a significant increase in reports. It is notable that the State of California, which enacted its law in 1963, was a party to a court settlement in 1970 that involved the establishment of a $600,000 trust fund by insurers of four physicians and a police chief who had been accused in a $5 million damage suit for failing to report a "battered child syndrome" that resulted in permanent brain damage of a 3-year old boy.

These various efforts crystalized in the passage of national legislation on January 31, 1974 —The Child Abuse Prevention and Treatment Act (P.L. 93-247). It established a National Center for Child Abuse and Neglect in the Department of Health, Education, and Welfare to (1) compile, analyze, and publish an annual summary of research on child abuse and neglect; (2) act as a clearinghouse for information; (3) publish training materials for personnel in fields dealing with child abuse programs; (4) provide technical assistance (by grant or contract) to public and nonprofit organizations; and (5) conduct research in the area of child abuse. The Center is also authorized to make grants and contracts for state and local demonstration programs designed to identify, prevent, and treat child abuse and neglect.

Obviously others than physicians and health and welfare agencies have important roles to play with reference to the abused or battered child. Murdock[25] has made the following points with reference to the responsibility of school systems, based on his experience in Syracuse, N. Y.:

1. The reluctance of school personnel to report suspected cases (of child abuse) for fear of legal involvement and court appearances can be overcome by a proper presentation of the problem, especially in those states where reporting is mandatory.

2. Maximum cooperation between the school systems and the investigating agency is of extreme importance. A frequent exchange of information between the two organizations should be encouraged, not only in the initial reporting but also in the continued observation of these cases.

In addition, of course, is the extremely important contribution made by many of the social service agencies throughout the nation. It is obvious, however, that none of the professions or organizations alone—health, legal, social service, education, or any other—can solve this tragic problem. It presents a classic example of the necessity of interdisciplinary teamwork. This is emphasized by Gray,[26] "The problems of the battered child and his family are multiple and varied, and, therefore, hospital personnel who become involved in their solution must have varying backgrounds, abilities, and assets. This concept has led to the establishment of hospital-based battered child teams so that physicians, medical social workers, and public health nurses are all available for consultation regarding the most beneficial manner to help a battered child and his family."

## JUVENILE DELINQUENCY

A few comments should be made about delinquency in youth. It has always occurred. Unrest, it has been pointed out, is part of youth. The problem is the degree of unrest in relation to the social mores of the times, and when unrest and dissension in youth passes a certain point, it becomes labeled juvenile delinquency. On the basis of police reports juvenile delinquency rates are highest in cities, lower in suburbs, and lowest in rural areas. In 1968, for example, the rate for urban areas was three times that for rural areas. As would be expected, slums of large cities produce the largest number of offenders. It appears, however, that where the individual lives is more significant than whether he comes from a broken, poor, or socially deprived family. During recent years there has been a dramatic rise in delinquency rates in all types of communities. There is probably a triple reason for this—improved detection and reporting systems, the increase in the number and proportion of the population under 18 years of age, and the peculiar conflicting interplay between the material benefits to today's youth combined with certain social limitations and restrictions placed on them. As a result, the increase in arrests of juveniles has outstripped the increase in their population increment. In 1958, with 23.5 million individuals between the ages of 10 and 17 years, there were 500,000 cases of juvenile delinquency handled by the courts in the United States. A decade later the population of this group had risen about 33%, whereas the cases increased about 80%.

Boys are referred to juvenile court four times as frequently as girls. It is predicted that 1 out of every 6 boys today will end up in court for other than a traffic offense some time before his eighteenth birthday. The charges at present consist of theft, 25%; breaking and entering, 11%; violation of curfew, loitering, and runaways, 16%; vandalism, 9%; auto theft, 4%; violation of liquor laws, 2%; violation of drug laws, 1%; and all other charges, 32%. Girls are most often sent to juvenile court for running away, ungovernability, larceny, and sex offenses. These differences indicate that in the United States people refuse to recognize certain basic physiologic and psychologic differences between boys and girls. Most schoolbooks deal with "children" rather than "boys" and "girls." Children through their teens are consistently put into the same school classes, presented with the same curricula and teaching methods as well as behavior requirements, ideals, systems of rewards and punishments that in general are geared to the girl and not to the boy. Certain shared experiences are certainly important, but insistence on uniformity "across the board" has resulted in ten times as many behavioral problems among boys as girls—stammering, bed-wetting, reading problems, and delinquency. Comparatively speaking, few youths are involved in violent offenses against the person such as murder, assault, and robbery, although recently this appears to be changing somewhat for the worst.

The attitude of youth itself toward delinquency is interesting. A comprehensive study,[27] the first of its kind, of an entire birth cohort involving almost 10,000 boys who were born in Philadelphia in 1945 revealed the following. By the time they reached 19 years of age about 35% had at least one officially recorded contact with the police for delinquent behavior. However, a group of only 627 boys (6%) accounted for more than one half of all of the delinquent acts and about 70% of the robberies, aggravated assaults, and homicides committed by the entire cohort. It was also notable that the juvenile justice system apparently had no subsequent effect on reforming the chronic offenders. It is especially significant that 90% of the teen-agers interviewed confided that they had committed an act for which they could have been brought before a juvenile court. Fewer than 3% of the acts were detected by the police, and fewer than 1% of these were recorded as delinquent. It appears that teen-agers themselves apply more rigid standards to their behavior than do the police or the courts.

Wolfgang,[28] a renowned sociologist who served as Director of the Center for Studies in Criminology and Criminal Law at the University of Pennsylvania, in discussing delinquency in youth emphasized that relatively few commit serious acts of violence compared to adults. He stated "Not yet arrived at positions of power where responsibilities are shared, youth cannot be blamed for a society that yields violence because it fails to make automobiles and highways safer, fails to reduce inordinately high rates of infant mortality, to move more vigorously to reform cities of blight and organized crime, or to control the manufacture and sale of guns."

Whether it is boys smashing windows and telephones in the slums or their campus counterparts seizing university facilities, each group is expressing through action that they are attacking what they consider is not of fundamental value, especially since they are not allowed to participate in the conduct and rewards of the system. The delinquent in the slums wants to obtain by whatever method at least some part of what he is being deprived; whereas the student, although desirous of education, is opposed to the manner in which he must obtain it and the purposes for which he sees it being presented. Each group is deliberately and delinquently disruptive as a means of showing his disdain. In a sense Wolfgang indicates that "For all their protest against their established elders, youth in a sense relies on the patience, understanding, tolerance, and responsibility of the older generation to check their escalating demands." Unfortunately, all too often in recent years well-considered checks have tended to be absent. "It is the task of those in power," says Wolfgang, "to be alert, to listen to the messages from the mouths of those once in our wombs. The older generation cannot retreat into the pit of their age. The education we offer youth must link the best of our traditions with the imagination and humanity needed to cope with the future." However, "Our model has been faulty and youth today will not trust our advice like a child who takes refuge in obedience. We should respect their caution, yet learn how to warn them."

The question still remains: How should society meet the challenge of the delinquent acts of youth? The traditional approach has been arrest and arraignment before a juvenile court. However, the juvenile justice system as it now exists has been described at its best as having no effect on the subsequent offensive behavior of youths, and at its worst it has a deleterious effect. "Not only do a greater number of those who receive punitive treatment . . . continue to violate the law, but they also commit more serious crimes with greater rapidity than those who experience a less constraining contact with the judicial and correctional systems."[27] It is shocking to note that the President's Crime Commission reported in 1967 that one half of the juvenile court judges in the United States have not even graduated from college and one fifth had no college-level education at all.[29] There is good reason, therefore,

not to expect too much from many juvenile courts as now staffed. The uniqueness and potential value of juvenile courts, however, is that they are based on the philosophy that children are not to be considered criminals but rather immature individuals in need of help and guidance. Ordinarily the courts have access to consultation from psychiatrists, clinical psychologists, pediatricians, social case workers, and other professional specialists. Unfortunately in many places these resources have been minimally used.

Juvenile courts usually hold hearings in conference rooms with the proceedings essentially conversational. Pleas of guilty, not guilty, or nolo contendere should not be made or permitted in a juvenile court, and the proceedings should not lead toward a conviction or acquittal. The privacy of the juvenile should be respected, with the public excluded, and publication of names and photographs prohibited. He should be advised of his right to have legal counsel. Often the juvenile is not told of his rights and does not even know what legal counsel means. If the juvenile or the court wishes, representation by counsel should be provided. The youth has the right to face his accusers, to cross examine them and witnesses, and to introduce evidence that he believes might be pertinent. Disposition of juvenile delinquency cases varies from institutionalization, placement in a foster home, assignment to relatives, but usually return to the home of his natural parents. Frequently, since so many juvenile offenders come from homes where their parents are failing in their roles and where other social and mental problems may exist, this represents in far too many instances the development of "revolving door cases."[30]

Health personnel and facilities have a far greater role in the field of juvenile delinquency than they have recognized or practiced. The physician and health officer should regard it as a public health problem, an endemic disorder that constantly threatens the community. Just as they would not hesitate to provide or seek action with a case of communicable disease, they should in behalf of the youth, his family, and the community take the responsibility for assuring that available health resources are brought to bear on a family with a problem of delinquent behavior. Frequently in attempting to direct the delinquent child into the proper hands, they will find that necessary facilities will be inadequate or absent in the community.

It is here that his responsibility as a citizen will become an important aspect of the physician's or health officer's role. A special characteristic of American psychiatry beginning in the late nineteenth century was the child guidance movement and its offspring child psychiatry. "In this area," said Campbell,[31] "the emphasis has shifted to a study of the child's instinctive and emotional life, of his groping for satisfaction and for a grasp of the outside world and his urge towards self expression." This philosophy led to the establishment first at the University of Pennsylvania in 1896 by Witmer of a clinic where children with behavioral, emotional, or social problems were examined psychologically and medically. Subsequently the idea spread to Chicago, Boston, Allentown, Pa., and elsewhere where a psychiatric perspective was brought to bear on juvenile delinquency not only from the standpoint of treatment but especially with an eye toward understanding and possibly prevention.[32] In addition, there has been a growing recent trend for more enlightened juvenile courts to refer delinquent children to new types of foster homes with small groups of children (six to eight) living together essentially normally under the guidance of substitute parents who are responsible to the court and backed to the extent necessary and available by community mental health centers, child guidance centers, and visiting health and social workers.

## CONCLUSIONS

From what has been presented hopefully it is clear that much or most of crime, delinquency, and violence are essentially mental health problems and have their genesis within the family.[30,33] In an essay on the family and mental disorder Cumming[34] provides an excellent basis for this viewpoint in his delineation of family roles.

All families are divided along two great axes. Because of the generational differences which exist in any family, and because of the state of helplessness of the human infant, it is obvious that the father and mother can be designated as having more power than the children. A second axis of role differentiation corresponds with sex-categories. The male members play predominantly instrumental roles, that is, they provide for the family's needs in a practical way and relate the family to the surrounding community. They represent the family as it strives to achieve its goals, and defend it from any threat from outside. The women of the family play predominantly socio-emotional roles and are primarily responsible for dealing with the tensions which arise within the family and thus with defending the system against internal threats to its integrity. These two axes, taken together, yield four descriptions of the roles within the family. They give us the dominant role characteristics of the father, instrumental and powerful; the mother, powerful and socio-emotional; the son, less powerful and instrumental; and the daughter, less powerful and socio-emotional. According to this scheme, important disruptons in family functioning would occur if one or another member did not fulfill his or her appropriate function, or if competition for roles arose between family members.

This statement appears to describe well what is occurring today along both axes, not only in the United States but in many other nations as well. Both the respective age-related and sex-related roles are undergoing considerable change, giving rise to significant unaccustomed familial and social stresses manifested by marital discord, increased divorce and separation rates, jealousy, suspicions, and fears, sexual aberrations, youthful revolt, and increased delinquency both juvenile and adult. Urban life today with its complexity and demands for conformity, yet rapid role change, places great stress on all participants but especially on those who are basically rigid and those who for socioeconomic reasons are not able or not permitted to cope. The frustrations of such groups result in threats to self-esteem and meaningful existence. This in time produces deep and continuing anxieties, which perhaps is the most fundamental or ultimate base on which antisocial behavior rests. This is especially likely to be true of those entrapped in the poverty "syndrome." As Chilman[35] indicates, many of the very poor can find even temporary escape only in fantasy, dramatic behavior, psychosomatic illnesses, impulsivity, alcohol, and drugs. Yet she points out that the higher rates of child neglect and abuse, delinquency, crime, vandalism, and general social deviancy among the lower socioeconomic classes cannot be merely accepted in a society that values the rights of the individual to protection from and for himself. She continues,

These behaviors especially cannot be accepted in an urban society where, for instance, one man's undisposed garbage becomes the neighborhood's rat problem, or where one impulsive, hostile, aggressive youth can become a menace to his family, neighborhood, community, and—with the aid of a gun—the nation. And, where a neglected, abused child can grow into such a youth. Of course, such behaviors pose a danger to the individual and to society in whatever social class they occur; these behaviors simply are—or appear to be—most prevalent in very poor groups.

This relates to much of what was discussed in Chapter 6 on social pathology and public health. Poverty is indeed the germ of many social and biologic diseases. (And is there really any difference?) In view of this there is ample justification for members of the health and social professions to address themselves to this complex of problems; but to do so successfully requires the development of deep and genuine empathy and understanding to look beyond the antisocial manifestations and see the social causes.

## REFERENCES

1. Matthews, A. R.: Mental illness and the criminal law: is community mental health an answer, Amer. J. Public Health **57:**1571, Sept. 1967.
2. Solomon, P.: The burden of responsibility in suicide and homicide, J.A.M.A. **199:**99, Jan. 30, 1967.
3. Hall, W. W.: Amer. Med. News **14:**4, April 17, 1971.
4. Crime and medicine, M.D. **9:**120, Nov. 1965.
5. Saul, L. J.: The hostile mind, New York, 1956, Random House, Inc.
6. Freud, S.: Civilization and its discontents (1931). In Strachey, J., et al.: The complete psychological works of Sigmund Freud, London, 1955, Hogarth Press, Ltd.
7. Cannon, W. B.: Bodily changes in pain, hunger, fear and rage, New York, 1929, Appleton-Century-Crofts.
8. Allee, W. C.: Cooperation among animals, New York, 1951, Henry Schuman, Inc., Publishers.
9. Committee on Economic Development: Reducing crime and assuring justice, New York, 1972, The Committee.
10. Gillin, J. L.: Murder as a sociological phenomenon, Ann. Amer. Acad. Pol. Soc. Sci. **284:**20, Nov. 1952.
11. Pizer, V.: Murder and the tyranny of fear, Washington Star, May 7, 1972.
12. Banay, R. S.: Study in murder, Ann. Amer. Acad. Pol. Soc. Sci. **284:**26, Nov. 1952.
13. Washburn, S. L.: Aggressive behavior and human evolution. In Coelho, G. V., and Rubinstein, E. A., editors: Social change and human behavior, DHEW pub. no. (HSM) 72-9122, Rockville, Md., 1972, National Institute of Mental Health.
14. Endleman, S.: Violence in the streets, Chicago, 1968, Quadrangle Books, Inc.
15. National Institute of Mental Health: The impact of televised violence: Report of the Surgeon General's Advisory Committee on Television and Social Behavior, DHEW pub. no. (HSM) 72-9090, Rockville, Md., 1972.
16. Bandura, A.: The impact of visual media on personality. In Rubinstein, E. A., and Coelho, G. V., editors: Behavioral sciences and mental health, PHS pub. no. 2064, Rockville, Md., 1971, National Institute of Mental Health.
17. Psychogenic death rates, Amer. J. Public Health **60:**790, April 1970.
18. Bakal, C.: The right to bear arms, New York, 1966, McGraw-Hill Book Co.
19. Adelson, L.: Slaughter of the innocents, New Eng. J. Med. **264:**1345, June 29, 1961.
20. Kempe, C. H., et al.: The battered child syndrome, J.A.M.A. **181:**17, July 7, 1962.
21. De Francis, V.: Child abuse, Denver, 1963, American Humane Association.
22. Sanders, R. W.: Resistance to dealing with parents of battered children, Pediatrics **50:**853, Dec. 1972.
23. Children's Bureau, U. S. Department of Health, Education, and Welfare: The abused child—principles and suggested language for legislation on reporting of the physically abused child, Washington, D. C., 1963, Government Printing Office.
24. Maltreatment of children: recommendations of Committee on the Infant and Preschool Child of the American Academy of Pediatrics, Pediatrics **37:**377, Feb. 1966.
25. Murdock, C. G.: The abused child and the school system, Amer. J. Public Health **60:**105, Jan. 1970.
26. Gray, J.: Hospital-based battered child team, Hospitals **47:**50, Feb. 16, 1973.
27. Wolfgang, M. E., Figlio, R. M., and Sellin, T.: Delinquency in a birth cohort, Chicago, 1972, University of Chicago Press.
28. Wolfgang, M. E.: Aggression in youth, lines of communication, Philadelphia, Jan. 1973, Mental Health Association of Southeast Pennsylvania.
29. Curran, W. J.: Due process, jury trials and juvenile justice, Amer. J. Public Health **61:**1901, Sept. 1971.
30. Eisner, V.: Effect of parents in the home on juvenile delinquency, Public Health Rep. **81:**905, Oct. 1966.
31. Campbell, C. M.: Destiny and disease in mental disorders, New York, 1935, W. W. Norton & Co. Inc.
32. Rosen, G.: Madness in society, Chicago, 1968, University of Chicago Press.
33. Violence and the family (special issue), J. Marriage Family, vol. 33, Nov. 1951.
34. Cumming, J. H.: The family and mental disorder: an incomplete essay. In Causes of mental disorders, New York, 1961, Milbank Memorial Fund.
35. Chilman, C. S.: Growing up poor, SRS pub. no. 109, Washington, D. C., 1969, U. S. Department of Health, Education, and Welfare.

# PART NINE

# The substance
# of public health—
# health and environment

"What is this thing called health?" once asked the journalist-commentator, H. L. Mencken. "Simply a state in which the individual happens transiently to be perfectly adapted to his environment." But what is meant by man's environment. Events of recent years make the former definition appear incredibly simplistic. Until recently, most people considered their environment limited to some of the visible, tangible, inanimate aspects of their surroundings. For long, public health workers' interpretation of environmental health did not go much beyond insanitation. But a revolution has occurred, complete with speeches, marches, legal actions, and even occasional mild violence born of frustration. We have come to learn and understand the word and concept *ecology*. The age-old egocentric concept has been put aside that the planet and everything on it was ours to exploit and despoil without danger of repercussion. But nature has begun to strike back.

The widening gap between technologic developments and the ability of man-devised institutions (of which we are a part) to adapt, is at the root of the plethora of environmental problems that confront us—in our homes, at work, on the street, at play. Increasingly there seems to be nowhere to hide. And all of these environmental and institutional problems in turn are intertwined with and form a part of most of the social problems of the day. The situation was well put by C. P. Snow in his book, *The Two Cultures and the Scientific Revolution*. His most telling point is that "as history routinely and regularly records, because the engineering community and the political community could not get sufficiently on each other's wavelengths, one advanced civilization after another, sooner or later, collapsed." So now, man's only recourse is to "join the rest of the world," to live in it with greater wisdom than before, and to anticipate and guard against those environmental forces, natural and man made, that may mitigate against man's health, well-being, and continued existence.

*I brought you into a plentiful country, to eat
of the fruit thereof and the goodness thereof;
but when ye entered, ye defiled my land, and
made mine heritage an abomination.*

JEREMIAH, 2:7

CHAPTER 28

# Ecology, environment, and health

## A TIME OF CHANGE

A rising wind of unease and concern blows across the land, around the earth, shaking all the leaves and already felling some erstwhile mighty trees. Necessarily caught in this relentless movement is the field of public health with all its various manifestations—its professional schools, its established disciplines, its traditional programs, its timeworn approaches to planning, public relations, and service. New agencies based on new and broader concepts appear to pose genuine threats to the very continuance of public health as an entity. Dissatisfaction with the adequacy of the various professional schools and their products is causing a reexamination of and a return to the fractionation and a multiplicity of training approaches, institutions, and types of personnel. It is ironic that the field of public health, which accomplished so much with so little in such a short time, has now been weighed in the balance and seems to be found wanting as it enters the final quarter of the twentieth century.

This is an exciting period in which to live and work. It is marked by simultaneous and interlocking revolutions in science, transportation, education, communications, agriculture, biomedical research, demography, and the relationships among human beings. In nearly all respects it is most characterized by change. It is a period fraught with problems, since not only the magnitude but especially the rapidity of change threatens the very survival of man.

Yet for those who must deal with the untoward consequences of the changing man-environment relationship, it is also a period that is challenging in its opportunities and expectant of new approaches, intolerant of obsolescence and inadequacy, rich in opportunities for studies and experiments, alive with interest and concern, but woefully deficient in new concepts of health and well-being deriving from man's continually changing interaction with his environment.

For those charged with the preservation and enhancement of the public's health, their conceptual approach to the man-environment relationship and the quality of it that can lend perspective to what is wrong, how it went wrong, and what ought to be done to right it is of critical importance. The conceptual approach of public health workers is emphasized as the key because although it is all too often ignored in favor of busy action for action's sake, it is public health concepts that in the final analysis shape public health efforts. They determine how correctly public health workers view problems, how they propose to grapple with them, and how they develop and allocate their resources.

In many quarters outdated or fundamentally irrational concepts have caused public health workers to perpetuate many actions, as though the existing and potential external hazards to man's health were fixed and isolated phenomena related to one or another specific environmental element such as air, water, or waste. Admittedly this approach produced dramatic results in the past when people were confronted with widespread communicable diseases that superficially appeared to exhibit simple, single, specific cause-and-effect relationships. Unfortunately this viewpoint is dangerously unsuited to deal with illnesses and disorders that have multiple causes arising essentially out of an increasingly complex revolution in the environment. Such concepts ignore the convergent complexity of the relationship of *total* man to his *total* environment. This relationship merits closer examination.

## MAN AND HIS ENVIRONMENT

As an animal, a mammal, man is not particularly distinctive, except perhaps for certain physical developments, some of which appear rather ludicrous when viewed objectively. But as the end product of hominid evolution, possessed of cultural and technologic capabilities, man is unique. His environment in reality is a multienvironment system that encompasses the physical and biotic realms and the cultural setting fashioned by his unusual cerebral capabilities. Thus man, the organism, can be viewed simultaneously relating to the biophysical and to the sociocultural components of his environment. These interrelations between *total* man and his *total* environment are dynamic. Each makes aggressions on the other. Each, in return, responds to these aggressions. To support his biologic, cultural, and uniquely technologic needs, man boldly and continuously alters his naturally occurring environment and creates ever new environments. Often this is done with inconsistency and without a thought to the total or ultimate consequences. Thus man presents the incongruity of standing almost knee-deep in refuse, while he shoots rockets to the moon. Thus, he bequeaths to his descendants waters laced with nondegradable detergents and pesticides and lands littered with imperishable aluminum cans.

Until now, man could respond successfully through biologic evolution. This, of course, took time, but man had lots of time. Today the situation is different. Within recent decades man himself has set in motion forces of such magnitude and rapidity as to challenge seriously his own adaptive abilities. It is to this adaptive ability of man that attention is directed. The ability of the human organism to maintain internal integrity in the face of changing external

forces is one that is largely *past oriented;* that is, the internal integrating properties of man evolved and matured over many hundreds of thousands of years during which stimuli were occurring slowly and naturally. Thus the regulatory mechanisms to achieve homeostasis are genetically linked to a lengthy era in man's evolutionary history unlike that which he faces today. In other words, man is the product of past environmental circumstances with their homeostatic-upsetting forces to which he had the ability and, very importantly, the time to adapt.

In this era of burgeoning populations, and especially of rapid change, there is no longer time for leisurely adaptation and evolution. As a consequence, there can be no assurance and in fact there is considerable doubt that this limited natural adaptive capacity will suffice to carry him through all future experiences. Present man-induced drastic alterations and disturbances in his total environment are resulting in insults, excitants, and stresses that necessarily evoke responses from the human organism. Such responses may be physiologic, morphologic, behavioral, or social, or a mixture of all of them. Through these responses the organism seeks to reach a modus vivendi, seeks to maintain or to regain homeostatic compatibility. The complexity of this adaptive effort is readily apparent, since it includes the *total* human organism and its whole nature as it relates to its *total* environment. Furthermore, simultaneous insults that arise out of both the biophysical and sociocultural components, and often exhibit synergism or potentiation, can evoke human adaptive responses to threats that are so unequal, inadequate, or inappropriate as to be disruptive in their own right. Thus an individually acceptable amount of water pollution, added to a tolerable amount of air pollution and combined with a bearable amount of noise and congestion, can produce a totally unacceptable health environment.[1]

The implications of this have been dramatically emphasized by the deliberations and conclusions of the so-called "Club of Rome," which is composed of an informally related group of several hundred outstanding scientists, sociologists, industrial managers, and educators from several countries. Because of shared concerns for the future of mankind, beginning in April 1968, they arranged to have a large amount of data on land use, resource consumption, energy production, births, deaths, and many other things transmitted to the Massachusetts Institute of Technology, where it was put in a computer for the development of predictive mathematical models. They decided on five critical areas for measurement: population growth, the rate of industrialization, the ability to increase food supplies, the rate of depletion of natural resources, and the extent of environmental pollution. Obviously these are all interrelated. The result of the investigation so far[2] by this highly reputable group is that no matter what combination of events is fed into the computer, a satisfactory conclusion is yet to appear. They conclude that earlier individual warnings by population and agricultural specialists, ecologists, and students of natural resources fall short of the mark. They predict that if the current course of continued growth and depletion of resources is followed, although things may continue to look good for some for a while, a sudden cataclysmic collapse of industrial civilization will occur accompanied by widespread famine, disease, and strife—probably within 100 years. They liken the situation to a spent light bulb that glows ever brighter before it suddenly blows out. The only hope they see is the achievement as rapidly as possible of a "steady state society" on a worldwide partnership basis, in which there is collective action to stabilize all five of the basic areas at the same time—population food supply, industrialization, natural resource consumption, and pollution. That, of course, expects a great deal from human nature.

An attempt to illustrate the potential consequences of man's ecologic ignorance is provided by the work of Calhoun,[3,4] of the National Institute of Mental Health, with colonies of mice and rats. In a series of long-term studies he has illustrated the ultimate effects of uninhibited breeding and excessive crowding. He begins with a limited number of healthy laboratory animals, provided with constantly ample supplies of food, water, and nesting material and unhampered opportunity to propagate in quarters carefully designed to be spacially adequate for 144 animals. Well before reaching the eventual naturally imposed ceiling not of 144 but of about 2,500 animals, there develops a breakdown of almost all aspects of normal behavior. Laboratory mice are naturally clean about themselves and their environment. When limited in numbers, they typically avoid soiling each other or their nesting places. Under the conditions allowed in these experiments, however, gross insanitation from bodily discharges becomes ubiquitous, and the tendency for personal grooming is lost. Territorial prerogatives are ignored. The strong attack the weak, and groups of the strong drive off groups of the weak. As a result, in each large experimental pen, masses of essentially outcasts that Calhoun refers to as "behavioral sinks" appear. The members of the outcast behavioral sinks become excessively violent, but only among themselves—not with the strong overlords. Markedly aggressive behavior appears among many of the females. Scattered throughout may be seen individuals who clearly demonstrate various signs and symptoms of regression, confusion, and mental disturbance. Throughout, and even among the dominant animals, sexual desire and the ability to mate decline significantly. Homosexuality appears with males trying to copulate with males and females with females. Increasingly the group becomes nonproductive. Such normal mating as does occur becomes increasingly infertile; such cubs as are born are typically premature and weak and are typically ignored and cannibalized. It is of more than incidental consequence that once arriving at this state, transfer of animals, even the few dominants, to more "normal" circumstances does not typically result in recovery. Permanent physiologic damage, probably through endocrine glandular change, has resulted.

One has only to read the newspapers of American cities to recognize that a reasonable amount of interpolation from such studies to man, his numbers, concentration, living circumstances, and total environment may be valid. As the cities become more densely crowded, as people pave over their farm lands and abuse and neglect the urban environment at an ever more rapid rate and as in the process people place ever more physical, chemical, biologic, and psychologic hazards and stresses on those who live in the cities, one has ample cause for concern about the immediate and long-range results.

The British historian Arnold Toynbee, in a paper on "The Coming of the Worldwide City," stated that the most formidable of all problems man faces today is "the accelerating pace of change in our man-made environment within the span of a single lifetime. It is formidable because it is psychological. Here we are in a field in which technology cannot provide even a partial solution for a problem that technology has created. Here the human spirit has to fight its own battle, spiritually naked."

These concepts have been crystallized by

McCue and Ewald[5] into two basic forces of change: *macro-impacts* of the environment on the individual, including such factors as population, time, space, technology, and free-will expectations; and *micro-impacts* of the individual on the environment, including physiologic, psychologic, cultural, social, and ecologic factors, plus spiritual free will. In viewing their synthesis they observe that just thinking about the first can be depressing "because we seem so impotent to influence them." But it is pointed out that although they are certainly real forces, they are not the only ones. Accordingly they say that if man would accept the projection of the past into the future as a smooth predictable curve or the uncontrollable impacts of society on man, he would have no need for the projection of the individual's impact on the environment, either singly or in the aggregate, or would he be concerned with the human meaning of technologic systems to man. But the authors emphasize, man does not necessarily have to accept such a deterministic or fatalistic view. Man finds himself, then, with the uncomfortable understanding that human beings as individuals and in groups have their own impacts, therefore their own responsibilities, concerning the creation of the future environment through the proper application of the factors that make up the balancing micro-impacts. And the single most decisive factor in deciding the future, they believe, is the will of people, not technology. The more aware, the more comprehensive this understanding the greater will be the individual and group responsibility. What pertinent food for thought!

In the study of man, in health and disease, there has been much less interest shown in a better understanding of the *total* human organism's *total* response to the *total* environment than in the separate biochemical activities of its components. This narrow, parochial, and fractional approach, although highly productive of detailed particles of knowledge and techniques, has not increased greatly man's understanding of the interplay between the entire human organism and its environment. This caused Dubos[6] to observe that ". . . the time has come to give the study of the responses that the living organism makes to its environment the same dignity and support which is being given at present to the study of the component parts of the organism." And he predicts that ". . . exclusive emphasis on the reductionist approach will otherwise lead biology and medicine into blind alleys."

A classic example was the flurry of emphasis and publicity given to expensive heart transplants that enabled a rare few individuals to survive inadequately for a few additional months or years. This does not really represent science applied to the welfare of mankind. It is merely a technical contest with nature that involves an almost anonymous individual who is essentially selected by a whim of circumstance as a convenient subject. Consideration should also be given to the cost-benefit aspects of such procedures. The cost of just one such operation would suffice to train several medical students, each of whom, during their professional lives, could provide much needed basic health and medical care to many thousands of individuals. From this viewpoint the morality of this current emphasis on organ transplants and similar procedures appears somewhat questionable.

A consequence of the inadequacy of the reductionist approach to environmental health hazards has been a gradually growing recognition of the need for a new conceptual framework to study and deal with the complex and ever-changing interface between *total* man and his *total* environment. Such a framework, growing out of a synthesis of many disciplines and fields, would include within its purview the study of cause-and-effect relationships on the bases that man *is* a whole organism and reacts as a unit; that life *is* dynamic, and its infinite variations are primarily the result of reaction to specific and often compounded identifiable environmental factors, modified by individual tendencies of inheritance and qualities of resistance; and that disease or dysfunction, in any part, *is* the result of overall loss of ability to adapt successfully.

The emphasis that must be given to establish such a new basis for public health is, in essence, the application of the principles of ecology to the human circumstance. It is based on a recognition that the health status of man is the outcome of the interplay between and the integration of two ecologic universes: the internal environment of man, the biosocial organism, and the external multienvironments in which he exists. As it is with the individual, so it is with the community. Human ecology is thus concerned with the broad setting of man in his environment, that is, with all aspects of man and his nature, his interpersonal and intergroup processes associated with culture, technology, and social organizations, and the basic personality drives that are expressed in behavior and emotion. It strives to develop a conceptual framework wherein the public health and medical needs of mankind, as individuals, in groups, and as communities, may be approached not merely in a reductionist fashion—that is, viewing only a disease entity of specific etiology affecting a specific organ or system—but rather in a holistic manner wherein the integrated responses of man to environmental forces find expression on a *health-disease-death* continuum.

The human ecologic approach, of necessity and by definition, calls for an interdisciplinary effort wherein the natural, physical, and social sciences, in company with engineering, combine to study the adaptive responses of man, and especially the effects of unsuccessful adaptation on his health. The theologian, Paul Tillich, put it aptly when he said: "... to speak of health one must speak of all dimensions of life which are united in man. And no one can be an expert in all of them." The field of environmental health has been described by Lee[7] as "having its basis in the efforts of the total human organism to adjust, survive and thrive, through its continually changing interactions with its total environment, and to the extent that it fails, health hazards result, which ultimately require control efforts in the environmental component of this relationship."

If health and well-being are states in which man exhibits full adaptive capacity, the question arises as to the nature of the environment best suited to him. Increasingly these days people hear concern about the quality of the environment and the need to restore it. Restore it to what and for what purpose? Where is the blueprint for this restoration? Who drew it up and on what basis? Although there are many ideas and suggestions about the nature of a desirable or undesirable environment, there is little in the way of an intelligent comprehensive master plan. Indeed, for the most part environmental health is strangely underplayed if not ignored in most of the current so-called urban and national planning as well as in comprehensive health-planning activities on all levels of government. One of the problems is that man simply does not know all the circumstances under which his adaptive capacity can be pushed beyond the norm of adequate response. This is a fertile and critical field for inquiry.

## HAS MEDICINE FAILED?

Despite an increasing recognition that the disease process is best understood in terms of its demonstrated overall causation, body-centered etiology and specific chemotherapy, directed at altering particular body processes, continue as the focus of contemporary medicine. In view of this the charge may be made with some justification that contemporary medicine has failed. Now to contend that modern medicine has failed, at a time when it daily achieves great and dramatic wonders, may appear to pose a paradox and to be perversely incongruous. Who can deny the triumphs of vaccines and antibiotics, the great advances in surgery, and the technologic developments that take place daily in the great hospitals? But medicine should be concerned with health and well-being in addition to disease and disability. In fact, it still is almost entirely preoccupied with the latter and very little with the former. It is interesting to observe in this regard that the establishment of the National Institute of Child Health and Human Development came almost as an afterthought, following years of establishment of a series of categoric institutes concerned with the diagnosis and treatment of specific diseases. To say that health merely means not to have a disease is a bit like that classic definition of sanity as "the art of staying out of an asylum."

It is interesting to retrace the development of public health in this same sense. Public health derived from a concern about the environment. Through time, action in the environmental field has also tended to be fragmented into categories of special interest: air, water, housing, refuse, and numerous others, each with its own group of specialists. Eventually some of these even became competitive, as in the case of refuse disposal programs based on incineration coexisting with attempted air pollution programs. Interestingly, the funds and stimuli for both sometimes derive from the same agency. Meanwhile concern over the various biologic impairments of man received increasing emphasis. This became reflected in the training provided to professionals as well as in their practices. Thus a catalogue of medical and allied professions developed, each in turn further subdivided, amoeba-like, into spectra of clinical specialties. The end result was the ideologic separation of man, the subject, from his environment, and an inadequate appreciation of the effect of the one upon the other. Hence, we have arrived at the unfortunate place where man is chopped up, his environment is chopped up, and little, if any, interface between the two has been recognized, trained for, or allowed to develop.

It would appear, then, that both medicine and public health have become inadequate for the health needs of today and the future. Medicine, in the training of its clinicians and in its practice, has paid scant attention to the broad environmental causation of disease and has demonstrated little interest in the promotion of positive health. Public health, in turn, has ignored the convergent complexity of the man-environment relationship and has been content with categoric approaches to problems that now approach crisis dimensions. Both are inadequate because they have demonstrated surprisingly little interest in the social etiology and ecology of illness and health.

It is not suggested that ecology in itself is a panacea for the solution of man's health problems. Ecology does not possess a body of knowledge peculiar unto itself. It does not possess well-ordered techniques or methodology for solving the complexities of man's environmental relationships. Even the principles derived from extensive studies in terrestrial and aquatic ecology are found significantly wanting when applied to the human organism that has been modified by society and culture. Of what value, then, is human ecology to public health? Its principal value lies in the manner in which it looks at the man-environment system. Ecology forces the health worker to look at the whole human organism, not just its organs and organ systems, much less in terms of the interests of particular professions or societal groups. It forces health workers to view the environment as being, in reality, multienvironments integrated into a remarkable system. It forces them to look at the coinfluential relationships that exist between the two principals and among their complex parts and to realize that alteration or manipulation in one part of the system is necessarily reflected in other parts. It forces health workers to realize that the whole of the man-environment relationship is considerably more than the sum of its parts. It forces them to recognize that whereas specialists who pursue indepth studies of particular parts of the system contribute much to particulate understanding, they do not help health workers to understand the interplay between the *total* man and his *total* environment.

Human ecology, by contrast, places man at the center of concern. It views him as the ecologic dominant and recognizes that although he is a biologic organism, his position in the scheme of things is greatly accentuated by the uniqueness of his cerebral capacities, by the culture and society of his fashioning, and by the entirety of his surroundings, which as indicated, he has profoundly altered. Human ecology sees man at the interface of his two basic environments, the biophysical and the sociocultural, being at once in both, interacting reciprocally with both, affecting and being affected by both. It is out of conflicts which arise from this dynamic complex of interactions that insults to the integrity of the human organism arise. The result of this ecologic interplay determines man's place at any given time on the health-disease continuum, as indeed it will determine his ultimate fate.

Perhaps the health worker can think of the biosocial organism called man as an open-ended system through which the energy, resources, and influences of the environment flow, are transformed for good or ill, and which transform man in the process. From many sources in the physical environment come hazards to health in the form of biologic organisms, toxic chemicals, radioactivity, noise, physical forces; they run the gamut of ecologic exposures. From the sociocultural component comes the never-ending stream of informational stimuli, which require correct decisions or adaptive strategies that too often pose a threat to psychologic and social integrity and trigger emotional and behavioral patterns inimical to self and others. And the synergistic potential, the additive effect of these, elicits even greater maladaptive responses that manifest themselves as disease and disability. These become the clinical signs of an unsuccessful struggle.

How strange that man, who evolved as an integral part of his environment, with the appearance of a culture, has perversely adopted an attitude of environmental apartheid. The many terms that reflect the antagonistic attitude of man's culture toward its environment are noteworthy. Man *conquers* the environment. Man *subdues* nature. Man *pushes back* the frontier. Man views it as a *threat*, as an *enemy*, instead of cherishing, protecting, and conserving it, instead of recognizing that man himself is in fact part of it, instead of saying "I am myself and my circumstance." Somehow the environment is seen as something to be shaped, molded, and transformed to meet man's short-term preferences, or merely as the stuff that through exploitation, serves his transient needs in preparation for an anticipated "real" afterlife. That out of the manipulation and alteration of this natural bounty, and the societal institutions which make it possible, could come sickness and unhappiness, is a thought foreign to an organism that has a Ptolemaic view of itself.

## HEALTH OR SICKNESS—THE CHOICE

If the public health profession is to continue to be meaningful, it can no longer limit its concern to the causes of sickness. It must consider more deeply the causes of health. Has this not been the ultimate interest and goal of public health? Has not everything that has been accomplished so far been only a prelude to this greater concern? It may be that public health as a social concept is too complex and too important to be entrusted to traditional public health professionals any longer, that is, unless they discard their specialized and categoric interests and begin to think, plan, and act in the broader and time-dimensional context of ecology. The public health profession finds itself in a critical transitional period of history when traditionalists will be left behind while others, more perceptive, surely will move into the resulting vacuum. In this regard the current situation has been described as representing a kind of truce that might collapse at any time because the public health profession has not gone far enough.[8]

Some may say that the public health profession does not know enough. But the critical need at this time is not for more knowledge and data. Actually the public health profession presently has more available than it can properly catalogue and digest, much less apply. It may sound intellectually heretical, but the public health profession must avoid the cult of a search for complete answers to the pressing human ecologic problems before it takes action against them. To do otherwise is to erect a barrier to timely and intelligent action. There are too many timid or puristic souls who decry action until some distant unreachable day when the ultimate in scientific proof will assure foolproof action. The theory is attractive, so much so that is has resulted in investments of billions of dollars for more and more research, while support of action programs to apply existing knowledge to the benefit of man has languished. One does not need a horsepower-per-pound study before changing dirty spark plugs. It is not honest science but a misplaced martinet

distortion of the purpose of science that precludes the practitioner from the application of his professional judgment to whatever knowledge exists. The old hospital quip, "The clinical chart is now complete but the patient has died," could become the epitaph of the human society and species.

## CONCLUSION

Attention may be pertinently directed to a presentation, several years ago, by the Director-General of the World Health Organization.[9] Speaking from an ecologic point of view, he closely identified public health interests with the interests of conservationists. He said:

The ecologist conceives the term "conservation" as the wise management and utilization of natural resources for the greatest good of the largest number. One may debate the position of man in such a universe, but only as to what level of hierarchy he may allocate himself. That he exists and affects his own kind and all else in the world is not debatable. . . . man's history justifies the claim that he, like most other animal and plant life, is "an endangered species." . . . Man, in his struggle for survival, poses as many true ecological challenges as the more familiar lion, rhinoceros or whooping crane. The environment truly may be his friend or enemy.

This is a timely warning. Perhaps one of the greatest limitations of the public health profession is the extent to which it has alienated itself from ecologically oriented conservationists. Fundamentally, public health workers and conservationists have much more in common than either group appears to realize.

In a more positive vein, public health is the only field of endeavor with a built-in potential to deal with the interface between total man and his total environment. It had its roots in the environment, and its workers promptly developed a deep social concern. Many of its early practitioners were environmentalists. It has attracted a truly multidisciplinary personnel, and it has demonstrated a willingness based on constant introspection to adapt and change itself. Now, certainly, is a time for considerable introspection. There is much dust to shake out. Fundamental changes are called for, especially in how the public health profession views itself in relation to this limited closed system it calls its world or what Fuller[10] refers to as "Spaceship Earth." The health profession must call forth men and women with the foresight and courage to accept the new and broader philosophic base of human ecology, as applied to human welfare and, on accepting it, to act upon it. Only then may the public health profession make its true potential contribution to the development of a new society and a better world.

## REFERENCES

1. U. S. Department of Health, Education, and Welfare: A strategy for a livable environment. Report of the Task Force on Environmental Health and Related Problems, Washington, D. C., June 1967, Government Printing Office.
2. Meadows, D. H., Meadows, D. L., Randers, J., and Behrens, W. W.: The limits to growth, Washington, D. C., 1972, Potomac Associates.
3. Calhoun, J. B.: Population density and social pathology, Sci. Amer. **206:**139, Feb. 1962.
4. Calhoun, J. B.: Ecological factors in the development of behavioral anomalies. In Zubin, J., editor: Comparative psychopathology, New York, 1967, Grune & Stratton, Inc.
5. McCue, G. M., Ewald, W.R., Jr., and the Midwest Research Institute: Creating the human environment; Report of the American Institute of Architects, Urbana, 1970, University of Illinois Press.
6. Dubos, R.: Environmental biology, BioScience **14:**11, Jan., 1964.
7. Lee, J. A.: The environment in environmental health program, Boulder, 1964, Ecological Society of America.
8. Kartman, L.: Human ecology and public health, Amer. J. Public Health **57:**737, May 1967.
9. Candau, M. G.: Man's health in relation to the biosphere and its resources: scientific basis for rational use and conservation of the resources of the biosphere, Paris, France, Sept. 1968, UNESCO House.
10. Fuller, R. B.: What quality of environment do we want? Arch. Environ. Health **16:**685, May 1968.

*Our orientation must be to the total man in his
total environment, to the cumulative effects
of a growing number of environmental
hazards on a receptor—man—who can respond
to them in an incredibly complex manner.*

A Strategy for a Livable Environment

CHAPTER 29

# Environmental hazards*

## MAN AND HIS ENVIRONMENT[1-5]

Human health has always been dependent on the relationship of man to his environment. The human being, like other animals, is constantly being transformed by natural forces in the environment that act on him, and he is continuously transforming his environment. Human beings, other animals of all sizes and shapes from the sizable whale to the microscopic amoeba, bacteria that are smaller than the smallest animal, viruses tinier even than bacteria, and all plants of different sizes and shapes —all these living organisms are part of a dynamic system in which they continuously interchange matter and energy with the world about them (their environments). The human being, for example, takes into his body solid and liquid matter from his environment and puts solid, liquid, and gaseous waste into his environment; he exchanges gases with his environment, and he even contrives machines and gadgets that also exchange matter and energy with their environments. Other living organisms may get into man's body. Some act for his physiologic benefit, whereas others cause trouble. In addition, man both benefits from and becomes afflicted by the nonliving forces of his world. *All* of these interactions with the environment, including the great changes in the past 30 years, are involved in the relationship of man's environment to man.

Man's relationship to his environment neces-

sarily must be regarded in two contexts: (1) the elements of the natural environment that are hazardous to his health and safety, and (2) man's actions within his environment that themselves threaten his health. Within the first context are biologic agents of disease or injury, including microorganisms, noxious plants, and toxic or physically harmful animals; weather, including violent storms, cold, and thermal stress; natural radiation from the soil or from the atmosphere; geologic perturbations such as earthquakes, volcanic eruptions, and floods; and certain naturally occurring chemical substances. The second context consists of hazards to man's health that result from his own actions and maladaptations of the natural environment. This second context of human hazards brings the biologic scientists into a confrontation with conditions even more complex than those that comprise health threats of "natural" origins.

Man-made hazards include such things as accidental injury, suicide, and homicide; injury and genetic damage from ionizing and nonionizing radiation; poisoning from industrial, agricultural, and therapeutic chemicals; noise-induced hearing loss; and health threats from polluted air, land, and water. These health problems are direct although unintended results of social and technologic advancement or aberrant human behavior or both.

The automobile is an outstanding example of a social and technologic advancement that has brought with it a staggering toll in accidental death and injury, pollution of air, water, and land, and unmeasured hearing loss from noise as well as some of the most hazardous occupa-

---

*From Proceedings of the Federation of American Societies for Experimental Biology, Part II, 31, Nov.-Dec. 1972. (Reprinted with permission.)

tional environments such as oil drilling and highway construction. Elimination of the automobile as a threat to health and life cannot be achieved either by its removal from society or by "immunizing" mankind against its effects. Inevitably, a trade-off must be reached when man's chosen systems of transportation provide sufficient benefits to justify whatever toll results in terms of health effects. Similar acceptable cost–benefit decisions will have to be made with respect to radiation, pesticides, drugs, industrial chemicals, and most other hazards in this category.

Aberrant human behavior underlies many health hazards. Obvious examples are the steadily rising incidence of death from suicide and homicide. More subtle but significant is the inexplicable risk taking associated with misuse of narcotics and alcohol, exposure to venereal diseases, and many sources of accidental injuries. An ever-increasing number of people in American society seem willing—even eager—to risk the almost certain health threat of addiction or accidental death or injury so as to achieve whatever the benefit that risk offers them. There is much fancy and little fact to aid the life scientists in reducing health threats related to such behavior.

The unique nature of human and environmental hazards, especially those generated by man, is such that many complex social, economic, and political factors bear heavily on them, their genesis, their study, and their solution. Although the net result of such hazards is an unwanted effect on man's health and well-being, the traditional training and experience of the life scientist is insufficient to cope with these problems single-handedly. By introducing the element of human action—either purposeful or by indirection—the health scientist finds it necessary to form an alliance with engineers, physical scientists, behavioral scientists, economists, educators, and political scientists if prevention or control of these human hazards is to be achieved.

The successful development of the antipoliomyelitis vaccine against a biologic hazard was an excellent example. Health scientists recognized the health hazard and the need to eliminate it. They conceived of and successfully pursued the biologic means of accomplishing this. But the actual fulfillment necessitated working with physical scientists to develop the production equipment; with engineers and industrial designers to develop a high-speed hypo-

spray for safe, sterile, rapid, mass application of the vaccine; with behavioral scientists and educators to motivate individuals and groups and to understand and overcome the objections and misunderstandings of some; with economists to obtain the significant amounts of funds required for poliomyelitis research and application of its results; with lawyers to provide legal protection; and with various elected and employed practical political scientists and public administrators to secure the necessary social and community sanctions. Throughout, from conception to successful application, the biologic or health scientist was fundamental, but assistance was needed from the others. The total cost was great, but the benefit in lives and dollars was tremendous.

If one accepts the conditions of trade-off improvements as opposed to absolute prevention and need for multidisciplinary involvement, it is necessary to reexamine the criteria by which program priorities are established. Eight such criteria may be listed: (1) mortality rates, (2) morbidity rates, (3) financial impact on national economy, (4) utilization of hospital space, (5) numbers and availability of health personnel, (6) types of control measures available for attacking the problem, or the ease with which they can be attained, (7) available or obtainable human and financial resources, and (8) public receptivity to the idea and method of controlling the hazard.

None of the hazards to health considered here meets all of these criteria. Thus accidents and occupational injury and illness should receive high priorities in terms of the first four and possibly the fifth criteria but should probably be rated low on the last three.

With respect to scientific breakthroughs the widest possible variance exists among the hazards considered. They range from vast strides and control over many communicable diseases to meager beginnings on the subject of noise. In a real sense accomplishments serve as a measurement of both society's concern for the problem and its willingness to invest in its solution. Even more specifically, progress in controlling human and environmental hazards reflect the extent to which political leaders are motivated by physicians, scientists, and the general public who may believe that a particular hazard can and must be controlled and eliminated.

History describes the sequence: The first step is taken by a scientist who believes that a hazard might be understood and controlled. Then, after successful research has shown what can be done, concerned citizens and their political leaders are prompted to apply the results.

## CHANGING NATURE OF HAZARDS

The past three decades have witnessed tremendous advances in medicine, science, engineering, and technology. In the United States varying degrees of affluence and high standards of living have been achieved for a large proportion of the population. The chief health problems of the past—yellow fever, plague, malaria, cholera, typhoid, dysenteries, and many others—have all succumbed to the application of research. Unfortunately many of the recent technologic advances have given rise to new and unfamiliar limitations to human life and happiness. Population increase, road construction, and transportation improvement have led to grotesquely increased crowding and its accompanying stresses.

An ever-increasing barrage of new chemicals reaches man's body through food and water consumed, air breathed, and drugs taken therapeutically or otherwise. Streams and lakes have become contaminated with biologic, agricultural, industrial, and mining wastes. Rapidly increasing amounts of garbage, solid wastes, and discarded vehicles multiply the opportunities for insect and rodent breeding. A crescendoing cacophony is affecting the auditory perception of an increasing number of persons. Ionizing and nonionizing radiation are a growing part of man's environment. It is used not only in nuclear testing but also in industry, in laser and microwave technology, in electronic products in the home, and in devices for medical diagnosis and treatment. Each of the various environmental hazards is becoming increasingly significant in its own right, but the implications in terms of total "body burden" are yet to be comprehended.

Thus the modern environment is dangerous on two accounts: it contains elements that are clearly noxious and stressful, and it has been changing so rapidly that man appears unable to make proper adaptive responses to it. The rate of technologic change is accelerating every year; most changes demand a human adaptation. A complex of physical, mental, and emotional stresses of human life are resulting from increasing urbanization. Small but long-term exposures to many environmental stresses, hazards, and contaminants cause many previously little understood chronic ailments, disabilities, and even death. There is only now a beginning realization of the complexity of the environment and of the various factors within it that may act together to reinforce each other (synergism) or to oppose each other (antagonism). Those who are today concerned about human health and welfare must learn more and more to assess the problems of their own special areas of interest from an overall, a total, a holistic viewpoint. It will no longer do for the problems of one area to be considered in isolation or separately from the problems of related areas.

Little has been learned about the interactions within the human body and human mind of the various environmental stresses, although it is known, for example, that the intended effects of certain medications may be initiated, intensified, or otherwise transformed by certain other factors in the environment. Similarly it is known that radiation, cigarette smoking, certain air pollutants, and various chemicals encountered in the occupational setting can have a multiplying effect in the development of pulmonary cancer. The little that is known about multiple hazardous impacts merely highlights the vast amount still to be learned about human response to the environment. Most of the vast and ever-increasing array of physical, chemical, biologic, and psychologic stresses to which modern urbanized humans are now being subjected did not even exist in their grandparent's time.

In the late nineteenth century, the sociologic and hygienic leaders were primarily concerned with malnutrition, overwork, filth, and microbial contamination. Today's characteristic diseases result from economic affluence, chemical pollution, and high population densities. The increase in chronic and degenerative diseases is due in part to these environmental and behavioral changes and not, as often mistakenly supposed, due to an increase in human life expectancy. Most people do not realize that life expectancy after the age of 45 years has not increased significantly. A person 45 years or older is little better off than he would have been in 1900 or before, even if he can afford good medical care. It can be assumed that medical science will continue to develop useful techniques for ameliorating cancers, vascular disease, and certain other degenerative disorders. Undoubtedly it will refine methods for organ transplantation and for artificial prostheses. But most of the conditions to be treated need not have occurred in the first place. Greater knowledge of environmental determinants, provided by more biomedical research, is the path to prevention and control—a better and less expensive way.

The protection of the public from hazards involves skills and knowledge far more extensive and varied than seemed sufficient even in the recent past. To accomplish this requires sound scientific understanding resting on intensive and extensive biologic and biochemical research. Fortunately there is a growing public awareness of the need for improved environmental quality. Increasingly, as environmental deterioration has affected more and more citizens, their uneasiness has produced demands for safer and more sensible use of the environment and an increasing willingness to provide whatever support is necessary for its restoration and preservation. This implies involvement, which in terms of universities and similar concentrations of expertise, brings one back to the subject of research. In the absence of increased attention to the study of the effects of environmental hazards on man, increases in disease rates and greater expenditures for avoidable therapy are inevitable.

## A VIEW AHEAD

The population of the nation is projected to increase to 250 million people by 1980 and over 300 million by A.D. 2000. Metropolitan areas probably will absorb nearly all the increase, and environmental problems will be intensified geometrically. Moreover, new and presently unsuspected environmental hazards will be identified. Without corresponding growth in environmental health protective activity, the future can only bring mankind increased physiologic and psychologic suffering.

An overview of where the public health profession stands and how it must proceed is pertinent. Guidance is provided by successes in in the combined areas of environmental biology and aerospace physiology. Man's space travel provided the impetus to bring together the knowledge of several disciplines in a new, more positive approach to human health. Thus research on space vehicles has provided facts that are useful in occupational health programs and radiation protection procedures. Already these breakthroughs have begun to result in

improved health through the establishment of realistic criteria for technologic assessment. They have increased substantially the awareness of the holistic approach to the solution of environmental problems at every segment of society, encompassing both professional and and general citizenry. Among the "spin-offs," the many specialists in environmental health have necessarily become broader professionally and are now more effectively bringing together the health scientist and the urban planner, and the lawmaker and the toxicologist, to mention only two of innumerable examples. Other spin-offs worthy of mention are in the area of therapeutic medicine. Better health care delivery systems have evolved, and the need for comprehensive health programs has been more clearly defined.

Against this background two major breakthroughs during recent decades are worth special note. The first was the appreciation that small amounts of chemicals may become toxic after periods of accumulation or latency. The kind of biologic and toxicologic research that was carried out on beryllium, asbestos, benzene, and mercury exemplifies this. It demonstrated some of the fundamental enzyme systems involved and showed that the rate at which the body acted on a chemical affected its toxicity. As a result, the basic mechanisms of toxicity became better understood as these biologic and chemical processes were probed in depth. Safety evaluation techniques were improved, and the methods for studying the potential of chemical carcinogenesis, teratogenesis, and mutagenesis were and are still being developed as a result of these research efforts.

The second major and concurrent breakthrough was that the scientific community became aware that there was inadequate information on the effects of these widespread chemicals (air pollutants, metals, persistent pesticides, additives, pharmaceuticals, and the like) in the biosphere. As a result, the research community is now expressing its concern that the total ecologic threat may in some instances be more important than any direct toxic effect on humans. In sum, the major breakthrough was to appreciate the latent, insidious, and chronic effects of small amounts of chemicals in the environment, often over prolonged time periods, and their potential threat to future generations through their effects on the biosphere. Even this breakthrough is inadequate unless consideration goes beyond acute, easily recognized, clinical responses to chemical toxins, to consideration of genetic potentials.

The number of factors in the environment that may affect man are presented in the following outline:

*Life support*
  Food
  Water
  Oxygen

*Physical factors*
  Mechanical
  Acoustic
  Electrical
  Magnetic
  Thermal
  Particulate
  Ionizing radiation

*Biologic factors*
  Microorganisms
  Toxins
  Biologic wastes
  Biologic antagonists
    Animal
    Plant
  Allergens

*Psychosocial factors*
  Crowding
  Demands
  Physical time
  Biologic time
  Cultural time

*Chemical factors*
  Inorganic
    Light metals and their compounds
    Transitional and rare earth metals and their compounds
    Heavy metals and their compounds
    Nonmetallic elements and their compounds
  Organic
    Acyclic hydrocarbons including alkyl compounds
    Carbocyclic compounds
    Halogenated acyclic hydrocarbons
    Heterocyclic compounds
    Organic phosphorus compounds
    Organic sulfur compounds
  Product complexes
    Combustion products
    Macromolecular products
    Industrial wastes
    Agricultural wastes (including fertilizers, pesticides, and herbicides)

Some of these factors in proper form or amount are helpful or even necessary to life; others are hazardous. Consideration of several of them, with some consideration of significant breakthroughs and further needs, follow under three categories of hazards—biologic, chemical, and physical.

## BIOLOGIC HAZARDS TO MAN[6-10]

The biologic hazards to human health are mostly those posed by bacteria, viruses, and other microorganisms and parasites. Since the advances against them have been discussed in other chapters, they will be considered here in a general way. Those microbiologic accomplishments directly related to human health include modifications of man's susceptibility to disease or of his recuperative ability (better diagnostic and immunizing methods and better antimicrobial drugs) and modification of his environment or of his relationship to his environment (more knowledge of the agents that cause or induce infectious disease and how to control them; better methods of ensuring that food, milk, and water are free of disease-producing microorganisms; more aseptic homes, public institutions, and food distribution industries; better understanding of community health problems; and better control of disease in domestic and wild animals). Those accomplishments that have an indirect relation to human health include, for example, improvement in worker productivity with consequent increase in plant and animal food production. During the past 30 years microbiologic research could have been even more effective had there been more complete communication between scientists, administrators, and agency representatives and less unnecessary duplication of research activities, whether funded by federal, local, or private sources.

Information exchange is vital to success and economy of applied research in the field of microbiology as related to health and disease. There has been little planned exchange of information other than through publication of scientific papers and presentations at scientific meetings. One notable exception is the Arbovirus Information Exchange, which is issued three or four times a year to scientists in 235 institutions. This plus an annual meeting in conjunction with the Society of Tropical Medicine and Hygiene minimizes unnecessary duplication and directs attention toward critical problems.

Microbiologic research in the past might have been more effective if there had been a nationally sponsored expert committee for each of the major diseases such as malaria and tuberculosis. The U. S. Armed Forces Epidemiological Board has had outstanding success with this kind of system, providing an example that should be followed by other organizations and governments. Another deficient area of communication lies between the researcher and the tax-paying citizen, whose support for research could be retained if he had understandable information on research activities and accomplishments.

The following achievements may be anticipated during the next decade in this fight against microbiologic hazards: (1) more effective and less expensive methods for disposing of human wastes, thereby reducing water pollution from this source and reducing the biologic usage of oxygen in rivers; (2) better methods of controlling disease caused by microbes in agricultural products (plants and livestock) leading to an increase in quality and quantity of food; (3) more specific drugs for use against microbes, fungi, and certain viruses that cause human disease and disorders; (4) more effective immunizing agents for human and animal use, including attenuated live virus vaccines administered orally or into the nose–throat region; (5) determination of the causative agents of various types of cancer and their role in the pathologic origin of cancer; (6) improvements in the control of those diseases transmitted from animals to man, diseases such as Rocky Mountain spotted fever, plague, brucellosis, hemorrhagic fevers, encephalitis, rabies, and the like; (7) more accurate and less expensive diagnostic microbiology by means of automation and reducing the size of clinical diagnostic samples; (8) better understanding of immune mechanisms leading to significant improvement in the prevention and management of disease problems of the very young and the very old, particularly problems such as multiple sclerosis, rheumatoid arthritis, and disease states of the blood (blood dyscrasias).

Although improvements in man's control of the biologic hazards of his environment can be expected to continue, these advancements should be accelerated and made more effective by similar improvements in the kinds of communications needed for planning and coordination of research and development activities.

## CHEMICAL HAZARDS TO MAN

### General[11-14]

The chemical hazards to which man is exposed exist in all three aspects of the environment—air, water, and soil. Although a particular chemical hazard initially may be limited to one of these, dispersion to one or both of the others may occur. This is especially likely to be the case for persistent pollutants. Agricultural chemicals present a classic example. As a result, a fourth source of environmental chemical hazard should be considered in the form of food, in the sense that it may reflect possible concentrations from air, water, or soil.

With reference to chemical hazards in terms of implications to human disease perhaps the major advance of the last three decades has been the realization that spontaneous diseases, for which no cause can be found, are in fact induced by environmental pollutants. Thus certain cancers and deformities may be largely explicable in terms of exposure to certain specific environmental pollutants. More recently there has beeen a growing realization of the importance of chemical induction of genetic changes. Apart from preformed agents that may cause cancer (carcinogens), induce morphologic abnormalities (teratogens), or bring about genetic changes (mutagens), there is a growing interest in the possibility of their synthesis in the body from simpler chemical compounds normally present in the environment.

Although the word *pollutant* is often restricted to synthetic industrial chemicals, there are four broad categories of other important chemical pollutants: The first group consists of natural chemicals in excess, and includes nitrates that are normal dietary components. At high concentrations in food or water, nitrates can cause a blood disorder (methemoglobinema) in infants. Also, nitrites, as reduction products of nitrates, may interact with secondary amines to form nitrosamines. Some of them are carcinogens, teratogens, or mutagens.

Toxic chemicals in fungi on plants or in crop plant products comprise the second group, of which aflatoxins and cycasins are notable examples. The yields of these toxins can generally be considerably influenced by technologic factors, such as conditions of harvest, storage, and processing. The third group consists of complex organic and inorganic mixtures, such as air and water pollutants, which comprise a wide range of undefined and defined components.

Finally, there is the group of synthetic chemicals—agricultural chemicals, notably pesticides and fertilizers; food additives; fuel additives; household chemicals; industrial chemicals; and in a somewhat specialized class therapeutic and prophylatic pharmaceuticals, as well as habituating and addicting drugs.

Pollutants may have a wide range of adverse biologic effects, from health impairment to death. The possibility that chronic toxicity is also manifested in immunologic impairment or psychologic disorders has yet to be determined, although there is already suggestive evidence to incriminate carbon monoxide in these regards.

Some pollutants produce any one or more of these types of reactions and may interact with one another outside the body as well as inside the body to produce otherwise unanticipated synergistic toxicity.

### Naturally occurring chemicals[15-17]

There are many naturally occurring chemicals that are hazardous to man. The toxicity of some, mercury and arsenic, for example, was known in ancient times. In recent decades information from a variety of research investigations had indicated that many others play a role in human health and disease. Some trace elements play an important part in human nutrition and in many physiologic reactions. But excesses and deficiencies of certain metals such as cadmium, selenium, chromium, lead, copper, zinc, lithium (or of radiation) may be related to major degenerative diseases such as heart disease, muscular dystrophy, diabetes, multiple sclerosis, cancer, mental illness, or congenital malformations. There is a growing awareness that many diseases have geographic patterns that seem to relate somehow to the physical environment and its different geologic metal-containing areas. This awareness has led to a corresponding recognition of the need for interdisciplinary teamwork among the geochemists and the medical scientists. Some of the observations that have resulted from this multipronged investigative effort are described briefly in the following discussion.

For a long time *arsenic* was believed to produce cancer, but recent research with animals and lack of evidence in man has dispelled this notion in the United States. Major sources of arsenic intake are food, especially crustacea, and beverages, particularly wines. Except for some isolated sites, the arsenic content of water supplies is extremely small. But in Europe there have been claims that arsenic does induce cancer. Arsenic has long been known to counteract selenium toxicity, and it

has been added to poultry and cattle feeds to suppress selenium toxicity in areas where selenium content of soil and water is high. However, in hamsters selenium does not suppress the monster-forming effect of high levels of arsenic. It is possible that the different United States and European views of arsenic as a cancer-inducing agent may result from differences in exposures to these two antagonistic elements in the two regions of the world and to the quantities and chemical forms of these substances taken in.

Certain tumors (mesotheliomas) have been known for decades but it was not until 1965 that *asbestos* was found to be a causative agent. Its carcinogenicity appears related to certain trace metals and certain chemical compounds such as benzpyrene. Benzpyrene is a ubiquitous air pollutant, a prominent constituent of tobacco smoke and of charred and smoked foods. Asbestos workers who smoke cigarettes have three times greater risk of developing lung cancers than do nonsmoking fellow workers. The trace metals (Ni, Cr, Fe) are associated with certain types of asbestos fiber (chrysotile). There is some indication that the cancerous growths are brought about by an interaction between benzpyrene or benzypyrene compounds, an enzyme, and the particular trace metals. The chief source of nonoccupational asbestos exposure is not yet known; possible sources are asbestos water pipes, asbestos filters for beer, asbestos brake linings, asbestos household iron-holders, asbestos used in some cigars, and asbestos in water supplies (possibly the most continuous source).

*Beryllium* causes a serious disease, berylliosis, a name only about 30 years old. Also it is known to induce tumors in animals but has not been found to do so in man, although vigilance is being maintained regarding this. Beryllium poses no threat to health from water or food sources, since it is poorly absorbed from the gastrointestinal tract and is highly insoluble in water either inside or outside the body. The potential environmental threat is from air and dust around beryllium production plants. The use of beryllium as an industrial material is increasing rapidly.

Another chemical hazard is the trace element *cadmium*. In 1965 it was shown that the kidneys of persons dying from hypertensive complications had increased amounts of cadmium or increased ratios of cadmium to zinc, as compared with persons dying from other major diseases. This discovery has been substantiated experimentally in animals. The chief sources of cadmium are believed to be drinking water and food grown in soils containing cadmium from certain fertilizers; from beverages that have been in contact with galvanized zinc (container coatings), which contains small amounts of cadmium; and from vegetables, coffee, and tea (all of which usually contain small amounts of cadmium). Drinking water is not thought to be a large source. Whether or not cadmium induces renal hypertension seems to depend also on the intake of zinc and selenium, antagonists to cadmium. In hamsters monster formation induced by cadmium is antagonized by selenium. The highly lethal effect of cadmium on fish is increased (synergized) by cyanide.

A highly significant advance was made in 1960, when it was found, in many locations throughout the United States, that water with relatively more dissolved salts, so-called "hard water," was associated with lower death rates from cardiovascular and coronary heart disease. Not all states showed this correlation, and the correlation was somewhat better for coronary heart disease in white men 45 to 64 years old, by state and in the 163 largest cities that had about 58% of the total national water supplies. Mortality from all other causes showed no such correlation. Prior to this discovery, state-to-state variations in cardiovascular deaths were unexplained on either a dietary, racial, or social basis. Evedently something in hard water, or the lack of something in soft water (relatively low in dissolved salts), influences the death rate. Of the various trace elements for which correlations have been worked out, only cadmium and *chromium* ($Cr^{3+}$) have been revealed as trace elements affecting cardiovascular disease. This raises the possibility that perhaps in time the prevalence of cardiovascular disease may be decreased by adding certain trace elements to water supplies.

*Lead* poisoning has been known from ancient times, but its clinical manifestations were classified only 110 years ago. Lead exists in many forms in man's environment, and its industrial use is practically ubiquitous. Occupational safeguards have limited its harmful effects, but a special hazard is the use of tetraethyl lead as an antiknock and power-increasing agent in gasoline. Tetraethyl lead is highly toxic when inhaled or absorbed through the skin and predominantly causes cerebral or central nervous system symptoms. It pollutes the atmosphere. The toxic lead-bearing household paints have been largely eliminated, but still in the United States, thousands of small children eat dangerous amounts of flaked household lead paint, mostly in the older and poorer parts of large cities; some die and others develop mental retardation, cerebral palsy, convulsive seizures, blindness, and various other disorders. Research is being directed toward safe and effective physiologic deleading procedures, and recently chromium as a trace element in food appears to decrease lead toxicity in some animals—and presumably in man. Evidence suggests that chromium (trivalent) acts as an antidiabetic and antiatherosclerotic agent through its role in sugar and fat (glucose and lipid) metabolism.

Inorganic *nitrates* and *nitrites* are a health concern because they contaminate drinking water. They are a special hazard to infants up to 6 weeks of age and also to Alaskan Eskimos and Indians, those who have a genetically transferred methemoglobinemia. The young infants are susceptible because they have not yet developed certain metabolic enzymes, they have a more readily reactive hemoglobin that decreases after birth, and they have a small blood volume relative to fluid intake. Milk from cows that drink nitrate-polluted water can be an added threat to children. Although nitrates are used in preservation of some meats and fish, such food is not a common part of infant diet. Continued intake of nitrates may result in death. Although in the United States community water supplies are monitored in accordance with standards set by the Public Health Service, well water on farms has no such surveillance. Any increase in the use of nitrate fertilizers and superphosphate wastes, both being sources of nitrites and produced by bacterial action, will necessitate even greater surveillance and increase the hazard of nitrates and nitrites in well water on farms.

## Toxic chemicals in fungi and plants[18,19]

Substances produced in the process of growth and development of certain forms of fungi, more commonly called molds, represent another group of toxic chemicals. Molds cause economic loss through deterioration of food fiber, induce plant diseases, and cause certain pulmonary and invasive diseases in man. Mold-damaged foods were once considered harmless and used as animal feeds. It is now known that a few molds of grain and other foodstuffs produce toxic chemical substances (metabolites) called mycotoxins.

The oldest mycotoxin is ergot, from a fungus that infects cereal grasses, especially rye. Ergot has been the cause of serious epidemics in Western Europe and parts of the USSR since the middle ages. The most recent outbreak of ergotism occurred in 1951 in southern France. Many people were stricken and some died; a large proportion showed central nervous system symptoms such as hallucinations, depression, and self-destruction manias.

Among the substances (alkaloids) identified in ergotized grain are some related to LSD (lysergic acid diethylamide). One of these substances, ergotine, cause contractions of blood vessels (arterioles) and smooth muscle fibers and is used medically to stop hemorrhage, especially after childbirth, to stimulate labor, in spinal and cerebral congestion, in paralysis of the bladder, and in diabetes (diabetes mellitus). Ergotamine tartrate inhibits certain nerve endings (sympathetic) and has been used to treat migraine.

Other mycotoxins include the aflatoxins, produced by molds on peanuts and other agricultural products. Even in low concentrations aflatoxins cause acute intoxication, liver damage, and cancer of the liver (hepatoma) in animals. Certain molds on wheat allowed to remain in the fields during the winter produce poisons that cause a blood disorder (alimentary toxic aleukia). In 1944, in a district of the USSR, this disorder affected about a tenth of the population. Another mold that grows on millet has caused epidemic polyuria (excessive urinary excretion). The paucity of knowledge regarding these types of hazards indicates the great need for future research efforts.

## Complex organic and inorganic chemical mixtures[20-29]

In addition to naturally occurring chemicals and plant and fungal poisons, complex organic and inorganic chemical mixtures make up a third group of environmental hazards. They arise as a result of the pollution of air and water by combinations of community and industrial wastes. Man is now beginning to learn that the atmosphere and waters of this earth, although extensive, are not limitless and cannot with safety be used as sewers and disposal dumps. Air, water, and consequently food cannot continue to be mistreated in this way without rapidly increasing danger to a rapidly increasing population in a limited world.

Most people do not realize that the average person in the United States takes into his body each day about 30 pounds of air, in contrast with only 4 pounds of water and 3.5 pounds of food. The unused remains of these are returned to the environment as contaminants or as potential contaminants.

## Air pollutants

There has been a belated recognition that air pollution is one of the most important sources of chemical hazards, especially in highly urbanized and industrialized societies. More than 200 million tons of toxic material are released into the air above the United States each year, about 1 ton per person. About 60% comes from approximately 100 million internal combustion engines, the other 40% from sources such as factories, power plants, municipal dumps, and private incinerators. The pollutants include carbon monoxide, sulfur oxides, nitrogen oxides, hydrocarbons, and particulates. They produce ill effects in people either by short-term, high-level or by long-term, low-level exposures (Table 29-1).

Short, high-level exposures cause acute reactions with increased mortality, especially among the elderly and the chronically ill. There may be increase of respiratory infections, irritation of ear, nose, and throat, and impairment of physiologic functioning. The more serious effects that may lead to death include an increase in the severity of chronic illnesses such as bronchitis, emphysema, asthma, and heart attacks (myocardial infarction). In the United States more than 6,000 communities are considered to be affected by varying degrees of air pollution. Inhabitants who show asthma-like responses, the most frequent response to polluted air, tend to have an increase in $\beta$- and $\gamma$-globulins in their blood, and biochemical studies have shown that asthma patients also have increased $\gamma$-globulins.

The insidious long-term effects of low-level exposures to polluted air perhaps are even more significant, since these exposures result in slowly developing difficulties that are hard to define or measure. Chronic diseases of several kinds, including cancerous growths and genetic mutations, may be initiated, general body defense mechanisms impaired, and physiologic function interfered with. The protective cilia of the respiratory tract, for example, may be slowed down or destroyed by atmospheric sulfur oxides, nitrogen oxides, and ozone, and this injury may be associated with and followed by other re-

**Table 29-1.** Estimated atmospheric emissions, United States, 1968, $10^6$ tons per year

| Source | Carbon monoxide | Particulates | Oxides of sulfur | Hydrocarbons | Oxides of nitrogen |
|---|---|---|---|---|---|
| Transportation | 63.8 | 1.2 | 0.8 | 16.6 | 8.1 |
| Fuel combustion in stationary sources | 1.9 | 8.9 | 24.4 | 0.7 | 10.0 |
| Industrial processes | 9.7 | 7.5 | 7.3 | 4.6 | 0.2 |
| Solid waste disposal | 7.8 | 1.1 | 0.1 | 1.6 | 0.6 |
| Miscellaneous | 16.9 | 9.6 | 0.6 | 8.5 | 1.7 |
| Total | 100.1 | 28.3 | 33.2 | 32.0 | 20.6 |

spiratory disorders and diseases. In the United States chronic bronchitis and emphysema are among the most rapidly increasing causes of death. One in twenty asthma patients is severely affected by air pollution. Lung cancer has been correlated with air pollution as well as with certain other factors, such as smoking habits.

Deaths from pulmonary carcinoma have been correlated with air pollution, taking into consideration several pertinent socioeconomic variables, such as smoking habits, economic status, and degree of urbanity. For example among English nonsmokers, a ten-fold difference was found between the death rates for cancer of the lungs for rural and urban areas. Adult British immigrants to New Zealand and to South Africa have been found to suffer a higher incidence of lung cancer than individuals of the same ethnic stock who were born in those two locations. Among Norwegians living in Norway, where air pollution is low, the lung cancer rate is also low. Among Americans living in the United States, where air pollution is heavy, the rate is twice as high. For Norwegians who have migrated to the United States the rate is halfway between.

Correlations have also been found between air pollution and carcinomas other than pulmonary, such as of the stomach. In addition, deaths for cirrhosis of the liver have been observed to be higher in heavily air-polluted areas, probably because livers already damaged by alcoholism decompensate when exposed to toxins of polluted air. In the laboratory, injection of animals with trace amounts of extracts of urban atmospheric pollutants from some cities, especially those using predominantly solid fuel, produced a high incidence of tumors of the liver, lymphatic system (lymphoma), and lung (multiple adenomas). Such amounts would be inhaled in about 3 to 4 months by a resident of the cities involved.

Apart from frankly evident air pollution and smog, specific gases may be harmful to health. A study in Chattanooga, Tenn., has linked relatively low levels of nitrogen oxides to the susceptibility of children to the Asian influenza. Evidence from California indicates that a concentration of carbon monoxide in the air of as little as 10 parts per million for about 8 hours may result in impaired performance because of reduction of ability of the blood to carry sufficient oxygen to the brain. Such levels are common in many cities around the world.

Elevated levels of carbon monoxide have also been associated with the increased probability of motor vehicle accidents and with the inability of individuals to survive myocardial infarctions. Although admittedly several other factors are involved, it is notable that death rates from coronary heart disease are 37% higher for men and 46% higher for women in metropolitan areas with high atmospheric pollution levels than they are in nonmetropolitan areas. Cardiovascular death rates are more than 25% higher for male Chicagoans between 25 and 34 years of age than for their counterparts in rural areas. The difference is 100% for men between 35 and 54 years old and nearly 200% for men between 55 and 64 years old. Since 1940, genetically determined coronary artery patterns have been recognized as playing a significant role in vulnerability to coronary atherogenesis and myocardial infarction. Of the three branching patterns identified, hearts with a left coronary artery pattern are considered most vulnerable to fatal coronary artery occlusion, and those with balanced patterns, least vulnerable. These and similar findings, combined with those that associate atherosclerosis with carbon monoxide, indicate the inadvisability of certain types of individuals residing in areas of high pollution.

In the earlier discussion of lead as an environmental chemical hazard, passing mention was made of the special problems presented by the addition of tetraethyl lead to gasoline for anti-knock and extra power purposes. The consumption of leaded fuels has increased tremendously —from 100,000 pounds in 1940 to 450 million pounds in 1967, an increase of 4,500-fold in 27 years. If a uniform distribution throughout the country of its 90 million cars and trucks is assumed, the potential exposure to each of the country's individuals (200 million) approximates 2.25 pounds per year—certainly a frightening thought, particularly when lead distribution is not uniform but is concentrated in areas of heavy traffic.

Confronted with the facts, several investigators made worldwide comparisons of lead concentrations in the blood and urine of man. These comparisons showed: (1) variations in body concentrations did not exceed 3.5-fold anywhere in the world; (2) lead values in primitive societies often equaled those in the metropoli; (3) lead values had not changed in three decades; and (4) there is no evidence that at current lead levels adverse effects of the health of man occur; urinary D-aminolevulinic acid levels of normal populations are well below response levels.

Inferences from the foregoing blood and urinary lead levels are somewhat misleading unless one notes that they are average values. Blood lead values were measurably higher in certain groups such as traffic policemen and persons living adjacent to busy highways. In none of these individuals, however, did lead values approach levels considered hazardous.

Nevertheless, the measurable elevations in blood lead found by repression analysis are interpreted as evidence of a measurable contribution to the body lead burden from the atmosphere, heretofore not considered possible of attaining significance in comparison with the daily intake from food and beverage. The evidence is made plausible by the postulation of body absorption of up to 50% of atmospheric lead generated in submicron particle size from motor exhausts. Experiments with animals suggest a need for the larger cities to establish an air standard for lead. Several communities such as Philadelphia and New York City set limits on atmospheric lead concentrations. However, this limit (5 $\mu$g/m$^3$) may prove not to be too conservative, in light of increased toxicity of lead in certain deficiency states observed in advanced age groups and the demonstration in man of the interference of lead in various endocrine functions.

Whereas many other examples of the relationship between general atmospheric pollution and ill health might be presented, the seriousness of the situation is perhaps most succinctly illustrated by the recommendation of the California Department of Health that physicians should estimate the contribution that local air pollution conditions may make to the outcome of a patient's illness and that in areas with high air pollution some patients may benefit from a preoperative period in a clean-air room or chamber before receiving general anesthesia.

**Water pollutants**

Water is one of the prime necessities for life. Without it survival beyond a few days is impossible. In addition to oral consumption modern man has another use or misuse of water: as a vehicle for the removal of human wastes, as a great cesspool, for an ever-increasing complex mixture of industrial and related waste materials. As a result, there have been repeated, extensive water-borne epidemics of bacterial diseases, such as cholera and typhoid fever. In the late nineteenth and early twentieth centuries technologic means were developed to remove these hazards from water with notable declines in case and death rates. Yet even today epidemics of enteric diseases occur with alarming frequency.

The hazardous aspect of water has been recognized of late as being greater also because of its contamination by viruses. Thus current levels of bacterial purity of water must be maintained and improved, practical methods of removing disease-producing viruses must be developed, effective means of surveillance and control of chemical pollution must be developed and put into practice.

Man is beginning to realize that he is living in an environment replete with agents that induce, promote, and accelerate cancerous growths and genetic mutations. Such substances contaminate man's drinking water as well as urban air and other parts of his environment. Water pollution with hazardous chemicals may be expected to increase as a result of the development of new industrial plastics, chemical sterilizing compounds for use against pests, missile fuels, and other substances. Many of these substances are unstable; they may break down in water before they become a significant health hazard. But a threat may be posed, according to some epidemiologic evidence, by a combination of potentially mutagenic chemical agents with radioactivity in water sources.

The National Community Water Supply Study, completed in 1970, made a wide variety of recommendations for the delivery of an adequate supply of potable and safe water. Strengthened legislation, forthrightly enforced, is required to limit or prevent the discharge of untreated human and industrial wastes into the streams and lakes of the nation.

With specific reference to chemicals, inorganic and organic, the study clearly evidences the need: (1) to simplify and lower the cost of removing excess chemicals known to be dangerous to the public health; (2) to improve systems to control undesirable concentrations of iron, manganese, hydrogen sulfide, and color as well as organic chemicals causing unpleasant taste and odor; and (3) to develop surveillance techniques or conditioning procedures to eliminate the deterioration in water quality between the time that the water leaves the community water treatment plant and the time it reaches the consumer's tap.

A first step is better monitoring of water quality. Instrumentation for routine continuous monitoring with computerized interpretation must be developed. The bacteriologic monitoring of drinking water of the United States employs satisfactory but inefficient methods. A tremendous investment will be necessary, however, if the proper tools and skilled personnel are to be provided so that the presence of potentially toxic materials in the environment can be identified. Only then can the epidemiologic studies necessary to identify the significance of various toxic substances in water be started.

The outstanding breakthrough of recent years in instrumentation has been the development of membrane filters for the collection of microorganisms and large molecules. The membrane filter has permitted many research workers to adapt the filter to a wide range of problems, and the uses to which this type of membrane can be put are still being explored. A similar development might come from the application of other kinds of membranes, particularly the cellulose acetate membranes being used in desalination technology, which have possibilities for the concentration of microorganisms and other contaminants. There are numerous voids in existing technology that do not allow measurement of current procedures. Current

drinking water standards do little more than mention viruses, neglect numerous inorganic chemicals, and identify only the index that is to cover the entire family of organic compounds. A breakthrough required in the next decade is the development of similar concentration and identification techniques for viruses, and particularly the ability to grow the infectious hepatitis viruses in vitro.

With the trend toward multiple use of water sources, plus the complex types of chemical contaminants, new methods of surveillance and treatment are required. Among the new contaminants that must be dealt with are fertilizers, herbicides, fungicides, irrigation residues from agriculture, detergents from homes and industry, radioactive wastes from power plants, industrial, and research installations, a spectrum of heavy metals, a wide variety of salts, and numerous other materials. Many of these are not readily biodegradable, and unaffected by conventional treatment methods, and build up in water supplies. This makes necessary continuous spot-testing techniques based on a variety of approaches. Some measure particular characteristics such as biologic or biochemical oxygen demand and acid concentration. Kits for determination of more than 100 different physical, chemical, or biologic characteristics or contaminants are now available. There are also more versatile instruments such as the direct-reading colorimeter with which 20 or more different tests can be made. The gas-liquid chromatograph has proved its value in identifying traces of organic materials in water. Continuous water pollution monitoring of effluents from industrial plants can be carried out by ion-selective electrodes, consisting of an ion-selective membrane sealed onto the end of an insulating glass or plastic tube containing an internal reference electrode of silver chloride or calomel. The solution to be measured is placed in the tube, and a voltmeter measures the electrical potential developed between it and an external reference electrode when both are immersed in a solution.

The need for knowledge about the health effects of water-borne contaminants will require thorough investigation. The concentration levels at which numerous contaminants, such as mercury, molybdenum, or selenium, cause adverse health effects must be determined. Similarly the effect of the long-term ingestion of low-level concentrations of toxic, organic materials in water must soon be determined.

Some of these toxic materials are carcinogenic, some teratogenic, and some have other toxicologic effects. Some of these effects are only identifiable after many years of exposure, and because the effects are little different from other types of exposure and deterioration, the cause-and-effect relationship is not easily established. This research will be exceedingly expensive.

Recognizing the relatively fixed amount of ground and surface water supply, the increasing water needs of the general population and industry, and the need to reuse the available supply to satisfy future demands, the public health and related professions can no longer afford to wait and see what happens.

The types of research mentioned are essential and minimal, but this generation also bears a responsibility for the health and well-being of future generations. Realistically, answers to many of the currently identifiable research problems must be obtained quickly so that planners of the environment can formulate rational, economical, and effective plans for the continued growth, development, and survival of society.

### Synthetic chemicals[30-36]

A most important achievement in the past three decades has been the development of longer lasting, more effective, and more toxic organic insecticides, a breakthrough the significance of which in terms of human health has been of the highest order. It was one of the most spectacular advances in improving man's health the world has ever seen, but in terms of certain problems engendered by them, they became a mixed blessing.

It is impossible to say just how many hundreds of thousands of individuals have had the opportunity to live out their life-span or, at least, die of accident, chronic disease, or starvation rather than to die of malaria, typhus, or some other arthropod-borne disease, probably at an early age. The advent of these longer lasting or more toxic compounds also made possible the control of vectors of diseases such as shigellosis, which, particularly in the neonatal phase of life, has produced so much misery and death. Although resistant strains of arthropods were developed rather quickly and chemical control was not permanently effective, the few years of its effectiveness removed the apathy and the general acceptance of these diseases as routine risks in many parts of the world. Chemical control

of flies, for example, is not as effective or as desirable as improved sanitation, but the latter had been hard to sell prior to the demonstrated benefits of flyless life through pesticides. The real impetus to the increased use of pesticides, of course, has been the tremendous benefits they have brought in production of food and fiber.

Researchers are now faced with the necessity—not merely the desirability—of evaluating the unanticipated effects of the host of chemicals that have been in widespread use in ever-increasing amounts since World War II. These chemicals are not limited to pesticides—pesticides comprise only a small part of the problem. Many more chemicals are used as food additives, drugs, other household materials, and a complex of industrial effluents that get into the air, food, and water on which man depends. The enormity of the task is not only beyond economic ability, but almost beyond comprehension, when it is known that hundreds of these substances have the potential for interaction with one or more other substances. With limited talents and resources, problems must be selected that are representative of many others and attempts made at their solution.

An illustration is provided by the antibiotic griseofulvin. This pharmaceutical is administered by mouth over long periods to humans with certain fungal skin infections. In the laboratory, griseofulvin produces a high incidence of liver tumors in mice at proportionate doses less than used therapeutically in man. Meanwhile, a comparatively inert and nontoxic compound, piperonyl butoxide (PB), used in agricultural pesticidal formulations to augment or synergize the effects of pyrethrums has been developed. The action of PB appears to inhibit detoxifying enzymes in the insect; thus the insect becomes more sensitive to the insecticidal effects of pyrethrum. Piperonyl butoxide administered alone to infant mice was neither toxic nor carcinogenic. However, when administered together with a variety of other agents at nontoxic levels, including griseofulvin, 3,4-benzpyrene (a polycyclic carcinogen widely distributed in the environment), and certain Freons (fluorocarbons with a wide range of domestic and industrial uses), the combination produced a significant synergistic toxicity. Additionally, in the case of Freons, combined administrations with PB also produced liver tumors. These results suggest the need to consider interactions, synergistic and otherwise, between unrelated and related agents when testing for effects of environmental pollutants.

One of the most serious problems is not generally recognized, that is, measuring the long-term hazards of popular materials. Pesticides, for instance, are usually evaluated for acute toxicity. The upper limit of tolerance is established in test animals by administration of high dose rates over short time periods. Often acute toxicity levels are far above exposures man would ever encounter, but more and more chronic hazards—problems resulting from long-term exposure to low concentrations of these chemicals—are being recognized. Thus acute or short-term effects are no accurate measure of chronic or long-term hazards. Methods of evaluating both acute and chronic hazards must be developed before irreparable damage is done to mankind or his environment.

It may prove to be true that some substances are carcinogenic, irrespective of dosage, but since so many known carcinogens are widespread in the environment, investigators must develop means to assess the risks. The idea of identifying carcinogens by high dosages administered to exquisitely sensitive animals was predicated on the hope that if such substances were so identified, perhaps man could avoid them and, furthermore, that unless a no-effect level could be identified, investigators should assume that none existed. Carcinogenic food additives and pesticides could be banned and naturally occurring carcinogens could be avoided. This idea developed before human analytical capabilities had included a capacity to recognize the wide distribution of minute amounts of known carcinogens.

It is now known that they cannot be avoided entirely. The relative risks entailed must be assessed to guide future actions. Unless this is done, an early demise of the industrial research and development of pesticides, food additives, and other useful chemical compounds is a possibility. The already high cost of such research is being driven to new heights. Many companies are sharply curtailing development of new products simply because their research resources are wholly engaged in defensive research to prove the safety of established products. This is the dilemma—not only benefit as opposed to cost but also benefit as opposed to risk. These companies are committed to the premise that products must be as safe as is possible, that risks should be minimal. They

firmly believe that a long record of wide usage has proved the safety demanded.

The alternatives are not simple, but they suggest that the federal dollar must be spent either (1) to develop and safety test new compounds (after which companies will vie with each other in efficient production) or (2) to develop protocols for testing that are reliable and feasible for the companies to undertake or to contract for with commercial research laboratories. Otherwise, these extra costs will greatly increase product prices. Another approach might be legislation to permit industrial collaboration that otherwise could be viewed as industry-wide price fixing, outside the public interest. Science can study, but only the public can make such decisions.

A new approach to research must be developed. Although federal laboratories have increased tremendously in scope and ability during the past two decades, and additional federal funds have been devoted to the development of research potential and manpower in American universities and nonprofit research institutions, these growth curves have lagged behind the growth of research and development in industry. Today this trend is being reversed. Even when allowances are made for the promotional aspects of the "D" in "R and D," industry has provided the bulk of the funds. In some segments of industry, however, such as aerospace, tax dollars support much of these industry expenditures.

With decreasing federal support it was hoped that industry, through product sales, would take over. However, the Food and Drug Administration has the policy of requiring industry to pay the bill for testing—a cost passed on to the consumer, who is also the taxpayer. In this application this policy appears sound. However, regulatory demands for more elaborate testing to ensure safety are adding unprecedented costs to industry's research effort.

These alternatives are based on present methods of requiring industry expenditures for safety testing. However, if a new factor could be introduced into safety testing, that is, industry, government, and academic cooperation, if tax dollars could be used to develop, test, and evaluate protocols for establishing safety, the cost to both industry and the consumer who pays the taxes, directly or indirectly, could be reduced. This can be accomplished only if communications among industry scientists, regulatory scientists, and academic scientists are vastly improved and a concerted effort made to coordinate existing knowledge as well as discoveries derived from research.

At this moment there is great need for reliable methods of extrapolating from animal experiments to man. Although one could hardly expect this extrapolation to be either direct or simple, it would help tremendously if investigators could determine with repetitive reliability the dosage levels at which no chronic adverse effect can be expected in man. How this can be done is a subject of much discussion at present. From this discussion will emerge theoretic approaches to the solution. Federal funds are needed to test these approaches. Once reliable methods have been demonstrated, industry risk funds again will be expended. The probability of this will be vastly enhanced if the scientific community, government, industry, and academic, can become cooperatively involved. Such cooperation might be regarded as the outstanding hoped-for breakthrough in the future, since it is the essential ingredient to the success of developing safety standards. Now, no proof of safety exists; people only assume safety in absence of evidence to the contrary.

Meanwhile, it is reasonable to expect the following specific advances to take place:

1. Continued development of biologic pest control. Research on pest predators, radiation sterilization, and chemical sterilants has increased the potential of control through means other than conventional pesticides and thus has reduced the risk that they offer to human health.

2. Continued development of specific pesticides. The development of agents that have control effects on specific pests permits more precise use of pesticides and reduces the necessity for widespread coverage of agricultural areas with a general purpose agent irrespective of local essential requirements.

3. Development of relatively safe, nonpersistent pesticides. The nonpersistent pesticides in current use are, for the most part, toxic to man in the form in which they are used. Fatalities are not uncommon in children who have access to material, and accidental poisonings occur in the applicators and other workers in recently treated crops. Safe forms of nonpersistent pesticides should be under development.

4. Development of integrated chemical and biologic control programs. The most effective and safest combinations of chemical and biologic control agents for various crops are under investigation and should lead to optimal combinations in the next decade.

5. Development of presently unavailable data on the more subtle and slowly produced effects of synthetic chemicals and pharmaceuticals individually and in combination on the basis of epidemiologic retrospective and prospective studies of extremely large samples of humans.

6. Development of more effective and time-compressing methods of laboratory animal assays of synthetic chemicals and pharmaceuticals.

The principal effect of these developments just mentioned would be reduction of the chances for the initiation or the promotion of long-term degenerative disease processes such as carcinogenesis. To this should be added a corresponding reduction of the chances of teratogenesis and mutagenesis from the action of certain agricultural and household chemicals, as well as pharmaceuticals, on the human reproductive system.

### Summary and conclusions

The overall picture of significant environmental chemical pollutants and the disease states that either have been proved or are highly suspected to be related to them has been summarized by Stokinger[11] (Table 29-2). It is noteworthy that these diseases head the list of causes of morbidity and death as well as of shortening of life expectancy. He draws the following important conclusions with reference to chemical hazards to man:

1. Airborne pollutants possess greater potential for contributing to man's deteriorating health with age than do water-borne and food-borne contaminants together.

2. As a rule, pollutants express their effects only through interaction with other agents or with some preconditioning factor(s) within the host (a natural consequence of their extremely low ambient levels), be they infectious agents, trace-element deficiencies, or genetic defects of metabolism. Thus environmental pollutants must definitely be included among the multiple factors in the causality of chronic degenerative disease.

3. Acceleration of aging is the dominant characteristic of the effect of many of the top eight of the environmental pollutants. The imposition of such effects on the normal process of aging, whose complexities are only beginning to be understood, compounds the difficulties

**Table 29-2.** Disease states for which evidence points to environmental pollutants as either direct or contributing causes*

| Disease | Geographic distribution | | Relative incidence index† | Etiologic pollutants and associated conditions | Direct | Contributing |
|---|---|---|---|---|---|---|
| | General | Localized | | | | |
| Accelerated aging | + | | High | Ozone and oxidant air pollutants | + | |
| Allergic asthma | | + | High | Airborne denatured grain protein and other | + | |
| Cardiovascular and atherosclerotic heart disease | + | | High | "Soft" waters and hereditary tendency, Cr-deficiency states, CO(?) | | + |
| Berylliosis | | + | Very low | Airborne Be compounds | + | |
| Bronchitis | | + | High | Acid gases, particulates, respiratory infection, inclement climate | | + |
| Cancer of gastrointestinal tract | + | | Medium | Carcinogens in food, water, air and hereditary tendency | | + |
| Cancer of respiratory tract | + | | Medium | Airborne carcinogens and hereditary tendency | | + |
| Dental caries | | + | Low | Se | + | |
| Emphysema | + | | Medium | Airborne respiratory irritants and familial tendency | + | |
| Mesotheliomas | + | | Low | Asbestos and associated trace metals and carcinogens (air, water) (other fibers?) | + | |
| Methemoglobinemia infant death | | + | Low | Water-borne nitrates and nitrites | + | |
| Renal hypertension | | + | Low | Cd in water, food and beverage in As and Se-low areas(?) | | + |

*From Stokinger, H. E.: The spectre of today's environmental pollution, Amer. J. Industr. Hyg. Ass. J. **30:** 195, May-June 1969.
†A composite index derived from an estimate of incidence, geographic extent, and seriousness of effect.

in either determining causal relationships or assessing the degree of contribution from environmental pollutants.

4. Finally, decidedly in the overall evaluation are the counteractants, the natural antagonists existing both in the environment and within the host. To measure only the pollutants without the counteractants can lead to an overestimation of the health problem,. The homeostatic mechanisms leading to adaptation provide the balance to counteract the effects of pollutants at existing levels in the United States among the majority of the population. It is only when this balance is upset through predisposing disease or genetic fault (susceptibility) that environmental pollutants exert effects on man.

Major difficulties militating against the adequate solution of these environmentally induced disease problems include an inability to isolate the effects of any one chemical pollutant from others to which people are exposed, the long latent period for some cancers (e.g., 18 years for aromatic amine-induced bladder cancer), the longer latent period for genetic effects (e.g.,

more than one generation), the grossly inadequate base-line data because of the lack of national registration systems for cancer, birth defects, genetic defects, occupational disease, and the like, and the gross insensitivity of animal testing procedures.

Realization of these concepts and also of the high total costs of human disease clearly indicates the need to strengthen anticipatory and preventive approaches, apart from improving techniques for testing, recognition, and measurement.

What is required is an adequately supported interdisciplinary investigation to determine the distribution of the respective chemical hazards in the environment and their availability to and effects on plants, animals, and man; to consider ways and means of standardizing data collection and analysis and computer storage and retrieval; to establish avenues of communication and ways of disseminating information among the interdisciplinary groups; and to promote interdisciplinary national and international education in regard to the chemical environment and its effect on health and disease. The efforts of such an investigating group would provide an extremely important start toward the hoped-for identification on a statistically sound basis, those correlations between geochemical and disease patterns that do, in fact, exist.

## PHYSICAL HAZARDS TO MAN

Physical hazards in the environment probably represent the oldest recognized by man. The impact of various geologic perturbations such as earthquakes, volcanic eruptions, floods, and tidal waves must have been dramatically evident. Yet although natural disasters represent one of the major areas of threat to the existence of man, civilization and its resulting urbanization and industrialization has brought with it several physical threats that make the natural hazards appear minor. Three outstanding manmade threats to himself are radiation, noise, and accidents.

### Radiation[37-46]

Man has always been exposed to radiant energy from the sun and from minerals. The extent of the role natural radiation has played in the evolution of man is a conjecture. The discovery of artificially produced x rays by Roentgen in 1895 and successful nuclear fission in the 1940s significantly added to the problem of radiation.

The new sources of radiant energy range from large-scale applications of nuclear energy, especially for electric-power generation, through lasers and microwave technology in industry, to the use of radionuclides and x rays in the healing arts, the rapidly increasing use of microwaves by the communications industry, and in electronic equipment in the home. Scientific knowledge and protection against this radiation is still at a very early stage. The extensive use of x-ray and other devices based on radiant energy has added appreciable exposure loads to large numbers of patients. Between one third and one half of all critical medical decisions are dependent on radiologic information. However, only one sixth of the world's population has access to modern radiology. As a result, throughout the world, including the United States, a large proportion of diagnostic x-ray films are inferior, uncertainly exposed, insufficiently collimated, poorly developed, and therefore difficult to interpret.

There are great disparities in the amount of radiation exposure used for comparable procedures and in the levels of genetic radiation doses. Even one x-ray during pregnancy has been found to increase significantly the chances of a child developing cancer during the first 10 years of life. This risk is greatest during the first trimester but exists throughout the pregnancy of the mother. Thus in a study at the University of Oxford of 15,298 children born between 1943 and 1965, one half had died of malignancies before the age of 10 years. The other one half served as matched controls. Almost twice as many of the children who developed cancer had been exposed to x rays before birth as had the children in the control group. If only one x ray had been taken, the increased cancer risk was 1.26 to 1. If five films had been taken, the increased risk was more than double, 2.24 to 2. X rays taken during the first trimester of pregnancy led to more than an eightfold increase in risk of childhood cancer.

An Expert Committee of the World Health Organization found that "the types of cancer in man that are directly or indirectly due to extrinsic factors are thought to account for a large percent of the total cancer incidence." It concluded, "Therefore, the majority of human cancers are potentially preventable."

The rapidly expanding use of ionizing and nonionizing radiation for weapons manufacture, power development, industrial uses, communications, and other purposes introduces to the air, water, and land a pollutant awesome in its potentials and implications. Merely the problem of safe disposal of the large amounts of radioactive wastes is beginning to appear overwhelming. Added to this are the dangers of leakage from stored materials, of radioactivity transmitted to cooling waters, and the problem of thermal pollution of streams and lakes, possibly eventually of even the ocean itself.

Of the total radiation exposure to which people in the United States are subject, 45% is from natural sources, such as from minerals and from the sky (cosmic); 55% is from manmade sources, most of which (45% of the total) is from medical equipment. Industrial and occupational sources account for 7% of the total, and television screens, luminous clock-watch dials, and fallout plus fission testing account for 1% each. It is important to remember that radiation cannot be directly detected by the senses and that the effects of radiation are irreversible. There is no immunity against radiation; parts of the body escaping damage from one exposure do not have an increased tolerance for future exposures.

Radioactive minerals provide real radiation hazards for the men who mine them. Among a group of 907 white uranium miners with more than 3 years of underground experience, death rates were 17.8 times the normal rate for heart disease, 5 times the normal from respiratory cancer, and 4.5 times the normal from nonautomotive accidents; of 6,000 men who have been uranium miners, it is estimated that 600 to 1,100 will die of lung cancer in the next 20 years.

Two outstanding achievements of recent decades in the field of radiologic health have been the development of an understanding of the genetic effects of ionizing radiation and the development of a logical basis for standards in radiation protection. The development of standards in radiation protection has resulted from the cooperative efforts of many people and several different organizations. In radiation standards development perhaps the best references are found in the published reports of the Federal Radiation Council, the National Committee on Radiation Protection and Measurements, the International Commission on Radiological Protection, the United Nations Scientific Committee on Atomic Radiation, and the standards hearings of the Joint Commission on Atomic Energy.

Research on the genetic effects of radiation provided an experimental basis for determining the limits of radiation exposure to large groups of people and for improving national and international standards. A nuclear test ban treaty was stimulated by the data accumulated. Although human health was not improved in the sense of curing radiation sickness, it was improved in a preventive sense. Undoubtedly millions of people are enjoying better health today because of the improved standards that have been developed.

These research developments and higher standards have, from a preventive standpoint, led to a better basis of control in the nuclear industry, in military applications of nuclear energy, and in the medical use of radiation, as in x-ray machines. For the most part, the scientific community and the government agencies involved deserve great credit and recognition for meeting this important problem in a most orderly way. Yet even more could have been achieved more effectively if organized medicine had taken a more constructive approach toward a critical review of its practices and had encouraged a greater effort in establishing medical

x-ray standards and techniques for compliance with them. Many physicians provided real leadership in the effort, but more valuable human data could have been obtained if physicians had participated to a greater extent. Had it been possible earlier to have openly and freely discussed such things as plutonium, tritium, iodine, and krypton from the standpoint of radioactivity, earlier recognition could have been given to the problems involved in the use of these and other radioactive substances in the medical and bioscientific areas.

Although there continues to be some criticism of the established standards, most of the knowledgeable scientists and organizations find them acceptable, while continuing periodically to re-evaluate them relative to necessary improvements. The adequacy of ionizing radiation standards could be made better in the future if additional information were available on the long-term effects of the radiation on animals and man, obtained through long-term animal studies and epidemiologic studies of human populations. Such studies would require long-term investments, best assured as a national commitment to this purpose.

Because of the extensive work already done in the field of ionizing radiation, dramatic breakthroughs in this area are not unlikely to occur in the near future. It is anticipated, rather, that painstaking research will produce new information in regard to such things as the genetic effects of radiation, the problem of radiation exposure during pregnancy, and radiation problems related to tritium. It is more likely that breakthrough types of advancement may occur in the field of nonionizing radiation, which has been investigated to a lesser extent, or perhaps in the area of sonic radiation (ultrasonics) and its biologic effects. Perhaps the achievements to date in the field of ionization radiation and the ionizing radiation standards will serve as a stimulus and a model for advances in the more slowly developing field of nonionizing radiation.

A system should be established that makes it mandatory to allow scientists within the government or working under government contract to publish their findings without restriction in appropriate scientific journals irrespective of administrative clearance (other than national security). This would help the scientists and would provide a forum for discussion in the scientific community. It would also protect those administratively responsible because it would minimize the import that scientific papers represent on agency position. The scientific efforts of the personnel of an agency should not become automatic determinants in the development of policy, and administrative considerations should not be allowed to prevent the results of scientific research efforts from reaching the appropriate scientific community.

## Noise[47-54]

Another of man's environmental physical hazards is noise. This immediately gives rise to perplexing questions: What is noise? Can it actually produce ill effects? If so, how, under what circumstances, and with what other factors? Are any ill effects reversible? How might they be prevented? These questions indicate noise to be the least understood of the environmental hazards. The only way to delineate the noise problem of a community is to note the sociologic changes that might occur. If this could be done, it might be possible to judge whether noise is totally, partially, or not at all responsible for any changes. Noise is more difficult to deal with than most other nuisances or environmental factors because it is partly subjective. In any society each individual must necessarily accept a certain amount of annoyance, inconvenience, and interference. The essential question is how much and at what point may actual harm become a possibility.

There are three measurements of noise as a hazard to health: its intensity, its frequency, and the length of exposure. Depending on these, the environmental circumstances, and the individuals involved, the effects of noise fall into four general categories: annoyance, disruption of activity, loss of hearing, and physical or mental deterioration. Annoyance is the most widespread response to noise. Some claim that annoyance is not related to health, but the issue is academic since noise abatement can be justified from either standpoint. An annoyance condition may aggravate existing physical disorders. Noise that disrupts sleep can lessen the body's resistance to disease or physical stress, and noxious noise generally disturbs one's feelings of well-being. Excessive sound can lead to somatic manifestations such as stomach problems, including ulcers, and allergies such as hives. In certain instances excessive noise is thought to aggravate mental illness. Evidence has also been found that exposure to certain types of noise causes constriction of the blood vessels near the skin surface, an effect that does not disappear with adaptation to the noise.

Noise can cause the blurring or masking of speech and other wanted sounds. Thus noise from machinery may interfere with instructions to a worker. Several hospitals, especially near airports, have noted an apparent effect on the ability of patients to convalesce. In the field of education noise disrupts attention and hinders concentrated mental effort.

The greatest physiologic effect of noise is hearing loss, temporary or permanent. Temporary impairment of hearing, called auditory fatigue, occurs after short exposure to intense noise. Exposure to a continuous high level of sound with inadequate recovery time between exposures may lead to permanent hearing damage.

In terms of the measurements of intensity, frequency, and length of exposure, their effect on hearing loss is as follows: Intensity—exposure to sound pressure levels of over 80 decibels is hazardous, but there appears to be no permanent hearing hazard for levels below 80 decibels. Frequency—the inner ear is more susceptible to damage at middle and especially higher frequencies in the audible range than at low frequencies, and damage increases with increased exposure time. In addition, a fourth factor is the susceptibility of an individual's inner ear to noise-induced hearing loss. Individuals vary in this regard, but about 3% of the general population may be classified as highly susceptible. A survey between 1959 and 1961 by the Public Health Service of the population of the United States showed that the rate of hearing impairment per 1,000 persons was 7.6 for those under 25 years of age, 22.2 for those aged 25 to 44 years, and 51.2 for those between 45 and 64 years. Continued exposure to loud noise was believed to be the major cause of the increase as years of life passed. This is in agreement with the estimate that about 18 million Americans suffer total or partial deafness and that among working males two thirds of the hearing loss is caused by noise. The progressive loss of hearing as age progresses is known as presbycusis.

Research on hearing acuity has been carried out among the Nilitic tribes in the Sudanese desert. These people live in probably the most noise-free area on earth. They have no musical instruments and apparently do not even sing. Remarkable hearing acuity has been observed, exemplified by their ability to communicate with a normal speaking voice over long distances and a sustained hearing acuity not only among the adults but also in the aged.

However, in the field of noise as an environmental health hazard, the progress made is the result of patient studies that often appear pedestrian but are necessary if realistic damage-risk criteria are to be established. To assess the physiologic effects of noise one must either find a population of persons whose necessary noise exposures can be measured in detail or expose experimental animals under controlled conditions. Because of individual differences in susceptibility to damage by noise, either course involves a large number of subjects and is therefore expensive.

Although no breakthroughs can be indicated, progress has been steady. It is now known how much steady 8-hour per day, 5-day per week noise can be endured with negligible risk to hearing. Scientists are on the way toward determining equally reliable damage–risk criteria for intermittent noise exposure and for impulsive noises such as gunfire. The quantification of the relations between the physical and temporal characteristics of intense sound and the degree of both temporary and permanent losses in hearing thus induced has been a significant accomplishment in the past 30 years. Now there is some agreement that hazards to the hearing from exposure to noise can be predicted with confidence. As a result, it has been possible to set tolerable limits of noise exposure in both industry and in the community. Noise-induced deafness is a pervasive disease and social handicap that is now suffered by millions.

Once it could be shown that a level of 80 decibels or higher was hazardous, it was easier to convince workers that the use of ear protection devices was good sense. This, of course, is more of an educational achievement than a research one, but there now are young drop-forge operators, riveters, jet mechanics, and policemen who still have normal hearing because they use these ear protectors.

Perhaps the most significant results achieved in the past three decades have been the *negative* ones—that is, studies which show that some of the effects attributed to noise on an anecdotal basis are not folklore. Research on the effects of noise on sleep and on the neurovegetative system continue, and should continue, even though results are ambiguous. Study of the physiologic changes in the cochlea associated with noise damage should also continue, even though there seems to be little hope that any

sort of ameliorative agent will ever be uncovered that will reduce significantly or partially restore the damage done by noise.

In the future some of the more subtle effects of noise on mental and physiologic stress may be discovered and measured. This would permit the specification of tolerable limits and the exercise of noise control. Present research data are highly controversial and need clarification.

1. How much noise energy is tolerable as a daily dosage if the exposure is intermittent instead of continuous?

2. Are very young or very old people more susceptible than others to damage from noise?

3. In the case of persons with noise-induced hearing losses so severe as to cause trouble understanding ordinary conversation, how can the information in the speech signal be recoded so that understanding is restored?

4. Is hearing loss, as measured by changes in auditory threshold, really an adequate measure of the damage actually done by noise? (Recent animal research has indicated that extensive irreversible damage to the hair cells of the cochlea may occur without affecting threshold significantly; if this is confirmed, it could be considered a genuine breakthrough.)

5. Is an ear that has already been moderately damaged more susceptible to further insult than an unsullied one?

6. Are there any long-range consequences of repeated autonomic excitation by noise?

In addition to progress in the acquisition of physiologic and anatomic knowledge there is need, of course, for significantly improved technology in noise abatement with reference to heavy industry, housing, streets, highways, and planes. This appears to be coming to a head rapidly as a result of the burgeoning aerospace industry and its present and potential effects on the environment of man and other creatures.

**Injury**[55-65]

With the decline in mortality rates from communicable diseases the relative importance of injury as a cause of death has increased. Accidental injury, suicide, and homicide rank fourth, twelfth, and fourteenth, respectively, among the leading causes of death. These are subjects considered in detail in Chapters 32, 24, and 27. A few general observations concerning them as physical hazards may be useful here. The 10-year trends (1958-1967) shown in Table 29-3 make it clear that little recent progress has been made in reducing these hazards.

**Table 29-3.** Death rates in United States from accidental injury, suicide, and homicide between 1958 and 1967*

| Cause of death | Death rate | | | | | | | | | |
|---|---|---|---|---|---|---|---|---|---|---|
| | 1967 | 1966 | 1965 | 1964 | 1963 | 1962 | 1961 | 1960 | 1959 | 1958 |
| Accidental injury | 55.2 | 58.0 | 55.7 | 54.3 | 53.4 | 52.3 | 50.4 | 52.3 | 52.2 | 52.3 |
| Suicide | 10.8 | 10.9 | 11.1 | 10.8 | 11.0 | 10.9 | 10.4 | 10.6 | 10.6 | 10.7 |
| Homicide | 6.8 | 5.9 | 5.5 | 5.1 | 4.9 | 4.8 | 4.7 | 4.7 | 4.6 | 4.5 |

*From Vital statistics of the United States, Washington, D. C., 1967, Government Printing Office.

Although morbidity data have no real meaning with respect to homicide and suicide, the attack rate for accidental injuries is approximately 25%—exceeding the common cold in frequency. Some 52 million annual injuries require medical care or at least 1 day of restricted activity. Injury victims require more general hospital beds than any other class of patient (20 million bed days per year) and require 80,000 man years of professional care.

The sophisticated statistics of the injury problem are not matched by the availability of control measures. Research on behavior, both aberrant and delinquent, has not yet provided enough information to move confidently with preventive programs. Research on injury epidemiology, agent modifications, and environmental adaptation, coupled with safety education, has produced some tangible benefits for injury control.

A more important development has been in precise methods of analysis of the causes of accidents. The epidemiologic and biostatistical methods used in the study and control of disease have been applied to accidents. Valuable information is now obtained on the major categories and specific kinds of accidents and injuries, those experiencing them, conditions of occurrence and the interrelationship between persons, environmental factors and specific agents producing the injury. This information is useful in designing methods to reduce accidents.

Another advance has been the development of the field of human factors engineering (ergonomics), the major objective of which is to reduce accidents and injury by better integration between man and the equipment he uses, paying attention to biologic and psychologic factors as well as physical factors. Originally developed in relationship to safer design of complex military and aerospace equipment, the ergonomic principles have been applied increasingly to civilian transportation and industrial operations.

Advances have been made in the development of greater protection of an individual from injury by redesigning equipment, such as machine-tool guarding, the padding of automobile instrument panels, recessing knobs and strengthening door locks on cars. Air-bag restraints are now being developed. However, illustrating the great need for behavioral research, only one in three drivers actually uses seat belts even when the law requires them.

Over the past 30 years there has been a gradual improvement (decrease) in accidental death rates on a population basis. But improvements can be definitely cited only in the rates of injury in industrial work situations, and here the improvements seem to be getting less. The outstanding exception to improvement has been in the death rate due to motor vehicle accidents. The death rate remained the same for 20 years until 1960, but since then it has increased, possibly due to increased exposure to hazard and inadequate controls.

Much useful information on fatal and nonfatal accidents has been provided by the National Health Survey. Home accidents have been found to result in about half as many deaths as motor vehicle accidents, but they account for more than twice as many disabling injuries and about seven times as many less severe nonfatal injuries.

Significant advances in accident prevention and injury control have been made by the application of biologic and human factors information in air transportation and military flying. This information has been obtained by studies on human factors in relation to equipment design, from research on flight physiology and aerospace medicine, from the development of criteria for the medical and psychologic selection of flying personnel and for maintaining their health and efficiency, and from especially intensive and extensive analyses, including autopsies, of accidental occurrences. The armed services schools of aviation medicine and the universities have helped to train the personnel for this work. No corresponding trained group exists for the control and treatment of highway injuries.

In automobile accidents the impact of the steering wheel and column is a major source of injury and death. A substantial reduction in driver injury has been achieved by designing steering wheel rims and spokes so that they would deform rather than break under impact and by using larger steering wheel hubs that would spread the impact forces. Another important development has been the seat belt, developed when studies showed that ejection from the car was a frequent factor in producing death or serious injuries. Seat belts reduce injuries and deaths, yet efforts to induce the majority of car occupants to use them have been unsuccessful. More recently combined lap–and–shoulder belts have been developed to both prevent ejection and reduce injuries inside the car, and they have proved highly effective for those who use them. In Sweden, in 28,000 accidents analyzed, no deaths of lap–shoulder belt wearers occurred at impact speeds less than 60 miles per hour, whereas fatalities did occur among nonwearers beginning at a 26-mile-per-hour impact speed.

In the United States educational programs have helped reduce other types of injury by changing human behavior. In one Arkansas county within 1 year the incidence of burn injuries requiring hospitalization was cut to one half of the 5-year average. The injuries were caused by improper wiring in the home, misuse of petroleum products, and proximity of flammable materials to heating units. In one county in South Carolina hospitalization for poisoning accidents was reduced by 29% as a result of a 3-year educational project for parents of young children. In a Philadelphia area a small-group educational program was carried on for a year relative to injuries occurring to members of the several groups or their families. In 1 year inpatient admissions to the hospital had decreased by 17%, and admissions from the areas in which the members of the discussion groups lived decreased by 26%. Some studies in the circumstances relating to injuries from falls of older persons, accidents with a high death rate, have provided helpful information relative to the severity of skeletal degeneration (osteo-porosis) in these people, frequency of bone fractures, some of which were found to have preceded the accidental fall, and the like. Other studies have indicated that fluoridation of water supplies may retard the skeletal degeneration and perhaps decrease the frequency of bone fracture injuries in the elderly. A Swedish study showed that the rate of fractures was much higher in postmenopausal women than in men of comparable age.

Accidents lead all diseases as a cause of death between the ages of 1 and 37 years, yet research on the causes of accidental death has been relatively unsophisticated. Opportunities for the necessary professional training for accident research have been limited. In 1969 only 2 of 10 schools of public health offered training for this area. Neither have sustained funding patterns for nontransport accident research and control been developed. Currently only $1 goes for research on accidents as compared with $300 for medical research. There is no basic reporting system to provide data for the evaluation of community programs; systems for epidemiologic intelligence or surveillance have not been developed on a geographically balanced basis. No central repository exists for information on injuries, and rapid retrieval systems for data are only in development stages.

A significant reduction in the total number of accidents in the near future is unlikely, but recent developments may eventually bring improvements. New concepts from the fields of biostatistics, medicine, engineering, and psychology are providing impetus for experimental studies and the design of safety programs. Work is underway to determine injury thresholds of the human body relative to impact forces, data important to the design of protective devices. Neurosurgeons have studied head injuries from a variety of high impact accidents. Public interest has increased somewhat, and there has been national legislative activity such as the highway safety acts of 1966, legislation relating to fabric flammability and other hazards to child safety, product safety, and consumer protection; these can provide impetus for increased attention to accident potentials in private and industrial sectors.

As discussed in Chapter 33, health personnel and the medical profession seek to improve emergency medical services, but there is an urgent need for a strong centralized national accident prevention program to (1) conduct research, (2) provide technical assistance to states and communities, (3) train personnel, and (4) supply financial support. In the long run the savings could be enormous. An effective prevention and control program for accidents could result in (1) an annual prevention of 30,000 fatal injuries, (2) the saving of 60,000 people annually through prompt medical care, (3) the prevention of 10 million accidental injuries each year, (4) the annual savings of 2 million hospital bed days now needed for accident victims, (5) the annual savings of 8,000 man years of medical care services, and (6) an annual $3 billion reduction in direct costs to accident victims. Accidental death and disability truly represent the "neglected disease" of modern industrialized society in this country.

## SUMMARY AND CONCLUSIONS

These are only some of the environmental hazards with which modern man must contend. They have given rise to the rapidly growing field of environmental medicine, which applies the principles and knowledge of biologic and epidemiologic research to an understanding of a complex of physical, physiologic, and psychologic disturbances. The results of these disturbances now constitute the major portion of conditions that come to the attention of the medical practitioner, unfortunately too often too late.

Patterns of morbidity and mortality are changing. Evidence from data obtained from past efforts may not be relevant to future events. People, their hazards, and their diseases are changing. The illnesses that will be experienced within a few decades will not be the same as those of today, much less of yesterday. Environmental factors certainly enter into their causation, but to what extent and in what manner is still largely to be determined, and only by means of research.

Environmentally induced chronic diseases are now known to have certain characteristics as follows:

1. Typically they result from low-level exposures, insufficient to produce acute reactions.

2. They tend to develop insidiously over long periods of time.

3. By the time they are clinically recognizable the conditions are often irreversible. Emphysema, absestosis, some cancers, teratogenic anomalies, and environmentally induced hearing loss are good examples.

Several years ago the direct health effects of environmental hazards on man were summarized by the President's Science Advisory Committee. Five categories of increasing severity were listed as follows: (1) annoyance, irritation, and inconvenience, which although certainly real, produce effects that are uncertain and almost impossible to measure; (2) physiologic effects of unknown clinical significance, which occur on a transient basis and the cumulative effect of which is uncertain; (3) worsening of existing diseases or disability and increasing the general level of sickness, the determination or evaluation of which is open; (4) effects of a general increase in the death rate, again open; and (5) the initiation of specific progressive disease, an area also with many questions unanswered.

The general conclusion was that the human effects of environmental hazards were poorly understood, but because of the obvious importance of the effects, delay in intensive and extensive study could not be avoided.

In any consideration of most needed research in this field, the following fundamental characteristics of environmental hazards stand out:

1. They tend to be ubiquitous.

2. They tend to be multifaceted as to sources and effects.

3. They are generally insidious in their action time frame.

4. They often act in concert and may potentiate one another.

Despite these characteristics, it has been customary for science, industry, and government to study and deal with environmental hazards separately. For example, is mercury hazardous, in what physiologic way, at what levels, and with what effects? The same question is asked about lead, pesticides, individual pharmaceuticals, sulfur oxides, and so on, each separately, each usually in terms of acute effects, and each in terms of toxicity alone, ignoring possible carcinogenic, teratogenic, mutagenic, and psychic effects. This approach has led to the fallacious tendency to decide that X is the toxic or dangerous level of a particular substance or hazard and that to be conservative perhaps one tenth of that amount should be designated as the minimum toxic level. This ignores the fact that humans are not exposed to one substance alone but to an extensive and cumulative spectrum of hazards, each of which might even be minimal but the total burden or effect of which might be critical or overwhelming.

From an overall viewpoint present efforts for

the study of environmental hazards to modern man may be considered to fall into these categories: (1) the search for and application of new experimental and clinical methods of defining health risks for known or potential environmental contaminants and hazards; (2) more intensive studies of synergistic potentials of the innumerable combinations of environmental hazards with particular consideration of the development of toxicity, carcinogenicity, tetragenicity, mutagenicity, physical injuries, and psychic stress; and (3) the categorization of physiologic and biochemical hazards in terms of human population and risk.

Obviously any sound approaches to eventual protective measures must be based on the results of such essentially biologic research.

## REFERENCES

1. U. S. Department of Health, Education, and Welfare: A strategy for a livable environment, Report of the Task Force on Environmental Health and Related Problems, Washington, D. C., June 1967, Government Printing Office.
2. President's Science Advisory Committee: Restoring the quality of the environment: Report of the Environmental Pollution Panel, November 1965, The White House.
3. Health hazards of the human environment, Geneva, 1972, World Health Organization.
4. Cleaning our environment: the chemical basis for action: Report by the American Chemical Society, Washington, D. C., Sept. 1969, American Chemical Society.
5. U. S. Department of Health, Education, and Welfare: Man's health and the environment—some research needs; Report of the Task Force on Research Planning in Environmental Health Science, Washington, D. C., March 1970.
6. Starr, M. P., editor: Global impacts of applied microbiology, New York, 1964, John Wiley & Sons, Inc.
7. Communicable Disease Center: Annual supplements, morbidity and mortality weekly reports, Atlanta, Summaries for 1951, 1960, and 1969, U. S. Department of Health, Education, and Welfare.
8. May, J. M., editor: Studies in disease ecology, New York, 1961, Hafner Publishing Co., Inc.
9. Sartwell, P. E., editor: Maxey-Rosenau preventive medicine and public health, New York, 1965, Appleton-Century Crofts.
10. U. S. Department of Health, Education, and Welfare, National Center for Health Statistics: Vital statistics rates in the United States 1940-1960, Washington, D. C., 1968, Government Printing Office.
11. Stokinger, H. E.: The spectre of today's environmental pollution, Amer. Industr. Hyg. Ass. J. **30:**195, May-June 1969.
12. Epstein, S. S.: Control of chemical pollutants, Nature **228:**816, Nov. 28, 1970.
13. Singer, S. F., editor: Global effects of environmental pollution, New York, 1970, Springer-Verlag New York, Inc.
14. Clinical handbook of economic poisons, Washington, D. C., 1963, Government Printing Office.
15. Hemphill, D. D. Trace substances in environmental health, Columbia, 1969, University of Missouri Press.
16. Dixon, J. R., Lowe, D. B., Richards, D. E., Cralley, L. J., and Stockinger, H. E.: The role of trace metals in chemical carcinogenesis—asbestos cancers, Cancer Res. **30:**1068, April 1970.
17. Selikoff, I. J., Hammond, E. C., and Churg, J.: Asbestos exposure, smoking and neoplasia, J.A.M.A. **204:**106, April 8, 1968.
18. Wogan, G. N., editor: Mycotoxins in foodstuffs, Cambridge, 1964, Massachusetts Institute of Technology Press.
19. Russell, F. E., and Saunders, P. R., editors: Animal toxins, New York, 1967, Pergamon Press, Inc.
20. Goldsmith, J. R.: Effects of air pollution on human health. In Stern, A. C., editor: Air pollution, ed. 2, New York, 1968, Academic Press, Inc.
21. Anderson, D. O.: The effects of air contamination on health, Canad. Med. Ass. J. **97:**528, 585, 802, Sept. 23, 1967.
22. Morrow, P. E.: Some physical and physiological factors controlling the fate of inhaled substances, Health Phys. **2:**366, Feb. 1960.
23. Kuschner, M.: The causes of lung cancer, Amer. Rev. Resp. Dis. **98:**573, Oct. 1968.
24. Toxiocologic and epidemiologic bases for air quality criteria (special issue), J. A. Pollution Control Ass. **19:**629, 1969.
25. Shubik, P., Clayson, D. B., and Terracini, B., editors: The quantification of environmental carcinogens, Geneva, 1970, International Union Against Cancer, vol. 4.
26. Hartwell, J. L. (1951); Hartwell, J. L., and Shubik, P. (1957); Peters, J. (1969): Survey of compounds which have been tested for carcinogenic activity, PHS pub. no. 149, Washington, D. C.
27. Boren, H. G.: Pathobiology of air pollutants, Environ. Res. **1:**178, Jan. 1967.
28. Hanna, M. G., Jr., Nettesheim, P., and Gilbert, J. R., editors: Inhalation carcinogenesis, Proceedings of the Biology Division Conference, 1970, Oak Ridge National Laboratory, Oak Ridge, Tenn.
29. Epstein, S. S., and Shafner, H.: Chemical mutagens in the human environment, Nature **219:**385, July 27, 1968.
30. Moser, R. H.: Diseases of medical progress, ed. 3,

Springfield, Ill., 1971, Charles C Thomas, Publisher.

31. Selye, H.: Adaptive steroids—retrospect and prospect, Perspect. Biol. Med. **13:**343, Spring 1970.

32. Report of the Secretary's Commission on Pesticides and Their Relationship to Environmental Health, Washington, D. C., 1969, Government Printing Office.

33. Report of the NCI/Bionetics study of pesticides, J. Nat. Cancer Inst. **42:**1101, 1969.

34. Conney, A. H.: Drug metabolism and therapeutics, New Eng. J. Med. **280:**653, March 20, 1969.

35. Jillette, J. R., editor: Proceedings of symposium on microsomes and drug oxidations, New York, 1969, Academic Press, Inc.

36. Mannering, G. J.: Significance of stimulation and inhibition of drug metabolism. In Burger, A., editor: Selected pharmacological testing methods, New York, 1968, Marcel Dekker, Inc.

37. Ingraham, S. C., Terrill, J. G., and Moeller, D. W.: Concepts of radiological health, 1953, PHS pub. no. 336, Washington, D. C.

38. Gitlin, J. N., and Lawrence, P. S.: Population exposures to x-rays, U. S., 1964; Report on the Public Health Service x-ray exposure study, PHS pub. no. 1519, Washington, D. C.

39. U. S. Public Health Service: Report of the Medical X-ray advisory Committee on Public Health Considerations in Medical Diagnostic Radiology, Washington, D. C., Oct. 1967.

40. U. S. Public Health Service: Radiation exposure overview: diagnostic dental x-rays and the patient, Washington, D. C., July 1968.

41. Carpenter, R. L., and Clark, V. A.: Responses to radiofrequency radiation. In Altman, P. L., and Dittmer, D. S., editors: Environmental biology, Bethesda, 1966, Federation of the American Society of Experimental Biology.

42. U. S. Public Health Service: Radiation bio-effects, summary report, Washington, D. C., 1968.

43. Proceedings for the symposium on public health aspects of peaceful uses of nuclear explosives, Springfield, Va., 1969, Clearinghouse for Federal Scientific and Technical Information.

44. Moore, W.: Biological aspects of microwave radiation—a review of hazards, Washington, D. C., July 1968, U. S. Public Health Service.

45. U. S. Public Health Service: An annotated bibliography of regulations, standards and guides for microwaves, ultraviolet radiation, and radiation from lasers and television receivers, Washington, D. C., April 1968.

46. A study of the radiological health aspects of agents modifying the biological effects of radiation, Bethesda, June 1969, Federation of the American Society of Experimental Biology.

47. Burns, W.: Noise and man, London, 1968, John Murray Publishers, Ltd.

48. Ward, W. D., and Fricke, J. E., editors: Proceedings of the conference on noise as a public health hazard, Washington, D. C., June 13-14, 1968, Amer. Speech Hearing Ass. Rep. no. 4, Feb. 1969.

49. Kryter, K. D.: The effects of noise on man, New York, 1970, Academic Press, Inc.

50. Noise: An occupational hazard and public nuisance, WHO Chron. **20:**191, June 1969.

51. Rosen, S., et al.: Presbycusis study of a relatively noise-free population in the Sudan, Ann. Otol. **71:**727, 1962.

52. Engineering control, industrial noise manual, ed. 2, Detroit, 1966, American Industrial Hygiene Association.

53. Cohen, A.: Noise effects on health, productivity and well-being, Trans. N. Y. Acad. Sci. **30:**910, 1968.

54. Farr, L. E.: Medical consequences of environmental home noises, J.A.M.A. **202:**171, Oct. 16, 1967.

55. Backett, E. M.: Domestic accidents, Public Health Paper no. 26, Geneva, 1965, World Health Organization.

56. Gallagher, R. E., and Marland, R. E.: The effect of federal legislation on burn injuries involving flammable fabrics, Proceedings of the First Annual Meeting, Atlanta, March 1969, American Burn Association.

57. Gordon, J. E.: The epidemiology of accidents, Amer. J. Public Health **39:**504, April 1949.

58. Haddon, W., Suchman, E. A., and Klein, D.: Accident research, New York, 1964, Harper & Row, Publishers.

59. Iskrant, A. P., and Joliet, P. U.: Accidents and homicide, Vital and Health Statistics Monogr., Cambridge, 1968, Harvard University Press.

60. Marland, R. E.: Injury epidemiology, J. Safety Res. **1**(3):17, Sept. 1969.

61. Marland, R. E., and Burg, F. D.: The injury control program of the U. S. Public Health Service, Pediatrics **44**(supp.):888, Nov. 1969.

62. McFarland, R. A.: Injury—a major environmental problem, Arch. Environ. Health **19:**244, Aug. 1969.

63. McFarland, R. A., Moore, R. C., and Bertrand, W. H.: Human variables in motor vehicle accidents: a review of the literature, Boston, 1955, Harvard School of Public Health.

64. Norman, L. G.: Road traffic accidents: epidemiology, control and prevention, Public Health Paper no. 12, Geneva, 1962, World Health Organization.

65. Suchman, E. A.: Cultural and social factors in accident occurrence and control, J. Occup. Med. **7:**487, Oct. 1965.

*Is ecology a phase of science of limited interest and utility? Or, if taken seriously for the long-run welfare of mankind, would it endanger the assumptions and practices accepted by modern societies, whatever their doctrinal commitments?*

PAUL B. SEARS

CHAPTER 30

# Environmental health programs

## SANITATION, SINE QUA NON

Activities aimed at the preservation and improvement of the environment will always represent a major part of community health programs. In Chapter 2 mention was made of the many sanitary installations that remain as evidences of the degree of sanitary consciousness attained by Minoan, Grecian, Roman, and other early civilizations. Similar reference was made to the problems that concerned the early public health organizations of the United States. It will be recalled that most of them related to problems of the physical environment, particularly of the growing urban communities. The essential similarities among the sanitary concerns of ancient civilizations, those of the founding fathers, and those of the present time are striking. Whatever the reason, activities in environmental health tend to be the most firmly established, most readily supported, and most vigorously demanded of the many constituent parts of the community health programs. Because of this, newly established local health departments have often begun operation with various phases of a sanitation program before proceeding to some of the other aspects of a well-rounded health program that might be less readily understood, less evident in results, or more controversial.

Many of the public health or epidemiologic accomplishments in the United States and certain other countries can be attributed to the sanitary measures that have been instituted. Included among these have been the spectacular reductions in typhoid fever, cholera, dysenteries, summer diarrheas, the control of many of the milk-borne and food-borne infections, the control of malaria, and the elimination of yellow fever. It was not until the beginning of the present century that the chains of events involved in the transmission and perpetuation of these diseases became unraveled. Prompt steps were taken to break links in these chains. At first, activities in the field of sanitation were concerned primarily with the abatement of noisome nuisances. Gradually the provision and supervision of sanitary water supplies and sewage disposal facilities were added as the first well-defined and scientific measures. Meanwhile the Rockefeller Sanitary Commission, established in 1909 to combat hookworm disease, led to programs by state health departments with emphasis on the eradication of hookworm and other enteric infections in the rural population. These activities laid the foundation for the eventual establishment and spread of full-time county health departments in the United States.

In this regard the noteworthy surveys, demonstrations, and epidemiologic investigations of the Public Health Service, particularly those by Lumsden, should not go unmentioned. Throughout this formative era of the modern sanitation and public health program much emphasis was placed on the construction and use of sanitary privies as a practical means of preventing the spread of enteric disease, and it was one of the chief functions of public health workers of that period to assure the sanitary disposal of human excreta. This has prompted

**545**

some to indicate the sanitary privy as a primary factor in the development of the tremendously significant public health movement.

## CONTENT AND PURPOSE OF ENVIRONMENTAL CONTROL

It is essentially true that the initial phases of sanitation activities centered on keeping human excreta out of the diet. By comparison the field today covers an imposing spectrum of responsibilities and activities, for most of which sound technical and scientific reasons have been demonstrated. This has been emphasized by numerous recent groups, particularly notable among which are the Task Force on Environmental Health of the National Commission on Community Health Services[1] and the Program Area Committee on Environmental Health of the American Public Health Association. In discussing the present definition and scope of the field, the latter group has indicated that the administration of today's environmental health programs has become so complex that it must weigh, balance, and take action on situations involving, in varying proportions, air pollution, water pollution, surface-water and ground-water disposal; food and dairy product protection; occupational health and safety; solid waste managment—its collection, transportation, disposal and recycling; housing and neighborhood planning, conservation, and rehabilitation; noise abatement and prevention; radiation protection; insect and rodent control; institutional sanitation, hospital sanitation, accident prevention, sanitation and safety supervision of swimming pools; participation in planning and supervision of recreation, flood control, topography, highways, transportation and traffic; and concerns about budgeting, tax jurisdictions, and neighboring communities and special districts. It must also place the economic, legal, sociologic, and political factors in their proper perspective in relation to the technical factors.[2]

The trend has been to draw health agencies away as much as possible from activities that involve physical operation, repair, correction, and enforcement, toward programs of a positive or promotive nature. This philosophy has been put increasingly into practice as a result of functional reorganizations on the national, state, and to some extent local levels of government. In other words, until relatively recently, public health activities have been based on negative concepts, on definitions of ills, environmental as well as human. This resulted in programs

designed to attack things that have gone wrong, that is, the isolation of an infected person, the filling of a decayed tooth, the purification of polluted water. The public health profession has now reached the point in many areas where its workers can begin to think and act in positive terms. They can begin to base their planning on a definition of good health rather than of illness, on the maintenance of cleanliness and salubrity instead of continually cleaning up an environment allowed to become insanitary.

This trend has led to the consideration of man, his environment, and their interrelationships in both a positive and total sense.[3-5] In other words it is a recognition of the fact that man is affected by his environment and his environment can affect him and that preventive and promotive measures may be applied to all aspects of man's environment as well as to man himself. Thus a task force[6] established by the Secretary of Health, Education, and Welfare in 1967 to consider the broad problem recommended that the purpose of environmental control be regarded as the assurance "that every American can thrive in an attractive, comfortable, convenient, and healthy environment by controlling pollution at its source, reducing hazards, converting waste to use, and improving the aesthetic value of man's surroundings."

It should also recognize that man, his psyche as well as his physical being, is inseparable from his total environment and that much more emphasis must be placed on the total ecology of man. For this reason the task force referred to, recognizing the considerable dispersal of environmental interests, authorities, and responsibilities, not only recommended some practical degree of consolidation but also urged that there be established a Council of Ecological Advisors on the federal level, as a supracabinet organism advisory to the President on all problems, proposals, or activities that relate to the complex interrelationship of man and his total environment.

Finally the trend is a recognition of the synergistic and cumulative effects of a spectrum of environmental hazards. Because of the usually slow development of the consequences of environmental abuse, society has failed to recognize the full impact of environmental hazards on human health and welfare. This has led to sporadic and fragmentary efforts to meet only some of the most flagrant of environmental problems. Thus not only should the rate and direction of environmental pollution be changed but the citizenry also needs protection from a conglomerate total of environmental health threats. These threats include not only air and water pollutants but also combinations of these, plus noise and crowding, safety hazards, and other factors. It must be recognized that an individually acceptable amount of water pollution, added to a tolerable amount of air pollution, added to a bearable amount of noise and congestion can produce a totally unacceptable health environment.

It is entirely possible that the biologic effects of these environmental hazards, some of which reach man slowly and silently over decades or generations, will first begin to reveal themselves only after their impact has become irreversible. Because of this, the Task Force on Environmental Health and Related Problems insisted that an effectively coordinated environmental health protection system was necessary. It should be predicated on the basic premise that the environment affects man's mental and physical health and welfare. Any approach toward environmental health protection that is limited to concern for less than the total range of hazards that do or may exist in man's environment must be viewed as inadequate. These recommendations bore fruit in the passage of the National Environmental Policy Act of 1969, which declared a national policy on the environment for the first time, established a Council on Environmental Quality and prepared the way for the formation of the Environmental Protection Agency at the end of 1970. This consolidated in one agency the major federal programs dealing with air and water pollution, solid waste disposal, pesticide regulation, and radiation and noise control. Subsequently, as already indicated, some states and large municipalities followed suit. Despite complaints by some to the contrary, this does remove health agencies from the environmental scene. This could and should never occur. Their roles, responsibilities, and challenges have merely changed. As will be brought out later, health agencies still retain and are continuously active in a great many environmental functions.

The concept of a coordinated, total environmental health protection system has also been presented by Stead[7] in a clear and perceptive manner. In line with the thinking of the APHA Program Area Committee on Environmental Health he subdivides the field into four basic sectors: water sanitation, food sanitation, air sanitation, and shelter sanitation.

Water sanitation includes consideration of the quantity, quality, and safety aspects of water from the stages of planning, development, transportation, storage, treatment, distribution, and use on through the stages of treatment and disposal or conservation, reclamation, and reuse of waste water for sewage. As Stead indicates, public health concern must go beyond the provision of potable water. It must also extend to the use of water for recreation, irrigation, and food processing as well as the potential for vector breeding.

Food sanitation encompasses the entire chain of events from production of food on land or sea, its processing, distribution, storage, and marketing down to the actual preparation and serving of meals and the disposal of wastes. Stead summarizes this sector with the neat phrase that the food sanitation program must "follow the food" back to its source and forward to its ultimate consumption.

Air sanitation is concerned with the physical, chemical, and biologic quality of air as a natural resource. Problems vary from its transparency to its radioactivity and its pesticide and allergen content, and programs should be alert to air quality at home, at work, during travel and recreation, and outdoors as well as indoors.

Shelter sanitation is regarded as encompassing not only the field of housing as related to separate dwelling units, apartments, hotels, public buildings, mobile homes and trailers, and camps but also the general artificial and natural environment for work, play, and general living. It includes the whole field of protection of human beings from rigors of the elements as well as the onslaught of insects, rodents, dust, dirt, odors, noise, radiation, accident hazards, and other detrimental impacts of the environment on man. Stead properly considers that omission of any of the four sectors briefly described results in an unbalanced environmental health program.

The four basic levels of concern with the environment are listed in the order of program preference:

1. Ensuring the elements of simple survival
2. Prevention of disease and poisoning
3. Maintaining an environment suited to man's efficient performance
4. Preservation of comfort and the enjoyment of living

As Stead analyzes it, each of the four levels

of concern (survival, disease prevention, efficient performance, and enjoyment) necessitates programs in each of the four program sectors (water, food, air, and shelter), which requires four program stages (research, field investigation, analysis and planning, and the action program).

To assist in the planning of broadly comprehensive environmental health programs the Public Health Service has developed a useful Environmental Health Planning Guide,[8] which if used as extensively as is merited, is certain to contribute to the improved development, performance, and evaluation of programs in this field.

## REGIONAL DIFFERENCES

Although the basic objectives are universal, the details of the environmental health program have not developed uniformly throughout the communities and states of the nation. Furthermore, as will be discussed later, all activities in this field have not necessarily been centered in health departments. The more rural agricultural South and Midwest are faced with problems rather different from the urban industrialized Northeast, the fringe of the lower Great Lakes, or the West Coast. As a result, certain activities are stressed more in one area than in the other, and dependence is placed on somewhat different categories of personnel. The congregation of large numbers of people in the many cities of the northeastern, western coastal, and Great Lake states necessarily has led to their emphasis on the construction and operation of sanitary engineering facilities and to the employment of many sanitary and public health engineers.

In other more rural parts of the country, particularly in the southern states, the opportunity for centralized sanitary control has been limited essentially to a few moderately sized towns and a handful of larger cities. Chief emphasis in this area, therefore, is placed on a somewhat simpler and more individualized approach. Here much more patient and persistent attention had to be given to such matters as privy and well location and construction, dairy barn sanitation, screening, and the like. To many health workers these may appear prosaic, elementary, and nontechnical. However, a background of technical knowledge of no small degree is necessary for the solution of such environmental problems. Furthermore, they provide a measure of community health

protection comparable to that resulting from the more complex and sophisticated structures of municipal sanitary engineering. For example, a Federal Community Sanitation Program, in cooperation with state health departments, during the period from December 1933 to July 1942, made possible the construction of about 3 million sanitary privies in 38 states and in Puerto Rico. This figure does not include the many others constructed privately or under the sponsorship of the agricultural and farm agencies. The sanitary and public health impact of this effort should not be underestimated.

A point to be realized is that whereas the turning of a valve in a water treatment plant or the flushing of a toilet in urban or suburban areas involves no particular educational impact for the individual citizen, this is not true on the rural scene. The development of several million sanitary privies made it necessary to explain to at least 15 million persons the reasons for sanitary disposal of excreta. It cannot be doubted that this program during the 1930s contributed significantly to the public understanding of this and, in fact, of several other important phases of environmental sanitation and public health. In fact this provides an excellent example of what might be termed the potentiation effects of seemingly simple social actions. During the economic depression of the 1930s, the federal government wanted to provide some gainful employment to the rural population. Among other things they built much-needed sanitary privies, which led to extended sanitary information as well as practice, which led to improved health, which led to improved education, which led to the wish for broader public health programs.

One of the great difficulties, of course, is in the differences in means, abilities, and willingness to finance sanitary improvements. Thus as Hollis[9] pointed out some years ago:

Government is ordinarily held responsible for financing public health services in the city. This is not so in the country. Sanitation of food and premises is clearly a public problem in the village and other rural centers such as the school, church, and grange or community hall. But in most rural areas in the United States, sanitation is ordinarily regarded as an individual or private concern, even though many individual rural families cannot finance sanitation by themselves. If there is the will to bring rural demands for environmental improvement into balance with the demand for cars and electricity, however, the economic devices that provide cars, telephones, and power are capable of financing pipes and drains as well.

In the city, the danger of contagion has created awareness of community responsibility. In rural areas, the danger of contagion is less apparent. It is recognized mainly in the enforcement of sanitation on dairy farms, in the effort to protect the safety of fluid milk produced for the urban market. Hygienic milk production is probably the heaviest single contribution of its kind to rural environmental health in the United States.

He concluded therefore:

Three major factors in the lag in rural sanitation are the relatively high cost of water and sewage systems for isolated structures, the usual necessity to finance each installation individually at relatively high rates, and the absence in many rural areas of a strong public health authority. These factors have less force in the village than on the farm.

An administrative benefit for which the rural sanitation program may be given credit has been the development of a spirit of cooperation among the officials of the health agencies on the various levels of government. Thus it may be said with little exaggeration that it was in this field that the state health departments and the federal Public Health Service first learned to work together as did, to a considerable degree, the state and local health organizations. Furthermore, the successful pursuance of the program necessitated the integration of activities and therefore cooperation among public health departments and other agencies on the same governmental level such as the agricultural and farm organizations.

## SANITATION NEEDS

Although the United States is one of the most sanitized nations in the world, much unfinished business remains. Numerous surveys and evaluations of environmental health needs have been made by various organizations and agencies. They have resulted in several useful reports that have influenced to varying degrees public opinion, legislation, programming, and organization in the field.[1,6,10 15]

Although it is true that significant strides have been made during the past two decades, the combination of population growth, continued urbanization and suburbanization, and industrial expansion has easily offset any additions and improvements in sanitary facilities. As merely one example, there are still many communities, including some of large size, with inadequate or no sewage treatment facilities. The cost of remedying just this problem is estimated at many billions of dollars. Similarly it is questionable if the air and water pollution problems and the housing problem have improved significantly if any since the survey was made. With reference to dental health there are still only about 88 million people in about 7,500 communities in the United States with adequate natural or added fluoride in their public drinking water.

With this general background and the statement of sanitation needs, a consideration of the most important present concerns in environmental health is indicated.

## WATER SUPPLIES

Water is one of the prime necessities of human existence, so much so that, given dire enough circumstances, even the most educated individual will resort to the consumption of water from grossly polluted or dangerous sources. Beyond its importance for human consumption water serves many purposes: as a source of fluid for animals; as a medium of transportation; as an agent for cleansing and cooling the body, objects, or the environment; as a means of recreation for swimming, boating, and fishing; as an agricultural irrigant; as an adjunct to innumerable industrial processes; as a conveyor for the disposal of human and industrial wastes; as a means of air conditioning; as a fire extinguisher. In the United States per capita domestic use of water from public supplies has grown from about 90 gallons a day in 1890 to approximately 180 gallons a day at the present time. With regard to total use it is estimated that municipal water consumers use almost 24 billion gallons of water each day, rural consumers use about 4 billion gallons, industry uses about 152 billion gallons, and irrigation uses about 130 billion gallons.

The chief concern here is with the consumption of water by humans for domestic purposes. At the moment most of the other uses of water are of interest insofar as they affect the salubrity of the water that humans drink. Water supply systems may be classified as public and private. About three fourths of the American population are served by public water systems. However, about 10% of the families living in about 7 million homes in communities so served do not have water outlets readily available. In addition, there are still an estimated 2.5 million people living in communities of 200 to 500 population without a public water system. Federal assistance programs are under way to provide safe water for many of these. In rural areas about 27 million people need improved pure water facilities.

Public water supplies are derived from various sources, that is, streams, lakes, deep wells, and springs, and their nature differs according to their source. Surface waters such as streams and lakes, which depend for replenishment on repeated runoffs, under most circumstances do not have as high a natural chemical content as do ground waters from deep wells and springs. On the other hand, increasingly surface waters are contaminated by dangerous industrial wastes and agricultural runoffs. Underground waters generally are clear, whereas surface waters ordinarily contain considerable amounts of suspended matter, which must be removed before they can be considered suitable for human consumption. These differences in source, hence composition, necessarily give rise to differences in approach to administrative control. Streams and lakes in general do not lend themselves to adequate control of the watershed. On the other hand, some impounding reservoirs are subject to control from the standpoint of prevention of further pollution of the water. Increasing public pressure for recreational facilities is resulting in more liberal access to both the reservoir and the surrounding watershed. In any case, in view of the high factor of safety in relation to cost, surface waters should probably always be subjected to filtration, chlorination, and fluoridation. Rapid sand filtration is the usual method of choice. Recent improvements in sanitary engineering have resulted in filters with rates up to 4 gallons per square foot per minute, about double the previous usual rate, and when properly operated, do not sacrifice any safety.

The provision of a safe and satisfactory public water supply to a community involves the following procedures:

1. If a surface water, the watershed should be protected and controlled insofar as is practical.

2. The intake should be located properly with regard to all possible sources of contamination and pollution.

3. Provision should be made for primary sedimentation and clarification by means of storage reservoirs and exposure to air and light.

4. Bacteria, algae, and any residual turbidity should be removed by the addition of a coagulant (usually alum) and settling out of the coagulated particles, and then passage through a rapid sand filter.

5. Residual and subsequent bacterial contaminants are combated by the addition of a disinfectant, usually chlorine, to a concentration of from 0.2 to 0.5 parts per million. This is a most important procedure.

6. A concentration from 0.7 to 1.5 parts per million of fluoride should be achieved by the addition of sodium fluoride, sodium silicofluoride, or hydrofluosilicic acid for the prevention of dental caries. The ultimate concentration will depend on the average water consumption per individual.

7. Use of the water by all the population of the community should be assured by reasonable water rates, adequate distribution systems, and housing requirements.

8. Contamination of the purified water should be prevented by residual disinfection of the distribution system pipes and by prevention of cross connections and back siphonage.

To achieve these ends the cooperative action of several community agencies is necessary. Among these are the health department, the department of public works or the water department, the tax or finance office, possibly the park police, the plumbing department, the housing commission, the dental society, and possibly others.

The assurance of safe water to the rural population poses a completely different set of problems. The sources are usually relatively simple and primitive wells, often shallow and unprotected. Hence they are easily subject to pollution not only from the surface but also through seepage from poorly placed privies, improperly constructed septic tanks, or nearby barnyards. Contamination over greater distances may occur if fissures or other subterranean passages exist in the substrata. Offsetting these hazards is the fact that the use of each small rural water supply is usually limited to a small group of people, often one family.

The solution of this difficult problem lies essentially in persistent rural health education programs coupled with sanitary consultation from the local health department. The objectives of these efforts should be encouragement of proper locating of wells and excreta disposal facilities, proper construction of wells, and installation of a pump in a tightly sealed, curbed, and drained well top.

## STREAM POLLUTION CONTROL

Although pure water for drinking purposes is of paramount public health concern, the many other uses of this precious commodity make it desirable to regard the development, protection, and use of water resources as a unit. By now 75% of the population in the United States lives and works in metropolitan centers with resultant concentration of tremendous burdens of human and industrial wastes on the bodies of water to which they are related. The magnitude of water pollution was first established on a systematic basis in 1950 by studies that covered 226 river basins in the United States, of which 146 were interstate. The summary of these studies[16] indicated that there were more than 22,000 sources of stream pollution in the country, including 11,800 municipal sewer systems and 10,400 industrial waste outlets. Of the latter, one half produced organic wastes that greatly increased the biologic oxygen demand and infectious material, whereas others discharged wastes that were toxic or gave rise to tastes and odors that detracted from the subsequent usefulness of the water by humans.

Concern with the problem led to the enactment of the federal Water Pollution Control Act of 1956. Whereas Congress recognized the primary responsibility of the states in the matter, the Water Pollution Control Act authorized and directed the Public Health Service to take the initiative in developing or adopting comprehensive programs for the solution of water pollution problems in cooperation with the states, interstate agencies, municipalities, and industries. The act stated that comprehensive programs were to be developed for surface and underground waters, giving due consideration to all water uses—public water supply, propagation of fish and aquatic life, recreation, and agricultural, industrial, and other legitimate uses. The act provided federal grants to the states and interstate agencies to help them carry out industrial waste studies, and loans to municipalities to assist in the construction of needed abatement work. The act further provided federal research and technical and consultative assistance to state and interstate agencies, municipalities, and industries, and the encouragement of uniform state laws, interstate compacts, and cooperative state activities in the field of water pollution control. Initial responsibility for enforcement of pollution control measures was left with the states; federal authority was to be exercised only on interstate waters, only after the efforts of the states had been exhausted, and only with the consent of the states.

To carry out its responsibilities the Public Health Service instituted a water pollution control program with field units in each of the ten large drainage basin areas. Each unit was staffed with engineers and scientists with extensive experience in water pollution control to work closely with officials of the various state governments. The Robert A. Taft Sanitary Engineering Center in Cincinnati served as the research center for the work. In 1962, Congress further supplemented this program by providing for the establishment of a series of water pollution research laboratories throughout the nation. As indication of its growing concern and impatience, Congress subsequently passed the Water Quality Act of 1965, the Water Resources Planning Act of 1965, the Public Works and Economic Development Act of 1965, and the Clean Water Act of 1966. In the process it established a Federal Water Pollution Control Administration in the Department of the Interior and transferred the water pollution control responsibilities of the Public Health Service to it. Subsequently in late 1970 the program became part of the newly established environmental Protection Agency. Despite the efforts made over the years, a report to the Congress[17] in 1970 indicated unfulfilled water pollution control needs in 1,008 communities with 89 million people. The remedial cost was estimated at about $20 billion.

There are two particularly important conditions for successful control of stream pollution. The first is planning on a regional basis, since few situations involve only one state. Although it is important that each state develop its own programs based on its own legislation, it is fundamental to plan and coordinate the various state water pollution control programs and, insofar as it is possible, the laws on which they are based, to bring about a practical program that will serve the needs of the drainage basin in question.

The second condition is a recognition of the fact that although the chemical and physical characteristics of human wastes do not vary significantly, it is rare that industrial wastes, even those from similar enterprises, are the same. Hence each stream pollution problem, especially if it involves industrial wastes, is a case study in itself. Hunter[18] points out that current policies on which water pollution control programs are based rest on (1) financial support for treatment plant construction and (2) the establishment of water quality standards. These policies are actually responsible in large part for the unsatisfactory rate of water quality improvement. They offer no economic incentives to institute satisfactory measures. In fact they make it less costly or more economical for industries and municipalities to continue to pollute. Added to this is the inability of current enforcement procedures to respond quickly enough because of inadequate monitoring staffs and usually overburdened and inefficient judicial procedures. One suggested approach is to levy "effluent charges." However, this is tantamount to a license to pollute, which could be tax deductible as well as passed on to the purchaser of the product made. Hunter suggests as more practical the combination of (1) establishment of effluent standards, (2) the imposition of prorated fines, and (3) a thorough monitoring system. To these one must add a greatly improved judicial system, perhaps with special courts with built-in environmental expertise.

## WASTE DISPOSAL

Closely related to the problems of water sanitation and stream sanitation is that of satisfactory waste disposal. The waste materials of present-day households consist of human excreta, garbage, and refuse. In urban areas there is also added an increasing amount of industrial wastes. Until recently each of these was considered to be a somewhat separate problem. In urban communities, however, they have become increasingly interrelated. In some instances garbage and refuse are collected and disposed of together. In addition, many households now grind garbage, which is disposed of with excreta and other household wastes through the plumbing and sewerage system. Industrial wastes may also be discharged into the sewerage system or directly into bodies of water which also receive raw or treated sewage.

There are various methods of disposal of waste products of human societies. These may be listed as: (1) discharge into bodies of water, with or without treatment, (2) discharge onto the surface of the ground in either a sanitary or insanitary manner, (3) burial in the ground, (4) incineration, (5) composting, and (6) recycling. No one of these offers the perfect solution, since each has some disadvantages or hazards and each may be more applicable than the others in specific situations. In general, the following principles should be applied to the choice of disposal methods:

1. There should be no contamination of ground water that may enter springs or wells.
2. There should be no contamination of surface water.
3. The surface soil should not be contaminated.
4. Excreta or other organic material should not be accessible to flies or animals.
5. There should be freedom from odors or unsightly conditions.
6. The method used should be simple, reasonable in cost, and require a minimum of maintenance.

It is not within the province of this book to describe and assess the various methods of waste disposal, since those details are readily available in several excellent books devoted specifically to the field of sanitation and sanitary engineering. An excellent overview of the complexities, needs, and methodologies in this field is available in a report by the National Academy of Sciences and the National Research Council.[19] The intent here is merely to present a general background picture of certain factors that must be considered with regard to a public health agency's interest and responsibility in the problem.

Social and environmental circumstances are of particular significance with regard to the disposal of human excreta, which is by far the potentially most dangerous type of waste material. The pertinent situations, hence the methods of approach, are three in kind. The simplest situation is that in which no water carriage is possible. Typically this applies particularly to rural areas. Under such circumstances resort may be made to the pit privy, the bored hole latrine, the vault privy, the chemical toilet, the septic privy, or the box and can toilet. A second situation may be observed in suburban areas and some small communities where no public sewerage system exists. Under such circumstances individual cesspools or septic tanks are commonly used. Finally, there is the situation where both a public water supply and a public sewerage system make possible not only water carriage but also water disposal of human excreta. Here new problems arise in that there is a concentration of tremendous amounts of human wastes, the complication of plumbing hazards in the form of possible cross connections and back siphonage, and the frequent addition of garbage and industrial wastes. Some attempts have been made to dispose of sewage by making use of it for irrigation purposes in so-called sewage farms. The success and practicability of this approach have been limited in the United States.

Generally speaking, therefore, and because of the large amount of water it contains, sewage is usually disposed of in a body of water. Unfortunately this is sometimes done without treatment. The dangers of the discharge of raw sewage into streams or lakes are obvious, and increasingly it is important and necessary to treat sewage for the following reasons:

1. Public health reasons—to prevent the pollution of drinking water, fish and mollusks, and bathing places
2. Aesthetic reasons—to prevent the formation of foul odors and the development of streams and shorelines made unsightly by solid or suspended waste matter
3. Economic reasons—to prevent the killing of commercially valuable fish life, the infection of livestock and other animal life, and the deterioration of land values
4. Salvage reasons—to make possible the recovery of commercially valuable fertilizer, grease, gases, and other products

The objectives of the various methods of sewage treatment may be summarized as follows:

1. To diminish the amount of solid materials discharged into a stream to lessen the demands on its purifying properties and to prevent the formation of sludge banks and the appearance of objectionable floating materials
2. To decompose, through the agency of biologic methods, the organic matter in sewage and to transform it into simpler organic compounds, and into gases and liquids, thus greatly diminishing the burden of the final purification that takes place in a stream
3. To stabilize the organic matter in sewage through the agency of biologic methods operating under aerobic conditions so that the purifying properties of a stream into which the treated sewage is ultimately discharged will be taxed to a minimum
4. To diminish or destroy the bacteria present in sewage, particularly the pathogenic varieties capable of producing disease
5. To remove by chemical or other processes

industrial or related wastes that may be toxic or otherwise affect the subsequent use of the receiving body of water

These objectives are accomplished in different situations by combinations of the following procedures: (1) screening and/or sedimentation; (2) anaerobic digestion of settleable solids in a septic tank, Imhoff tank, or separate sludge digestion tank; (3) oxidation of nonsettleable organic matter by filtration, activated sludge, or irrigation methods; (4) disinfection with chlorine or other disinfectants; and (5) chemical or other neutralizing procedures.

Although the operation of public sewerage as well as water systems is a local responsibility,[20] the overall supervision of these facilities is largely a state concern. In most instances the state health department is the official agency with major responsibility, but in nearly three fourths of the states the responsibility is shared with other departments or special commissions.[21] Among these are departments of public works, labor, education, and industry; special state sewage, stream pollution, or sanitary boards or commissions; state universities and laboratories. Currently there is an increasing trend for states to follow the federal lead and establish separate environmental control agencies with the regulatory powers. In such instances, however, the state health departments usually retain authority for establishment of hygienic criteria and standards. Among the functions for which the state commonly has responsibility are the promulgation and enforcement of laws, rules, and regulations; approval of plans and installations; examination and licensure of treatment plant operators; periodic inspection of installations; provision of consultation services to localities; provision of grants-in-aid to local sanitation units; and the promotion of satisfactory local facilities.

Authority for the supervision of semipublic waste disposal systems is more likely to be shared among several agencies than in the case of public supplies. Thus if the system involves educational institutions, parks, or industries, for example, the departments of education, parks, industry, or labor are almost certain to be involved in most instances. This shared responsibility and authority, however, does not alter the fact that the state health department must play the primary regulatory and supervisory role with respect to the sanitary aspects of the situation. Often, of course, these responsibilities are met in collaboration with or through the local public health structure if it is adequately staffed.

The weakest link exists in relation to supervision and control of individual private waste disposal systems in rural areas. In places where a local public health department exists, it almost invariably includes some form of activity in the field of human excreta control. The basis of the activity usually consists of a persistent health educational approach on a personal visit basis, augmented by general educational measures, consultation from the state health department, and sometimes actual assistance in the financing and construction of private sanitary privies or septic tank systems.

## FOOD AND MILK SANITATION

The majority of the cases of epidemic gastrointestinal infections that occurred up through the first fourth of this century were attributable to impure water. Because of the remarkable strides that have been made since that time in providing safe water to concentrations of people in urban centers, water no longer plays an outstanding role as a transmitter of disease in the United States. Between 1938 and 1960 the Public Health Service compiled and analyzed reports of water-, milk-, and food-borne epidemics from data submitted by local and state health departments. An analysis of these data (Table 30-1) is illustrative.[22] Between 1938 and 1942, water not only caused many outbreaks but was most important in terms of persons affected. Although the average annual number of outbreaks caused by water and milk was roughly the same and in each case only about one fourth of the number caused by other foods, the number of persons affected by water-

borne epidemics was about three and one-half times the number affected by other foods and about eleven times the number affected by milk and milk products.

However, when the data for the period since 1942 are considered, a significant shift is seen to have occurred. Comparing the two periods, although the average annual numbers of epidemics attributable to water and to milk and milk products have been cut in half, those due to other foods have doubled in number. Furthermore, although the average annual number of persons affected in the recent years by milk and milk products was one half of what it had been and for water only one sixth of what it had been, with regard to outbreaks due to other foods the number of persons affected doubled. The figures for the period 1953 to 1960 indicate a decline in all three types of epidemics. However, the decline was greatest in the instances of water-borne and milk-borne epidemics, which declined both in number of epidemics and number of persons affected. Indeed, although the average annual number of epidemics borne by foods was about one third less in the period from 1953 to 1957 than in the period from 1943 to 1951, the number of persons affected remained essentially the same.

The figures, however, are deceptive and must be interpreted with caution. Whereas data for water-borne disease in the United States for the year 1971 is not available and would probably be low, there were reported to the federal Center for Disease Control 320 food-borne outbreaks of which only 7 were attributed to milk and other dairy products. A total of 13,453 persons were affected. However, the center's report[23] makes this important observation. Food poisoning in the United States is grossly underreported. In

**Table 30-1.** Changes in food-borne and water-borne disease outbreaks, United States, 1938 to 1960*

| Time period | Water | | Milk and milk products | | Other foods | |
|---|---|---|---|---|---|---|
| | Outbreaks | Cases | Outbreaks | Cases | Outbreaks | Cases |
| 1938-1942—Number | 247 | 103,441 | 208 | 9,114 | 902 | 29,095 |
|            Annual average | 49 | 20,688 | 42 | 1,823 | 181 | 5,819 |
| 1943-1951—Number | 208 | 32,342 | 205 | 7,259 | 2,769 | 101,466 |
|            Annual average | 23 | 3,594 | 23 | 806 | 308 | 11,274 |
| 1953-1957—Number | 33 | 3,043 | 55 | 1,539 | 1,081 | 53,469 |
|            Annual average | 7 | 609 | 11 | 308 | 216 | 10,694 |
| 1958-1960—Number | 22 | 2,535 | 29 | 538 | 740 | 27,954 |
|            Annual average | 7 | 845 | 10 | 179 | 247 | 9,318 |

*From Dauer, C. C.: Summary of disease outbreaks and a 10-year résumé, Public Health Rep. **76:**915, Oct. 1961.

the state of Washington, where food-borne disease surveillance has been developed to a high degree, 57 outbreaks were reported to the Center for Disease Control in 1971. Projecting from this figure, the estimated number of outbreaks for the entire United States was about 3,100 in 1971; however, only 320 outbreaks were actually reported to the center. The fact that only 10% of the "expected" number of outbreaks were reported for the country serves to emphasize the need for improvement in both surveillance systems and investigations. In 1971, for the second time in 5 years, the number of reported outbreaks (320) decreased when compared with the number for the previous year (366). This decline probably does not reflect a decrease in the number of outbreaks of food-borne illness. Rather, it suggests that food-borne disease surveillance may occupy a position of low priority relative to competing health problems.

Despite their limitations, the figures illustrate two facts with regard to the present time: (1) Foods are easily the most important and an increasing cause of gastrointestinal infections in the United States. (2) Although milk and milk products are potentially the most perishable and most dangerous foods and despite their ever-increasing use, they now are a relatively unimportant cause of disease when compared with other foods. This is explainable on the basis that their very perishability has focused so much attention on means of ensuring their safety.

To promote scientifically sound standards and uniform legislation the Public Health Service in 1924 developed a recommended standard milk ordinance, which has since been revised numerous times.[24] It represents the pooled opinions and experience of public health officials, the milk and dairy industry, veterinarians, agriculturists, scientists, consumer representatives, and others. By now it forms the basis for regulation and practice in 49 states and is enforced statewide in 26 states. Also adopted separately by 107 counties and 120 municipalities the ordinance and its accompanying code now protect a majority of the urban and much of the nonurban population. It is recognized as the only fluid milk regulation approaching a national standard. For use in conjunction with it, procedures relating to the interstate shipment of milk[25] and methods for rating milksheds[26] have been developed. In addition, the Public Health Service has developed widely used standards for community infant formula services,[27] automatic vending of foods and beverages,[28] and food service sanitation.[29] With specific reference to market milk, of special significance in the maintenance of the safety of milk and milk products is the widespread application of the pasteurization process. Pasteurization of all market milk is compulsory in almost all the states, counties, and municipalities of the nation. As a result, well over 90% of the fluid milk consumed by the urban population in the United States is protected by pasteurization.

Important in the successful supervision and control of the many complex factors involved in the production, processing, and sale of milk and milk products has been the cooperative action on the part of public health agencies, departments of agriculture, and representatives of the milk and dairy industry. The actual control programs are administered by sanitarians and veterinarians on the local level supported by the state departments of health and agriculture and by the industry. On the state level, authority may be vested in either the state health department or the department of agriculture, and sometimes in both.

From the analysis of epidemics presented it is obvious that foods other than milk are a matter of considerable concern to public health agencies as an increasing source of preventable disease. The food-borne outbreaks during 1971 give a picture of the problem. Of those reported, the diseases involved were staphylococcal food poisoning, 92; salmonellosis, 30; shigellosis, 7; botulism, 9; noxious plant illness, 4; chemical poisoning, 30; trichinosis, 4; *Clostridium perfringens*, 51; streptococcal infection, 2; hepatitis, 4; others, 10; and unknown, 81. The types of establishments known to be involved were food service establishments, 96; schools, 22; homes, 123; camps and picnics, 13; and churches, 10. It is epidemiologically important to note that the last three types of situations that accounted for 146 (or 55%) of the outbreaks are of a private nature, compared with 118 (or 45%) of the outbreaks attributable to public or semipublic food places that should be subject to control by health authorities.

The first efforts of the federal government to bring about control and supervision of the quality of foods occurred in 1879, when a bill was introduced in Congress to prohibit the adulteration of articles of food and drink. This and several subsequent efforts came to naught, and 27 years passed before June 30, 1906, when

Theodore Roosevelt signed a bill that prohibited the manufacture and sale of adulterated and misbranded food. For 20 years it was administered by the Bureau of Chemistry of the Department of Agriculture. During this period several other acts were passed relating to proper weights, packaging, labeling, food purity, meats, and standards for butter. In 1927 the Secretary of Agriculture recommended the establishment of a Food and Drug Administration to administer all of these various acts. Between 1927 and 1933 additional legislation was passed dealing with canned foods and inspection of seafood plants on invitation. Meanwhile attempts were made to revise and bring up to date the original Food and Drug Act of 1906. On June 25, 1938, President Franklin D. Roosevelt signed a bill that established the present Federal Food, Drug, and Cosmetic Act. Two years later the Food and Drug Administration was transferred from the Department of Agriculture to the Federal Security Agency (now the Department of Health, Education, and Welfare).

The situation on the federal level is somewhat complicated by the retention of meat inspection responsibilities by the Department of Agriculture and by the obvious concern of the Department of Health, Education, and Welfare for all matters dealing with the salubrity of foods. Actually, these two federal agencies are concerned with different aspects of the food problem and work in close collaboration, each fulfilling certain responsibilities. On the state level the situation is more confused. All states have some agency or agencies responsible for food control, but there is no uniformity. The agencies involved are departments of agriculture, 23 states; departments of health, 43 states; and others, 4 states. From the numbers it will be noted that in some states responsibility is shared.

Almost all municipalities and a great many counties carry out some form of food control activities, usually by personnel of the local public health agency. The personnel vary in quality from untrained inspectors to well-qualified sanitarians and veterinarians. In general the activities consist of inspection, rating, and certification of food processing and dispensing establishments, sampling an analysis of foodstuffs, physical examination and training of food-handlers, and local prosecution of infringements of food ordinances and laws. In carrying out these activities the local personnel work closely with and are supported by personnel of the various interested state and federal agencies.

Particular attention is given by local public health authorities to sanitary conditions in restaurants and taverns and bars. Many different types of inspectional and rating forms have been developed, and many types of action such as certification, licensing, and awards of merit have been used. Since obviously there is no justification for variance in basic food safety requirements in different jurisdictions, the Public Health Service in 1934 began the development of a suggested procedure that eventually took the form of a *Food Service Sanitation Manual*. It includes a model food sanitation ordinance and code, which has been adopted widely.

In several fields public health interests and private enterprise have found themselves in the same arena. In some instances they have unfortunately acted at cross-purposes. Sometimes business and industry have looked on public health workers as interfering, unrealistic, and restraining and have pointed, with considerable right, to the maze of conflicting requirements, ordinances, codes, and standards with regard to the same article or process in different communities or states. Public health workers, on the other hand, have sometimes accused private enterprise of being completely mercenary and without social conscience.

Fortunately in recent years industry and public health have made several sincere attempts to get together in an amiable and intelligent manner to arrive at mutually satisfactory conclusions and recommendations in the public's interest. In the field of environmental health, and especially with regard to food sanitation, the National Restaurant Association and the National Automatic Merchandising Association have long supported the goals of the Public Health Service by preparing and promoting training classes and training materials. In 1944 the National Sanitation Foundation was established. This is an independent, nonprofit corporation financed entirely by business and industry and governed by a board of directors comprising individuals from private enterprise and public health. Its purposes are (1) to bring together representative industrialists, businessmen, and public health workers to define and outline mutual problems, (2) to finance research in fields of mutual concern and interest, (3) to promote a program of personal and community health to acquaint employees and the general public with the needs for good sanitary practices and community cleanliness, and (4) to provide a testing laboratory, similar to the Fire Underwriters Laboratory, for materials of sanitary and health-promoting value.

The National Sanitation Foundation sponsors Joint Committees on Standards with representatives from interested national professional organizations. "Task committees" set up by industry prepare preliminary standards for consideration with the joint committees. After repeated conferences and revisions, if agreement is reached, the standards may be approved by the joint committee. After final review and approval by the foundation's Council of Sanitation Consultants the standards are published. Equipment that meets the standards is then awarded the foundation's seal of approval. The procedure, although long and complex, assures the careful study and consideration of all aspects of the problem at hand and when completed, concurrence of public health workers, scientists, and industrialists is almost certain. So far the National Sanitation Foundation has developed 12 sets of recommended standards for the food service field, including standards for soda fountain equipment, general food service equipment, dishwashing equipment, and other items. In addition, it carries out significant activities in public sanitation education and has conducted several worthwhile symposia and in-service training courses for representatives of public health agencies, business and industrial groups, and public officials.

Somewhat similar to these efforts are the increased activities on the part of business and industry toward "self-policing." Among the examples of this are the programs of the National Canners' Association, the Ice Cream Merchandising Institute, the Food Industries Sanitarian Association, the National Automatic Merchandising Association (food and beverage vending machines), and the American Institute of Baking. These are all good signs that point toward a more fruitful and mutually more agreeable method of cooperative action from which the public cannot help benefiting. This is in conformity with one of the recommendations of the National Commission on Community Health Services,[1] which states, "Industry and commerce [should] assume more responsibility for self-policing and control of their products, services, and operations in relation to associated environmental health problems; and health agencies [should] encourage and assist them in so doing."

## ATMOSPHERIC POLLUTION

The nature, magnitude, and biologic ill effects of atmospheric pollution have been presented in the preceding chapter on environmental hazards. Emphasis here will be placed on what should be and what is being done. During recent years public and health officials have become increasingly aware of the atmosphere as the important medium in which mankind lives and of the possibility and consequences of overloading it with waste products of human activity. Thus concern has been mounting in relation to air pollution similar to that which exists in relation to stream pollution. Increasingly it is recognized that the layer of air above the earth surface is thin, is not limitless, and must stop being used as an aerial sewer. Pound for pound man consumes at least ten times as much air as water. Although there has been concern for many years over the purity of the water used by human societies, little attention has been given to the quality of the air that constantly is breathed into the lungs and absorbed into the bloodstream. Even now, despite the mass of literature about the serious health effects of air pollution, most public reaction relates to the unesthetic effects of smoke, dirt, and odor. This is clearly an area in which science and government together must provide not only the facts but more importantly the initiative and leadership to solve one of the world's most critical problems.

Historic records do exist, however, that indicate at least momentary concern with the problem and even legislation in earlier times. As a result of the widespread use of soft sea coal for fuel in English towns and cities, a smoke-abatement law was passed as early as 1273 by King Edward I. He banned the use of coal as being prejudicial to the public health. Shortly after, Parliament in 1306 formed a smoke-abatement group whose recommendations resulted in a royal proclamation that prohibited the use of coal in the furnaces of artificers. Record has it that in 1307 one offender was actually executed for violating the regulations. In 1661 a report entitled *Fumifugium* claimed that almost one half of the deaths in London were "phthisical and pulmonic distempers" resulting from polluted air.[30]

The atmosphere may be polluted from many sources. Smoke results whenever fuel or other material is incompletely burned, that is, industrial, commercial, or domestic heating facilities, incinerators, brush fires, dumps, and automobile motors. In urban areas especially, automobile motors are a major generator of toxic gases. In rural and suburban areas irritating pollens and toxic agricultural sprays and dusts are likely to be particularly prevalent. Industrial contaminants represent a particularly complex and important source of atmospheric pollution.

In general, air pollutants consist of particulate matter, aerosols, gases, and vapors. The most common forms are condensed organics such as fly ash and tar; oxides of sulfur, carbon, and nitrogen; metallic oxides and fumes; minerals such as asbestos; vegetable matter such as pollens; and mists and fogs. Carbon monoxide and sulfur dioxide are probably the most common of the gases. In addition, ozone produced by photochemical reactions can give rise to irritating proportions as well as aid in the development of additional irritants by its oxidizing action on other pollutants. The complexity of industrial, automotive, and other sources that may pollute air is illustrated by studies of smog samples from Los Angeles.[31] Among the contaminants found were the following:

*Aerosols*

| | |
|---|---|
| Ether-soluble aerosols | Lead |
| Sulfuric acid mist | Aluminum |
| Carbon | Calcium |
| Silicon | Iron |

*Gases and vapors*

| | |
|---|---|
| Acetylene | Methyl chloride |
| Aromatics | Nitric oxide |
| Benzene | Nitrogen dioxide |
| Isobutane | Nitrous oxide |
| n-Butane | n-Pentane |
| Butenes | Phosgene |
| Carbon tetrachloride | Propane |
| Ethane | Propylene |
| Ethyl benzene and xylene | Sulfur dioxide |
| Formic acid | Toluene |
| Methyl cellosolve | Trichlorethylene |

Unsaturated hydrocarbons ranging from $C_5H_8$ to $C_{12}H_{24}$

Products of oxidation of the above unsaturated hydrocarbons (aldehydes, peroxides, ketones, and organic acids)

This list is by no means all inclusive in terms of the total possible pollutants that might occur in various locations or circumstances.

In addition to the discharge of contaminants into the atmosphere certain fixed or variable meteorologic and topographic factors may determine whether or not an air pollution problem will develop, the degree of its concentration or extension, and the acuteness and severity of its result. If a community is situated within a topographic bowl, natural dispersal of atmospheric pollutants will be limited and concentrations of dangerous substances may result. In addition, depending on the location and nature of the emissions, localized or neighborhood areas at risk may develop. The interrelationship of these factors has been summarized as follows[32]: "The average distribution of contaminants in a city is governed by wind, rain, atmospheric stability, and topographic features. The contaminants in their turn influence rainfall and fog occurrence and persistence."

Typically, insufficient attention is given to these factors until they combine under special circumstances to cause dramatic disastrous situations such as those that occurred at Donora, Penn., the Meuse Valley in Belgium, and elsewhere. Any program relating to atmospheric pollution must take into account a study of winds, atmospheric stability, and precipitation as they are related to seasonal variation, diurnal variation, surface temperatures, and many other meteorologic factors. This accentuates the need to consider air pollution control measures from three viewpoints: (1) local or neighborhood problems that are only partly related to topographic and meteorologic factors and more related to proximity, nature, and concentration of the polluting source; (2) air conservation in an urban area; and (3) ecologic conservation of broad areas that might be affected by acid rains, atmospheric dissemination of lead, and the like, where even if the concentrations of such materials in urban areas may be low, their cumulative broadcast emission may become significant in the large, longer range context.

Pollution of the atmosphere may result in economic loss to individuals and to the general population in a variety of ways. Losses may take the form of damage to livestock and vegetation, corrosion of metals and structural materials, damage to clothing and other fabrics, damage to the finishes of automobiles and houses, disruption of communications and increased artificial lighting requirements, depreciated real estate values, and last but by no means least the acute and chronic harm done to humans. Not including the effect on humans, the national economic loss caused by atmospheric pollution has been estimated variously as between $4 billion and $10 billion. On the other hand, one can cite many examples of industrial establishments that, by installation of control procedures, have actually netted from modest to substantial profits from the recovered materials. For example, one chemical company in Los Angeles spent $40,000 for the installation of equipment to prevent atmospheric contamination. As a result, it is now recovering 15 barrels per day of lead oxide worth $90,000 per year. Furthermore, if permissible tax benefits are applied to equipment purchase and operation, the savings are even more substantial.

For health purposes, of course, it is the effects on human life that are of greatest interest and importance. The effect of air pollution on the health of the individual or of a community under ordinary circumstances is so insidious that a cause-effect relationship is difficult to demonstrate. Nevertheless it can be done, as was true in the similar problem presented by cigarette smoking and cancer. Admittedly, base lines, standards, and methods of measurement necessary to determine adequately the physiologic or histologic effects of substances in the air still leave much to be desired. Even when a relatively severe short-term exposure occurs, such as that at Donora, conclusive answers are usually not obtained because the investigations take place after the fact and not before and during the incident. Nevertheless, much has been learned during recent years as a result of studying "epidemics" of air pollution, continuous smog situations, long-term effects on workers constantly exposed to certain substances, and laboratory experiments.[33]

The "epidemic" situation, of course, is the most dramatic, and several facts of value have resulted from their investigation. Four of these occurrences merit special mention. During 1930 the heavily industrialized area in and around Liege in the Meuse Valley of Belgium was subjected to 4 days of continuous fog saturated with industrial smoke and fumes. Many thousands of people died. Although studies indicated significant amounts of sulfur dioxide, sulfuric acid, and other chemicals in the air, no single substance was found in a concentration sufficiently high to have caused the damage by itself.[34]

A similar tragedy occurred in 1948 in Donora, Penn., a small town of about 14,000 inhabitants. Because of its location in a valley and because of its industry, polluted fogs are extremely common in Donora. Usually the sun and wind dissipate the fog during the early hours of the day. Occasionally, however, it may remain throughout a day. On October 27, 1948, a thick fog settled down in the valley and remained for 4½ days, meanwhile becoming more and more polluted by the smoke, fumes, and gases from the town's industrial plants. During the period, 20 individuals died and about 6,000 others, or 43% of the population, became ill in varying degrees. The episode and the circumstances were studied exhaustively for a year by the Pennsylvania Department of Health assisted by the United States Public Health Service.[35,36]

As with the Meuse Valley disaster, although a large number of gases and fumes were identified in the atmosphere, it was concluded that no single contaminant was responsible. In both instances it was believed that a combination of irritating and toxic materials, of which sulfur dioxide undoubtedly was one, acted synergistically to produce the illnesses and deaths. In both instances the deleterious conditions were observed to affect the population selectively. Almost all the victims who were affected fatally and many of those who became ill but did not die suffered from respiratory or cardiac difficulties. The intensive pollution of the air harmed the aged, the infirm, and enfeebled infants earlier than it affected the remaining more vigorous fraction of the population. Among other things this indicates the need for a completely different set of tolerance levels of toxic substances for a community as a whole as against those used heretofore. Most of the latter are based on the tolerance of industrial workers.

A third disaster of this type occurred on November 24, 1950, at Poza Rica, Mexico, where 320 persons were hospitalized, 22 of whom died.[37] This case differed from the Meuse and Donora episodes in that it was possible to point to a single toxic agent. A petroleum refinery at the site discharged a number of aerial contaminants, one of which was hydrogen sulfide. A combination of relatively localized unusual meteorologic phenomena, combined with an operational breakdown that caused more venting than usual, resulted in an extremely high concentration of hydrogen sulfide gas around the plant.

The city of London, England, has experienced several sudden increases in the death rate because of atmospheric pollution. Its situation is somewhat different from the others described in that the problem is not primarily related to industrial contaminants. Severe fogs with stasis and lethal concentration of atmospheric pollutants occurred particularly in 1873, 1880, 1892, 1948, 1952, and 1962. In the 1880 incident the death rate of 896 per million was about 50% above normal expectancy. In fact, it was significantly higher than the rate of 876 recorded for the worst week of the great London cholera epidemic of 1866. Despite this, the events of December 1952 and especially of the 5 days from December 5 to 9 were even more spectacular. It has been shown conclusively that during the total period of the first 3 weeks of December about 4,000 deaths were caused by the polluted fog. Although the very young, the aged, and the infirm were affected most, it is interesting that all age groups contributed to the increased mortality. The mortality of infants doubled, deaths of children 10 to 13 years of age increased by one third, and deaths of young adults increased by almost two thirds. Deaths from bronchitis, which were eight times normal, and deaths from pneumonia, which were three times normal, accounted for about one half of the total increase in mortality. Other causes of death for which significant increases were observed were pulmonary tuberculosis and cancer, coronary disease, and myocardial degeneration.

The cause of the phenomenon in London was a prolonged absence of wind and a low temperature, which produced a low altitude inversion whereby the normal upward air currents came to a stop. As a result, the usual air contaminants of the area accumulated to extremely high concentrations. For example, the concentration of smoke rose thirty-six times and of sulfur dioxide 19,000 times the summer daily average.[38,39] In December 1962 during 4 days, 1,000 persons were hospitalized and about 100 persons died from the effects of a similar but shorter episode.

More difficult than "epidemic" situations is the problem of determining the chronic effects of atmospheric contaminants. Attempts have been made to study this problem, but inherent difficulties have made them incomplete and inconclusive. Nevertheless, this is a highly active research field,[40] some of the results of which have been presented in the preceding chapter.

By its very nature atmospheric pollution is difficult to control. Its causes are many and complex; adequate criteria, standards, and means of measurement have been developed only relatively recently; and an extensive number of public and private agencies, businesses, and industries have important interests in anything that is done. The atmosphere surrounding a present-day community is bound to be contaminated. A completely pure atmosphere is unattainable. Some trade-offs must be considered. It would seem that control must depend on legislation, public and industrial education, the fur-

ther improvement of criteria, standards, and measurement techniques, the further development and application of practical devices for controlling automotive and industrial emissions, and the development and application of new sources of heat and power. Recognition of air pollution as a health and social problem has resulted in the enactment of legislation at all levels of government. Enabling legislation to permit local jurisdictions to act against specific problems was passed in California in 1947. This was followed in 1955 by legislation that permitted regional control programs. In addition to establishing a control authority and providing for continuous study and research, it placed a limit on the dusts, fumes, and sulfur that may be discharged by industry and required approval of plans for any installation that might add to the pollution of the atmosphere. Numerous local communities have since followed the example of Los Angeles and California.

In 1959 the California legislature required the promulgation of ambient air quality standards and emission standards for motor vehicles. This led to the California Motor Vehicle Pollution Control Act of 1960, which required the installation on motor vehicles of devices to reduce emissions. This affected the entire automobile industry, and exhaust control devices became applicable on all new cars in the United States in September 1967.

Federal legislation in 1955 authorized and supported research and technical assistance on the federal and state level. The federal role was strengthened by the passage of the Clean Air Acts of 1963, 1965, 1966, and 1967. These were administered by the National Air Pollution Control Administration, of the Environmental Health Service, Department of Health, Education, and Welfare, until December 1970, when the program became one of the basic units of the new Environmental Protection Agency. The past few years have witnessed an acceleration of research and legislative action with the establishment of increasingly exact and strict criteria and standards. On the basis of these, many large industries, especially those concerned with automobiles and energy sources, have been given tight time limits within which to comply. As one leader in the field of air pollution control has stated, "The automobile was recognized as a problem in 1950. We began to do something about it in 1960, the industry finally agreed that the problem existed in 1970. If we are lucky, we will have the technology for a true cleanup by 1980, and maybe there will be a 'clean car population' by 1990. Meanwhile the condition of the earth's atmosphere is getting more critical all the time."

## RADIOLOGIC HEALTH

One of the newest and very important aspects of environmental health relates to problems arising from the use of fissionable materials.[41] Increasing amounts of radioactive isotopes are being used for medical diagnosis and treatment and for industrial research and materials testing.[42] Already several ships and electrical power plants using nuclear energy have been constructed. The potential of fallout from nuclear weapons testing or attack compounds the situation. In several instances accidental spillage of fissionable material has presented health agencies with new challenges.[43]

The chief concern of the public health agency in this field is protection of the community and the nation from damaging radiations, whether due to misuse, accident, improper disposal of fissionable waste materials, weapons testing, or military attack. Understandably the last two possibilities are dominant in the public's mind, largely because of extensive discussion in the public information media. It is important to realize, however, that they do not represent the major threats. Bugher[44] pointed out that studies by the National Academy of Sciences and the National Research Council have shown that fallout from weapons testing in the atmosphere represents only a small fraction of the total radiation exposure of the public in contrast with the large part of the total exposure from the diagnostic and therapeutic uses of x rays. He went on to predict that "With the rapid development of nuclear power and the expanding employment of radioactive materials and nuclear reactions in industry, agriculture, and medicine, we may anticipate that maintaining control over these potential hazards will become more complex rather than less."

Among the radiologic control activities in which various health agencies have become involved are the determination of the amounts and effects of natural or background radiation; the prohibition of shoe-fitting fluoroscopic machines; the testing of x-ray and fluoroscopic equipment in medical and dental offices, hospitals, and clinics as well as in industry; the surveillance of fluctuations in atmospheric radiation; the testing of milk, water, and other substances for levels of radioactive contamination; consultation in the construction of nuclear-powered ships

and electric power plants; planning for civilian protection in case of nuclear attack; and the disposal of radioactive wastes.

These new responsibilities have made it necessary for increasing numbers of public health workers to familiarize themselves with totally new areas of knowledge. To facilitate this the Division of Radiological Health of the Public Health Service, the Atomic Energy Commission, the Department of Defense, and many universities have provided special continued education and in-service training courses and have engaged in the development of various specialized technologists in this field. Of assistance to the general health worker is a handbook by the American Public Health Association.[45] In addition, because of the extensive geographic, social, political, and biologic ramifications of this field, it has become increasingly necessary for public health workers to involve themselves in interdisciplinary, interorganizational, and intergovernmental relationships quite different from the past.

Governmental concern about radiation is not new. Its history in the United States began with the standardization by the National Bureau of Standards of radium for medical uses in 1913, the concerns in relation to radium poisoning of watch-dial painters as well as radium water tonics and rejuvenators, leading eventually to the formation in the late 1920s of the Advisory Committee on X Ray and Radium Protection, later renamed the National Committee on Radiation Protection. In 1946 the Atomic Energy Act was passed, which provided for the distribution of radioactive isotopes on the basis of strict health and safety standards. In the late 1950s the Public Health Service established a Division of Radiological Health and designated an Advisory Committee on Radiation. It has cooperated with the Atomic Energy Commission, the Food and Drug Administration, the Department of Defense, and various other agencies. In the process it has carried out many studies on the decontamination of radioactively contaminated waters, the treatment and disposal of radioactive wastes, the standards necessary in the industrial and transportation uses of atomic power, the evaluation of varying degrees of hazards associated with radioactive elements and the biologic effects of radiation. In 1960 a further step forward was taken by the enactment of P.L. 86-373, which established the Federal Radiation Council. A major purpose has been to examine all scientific evidence, as it develops, regarding the biologic effects of radiation, leading to the development of broad guidelines for national policy. Federal efforts were later strengthened by the passage of the Radiation Control for Health and Safety Act of 1968.

Accompanying national action and greatly stimulated by it has been the development of programs of varying degrees of extensiveness throughout the states and major cities of the nation.[46] In the process of developing and carrying out these programs one of the most difficult problems that confronts the public health worker is the maintenance of an appropriate balance between the benefits that may result from the use of radioactive materials and radiation-generating equipment and the risks that might possibly be entailed.[47] No one would suggest that the use of x rays be ceased because of some measure of risk. Similarly it would be ill-advised to deprive man and his societies of the tremendous benefits to be reaped from the application of radiation to industry, food preservation, power development, and the like. Bugher[44] has put the question well:

Nearly all of us of this scientific generation have been brought up on the concept that all changes produced by ionizing radiation are deleterious in general and that in the genetic sense any biologically beneficial effect is outweighed by the handicaps that are introduced. We find it difficult to conceive that absorption of radiation may not be followed by permanent cell changes. It is possible that we neglect to consider that all life on this earth has come to its present state through continuous contact with a radioactive environment. There has been not a single living cell in all the history of life on this planet that has not been subjected to radiation from both without and within its substance.

The challenge then is for public health workers to deal with problems of radioactivity with a balance of respect and reason based on sound proved scientific data and not emotion or fear of the unknown. To provide a practical measure of protection from unnecessary emissions from x-ray equipment, television sets, and other electronic devices, Congress passed the Radiation Control for Health and Safety Act in October 1968.

## HOUSING AND COMMUNITY PLANNING

In discussing the need for public health interest in housing Winslow[48] commented as follows:

The filth epidemics of the Nineteenth Century have been conquered in civilized and relatively prosperous lands like ours. We can now think in terms of health rather than in terms of disease; and, from this standpoint, such problems as nutrition and housing come

to the forefront. The slum of today is no longer a hot-bed of cholera and typhus fever as it was seventy-five years ago. It remains, however, one of the major obstacles to that physical and emotional and social vigor and efficiency and satisfaction which we conceive as the health objective of the future.

Many attempts have been made to establish a conclusive relationship between unsatisfactory housing and ill health. Several of these have been referred to earlier in the discussion in Chapter 5 on the sociologic aspects of public health. However, because the dwellers in poor housing are subjected to so many other undesirable factors such as low economic income, malnutrition, limited education, and the like, it is impossible to determine with exactness what is cause and what is effect. The difficulty and its proper interpretation has been well summarized by Anderson[49] as follows:

Of the many newer aspects of environmental sanitation, the standards of housing seem to rest on an especially insecure epidemiological foundation. I would not question the potential health significance of housing, and yet epidemiological data on which to base this belief are virtually nonexistent for poor housing cannot be separated from other attributes of poverty.

This inability to secure epidemiological support for housing standards should not discourage us from attempts to improve housing conditions or even to do so by regulation. Almost every community has houses that by no stretch of the imagination can be defended as desirable for human habitation. An appreciable fraction of our population lives under conditions that are undesirable socially, morally, and hygienically. Housing needs no defense nor need await epidemiological support.

The history of the movement to provide decent housing for people has been briefly traced by Bauer[50] on a basis that should not be disregarded by public health workers. She reminds us that the housing movement may be viewed not only as a significant chapter in scientific and public health history, "but also as a very lively and important chapter in political history." She points out that without exception "every major step in housing progress in the past century has involved some public action," and suggests that "political philosophy—the motivating forces behind public action and the application of scientific knowledge—is not secondary or incidental, but paramount." Of particular significance to our present consideration, she traces the gradual development of enlightened political philosophy, dating from the English Poor Laws of the early nineteenth century, with its expanding concepts of individual rights—to due process of law, to health, to education—to the more recent concept of the right of individuals to a decent home. She proceeds then to provide public health workers with a sound basis for future thought and action in proposing that henceforth their interest is "not just a question of 'minimum standards,' to allay disease or prevent divorce or save the taxpayers money, or of sporadic housing programs tied to one emergency kite or another, to provide employment or increase the birthrate or improve the physical qualities of soldiers or lessen the danger of revolution, but good housing for all, to be provided by public action where private enterprise could not do the job, on the fundamental democratic principle of equal opportunity."

The production of housing in the United States has depended essentially on the law of supply and demand. The demand, however, has been closely linked to the economic ability of individuals and families to afford the product. Budget experts believe that a family should not expend more than about one fifth of its income for housing.

An important consideration is that private housing is constructed largely during periods of economic upswing when building costs are also going up. Furthermore, during periods of economic depression, the cost of houses does not go down to the extent that salaries and incomes decline. During the depression years of the 1930s, despite ever-growing needs because of population increase and continued movement toward cities, construction of homes lagged considerably. The postdepression spurt was then thrown off balance by the resource requirements of the war effort. By the end of World War II a tremendous backlog of housing needs had developed. Since that time, the greatest building boom in United States history has occurred. This combined with extensive slum clearance and suburbanization has resulted in only a few percent of dwellings with basic health deficiencies. In 1970, out of almost 68 million occupied housing units 94% had complete plumbing facilities including hot and cold piped water, flush toilet, and bathtub or shower. Less than 1% of vacant housing units were rated dilapidated. Overcrowding and deficient lighting, ventilation, and heating were not included among the criteria.

The components of healthful housing have been studied over several years by the Committee on the Hygiene of Housing, which was estab-

lished in 1937 by the American Public Health Association. In the course of its work the committee has issued a series of important documents on the subject that have filled an important need not only of public health but of other disciplines. Prominent among these have been *An Appraisal Method for Measuring the Quality of Housing,*[51] *Housing—Basic Health Principles and Recommended Ordinance,*[52] and *Guide for Health Administrators in Housing Hygiene.*[53] Under four broad headings the committee has listed the following thirty basic principles that must be considered with regard to healthful housing:

*Fundamental physiologic needs*
1. Maintenance of a thermal environment which will avoid undue heat loss from the human body
2. Maintenance of a thermal environment which will permit adequate heat loss from the human body
3. Provision of an atmosphere of reasonable chemical purity
4. Provision of adequate daylight illumination and avoidance of undue daylight glare
5. Provision for admission of direct sunlight
6. Provision of adequate artificial illumination and avoidance of glare
7. Protection against excessive noise
8. Provision of adequate space for exercise and for play of children

*Fundamental psychologic needs*
1. Provision of adequate privacy for the individual
2. Provision of opportunities for normal family life
3. Provision of opportunities for normal community life
4. Provision of facilities which make possible the performance of tasks of the household without undue physical and mental fatigue
5. Provision of facilities for maintenance of cleanliness of the dwelling and of the person
6. Concordance with prevailing social standards of the local community

*Protection against contagion*
1. Provision of a water supply of safe, sanitary quality, available to the dwelling
2. Protection of the water supply system against pollution within the dwelling
3. Provision of toilet facilities of such a character as to minimize the danger of transmitting disease
4. Protection against sewage contamination of the interior surfaces of the dwelling
5. Avoidance of insanitary conditions in the vicinity of the dwelling
6. Exclusion from the dwelling of vermin which may play a part in the transmission of disease
7. Provision of facilities for keeping milk and food undecomposed
8. Provision of sufficient space in sleeping rooms, to minimize the danger of contact infection

*Protection against accidents*

1. Erection of the dwelling with such materials and methods of construction as to minimize danger of accidents due to collapse of any part of the structure
2. Control of conditions likely to cause fires or to promote their spread
3. Provision of adequate facilities for escape in case of fire
4. Protection against danger of electrical shocks and burns
5. Protection against falls and other mechanical injuries in the home
6. Protection of the neighborhood against the hazards of automobile traffic

The achievement of these goals involves action on three fronts: first, *prevention* of accelerated rates of deterioration of dwellings and their environment, thereby forestalling the formation of new blighted and slum areas; second, *rehabilitation* of existing substandard housing, if salvage is economically feasible, and demolition—which is part of rehabilitation in its broader sense—of substandard dwellings that are beyond repair; and third, *production* of enough new housing to provide for population increase, for families now overcrowded, for replacement of demolished and decayed structures, and for the normal vacancy cushion.

As is indicated by several of the preceding criteria, adequate housing is now considered to involve circumstances that extend beyond the physical structure of the dwelling. Many of the objectives are unattainable if the surrounding neighborhood or indeed the entire community is allowed to develop in a completely hit-or-miss fashion. It is necessary therefore to give consideration to the overall living needs of the neighborhood and to the planning of the community as a whole. This involves the development of long-range programs of neighborhood and community improvement, land use and traffic planning, with attention to street and freeway layouts, parks and playgrounds, sites for schools and other public buildings, shopping center, and the location of business and industrial enterprises. A serious mistake would be to consider the dwelling alone without reference to its use, its surroundings, and its community service connections. Thus the following factors have been listed as important if an optimum residential environment is to be achieved[54]:

1. Space for light, air, and recreation
2. Adequate water supply

3. Proper sewage and waste disposal facilities
4. Drainage
5. Freedom from accident hazard
6. Clean air
7. Freedom from unnecessary noise and disturbances
8. Insect, rodent and nuisance control
9. Suitable recreational facilities
10. Building codes
11. A land use plan
12. Zoning

Beyond this is the need for increased attention by public health workers and others to suburban areas that surround municipalities. Here, in addition to many structural signs of affluence one can find some of the worst housing problems. There are three reasons for suburban subdivisions going sour and giving rise to difficulties. In the first place they may be premature, with land subdivided before there is a real need. Beyond the economic loss that results from much of the land lying unused the situation invites the development of suburban squatter slums. A second reason for failure is that subdivisions may be poorly designed by promoters butchering the land into inadequate-sized lots in an uncompromising grid-iron pattern, with no concern for recreation, parking, or other public spaces. Finally, subdivisions and fringe areas are very likely to suffer because of inadequate plans for water, sanitary or storm sewers, street lights, fire hydrants, or grading and surfacing of streets. Woodbury[55] insists that the dispersal of people and their housing is not basically at fault. To the contrary, he points out that the nineteenth century city, which still determines much of American urban thinking and planning, was a product of a time, culture, and technology quite different from that of today. As he says, "Nothing could be more illogical and more disastrous for our increasingly metropolitan civilization than to let the problems of urban sprawl drive us back to a pattern of city building that, on balance, is definitely worse, even if the new version of that pattern would be largely in metal and glass in place of brink, stone, and wood." The problem then is twofold—the inadequacy of archaic cities and the unplanned manner in which suburbs are being allowed to develop.

Any reasonably adequate solution of the tremendous and complex problem of housing obviously requires the combined and coordinated efforts of private enterprise, the local, state, and federal governments, and various professional and civic groups. Governmental action on all levels involves participation by many different agencies and departments, including those concerned with health, building inspection, plumbing, water, legal counseling, schools, recreation, traffic engineering, fire protection, public works, tax enforcement, public welfare, public housing, and redevelopment. This is not a job for the official health agency alone.

Several administrative approaches have been tried. Traditionally in the United States responsibility for the quality of new housing has been vested in housing officials who have been primarily concerned with protection against fire and structural collapse. Of somewhat secondary interest have been requirements relating to the water supply, plumbing, heating, lighting, and ventilation. Once housing is constructed and occupied, responsibility for the supervision of its quality is generally transferred to the local health department. This is perhaps because the health department is in the best position to use effectively the police power and other legislative measures[56] and because of the multiplicity of interests of public health agencies. Thus many local health departments have long been active in various fields directly related to housing. Among these are the enforcement of requirements with regard to heating, lighting, and ventilation, control of atmospheric pollution, supervision of water supplies and of plumbing and sewerage systems, rodent and vermin control, nuisance abatement, accident prevention, and sanitary education.

The contributions of the local health department to the solution of the broad problem of housing may be in several fields, which include the following:

1. Development and promotion of the acceptance of local desirable housing and neighborhood standards
2. Participation in the enactment and enforcement of proper building codes and housing ordinances
3. Measurement of the quality of existing housing and neighborhoods
4. Participation in the remedying of existing housing deficiencies through rehabilitation and slum clearance
5. Participation in the proper control and direction of new housing through zoning, city planning, and the issuance of various permits and licenses

6. Education of the public in the hygiene of housing

Mood[57] cautions, however, that in assuming a leadership role public health officials should realize that the involvement of health agencies in housing programs is not revolutionary in nature but rather, that it is evolutionary. In this regard it should always be remembered that whereas laws and regulations may provide a basis and a legal means of requiring conformance to housing standards, they have never in themselves provided or maintained a decent dwelling. One of the greatest areas of neglect has been in health education as it relates to housing. If adequately pursued, it would undoubtedly bring about the correction of more housing deficiencies than could ever be accomplished by laws.

For practical reasons major consideration has been given to the situation and possibilities on the local level. Mention should be made about the position of the state and federal governments. They may provide types of assistance and service that individuals, communities, and organizations are unable to provide for themselves. State governments may provide funds and consultation for the planning and construction of public housing, for slum clearance and redevelopment, and for regional planning. In a few instances statewide housing legislation has been enacted and enforced. The federal government through legislation may assist by the insurance of mortgages and of deposits in home loan banks, by the subsidization of slum clearance, redevelopment and low-rent public housing, by rent controls, by grants for farm housing, by research, and by the collection of statistics on housing, labor, and materials.

In 1949 Congress passed the Federal Housing Act. It established a Housing and Home Finance Agency as part of a major national housing instrument, the Federal Housing Administration. The functions of the agency were gradually expanded by subsequent amendment. The agency establishes standards and requirements that qualify local governments for grants and loans for surveying, planning, and correcting substandard housing and environmental living conditions. To qualify, the local government must submit a plan of action designated as the "workable program." It should give consideration to seven basic elements:

1. Enforcement of sound local housing and building codes; an end to tolerating thousands of illegal, degrading, unhealthy,

substandard structures and areas where many people have to live
2. General master plan for the community's development; an end to haphazard, thoughtless planning and growth; a road map for the city's future in a planned framework for the region, metropolitan, or intercity urbanization of which it is a part
3. Basic analysis of neighborhoods and the kind of treatment needed; an inventory of blighted and threatened areas to form the basis of a plan of treatment to stop blight in its tracks
4. An effective administrative organization to run the program; coordinated activity toward a common purpose by all officers and arms of the local government
5. Financial capacity to carry out the program, using community revenues and resources to build a better city for the future instead of continuing to pay heavily for past mistakes
6. Rehousing of displaced families; expanding the supply of good housing for all income groups through new construction and rehabilitation so that families paying premium prices for slums can be rehoused
7. Full communitywide participation and support; public demand for a better community and public backing for the steps needed to get it.

In 1965 the functions of the Federal Housing Administration became the nucleus of a new Cabinet entity, the Department of Housing and Urban Development.

## VECTOR CONTROL

As indicated in Chapter 21, those pathogenic organisms that involve nonhuman hosts or vectors at any stage of their life cycles offer an additional point of potential control. The number of such diseases is substantial and the numbers and types of vectors impressive. Vectors of public health concern are rodents and arthropods. Increasingly, wild rodents have been found to be the true reservoirs of plague and widespread epizootics with commensal rodents being merely side or incidental aspects of the particular biologic cycles. Among rodent vectors, rats, ground squirrels, and prairie dogs are most important, especially in view of their role in the spread of plague. Among the innumerable arthropods, certain mosquitoes, flies, fleas, roaches, lice, mites, and ticks are of

impressive significance. It is all too easily overlooked by residents of the United States that insects exact a far greater toll of health and life than any other thing. Malaria is still one of the world's leading causes of death, and other insect-borne diseases are far from rare. Furthermore, considerable numbers of the insect vectors of many of those diseases are present in certain areas of the United States. Accordingly the control of insect vectors of disease is still and will long continue to be an important phase of environmental health programs.

The possibility of controlling disease-transmitting insects became a reality at about the turn of the century. Life cycles of many organisms and of many vectors became known. Experiments and demonstrations of various methods of control of breeding places and of protection against adult insects were carried out. The use of courageous administrative procedures for the widespread use of these methods established Havana and Panama as famous landmarks in public health history. Elimination of mosquito breeding places was accomplished by drainage and fillings; larvae were killed by fish and by the spreading of oils; adult insects were destroyed or repelled by fumigants and smudges and were excluded from living and sleeping quarters by screening and bed nets. Subsequent decades brought cheaper and easier larviciding with Paris green, and pyrethrum became widely used as in insect adulticide. It was not, however, until World War II presented the terrible risk of action in far-flung disease-ridden areas that insect control really came into its own. Some of the older materials like pyrethrum were made more effective by refining their insecticidal principles and applying them with aerosols as the medium. Remarkably efficient new repellents were also developed. It was the development of DDT and other potent insecticides and their widespread use against mosquitoes, lice, and other disease vectors, however, that really opened a new epidemiologic era. The numerous successes of these compounds against the vectors of a large number of diseases in many places represent a real triumph of man over his environment. Offsetting this, however, is the disturbing combination of increased resistant strains of insects and increased human and ecologically undesirable side effects of pesticides. One of the most interesting and potentially important approaches to the solution of these problems is the large-scale breeding and dissemination of insects that have been sterilized artificially.

The control and destruction of rodents is of importance because of two diseases in particular, that is, plague and murine typhus. In the United States, plague-infected wild rodents appear to have been spreading eastward from the West Coast at a rapid rate, necessitating intensified control procedures to prevent epidemics. However, the ecologic distribution of plague is inadequately understood. The density of positive recovery sites seems to represent the degree of intensity of surveys as much as geographic involvement of rodents and fleas in nature. Murine typhus is endemic in several southeastern and some western states. In this instance rats and mice that infest households are the rodents of consequence. Other mammalian hosts of diseases dangerous to man that in certain areas assume importance are wild monkeys and some ruminants (in relation to yellow fever) and dogs, wolves, foxes, and bats (in relation to rabies).

Many urban and rural local health departments, as well as state health departments, have established vector control activities, usually in conjunction with their environmental health programs. Activities that are variously included are educational and promotional activities, vector surveys, research with regard to vectors, materials, and control measures, direct application of insecticides and rodenticides, licensure and supervision of pest eradicators, studies on or supervision of garbage collection, storage, and disposal, rat proofing in relation to the housing program, and elimination of mosquito breeding by spraying, drainage, filling, or variation of impounded water levels. To perform these various functions adequately a variety of types of personnel is required, that is, sanitary engineers, laboratorians, sanitarians, sanitary inspectors, and sometimes biologists, zoologists, and chemists. Of particular importance are entomologists and ecologists, to whose services and abilities increasing attention is being given by public health agencies.

## MISCELLANEOUS SANITATION ACTIVITIES

In addition to the areas of environmental health already discussed, a varied array of miscellaneous activities and programs may be carried out by health agencies. No more than passing mention will be made of them here, since most of them are of specialized and restricted importance, interest, and responsibility.

Of specific federal concern is the supervision of the salubrity of vehicles of interstate and international traffic, that is, buses, trains, boats, and airplanes. The Public Health Service, which is responsible for these activities, has developed standards for each. The maintenance of a sanitary environment in connection with parks, recreation areas, and trailer camps may be a concern of a local, state, or federal health agency, depending on the particular situation. Usually the responsibility is shared with another branch of government, such as those concerned with highways, recreation, or conservation. Related to these problems but more exclusively the responsibility of the public health agency is the supervision of the quality of swimming pools and bathing places.

## ENVIRONMENTAL HEALTH MANPOWER

In 1970 a total of 243,000 people were employed in some aspect of environmental protection in the United States—over 35,000 engineers; 37,000 scientists, sanitarians, etc; 69,000 technologists; and 101,000 environmental aides.[58] A characteristic of the persons who make up the pool of environmental health manpower is their diversity, both in disciplines and functions. They represent a wide range of the physical, biologic, and social sciences. In the physical sciences, representation extends from classic physics and chemistry through meteorology and radiation physics to hydrology, oceanography, and engineering. In the biomedical sciences, requirements extend from molecular biology, botany, and microbiology through biochemistry, pharmacology, and radiology to ecology, epidemiology, veterinary medicine, toxicology, genetics, and several clinical medical specialties. To these may be added individuals versed in mathematics, statistics, law, sociology, anthropology, political science, management, and economics. The roles and functions of the specific professional and subprofessional environmental health occupations have been evolving rather haphazardly, and for most occupations clear definition is still lacking. This is reflected in the absence of coherent and reasonably stable and agreed-upon training programs for work in the field, despite the important initiating role that insanitation played in the early development of public health efforts. Ironically, writing in 1972, Grupenhoff and Stickland[59] point to the newness of "environmental education" as a delimited subject as explaining why environmental education programs of the several federal departments and agencies are carried on in such a disjointed manner.

The foregoing list of specialties and professions is subject to some simplification. Actually it consists of some who are concerned with environmental health effects research, with environmental health technology development, and with environmental health policy and finally those involved in what might be termed *applied environmental health*. This last group is the chief concern here and comprises essentially individuals employed by public health or environmental protection agencies on the several levels of government. Aside from veterinarians, who play extremely important but somewhat specialized roles in epidemiology, and food and milk control, the majority of those involved in "action" programs are engineers, sanitarians, and environmental technologists.

Because of regional differences that exist with regard to types of problems, degree of urbanity, and availability of funds, facilities, and trained personnel, there is some difference of opinion concerning the type of training needed to direct and conduct environmental control programs. Generally rural areas and small towns have found it necessary to depend on nonengineering personnel, sometimes with no training except perhaps for a few weeks' indoctrination and orientation provided by the state health departments. In contrast, because of the complexity of their problems, urban centers have characteristically employed civil or sanitary engineers to provide the leadership for their environmental control programs. These, of course, must be augmented by a cadre of qualified sanitarians and other types of environmentalists. Engineering is concerned essentially with design, construction, and operation. Although benefits of great significance to public health result from sanitary and civil engineering, their practitioners are primarily interested in the design and construction of a waterworks system, a sewage treatment plant, air pollution control equipment, or an incinerator. They tend to focus their attention much more on construction materials, hydraulics, rates of flow, and heat losses rather than on potential morbidity decreases and other responses of those served.

Sanitary inspection, as has been pointed out, antedated sanitary engineering by a considerable period. Its efforts have been directed toward more local and personal environmental factors that were thought to exert a possible deleterious or unpleasant effect on living. During much of its development, sanitary inspection was and still is based on supposition rather than scientific knowledge, and to a considerable degree it may be regarded as largely concerned with esthetics. For a period this concern was downgraded, but interestingly both the public and health professionals in recent years are again giving it more attention on the bases of mental health and the quality of life. During recent decades, the horizon of sanitarians has been extended in many ways.[60] Substantial qualifications and detailed curricula have been developed that have been accepted and used widely by educational institutions, health agencies, and industry.[61] Increasingly the unqualified have been either upgraded or winnowed out. A certification system has been established, and sanitarians now represent a large and growing cadre of important health professionals. They may be found making significant contributions to all aspects of environmental health work.[62] It is difficult to visualize a viable public health program without them.

Under either rural or urban circumstances local health departments that provide direct service must for economy and efficiency supplement their professional engineers, veterinarians and sanitarians with auxiliary workers, commonly referred to as environmental technologists and environmental aides, to perform specific tasks under supervision. Such tasks may include obtaining samples of air, water, food, or other materials, assisting in the operation of various environmental protective facilities, and inspection and evaluation to determine compliance.[58] As in medicine, dentistry, and nursing, such individuals in significant numbers serve as valuable professional-extenders. Originally trained "on the job," in recent years these workers have had well-designed training programs developed to improve their ability and status.[63.64] Severe shortages exist in all personnel categories. There are about 14,000 environmental engineers but 24,000 needed, 18,000 sanitarians but 30,000 needed, 110,000 environmental health technologists but 138,000 needed, and 123,000 environmental health aides but 154,000 needed.

The question is sometimes raised concerning supervision. In a sense this seems academic.

Much depends on the size and nature of the community and its health program, the responsibilities placed on the latter, the availability of manpower, and sometimes custom. Smaller jurisdictions often cannot afford or make efficient use of an engineer. In such circumstances, when needed, assistance may be sought from the state. Larger jurisdictions with problems involving water and sewage treatment, air pollution, and the like must have engineering competence, but they also need sanitarians. The question of who supervises what should depend on the program. On the national and state levels this does not usually present a problem, since most environmental advisory and policy-making functions on those levels imply the employment of engineers. The difficulty arises chiefly on the local level. Many municipalities of significant size employ engineers who may plan and supervise the total environmental control program, including its inspectional phases as well as those of a more complex engineering nature. Some municipalities, on the other hand, split the functions and responsibilities into those of a true engineering nature and those that deal with sanitary standards, surveillance, and enforcement. In small communities and rural areas that are served by the usual county health department, the employment of engineering personnel is relatively rare. As a result, the environmental health program depends entirely on sanitary inspectors or increasingly and far better on sanitarians who have received formal training to qualify them as registered sanitarians.

In areas where needed professional personnel does not exist on the local level, supervision, planning, and direction should be provided by the state health department. Fortunately there is an increasing appreciation by engineers on the staffs of state health departments of their responsibility for the importance of their involvement in guidance and of assistance to local sanitation programs. This makes for a more comprehensive program in the field and enables the local sanitarian to assist with certain difficult and technical activities that formerly were handled exclusively by the state. Among these may be named the supervision of water supplies and sewage disposal systems of towns and small cities, the surveillance of milksheds, participation in programs of occupational health and safety, and the prevention of stream pollution. When the state health department endeavors to fulfill these functions alone, it is essentially an attempt at remote control. By bringing the local staff into the program the supervision and services are rendered on a day-to-day basis rather than at monthly or yearly intervals. This acknowledgement by the state of the responsibility to provide the local personnel with technical assistance and direction is expanding the usefulness of the local sanitarian considerably and is making it possible for small local health departments to provide much more adequate service to the public than would otherwise be possible.

Theoretically some of the need for supervision of the local environmental control personnel should be met by the local health officer who, after all, is ultimately responsible for all phases of the community health program. In some instances, however, this is neither attempted nor possible, since many local health officers unfortunately appear to lack the inclination, interest, or ability to assist their environmental control staffs with their problems. This provides further evidence of the need for rather extensive postmedical training in public health for physicians who aspire to become directors of public health programs.

Recent trends indicate more and more reason for closer association between the health officer and the sanitation staff and for mutual attack on problems that are really of common concern. Where formerly sanitarians may have restricted their activities to the inspection of wells, privies, and restaurants, they now, in addition, engage in many functions that cut across the direct interests of the medical health officer. Among these are intensive programs of school sanitation and education, typhus fever and malaria control, and the epidemiologic control of food and milk. Attention is called in Chapter 36 to the recent introduction in some schools of public health of courses for medical health officers in the administration and supervision of public health nursing. Under the circumstances the development of similar courses relating to the responsibilities of the health officer in the field of environmental control would also appear to be indicated.

## PRESENT ORGANIZATION OF ENVIRONMENTAL CONTROL PROGRAMS

As implied by previous comments, responsibilities and functions in environmental control are divided among the different levels of government in a variety of patterns. Generally speaking the supervision of public water supplies and sewerage systems and the prevention of stream pollution are responsibilities of the federal and state governments. The federal concern, until recently through the Public Health Service and now through the Environmental Protection Agency, is based largely on responsibility for interstate sanitation and for interstate and international public carriers, water, and air sheds. In recent decades federal grants-in-aid to states and localities have become a factor of great potential significance. State precedence over local communities in these matters results from legislative direction, the potentiality of intercommunity problems, and the availability of professionally qualified personnel in the average state health department.

In general, federal interests are concerned with research, the development of criteria and standards, and the promulgation and enforcement of various laws relating to foods, wastes, and the like. The states in turn are responsible for the establishment of state standards, the formulation and enforcement of state policies and regulations, and the promotion and general supervision of local programs. In some instances state agencies engage in the field inspection activities necessary for the implementation of the standards and regulations, but more often this is left to the local health department.

The developmental history of local health units in a state has much to do with the functional relationship that exists between the state and local agencies in matters of environmental control. Those states that were slow to promote the establishment of local health units still tend toward the centralization of sanitation activities in the state health department, even though they may now contain ample city and county health departments.

In contrast with public water and sewerage systems those private facilities that are designed to serve single or small groups of families are almost always left to the supervision of the local health department. In many instances these small private facilities are inspected only on request or complaint or when they are related to epidemiologically significant circumstances such as dairies or food processing or handling establishments. Between these two types of facilities, public and private, are some that are called semipublic facilities. These are found in tourist camps, roadside parks, comfort stations, rural schools, hospitals, and other institutions. Since they serve a number of unrelated persons

of diverse origins, they constitute an obvious public health responsibility. In some areas this is met primarily by the state, whereas in other areas the local health departments provide most of the supervision.

Aside from the variations in responsibilities for environmental control that relate to the different levels of government, the organizational and administrative picture is further complicated by the spreading of health functions, and especially environmental control functions, throughout several agencies of government on each level. Although true on all levels, it is most evident in the states. Usually the state health department has been designated as the regulatory agency responsible for public water and sewerage systems, although in some instances other departments of government, particularly state universities and special sanitary authorities, commissions, or boards, enter into certain phases of the program. The situation is more confused in some other areas of environmental control. In fact things are not much different from when they were described by Mountin and Flook[65] in the following terms:

> The acme of complexity in sanitation activities occurs in that portion of the program which involves food and drug control (including milk and shellfish sanitation) and restaurant supervision. Confusion is due to disagreement regarding what should be covered, who should be responsible and how the desired results should be attained. As a result, the division of authority and variation in procedures are so heterogeneous that they almost defy classification and description in accordance with any pattern that could be devised. Functional overlapping and interweaving apply principally to the health departments and the departments of agriculture. To a lesser degree, they involve many other State agencies among which the dairy and food commissions, hotel and restaurant commissions, livestock sanitary boards, departments of labor, departments of conservation, boards of pharmacy, state universities and colleges, and independent state laboratories are outstanding. Control methods of agencies other than the health department are usually limited to inspections, laboratory analysis of suspected products, and law enforcement.

Similar variation is found in connection with most other sanitary activities, including the control of stream pollution, industrial safety and health, insect and pest control, resort sanitation, and many others.

A common complaint therefore among public

health workers today is that environmental health concerns and authorities are being bled away by other agencies. Areas of particular concern are air pollution control, radiologic health, solid waste management, occupational health and safety, water hygiene, food and milk sanitation, housing, vector and rodent control, injury control, recreation safety or sanitation, pesticides, and hazardous product and drug surveillance. A study[66] of primary responsibility in these areas produced results shown in Table 30-2. In cases where no information was provided there is probably no program activity in a particular category. Several exceptions to that assumption may exist, such as in drug surveillance and food and milk sanitation. Similarly the 13 states and 13 cities that provided no information on injury control activities probably contain some agencies active in this area. Interestingly enough, the four program areas where "no activity" was specifically stated dealt with the problems air pollution, radiation, solid waste, and occupational health. This may indicate, at least, awareness, urgency, and need for action.

The data show that despite current trends and fears, health agencies are still, for the most part, the responsible or lead agency in the various problem areas considered. Areas where primary responsibility appears most diffused are air pollution control, solid waste management, water hygiene, food and milk processing, sanitation, and pharmaceutical surveillance. In these areas special pollution control authorities, departments of public works, public service, or sanitation, water departments or water development boards, departments of agriculture, and boards of pharmacy play significant roles. It is notable, however, that even in these instances, health agencies tend to be the most common responsible or lead agency.

The complexity of the problems encountered in these various fields is such as to regard multiple agency involvement and interagency cooperation as inevitable, if not necessary, provided respective responsibilities and authorities are carefully spelled out. Certainly public health workers may be expected to contend, and rightfully so, that each one of the program areas considered has an important health component which should be carefully considered regardless of who has primary authority for the program.

The confusion and diffusion in the face of accelerating and mounting environmental problems has brought about the beginning of a much needed trend toward consolidation of environmental planning and effort. Several references have been made to actions on the national level that resulted in the bringing together in the Environmental Protection Agency many of the responsibilities, authorities, and resources of several previously separated agencies. As of this writing, about one fifth of the state governments and a few large municipalities have followed suit. This trend has been disturbing to many in the field of public health. Some of the concern is justified and some is not. Walker[67] states the case well: "Few would venture to criticize this direction nor is the public health profession alarmed because new administrators, political and nonpolitical, and new organizations are entering the field of environmental quality control as it relates to community health." All the help possible is needed. What is disturbing, however, is a dangerous tendency in such reorganizations to underestimate the important partnership role that public health must be allowed to play in all aspects of this broader approach. Although it is certainly true that the environment has many facets, of which public health is only one, nevertheless in the final analysis it is the effect of environmental abuse and mismanagement on man and his health that constitutes the ultimate concern.

In many ways the organization of environmental control activities in the United States appears best described as disorganized. On the federal and state levels, especially, it is difficult to find any agency of government that does not have some direct or indirect concern or involvement. The remarkable extent to which this is true has been well documented by Roemer and associates,[68] who list the multitude of agencies involved in one way or another on each level of government. And this, of course, cannot begin to convey the complexities of the interagency-intergovernmental relationships required to solve a problem or to activate a program. By like token an increasing array of types of workers are involved. As indicated by Sargent,[69] the problems of environmental health are really adisciplinary; that is, they relate to no particular discipline, yet at the same time involve many disciplines, as was noted in the brief discussion of manpower. The major problems of the sciences concerned with environment, Sargent says, makes meaningless the traditional boundaries that have separated man's compartmentalization of knowledge and methodology. To paraphrase his thoughts, be-

**Table 30-2.** Agencies with sole or primary responsibilities in environmental health management in 53 states and territories and 45 major cities, United States, 1969

| Agencies with sole or primary responsibility | Air pollution control | Radiologic health | Solid waste management | Occupational health and safety | Water hygiene | Food service sanitation | Food process sanitation | Milk sanitation | Shellfish sanitation | Housing hygiene | Vector control | Injury control | Pesticide surveillance | Recreation sanitation | Hazardous products | Drug surveillance |
|---|---|---|---|---|---|---|---|---|---|---|---|---|---|---|---|---|
| *53 states and territories* | | | | | | | | | | | | | | | | |
| Health agencies | 37 | 48 | 44 | 23 | 37 | 46 | 23 | 22 | 9 | 15 | 33 | 35 | 3 | 11 | 13 | 15 |
| Health plus other agencies (see footnote) | 14[a], 1[b] | 1[c], 1[m] | 4[d] | 4[e] | 8[a], 7[b] | | 1[g] | 3[g] | 2[i] | 2[l], 3[n] | 1[g], 1[o] | 4[p] | | 1[b] | | 2[g] |
| Other agencies (see footnote) | 1 | 2[c] | 3[a], 1[b] | 5[e] | 1[a] | 5[g], 1[i] | 26[g], 1[k], 1[i] | 13[g], 1[b] | 1[g] | 5[l] | 1[g] | 1[p] | 4[g], 1[i] | | 4[g], 1[i] | 15[q], 3[g], 3[i,m] |
| Reported no activity | 1 | 1 | 1 | 10 | | | | | | | | | | | | |
| No information | 11 | 1 | | 11 | | 1 | 1 | 14 | 40 | 28 | 17 | 13 | 45 | 41 | 35 | |
| *45 major cities* | | | | | | | | | | | | | | | | |
| Health agencies | 23 | 22 | 11 | 8 | 16 | 37 | | 31 | 6 | 10 | 19 | 15 | 2 | 8 | 2 | 10 |
| Health plus other agencies (see footnote) | 14[a], 4[m,r] | | 5[d] | 1[e] | 12[f], 4[d,k,m] | 7[g] | | 4[g] | | 1[i], 2[s] | 1[i], 1[s] | 1[d,e] | | | | |
| Other agencies (see footnote) | 4 | 1[c] | 23[d] | 1[e] | 7[f], 2[a] | | | 3[g] | | 6[l] | 1[d], 1[s] | 1[t] | | | | |
| Reported no activity | | | | 19 | | | | | | | | 15 | | | | |
| No information | | 22 | 6 | 16 | 4 | 1 | | 7 | 39 | 26 | 22 | 13 | | | | |

Key: a, Special pollution control authority; b, Department of Natural Resources; c, Nuclear energy agency; d, Department of Public Works, Public Service, or Sanitation; e, Department of Labor, Labor and Industry, Industrial Relations, or Compensation Board; f, Water Department Board; g, Department of Agriculture; h, Consumer Protection Agency; i, State Laboratory or State Chemist; j, Fisheries Department or Commission; k, Department of Commission; l, Department of Housing; m, Department of Licenses and Inspection; n, Department of Community Affairs; o, Vector Control Commission; p, Department of Motor Vehicles, Police, or Public Safety; q, Board of Pharmacy; r, Building Department; s, Department of Neighborhood Improvement; t, Safety Council.

cause the problems are adisciplinary, it is necessary to develop institutions wherein problem-oriented configurations can be brought together to work effectively and efficiently. Such institutional formulations, he notes, are being explored in government at the federal and state levels, in professional organizations, and in educational institutions. Progress is slow, however, because innovation disturbs traditional values and alignments and creates insecurity in established federal baronies. What is disturbing is that the field of public health and its environmental health component appears to be included in this last category. Instead of anticipating and preparing to react to problems that are essentially of a public health nature, there seems to have transpired a period of nonresponsiveness.

In observing this with distress, Sargent concludes: "The essence of the challenge to public health is to establish itself as a significant force in planning for and in implementing meaningful action-oriented programs aimed at solving important environmental problems. To achieve such a goal, public health must develop unifying concepts that allow identification of the real problems and operationally-meaningful approaches to the solution of those problems."

## UNITED NATIONS CONFERENCE ON THE HUMAN ENVIRONMENT

It is appropriate to close this chapter with a few words about the international conference held in Stockholm by the United Nations in June 1972. By the end of the 1960s concerns about the ecologic consequences of environmental abuse reached a point where several nations suggested that a large meeting be called to discuss the problem and hopefully lay the groundwork for an international effort. The proposal was overwhelmingly approved. Meticulous planning took place through a preparatory committee, which sponsored four preliminary regional meetings that developed reports and recommendations to form part of the agenda material for the larger meeting. The World Health Organization published a book[70] on the health hazards of the human environment, prepared by some 90 specialists in 15 countries. The 10-day conference in Stockholm was in effect a double meeting. The formal sessions were attended by 1,250 official delegates from most nations. Delegates consisted of diplomats, economists, and professionals from the health and related fields. In addition to the formal delegates the meeting was attended by about 3,000 interested individuals, some of whom represented professional or conservation organizations, but a great many of whom came on their own initiative because of personal concern. In the course of the sessions these "unofficial" participants developed and held sessions of their own. There was worldwide news coverage by about 1,500 journalists.

It was and still is difficult to determine the ultimate effect of this momentous and unique international conference. It was not without problems. Several important nations did not attend for political reasons. Perhaps the most difficult problem was a difference of opinion that arose early between the more affluent industrialized nations, who urged a slowing down of development and resource use, and the developing nations, who understandably insisted on their opportunity for economic and industrial progress. The answer to this dilemma is yet to be found. Despite such limitations, the outcome was 106 recommendations that related to three major decision areas:

1. A Declaration on the Human Environment containing a set of principles designed to guide nations toward a safer environment
2. A resolution calling for the establishment of a United Nations mechanism, including a voluntary Environmental Fund to support international action on global problems
3. A recommendation for an Action Plan to attack global environmental threats through a combination of governments and international organizations

Action on each of these followed promptly. A widely publicized declaration was developed, a Secretariat for the Environment with a Governing Council of 54 members has been established within the United Nations, and the goal of $100 million in commitments to finance the first 5-year program has been fulfilled. A permanent implementing agency has been established with headquarters in Nairobi. In commenting on the conference, Maurice F. Strong of Canada, who served as the Secretary-General of the conference and who was overwhelmingly selected as the first Director of the permanent Secretariat, declared: "We have taken the first steps on a new journey of hope for the future of mankind. The fundamental task of the Stockholm Conference has been to take the political decisions that will enable the community of nations to act together in a manner consistent with the earth's physical interdependence."

## REFERENCES

1. U. S. Department of Health, Education, and Welfare: Changing environmental hazards, challenges to community health, Report of the Task Force on Environmental Health of the National Commission on Community Health Services, Washington, D. C., 1967, Government Printing Office.
2. Description of environmental health, Amer. J. Public Health **65:**928, June 1965.
3. Environmental determinants of community well-being, Scient. pub. no. 123, Washington, D. C., 1965, Pan American Health Organization–World Health Organization.
4. Marquis, R. W., editor: Environmental improvement, Washington, D. C., 1966, Graduate School, U. S. Department of Agriculture.
5. Kates, R. W., and Wohlwill, J. F., editors: Man's response to the physical environment, J. Social Issues, vol. 22, no. 4, Oct. 1966.
6. U. S. Department of Health, Education, and Welfare: A strategy for a livable environment, Report of the Task Force on Environmental Health and Related Problems, Washington, D. C., 1967.
7. Stead, F. M.: Levels in environmental health, Amer. J. Public Health **50:**312, March 1960.
8. U. S. Public Health Service: Environmental health planning guide, PHS pub. no. 823, Washington, D. C., 1967.
9. Hollis, M.: Environmental health in a rural economy, Public Health Rep. **68:**1108, Nov. 1953.
10. U. S. Public Health Service: Report of the Committee on Environmental Health Problems, PHS pub. no. 908, Washington, D. C., 1962.
11. Man—his environment and health. Report of a conference, Amer. J. Public Health **54:**(supp.), Jan. 1964.
12. Special report on water supply and pollution control—are we ready for the future? Water Works and Wastes Engin. vol. 2, 1965.
13. U. S. House of Representatives: Environmental pollution, a challenge to science and technology, Report of the Subcommittee on Science, Research and Development, to the Committee on Science and Astronautics, 89th Cong. sess. Serial S, Washington, D. C., 1966, Government Printing Office.
14. President's Science Advisory Committee: Restoring the quality of the environment, Report of the Environmental Pollution Panel, Washington, D. C., November 1965, The White House.
15. Research needs in environmental health, Washington, D. C., 1966, National Academy of Science.
16. A water policy for the American people, Report of the President's Water Resource Policy Commission, Washington, D. C., 1950, Government Printing Office.
17. Muskie, E. S.: Water pollution control needs for next 6 years, Congressional Record, E6377, July 8, 1970.
18. Hunter, J. S.: Shortcomings and remedies for the water quality improvement programs of the United States, Amer. J. Public Health **63:**345, April 1973.
19. Waste management and control, Report to the Federal Council for Science and Technology, Washington, D. C., 1966, National Academy of Sciences–National Research Council.
20. U. S. Public Health Service: Statistical summary of 1962 inventory of municipal waste facilities in the U. S., PHS pub. no. 1165, Washington, D. C., 1964.
21. 1972 Inventory, health programs in the states and territories, Washington, D. C., 1973, Association of State and Territorial Health Officers.
22. Dauer, C. C.: Summary of disease outbreaks and a 10 year résumé, Public Health Rep. **76:**915, Oct. 1961.
23. Center for Disease Control: U. S. Department of Health, Education, and Welfare: Foodborne outbreaks, annual summary, DHEW pub. no. (HSM) 73-8185, Atlanta, 1972.
24. U. S. Public Health Service: Grade "A" pasteurized milk ordinance, 1965 recommendations of the U. S. Public Health Service, PHS pub. no. 229, Washington, D. C., 1967.
25. U. S. Public Health Service: Procedures governing the cooperative state-public health service program for certification of interstate milk shippers, PHS pub. no. 1046, Washington, D. C., 1967.
26. U. S. Public Health Service: Methods of making sanitation ratings of milksheds, PHS pub. no. 678, Washington, D. C., 1966.
27. U. S. Public Health Service: Minimum sanitary standards for community infant formula services, PHS pub. no. 1625, Washington, D. C., 1967.
28. U. S. Public Health Service: The vending of food and beverages, a sanitation ordinance and code, PHS pub. no. 546, Washington, D. C., 1965.
29. U. S. Public Health Service: Food service sanitation manual, including a model food sanitation ordinance and code, PHS pub. no. 934, Washington, D. C., 1967.
30. Isaac, P. C.: Air pollution and man's health—in Great Britain, Public Health Rep. **68:**868, Sept. 1953.
31. Larson, G. P.: Air pollution and man's health—in Los Angeles, Public Health Rep. **68:**873, Sept. 1953.
32. Proceedings of the United States Technical Conference on Air Pollution, New York, 1952, McGraw-Hill Book Co.
33. Heimann, H.: Status of air pollution health research, 1966, Arch. Environ. Health **14:**488, March 1967.
34. Firket, J.: Sur les causes des accidents survenus dans la vallée de la Meuse, lors des brouillards de décembre 1930, Bull. Acad. Roy. Med. Belg. **11:**683, 1931.

35. Townsend, J. G.: Investigation of the smog incident in Donora, Pennsylvania, and vicinity, Amer. J. Public Health **40**:183, Feb. 1950.

36. Ciocco, A., and Thompson, D. J.: A follow-up of Donora ten years after, Amer. J. Public Health **51**:155, Feb. 1961.

37. McCabe, L., and Clayton, G.: Air pollution by hydrogen sulfide in Poza Rica, Mexico, Arch. Industr. Hyg. Occup. Med. **6**:199, Sept. 1952.

38. Logan, W.: Mortality in the London fog incident, 1952, Lancet **7**:336, 1953.

39. Scott, J.: Fog and deaths in London, December, 1952, Public Health Rep. **68**:474, May 1953.

40. Ludwig, J. H., and Steigerwald, B. J.: Research in air pollution: current trends, Amer. J. Public Health **55**:1082, July 1965.

41. Policy statement on radiological health, Amer. J. Public Health **50**:885, June 1960.

42. Eisenbud, M.: Industrial uses of ionizing radiation, Amer. J. Public Health, **55**:748, May 1965.

43. Longood, R. J.: Radiation accidents—the public's right to know, Amer. J. Public Health **56**:1751, Oct. 1966.

44. Bugher, J. C.: Health perspectives of our radioactive world, Amer. J. Public Health **52**:727, May 1962.

45. American Public Health Association: Ionizing radiation, New York, 1966, The Association.

46. Committee on Local Control of Ionizing Radiation of the Conference of Municipal Public Health Engineers: The responsibility of local health agencies in the control of ionizing radiation, Amer. J. Public Health **53**:1136, July 1963.

47. Brodsky, A.: Balancing benefit versus risk in the control of consumer items containing radioactive material, Amer. J. Public Health **55**:1971, Dec. 1965.

48. American Public Health Association Committee on the Hygiene of Housing; Winslow, C.-E. A., chairman: An appraisal method for measuring the quality of housing. Part I. Nature and uses of the method, 1945, The Association.

49. Anderson, G. W.: The present epidemiological basis of environmental sanitation, Amer. J. Public Health **33**:113, Feb. 1943.

50. Bauer, C.: The provision of good housing, Amer. J. Public Health **39**:462, April 1949.

51. American Public Health Association: An appraisal method for measuring the quality of housing. Parts I, II, III. Washington, D. C., 1945, 1946, 1950, The Association.

52. American Public Health Association: Housing—basic health principles and recommended ordinance, Washington, D. C., 1971, The Association.

53. American Public Health Association: Guide for health administrators in housing hygiene, Washington, D. C., 1967, The Association.

54. Molner, J. G., and Hilbert, M. S.: Responsibilities of public health administrations in the field of housing. In Housing programmes: the role of public health agencies, Geneva, 1964, World Health Organization.

55. Woodbury, C.: Impact of the urban sprawl on housing and community development, Amer. J. Public Health **50**:357, March 1960.

56. Ascher, C. S.: Regulation of housing: hints for health officers, Amer. J. Public Health **37**:507, May 1937.

57. Mood, E. W.: Health and housing programs in large cities, U.S.A., 1965, Amer. J. Public Health **56**:1540, Sept. 1966.

58. Graber, R. C., Erickson, F. K., and Parsons, W. B.: Manpower for environmental protection, Environ. Sci. Technol. **5**:314, April 1971.

59. Grupenhoff, J. T., and Strickland, S. P.: Federal laws: health/environment manpower, Washington, D. C., 1972, Science and Health Communications Group.

60. Goldsmith, F. J.: Professional development program for the sanitarian, J. Environ. Health **31**:487, March-April 1969.

61. Hatlen, J. B.: Basic academic preparation for a professional sanitarian, J. Environ. Health **33**:33, July-Aug. 1970.

62. Goldsmith, F. J.: Sanitarian's practice becomes more complex, J. Environ. Health **32**:579, March-April 1970.

63. Koren, H.: Environmental technician curriculum guidelines, J. Environ. Health **33**:155, Sept-Oct. 1970.

64. Austin, J. H., McLellon, W. M., and Dyer, J. C.: Training the environmental technician, Amer. J. Public Health **60**:2314, Dec. 1970.

65. Mountain, J. W., and Flook, E.: Distribution of health services in the structure of state government, Public Health Rep. **57**:948, June 19, 1942.

66. Hanlon, J. J.: Who manages the environment, J. Environ. Health **32**:409, Jan.-Feb. 1970.

67. Walker, B.: Environmental quality and the local health agency—a re-examination, Amer. J. Public Health **63**:352, April 1973.

68. Roemer, R., Frink, J. E., and Kramer, C.: Environmental health services, multiplicity of jurisdictions and comprehensive environmental management. In Zela, I. K., and McKinlay, J. B., editors: Organizational issues in the delivery of health services, New York, 1974, Milbank Memorial Fund.

69. Sargent, F.: Man-environment-problems for public health, Amer. J. Public Health **62**:628, May 1972.

70. Health hazards of the human environment, Geneva, 1972, World Health Organization.

CHAPTER 31

# Occupational health and safety *

## HEALTH AND THE WORKPLACE

The existence of a common ground of concern and responsibility between public health and private enterprise has become increasingly evident in recent years. Public health's concern with private enterprise is based on several factors. A fundamental consideration is that health is everybody's business. Actually, occupational health is a link between the threefold considerations of the environment, health care delivery, and consumer protection. Perhaps the most obvious interest of public health agencies in the affairs of private enterprise relates to products manufactured and sold. Certain industrial products have far-reaching potential consequences for the buying public; therefore tax-supported public health agencies bear a responsibility. The production, handling, processing, and circumstances of sale of a large number of food products are well established as big business. The paths of public health workers and private entrepreneurs therefore have long since crossed in relation to the supervision of the sanitary aspects of these products. This subject is considered elsewhere.

Another obvious and early reason for public health interest in private enterprise relates to problems brought about by the conditions of work in industry. At times workers have been exposed to grievous physical and chemical risks. There are four types of recourse against undesirable conditions of work: strikes, dis-

ability compensation, labor-management arbitration, and cooperative preventive planning and action by public health agencies, labor, and industry. The latter has led to the development and use of safety devices and to provision for the diagnosis, treatment, and prevention of occupational diseases and injuries. It is this phase of the problem that constitutes the chief concern of this chapter.

A further reason why public health agencies should be concerned with conditions of employment is the fact that a large segment of the population, in fact about 40%, spends a significant amount of their time in the work environment. In view of this the hazards of the work place cannot be looked on as if they existed in a vacuum. Not only may workers be affected by it but they may also be reached and influenced for public health purposes through their place of employment. This circumstance has been used to considerable advantage in preservice and in-service physical examinations, health education and nutrition programs, mass diagnosis, and illness and disability surveys. People are employees and employers only part of the day. The remainder of the time they are plain everyday citizens. Their influence on community health and action can be great and worth consideration in planning and providing total community services essential to the maintenance of health. Hence in any community planning for health all groups should be represented. Moreover, this planning should be for total community health and not merely for health services in the place of employment. The greatest opportunity for lifesaving and the

---

*For a series of interesting presentations of various aspects of the subject, see "Occupational Health, 1914-1964," *Public Health Reports.*[1]

prevention of disease and disability lies, at the present time, in the age and social class represented by the wage earner. This is also the point of greatest social and economic productivity and potential. The approach through industry, business, and labor unions to the health of the wage earner offers the same administrative advantages inherent in school health programs, that is, large numbers readily accessible and, from the community standpoint, a group whose health is vitally important and peculiarly at risk.

This raises a question that must be faced up to by the nation—whether it is proper to provide preventive, diagnostic, and therapeutic medical services for any and all illnesses, regardless of their source, within the place of occupation where so many people are concentrated and where facilities are or could be made conveniently available. Large centers of employment are community assets, and many of them are already involved in a variety of group health plans.[2] It would seem logical to regard and use them as an important part of the total community health care system with their staffs augmented or backstopped by the private practitioners and medical institutions of the community. This would be especially feasible when a national health care program comes into existence.

Finally, if proper relationships are developed, support of the general public health program of no small magnitude and significance may be obtained from those in positions of responsibility and authority in private business and industry, as well as in labor unions. The nature of occupational health activities requires accessible service and a close relationship between the public health administrator and the industrialist. Through an effective and profitable program of occupational health and safety and product sanitation the health officer is in a position to meet and influence the industrialists and businessmen of his community on their own terms with the importance of the total public health program. The health officer should always bear in mind that businessmen and industrialists are citizens too and that business and industrial enterprises produce the economic lifeblood of the modern community.

Programs and activities concerned with the well-being of workers exist under numerous labels in various times and places, that is, industrial or occupational health, hygiene, safety, engineering, welfare, or medicine. As a result

of the gradual coming together and synthesis of the various interests implied by these designations and the ever-broadening view of the many factors that are involved in the well-being and efficiency of workers, a tendency to refer to the entire area of interest as occupational health has come about. In general it appears that the label and definition given to the field has depended essentially on the profession of primary interest or background of the discussant. In this regard Hussey[3] appropriately wrote the following:

This whole subject of occupational health and medicine is analogous to a three-legged stool, one leg representing medical science, one representing engineering and chemical science, and one representing the social sciences.... Up to the present we have been trying to balance ourselves on two legs and in some instances on one leg. It is a very uncomfortable position and one that cannot get us very far and certainly will lead, as it has, to fatigue.

A Joint Committee of the International Labor Office and the World Health Organization has defined the objectives of occupational health as follows[4]:

... the promotion and maintenance of the highest degree of physical, mental and social well-being of workers in all occupations; the prevention among workers of departures from health caused by their working conditions; the protection of workers in their employment from risks resulting from factors adverse to health; the placing and maintenance of the worker in an occupational environment adapted to his physiological and psychological condition.

## BACKGROUND

Ramazzini is usually considered to be the father of occupational health, based on the publication in the early eighteenth century of his treatise *Diseases of Tradesmen*. Modern occupational health is an outcome of the industrial revolution in nineteenth century England. As a result of the rapid development of deplorable work conditions, in general, and the exploitation of women and children, in particular, numerous laws were passed for the protection of workers. After a short lag period there came about what Legge[5] referred to as the "American Industrial Renaissance." During this period America profited by the events, researches, and measures that had previously occurred in England, even to the extent of adoption by some states of some of the earlier English legislation. In 1908 Congress passed the Federal Employers' Liability Act, which made railroads and other interstate carriers liable for industrial injuries sustained by their employees. At that time the Wainwright Commission in New York showed that only 1 out of every 8 injured men was awarded any compensation and that he actually received only about a third of what was awarded. The other two thirds went for insurance adjusters, legal advice, and commissions. Various states had previously enacted workmen's compensation laws, but these early laws were declared unconstitutional by the courts. The year 1911, however, marked the beginning of the first valid state workmen's compensation laws, and no less than 10 states passed legislation in that year alone. There followed an era of compensation medical service, and employers were made increasingly responsible for the medical and surgical care of workers who became injured or ill at their jobs and for payment of accident and disease compensation.

Meanwhile increasing attention was being given to the identification, definition, and diagnosis of occupational diseases, that is, silicosis, plumbism, anthrax, benzol and radium poisoning, and many others. A separate development of occupational disease compensation laws resulted, among the earliest of which were California and Wisconsin (1919), North Dakota (1925), and Minnesota and Connecticut (1929). Unfortunately many of these compensation laws were hastily promulgated during a period of considerable public stimulation and concern, with the result that many were extreme, ill advised, and impractical. Under the circumstances extensive subsequent amendment is not surprising. At the present time workmen's compensation laws exist in all 50 states.

As Hatch[6] has indicated, the period 1910 to 1920 witnessed the firm establishment of occupational health as a specialty. The Department of Labor was established as a separate Cabinet entity, the Bureau of Mines of the Department of the Interior and the Office of Industrial Hygiene and Sanitation (later the Division of Occupational Health) of the Public Health Service came into existence, an Industrial Hygiene Section was established in the American Public Health Association, and the National Safety Council was organized. Two of the most significant events were the organization in 1915 of the American Association of Industrial Physicians and Surgeons (now the Industrial Medical Association) and the

adoption of minimum standards for medical service in industry by the Committee on Industrial Medicine and Traumatic Surgery of the American College of Surgeons. Some years later, in 1937, the American Medical Association created the Council on Industrial Health to coordinate all medical efforts in the industrial health field. The *Journal of Industrial Hygiene* and the first specialized teaching of the subject appeared in schools of public health at about the same time.

Prior to the passage of the federal Social Security Act in 1935 little progress had been made by state health agencies in occupational health. Up to that time only 5 states engaged in any activities designed for the benefit of industrial workers. The first were instituted in 1913 in New York and Ohio. The act made funds available for the expansion of state and local programs as well as other forms of activity, with the result that by 1950 all of the states and Alaska, Hawaii, Puerto Rico, and the District of Columbia were engaged in some type of activity for the improvement of health and safety of workers in gainful occupations.[7] These are only a few of the many landmarks in the development of this important field.[8,9]

## NATURE AND SCOPE OF THE PROBLEM

The hazards to the work force may be looked at in terms of injuries, illnesses and deaths from accidents, and occupational diseases caused by the work place. Valid national statistics on the nature and causes of occupational diseases and industrial accidents do not exist. Detailed statistics are compiled by several state workmen's compensation and labor authorities, but these are not strictly comparable because of substantial variations in sources of data and tabulation procedures. Individually they contribute little to national programs for prevention and control. Nevertheless, some statistics on injury and disease are available.

For occupational injuries and deaths caused by work accidents some data are available from the Federal Bureau of Labor Statistics, the National Safety Council, the National Health Survey, and individual states. It should be pointed out, however, that of all the 52 major jurisdictions in the United States (the 50 states, District of Columbia, and Puerto Rico) only 33 require the keeping of accident reports by the employer. Because of increased emphasis placed on occupational safety since the Korean War, accidental deaths on the job have stayed remarkably constant at around 14,200 per year from 1955 to 1969, despite a 34% increase in the number of workers (from 59.4 million to 80 million). This means a reduction in the death rate from 24 per 100,000 workers in 1955 to 18 per 100,000 workers in 1969. If continued emphasis on worker safety is assumed, the number of on-the-job deaths should remain at the 14,220 mark during the next decade, despite the 25% projected increase in the number of workers in that period. A death rate therefore of 14.2 per 100,000 workers is expected.

In the period 1958 to 1966 injuries on the job rose steadily from a low of 1.8 million to a high of 2.2 million. The injury rate per worker per year remained steady at 3.03%. Since 1966, however, the number of injuries has remained constant at 2.2 million per year for a rate of 2.75% in 1969. In the absence of desirably exact definition and analysis, it can be said that a large proportion of these injuries are of minor consequence. As with the accidental deaths, it is reasonable to assume that the number of injuries should hold steadily at 2.2 million for the next decade. By 1980 therefore an injury rate reduced to 2.2% would be expected.

When occupational disease and illness are considered, however, the available data are poor. Of all the states, California may be considered the only one with any reasonable occupational disease data. If the California data are assumed to be valid and reflect conditions nationally, one can project that approximately 390,000 cases of occupational disease occur annually in the United States. This is probably an underestimation, but even if correct, it represents a significant problem.

There are several reasons for poor occupational disease data. Nonrecognition and nonreporting of diseases are probably paramount.[10] In addition, there are long development times of exposure before disease is manifested. For example, silicosis does not occur usually until after about 15 years of exposure. Other dust diseases, such as byssinosis and asbestosis, also have prolonged developmental periods. In addition, there is a lag time between the onset of the disease process in the body and clinical evidence of frank disease. This holds true even though exposure may have long since ceased. Cases of beryllium poisoning, for example, have become manifest as long as 20 years after the last known exposure.[11]

Despite their inexactness, some examples

of the incidence of various occupational diseases may be illustrative. It has been estimated that 125,000 active or former coal miners have radiographic evidence of pneumoconiosis; nearly 50,000 men may be disabled, and about 4,000 men die annually as a result of it.[12] Three and a half million American workers are exposed to asbestos on the job. Significant numbers of them develop asbestosis, which often leads to mesothelioma, or cancer of the lung pleura. Studies of asbestos insulation workers indicate that half of the men who had worked in the trade for 20 years had x-ray evidence of asbestosis, and 1 in every 10 of their deaths was due to mesothelioma, in contrast with 1 in 10,000 in the general public.[13] Byssinosis, a lung disease caused by cotton mill dust, was long said not to occur in America. Studies in recent years give estimates of about 17,000 cases in the industry.[14] Talc, diatomite, sugarcane fiber, and dust from moldy silage all produce various forms of respiratory diseases among workers. Of the 6,000 men who are or have been uranium miners, an estimated 600 to 1,100 will die of lung cancer within the next 20 years because of radiation exposure on the job. Large numbers of workers are exposed to heavy metals, each of which exacts its toll—lead, mercury, arsenic, beryllium, to name only a few (see Gafafer[10] for details of substances, workers, and industries). Hundreds of thousands of workers each year suffer skin diseases from contact with materials used in their work. Dermatoses are the most common of all occupational diseases. An estimated 7 million industrial workers are exposed to noise levels that cause impaired hearing among many.

Another important aspect of occupational health and safety is the additive effect of mental stresses the worker brings from his home to the work place. These may be domestic or neighborhood problems, concerns about economics or illness in the family, the use of drugs or alcohol, or other forms of delinquency. Such stresses cannot but affect the worker's safety on the job, and it is reasonable to expect them to exacerbate work-generated stresses. In the same way stresses in his work environment can affect an employee's health and safety off the job. Such terms as *ulcerogenic jobs, crawling up the walls,* and *the daily grind or rat race* are based on much more than apparent humor. A worker subjected to the stresses of noise, vibration, solvents, speed-ups, or overbearing supervisors can become occupational casualties just as much as if they inhaled dust or were exposed to toxic chemicals.[15] Occupational health and safety programs are not complete without consideration of these psychologic considerations, but unfortunately few have given them significant attention.[16]

## BENEFITS

Serious attention to and support of occupational and public health activities carry with them many benefits to private enterprise. Three of the greatest items of loss to business and industry are labor turnover, absenteeism, and liability compensation for occupational illness and injury. Among the tangible profits of good community and occupational health programs are remedies against these three sources of loss. A healthy worker is a happier, more dependable worker with high morale and pride in his work. He will tend to remain in his position rather than search for another.

According to statistics of the National Safety Council[17] for the year 1970 there occurred 2.3 million work-related disabling injuries. Of these, 14,200 resulted in death, and about 90,000 resulted in permanent disability. In addition to the liability compensation involved, this constituted a work loss to industrial production and an estimated total economic loss of over $4 billion. Manufacturing industries have gained the most, with a reduction in their occupational death rate of about 40% during the past 20 years. In fact, it is interesting that the work-related death rate for manufacturing occupations was only 10 per 100,000 workers in contrast with 23 per 100,000 workers in nonmanufacturing employment. It is further significant that the overall on-the-job death rate was 20 per 100,000 workers in contrast with an off-the-job death rate of 54 per 100,000 workers. The improvements noted have been largely due to the efforts of the National Safety Council, the National Association of Manufacturers, and the Industrial Conference, which comprises 160 top safety experts. In return a reduction in absenteeism of 20% to 30% has been noted.

Several factors are involved in such striking results from occupational health and safety programs:

1. Occupational health personnel have done much to control environmental hazards, thereby providing built-in safety measures, which in turn result in a greater sense of security and employment satisfaction in the worker.

2. Occupational health personnel are more likely to make the worker realize that his welfare and employment career are partly dependent on his own sense of responsibility for maintaining his health, safety, and working ability.

3. A sound occupational health program makes possible a gradual and selective return to work consistent with the degree and speed of recovery.

4. Competent occupational medical and nursing personnel have had a desirable persuasive effect on patients and their physicians, which often results in the seeking of early preventive and curative private medical care and in a demand for private medical service of high quality.

5. Occupational health personnel have developed effective and appropriate techniques for the detection and handling of occasional malingerers.

6. Occupational health services form a link between the workers' total health problems and the community health and social services.

Other benefits to business and industry are a diminution in employee grievances, improved employee relations and consequently improved public relations, increased worker and community pride in the company and its products, and the enhanced appeal and advertising value of a clean plant, healthy, contented employees, and a sanitary product. Out of 1,625 companies completing questionnaires concerning the value of industrial health programs, only 5 companies failed to report to the National Association of Manufacturers that they considered their health program a paying proposition.

The important point is that health problems and resonsibilities are always present in the plant or in the office, whether or not industry and business want to recognize them and whether or not they wish to do anything about them. If they do accept these responsibilities, they not only perform an important public service but, as already pointed out, may also turn that recognition and action to their own financial advantage. On the other hand, if they refuse to recognize their health problems and responsibilities, it automatically becomes incumbent upon official public health agencies, acting in the public interest, to step in and do something about the situation. However, from the standpoint of official agencies there is much to be gained by interesting private enterprise in meeting its own problems.

In the past private enterprise, business, and industry traditionally have been highly regarded by the public. During recent years, the public has also developed an intense interest in matters of personal and community health. This is indicated by studies of shifts in social prestige over the past three decades. The most notable change has been the replacement of the banker and businessman by the physician as the individual enjoying the highest prestige in America today. Here, therefore, is a situation in which business and industry may work with another high prestige group to mutual advantage in providing valuable community leadership and achieving even greater public esteem as well as efficiency in the process. Many large companies and industrial concerns have already seen the value of following this line of action and not only are cooperating actively with official public health agencies but, in addition, on their own initiative are engaging in employee health programs, plant safety, and product sanitation activities of considerable consequence.

Occupational health programs therefore bring many benefits—to the employee, to the employer, and to the community. For the employee and his dependents it means better personal health and sustained earnings, lower personal medical and hospital expenditures, increased and prolonged productive capacity, and the enjoyment and security that comes with good health and job satisfaction. For the employer it means decreased production costs because of lower labor turnover, less absenteeism, fewer disability payments, lower insurance, and more capable and more alert workers. It also brings higher worker morale and desirable labor-management relations. All of these result in diffused but extensive benefits to the community in increased prosperity, decreased welfare costs, less labor-management strife, and increased pressures for and support of high quality medical, hospital, and public health services.

## OCCUPATIONAL HEALTH AND SAFETY PROGRAMS

It is appropriate to preface a discussion of the objectives and content of occupational health and safety programs by a pertinent comment made some years ago by the Director of Industrial Hygiene of one of the world's largest industrial corporations.[18] It is fairly representative of the basic approach and attitude of the private sector. "Business," he pointed out "is conducted on a practical, or profit and loss, basis and when losses equal or exceed profits, you do not stay in business long. Industrial hygiene programs that are not basically sound are not likely to survive the test of time." On the other hand, from the viewpoint of the public an occupational health program is designed primarily for the benefit and welfare of the workers. Its objectives are the following[19]:

1. Assessment of a worker's physical and psychological assets, as well as his liabilities, to facilitate proper selection and placement
2. Prevention of occupational and nonoccupational illnesses
3. Provision of treatment, the type and extent of which depends on the policy of the organization
4. Fostering of a personal, physical, mental, and social ability to work and enjoy life beyond the mere absence of disease or infirmity

The inclusion of psychologic, mental, and social factors merits particular note. There are indications that up to 30% of absenteeism is due to emotional disturbances resulting from interpersonal problems in the plant, in the home, and in the community.

Many factors influence the nature and extent of an occupational health and safety program that a business or an industry may find it worth while to carry out. Among these are the type of industry or business; the nature of its product and of the ingredients and equipment used in its manufacture; the disposition of the product; the size and location of the establishment; the complex attitudes and relationships among top management, labor unions, the community and its medical profession, public health agency, and government; and the organizational status of the unit responsible for the activities. For these reasons it is obvious that a detailed standard pattern is impossible. To the contrary, each program must be more or less tailored to fit the needs and circumstances of the particular situation. It is possible, however, to state certain fundamental principles that should apply in general. Thus the Council on Industrial Health of the American Medical Association[20] lists the objectives of an occupational health program to be (1) to protect individuals against health hazards in their work environment, (2) to ensure and facilitate the suitable placement of individuals according to their physical capacities and their emotional makeup in work that they can perform with an acceptable degree of efficiency and without endangering their own health and safety or that of their fellow employees, and (3) to encourage personal health maintenance.

The scope of services that should be provided by the medical department of an industry, should include the following:

1. Regular appraisal of plant sanitation
2. Periodic inspection for occupational disease hazards
3. Adoption and maintenance of adequate control measures
4. Provision of first aid and emergency services
5. Prompt and early treatment for all illnesses resulting from occupational exposure
6. Reference to the family physician of individuals with conditions needing attention, cooperating with the patient and physician in every practical way to remedy the condition
7. Uniform recording of absenteeism due to all types of disability
8. Impartial health appraisals of all workers
9. Provision of rehabilitation services within industry
10. The conduct of a beneficial health education program

Adequately expanded, developed, and adapted to the particular circumstances, these areas of activity would provide a satisfactory occupational health program in most situations.

Because of the large numbers of employees involved, many of the larger business and industrial concerns find it practical to operate most or all of their employee health and safety programs themselves. One of the greatest problems relates to small plants and businesses, which are in the majority and which taken together employ the major proportion, 60%, of workers. Individually they are usually too small to afford or justify the employment of even a single full-time nurse, much less a physician.[21] Unfortunately they have been largely left out of the picture except for essentially token services rendered by state and occasionally local health departments. To overcome the problem there has been a trend toward the joint employment, by groups of small industrial plants, of full-time health personnel who devote the necessary number of hours a week to each plant in the group. This plan has proved of value in several locations. For the supervision of the environmental hazards of small plants various types of portable or mobile equipment have also been used to advantage.[22]

## ROLE OF GOVERNMENT

Since the occupational environment is part of the total community to which the public health agency is responsible, it is to be expected that the latter have appropriate interest in the field. Reference has been made to the relatively slow growth of occupational health programs in governmental agencies, beginning with the initiation of activities in 1913 in New York and Ohio. Activity and interest accelerated with the passage of the Social Security Act in 1935 and again during the period of the World War II. In 1940 more than one fourth of the state health agencies had no occupational health activities. By 1950, however, all but 8 agencies had at least one professional employee assigned to this field on a full-time basis.[6] The overall picture in 1960 was 51 state and territorial health departments, 42 labor departments, 16 departments of mines, 15 industrial accident boards or commissions, and several other agencies participating in some manner in occupational health activities. In addition, an ever-increasing number of local jurisdictions, especially those of an urban nature, are engaged in occupational health activities to some extent.

In general, the function of government agencies on the state and local levels in occupational health and safety[23,24] includes surveys and field investigations of environmental conditions in industry; the collection and analysis of data relating to occupational ills and injuries and to absenteeism; the surveillance of atmospheric pollution and radiation in industrial plants; the development of techniques for the detection of occupational disease, methods of prevention and control, and the development of specific treatment. Health departments concentrate on the supervision of environmental conditions conducive to employment-related illness. They suggest measures for control, promote in-plant sanitation and medical services, provide advisory engineering and nursing services, and conduct health educational activities. Departments of labor and mines are primarily concerned with safety measures and the regulation of working conditions. The industrial or occupational health units of these agencies, in addition to their specific functions, coordinate their activities and services with those of units concerned with sanitation, health education, and preventable and chronic disease, thereby attempting to bring to industry a well-rounded health program. In addition, they usually maintain cooperative working relations with labor, management, and various pertinent professional societies.

To varying degrees state agencies are charged with the enforcement of laws relating to the field of occupational health. It is interesting, however, that whereas state health departments are the agencies most frequently responsible for general occupational health and safety functions, labor departments are more often charged with enforcement powers.[25]

On the basis of the considerable experience of the California State Department of Health, Abrams[26] warns that a governmental occupational health and safety agency must observe certain basic principles if its work is to be successful:

1. It has primary responsibility to safeguard the health of workers.
2. Its technical work and its policies must be unbiased.
3. It must be able to speak authoritatively regarding health hazards and the adequacy of measures for protecting the health of employees.
4. It must be able to interpret intelligently its program to labor and management and to the health professions.
5. It should endeavor so to conduct studies that not only the plant's previous methods and programs but also its own are improved thereby.

It is of interest to compare these with the characteristics which a representative of industry said at the same time that industry expects of health agencies.[27] They may be summarized as follows:

Availability of services—speed, quality, and quantity balanced

Uniformity—of advice, standards, methods

Accuracy—evaluations based on technical data or mature experience

Clarity—clear reports with understandable terminology

Practicality—recommendations economically feasible

Palatability—recommendations couched in persuasive language

Tact—in the conduct of investigations to prevent fears, suspicion, or misunderstanding

Balance—representation of pertinent professions needed for an adequate program

It is obvious that the problem of occupational health and safety is large and complex. Furthermore, it is certainly destined to become even more complicated and to require the services of still more types of specialists including the nuclear physicist. Because of its complexity and its many ramifications, it is impossible for any single group or agency to provide a complete solution. This can be achieved only by sincere teamwork on the part of all groups concerned. Thus management must accept moral and legal responsibility for the provision of safe and healthy work conditions. Labor must accept the responsibility of convincing its members that they should cooperate with measures taken in good faith in their behalf. Industrial and public health workers must fulfill their legal responsibilities to ensure a safe and sanitary environment for industrial workers. Finally, the community must accept its responsibility to provide continuing and contiguous safeguards and services for the nonindustrial environments and hours of the worker.

On the national level occupational health and safety programs are conditioned by the stage of social and educational development and the spectrum of bases of the economy of the particular nation involved. The form of political system and health organization, of course, also play key roles. Generally speaking, what has been described would apply to greater or lesser degrees in most of the developed nations. Occupational health and safety programs in the developing nations, however, are hampered by several additional problems, among which may be found extensive communicable illness, malnutrition, inadequate manpower, managerial inexperience, and careless exploitation of human and natural resources. Many obtain assistance toward the solution of such problems from the World Health Organization, the International Labor Office, the International Bank for Reconstruction and Development (World Bank), various bilateral technical assistance agencies, foundations, and universities.[28]

In the United States several important forward steps have been taken in the past few years.[29] One of them was the passage of the Federal Coal Mine Health and Safety Act of 1969 (P.L. 91-173), which placed significantly increased responsibilities on the Secretary of Health, Education, and Welfare and the Secretary of the Interior. For the first time in this country a federal law recognized a specific disease, coal workers' pneumoconiosis or "black lung," required radiographic examination of all exposed workers, and provided federal funds to pay some remuneration to its victims as well as to survivors of deceased miners. By the end of the first quarter of 1973 over 73,000 of the

90,000 coal miners in the United States had been x-rayed, and files including diagnoses were complete on about 65,000. Between 12% and 13% of them were found to be affected. The legislation also provided for stringent dust standards and penalties for failure to comply. Of great potential was the enactment of the Occupational Safety and Health Act of 1970 (P.L. 91-596). This elevated the existing program to the status of the National Institute for Occupational Safety and Health. Among the responsibilities given to it were research on occupational safety and health problems, hazard evaluation, toxicity determinations, manpower development and training, industry-wide studies of chronic or low level exposures to hazardous substances, and research on psychologic, motivational, and behavioral factors as they relate to occupational safety and health. Several field stations are used in Cincinnati, Salt Lake City, and Morgantown, W. Va.

A quarter century ago, Winslow[30] editorialized in the following manner:

There is no single, perfect solution of this problem now in sight. There is rather a challenge to the inventiveness of management, labor, the medical profession, and the public to find empirically the best plan that will fit a given local situation. For management and labor, the need for cooperation in the meeting of a common problem is called for rather than insistence on vested interests. For the medical profession, it seems certain that the principles of group payment and group practice must be essential to any sound solution. For the public health authorities, leadership in research, formulation of reasonable standards of attainment, and assistance to small industries, where desirable, would appear to be the appropriate role.

More recently, in discussing the considerable challenges presented in the field and the extensive personnel needs to meet them, Kehoe[31] noted that (1) the industrial population of the United States is more than 60 million persons (it is now about 80 million), (2) technologic developments in industry now expose workers to countless numbers and types of inadequately explored chemical and physical hazards, and (3) the incidence of known varieties of occupational disease within the industrial population is unknown and the unrecognized, nondisabling impairments of health that occur have yet to be explored. It would appear therefore that Winslow's comment is destined to remain valid for many more years.

**REFERENCES**

1. Occupational health, 1914-1964, Public Health Rep. **79:**941, Nov. 1964.
2. Colwell, M. O.: The balance sheet in employee health conservation, J. Occup. Med. **13:**103, March 1971.
3. Hussey, R.: In discussion of an article by Hemeon, W. C. L.: Engineering in industrial health education, J. Occup. Med. **4:**201, Aug. 1947.
4. Occupational health, W.H.O. Techn. Rep. Ser. no. 66, Geneva, 1963, World Health Organization.
5. Legge, R. T.: Progress of American industrial medicine in the first half of the twentieth century, Amer. J. Public Health **52:**904, Aug. 1952.
6. Hatch, T.: Major accomplishments in occupational health in the past fifty years, Industr. Hyg. J. **25:**108, March-April 1964.
7. U. S. Public Health Service: Distribution of health services in the structure of state government, PHS pub. no. 184, 1950, Washington, D. C., 1954.
8. U. S. Public Health Service: Man, medicine and work, PHS pub. no. 1044, Washington, D. C., 1964.
9. U. S. Public Health Service: Fifty years of occupational health, PHS pub. no. 1171, Washington, D. C., 1964.
10. Gafafer, W. M., editor: Occupational diseases, a guide to their recognition, PHS pub. no. 1097, Washington, D. C., 1966.
11. Johnstone, R. T., and Miller, S. E.: Occupational diseases and industrial medicine, Philadelphia, 1960, W. B. Saunders Co.
12. Kerr, L. E.: Coal workers pneumoconiosis in an affluent society, Public Health Rep. **85:**847, Oct. 1970.
13. Selikoff, I. J., Churg, J., and Hammond, E. C.: Relation between exposure to asbestos and mesothelioma, New Eng. J. Med. **272:**560, March 18, 1965.
14. U. S. Public Health Service: Byssinosis, a review of the problem with recommendations for action; Report prepared by Bureau of Occupational Safety and Health, Rockville, Md., Dec. 1969.
15. The psycho-social environment in industry, WHO Chron. **14:**276, July 1960.
16. Hirschfeld, A. H., Wagenheim, H. F., Hagen, D. Q., et al.: Interpersonal relations in industry: a positive approach to industrial mental health, Amer. J. Public Health **60:**2094, Nov. 1970.
17. Accident facts, Chicago, 1971, National Safety Council.
18. Patty, F. A.: The industrial hygiene program in industry, Amer. J. Public Health **41:**971, Aug. 1951.
19. Cameron, D. C.: Human relations in occupational health, Public Health Rep. **67:**686, July 1952.
20. Council on Industrial Health of the American

Medical Association: Scope, objectives, and functions of occupational health programs, J.A.M.A. **164:**1104, July 6, 1957.

21. Howe, H. F.: Preventing occupational health and safety hazards in small employee groups, Amer. J. Public Health **61:**1581, Aug. 1971.

22. Small plant health services—conference report, Public Health Rep. **75:**615, July 1960.

23. U. S. Public Health Service: Occupational health services for employees, a guide for state and local governments, PHS pub. no. 1041, Washington, D. C., 1963.

24. American Public Health Association: Local health official's guide to occupational health, Washington, D. C., 1968, The Association.

25. 1972 Inventory, health programs in the states and territories, Washington, D. C., 1973, Association of State and Territorial Health Officers.

26. Abrams, H. K.: Labor, management, and the official agency, Amer. J. Public Health **42:**38, Jan. 1952.

27. Newman, L. E.: What industry expects of the official industrial hygiene agencies, Amer. J. Public Health **43:**330, March 1953.

28. Occupational health programmes, WHO Chron. **26:**537, Dec. 1972.

29. Key, M. M. New horizons in industrial health, Health Services Rep. **88:**195, March 1973.

30. Editorial: Administrative problems of industrial medicine, Amer. J. Public Health **37:**1338, Oct. 1947.

31. Kehoe, R. A.: Occupational medicine and public health, Public Health Rep. **76:**645, July 1961.

*There is no such thing as an accident.
What we call by that name is the effect
of some cause which we do not see.*

**VOLTAIRE**

CHAPTER 32

# Consumer protection and accident prevention

## EMERGENCE OF THE PROBLEM

In the discussion of the philosophy and content of public health, its ever-broadening vista and the constant extension of its activities were described. It was pointed out that the present-day public health agency must be interested in the well-being of the total individual and the total community life. Accordingly it concerns itself wherever feasible with all factors that may adversely affect any phase of the physical and mental health of the community and its population. As a result, the public health worker finds himself involved more and more in what some might consider fringe activities. Actually to consider them as such is erroneous. Merely because certain problems require joint action with other community agencies or groups, they are not necessarily of a fringe or tangential nature. Indeed, it should be realized that joint or community action is the essence of public health programs. Accident prevention represents a good example.

If there is ever a tendency for people to consider disease or disability fatalistically, it is most likely to be in relation to accidents.[1] In fact, the average person in even the most advanced societies tends to define the word *accident* as something due to chance, over which the individual has little if any control. This negative attitude explains to a considerable degree why so little concerted attention has been given to the problem until recent years. Gradually, however, several factors have captured the attention of certain groups in society. Each has attempted in its own way and for various reasons to explore approaches to solution. Some partial progress has resulted. The large life insurance companies were perhaps the first to give attention to this problem. With a major portion of the population in the United States now covered by some type of life or disability insurance it has become increasingly important to these companies that everything possible be done to decrease the extent of accidental disability or death. At the same time it is of importance to the policyholder, not only from the standpoint of avoiding suffering or death but also in terms of lowering the costs of policies. As a result, some of the best health educational work and promotion of home safety has been conducted by the large insurance companies. For somewhat similar reasons, although companies that ensure against losses due to fire have the reduction of material losses as their primary interest, they nevertheless have also been involved in the prevention of fire injuries and deaths. Industries, particularly the large industries, have carried out safety programs of considerable magnitude involving the installation of various safety devices and careful worker selection, placement, and education. Increasing costs of tax-supported service for fire prevention, emergency care, and hospitalization have caused public officials to look for means of re-

586

ducing the extent of accidents from all causes. Finally, as just mentioned, public health workers have become aware of the ever-growing threat of accidents to well-being and of the relationships of certain types of accidents to various mental or physiologic factors with which they were already concerned. Gradually therefore the fatalistic attitude that accidents are events that just happen has been changing. Increasingly individuals and agencies have been getting together to see if something positive could be done about the problem.

## EXTENT OF THE PROBLEM

Currently about 114,000 people are killed each year by accidents in the United States. This amounts to about 13 deaths each hour. The number of nonfatal accidents is more difficult to determine, since many of them never come to official attention. On the basis of reports, insurance claims, and the like the National Safety Council has estimated that there are about 100 injuries for each fatality, or a total of almost 11 million.[2] However, the National Health Survey,[3] through its household interviews, determined a total of about 50 million nonfatal injuries of all types and degrees of severity during the year July 1967 to June 1968. (In 1967 almost 52 million injuries were estimated.) Slightly more than half, or 27.6 million people required restricted activity; 11 million of these required convalescence in bed, 2 million of whom were hospitalized. These accidents resulted in 550 million days of restricted activity, including 141 million spent in bed at home or in a hospital. Altogether the cost of accidents in terms of lost wages, medical expenses, and other factors has been estimated by the National Safety Council to amount to a staggering total of about $22.7 billion in 1968. Although three fifths of all the accidents involved males, there is an interesting sex variation by age. Male accidental death rates exceed those in females of all ages except the most advanced. Accidental death rates for males are only slightly in excess of rates for females up to about the fifteenth year of life, after which male accidental death rates increase sharply and remain high from then on. By contrast, accidental death rates for females remain relatively low until about the sixty-fifth year, after which they rise sharply and exceed those in males at age 85 years. An unusual study[4] of 50,000 child years of accidental injury in which 8,874 children were followed for 16 years

showed that the rate for all medically attended nonfatal injuries was 246 per 1,000 children per year. Boys had more injuries than girls at all ages, and their injury rate increased with age, whereas for girls it went down. It was also noted that children with high rates at one age tended to have high rates in subsequent periods of childhood.

The carnage occurs in all parts of the environment—in automobiles, on the streets, in the home, at work, and on the farm as well as in the city. About five eighths of nonfatal accidents are urban, two eighths are rural nonfarm, and one eighth is rural farm. Because of their dramatic nature, accidents involving public or private vehicles tend to monopolize the public attention. These, however, are only a part of a much larger problem. Accidental injuries and deaths by place of occurrence present an interesting picture (Table 32-1). Whereas the home is the most dangerous locale in terms of frequency of accidents, motor vehicles are most dangerous in terms of serious injury or death.

Motor vehicle accidents rose sharply after World War I and have continued high. Annual deaths from this cause were about 12,500 in 1920 but by 1930 had risen to about 33,000. They have continued to climb more slowly but constantly, except for the tire and gasoline rationing period of World War II. By 1971 motor vehicular deaths reached 55,000. During the period since World War I, however, the death rate from motor vehicle accidents per 10,000 motor vehicles registered has dropped significantly. Thus in 1920 it was about 13.5 deaths per 10,000 cars registered, whereas now it is only about 5.5 deaths per 10,000 cars registered. Similarly in terms of vehicular deaths per 100 million miles traveled, the rate has dropped from about 14.0 in 1925 to 5.6 in 1971. Nevertheless, both in terms of absolute numbers of deaths and deaths per 1,000 injuries, motor vehicle accidents are by far the most serious part of the problem.

Occupational injuries and deaths have been subjected to a considerable reduction. For example, in terms of injuries per million man-hours, the frequency in 1926 was 32 injuries as against about 7 now. Work-related accidents do not appear to be as severe in terms of fatalities as do motor vehicle accidents, deaths per thousand injuries for the former being about one sixth those of the latter.

Accidents in the home are particularly important because of their frequency, which ap-

**Table 32-1.** Annual distribution of accidental injuries and deaths by location

| Location | Injuries | | | Deaths | Deaths per 1,000 injuries |
| | Total | Activity restricted | Hospitalized | | |
|---|---|---|---|---|---|
| Motor vehicle | 4,702,000 | 3,004,000 | 890,000 | 40,000 | 8.5 |
| Home | 19,137,000 | 10,974,000 | 469,000 | 27,700 | 1.4 |
| Work | 8,150,000 | 4,228,000 | 123,000 | 11,300 | 1.4 |
| Other | 14,930,000 | 9,408,000 | 233,000 | 16,000 | 1.1 |
| Total | 46,919,000 | 27,614,000 | 1,715,000 | 95,000 | 2.0 |

proaches one half of all accidents. However, in terms of severity, as measured by deaths per thousand injuries, they are on a par with occupational accidents. In recent years there has been considerable study of home accidents that has brought out numerous facts of interest. Of social significance is the fact that among females the highest home injury rate is in the lowest income group, whereas among males it is just the opposite, with the home injury rate in the highest income group being twice the rate for males in the lowest income group. It is interesting that, whereas the kitchen is the locale of the highest percent of all home accidents (26%), the bedroom is the most fatal place, accounting for 40% of all accidental deaths in the home. This is attributable to the many toxic drugs kept there plus the dangerous habit of some people to smoke in bed. Other fatal accidents in the home occur in living rooms, 10%; in kitchens, 12%; on stairs, 4%; in dining rooms, 3%; and in bathrooms, 3%. By type of home accident, falls are the most frequent cause of death, accounting for 40% of accidental deaths. Fires account for 23%, suffocation for 8%, and poisoning for 6%.[2]

Accidents should also be considered from the viewpoint of their relative position as a cause of death. Although more than 3,000 infants die accidentally each year, there are numerous other conditions that contribute more to the infant mortality. Once the first birthday is approached and passed, however, the picture changes dramatically. Accidents constitute the leading cause of death in age groups 1 to 4, 5 to 14, 15 to 24, and 25 to 34 years. From 35 to 44 years and from 45 to 54 years accidents are in second place; from 55 to 64 years, fourth place, and beyond 65 years, sixth place as a cause of death. Certainly a problem of this magnitude cannot be ignored.

During 1968, the Department of Health, Education, and Welfare conducted analyses of data from a wide variety of sources to obtain an estimate of the incidence of injuries from consumer products. It was not possible to refine the data in terms of severity of the events. The annual total for each broad source or type of injury is shown in the following list:

| | |
|---|---|
| Household appliances | 500,000 |
| Cooking devices | 150,000 |
| Kitchen and serving devices | 500,000 |
| Home furnishings | 500,000 |
| Home fixtures | 700,000 |
| Home stairs—falls | 1,800,000 |
| Heating devices | 175,000 |
| Home tools—power | 90,000 |
| Home tools—other | 785,000 |
| Cleaning/polishing products | 250,000 |
| Garden equipment | 500,000 |
| Hobbies and toys | 1,100,000 |
| Mobile sports equipment | 1,300,000 |
| Camping and fishing | 500,000 |
| Other recreational | 5,100,000 |
| Flammable liquids | 200,000 |
| Clothing injuries (not burns) | 200,000 |
| Firearms and explosives | 150,000 |
| Cosmetics and toiletries | 110,000 |
| Pesticides | 75,000 |
| Containers | 250,000 |
| Estimated total injuries from consumer products | 14,960,000 |

## CONSUMER PROTECTION PROGRAMS

Unfortunately no single government agency has general authority to prohibit, supervise, control or conduct programs with reference to the ever-increasing number of products that do or may present risks to the consuming public. Federal product safety legislation consists of a series of isolated acts that deal with specific hazards in generally narrow product categories. Usually legislation follows some unfortunate occurrence. Among other faults this approach results in both gaps and overlaps. The Department of Health, Education, and Welfare, for example, operates under certain general provisions of the Public Health Service Act; the Food, Drug and Cosmetic Acts of 1938 and 1959; the Hazardous Substances Acts of 1962 and 1966; the Child Protection and Toy Safety Acts of 1966 and 1969; the Fair Packaging and Labeling Act of 1967; the Flammable Fabrics Act of 1968; and the Electronic Products Act of 1969. This is only a partial list. Other departments have similar diffused categoric responsibilities.

Such limited federal authority as does exist therefore is incomplete and scattered among many agencies. In fact jurisdiction over a single category of products, of which pesticides is an excellent example, may be shared by as many as four or more different agencies. Moreover, as the National Commission on Product Safety observed, where it exists, federal product safety regulation is burdened by unnecessary procedural obstacles, circumscribed investigational powers, inadequate and ill-fitting sanctions, meager budgets, distorted priorities, and misdirected technical resources. Data collection and processing programs and early warning systems, to the extent they exist, leave much to be accomplished. In recent years there have been several attempts to establish effective and viable consumer advocacy and protection offices in several agencies and even in the Office of the President, but in view of the magnitude and complexity of the problem, combined with the confused uncoordinated arrangements to deal with them, such efforts have all been doomed to ineffectiveness. This will continue to be the case until proper and comprehensive organizational and legislative coordination occurs. It is regrettable but not surprising to note a similar situation on the state level.

## COST OF ACCIDENTAL INJURIES

It is difficult, of course, to determine with accuracy the economic loss due to accidents. The magnitude of estimates depends on the extent to which accidents and injuries are reported and the items that are included in the calculations. The National Safety Council[2] has carried out perhaps the most accurate analysis, which attempts to take into consideration all possible cost factors that might legitimately be involved. The result is summarized as follows:

| | | |
|---|---|---|
| 1. | Wages losses due to temporary inability to work, lower wages after returning to work due to permanent impairment, and present value of future earnings lost by those totally incapacitated or killed | $6,300,000,000 |
| 2. | Medical fees and hospital expenses | 2,400,000,000 |
| 3. | Insurance administrative and claim settlement costs | 4,900,000,000 |
| 4. | Property damage in motor vehicle accidents | 3,800,000,000 |
| 5. | Property destroyed by fire | 1,830,000,000 |
| 6. | Property destroyed and production lost due to work injury accidents | 3,500,000,000 |
| | Total | $22,730,000,000 |

The Governing Council of the American Public Health Association in 1960 put in the form of a policy statement[5] its growing concern about accidents as a public health problem and challenge equal in scope to the prevention of infectious diseases and the control of chronic diseases. It recommended that:

Accident prevention be recognized as a major public health problem and that all component units of the American Public Health Association cooperate to improve accident prevention activities at the local, state and national level;

State and local health departments, and the Public Health Service increase the size and scope of their accident prevention activities to be more commensurate with the magnitude of the problem and with the level of activity that has been or is being achieved in the field of infectious and chronic disease;

All state health departments and large local health departments provide that:

Their accident prevention programs be headed by a full-time administrator qualified by training and experience to discharge this responsibility adequately and that a wide range of consultant services be made available to the administrator and

Active educational efforts be designed to dispel ignorance about the basic causes of accidents and the role people play in their causation, devised and carried out in cooperation with other interested agencies and organizations, and

Research efforts be significantly increased in number, scope, and depth and embrace the study and control of all types of accidents regardless of their place of occurrence, and

Greater attention be directed to identifying the human factors involved in accidents, and to developing active methods of coping with them, and that in this concern full consideration be given to the structures, implements, and conditions created by man himself which make accidents more likely to occur, and

Increased efforts be made to enlist the cooperation of physicians and state and local medical societies in accident prevention activities;

Increased cooperation be promoted by official agencies with the National Safety Council and state and local safety councils, which have played so important a role in accident prevention; and

Additional funds be provided for the Public Health Service to encourage and support additional research efforts and to assist state and local health departments in developing more effective accident prevention programs.

There are many reasons why public health agencies and workers should be concerned with the problem of accidents. The absolute and proportionate magnitude of the problem that has been described is, of course, one reason for concern, as is also its economic significance. Beyond these, however, there are actually a great many activities of public health agencies that do or could impinge on the problem. Emphasizing this are several useful manuals that have been issued to assist the public health worker and others in the development of accident control and consumer protection programs.[6-8] The Department of Health, Education, and Welfare, the American Public Health Association, the National Safety Council, and the Departments of Transportation, Agriculture, and Housing and Urban Development are all useful sources of such materials. Among the various activities that may make significant contributions are public health statistics, health surveys and studies, community health and safety education, child health, occupational health and safety, housing, and mental health. The latter is mentioned specifically in view of the growing body of knowledge about accident proneness and the development of techniques for its determination.[9,10] Increasingly workers in the fields of public health and preventive medicine have been relating these general activities or methods of approach to accident prevention. In several communities accidental injuries and deaths are reported to the public health agency for study and analysis to determine improved and more fruitful avenues of attack. In many other communities surveys have been carried out for the same reason. In still others the recording of and educational activities about home accidents have been incorporated as part of the public health nursing function. Some excellent epidemiologic studies have been made of the problem.[11-14]

Of particular interest and value are some studies on program analysis and cost benefits carried out by the Public Health Service.[15] One of these relates to motor vehicle and passenger injury prevention. The problem was examined exclusively in terms of human factors. Three major factors in the vehicular accident complex—law enforcement, road design, and traffic engineering—were for the most part excluded. Thus the problem was limited to considerations traditionally within the purview of health agencies. Six alternative programs were examined in terms of the program cost per death anticipated to be averted if an effective program were adequately financed and carried out. The results were as follows:

| Program | Cost per death averted |
|---|---|
| 1. Seat belt use—to encourage people to use seat belts | $87 |
| 2. Restraint devices—to educate people to obtain and use additional safety restraining devices | 103 |
| 3. Pedestrian injury—to educate accident-prone pedestrians how to cross the street | 666 |
| 4. Motorcycle injury—to encourage motorcyclists to use helmets and eye shields | 3,336 |
| 5. Reduce driver drinking—to educate people not to drink and drive | 5,824 |
| 6. Driver licensing—to establish a medical screening program for licensing and to exclude drivers with certain conditions | 13,801 |

Through the efforts of workers in the field of environmental health more and more accident prevention measures are being built into the standards, specifications, and requirements for dwelling and city plans. Such measures coupled with persistent public educational measures form the core of the attack on home accidents. Reference has been made to the significant decline in occupational accidents. This has largely resulted from activities in industrial health and safety programs, involving inspections and surveys, improved plant and machine design, development and use of safety devices, preemployment examinations, and worker education (Chapter 31).

Many state health departments engage in some activities relating to accident prevention at the present time. Accident prevention educational activities are carried on by almost all state health departments. In addition, many of them are attempting to stimulate local accident prevention programs. Special conferences, short courses, and workshops are held for local health department personnel and for representatives of other official and nonofficial local agencies. Also various state health departments cooperate with other official state agencies such as those concerned with mines, industry, labor, and traffic safety in carrying out cooperative programs in those areas.

On the federal level increased interest and concern has been manifested by research, education, and encouragement of and grants to state and local health agencies. Some of the legislation that makes this possible has been listed previously as well as some of the needs in the national scene.

In the final analysis, of course, the prevention of accidents depends on the individual, and if efforts are to be fruitful, they must take place especially on the local level. "Public apathy to the mounting toll from accidents must be transformed into an action program under strong leadership. This can be accomplished by the methods employed to bring poliomyelitis and other epidemics under control, and to make frontal attacks to conquer cancer, heart disease and mental disease. . . . Basic to this unified approach is identification of the individual citizen with a means by which he can satisfy the inherent desire to serve his fellow man."[1]

No single satisfactory pattern has yet been devised or adopted. It is certain, however, that there must be involved some of the basic epidemiologic approaches and techniques that have proved to be effective in many diverse fields. Among these are (1) development and improvement of data on the prevalence and incidence of accidents through reporting, surveys, and studies; (2) education of the public through effective pertinent channels; (3) improvement and extension of safety devices in the home, public buildings, industry, vehicles, and farm machinery; (4) inclusion of training in accident prevention in schools of public health, public administration, and architecture; (5) improvement of structural safety through the general inclusion of accident prevention factors in building codes; (6) improvement of city planning, traffic studies, and highway design; (7) improved driver training, education, and supervision with consideration given to physical and mental factors that may indicate accident proneness; and (8) improvement of the functional design of toys, household equipment, and furniture with consideration given to the peculiar needs and behavior habits of the very young, of the handicapped, and of the elderly.

Only through the cooperative efforts of many community agencies, one of which is the health department, in attacking along all of these and many other fronts, will the toll of accidents be lessened eventually. In the process, because of its all-embracing interest in all aspects of safe and healthful living, it is the official public health agency that is best fitted to serve as a catalyst and rallying point.

## POISON CONTROL

A special type of accident hazard is presented by the extensive and increasing number of toxic materials to be found in the modern home.[16] In recent years industrial chemists and pharmaceutical research have developed many wonderful products that have contributed greatly to the American way of life. Their widespread availability, however, has not been without danger. No longer is it possible to use a "universal antidote." The highly complex nature of many new pharmaceuticals and household products requires a knowledge of their chemical constitution so that a quick and effective remedy may be used in case of toxic ingestion.

It is estimated that each year between 1 and 2 million individuals in the United States, many of them children, accidentally ingest a wide variety of household aids, and about 2,200 of them die, including 300 children under 5 years of age. This is about one ninth the number of deaths from stroke. The nature of the substances ingested is of interest. In a study of accidental poisonings in children under 15 years of age in New York City, Jacobziner[17] found the causes shown in Table 32-2.

**Table 32-2.** Accidental poisonings of children under 15 years of age, New York City, 1956

| Type of poisoning | Percent of total |
|---|---|
| Aspirin, barbiturates, and other internal medications | 26 |
| Bleach, furniture polish, lye, and other household preparations | 20 |
| Lead | 10 |
| Iodine and other external medications | 9 |
| Insecticides | 7 |
| Turpentine and other solvents | 6 |
| Cosmetics | 5 |
| Rodenticides | 3 |
| Miscellaneous | 15 |

Particular attention should be called to poisonings from lead. Most of these occur in young children from low-income families who live in old housing, the interiors of which have been painted with many layers of lead-containing paint. The problem is complicated by the frequent casual attitude of many parents who accept pica as normal behavior in young children and by the frequent absence of supervision of children in such socioeconomic circumstances.[18] An estimated 600,000 children between 1 and 6 years, mostly in inner cities, have significant blood-lead levels from these sources. Lead paint has been banned for interior household use. Increased awareness and concern about this problem, hastened by the development of improvements in diagnosis and treatment, resulted in the Lead-Based Paint Poisoning Act of 1971, which provides for research, education, diagnosis, and treatment.

As a result of the growing concern over accidental poisoning, an increasing number of communities have been developing poison control centers.[19,20] In 1957 a National Clearinghouse for Poison Control Centers was established by the Surgeon General to (1) disseminate data to centers on ingredients and toxicity of household products and medicines, (2) collect and tabulate data regarding poisoning incidents, and (3) provide and assist public information and education programs on the subject. There are now about 460 centers in all but 2 states and the District of Columbia. To varying extents they compile and keep up-to-date a readily usable file on pharmaceutical, household, industrial, and other substances with data about their composition, toxicity, and antidotes; they provide laboratory analytic service and treatment; they answer telephone requests for first aid information and carry out educational activities for the professions and the public. Some provide follow-up by means of public health nurses or other types of investigators or educators.

One interesting question that calls for more study is the relationship of mental health to so-called accidental poisoning. Unquestionably a certain number of such "accidents" actually represent either conscious or subconscious attempts at suicide or homicide. With regard to the latter is the possible factor of withheld or avoided supervision, warning, or prompt treatment by some parents, older children, or spouses. The reader is referred to Chapters 24 and 27 for discussion of this subject.

## SHEET PLASTIC

Another special problem has resulted from improvements in the packaging of goods. The development and inexpensive production of polyethylene plastic have prompted its widespread use for packaging many types of foods, household materials, and equipment and for use as a protective covering of clothing. Concurrent with its widespread use has been a rise in the number of young children who have suffocated as a result of having their faces covered by this material. Since the sheet plastic tends to build up a considerable amount of static electricity it is particularly likely to adhere tightly to the skin. Already several states and communities are exploring the possibility of limiting the use of the material or requiring vents in its surface. Meanwhile extensive programs are being conducted to educate parents concerning the potential dangers of sheet plastic.

## REFERENCES

1. Accidental death and disability, the neglected disease of modern society, Washington, D. C., 1967, National Academy of Sciences, National Research Council.
2. Accidents facts, Chicago, 1970, National Safety Council.
3. U. S. Public Health Service: Health statistics, persons injured by class of accident, U. S., July 1967-June 1968, PHS pub. no. 584-B8, Rockville, Md., 1969.
4. Manheimer, D. I., Dewey, J., Mellinger, G. D., and Corsa, L.: Fifty thousand child-years of accidental injuries, Public Health Rep. **81:**519, June 1966.
5. Policy statement on accidents—a public health problem, Amer. J. Public Health **51:**122, Jan. 1961.
6. U. S. Public Health Service: A guide to the development of accidental injury control programs in local health department, PHS pub. no. 1368, Rockville, Md., 1965.
7. Tiboni, E., editor: Development and operation of an accident control program through a local health department, Ann Arbor, 1967, School of Public Health, University of Michigan.
8. American Public Health Association: Accident control in environmental health programs, Washington, D. C., 1966, The Association.
9. Webb, W. B.: The illusive phenomena in accident proneness, Public Health Rep. **70:**951, Oct. 1955.
10. McFarland, R. A., and Moore, R. C.: Human factors in highway safety, New Eng. J. Med. **256:** 792, April 15, 1957; **256:**837, May 2, 1957; **256:** 890, May 9, 1957.
11. Haddon, W., Suchman, E. A., and Klein, D. L.:

Accident research, methods and approaches, New York, 1964, Harper & Row, Publishers.

12. Roberts, H., Gordon, J. E., and Fiore, A.: Epidemiological techniques in home accident prevention, Public Health Rep. **67:**547, June 1952.

13. McFarland, R. A.: Epidemiological principles applicable to the study and prevention of child accidents, Amer. J. Public Health **45:**1302, Oct. 1955.

14. Iskrant, A. P.: The epidemiological approach to accident causation, Amer. J. Public Health **57:** 1708, Oct. 1967.

15. U. S. Department of Health, Education, and Welfare, Office of the Assistant Secretary for Program Coordination: Program analysis, selected disease control programs, Washington, D. C., 1966, Government Printing Office.

16. The public health problem of accidental poisoning, a symposium, Amer. J. Public Health **46:**951, Aug. 1956.

17. Jacobziner, H.: Accidental poisoning among children, Amer. J. Dis. Child. **93:**647, June 1957.

18. Bradley, J. E., and Bessman, S. P.: Poverty, pica, and poisoning, Public Health Rep. **73:**467, May 1958.

19. Press, E., and Mellins, R. B.: A poisoning control program, Amer. J. Public Health **44:**1515, Dec. 1954.

20. Cann, H. M.: Control of accidental poisoning—a progress report, J.A.M.A. **168:**717, Oct. 11, 1958.

# PART TEN

# The substance
of public health—
health care delivery

Probably the single most regrettable event in the development of public health in the United States was the decision early in this century to separate it from the therapeutic and rehabilitative aspects of health care. The lack of realism seems triply ironic. Public health had its roots in the care of the sick. Then when the change of philosophy occurred, it was quickly recognized that true or complete "health" was ephemeral, an ideal, to attain it required some measure of treatment as well as prevention and promotion, and to the extent that it might be achieved it was destined to be temporary or transient. Where could one draw a distinction between the well and the sick? Ask anyone who was ever responsible for a "well-child" clinic and see what answer comes forth. Thus several generations of public health workers and physicians were practicing both public health and curative medicine without either recognizing it or being willing to admit it openly. So now at long last logic appears to be given increasing attention by both groups, albeit sometimes with apprehension and reluctance. But they are finally appreciating the fact that they are not really two groups—they are complementing components of the same group, the health team, striving for the well-being of people. In the following three chapters are presented some aspects of emergency medical services (the entry point for so many), medical care, and rehabilitation.

*The ancient word for "crisis" is made up
of two characters. One means "danger" and
the second means "opportunity."*

CHAPTER 33

# Emergency medical services

## BACKGROUND

The assurance of easily accessible, effective, and acceptable emergency medical services is currently and will certainly continue to be one of the most important responsibilities of health agencies. One of the most visible of the many critical areas in health care is the appalling amount of disability and loss of life from sudden catastrophic illness and accidents. With reference to highway accidents, if the current trend continues, the nation will experience its two millionth traffic fatality by 1976. Ironically this figure approximately equals the total population of the American colonies when they achieved their independence, 200 years before. About 55,000 such deaths now occur each year accompanied by almost 2 million highway injuries, one tenth of them resulting in permanent disability. The toll from nonhighway accidents in the home, at work, and at play is no less alarming. It totals over 60,000 deaths each year plus 9 million nonfatal injuries, 250,000 of which are permanently disabling.[1,2] On the other hand, some studies indicate that as many as 15 million children sustain significant accidental injuries each year and about 16,000 of them die.[3] Currently accidents kill more people in the productive age groups up to 39 years than any other single factor and are the fourth largest cause of death after that age. The costs of accidental death, disability, and property damage are phenomenal and are estimated at about $28 billion a year.[4] One of the most distressing facts about this carnage is that studies have demonstrated that 15% to 20%

of accidental highway deaths could be avoided if prompt, effective care were available at the scene of the emergency, on the way to the hospital, and within it.[5,6]

The situation with regard to sudden medical emergencies is no less disconcerting. Included in this category are coronary occlusions, cerebrovascular strokes, diabetic crises, precipitous miscarriages or deliveries, and various other sudden critical events. The American Heart Association estimates that approximately 10% to 20% of the 275,000 prehospital coronary deaths could be prevented if proper care were administered at the scene and in route to a medical facility.[7] In all, Huntley[8] estimates that prompt and proper emergency care could save about 60,000 lives annually, as shown in Table 33-1.

The amount of suffering, disability, lost income, and the like that could be avoided is impossible to estimate. Then there is perhaps the most ignored component of emergencies—

**Table 33-1.** Deaths preventable annually by proper emergency care, United States

| Medical emergency | Number of deaths |
| --- | --- |
| Myocardial infarction | 35,000 |
| Vehicular accidents | 12,000 |
| Other trauma | 6,000 |
| Stroke | 2,500 |
| Poisonings, drownings | 2,500 |
| Other | 2,000 |
| Total | 60,000 |

the psychiatric emergency,[9,10] which include suicidal and homicidal attempts, battered children and spouses, destructive manic states, drug and alcoholic crises—all of which cry for attention and help. This necessitates a broad definition of a medical emergency as an unforeseen event that affects an individual in such a manner as to require immediate medical care (physical, physiologic, or psychiatric).

Individuals in need of emergency medical assistance usually are confused about where to seek services and lose vital time in obtaining care. In many communities all emergency patients transported by public ambulance services are carried to the municipal hospital, frequently bypassing other hospitals that are adequate to provide the needed services. The patient is thereby denied prompt access to the service he needs. For the patient with a heart attack, severe respiratory distress, or extensive bleeding the difference in time may be a life or death matter. Robert Baker, Director of the Trauma Unit at Cook County Hospital, Chicago, claims that for every 30 minutes that elapse between the time of an accident and when the patient receives definitive care, the mortality rate increases threefold.

## THE PROBLEM

The status of all aspects of emergency medical care resources in general leaves much to be desired. There are gross inadequacies in planning, training, equipment, and especially coordination. To approach the problem perhaps backwards, there has been a duplicative and often wasteful proliferation of emergency rooms (not necessarily emergency departments) in most hospitals regardless of need, essentially to meet hospital accreditation standards and also as a means of providing a base of inpatients.

This, of course, does not assure quality. Thus three fourths of the 5,130 community hospitals with emergency facilities have fewer than 200 beds. Only 10% of these institutions are considered equipped to handle all medical and surgical emergencies, and only 14% are capable of effectively handling psychiatric emergencies, much less drug crises. Fewer than 50% have blood banks, and 58% are not equipped to handle cardiac emergencies; only 6% are able to communicate with the ambulances or rescue vehicles that serve them. As Seeley[11] of the National Academy of Sciences-National Research Council has emphasized, "Many of the smaller hospitals don't even have the emergency equipment we recommend for ambulances." Only 17% of these hospitals have 24-hour physician coverage, whereas many rely on "on-call" physicians who are theoretically available around the clock and presumably, but by no means always, qualified to handle properly the complex of emergency cases that might be brought in.[12] Regionalization and categorization of facilities with graded emergency capability would ameliorate many problems if, in addition, the public and ambulance services personnel are informed about which facilities are to be used and for what purpose.[13]

In any recent year there were more than 50 million patient visits to hospital emergency facilities in the United States. The number has been increasing at the rate of 10% a year. An extremely difficult problem is presented by the fact that one third of all such visits are not actually emergencies but, rather, occur because of the convenience of a known location where health care is accessible 24 hours a day or because those who come have limited funds or nowhere else to go. This situation or need is increasing as the costs of health care go up, access to private physicians becomes more difficult, home visits become more rare, and residential location becomes more changing. There is a serious need therefore to sort by triage those who come to emergency departments into three approximately equal groups and provide properly, efficiently, and separately for each. The three groups are (1) those who are true emergencies, in which immediate care to preserve life or diminish the effects of the patient's condition is needed, (2) patients who have urgent conditions and need care sooner than could be otherwise scheduled but who would not be harmed by several hours' delay in treatment, and (3) patients without immediate medical need who use the emergency facility as an ambulatory care clinic. Especially, alternative methods of providing access to care need to be developed for this latter group of patients to avoid diluting the quality of emergency care.

Some of the most glaring deficiencies in the emergency medical picture relate to lack of ambulance coverage, either or both geographic and around-the-clock, poor vehicular design, inadequate equipment for extrication of trapped accident victims and for on-the-site and in-transit, life-preserving treatment, and inadequate or more often a lack of means of communication with the professional persons and the institution that is to receive the patient.[7]

Brown[14] reasonably believes that an ambulance should be like an extension of a well-staffed and equipped hospital emergency department. He says, "More important than immediate transportation is the immediate life-saving care—control of hemorrhage, splinting fractures, keeping the breathing passages open. On-the-site care should be by trained emergency technicians and then the transportation should be deliberate and gentle." This is the theory, but what is practice? Of the 44,000 ambulances in the nation, only about 1,300 are operated by hospitals; 4,500 are operated by fire or police departments; 4,700 by commercial firms; 11,000 by volunteer groups; and 19,000 by morticians. One third of the morticians state they intend to give up the ambulance business when their states enforce the standards established by the National Highway Safety Administration. The term *ambulance* is often a euphemism. Almost one half of the vehicles were not intended for use as ambulances; one tenth are panel trucks or vans; one fourth are station wagons; many are actually hearses; and of the 36% that are conventional ambulances, many are too low and too cramped for space to allow an attendant to administer to a patient. Fewer than one third carry all the equipment recommended by the American College of Surgeons. Equipment on most ambulances consists merely of an oxygen tank and a mask, but fewer than one half have bag-mask resuscitators. Often there are not even splints, backboards, or equipment for keeping the windpipe open for intravenous therapy. Only a small percent carry cardiac defibrillators,[15] and telemetric equipment for long-distance monitoring of vital signs is rare indeed. In fact, less than 6% of the vehicles are equipped to communicate with a hospital, whereas 38% do not have two-way radio communications at all.[16]

## PERSONNEL

The 44,000 ambulances require an average of five attendants to cover their various shifts. This is a total of 220,000 individuals. The various professional organizations concerned have recommended that each ambulance be manned by two emergency medical technicians who have completed at least 70 hours of carefully planned and presented instruction plus 10 hours of emergency room training. Actually, by 1970 only about 5% of attendants had obtained this minimum recommended training; about 57% had achieved the advanced

first aid course; 33% had the standard 10- to 12-hour first aid course or equivalent; and 5% had no training at all.[8] Ambulance drivers especially are lacking in training. They are typically inadequately paid, hence the turnover tends to be great and the quality low. Under these circumstances it is not surprising that as estimated by the Ambulance Association of America,[7] about 25,000 persons are permanently injured or disabled each year by untrained ambulance attendants and rescue workers. It is also notable that the accident rate for ambulances at intersections is twice that of other vehicles. It is estimated that it costs approximately $90,000 to operate an ambulance on a 24-hour basis for a year. This includes capital investment, maintenance, repairs, garaging, equipping, and staffing. Used properly, the ambulance would return the investment in it many times over. Under the circumstances therefore it merits efficient and careful use. The many conscientious individuals involved in the rescue and patient-transport field have been taking ever-stronger steps to improve both equipment and personnel. The Ambulance Association of America in cooperation with professional groups and governmental agencies has been notable in this regard. With reference to personnel qualifications and training the recently established Registry of Emergency Medical Technicians-Ambulance, which already is developing a certification program, should be mentioned.

Consideration of emergency vehicle attendants focuses attention on the broader subject of related personnel. Several years ago it was estimated that there were about 300,000 allied health workers of various types in the emergency medical care field. This falls far short of the need, and much must be done to attract, develop, and hold desirable individuals in this important work. New types of personnel must be tried, legal barriers to their effective utilization must be removed, roles must be defined, appropriate curricula must be planned and presented, and positions must be established with proper career development opportunities.

One of the most difficult and costly problems to solve is the provision of a sufficient number of adequately trained and qualified physicians for this critical aspect of community medicine. Many medical graduates have had no formal training in emergency care. A survey in the late 1960s of 108 medical schools in the United States and Canada showed only 33 schools with courses in the subject. At present there are about 15,000 physicians devoting most if not all of their time to emergency medicine. Twice that number is needed. This is not a task for which every physician is qualified. Belatedly it has been realized that a special type of training is needed. Accordingly, as recently as July 1970, the first residency in emergency medicine was established at the University of Cincinnati Medical Center. Since then several other centers of medical education have followed suit. Several professional organizations deserve special mention for their leadership. Among them are the American College of Surgeons, the American Academy of Orthopaedic Surgeons, the American Association of Anaesthesiologists, the newer University Association of Emergency Medical Services, and the American College of Emergency Physicians (ACEP). The ACEP, now with about 3,000 members, has been working especially to improve specialty training in acute care and to make emergentology a board-certified specialty. Another important effort to improve the quality of care was the formation in 1971 of the Emergency Department Nurses Association (EDNA) with a fast-flying bird as its symbol.

## THE DETERRENT TO SOLUTION

All those who have addressed themselves to the problem are convinced that it need not exist—that the technology, the expertise, and even the resources currently are available to ensure efficient, effective, and acceptable emergency medical services to all American citizens. This is different from killers such as cancer, a field in which much more research is required before control becomes possible. In the final analysis the deficiency is in the unwillingness or inability of professions, institutions, agencies, and units of local government to coordinate and utilize their joint existing resources and capabilities and in the failure of the state and federal governments in turn to coordinate their resources and efforts to eliminate duplication, waste, and needless legal barriers. The question has been raised by many: Why is it possible to send men to another planet and back and monitor and protect their health literally by the second but not be possible to duplicate this feat within a radius of a few miles? The answer, of course, is clear. A tremendous amount of intensive planning and effort went into the former feat, and it was done comprehensively

and with a systems analytic approach. By contrast, examples of lack of planning, cooperation, and systematic approach in the emergency medical field are the rule rather than the exception. For example, hospitals may develop not only independently of each other but independently of and unrelated to ambulance services; satisfactory communications equipment may be in ambulances but not in hospitals, or there may be equipment without personnel trained to use it; all the foregoing services may be present, but no medical backup provided to give directions and guidance; satisfactory hospitals and ambulances may exist but no means of access to the system or no central dispatch; there may be good on-site and in-transit care but no preparation at the hospital; an ambulance transporting a cardiac patient may bypass a hospital with a coronary care unit to deliver the patient to an inappropriate or ill-equipped and staffed institution; there may be no ambulance service available beyond a city's limits or at night; either no ambulance or several may respond and their personnel argue as to who gets the patient. Examples of such gaps or duplications are legion and common knowledge.

## EMERGENCY MEDICAL SERVICES SYSTEM[17-21]

An emergency medical services system is an organized procedure for receiving and acting on requests for assistance when there is a likelihood of either trauma requiring rapid medical attention or an illness that poses conditions threatening to life or requiring immediate resuscitation to sustain life. It usually requires a communication system to receive requests for help from many sources and locations; a defined procedure for acting on the requests, including central dispatch and alerting actions; availability of an appropriately staffed transportation system or systems by land, air, or water, and with a capability for immediate on-site treatment and in-transit life support. There must also be available 24-hour, 7-day-a-week emergency care centers prepared to receive emergency patients from within a defined service area and staffed with appropriately trained professional and technical medical and surgical personnel and with supportive laboratory, diagnostic, and treatment facilities. Such centers may be either in large general hospitals as part of their emergency service function or in independent and free-standing specialized institutions for trauma care. Under certain circumstances mobile emergency treatment units have been

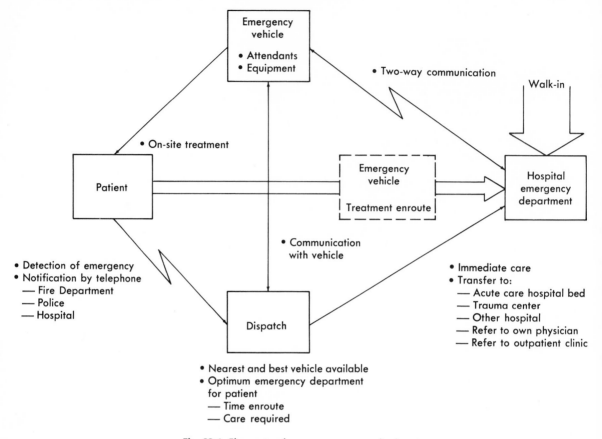

**Fig. 33-1.** Elements of an emergency medical system.

found useful as ancillary emergency care resources brought to the scene of accident or serious illness. All emergency treatment centers should be intimately related to appropriate specialized capabilities as might be needed. The emergency medical services system should be regarded as an integral part of the total health care system to assure proper medical, rehabilitative, and other follow-up services and assistance so that patients receive maximum opportunity for recovery of personal function after survival from a true emergency situation. Fig. 33-1 presents the elements of an emergency medical system and their interrelationships.

## PHASES OF AN EMERGENCY MEDICAL SERVICES (EMS) SYSTEM

The following outline presents in sequence the events that can follow occurrence of a damaging incident that produces emergency medical patients. It is recognized that not all those concerned with the subject would agree

with all of its aspects. Some would combine certain of these events, and others might subdivide the list further. However, it provides a reasonable enumeration of points where medical emergency system failures may exaggerate rather than prevent losses from damaging incidents. Many of these steps are not recognizable as separate entities in response to certain kinds of medical emergencies. Some may be ineffective in cases in which medical science cannot help the victim, regardless of where he is taken. However, the medical needs of the victim must determine the manner of system response.

*Pretreatment phase*
1. Occurrence
2. Detection
3. Notification
4. Dispatch of mobile emergency medical services
5. Travel to site

*Preliminary care phase*
6. On-site problem analysis
7. On-site treatment

8. On-site extrication
9. On-site stabilization
10. On-site loading
11. Selection of definitive care facility
12. Transport (continuing patient maintenance)
13. En route notification of receiving facility
14. In-transit transmission of patient's condition and receipt of necessary life maintenance instructions and their application
15. Facility preparation for receiving patient
16. Delivery to definitive care facility

*Definitive care phase at receiving facility*

17. Patient transfer
18. Information transfer
19. Patient evaluation (by facility staff)
20. Triage
21. Continuation of treatment
22. Second stage diagnosis
23. Emergency room treatment
24. Intensive care
25. Definitive diagnosis
26. Definitive treatment

*Recuperation phase*

27. Recuperative care

*Rehabilitation phase*

28. Transfer to extended care facility or home
29. Rehabilitative treatment
30. Discharge
31. Return to normal function

## CRITERIA, STANDARDS, AND REGULATIONS

One of the most basic problems in the delivery of emergency medical services in the United States is the absence or inconsistency of personnel qualification requirements or of criteria, standards, guidelines, and regulations for emergency medical services systems.[22] As has been indicated, until now responsibility has rested essentially with local communities with some assistance and support from state and federal governments. However, to achieve maximum utilization and efficiency and in the interests of high quality and continuous patient care, local systems must be compatible with those adjacent to them. To achieve these objectives uniform qualifications, criteria, standards, and regulations must be adopted. Specific subject areas in which needs exist are the following:

1. Categorization of emergency facilities
2. Criteria for ambulance design and equipment
3. Model ordinances for the regulation of ambulance services
4. Ambulance and emergency department report forms
5. Uniform standards for training

   a. Emergency medical technicians (ambulance)
   b. Emergency room personnel
6. Certification of emergency medical technicians

The Public Health Service and others have provided several recommended standards for reference and guidance. Some of them are summarized as follows[23]:

*State legislation*[24]

1. Should establish Divisions of Emergency Medical Services
2. Should specify duties and qualifications of personnel
3. Should require establishment of a system to supervise and regulate ambulance services and personnel
4. Should assist in establishment of a coordinated central communications and dispatch system

*Ambulances*[25,26]

1. Should meet the vehicle design specifications as recommended by the National Academy of Engineering and the National Research Council
2. Should have as minimal equipment those items recommended as essential equipment by the American College of Surgeons
3. Should exist in sufficient numbers and be so placed as to provide maximum utilization and effectiveness in the shortest possible response time

*Ambulance personnel*[27-29]

1. Should have have basic training of at least 70 hours' instruction, plus 10 or more additional hours of emergency room training
2. Should routinely maintain skills by observation and instruction in a hospital emergency department under the supervision of a physician, including regular critique by emergency room physicians with ambulance personnel of care administered to the patient prior to his arrival at the emergency room
3. Should meet or exceed requirements of the Registry of Emergency Medical Technicians-Ambulance
4. Should comprise two emergency medical technicians, one of whom may be the driver, for each emergency ambulance

*Hospital emergency facilities*[13,30]

1. Should promote the development of satisfactory plans for regionalization of services
2. Should be categorized using the National Academy of Sciences' recommended criteria
3. Should provide for ongoing self-improvement training for all emergency department staff, both clinical and administrative
4. Should meet or exceed the emergency department standards recommended by the Joint Commission on Accreditation of Hospitals

5. Should accept a leadership role in providing training for emergency medical technologists

6. Should base ambulance services at the hospital, wherever and whenever feasible

*Communications*[31]

1. A single telephone number for emergency medical services, that is, "911," instituted throughout the nation

2. Central dispatch provided for all emergency ambulances

3. Radio or environmentally secure communications should exist between
   a. Central dispatch center
   b. Ambulance
   c. Hospitals
   d. Law enforcement and fire units
   e. Emergency operating centers

*Supportive actions*

1. Toll-free public telephone services available for all emergency calls from pay telephones

2. Emergency medical identification[32]—to be carried by all persons with conditions or medical histories that should be known to anyone rendering emergency medical care

3. Medical self-help[33]—at least one member of every family trained in medical self-help and/or Red Cross first aid

4. Highway signs[34] (*coordinated with hospital categorization*) placed in adequate numbers and locations to identify emergency medical care facilities

Obviously, additional criteria, standards, and regulations are needed in other aspects of emergency medical services, and provision should be made for modification of existing qualifications, criteria, standards, and regulations when it is considered necessary.

## DATA COLLECTION AND ANALYSIS[35,36]

To introduce effective planning and systems changes that are economically sound, a national data collection and analysis system must be implemented. At a minimum the following information should be collected and analyzed prior to implementation of large-scale emergency medical services system efforts:

1. Epidemiologic data concerning medical emergencies

2. Geographic, demographic, and topographic data

3. Patient-flow patterns

4. Patient-demand patterns

5. Road networks

6. Travel times (ground and air)

7. Population densities

8. Distances from health care resources

9. Health care resources should be analyzed as follows:
   a. Type
      (1) Personnel—physicians and allied professionals and technicians
      (2) Emergency centers, hospitals, and related facilities
      (3) Ambulance services (ground and air)
      (4) Communications networks
   b. Category
   c. Location
   d. Distribution
   e. Services provided
   f. Capacity
   g. Capability
   h. Availability
   i. Manpower
      (1) Quantity
      (2) Training
      (3) Staffing patterns
   j. Equipment
   k. Administration and control
      (1) Government
      (2) Public
      (3) Private enterprise
      (4) Volunteers
   l. Response times

10. Needs

11. Priorities

All the aforementioned factors must be analyzed and evaluated to plan efficient and effective response systems that are suitably located and properly utilize, maximize, and expand existing resources. If this is not done, the resulting system could place a tremendous psychologic and socioeconomic burden on a community that would be a detriment to good patient care.

## PUBLIC EDUCATION

The education, understanding, cooperation, and intelligent action of the general public is essential to any successful emergency medical services system. The public must continually be made aware of what is being done, who is doing it, and for what purpose. In addition, the public must be informed of the services available, steps to take when a medical emergency is encountered or recognized, who and how to call for assistance. Extensive experiments have been conducted in the United States utilizing a common emergency telephone number. In places where such a number is available, the necessary assistance can be dispatched immediately because the central dispatcher knows current service load levels and the location of the closest appropriate and available medical facility and response vehicle. The common emergency telephone number can be distributed to the public in many ways, such as labels to attach to private telephones, mass mailings in utility and other bills, etc.

## EMERGENCY MEDICAL SERVICES COUNCILS[37]

As has been indicated, at present there is little coordination among providers of emergency medical services in the United States. Ambulance services operate essentially independently, often without direct communications to hospitals. Hence patients may be delivered to hospitals that have not been advised of their pending arrival, condition, or need for emergency treatment. Similarly there are few central dispatch facilities to coordinate ambulance usage and patient flow according to situational needs. Training and acceptance of emergency medical services personnel at all levels differ greatly from community to community and service to service. Communications and medical equipment differ considerably from vehicle to vehicle, and a few procedures have been established for exchange of equipment on delivery of a patient to a hospital so that ambulances can return promptly to further service. There is little or no uniformity in reporting forms and procedures either among ambulance services or hospitals. Essentially there exists no standard or uniform peer review or evaluation procedure with reference to the medical care provided to each patient. Few communities have established interhospital radio communications systems or interhospital agreements for systematic continuation of care in case of patient transfer.

Many of these problems could be and are in the process of being overcome by the establishment of community emergency medical services councils. Typically these councils comprise representatives from the community working with representatives from the various elements of the emergency medical services system, for example, hospital administrators, public health agencies, medical societies, law-enforcement and fire-protection personnel, private ambulance operators, disaster preparedness personnel, and others. The councils have the authority and responsibility for searching out the resources, bringing them together, and coordi-

nating the services provided by all elements of the system by virtue of new laws or local ordinances. In other words, emergency medical services councils offer the potential of establishing and implementing an orderly, efficient, and well-coordinated system for delivering emergency medical care.

## CURRENT STATUS ON THE NATIONAL LEVEL

At present there is no national unified system for planning, organizing, implementing, operating, and regulating emergency medical services in the total sense in the United States. There exists instead a variety of arrangements, each unique in character. Each attempts to meet the demands of the particular geographic area it serves, essentially through a somewhat loose interaction among its component parts (i.e., physicians, hospitals, rescue squads, private ambulance companies, law-enforcement and fire-protection agencies, etc.). Until recently, there have been few successful attempts to develop an effective, coordinated, and comprehensive emergency medical system that utilizes objective and scientific planning and management technology. Until now, the environment has not been receptive to deliberate total planning or to the provision of adequate public financial resources necessary to effect comprehensive emergency medical services delivery. Traditionally responsibility for the provision of emergency medical care has rested with the local community, most specifically with health care professionals and civic leaders. During recent years, however, stimulated by nationally sponsored comprehensive health planning programs and regional medical programs of the Department of Health, Education, and Welfare, the National Highway Traffic Safety Program of the Department of Transportation, the model cities program of the Department of Housing and Urban Development, and others, the components of local, regional, and state jurisdictions have begun to plan and work much more closely and effectively than before. Increasingly state and federal governments have recognized their responsibilities for providing professional and material support, coordination, and technical and financial assistance to local communities so that they might more adequately fulfill their responsibility.

In response to the recommendations of many individuals and nationally prominent groups and in recognition of the acute need for improved emergency medical services, the President of the United States in his State of the Union message of January 1972 directed the Secretary of Health, Education, and Welfare to develop new ways of organizing and providing comprehensive emergency medical care. This directive resulted in the initiation by the Department of Health, Education, and Welfare of a coordinated federal approach to meet the problem. The actions involved included the following:

1. The establishment in the Department of Health, Education, and Welfare of a national focal point for emergency medical services (EMS) to provide technical consultation and guidance to states, communities, professional organizations and facilities, citizen organizations, and others to assist them in developing quality emergency medical care

2. The establishment of a federal interagency committee for interdepartmental coordination to improve emergency medical services planning, funding, performance, and evaluation

3. The development of an emergency medical services information system with two primary duties:
   a. Information collection, storage, and retrieval
   b. Information dissemination, including the development and production of publications and promotional materials as well as response to inquiries

4. The development of an emergency medical services data collection, analysis, and evaluation system that will be coordinated with data systems of other governmental and nongovernmental agencies. This system should eliminate wasteful and confusing duplication of effort and provide data for meeting requirements of all participating organizations. It will include the following:
   a. The development of EMS computer models
   b. Research data for assessing the efficacy of local management approaches to EMS
   c. Research data for assessing the use of different types of equipment and procedures within an EMS system
   d. The collection of national data necessary for national decisions and policies relative to future programs and priorities

5. The sponsorship of a limited number of comprehensive emergency medical services systems for research and demonstration purposes that are intended to serve as models to demonstrate the systems approach to emergency medical services in different types of situations, combining the application of existing technology and good management

Since then, on September 12, 1973, the Congress overrode a presidential veto, thereby making possible a significant increase in federal assistance to state and local emergency medical service systems.

In addition to the aforementioned efforts, the Department of Transportation has developed, implemented, and funded training courses for medical technologists throughout the nation. This department has also provided funds for the purchase of ambulances and equipment in many localities. Both the training courses and the ambulances and their equipment meet the recommended standards of the National Academy of Sciences-National Research Council.

## MILITARY ASSISTANCE TO SAFETY AND TRAFFIC (M.A.S.T.)

Since July of 1970, three government agencies have co-sponsored a program known as M.A.S.T. (Military Assistance to Safety and Traffic). This program utilizes Department of Defense medical corpsmen and medical evacuation helicopters at various military installations' sites to supplement whatever local emergency medical services delivery system exists. Each is coordinated by a civilian emergency medical services committee according to a local plan. Initial community contact and continuing technical assistance are provided to the communities by regional representatives of the Departments of Health, Education, and Welfare and Transportation. The program is coordinated at the federal level by a three-man M.A.S.T. Interagency Coordinating Committee with representatives from the Departments of Defense, Transportation, and Health, Education, and Welfare. By means of this cooperative program, patients in critical condition, premature infants, human organs, blood, special medications, and medical personnel and equipment have all been transported by M.A.S.T. helicopters. Although many of the missions involve interhospital transfers of critically ill patients, M.A.S.T. also provides first response to medical emergencies and traffic accidents when use of a ground vehicle is not feasible.

## SUMMARY

On the basis of what has been presented it is clear that an effective, efficient, and acceptable emergency medical service program must be built on comprehensiveness and a systems approach that includes the following:

1. Clearly defined and delineated delegation of responsibility, authority, and procedures
2. Systematic planning, organization, administration, and operation
3. Uniform criteria, standards, regulations, and legislation
4. Coordination of efforts and resources
5. Increased skilled manpower
6. Uniform training programs for all levels of emergency medical services personnel
7. Increased and properly distributed quantities of equipment, vehicles, and facilities
8. Uniform communications networks and dispatching procedures
9. Uniform data collection and analysis
10. Public education
11. Implementation of standard evaluation and reporting systems

## REFERENCES

1. Division of Medical Science, National Academy of Sciences: Accidental death and disability: The neglected disease of modern society, Washington, D. C., 1969. The Academy.
2. World almanac, New York, 1973, Newspaper Enterprise Assn., Inc.
3. Izant, R. J., and Hubay, C. A.: The annual injury of 15,000,000 children, J. Trauma **6:**65, Jan. 1966.
4. Accident facts, Chicago, 1971, National Safety Council.
5. Frey, C. F., et al.: Resuscitation and survival in motor accidents, J. Trauma **9:**292, Feb. 1969.
6. Where minutes count, U. S. News and World Rep. June 26, 1972.
7. The crisis in emergency care, New York, 1971, Medical World News, McGraw-Hill Book Co.
8. Huntley, H. C.: National status of emergency health services. In Proceedings of Second National Conference on Emergency Health Services, DEHS pub. no. 16, Rockville, Md., 1972, U. S. Department of Health, Education, and Welfare.
9. National Institute of Mental Health: Emergency services: a service of the community mental health center, PHS pub. no. 1477, Rockville, Md., 1969.
10. Bellak, L.: The role and nature of emergency psychotherapy, Amer. J. Public Health **58:**344, Feb. 1968.
11. Seeley, S.: Quoted in Emergency medicine: emerging specialty, M.D. **16:**79, Sept. 1972.
12. U. S. Department of Health, Education, and Welfare: Ambulance services and hospital emergency departments: digest of surveys conducted 1965 to March 1971, DEHS pub. no. 11, Rockville, Md., 1971.
13. American Medical Association: Categorization of hospital emergency capabilities, Chicago, 1971, Commission on Emergency Medical Services, The Association.
14. U. S. Department of Health, Education, and Welfare: Emergency medical services communications systems, pub. no. (HSM) 73-2003, Rockville, Md., 1972.
15. Cardiac defibrillation can be performed by ambulance attendants, Mod. Med. **40:**57, July 10, 1972.
16. U. S. Department of Health, Education, and Welfare: Ambulance services and hospital emergency departments: digest of surveys conducted 1965 to March 1971, DEHS pub. no. 11, Rockville, Md., 1971.
17. Community-wide emergency medical services: recommendations by the committee on acute medicine of the American Society of Anesthesiologists, J.A.M.A. **204:**133, May 13, 1968.
18. Hampton, O. P.: The systematic approach to emergency medical services, Bull. Amer. Coll. Surg. **53:**231, Sept.-Oct. 1968.
19. American Medical Association: Developing emergency medical services; guidelines for community councils, Chicago, 1971, The Association.
20. Nahum, A. M.: Emergency medical care systems, J.A.M.A. **217:**1530, Sept. 13, 1971.
21. Flashner, B. A., and Boyd, D. R.: The critically injured patient: a plan for organization of statewide system of trauma facilities, Illinois Med. J. **39:**256, March 1971.
22. U. S. Department of Health, Education, and Welfare: State statutes on emergency medical services, pub. no. (HSM) 72-2017, Rockville, Md., 1972.
23. U. S. Department of Health, Education, and Welfare: Recommended standards for development of emergency medical services systems, DEHS pub. no. 4, Rockville, Md., 1971.
24. U. S. Department of Health, Education, and Welfare: Model act for emergency medical services, pub. no. (HSM) 72-2016, Rockville, Md., 1972.
25. National Highway Bureau: Ambulance design criteria, Report prepared by National Academy Engineering and National Research Council, Washington, D. C., 1970, U. S. Department of Transportation.
26. Essential equipment for ambulances, Chicago, 1970, American College of Surgeons.
27. Emergency care and transportation of the sick and injured, Chicago, 1971, American Academy of Orthopaedic Surgeons.

28. National Highway Traffic Safety Administration: Proceedings of national workshop on the training of emergency medical technicians, Washington, D. C., 1972, U. S. Department of Transportation.

29. National Highway Traffic Safety Administration: (a) Basic training program for emergency medical technician-ambulance, (b) Course guide and course coordinator program, (c) Instructor's lesson plans, Washington, D. C., 1969, U. S. Department of Transportation.

30. Hospital emergency services; and Hospital disaster plan. In Association manual for hospitals, Chicago, 1971, Joint Commission on Accreditation of Hospitals.

31. U. S. Department of Health, Education, and Welfare: Emergency medical services communications systems, pub. no. (HSM) 73-2003, Rockville, Md., 1973.

32. American Medical Association: Emergency medical identification symbol and emergency medical identification card, Chicago, 1967, The Association.

33. U. S. Public Health Service: Medical self-help training for you and your community, PHS pub. no. 1042, Rockville, Md., 1970.

34. American Medical Association: Highway directional signs for emergency medical facilities, Chicago, 1971, The Association.

35. Kraus, J. F.: Establishment of a national system for surveillance of injuries, HSMHA Health Rep. **87:**137, Feb. 1972.

36. Boyd, D. R., et al.: Computerized trauma registry: a new method for categorizing physical injuries, Aerosp. Med. **42:**607, June 1971.

37. Paetow, P. F.: Community emergency care advisory councils—how they work, what they accomplish, Bull. Amer. Coll. Surg. **55:**19, Jan. 1970.

*Accuse not nature! She hath done*
*her part. Do thou but thine.*

JOHN MILTON

# CHAPTER 34

# Medical care

The subject of the delivery of medical care has been controversial up to the present and undoubtedly will continue to be so for some time to come. It is not within the province of this book to discuss the details of the many legislative bills and proposals of the past and present. Events have been moving so rapidly that any such discussion would be out of date before publication. The intention, rather, is to present the general problem and the development of attempts at its solution, with emphasis on the dramatic forward movement of recent years.

## RELATIONSHIP BETWEEN PUBLIC HEALTH AND PRIVATE MEDICINE

Public health activities cut across a great many other phases of community life and involve contact with the members of most businesses and professions. Among these one of the most intimate contacts is with the medical profession. There are many reasons for this. To begin with, most of those engaged in public health work are themselves either members of the medical profession or of some other profession closely related to it. All public health workers and medical practitioners are concerned with the same ultimate goal,—health. Furthermore, many of the programs sponsored by health agencies require the active cooperation and participation of private physicians. In fact, it has been said that every private physician should be in effect a deputy health officer and that his office should represent, for the individuals and families he serves, a branch of the health department. The wish that some day most preventive and promotive as well as thera-

peutic medicine would be obtained from family or personal physicians seldom meets with argument. Finally, private medical practice and public health activities have a considerable effect on each other. Modern public health programs depend greatly on concurrent effective private practice. Every health officer realizes that the science and art of medicine are the foundations of public health. In turn, many public health activities such as laboratories and health education operate to the assistance of private practitioners.

To understand adequately the significance of this relationship, which in the light of recent trends is certain to become even more intimate, it is well to review briefly and jointly the development of these two fields, especially as related to and affected by the development of the modern industrial economy and social organization.

## EVOLUTION OF MODERN MEDICINE AND SOCIETY

Generally speaking, it is advantageous to consider these developments in three time periods: the period preceding the so-called Industrial Revolution, the period from about 1750 to 1850 during which the Industrial Revolution took place, and the time that has elapsed since. Before the Industrial Revolution, which is usually considered to have begun about 1750, the social and economic structure of the Western world was relatively simple. Few large cities existed, and the economy was essentially agrarian. Economic and social life was limited to the small local community or neighborhood,

**607**

and although these aspects of life were stable, they were on a rather low scale in comparison with the present and involved relatively little personal freedom. Social classes were rigidly stratified and adhered to by custom from one generation to the next. Only with great difficulty could a son pursue a way of life different from that of this father. Industry in the present sense of the word simply did not exist. The family was the unit of production, usually making for itself whatever goods it needed. Manufacturing, to the extent that it did exist, was carried on either through guilds, which provided for the continuous training of a limited number of apprentices by skilled craftsmen, or by means of the "putting-out system." This latter consisted of putting raw materials into the hands of individuals, who with all members of their families worked on them on a piece basis. Thus the individual craftsman was responsible for the entire process of manufacture and usually was personally acquainted with the source of his materials and the ultimate consumer of the product of his labors.

During this era, the practice of medicine was at one of its lowest ebbs. The scientific viewpoint was generally underdeveloped. Medical procedures were based largely on speculation and supersitition, and little experimentation or planned observation was engaged in. There were no standards of medical education or practice, and healers and physicians were often self-designated. Many of them were charlatans, often unworthy of trust not only with regard to competent medical care but also in terms of private possessions. Since surgeons worked with their hands and often performed surgery as an adjunct to barbering, they were held in particularly low esteem. Treatment consisted chiefly of the use of purgatives and leeches, and considerable attention was given to various aspects of cosmetology. The relatively few hospitals were essentially pesthouses, consignment to which usually signified impending death. At any rate the average member of society had little if any contact with physicians, since the latter, if not vagrant itinerants, were generally attached to the households of the noble and wealthy classes. They seldom received fixed payments for their services, usually depending on gratuities.

The provision of medical service in a public sense was in its most embryonic form. Social controls and requirements relating to the practice of medicine were either elementary or nonexistent. It is true that during the late Middle Ages the professional behavior and avarice of physicians in some urban centers occasionally led to the legal fixing of fees and to requirements that some arrangements be made for the care of the sick poor. At best, however, these requirements were rare and sporadic and of a highly unsatisfactory nature. As early as the thirteenth century, a few European towns employed town surgeons. Town physicians, on the other hand, are not encountered historically until the sixteenth century. From the fourteenth century on it became not uncommon to require surgeons and later physicians to submit public reports of all injuries they treated and cases of certain diseases, notably leprosy, plague, and syphilis. Very gradually physicians became concerned with sanitation and other aspects of public health.

Whatever care, medical or otherwise, provided for the sick, poor, aged, and homeless, the Church was its source. Charity by this time had become a dominant manifestation of acceptable Christian behavior, and medical, nursing, and hospital care became a major interest and activity of many monastic orders. Later, during the sixteenth, seventeenth, and eighteenth centuries these responsibilities gradually began to shift from the Church to the state. As pointed out by Shryock,[1] however: "This humanitarianism, like the clerical form of earlier centuries, largely expressed the benevolence of the upper classes rather than any demand for reform from below."

The Industrial Revolution brought with it tremendous changes not only in methods of manufacturing but also in the modes of transportation and facilities for the communication of ideas and information. Manufacturing was fractionated into component processes, and the laboring class became concentrated in industrial centers of population and organized to work in large factories for the greater profit of management. A new economic and political power came about in the form of the industrialist and economic royalist. To such a height did the desire for high profits soar that all consideration for human welfare and decency was forgotten. No longer were goods made by skilled guild members or craftsmen with pride in their workmanship. No longer was the consumer personally acquainted with the producer. The personal face-to-face relationship between employer and employee disappeared as well. Articles were now produced through the combined efforts of a great many individuals. As might have been expected, the social and economic center of gravity shifted from the agrarian to the urban scene. Rural areas themselves were directly affected. The populations of industrial cities were not self-maintaining because of their appalling death rates. They therefore required continuous replenishment from the rural population.

Interestingly enough it was during this period of cruel industrialization and economic interdependence that the search for scientific knowledge received a much needed impetus. Although it is true that the primary incentive was the development of new techniques for greater economic gains, the results were ultimately beneficial to society. The character of the practice of medicine began to undergo some improvement. A trend toward logical experimentation and observation developed. A system of medical training by apprenticeship came into vogue, and the physician changed his locale from the highway and the manor to take his place as a private entrepreneur in competition with other physicians. For a while this competition resulted in many abuses, which led eventually to the necessity for the reestablishment of a long-dormant code of professional ethics.

With some exceptions diseases were not considered as distinct entities but were classified in terms of their manifestations, such as swellings, fevers, and inflammations. The equipment of the physicians was still simple, and his only adjunct was the pharmacy, which in most instances he operated himself. Hospitals more than ever were pesthouses because of the tremendously increased incidence of communicable diseases for which the filthy centers of population served as breeding grounds.

During the nineteenth century the idea of corporate structures developed and resulted in the monopolistic control of each industry and not infrequently of several industries together. The intent, of course, was to achieve still greater industrial efficiency and, not incidentally, the ultimate in profits from the smallest possible cost or investment. Entire geographic regions as well as the workers themselves became specialized in function, and the social distance between producer and consumer was widened even more. Abuse of the laboring class became so flagrant that by 1850 a social reaction began to set in and slowly to swing the pendulum in the opposite direction. Notable in this respect were several prominent persons imbued, for that or for any period, with an unusual spirit of humanitarianism. A few among those who might be named were Edwin Chadwick, Robert Owen, Southwood Smith, John Stuart Mill, and Lord Ashley. These and others like them did their utmost to bring into the public consciousness an appreciation of the conditions under which the laboring classes were forced to live and work.

Gradually many social reforms got under way; these reforms dealt with working conditions, poor welfare, housing of the working classes, the care of orphans and the insane, education, and sanitary conditions. Scientific and technologic investigations that had formerly been conducted largely from the point of view of industrial development now began to be pursued for their own sake and for the benefit of humanity as a whole. Despite these trends, economic welfare was still insecure. More than ever, workers earned a living instead of making one. By this time the greatest handicap to industrial expansion was the fact that techniques of distribution of goods lagged far behind techniques of production. The subsequent solution of this was dependent on the invention of the steam locomotive, the internal combustion engine, and the construction of paved, all-weather roads.

During this period of social revolution, tremendous gains were made in the field of medicine, particularly in relation to scientific research and educational standards. There came about a great eagerness for new medical knowledge that eventually led, among other things, to the conclusive proof of the bacteriologic causation of many diseases. Spectacular discoveries followed one another at a breathtaking pace. One result of this was the foundation of preventive medicine and sanitary science. Medical education became formalized with the establishment of schools with increasingly higher standards. Although the general practitioner was still the prototype, many medical specialties began to appear. The construction and use of hospitals was expanded, and they gradually came to be looked on as places for the restoration of health rather than houses of death. Furthermore, they began to take their place as centers for teaching and research. Professionally trained nurses and scientific laboratories entered the ranks of auxiliary facilities on which both the public and the medical profession gradually became more dependent.

On the economic side of the practice of medicine some interesting changes were coming about. The itinerant physician became a thing of the past. Groups of physicians began to band together to form group practices or private clinics. Medical care was now offered to all components of the population on a competitive fee-for-service basis with a sliding scale as a means of adjustment for varying abilities to pay. A growth of free medical service in hospital wards appeared as one manifestation of the medical profession's acceptance of responsibility for the public welfare. In this manner medicine finally came to be regarded as a social science. Thus in 1847 Solomon Neumann of Berlin published his book *Public Health and Property,* in which he stated that medicine is fundamentally a social science and that as long as it does not correspond to this reality, we cannot taste its fruits and must content ourselves with the rind. A year later Rudolph Virchow declared that physicians were the counselors of the poor and that to a great extent medicine was the key to the social question.[2] Perhaps the most outstanding evidences of the influence of the changing social and economic structure on the form of medical practice were the widening of the breach between the discovery of medical knowledge and its application and the ever-rising cost of medical care resulting from the increased investment required for medical education and the rendering of modern medical services by skilled physicians and their auxiliary assistants.

It is interesting that despite the remarkable medical discoveries of the late nineteenth century such as improved diagnostic and therapeutic techniques, the development of anesthesia, antisepsis, and asepsis, and the study of cellular physiology and pathology, to mention only a few, medicine as practiced by average physicians was still scientifically backward. Until the close of the century, it was still common to consider illness as fevers, dropsy, inflammations, and the like, and treatment still consisted mostly of blood letting and the evacuation of "ill humours" by physicking, sweating, diuretics, vomiting, and the formation of blisters. Calomel, the leech, and the lancet were still the important contents of the physician's bag. In fact, leeches were used literally by the hundreds of thousands each year.

Characteristic of the American physician of this period was Dr. Hiram Buhrman, who practiced in small towns in Maryland and Pennsylvania in the 1870s. His regulation fee was 25 cents for an office call. This included medicines unless expensive drugs were necessary. A house visit within the township was 50 cents without medicine, 75 cents with medicine. The physician compounded his own prescriptions. In case of death there was a $3 fee, for which he did most of the work of the present-day mortician. All obstetric cases, regardless of the length of labor, were $5, as were abortions, whereas miscarriages were billed at $1.50. A search through his account books showed that in all but two instances he made only one house visit after delivery, and this on the following day. The fee for setting and caring for a fractured clavicle, including all material used in the dressing, was $5, whereas a fractured thigh cost $10. Lancing an abscess or a felon was 50 cents. Dr. Buhrman also functioned as a dentist. A tooth extraction cost 25 cents, except when several in a row were removed at the same time, in which case the fee per tooth was reduced. When chloroform was used for extractions, the total charge was $2. These were the charges, but they were not always collected. When money was needed, the physician set out in person as a collector of outstanding accounts.

As did other physicians of his day, to visit his patients he traveled on horseback with saddlebags or in a gig or buggy and carried a limited supply of fever medicine, sulfur, and molasses, obstetric forceps, and a bag of instruments for emergencies. His major expenses other than those of his home, involved the stabling and feeding of the horses and the purchase of saddles, horse collars, fly nets, and halters. In this unspecialized small town practice, conducted with few instruments and drugs, on a limited number of diseases, the hospital did not enter into the picture at all.[3]

As a matter of fact, as late as the 1890s much of the most advanced practice was usually carried on in an office that had as its equipment a medicine cabinet, a sofa or an examing table, and a table that could be used as a laboratory. The technical equipment consisted of a thermometer, a stethoscope, a prescription pad, and a sufficient amount of chemicals to determine the presence of albumin and sugar in the urine. A few particularly advanced practitioners had microscopes, and still fewer were able to examine a specimen of blood to determine the leukocyte count and the presence or absence of malarial parasites.

With the beginning of the twentieth century,

and especially as a result of the Flexner report on medical education, the practice of medicine began to mature as a science and as a result became much more effective. The speculative theories and traditional practices of the physician of the nineteenth century had failed to win the confidence of the public, and as a consequence many medical cults flourished. In fact it has been said that 1912 was a turning point in the United States when a patient finally had a 50% chance of a correct *diagnosis*. With the acceptance and application of the newer scientific knowledge by the orthodox physician in practice and as a result of more widespread public education and understanding, the medical profession has since risen high in the public esteem.

Unfortunately this has not occurred without accompanying complications. Improvements in diagnosis and treatment have required at the same time the development of highly trained specialists and costly diagnostic and therapeutic tools with a corresponding increase in the cost of medical care. Robinson[4] emphasized this by comparing two patients admitted to the same hospital with the same heart condition, one in 1913, the other 25 years later in 1938. The first patient was cared for by a visiting physician, an intern, and one specialist, the pathologist-bacteriologist. The completed record covered 2½ pages. The second patient was observed and described by 3 visiting physicians, 2 residents, 3 interns, 10 specialists, and 14 technologists, a total of 32 individuals, and although the record of the case was still incomplete, it already covered 29 pages. He concluded that the more recent case, in its sharp contrast with medicine of the past, presents one of the major social problems facing contemporary medical practice. The latter instance, it should be noted, occurred well before the current day of intensive coronary care units, electronic monitoring, and defibrillators.

## ECONOMIC FACTORS INFLUENCING THE NEED FOR MEDICAL CARE

Pertinent to the ability to obtain medical care are several related economic factors concerned with the distribution of wealth and its effect on the need for medical care and the distribution of medical facilities. It is obvious that the economic level of a community plays a significant role in determining the degree of its health and illness and in the extensiveness of its facilities to care for them. Since wealth is nowhere

**Table 34-1.** Distribution of families and unrelated individuals by total money income, United States, 1969*

| Total money income | Percentage of families |
|---|---|
| Under $3,000 | 9.3 |
| $3,000-4,999 | 10.7 |
| $5,000-6,999 | 12.3 |
| $7,000-9,999 | 21.7 |
| $10,000-14,999 | 26.7 |
| $15,000 and over | 19.2 |
| Median income = $9,433 | |

*Statistical abstract of the United States, Washington, D. C., 1971, Government Printing Office.

distributed equitably, it naturally follows that the state of health of a community or of a nation cannot be uniform. In a very literal sense health and the treatment of illness are purchasable, but the ability to purchase them is not always present. The use of average figures to depict the purchasing power of a community of people tends to be greatly misleading.

Thus although the median family income in the United States is high, about $9,590 in 1970, there is considerable variation by region, degree of urbanization, and other factors. For example, the mean family income for urban and rural nonfarm families is approximately twice that of the rural farm families. Table 34-1 presents the distribution of families by total money income, before taxes, in 1969 in the United States. It indicates, for example, a variation of from 9.3% of families with annual incomes less than $3,000 to almost 46% of families with annual incomes of more than $10,000.[5]

The inequity of the distribution of purchasing power is magnified still further when the nation is considered in terms of its constituent parts. It is well known, for example, that physicians tend to cluster in and around cities, especially the large metropolitan centers of population. They do this for many reasons—a better opportunity to develop large active practices; the availability of hospitals, laboratories, ancillary personnel, and other professional aid; opportunities for postgraduate education as well as for teaching; cultural attractions; living comfort; good schools, stores, and other essentials. The result is shown in Table 34-2. From it one can note not only the concentration of physicians but especially of specialists in the urban centers of the nation.

**Table 34-2.** Distribution of practicing physicians, hospitals, beds, population, and income by metropolitan and nonmetropolitan areas, United States, 1971*

| Resources | Total | Metropolitan | | Nonmetropolitan | |
|---|---|---|---|---|---|
| | | Number | Percent | Number | Percent |
| Total physicians in patient care | 263,730 | 225,651 | 85.6 | 38,079 | 14.4 |
| Office based | | | | | |
| General practice | 49,979 | 33,660 | 67.3 | 16,319 | 32.7 |
| Specialties | 144,953 | 127,641 | 88.1 | 17,312 | 11.9 |
| Hospital based | 68,798 | 64,350 | 93.5 | 4,448 | 6.5 |
| Number of hospitals | 5,749 | 2,819 | 49.0 | 2,930 | 51.0 |
| Hospital beds | 849,640 | 632,333 | 74.4 | 217,307 | 25.6 |
| Population | 205,017,100 | 150,907,300 | 73.6 | 54,109,800 | 26.4 |
| Income per household | $10,565 | $11,323 | | $8,422 | |

*From American Medical Association: Distribution of physicians in the U. S., 1971, Chicago, 1972, The Association.

**Table 34-3.** Distribution of practicing physicians by states per 100,000 population, United States, 1971*

| State | Physicians per 100,000 population | State | Physicians per 100,000 population |
|---|---|---|---|
| Alabama | 80 | Montana | 98 |
| Alaska | 75 | Nebraska | 99 |
| Arizona | 123 | Nevada | 100 |
| Arkansas | 82 | New Hampshire | 116 |
| California | 166 | New Jersey | 128 |
| Colorado | 148 | New Mexico | 101 |
| Connecticut | 163 | New York | 198 |
| Delaware | 121 | North Carolina | 94 |
| Dist. of Columbia | 344 | North Dakota | 85 |
| Florida | 122 | Ohio | 117 |
| Georgia | 96 | Oklahoma | 88 |
| Hawaii | 137 | Oregon | 124 |
| Idaho | 86 | Pennsylvania | 132 |
| Illinois | 122 | Rhode Island | 142 |
| Indiana | 90 | South Carolina | 85 |
| Iowa | 91 | South Dakota | 73 |
| Kansas | 103 | Tennessee | 104 |
| Kentucky | 91 | Texas | 105 |
| Louisiana | 107 | Utah | 122 |
| Maine | 98 | Vermont | 145 |
| Maryland | 157 | Virginia | 110 |
| Massachusetts | 171 | Washington | 127 |
| Michigan | 111 | West Virginia | 95 |
| Minnesota | 129 | Wisconsin | 109 |
| Mississippi | 75 | Wyoming | 89 |
| Missouri | 111 | U. S. | 128 |

*From American Medical Association: Distribution of physicians in the U. S., 1971, Chicago, 1972, The Association.

This factor combined with another, regional wealth, brings about a geographic variation of considerable dimension. This may be observed in Table 34-3, which presents for each of the states the physician-population ratios by specialty and hospital affiliation. It is obvious that the more affluent states have the lion's share not only of physicians but also of specialists. Beyond this the average age of physicians is significantly higher in the economically less privileged states and areas.[6]

The relative economic standing of the various geographic regions of the nation varies from the well-known disadvantageous position occupied by the southeastern states to the economically affluent northeastern and Pacific states. These economic inequities have a significant effect on the distribution of personnel and facilities for the treatment of illness. A direct

relationship is readily seen to exist between them and the purchasing powers of the respective regions. Thus the northeastern states, with an average household income in 1970 of about $11,700, have 194 physicians per 100,000 inhabitants, in contrast with the southeastern states, whose average household income of only a little more than $9,400 attracts and supports only 123 physicians for every 100,000 inhabitants. If the ages and qualifications of the physicians were considered, these discrepancies would become even greater. Similarly the more affluent northeastern states have about twice the number of dentists in relation to population as do the states of the southeastern region. With regard to the number of acceptable general hospital beds available the same picture holds true. However, a significant equalization has occurred in this regard as a result of the Hos-

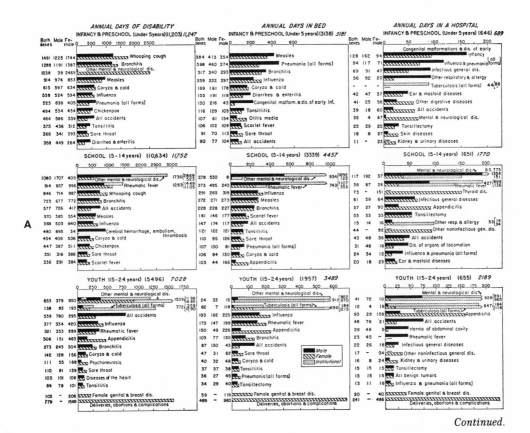

*Continued.*

**Fig. 34-1, A** and **B.** Twelve diagnoses with the highest annual rates per 1,000 population in each of six age groups for days of disability, days confined to bed, and days of hospital care—three household surveys with visits at intervals of 1 to 3 months, covering a total of 37,988 full-time person-years of observation for white persons. (From Collins, S. D., Lehmann, J. L., and Trantham, K. S.: Major causes of illness of various severities and major causes of death in six age periods of life, PHS pub. no. 440, Washington, D. C., 1955.)

**Fig. 34-1, cont'd.** For legend see p. 613.

pital Survey and Construction Act (Hill-Burton Act) of 1946.

Another factor that accentuates both the need for medical and hospital care and the disparities that exist among regional resources is the proportion of older persons in the population. Persons 65 years of age and over require more medical attention and hospitalization than any other age component of society. For example, this age group uses about 7 days of hospital care per capita per year as compared with less than 3 days per capita for all other age groups. Furthermore, this is a period of decreased or absent earning power, hence much less ability to afford the needed care. Regionally this works especially to the disadvantage of the northeastern, central, and northwestern states.

The unequal distribution of medical personnel and facilities would not be of such serious consequence if the socioeconomic factors causing it did not also have an adverse influence on the need for them. Numerous studies have shown

that the total illness experience of a population follows a more or less definite pattern. Although the average American suffers an injury or an illness about two and one half times a year, there obviously are some who go through the year unscathed, whereas others far exceed the average expectation. Accordingly, in any average current year out of each 1 million American people 470,000 will suffer no serious illness, 320,000 will have one illness during the year, 140,000 will have two illnesses, 50,000 will have three illnesses, and 20,000 will have four or more illnesses.

For the general population it is possible to know in advance not only the total amount of illness but also the type. Numerous studies have been carried out for this purpose during recent years. Among them, those of Collins and associates[7,8] are particularly classic. Some of the results of their analyses of five illness and household surveys in the United States are presented in Figs. 34-1 and 34-2. The charts

**Fig. 34-2.** Ten most frequent causes of surgery per 1,000 males and females of five broad age groups, and ten diagnoses with the highest percentage of cases in the same age groups that were treated surgically—white families canvassed periodically in five illness surveys covering 80,768 person-years of observation. (From Collins, S. D., Lehmann, J. L., and Trantham, K. S.: Surgical experience in selected areas of United States, PHS pub. no. 473, Washington, D. C., 1956.)

in Fig. 34-1 show annual days of disability, days in bed, and days in a hospital by age and sex for the predominant diagnoses. The charts in Fig. 34-2 show the incidence by age and sex of the most frequent causes of surgery.

The overall pattern of illness in the general population is predictable, whereas the forthcoming experience of the individual cannot be foretold. However, it is known that the lower the individual is on the economic scale the more likely he is to experience one or more serious illnesses during any year. This is not surprising, since purchasing power determines the amount

and quality of food consumed, the degree of exposure to or protection from the causes of illness or accidents, and the ability to obtain many medical as well as other types of services.

## EXPENDITURES FOR MEDICAL CARE

The combined effect of the unpredictability of illness in the individual and the influence of economic factors on the probability of illness and the distribution of medical facilities therefore has caused a relatively small proportion of a population to bear the major share of the economic burden due to illness at any given time. Furthermore, it is found that this unfortunate fraction of the population includes an unduly disproportionate number of those who are least able, because of their limited incomes, to meet the costs of adequate care.

When the factors of low income and increased tendency to become ill are considered together, it is found that the lower income groups not only have more frequent medical bills but they also must spend proportionately more of their income for this purpose than the higher income groups; this is true despite their greater tendency toward self-treatment or even their frequent failure to obtain care.

Considering the total picture, attention may be called to the fact that the nation suffers a loss of many billions of dollars each year because of illness. This is made up of expenditures for avoidable medical care, the value of the average 7 working days per year lost by the average wage earner because of illness, and the capital value of the lives that are lost because of causes that in the light of present medical science may be considered preventable. These seem like large sums, especially when the relatively small amount of money that would be required to avoid or at least reduce them is considered.

The amount of investment necessary for adequate preventive care and the early diagnosis and treatment of disease appears almost insignificant when compared with the sums expended by the nation for other purposes. Nations find it possible to spend enormous amounts in time of war for the destruction of life. It is a commentary on the human species that such expenditures are so willingly made at the same time that appropriations to provide inexpensive immunizations of children or examinations for cancer or heart disease are so often resisted.

Beyond the costs of waging war, expenditures for more routine needs and activities offer an interesting contrast to the amount expended for medical purposes. Table 34-4 presents a breakdown of personal expenditures of the American public in 1970. It will be observed that the amount spent for recreation is almost as much as the amount devoted to all aspects of medical care. Regretfully, the latter sum is only twice the amount spent for tobacco, which causes much disease and premature death.

It should be noted that whereas costs of medical care have increased in company with everything else, the major component of the increase has been in hospital costs.

**Table 34-4.** Personal consumption expenditures, United States, 1970 (in millions of dollars)*

| Item | Amount |
| --- | --- |
| Food, tobacco, and beverages (including alcoholic beverages) | 143,272 |
| Housing | 90,921 |
| Household operation | 86,629 |
| Transportation | 77,788 |
| Clothing, accessories, and jewelry | 61,966 |
| **Medical, dental, and hospital care** | **46,755** |
| Recreation | 40,197 |
| Personal business | 34,965 |
| Personal care (nonmedical) | 10,425 |
| Private education and research | 10,428 |
| Religious and welfare activities | 8,609 |
| Foreign travel and other | 4,806 |

* Statistical abstract of the United States, Washington, D. C., 1971, Government Printing Office.

How is the medical dollar spent? Table 34-5 presents the proportionate breakdown of medically related expenditures for the period between 1929 and 1970. Although in absolute terms the amount of money spent for all of the items has increased, significant shifts have occurred among them in relation to each other. By far the most striking change has been in connection with the cost of hospitalization. Although the proportion of the medical dollar devoted to payment of physicians and dentists has decreased during the past three decades, the proportionate amount expended for hospitalization has more than doubled. This is especially evident if the proportions for insurance, much of which represent hospitalization insurance, are added to the amounts designated for hospitals. In fact when this is done, the proportionate expenditures for hospitals and insurance combined show an increase from about one sixth of the total medical dollar in 1929 to about one third of the total medical dollar in 1970. Also of interest is the fact that whereas a large number of complex and valuable new drugs and medicines have been developed and put to use during this period, the proportionate expenditure for them has remained about the same. In fact in relation to percentage of disposable personal income, expenditures for medical drugs and appliances are now about one half of what they were in 1940. The changes that have occurred in expenditures for the various components of medical care, however, are most dramatically

**Table 34-5.** Changes in the percentage distribution of medical costs, United States, 1929 to 1970*

| Type of expenditure | 1929 | 1940 | 1950 | 1960 | 1970 |
|---|---|---|---|---|---|
| Physicians | 33 | 30 | 28 | 25 | 22 |
| Dentists | 16 | 14 | 11 | 10 | 8 |
| Hospitals | 14 | 18 | 23 | 26 | 42 |
| Drugs and appliances | 25 | 27 | 26 | 26 | 15 |
| All other | 12 | 11 | 12 | 13 | 13 |
| Total | 100 | 100 | 100 | 100 | 100 |

*Statistical abstract of the United States, Washington, D. C., 1971, Government Printing Office.

**Table 34-6.** Consumer price indexes, components of medical care, United States, 1950 to 1970 (1967 = 100)*

| Year | Total medical care | Physician's fees | Dentist's fees | Drugs and prescriptions | Optometric examination and eyeglasses | Hospital daily service charge | All consumer items |
|---|---|---|---|---|---|---|---|
| 1950 | 53.7 | 55.2 | 63.9 | 88.5 | 73.5 | 28.9 | 77.0 |
| 1960 | 79.1 | 77.0 | 82.1 | 104.5 | 85.1 | 56.3 | 101.6 |
| 1970 | 120.2 | 121.4 | 119.4 | 103.5 | 113.9 | 144.5 | 115.5 |
| Ratio, 1970 to 1950 | 2.24 | 2.20 | 1.87 | 1.17 | 1.55 | 5.00 | 1.50 |

*Statistical abstract of the United States, Washington, D. C., 1971, Government Printing Office.

indicated by a comparison of them with consumer price indexes. This is presented in Table 34-6, which shows that whereas between 1950 and 1970 physicians' and dentists' fees increased at a rate not much more than the general consumer price index and drug price increases were actually much less, hospital rates increased more than three times as fast. Several other points are of interest in relation to certain items not included in the figures. Expenditures for nursing are about one fifth of the amount paid to private physicians. Also the estimated amount paid to cultists is about equal to the per capita sum expended for public health work.

## ATTEMPTS TO SOLVE THE PROBLEM

By the end of the eighteenth century, if indeed not sooner, problems of health and disease were recognized as subjects of social and political concern. In fact by that time it was beginning to be realized that these problems were associated with and part of a social problem of much greater magnitude, that is, the emerging struggle for the expression of the rights of the common man. This struggle was destined to become a main theme of political appeal, and the health of the masses, particularly of the working classes, became one of the major talking points during the nineteenth century, not only of such humanitarians as Chadwick, Southwood Smith, Shattuck, and others like them, but also of the spokesmen for the new political ideologies exemplified by Engels and Marx. Thus the stage of recognition and orientation of the problem was reached. What to do about it, how to solve it, was yet another problem, the solution of which was not to be forthcoming for at least another century and a half.

To consider the preliminary attempts to find an answer it is necessary to retrace our steps to some extent. It has been seen that the eighteenth and nineteenth centuries were characterized by a shift from a rural agrarian society to an urban industrialized society, a growing insecurity of personal income, a great increase in the low-income population, a considerably increased risk of sickness due to the social and economic changes, and constantly rising costs of medical care. Rosen,[9,10] in his discussion of the early attempts to solve the problem, rightly highlights the propositions of three outstanding social thinkers of the times: Defoe and Bellers in England and de Chamousset in France. With the development of statistical methodology and the increasing accumulation and analysis of vital data it became possible, at least in a crude way, to calculate certain types of risks. Marine and fire insurance were fairly well established and used. Life insurance companies were in the process of acceptance. It is not too surprising therefore that even at a relatively early date some thought was given to the possibility of applying this valuable social technique to the risk of illness. Daniel Defoe was apparently the first to make the suggestion, in 1697. In an essay he proposed that the insurance principle be applied to the social problems of the poor, including medical and institutional care and disability pensions.

Shortly afterward, in 1714, John Bellers suggested a rather detailed plan for a national health service in England. He believed that the program should be sponsored by government, since "it is too great a burden to be left upon the shoulders, or to the care of the physicians alone, no private purse being able to bear the needful charges of it. Especially considering the necessity of many and the indifferency of others of that faculty, further than to procure a plentiful substance for themselves: And how much it concerns every other person, there is more reason to expect, the State should bear a good part of the expense of it."[10] He therefore proposed the establishment of governmental hospitals for teaching and research, a national health institute, and a plan to provide medical care to the sick poor. Going even further in his social thinking, de Chamousset in 1754 proposed a plan of hospital insurance with a broader population base. Here for perhaps the first time is encountered a concern for others than the traditionally dependent poor, that is, a concern for the bulk of the population comprising the so-called self-respecting middle class. He argued as follows[10]:

There are asylums available to the destitute, and that is a resource useful to those to whom it is not humiliating to accept the free assistance which charity offers. (But there is) the class of the greatest number of citizens, who not being rich enough to provide sufficient aid at home or poor enough to be taken to an almshouse, languish and often perish miserably, victims of the propriety to which they are subjected by their class of siciety. Such are the industrious artisans, merchants whose trade is limited, and in general all those valuable men who live daily by the fruits of their labor, and who often for that reason have no recourse to treatment when a disease becomes incurable. The start of a disease exhausts all their resources; the more they deserve help, the less can they bring themselves to profit by the only resources that remain to them, and to find themselves in public asylums.

Unfortunately little came of these suggestions. Eventually, with no action forthcoming from other directions, workers themselves in some parts of England and a few other countries began to inaugurate schemes at their own expense for protecting themselves against the risks of illness and injury. Trade benefit associations and societies were formed to contract with physicians and surgeons for the care of the members of the group, and each worker was assessed a fixed sum for annual dues or fees. How similar this is to recent events in the United States.

By the beginning of the nineteenth century there had been formed in England nearly 10,000 societies of this type with a total membership of close to a million workers. So common, in fact, had these plans become that in 1773 and later in 1789 bills were introduced in Parliament to provide sickness and old-age benefits for the laboring poor. In both instances the bills were approved by the Commons but rejected by the House of Lords. During the same period, there was much discussion in England concerning the possibility of requiring by law that all workers join privately operated benefit societies, and suggestions were even made that the government should bear part of the cost. Interestingly such ideas and proposals were vigorously opposed in England at that time with many arguments similar to those heard much more recently in the United States. Note the similarity between this idea and the third of the 12 points of the program suggested by the American Medical Association in early 1949.[11] It proposed that there be "further development and wider coverage by voluntary hospital and medical care plans to meet the costs of illness, with extension as rapidly as possible into rural areas. Aid through the states to the indigent and medically indigent by the utilization of voluntary hospital and medical care plans with local administration and local determination of needs."

Meanwhile the medical profession was not entirely inactive. Many steps were being taken to clean house by the development of standards, professional licensure, and the improvement of medical education. Public health measures, in the then ordinary but now narrow sense of state administration of quarantine and public sanitation, were generally supported by the medical profession. Opposition to public provisions for vaccination, however, was not unknown. Support was given to the extension of charity relief and medical care to the indigent. Beyond this, except for rare instances, little was attempted by the medical profession to solve the broader aspects of the medical care problem. Occasional private physicians engaged in a certain amount of contract practice whereby for a fixed prepaid sum they provided care to an individual or a family for a year or some other agreed-on period of time. Even this practice, however, was officially frowned on, as it still was in the United States only two decades ago.

The most significant attempt to solve the problem of providing adequate medical care for a large population was made in Germany during the second half of the nineteenth century. It took the form of a nationally sponsored and administered plan for compulsory, comprehensive social insurance. Although since frequently pointed to as an autocratic scheme to control the lives and behavior of a people and of the medical profession, it is interesting that the plan was not instituted and enforced merely by Bismarck's will. In all, the plan was the subject of 9 years of argument, debate, and struggle in the Reichstag and when finally adopted, represented a considerable compromise. It is also interesting that it met with relatively little opposition from German practitioners of medicine. The plan provided for sickness, accident, and old-age benefits, supported by contributions from employees, employers, and the state. Despite its past and present critics, so satisfactory was it to those involved that it was retained long after the downfall of the Bismarckian regime. In fact when Germany was defeated in 1918 and Alsace-Lorraine was returned to France, its population insisted that the German social insurance system be continued for them. Eventually in 1928 a similar nationwide plan was instituted for the rest of the French Republic.

Meanwhile recognition of the problem and attempts to solve it spread not merely throughout the European continent but beyond to many other parts of the world. One nation after another adopted some form of compulsory health insurance, and at the present time almost every major nation has some plan in operation. No two plans are identical, every major aspect of them showing some variation, whether in comprehensiveness of service, population served, type of administration and payment, or source of funds. Table 34-7 presents a listing of the years in which major compulsory health insurance plans were enacted.

**Table 34-7.** Dates of enactment of compulsory health insurance, 1883 to 1948

| | |
|---|---|
| 1883 | Germany |
| 1888 | Austria |
| 1891 | Hungary |
| 1901 | Luxemburg |
| 1909 | Norway |
| 1911 | Great Britain |
| 1911 | Eire |
| 1911 | Switzerland |
| 1912 | Rumania |
| 1917 | Estonia |
| 1918 | Bulgaria |
| 1919 | Czechoslovakia |
| 1919 | Portugal |
| 1920 | Poland |
| 1922 | USSR |
| 1922 | Yugoslavia |
| 1922 | Latvia |
| 1922 | Japan |
| 1922 | Greece |
| 1924 | Chile |
| 1925 | Netherlands |
| 1925 | Italy |
| 1925 | Lithuania |
| 1928 | France |
| 1933 | Denmark |
| 1936 | Peru |
| 1938 | New Zealand |
| 1940 | Holland |
| 1941 | Costa Rica |
| 1943 | Mexico |
| 1945 | Brazil |
| 1948 | England |

The National Health Service, which was initiated in England in 1948, attracted much worldwide attention. This plan, adopted by the government over the strong opposition of the medical profession, now claims 97% enrollment. From its inception it has been very comprehensive in its benefits and services. This resulted in considerable difficulty in its early years because of the public rush to remedy vast backlogs of dental and visual defects. Although it is still criticized on various counts by many outside as well as within the medical profession, there is general agreement that it has resulted in more widespread and generally better medical and related services for more people. It is interesting to note, however, that during the first decade of its existence membership in voluntary health insurance plans also increased tenfold, from 84,000 in 1948 to 834,000 in 1958. The National Health Services of both England and Scotland were significantly reorganized and modernized on April 1, 1974.

One basis of difference and disagreement among the prepaid medical care systems that have developed in various countries is the method of payment of physicians. As indicated by Evang,[12] no generally accepted system can be found in Europe at the present time, the following being currently in existence:

1. Payment on a capitation basis (panel system) as in England
2. Payment on a cash basis, as in Germany
3. Fee for service, as in Norway
4. Fixed salaries, as in the USSR
5. Basic salary combined with one of the preceding types listed

## DEVELOPMENTS IN THE UNITED STATES

The Western Hemisphere, perhaps because of the tardiness of its discovery and development and because of the usually extremely localized type of society and government during its early history, was slow to produce any specific thought or action with regard to the problem of the adequate provision of medical care. An exception to this was the provision made in the early years of the Republic for medical and hospital care of merchant seamen. Incidentally, the bill was the first introduced in the first session of the Congress of the United States, but because of some disagreements by ship owners who had to contribute part of the cost, along with the seamen themselves, the measure was not finally passed until July 16, 1798, when it was signed into law by President John Adams. As mentioned in Chapter 2, this was destined to be the precursor of the United States Public Health Service. In general, provisions for free medical services were scanty and simple and restricted to the very poor. The pattern that was followed varied from one town to another. In some instances a private physician would be engaged, perhaps because of a low bid, at a fixed stipend to provide care to the sick poor. In others stated fees were paid by the town treasurer when bills submitted by a physician were authorized. Not infrequently the fee for each particular case required a special vote. All of these three procedures are still resorted to in certain communities in the United States.

From this beginning there developed the provisions that have been followed for public medical care in the United States. These provisions are still essentially those of charity care of the sick poor, interrelated with and often administered in conjunction with other social welfare benefits such as subsidies for fuel, food, and housing. In most instances the application of some form of means test is required. This not too stimulating experience, in addition to being demeaning to the patient, necessarily adds considerably to the cost of administration. In contrast with this is the rather spectacular development of public health measures in the United States. Of most pertinent interest is the extent to which public health programs in this country have repeatedly found themselves in the position of having to assume responsibility for activities that ordinarily might be considered part of the private practice of medicine.

Over the years there has been demonstrated an unfortunate lack of interest on the part of many physicians to render certain types of services. As Davis[13] has stated, tax-supported medical care of the types referred to, for the nonindigent,

. . . has been furnished for a variety of reasons, of which the following have been most evident: (1) because, as in mental disease, only public funds can make the provision necessary for the large number of persons involved*; (2) because certain diseases, as tuberculosis, hookworm, and trachoma, frequently involve, or lead to, incapacity for self-support; (3) because only a public authority can provide care in a manner which will protect the rest of the community, as in the case of acute communicable disease; (4) because, as in poliomyelitis and some orthopedic conditions among children and in early tuberculosis among young adults, the diseases if untreated, are likely to make permanent dependents of those who, with proper care, could be self-supporting; (5) because, as in eye, ear, throat, and dental defects among children, the education and the usefulness of future citizens are threatened unless these conditions are corrected; (6) because, as with the diseases of babies and of the puerperal state, the widespread public interest in maternity and infancy devolves some responsibility for them upon a public agency; and (7) because, as in the case of syphilis or cancer, the relative costliness of diagnosis or treatment renders many self-supporting persons unable to meet the expense.

The public pressures on public health agencies to take the leadership for more complete protection and promotion of the health of all of the people have resulted in greatly expanded and more personalized programs. Unfortunately there never was a clear mandate given or sufficient funds and personnel provided to accomplish what was needed. Throughout,

---

*Note that only 2% of patients hospitalized for mental illness in the United States are in private hospitals.

public health has found itself caught in the middle of the forces of organized medicine, hospital interests, private enterprise, and political expediencies. The evolution of the process has been described in a statement of the Joint Committee on Medical Care of the American Public Health Association and the American Public Welfare Association[14]:

Public health has its historical roots in the long recognized necessity of invoking governmental authority to protect the community against the spread of communicable disease. From these limited beginnings, the increasing interdependence of individuals living in a highly industrialized and urbanized society has brought major advances in both areas of governmental responsibility for individual well-being. . . . Public health has also been undergoing a definite evolutionary trend toward a broadened concept of governmental responsibility. Whereas its earlier functions were primarily concerned with measures related to community sanitation and regulatory control of infectious diseases, public health activities have increasingly entered the area of services directly concerned with the personal health of individuals. With advances in medical science, the arbitrary line between prevention and treatment has narrowed and the distinction between community and individual health has become less sharply defined. Society has increasingly placed on public health an obligation to assure the availability of essential health services. This trend has been translated into broadened programs of prevention, diagnosis, and treatment for the principal communicable diseases; programs for the protection of the health of mothers and infants; school health programs; health education; and programs for the prevention, detection, and correction of dental, visual, hearing, and other defects.

Health Departments also provide an increasing range of services designed to help control such chronic diseases as cancer, heart disease, diabetes, arthritis and rheumatism, and to rehabilitate children crippled by orthopedic, cardiac, orthodontic, and other conditions. Programs have been developed in the fields of mental hygiene; hospital planning, construction and licensure; hygiene of the aging; as well as, in some states, general medical care for needy individuals.

In a brief but excellent review Anderson[15] has traced the development of interest in and agitation for medical care insurance in the United States. He divides it into three broad periods. The first, from 1910 to 1920, was notable for the activities of the American Association for Labor Legislation that were instrumental in bringing about the widespread enactment of workmen's compensation laws. On achieving this success the association selected medical care insurance as its next cause. It established a Committee on Social Legislation, which at first was supported by and participated in by the American Medical Association. Eventually, when several bills were introduced into state legislatures, many of the previously interested and cooperative groups including medical societies and pharmaceutical companies, as well as insurance companies and cultists turned against it. In 1920 the House of Delegates of the American Medical Association enunciated a basic policy of unequivocal opposition to any type of compulsory contributory insurance against illness.

The second period, from 1921 to 1933, is described by Anderson as "a quiet one devoted to the study of basic facts and problems only superficially comprehended in the first period." It saw the establishment of the Committee on the Costs of Medical Care, financed by six foundations and consisting of 42 persons representing medicine, public health, institutions, economists, and the general public. Its many studies and reports between 1928 and 1932 resulted in a final report, the conclusion of which has been summarized by Falk[16] in the form of five basic recommendations:

1. Comprehensive medical service should be provided largely by organized groups of practitioners, organized preferably around hospitals, encouraging high standards, and preserving personal relations.

2. All basic public health services should be extended to the entire population, requiring increased financial support, full-time trained health officers and staffs, with security of tenure.

3. Medical costs should be placed on a group payment basis through insurance, taxation, or both; individual fee-for-service should be available for those who prefer it; and cash benefits for wage loss should be kept separate.

4. State and local agencies should be formed to study, evaluate, and coordinate services, with special attention to urban-rural coordination.

5. Professional education should be improved for physicians, health officers, dentists, pharmacists, registered nurses, nursing aids, midwives, and hospital and clinic administrators.

A minority report was submitted. It agreed with recommendations 2, 4, and 5 but took strong exception to recommendation 1 on the organization of medical services and to recommendation 3 on group payment for medical service. How strange this seems in light of current events! The degree of concern of some of the opposition is illustrated by the tone of the editorial comment of the American Medical Association at the time.[17]

The alinement [sic] is clear—on the one side the forces representing the great foundations, public health officialdom, social theory—even socialism and communism—inciting to revolution; on the other side, the organized medical profession of this country urging an orderly evolution guided by controlled experimentation which will observe the principles that have been found through the centuries to be necessary to the sound practice of medicine.

Parenthetically it is interesting to note the repetition of the plea for "orderly and controlled experimentation" at the present time before proceeding further with such well-proved arrangements as health maintenance organizations.

The third period, beginning in 1933 and continuing into the present, represents again an action period similar to the first. Replacing the initiative of an unofficial labor legislation association, however, has been action by the federal government, strongly supported by well-developed and organized labor groups. Progress was triggered initially by the exigencies of the economic depression. The necessity to provide medical care as well as the other basic needs of food, clothing and shelter to the many individuals who were on unemployment relief was recognized and accepted of necessity by the American Medical Association (A.M.A.) as well as by other groups. However, this did not lead to inclusion of medical care insurance in the subsequent Social Security Act. The A.M.A. fought and defeated this, but as Falk[16] points out, "at the price of insuring the enactment in 1935 of Title VI of the Social Security Act which inaugurated federal grants to states for public health services and the federal funds for a research program out of which the National Institutes of Health burgeoned."

The passage of the Social Security Act was followed promptly by the 1935-1936 National Health Surveys of illness and underlying social and economic factors, and by the Presidential appointment of the Interdepartmental Committee to Coordinate Health and Welfare Activities. Its Technical Committee on Medical Care recognized the need for a general program of medical care and insurance against loss of wages because of sickness. A National Health Conference was called in July 1938 to consider the Technical Committee's findings and recommendations, with wide representation and discussion by all possibly interested parties. Legislation for a national health program was introduced the following year by Senator Robert Wagner, and

extensive hearings were held. In addition to federal grants to match state expenditures for public health the bill proposed to offer "services and supplies necessary for the prevention, diagnosis and treatment of illness and disability."

This prompted the A.M.A. to call an "emergency" meeting in St. Louis, as a result of which there was formed the National Physicians' Committee for the Extension of Medical Services. The subsequent history of action by this committee belied its name; whether because of great pressure from the National Physicians' Committee or for reasons of political expediency, President Roosevelt late in 1939 withdrew his support of the bill, and it died in Congress. Then the nation entered World War II. The large number of young men who were found unfit for military service because of physical defects obviously contradicted the claim that the American people were receiving adequate medical care. Furthermore, millions of young men and women who served in the Armed Forces were exposed to a system of medical care operated by the government that served their needs promptly and effectively. Beyond this, while the war was in progress, a public opinion poll by *Fortune* magazine in 1942 indicated that three quarters of the people of the nation were in favor of national health insurance.

Because of these and other factors, Senator Wagner in company with Senator James Murray and Representative John Dingell, Sr., in mid-1943 sponsored another bill more far reaching than the earlier bill. It proposed comprehensive medical, hospital, dental, and nursing home care for almost the entire population to be paid for out of a special fund based on equal contributions from employers and employees. The A.M.A. called it "the most virulent scheme ever to be conjured out of the mind of man," and again was successful in causing the bill to die in committee. As the war approached an end, President Truman asked that a new health insurance bill be prepared with careful consideration given to the rights of both the public and the medical profession. As a result a new Wagner-Murray-Dingell Bill was filed, which according to the A.M.A. would "mean the end of freedom for all classes of Americans." This bill, like its predecessors, was also killed.

In 1949 Governor Earl Warren of California unexpectedly sent to his state legislature a compulsory health insurance bill which was almost identical to one that had been proposed by the California Medical Association a decade earlier.

Now, however, the latter organization took a completely opposite stand and employed a public relations firm to carry the attack. Ironically the attack took the form of encouraging, as a substitute, membership in Blue Cross, Blue Shield, and commercial health insurance plans, programs that up to this time the A.M.A. had also been attacking as "socialized medicine." The idea behind this tactic was to prevent compulsory governmentally sponsored health insurance by offering voluntary insurance. An intensive propaganda campaign was conducted at a cost to the California Medical Association of $250,000, as a result of which the California bill was defeated.

In 1946, with the war at an end, Senator Robert A. Taft, widely known as a conservative, decided to solve the problem by means of a bill that would provide matching grants to states for medical care for those who on the basis of a means test could be proved to be indigent. The bill appealed to no one, and it is interesting that the A.M.A. called even this tame gesture "socialized medicine." A year later another Wagner-Murray-Dingell Bill was introduced. No one expected it to get any further than its predecessors. However, apparently on the basis of President Truman's reelection, the A.M.A. called it a crisis and assessed every member $25 to establish a $3.5 million "war chest" and to finance the largest lobby in American history. The assessment received wide publicity and was the subject of great criticism. More or less typical was the statement by Bishop G. Bromley Oxnam, "The assessment put upon every American doctor to raise a propaganda fund that today is being used to misinform a nation is a national disgrace." The A.M.A. engaged the same public relations firm that had been successful in California and the same approach was decided on— promotion of the appropriation of government funds for the purchase by individuals of private health insurance instead of governmental compulsory health insurance. On deciding to do this, it is interesting that the A.M.A. despite its earlier opposition, now claimed that it had been one of the first originators and supporters of the voluntary health insurance idea. Again the bill in Congress was defeated.

In 1948 another National Health Assembly was held, out of which came a statement of the principle that contributory insurance should be the basic method of financing medical care for most of the American public. Agreement was not reached, however, as to implementation. This was followed by a decade or more marked by (1) the continuation of the introduction of various types of medical insurance bills, (2) the acceptance and implementation of all of the recommendations of the Technical Committee on Medical Care of the President's Interdepartmental Committee with the exception of the general medical proposal, (3) a growing and great concern and awareness by the general public regarding problems of medical care, its distribution, and costs, (4) a considerable extension of group medical practice, (5) a significant development of labor and union medical care programs, and (6) a remarkable growth of voluntary medical and hospital insurance. With respect to the latter by 1970 in the United States 78% of the civilian population under 65 years of age was covered by voluntary hospitalization insurance. Slightly fewer, 76%, had medical and surgical insurance. Approximately 45% of all hospital coverage was by Blue Cross-Blue Shield plans, and about 16% of those so covered had additional coverage under one of the nearly 800 independent health care organizations.[18] Almost all persons past 65 years of age had Medicaid coverage. Unquestionably the interest and activity of government in the problems of medical care since the 1930s served as a major stimulus to the development and extension of voluntary prepaid medical care insurance plans and their acceptance and endorsement by organized medicine. However the growth of these plans was also undoubtedly indicative of a need and desire for action on the part of the public.

Meanwhile the American Dental Association began to address itself to the difficult problem of dental insurance. However, as noted in Chapter 20, by 1968 only 1.7 million Americans, or less than 2% were covered by any type of dental care insurance.

Experience has indicated that voluntary plans are not without their problems. They have several significant limitations. They are rarely comprehensive, being limited essentially to hospitalization and medical services while in the hospital. Only a few provide preventive and diagnostic services, and certain illnesses such as tuberculosis and mental disease are generally excluded from coverage. Frequent hospitalization for long-term catastrophic illness is not adequately provided. Much of the population, including a large part of the low-income group and the aged, those with the greatest need, are not covered.

As time passed, particular concern developed with reference to the older component of the population. It was increasing in numbers and percent. Because of their greater longevity, a disproportionate number of the aged were women; women seek medical and hospital care more than do men. Increasingly, older persons were forced to retire whether they wished to or not, thereby limiting their incomes severely. Not infrequently the combination of limited financial resources, increased medical needs, and aloneness have brought about the development of a vicious cycle wherein the older person delays obtaining necessary medical care, economizes on food, which in turn results in malnutrition, and thus has more medical problems, which require eventually more money.[19] From an actuarial viewpoint few voluntary insurance companies or plans have shown interest in trying to solve the problems of the aged, and from an individual viewpoint only a very small proportion of the elderly can afford effective voluntary medical insurance. The situation was unequivocally expressed by Basil MacLean[20] in 1960, when he retired as President of the Blue Cross Association, which had attempted to find some solution to the medical insurance needs of the aged. He commented:

A lifetime's experience has led me at last to conclude that the cost of care of the aged cannot be met, unaided, by the mechanisms of insurance or prepayment as they exist today. The aged simply cannot afford to buy from any of these the scope of care that is required, not do the stern competitive realities permit any carrier, whether non-profit or commercial, to provide benefits which are adequate at a price which is feasible for any but a small proportion of the aged.

It is interesting that although 78% of the population is now covered by some form of medical and hospital insurance, only about 25% of the total expenditures for medical care is in the form of insurance payments. Furthermore, as Reed[21] has pointed out, a significant amount of health insurance is written by companies on an individual basis, a form of insurance that results in about one half of the premiums going to selling costs and overhead rather than to medical service. This is a service to neither the patient nor members of the medical profession. Similarly, coverage by voluntary insurance has done nothing to prevent occasional excessively high medical fees or to effect economical hospital practice or to encourage sound hospital fiscal procedures.

The critical situation the nation was getting itself into was pointed out by Somers and Somers[22] in 1962, indicating the inability of insurance companies and private payment plans to provide in any adequate sense for the aged or other poor-risk groups. Presaging the events of the subsequent years, they observed that the atmosphere had become one of impending impasse and indecision—a clear reversal of the optimism and dynamism that had characterized private health insurance for several decades. They noted that this had led to various forms of public intervention already but that even here the problem had been found to be beyond the abilities of local and state governments alone to solve to any degree of satisfaction. Increasingly they noted that the public and local governments had been forced to look to the federal government for a solution.

Meanwhile, because of the lack of progress on the Wagner-Murray-Dingell Bill and the growing concern over the problems of the aged, Wilbur Cohen and I. S. Falk, who had drafted the preceding bills, decided on a more limited approach: a medical care plan for the aged that might possibly be acceptable. It took the form of a bill that was introduced in April 1952 by Senator Murray and Congressman Dingell to provide 60 days of hospital care each year as needed for all those on Social Security pensions. The number estimated to be eligible at that time was 7 million of the approximate 13 million people over 65 years of age. The financing would be by means of a slight increase in the Social Security assessments. Modest though it was, the bill was defeated, as it was again in 1953 and still again in 1955.

The latter year, however, witnessed the merger of the American Federation of Labor and the Congress of Industrial Organization. This resulted in a single union with more than 16 million workers, the vast majority of whom not only had family members who voted but also who tended to be liberal. Promptly the AFL-CIO adopted health insurance for the elderly as a major concern. One of the union's key officials, in company with a representative of the Social Security Administration and Cohen and Falk, cooperated in the preparation of a new and much broader bill to provide medical care for Social Security beneficiaries. Not only did it cover hospitalization costs but it also included costs of surgery and nursing home care. As had been true with all previous and subsequent bills, it was careful to allow for freedom of choice by both physician and patient. Again it was proposed that costs be financed by means of increasing the Social Security payments by employers and employees. Congressman Aimé Forand agreed to sponsor the bill and introduced it on August 27, 1957. Despite attempts to influence them by the A.M.A., both the American Nurses' Association and the American Hospital Association endorsed the principle on which the bill was based. Hearings on the bill were held both in 1958 and 1959, but still no legislation was forthcoming.

Growing concern, however, about the problems of chronic and degenerative diseases, especially among the older members of the population, caused the Senate Committee on Labor and Public Welfare to establish a Subcommittee on the Problems of the Aged and Aging. Senator McNamara was made chairman, and he proceeded to conduct public hearings in several cities throughout the nation. The attendance was considerable, and Senator McNamara followed a practice of first listening to experts and then making the microphone available to anyone in the audience. Large numbers of older citizens responded and told in dramatic and sometimes pathetic form of their problems. It became apparent to the nation through these firsthand statements that contrary to the avowals of the A.M.A. their needs were not being met. When the subcommittee submitted its report to the Senate in February 1960, its first recommendation was that the Social Security program be expanded to include health service benefits for all persons eligible under the program. Congress now began to be deluged by letters concerning the Forand Bill, 2 to 1 in favor. This forced the Ways and Means Committee of the House to vote on it. Nonetheless, contrary pressures led to its defeat.

By this time various political writers throughout the nation impatiently referred to medical insurance for the elderly as the most critical political issue in the nation. Mail overflowed the post offices of the House and Senate, 30 to 1 in favor of the Forand Bill. This forced its reconsideration by the congress. It also resulted in the Eisenhower Administration's finally presenting a bill of its own called the Medicare Program for the Aged. The name was borrowed from a previous measure that provided free medical care for dependents of servicemen. Viewed superficially, the administration bill seemed to go even further than the Forand Bill. However, when the various deductibles and exceptions were considered, few elderly people could benefit much. As a result it received little support from any quarter. Nevertheless, it served an unintended purpose: It indicated that by this time both political parties manifested an obligation on the part of the federal government to somehow provide medical care for the indigent and elderly. Meanwhile the Forand Bill was again defeated in Committee.

Soon afterward the House passed a bill introduced by Congressman Mills, which empowered the federal government to make grants to states to provide medical care for the elderly poor. It was not, however, to be financed through the Social Security system. This was quickly followed by a bill in the Senate under the sponsorship of Senator Kerr, the intention of which was to assist the aged who were neither poor enough to be on welfare nor wealthy enough to pay their own medical expenses. Again, financing would be by federal grants matching state expenditures. Wilbur Cohen, who drafted the bill for Kerr, adroitly included in it much of the intent of Congressman Mills' bill. It passed both houses with little opposition, and in mid-September 1960 the President signed what became known as the Kerr-Mills Act. It lacked many things. It was estimated that actually only about 2 million people would be assisted by it. Interestingly, whereas the A.M.A. did not oppose it, apparently on the basis of the lesser of two evils, it included many principles to which that organization had been objecting over the years. It consisted of two parts: (1) extension of the Old-Age Assistance Program, which had originated with the 1935 Social Security Act; the limit of federal participation was increased from $65 per person per month to $77 and later to $85. (2) A new section known as the Medical Assistance for the Aged Program; the intent of this was to provide medical expenses for elderly citizens who previously were ineligible for aid, in other words the so-called medically indigent who were over 65 years of age and who, although not on relief, could not meet the cost of medical services. The legislation placed no ceiling on federal support for this part of the act, the federal government paying a flat percentage of total outlays ranging from 50% for high-income states to 80% for poorer states. It was left entirely to the states to determine whether they wished to participate in the program. Furthermore, individual states could set not only their own income limits and deductibles but also all the conditions for the provision of care. The overall result was that many states did not elect to participate in the Kerr-Mills Act, and the conditions established by those that did presented all possible variations. Although the A.M.A. during the next several years spent large sums of money to try to convince everyone that the Kerr-Mills program was actually meeting the needs, it became apparent very shortly that this was far from the truth.

When Senator John Kennedy became President-elect, he let it be known that one of the first items on the agenda for his administration would be the enactment of a health insurance bill for the aged. Shortly after he took office Representative King and Senator Anderson served as co-sponsors of what became known as the Medicare Bill. Its provisions were extensive, and again it was proposed to be financed by an increase in Social Security assessments. It called forth the usual and expected accusations and cries of alarm from the A.M.A., which promptly established an American Medical Political Action Committee to raise several million dollars with which to fight it. The bill had great support, however, not only from the public but also from organizations such as the National Council of Churches, the Y.W.C.A., the American Nurses' Association, the American Hospital Association, and the American Public Health Association. In addition groups of physicians in several places in the nation disassociated themselves from the A.M.A. to form endorsing groups. Despite this, the bill was defeated in the Senate by a close vote. It was reintroduced in 1963 at President Kennedy's request, but his assassination brought hearings on the matter to a halt. As eventual successor to the Presidency, the then Senator Lyndon Johnson had already made clear his support of the Medicare idea. On his assumption of the Presidency, hearings on the bill were resumed in the Ways and Means Committee of the House, but progress was extremely slow. In the Senate the Social Security Act was the subject for amendment, and in the face of many obstacles the Medicare concept was attached to the bill that eventually was passed by the Senate, only to be held up in the Conference Committee by the representatives of the House.

After election in his own right, when President Johnson presented his State of the Union address on January 4, 1965, at the opening of the Eighty-ninth Congress, he made a strong call for action on a Medicare Bill as the first order of business. Promptly, Senator Anderson introduced S. 1, and Representative King introduced H.R. 1—identical bills that were very similar to those they had introduced in the previous Congress. In short order several other bills were introduced, among them one of Representative Byrnes that provided for subsidies to pay for private health insurance policies and one to expand and liberalize the Kerr-Mills Act. To the surprise of everyone Representative Mills, as Chairman of the Ways and Means Committee of the House, suddenly resolved the problem by deciding on a meld of the King-Anderson Bills, the bill to expand and liberalize the Kerr-Mills Act, and Representative Byrnes' bill. As he explained, this would provide a sort of three-layer cake: the expanded Kerr-Mills program making up the bottom layer to take care of those who were close to indigency; Medicare making up the middle layer to take care of the cost of hospital, nursing home, and home health care for the rest of the elderly; and the voluntary supplement making up the top layer to take care of physicians' fees, in and out of hospital. The bill that was drawn up by Wilbur Cohen at the Committee's request to accomplish this was finally approved by the House of Representatives by a vote of 313 to 115 and passed the Senate by a vote of 68 to 21.

On July 30, 1965, President Johnson flew to Independence, Mo., to sign the bill into P.L. 89-97 at the Harry S. Truman Memorial Library in honor of the former President, who had fought so valiantly for the principle of health insurance. Title XVIII of the Act (Medicare) provided everyone 65 years or older with 60 days' free hospital care after a $40 deduction to avoid unnecessary hospitalization and 30 additional days of hospital care at $10 a day; 20 days of free nursing home care with 80 more days at $5 a day; 100 home visits by nurses or other health specialists after hospitalization; and 80% of the cost of hospital diagnostic tests after a $20 deduction for each series of tests. This part of the act is paid for by raising the taxable wage base of the Social Security program to $6,600 a year and the tax itself by 0.5% for both employee and employer. The other, or voluntary part of the program, provides for the payment of 80% of "reasonable charges" for all physician services, after a $50-per-year deductible; another 100 home health visits whether the patient has been hospitalized or not; and the cost of nonhospital diagnostic tests, surgical dressings, splints, and rented medical equipment. This section of the act, known as Title XIX (or Medicaid), extends eligibility to all persons who are eligible for federally aided public assistance programs—the aged, the blind, the disabled, and families receiving Aid to Dependent Children assistance. States may also include medically indigent children under the age of 21 years. For the aged, Title XIX may serve as a supplement to Title XVIII, the basic Medicare section, since it allows states to pay both the deductibles and the voluntary medical insurance premiums for the aged who are wholly dependent on old age assistance. States may also elect to pay the deductibles for elderly persons whose Social Security payments are supplemented with old-age assistance payments. States were allowed until 1970 to adopt Title XIX, depending on their respective wishes. To pay for the voluntary or Title XIX supplements, people 65 years or older who wish to participate contribute $3 per month each. This is supplemented by about $500,000 per year from the general treasury. In 1972 the Social Security law was amended to provide greater and additional benefits.[23] These are financed by having raised the base income for Social Security deductions.

The Eighty-ninth Congress, as indicated elsewhere, passed a remarkable number of bills to strengthen the health of the nation. Several others that should be mentioned here are the provisions of Title V of the Social Security Amendments, which authorized a 5-year program of special grants to provide comprehensive health care and services to children of school age and preschool age, especially in areas with concentrations of low-income families. Grants are made to state and local health agencies, to medical schools and teaching hospitals affiliating with schools of medicine, and to state crippled children programs. In addition were amendments to the Economic Opportunity Act that made possible grants to local communities for the establishment of comprehensive medical centers to serve the needs of the economically disadvantaged. Elsewhere reference was made to P.L. 89-239, the Heart Disease, Cancer, and Stroke Amendments (Regional Medical Programs). This authorized substantial funds for a program of grants to encourage and assist the planning and operation of regional cooperative arrangements among medical schools, research institutions and hospitals for research, training, and related demonstrations of patient care in the fields of heart disease, cancer, stroke, and related diseases. The program is designed to enable states and communities to improve quantitatively and qualitatively the health manpower and facilities available in these fields.

## THE FUTURE

In his review of the history of attempts between 1910 and 1950 to achieve a practical and acceptable form of compulsory medical care insurance, Anderson[15] made the noteworthy point that the controversy over compulsion tended to obscure the significant points of agreement among all those concerned. All agree that everyone should have access to medical care regardless of income. All agree that the generally most satisfactory means is by insurance. Disagreement appears to be limited to the question of sponsorship and control. Finally, he emphasized that both sides share a basic faith in the present political and economic institutions. As he concluded, the proponents of compulsory medical care insurance are not necessarily revolutionaries, and the opponents are not necessarily reactionaries. The progress made in the implementation of Medicare and Medicaid appears at long last to have borne this out.

It must be recognized that a tax-supported plan for medical care is certain to have both advantages and disadvantages, potential dangers as well as benefits. Undoubtedly the outstanding advantages of such a plan would be the equalization of geographic and economic differences among states and regions and among the citizens of a community and the nation. This equalization would manifest itself, among other ways, in a more equitable distribution of medical personnel and facilities. Furthermore, and perhaps of greatest importance, would be the equalization through time of the costs to an individual of medical diagnosis and care. In addition, a comprehensive approach to health maintenance and health care, including prevention and rehabilitation, will become much more possible of achievement, as has been well demonstrated already by the several health maintenance organizations that have been operating for some time. These and other attempts to find workable and acceptable solutions are in the process of spreading and are the subjects of intensive study and research.[24,25]

Against the advantages are the potential dangers of political influence on the selection of patients, the appointment of administrative and professional personnel, and the methods of institutional management. Physicians and others might in some instances be poorly selected or poorly trained and practice under inadequate or no supervision. It may be pointed out, however, that in the complete absence of a plan these same poorly selected or trained persons would be engaged as they may be in private practice with no supervision. Similarly the cry has been heard that a publicly or governmentally sponsored medical care program will cause the quality of care to suffer. Objections on these grounds imply that all present physicians would be disenfranchised and an altogether new group would move in. It should be realized that the aim of all proposals has been control of the economic risks of illness and not of the manner in which those illnesses are treated. If under any plan, private or public, the quality of the care rendered decreased, the fault could be attributed only to those who render the service and not to the manner in which they received payment. Excessive charges could be made, as has occasionally occurred with the Medicare and Medicaid programs. Properly established and conducted peer and consumer review groups could guard against these dangers. Much depends, of course, on the structure of a plan and the manner in which it is administered. A tax-supported medical care program must involve some degree of governmental administration and supervision, but this does not necessarily imply dictatorial governmental control over technical and professional procedures and personal relationships.

The necessity of developing adequate mechanisms to ensure medical care and institutional service to high quality has been the subject of much discussion during the past few years, and most who have addressed themselves to the problem are optimistic that it can be solved.[26,27] A highly significant event was the enactment of P.L. 92-603 in October 1972, which requires the creation of Professional Standards Review organizations to monitor the quality and cost of all services provided under the Medicare and Medicaid programs. Under the law, state and local medical organizations have the first opportunity to establish Professional Standards Review organizations. They have 2 years after Jan. 1, 1974 during which to accomplish this.

That some form of general and comprehensive nationwide, tax-supported, medical, surgical, and hospital insurance plan will be eventually developed and put into effect in the United States is certain. The wheels of social progress grind slowly but inexorably. The increasing agitation and the concurrent stresses to which the nation has been and still is witness, the plethora of legislative bills introduced, discussed, and discarded during recent years, and the continuing propaganda for and against are only signs and symptoms of a social change already well under way and certain to run its course. Indeed, as this is written (May 1974), there appears to have developed a determination by all groups, professions, citizen organizations, and political parties in the United States to make whatever practical compromises necessary to bring about the earliest possible passage of a National Health Insurance Act.[28] The essential issue now is whether payments for service shall be by a spectrum of private insurance companies or by the social security mechanism. A secondary issue is the role to be played by the national, state, and local official health agencies. Whatever the decisions on these issues, it is now clear that the United States at long last is about to join the other nations that have national health service programs for all their citizens.

A quarter century ago an admirable and prophetic summary of this momentous social movement was made by Galdston.[29] It provides a most appropriate closing statement for this chapter.

When we study the history of social security legislation, we soon find that it follows a certain pattern, one that first became very clear in Germany. Increased industrialization creates the need, because it increases the social insecurity of growing numbers of the population. A second factor is found in the phenomenon that under the pressure of industrialization the working class organized into militant political parties that present a threat to the existing order. This was the case in Germany when the Social Democratic Party was founded in 1869 by Bebel and Liebknecht; in 1875 it absorbed the conservative Lassalle group. The Paris Commune of 1871 created a great scare in all conservative circles of Europe because it showed that socialism was not a parlor philosophy but might well become a tangible reality. A conservative statesman, Bismarck stepped in and with social insurance created a corrective mechanism to the system that he wished to perpetuate.

The very same pattern can be traced in England, the next large country that enacted national social insurance in the beginning of our century. At that time the impact of the second industrial revolution was being felt. The number of wage earners increased as a result of it and so did their insecurity. In 1900 the Independent Labor Party, the Fabian Society, and the Trade Unions joined to organize the Labor Party, which was in no way revolutionary but nevertheless had great potentialities in a highly industrialized country. In the election of 1906 the Labor Party won 29 seats and England changed from a two-party country to a three-party country. The

Russian Revolution of 1905 broke down as the Paris Commune had done thirty-five years before, but it again reminded conservative groups that socialism was not dead. Lloyd George and Winston Churchill began to promote social legislation, culminating in the National Insurance Act of 1911, which included sickness and unemployment benefits. Like the German system it had all the weaknesses of a compromise, was not comprehensive enough, and suffered from a considerable lack of uniformity, as it had to take into account the vested interests of a great number of private benefit societies and insurance companies.

World War I created a new and very strong stimulus to the enactment of social legislation. It was the first war in which the industrial potential of a group of countries proved to be the decisive factor. Industrialization was intensified in every warring country and the Russian Revolution of 1917 created a totally new situation. Not only France, but a number of other countries adopted systems of health insurance, and it was recognized that no nation could enjoy the benefits of industrialization without providing a corrective mechanism for the hardships and insecurity it created. This became particularly apparent during the protracted economic depression that followed the crisis in 1929 when all over the Western world millions of people were unemployed. At that time social insurance bills were introduced increasingly in the American republics. Chile introduced health insurance as early as 1924, and by 1942 nine Central and South American countries had some form of health insurance. In the United States, following the National Health Conference of 1938, various bills were introduced into Congress that had the purpose of completing the social security legislation of the Roosevelt era by developing a national health program that would include health insurance. So far no bill has been passed, but the need remains and some solution will have to be found because the attitude of medicine to society has changed and the view is generally accepted that in a civilized commonwealth the benefits of medical science should be available to all people.

## REFERENCES

1. Shryock, R. H.: In Galdston, I., editor: Social medicine, New York, 1949, Commonwealth Fund.
2. Sand, R.: Health and human progress, New York, 1936, The Macmillan Co.
3. Buhrman, H. M. F.: Leaves from a doctor's notebook of seventy years ago, Milit. Surgeon **86:** 547, June 1940.
4. Robinson, G. C.: The patient as a person, New York, 1939, Commonwealth Fund.
5. Statistical abstract of the United States, Washington, D. C., 1971, Government Printing Office.
6. American Medical Association: Distribution of physicians in the U. S., 1971, Chicago, 1972, The Association.
7. Collins, S. D., Lehmann, J. L., and Trantham, K. S.: Major causes of illness of various severities and major causes of death in six age periods of life, PHS pub. no. 440, Washington, D. C., 1955.
8. Collins, S. D., Lehmann, J. L., and Trantham, K. S.: Surgical experience in selected areas of United States, PHS pub. no. 473, Washington, D. C., 1956.
9. Rosen, G.: Provision of medical care—history, sociology, innovation, Public Health Rep. **74:**199, March, 1959.
10. Rosen, G.: In Galdston, I., editor: Social medicine, New York, 1949, Commonwealth Fund.
11. Editorial: J.A.M.A. **139:**529, 1949.
12. Evang, K.: Medical care in Europe, Amer. J. Public Health **48:**427, April 1958.
13. Davis, M. M.: Public medical services, Chicago, 1937, University of Chicago Press.
14. Editorial: Tax-supported medical care of the needy, Amer. J. Public Health **42:**1314, Oct. 1952.
15. Anderson, O. W.: Compulsory medical care insurance, 1910-1950, Ann. Amer. Acad. Polit. Social Sci. **273:**106, Jan. 1951; also in Committee on Medical Care Teaching of the Association of Teachers of Preventive Medicine: Readings in medical care, Chapel Hill, 1958, University of North Carolina Press.
16. Falk, I. S.: The committee on the costs of medical care—25 years of progress, Amer. J. Public Health **48:**979, Aug. 1958.
17. Editorial: J.A.M.A. **99:**1952, Dec. 3, 1932.
18. U. S. Public Health Service: Hospital and surgical insurance coverage among persons under 65 years of age in the United States, 1970, pub. no. (HSM) 73-1128, Rockville, Md., Dec. 18, 1972.
19. The aged and aging in the United States: a national problem; a report of the Subcommittee on the Problems of the Aged and Aging to the Senate Committee on Labor and Public Welfare, Washington, D. C., 1960, Government Printing Office.
20. Somers, H. M., and Somers, A. R.: Doctors, patients, and health insurance, Washington, D. C., 1961, The Brookings Institution.
21. Reed, L. S.: Group payment since the Committee on the Costs of Medical Care, Amer. J. Public Health **48:**992, Aug. 1958.
22. Somers, H. M., and Somers, A. R.: The paradox of medical progress, New Eng. J. Med. **226**(24): 1253, June 14, 1962.
23. American Medical Association: A guide to provisions relating to Medicare, Medicaid, and maternal and child health: enacted as Title II of Public Law 92-603, the Social Security Amendments of 1972, Chicago, 1972, The Association.
24. Battistella, R. M., and Weil, T. P.: Health care organization—bibliography and guidebook, Washington, D. C., 1971, Association of University Programs in Hospital Administration.
25. Aday, L. A., and Elchorn, R.: The utilization of health services: indices and correlates, pub.

no. (HSM) 73-3003, Rockville, Md., 1972, U. S. Public Health Service.

26. U. S. Public Health Service: Quality assurance of medical care, Proceedings of a conference held in St. Louis, Jan. 23-24, 1973, pub. no. (HSM) 73-7021, Rockville, Md., 1973.

27. Rutstein, D. D.: Quality control of medical care, Technology Review **76:**34, Jan. 1974.

28. National health insurance proposals: provisions of bills introduced in the 93rd Congress as of Feb. 1974, pub. no. (SSA) 11920, Washington, D. C., 1974, Government Printing Office.

29. Galdston, I., editor: Social medicine, New York, 1949, Commonwealth Fund.

*To every man his chance; to every
man, regardless of his birth, his condition,
his situation; to every man the right
to live, to work, to be himself.*

THOMAS WOLFE

CHAPTER 35

# Rehabilitation

## BIRTH OF CONSCIENCE

It is only relatively recently that the concept of community responsibility for the consequences of so-called acts of God, chance, and Mars has become a reality. One has to turn back only a few pages in human history to find an attitude of rather complete social irresponsibility even for disabled veterans who were accorded their day of acclaim, followed by a bitter lifetime as dependants or outcasts. Recent years, however, have brought increasing discussion of the problems of the handicapped and what might be done to make their lives personally more satisfying and economically more fruitful. It is only in the past few decades that the disabled began to be considered as fellow human beings, subject as any other to sensitivity, pride, and ambition, and as potential social and economic assets rather than liabilities.

Just how recent official interest and effort have been is well illustrated by the history of vocational rehabilitation.[1] With the entrance of the United States in World War I the Congress in 1917 began consideration of legislation to assist men disabled in military service to return to civilian life and employment. The original bills included provisions for the rehabilitation of industrially disabled as well as war disabled individuals. It was quickly decided to proceed separately with a bill for returning veterans and handle the problems of others separately. Considerable controversy arose in debates on the bills during the next few years. They were attacked as paternalistic and defended as humanitarian. When the constitutionality of spending federal funds for such purposes was challenged, supporters won the day by pointing to the precedent of federal appropriations for the attack on hog cholera. The narrowness of thought of some was epitomized by Senator Sherman of Illinois, who branded the measure as "2 percent bolshevist," then finally expressed willingness to go along with rehabilitation of the industrially disabled but opposed further extension saying, "Let such failures go to the poorhouse!" Finally, in June 1920 President Woodrow Wilson was able to sign into law "an act to provide for the promotion of vocational rehabilitation of persons disabled in industry or otherwise and their return to civil employment."[2] An authorization of $750,000 was allowed in 1921, and modest assistance and encouragement to states began. In May 1922 the First National Conference on Vocational Rehabilitation of Persons Disabled in Industry or otherwise was held in St. Louis, with 23 states represented by their state supervisors of vocational rehabilitation. Many of them constituted their entire staffs. In the years since, the program grew slowly but was nevertheless successful in restoring or developing the productivity of many of the otherwise chronically disabled population. It has never had sufficient resources, public enthusiasm, or legislative support, however, to address the total problem. As a result, its potential benefits have been made available only to a minor proportion of the estimated 3.7 million people in need of and eligible for services and the estimated 536,000 people who come into such need each year.

The problem of the definition of a handicap or a handicapped person developed early. Adequate definition, of course, is fundamental to the determination and conduct of a comprehensive and satisfactory program of rehabilitation. As might be expected, attention and effort were focused first on the visibly most obvious physical defects, that is, the traditional lame, halt, and blind. Gradually other physical handicaps began to receive attention in the public consciousness. Tuberculosis was established as an etiologic entity, and its physiopathology became understood. In the absence of other means, intensive rest and supportive care were instituted as a cure. Eventually it became evident that it was difficult to determine where cure ended and rehabilitation began. At any rate high relapse rates soon emphasized the importance of rehabilitation, at least in this and a few other diseases. Such circumstances provoked further reconsideration and redefinition. There resulted a realization that there also existed such conditions as mental, emotional, psychologic, or personality crippling which might be just as devastating to the individual and as costly to society as a physical defect. In addition, it has come to be appreciated that mental or psychologic handicaps and physical handicaps are frequently related. As a result, the present trend is to look on rehabilitation in extremely broad terms, as a need applicable to almost all types of ills and of as much concern to society as to the individual.

### SOURCE OF THE PROBLEM

There are many reasons why the field of rehabilitation should command attention at this time. For a long period it was ignored or overlooked because of the magnitude of other problems, many of which have been eliminated or abated, thereby allowing more time and effort for attention to other things. With the development of practical social and medical tools there occurred a movement away from the complacent fatalistic attitude that there were many conditions for which nothing could be done. The results of examinations for eligibility in the Armed Forces at the beginning of World War II came as a shock to most people and spotlighted the enormous numbers of ills, mostly chronic, among the supposedly most healthy segment of the population.[3] Despite the high standard of living in the United States, it was found that 40% of men called up for possible military service had to be rejected because they could not meet standard requirements. At the same time, because of ensuing manpower shortage it became necessary to draw on the reservoir of disabled persons who were not eligible for the Armed Forces. This brought out the surprising fact that many of all types of handicapped persons were capable of making significant social and economic contributions if they were given an opportunity to readjust themselves and their disability to the demands of working and living situations. In other words the rehabilitation needs of the nation and its communities represented a vast but diffuse frontier of preventive, therapeutic, and promotive medicine and community action that was waiting to be discovered.

Beyond this, however, is the fact that the number and proportion of disabled persons have increased considerably in recent years. American society has become more keyed up, more centralized, more industrialized, more complex, and faster moving, with an accompanying increase in accidents, cardiac and hypertensive disease, and mental illness. Recent wars have involved increasing numbers of people and have been more devastating, directly and indirectly, to the people on both the battle and the home fronts. Crippling diseases such as multiple sclerosis and, until recently, poliomyelitis, have increased. Finally, and despite the foregoing, the average life-span has increased remarkably during the past half-century. As a result, the population has been aging, with many more people reaching advanced years with accumulations of handicapping effects of chronic diseases, many of which had their origins in preventable illnesses that occurred earlier in life.

While all these events and changes were occurring, certain sociologic and cultural changes were coming about. Especially pertinent was society's gradual assumption of the responsibility for doing something about the needs and problems of the handicapped, which heretofore were considered to be essentially private burdens, responsibilities of the individual and his family. In the presence of such a vast vacuum, assistance to individuals began to be given by the many voluntary and philanthropic agencies that sprang up, often on the basis of very personal motivations. In recent years, however, governmental agencies have gradually entered more and more into the picture.

These various events and revelations necessitated the reexamination of existing concepts of physical fitness, disability, and rehabilitation. It has been realized that the term *physical fitness* must refer not only to the physical ability and endurance of the military man in combat but also to the ability of the worker and the family breadwinner to perform productive and continuous work. It is a term that is a key to the correct understanding of the whole problem of the crippled and disabled. False concepts of physical fitness have had an important influence on social, economic, industrial, and military life. *Fitness, disability,* and *rehabilitation* are now recognized to be terms with many political and economic implications. Vague and unsatisfactory standards and definitions have often been created, sometimes by law, that have in effect branded those with physical or psychologic defects as unproductive and socially useless and have committed them to the bleak outlook of permanent dependency.

Numerous attempts have been made to describe and define the field of rehabilitation. Rusk,[4] long a leader in the field, referred to it as the third phase of medicine, saying:

We now talk about the third phase of medical care, the first being obviously prevention, the second, definitive medicine and surgery, and the third, that phase between the bed and the job, what you do after the fever is down and the stitches are out to allow the chronically ill or the physically disabled person to live a self-supporting, self-respecting life with dignity.

Sensenich[5] viewed the field in terms of what should be done:

The problem of rehabilitation of an individual involves a twofold effort—on the one hand, to lessen and minimize through medical treatment his physical handicap, and on the other, to help the individual develop his strength and his abilities so that he is better equipped to meet and live on comfortable terms with the physically able of the community.

Another definition, succinct but useful, was developed by a group[6] who studied the field:

Rehabilitation is the process of assisting the individual with a handicap to realize his potentialities and goals, physically, mentally, socially and economically.

## MAGNITUDE OF THE PROBLEM

One strange aspect of the problem of the disabled is that the reaction of the public often appears to be that of seeing but not comprehending. This is to say that although in the majority of instances the disabled are visually very much in evidence, the public tends not to react by grasping the total significance to society of the implications of vast numbers of disabled individuals. Perhaps the reason is that to many the thought of disability is unpleasant, so they thrust it out of their consciousness. Yet even a cursory analysis indicates forcefully the great magnitude of the problem and the enormous economic loss to society that it entails.

In terms of impact on the public mind probably the first most effective picture of national disability resulted from the National Health Survey of 1935-1936.[7] Information was secured on illnesses that were present during the preceding 12 months in a sample of 800,000 families in 83 cities and 23 rural areas of 19 states. From the findings, which had been demonstrated to be reliable, the following national estimates were developed[8]:

1. 4.4% were disabled on the day of the survey visit
2. 1.2% were disabled the entire preceding twelve months
3. 17.7% were reported as having a chronic disease or impairment
4. 1.1% of workers (15 to 64 years of age) were reported to be "unemployable" by reason of disability

Not long afterward the nation became involved in World War II, and large numbers of young men were examined for military service. As previously mentioned, the nation was shocked by the high proportion with defects and in need of rehabilitation. Since the war ended, other surveys were conducted, in February 1949 and in September 1950,[9] followed later by the National Health Survey, which began in 1957 and has been continued since. Typically these surveys have all reported the number of persons between 14 and 64 years of age who were unable to carry on their usual activities because of some illness or other medical condition. The figures vary from about 3.6 million to about 5 million persons. Most of the variation is due to disabilities of short duration, 1 month or less, many of which are probably seasonal. On the other hand, the incidence of disabilities of 3 or more months' duration was generally similar in each of the various surveys.

In 1948 Rusk and Taylor[10] prepared a concise summary of the extent of the problem based on a review of recent literature. They reported about 2.6 million persons with orthopedic impairments of which 341,000 were incapacitating; approximately 900,000 amputees, almost one half of whom had major amputations; almost 400,000 registered crippled children; an estimated 336,000 persons with cerebral palsy; and somewhere between 500,000 and 1.5 million persons with epilepsy. Among additional impairments they called attention to between 9 million and 10 million persons suffering from diseases of the heart and arteries; an estimated 2 million diabetics; approximately 300,000 clinically significant, active cases of tuberculosis plus 150,000 convalescents who would benefit from rehabilitation services; an estimated 2.4 million persons in need of hearing aids, only one third of whom have them; and about 230,000 blind persons. These figures substantiated the statement that 88% of all disabilities were due to disease, 10% to accidents, and 2% to congenital conditions.[11]

A few years later, with specific reference to children, Lesser and Hunt[12] called attention to 500,000 persons under 18 years of age who suffered from rheumatic fever or its effects; about 64,000 children with cleft palate or cleft lip or both; at least 60,000 children with visual handicaps so serious as to need special educational help (with facilities at the time for only 8,000); from 250,000 to 500,000 children with serious hearing loss; and about 1.5 million children between 5 and 20 years of age with speech handicaps unrelated to hearing, cerebral palsy, or cleft lip or palate, of which about one half were functionally serious. An analysis[13] of those served by crippled children's programs in 1964 throughout the United States showed 276,297 children with only one condition and 55,274 with multiple conditions in need of rehabilitation. Overall there were 5.9 conditions requiring rehabilitation per 1,000 children under 21 years of age. The conditions for which children received rehabilitation services were as follows:

| | |
|---|---|
| 1. Congenital malformations | 27.3% |
| 2. Diseases of bones and organs of movement, excluding congenital malformations | 18.1% |
| 3. Cerebral palsy | 8.4% |
| 4. Poliomyelitis | 6.8% |
| 5. Diseases of the ears and mastoid | 6.1% |
| 6. Diseases and conditions of the eyes | 5.7% |
| 7. Accidents, poisoning, and violence | 4.5% |
| 8. Diseases of nervous system and sense organs (excluding 3, 5, and 6) | 3.3% |
| 9. Rheumatic fever and heart disease | 3.2% |
| 10. Other disorders | 9.8% |
| 11. Provisional or deferred diagnoses | 6.8% |

**Table 35-1.** Medical reasons for Selective Service rejection, 1953 to 1958*

| Diagnostic category | Prevalence per 1,000 examinees |
|---|---|
| Disorders of bones and organs of movement | 25.4 |
| Psychiatric disorders | 21.1 |
| Diseases of circulatory system | 19.1 |
| Eye diseases and defects | 18.3 |
| Anthropometric reasons (mostly obesity) | 11.5 |
| Diseases and defects of ear and mastoid | 10.0 |
| Diseases of digestive system | 9.2 |
| Allergic disorders | 8.6 |
| Infective and parasitic diseases | 7.1 |
| Neurologic diseases | 7.1 |
| Congenital defects | 6.2 |
| All other reasons | 25.1 |
| Total | 168.7 |

*From Karpinos, B. D.: Qualifications of American youths for military service, Washington, D. C., 1962, Medical Statistics Division, U. S. Department of the Army.

An indication of rehabilitative needs in the postchildhood or young adult period, supposedly the most healthy interval of life, was provided by the results of Selective Service or draft examinations for possible military duty during the period 1953 to 1958. The findings are presented in Table 35-1.[14] It should be noted that a large proportion of those not accepted because of "disorders of bones and organs of movement" had "flat feet." The other observation is the significant numbers of candidates whose impairments were preventable and/or correctable—some psychiatric disorders, hearing and vision defects, obesity, and others.

It is estimated that about 20 million people in the United States have some degree of chronic disability.[15] This is about 10% of the population. About 17 million of them are limited in their activities as workers, students, or housewives by their chronic ailments. Almost 5 million of them are confined to their living quarters and cannot move about freely or have trouble doing so without assistance. An estimated 4 million of them need and would profit from rehabilitative services. Disability related to military service is dramatic and tends to attract attention more readily than do handicaps that arise under other circumstances. However, it is important to realize that they constitute only a minor proportion of the problem, and indeed not all of them are attributable to combat wounds. Nevertheless, during World War II, as an example, there occurred about 17,000 amputations in the Army of the United States. During the same period there occurred 120,000 amputations in the United States civilian population due to accidents or disease. For this and other reasons it has been estimated that between 3 and 4 million civilian men and women of working age in the nation are so severely disabled by physical or mental impairments that they cannot support themselves or their families. Furthermore, a cause for great concern is the fact that not only the numbers but also the rates of most disabilities are increasing significantly in the United States, as is amply demonstrated in Table 35-2.[16]

Disabilities vary both in incidence and prevalence throughout life. The trend for most disabilities is to increase in prevalence as life progresses because of a combination of uncorrected ailments and injuries. The age variations for certain disabilities are illustrated in Fig. 35-1.

## ECONOMICS OF DISABILITY

Elsewhere the economic aspects of illness and death are discussed. It is pertinent to add at this point some comments on the economic implications of disability and what may be gained by rehabilitation efforts. Society pays in many ways for its failure to prevent and to care for disabilities among its constituents. A few of the more obvious ways are through insurance payments and therefore higher rates, wage losses, production losses, employees' disability compensation, and a significant part of the relief load. In terms of the present labor force, now estimated at about 86 million people fully employed, the loss due to compensable disability during 1 year approximates $5 billion.[17] Add to this the production loss of about twice the lost wages and the total is at least a staggering $15 billion per year. It must be recognized, of course, that much of this loss is because of temporary, self-eliminating disability and that it is dependent on fluctuating employment opportunities, strikes, and similar factors. However, a great deal of it represents needless and stupid loss. With reference to those between 15 and 54 years of age who have never worked because of severe chronic physical or mental disabilities, Allan,[18] using 1 million as the lower end of the estimated number, calculated a possible economic contribution. If only one half could be partially rehabilitated to a point where they could earn only $35 per week, they would add over $900 million to the purchasing power of the nation.

To approach the premise from the positive direction the economic returns from rehabilitative efforts are encouraging. For example, an analysis of handicapped people rehabilitated during 1955 showed that within a year they increased their earnings from $15 million to $105 million per year and added more than 100 million man-hours to the nation's productive effort. Almost 20% or about 11,000 of those rehabilitated had been receiving public assistance, which amounted to $11 million annually. These rehabilitated persons, after a year's work, contributed about $8.5 million in federal taxes. At this rate, within 3 years they repaid the total investment of $25 million made in them. In terms of their working life expectancy it may be considered that, on the average, they would pay $10 in federal income taxes for each dollar spent for their rehabilitation.[19] During 1959, state vocational rehabilitation agencies assisted 80,739 persons. Before rehabilitation their median annual wage was a mere $464, or a total of $61.4 million. After rehabilitation their median annual wage had increased to $2,292 and the total yearly earnings to $157.3 million.[20] It was estimated that within 4 years the cost of their rehabilitation was repaid in taxes. Beyond this, of course, they and their communities were spared the cost and the indignity of welfare existence.

Employment of handicapped workers therefore is far from a charitable proposition. It has been demonstrated repeatedly that many of the physically or mentally handicapped are able to perform efficiently about 3,500 different jobs or tasks, and in general they have better volume of production, higher attendance rates, and better stability and dependability than nonhandicapped workers. For example, one large industrial corporation with an enlightened attitude toward the disabled has the record shown in Table 35-3.[21]

## PROGRAM NEEDS AND GOALS

Many communities already have many rehabilitation services available for their handicapped citizens. Most of these, however, are scattered throughout many public and private agencies and often are unrelated. They have developed as part of the community-wide social services, beginning usually as isolated entities,

**Table 35-2.** Increases in rates per 1,000 population of selected impairments, United States, 1957 to 1965*

| Impairment | July 1957 to June 1958 | July 1959 to June 1961 | July 1963 to June 1965 |
|---|---|---|---|
| Visual impairments | 18.0 | 19.8 | 28.8 |
| Hearing impairments | 34.6 | 35.3 | 45.7 |
| Speech defects | 6.5 | 5.9 | 6.9 |
| Paralysis, complete or partial | 5.6 | 5.4 | 8.1 |
| Absence of major extremities | 1.7 | 1.5 | 1.4 |
| Absence of finger(s) or toe(s) only | 8.5 | | 9.1 |
| Other impairments of limbs, back, trunk, all sites | 58.6 | 74.9 | 94.8 |

*From U. S. Public Health Service: Prevalence of selected impairments, U. S., July 1963-June 1965, PHS pub. no. 1000, ser. 10, no. 48, Rockville, Md., 1968.

**Fig. 35-1.** Impairments per 1,000 persons by type and age, United States, 1958. (From U. S. Public Health Service: Health statistics, PHS pub. no. 584-B9, Washington, D. C., April 1959, p. 3.)

**Table 35-3.** Attendance and performance record of handicapped workers

| Disability | Attendance(%) | | Performance(%) | |
|---|---|---|---|---|
| | Average + | Average | Average + | Average |
| Vision | 66 | 32 | 28 | 65 |
| Hearing | 58 | 42 | 45 | 46 |
| Amputees | 53 | 45 | 40 | 52 |
| Neurologic | 43 | 45 | 40 | 52 |
| Musculoskeletal | 37 | 46 | 24 | 59 |
| Cardiovascular | 20 | 59 | 15 | 70 |
| Multiple | 40 | 40 | 20 | 65 |
| Miscellaneous | 29 | 55 | 13 | 65 |

for example, as programs for special handicaps or diseases or as services to particular age groups. As might be expected, more often than not a state of confusion in the field of rehabilitation, with some difficulty and inefficiency and a lack of services for certain types of cases or individuals, has resulted. Thus in one large city where the problem was studied preparatory to efforts toward coordination there were 37 agencies that were significantly active in some phase or other of rehabilitation. This did not include the various businessmen's service clubs or many of the church groups.

Rehabilitation is actually a complex of many component parts of which the physical or medical aspects of the handicap is only one phase. The individual's emotional acceptance or rejection of the handicap must be taken into account and treated, and his home and job environment, his mental attitude, his vocational skills, aptitudes, and training must also be considered. Attention must be given to all of these and other factors on a coordinated, interrelated basis with respect to the total individual so that he might become self-reliant and fill a useful place in society.

This philosophy requires a unified approach if it is to serve adequately the needs of all types of handicapped persons. It is just as important for the restoration of a patient with multiple sclerosis as for a double amputee. It applies equally to the less severely and to the more severely handicapped. It brings all the skills of several professions to bear on a common effort to restore the individual to a position of maximum usefulness and satisfaction in his society. It places each phase of the approach in its proper relationship to every other phase of treatment or education. The development of this philosophy is so recent that not many really adequate centers have yet been established.

Some, such as those at the Bellevue Institute of Rehabilitation and Physical Medicine, the Cleveland Rehabilitation Center, the Detroit Rehabilitation Institute, and the District of Columbia Hospital, provide excellent comprehensive rehabilitative care on an inpatient and outpatient basis. By following this approach of broad training for self-care these institutions have conclusively demonstrated the achievement of considerable economies in addition to far more successful patient care. Thus during the year prior to the formation of the department of rehabilitation of the District of Columbia Hospital, orthopedic patients spent an average of 55 days in the hospital. After the new program was instituted, the hospital stay of similar patients was reduced to 33 days, a saving of $122,000 for orthopedic patients alone.[22]

The challenge that faces at least the moderate to larger sized communities was indicated by Taylor[23] in a study he carried out in one of the major cities. He concluded that:

The greatest need . . . is the development of a single large center with sufficient staff and facilities to furnish rehabilitation services to all persons with physical disabilities regardless of the medical condition which has caused those disabilities.

He suggested that patients be referred to this community rehabilitation center from any physician, whether in private practice, industry, public agency, or elsewhere, and that the primary medical responsibility for the patient should remain with the referring physician. After evaluation, if the patient is accepted, the medical director of the center could assume the primary responsibility for the prescription and supervision of the physical medicine and rehabilitation services only. Such a procedure is similar to that customarily followed in the referral of patients for specialized care in other areas of medicine. A center of this type should have facilities for inpatients as well as out-patients. In fact, Taylor suggested that eventually a large proportion of the hospital beds in a city might gradually be allocated for convalescents and patients being rehabilitated, up to a level of 1 bed for each 1,000 of the population. This could be accomplished, at least in part, by the decreasing need for beds for communicable diseases and as a result of shortened hospital stays for many conditions.

The community rehabilitation center should operate under the leadership of a physician whose training qualifies him for certification by the American Board of Physical Medicine. The Baruch Committee on Physical Medicine recommends the organization of such a center under two primary divisions, that is, a medical services division and a vocational services division. The medical services division should include a physical medicine branch with an occupational therapy section, a physical therapy section, and a physical education section; and a psychosocial branch with a clinical psychologic section and a social service section. The second of the primary divisions, that dealing with vocational services, should provide branches for vocational testing and guidance and for special education. In addition, to meet the graded needs of various degrees of disability the vocational services division should conduct a sheltered workshop program, a curative workshop program, and a homebound program.

Sponsorship and support should be looked on, especially at this stage, as variable. In many communities the rehabilitation center may undoubtedly begin as a result of the initiative of a forward-looking public health agency in focusing attention on the total problem, drawing together all interested groups and perhaps providing the basic care of the center to which the others may make additions. There are few fields in which it is as easy to contemplate true community-wide interest and action involving public agencies, voluntary agencies, industry, and labor. It should be realized, however, that there is no single pattern that will be acceptable and successful everywhere. In the absence of a community rehabilitation center a few communities have developed central rehabilitation diagnosis and referral centers. This has usually been done under the sponsorship of health and welfare councils. The purposes are to provide preliminary screening and diagnosis, sometimes elementary therapy, social service, and referral and follow-up. Other aims

are to ensure that the patient neither gets lost among the several agencies that may contribute to his rehabilitation nor gets captured by any single one. The best of these agencies have multidisciplinary staffs available for the consideration of the various aspects of the patient's problem.

Commendable rehabilitation centers have been instituted and operated exclusively by voluntary agencies, industrial concerns, insurance companies, and labor unions. The goal, of course, should be a truly cooperative well-integrated and comprehensive program that serves all components of the community and for which all parts of the community have a responsibility and concern. It is in this regard that the official public health agency can bring into play its important role of catalyst. If many public health workers have not considered it, workers in other fields have. After considering the many community agencies interested in the handicapped, the director of a prominent voluntary agency[24] commented:

Some place major responsibility for leadership in community organization for rehabilitation on the hospital-medical school, others on the Bureau of Vocational Rehabilitation. The Health Department might logically be asked to exhibit leadership even in an area of health concern where its currect services are minor. A more realistic approach would seem to be one of accepting leadership where one finds it. This jibes with the nature of rehabilitation, a drawn-out process which uses many professional skills as it shifts emphasis from the original medical to the later vocational aspects.

In a similar vein, Notkin[25] stated:

In recent years, vocational rehabilitation and public health groups have been widely expanding both their ideas and the scope of their operations. Although autonomous operation is probably still desirable at this stage of progress, it may be wise to start thinking of vocational rehabilitation as part of the broader concept of public health which is prevalent today.

So it would appear that here is a public service frontier calling for effective coordinating leadership which some people outside the field believe might well be provided by a community's official health agency. Whether this frontier will be developed or lost by default will be interesting to watch and will be of intimate concern to many thousands of disabled persons who are waiting for an opportunity to live their lives properly.

## REHABILITATION PROGRAM CONTENT

For its part the American Public Health Association has expressed concern with the disparity between the high degrees of existing rehabilitative skills and the customary level of their application to those in need of them. It believes that rehabilitation should be everyone's concern, commanding the concentrated efforts not only of the public health field but all other major professional health and related groups.[26] With this in mind its Program Area Committee on Chronic Disease and Rehabilitation has enunciated the following general principles as a basis for a more effective national rehabilitation philosophy[27]:

I. **Local, regional, state, and national legislation and program planning should embrace all the disabled.**

Planning should be comprehensive in scope, embracing all categories of disability, all degrees of disability. It is recognized that rehabilitation work may be done by categories, special groups, and by priorities.

The skills, services, and facilities needed for independent living or for decreasing the disability of the chronically ill of all ages are very similar to those needed for rehabilitation of persons with foreseeable vocational goals. These include medical, psychological, and social (including educational and vocational) evaluations and a combined overall evaluation of these reports to determine a suitable goal for each disabled person.

II. **Significant data needed for planning.**

It is necessary to determine more accurately the nature and extent of disability in the population so that the scope of the problem can be appreciated and the magnitude of the measures needed may be foreseen. Resources for rehabilitation must be evaluated in each community and their actual availability to persons needing them documented.

III. **Services must be centered on the individual and his family, and all aspects of a given individual's disabilities and capabilities must be considered.**

Failure to look at any one individual's total situation—whether it be the medical, social, psychological, educational, environmental, or vocational facet—may allow an apparently reasonable program to proceed to the point at which all the efforts may have to be abandoned or reconstructed because of failure to reckon with limitations, lack of job opportunity, and so on. Individual-centered services also require the availability of comprehensive services. Particularly in smaller communities it is most unlikely that one

disability can be planned for and serviced satisfactorily by itself. Characteristically the chronically ill suffer from multiple disabilities. . . . The categorical appeal for funding and for educational efforts may have to be continued or strengthened, but the categorical approach should not necessarily apply to the rendering of service to individuals.

IV. **Services must be provided early in the course, or in anticipation, of disability.**

Early provision of services is a self-evident approach to avoidance of disability induced by prolonged bed rest or altered functions. It also serves to minimize psychological, social, and work pattern changes due to unnecessarily prolonged disuse, disability, and displacement. It avoids social and psychological dependency through unnecessary impoverishment of contact and feelings of productivity.

V. **Specific services must be under the appropriate responsible skill.**

Rehabilitation, involving a continuum and a variety of services and professional skills, requires careful teamwork and careful direction in order to insure the earliest and most effective result. In any phase, the decision as to the most desirable supervision must be based on the professional area of the patient's paramount problem at that time.

VI. **Recognition and mutual respect for the contribution of the various disciplines and public and private agencies that participate in this problem are essential.**

The three major national groups currently showing concern are health, vocational rehabilitation and social welfare. They have approached the field of rehabilitation from different viewpoints of their disciplines over the years. . . . For any one individual, no matter what his basic disability, both the medical and social-vocational skills are involved and innumerable other skills may be. The provision of rehabilitation services should not be the competitive, but rather the coordinated, use of the various services or skills, depending on the kind of rehabilitation problem involved.

VII. **Rehabilitation is such a large field that many agencies must share the responsibilities, for it is unlikely that any one agency can or will be given the authority to encompass all of the activities concerned.**

It is unreasonable to expect that all aspects of rehabilitation and all skills involved in the rehabilitation effort can or need be centered in one agency—be it voluntary or official. . . . The job is so huge that many agencies will be concerned, and many have already officially been given responsibility for different segments of the problem. . . . All agencies that have designated responsibility must develop their area of responsibility so their professed deeds are competently performed. When gaps appear at the local level in providing services to the individual, one of these agencies or even a new one may have to be created to fill this gap.

VIII. **Location, administration, and responsibility for rehabilitation services.**

If services are to be quantitatively and qualitatively adequate, responsibility must be clearly assigned. At least three levels of organizational pattern—national, state, and local—must be considered, whether the responsibility for services is to be governmental, voluntary, or professional. Local communities are where people live, and in so far as possible the community should provide the services required for rehabilitation of their citizens. . . . Some highly specialized or more expensive services may require support or even administration at the regional, state, or national level. . . . State and local organizations should also be responsible for providing consultation to help establish quality standards and to help the evaluation of locally provided services. . . . National responsibilities include appropriate financial support for other levels, recommendations relating to service standards, the provision of nationwide channels of communication and exchange of ideas, and the major burden of research, professional training, and establishment of facilities.

## REFERENCES

1. Social and Rehabilitation Service: Fifty years of vocational rehabilitation in the U.S.A., 1920-1970, Washington, D. C., 1970, U. S. Department of Health, Education, and Welfare.
2. Arneson, K. C.: Legislative perspective, Rehabilitation Record, p. 27, May-June 1970.
3. Britten, R. H., and Perrott, G.: Summary of physical findings on men drafted in the World War, Public Health Rep. **46:**41, Jan. 10, 1941.
4. Rusk, H. A.: America's number one medical problem, Proceedings of the Forty-Second Annual Meeting of Life Insurance Association of America, Dec. 9, 1948.
5. Sensenich, H.: Team work in rehabilitation, Amer. J. Public Health **40:**969, Aug. 1950.
6. Van Riper, H. E.: Rehabilitation interests of a voluntary agency, Amer. J. Public Health **44:**744, June 1954.
7. The National Health Survey, list of publications, Public Health Rep. **57:**834, May 29, 1942.
8. Britten, R. H., Collins, S. D., and Fitzgerald, J. S.: The National Health Survey, some general findings as to diseases, accidents and impairments in urban areas, Public Health Rep. **55:**444, March 15, 1940.
9. Woolsey, T. D.: Estimates of disabling illness prevalence in the United States, PHS pub. no. 181, Washington, D. C., 1952.
10. Rusk, H. A., and Taylor, E. J.: Physical disability: A national problem, Amer. J. Public Health **38:** 1381, Oct. 1948.
11. U. S. Senate: President's Health Recommendations and Related Measures; Hearings before Subcommittee on Health of the Committee on Labor and Public Welfare, 83rd Cong., 2nd sess., Washington, D. C., March 30, 1954.
12. Lesser, A. J., and Hunt, E. P.: The nation's handicapped children, Amer. J. Public Health **44:**166, Feb. 1954.
13. Children's Bureau: Crippled children's program: Statistical highlights, 1964, Washington, D. C., 1966, U. S. Department of Health, Education, and Welfare.
14. Karpinos, B. D.: Qualification of American youths for military service, Washington, D. C., 1962, Medical Statistics Division, U. S. Department of the Army.
15. U. S. Public Health Service: Chronic conditions and limitations of activity and mobility, U. S., July 1965-June 1967, PHS pub. no. 1000, ser. 10, no. 61, Rockville, Md., 1971.
16. U. S. Public Health Service: Prevalence of selected impairments, U. S., July 1963-June 1965, PHS pub. no. 1000, ser. 10, no. 48, Rockville, Md., 1968.
17. U. S. Public Health Service: Health statistics, Impairments by type, sex and age, PHS bull. no. 584-B9, Washington, D. C., April 1959.
18. Allan, W. S.: Rehabilitation, a community challenge, New York, 1958, John Wiley & Sons, Inc.
19. Annual Report—1955, Washington, D. C., 1957, U. S. Department of Health, Education, and Welfare.
20. Health, education and welfare trends, Washington, D. C., 1961, U. S. Department of Health, Education, and Welfare.
21. D'Alonzo, C. A.: Some philosophic concepts and experiences with respect to disease and disability, Bull. N. Y. Acad. Med. **41:**286, March 1965.
22. Rusk, H. A.: Rehabilitation in the hospital, Public Health Rep. **68:**281, March 1953.
23. Taylor, E. J.: Unpublished study, 1950, Health Council of the Council of Social Agencies of Metropolitan Detroit.
24. Wenkert, W.: Community planning for rehabili-

tation, Amer. J. Public Health **42:**782, July 1952.

25. Notkin, H.: Vocational rehabilitation and public health, Amer. J. Public Health **41:**1100, Sept. 1951.

26. American Public Health Association: Chronic disease and rehabilitation—a program guide for state and local health agencies, New York, 1960, The Association.

27. Rehabilitation—everyone's concern; Report of Program Area Committee on Chronic Disease and Rehabilitation of the American Public Health Association, Amer. J. Public Health **53:**294, Feb. 1963.

# PART ELEVEN

# The substance
# of public health—
# supportive services

It is all too easy when speaking of medicine to refer to the physician, or when discussing public health, to talk about the health officer. Each is basic, of course, to the enterprise of which he is a part. However, they must depend on the efforts of many other disciplines that make it possible for them to function. In the case of public health the debts of the health officer are many. Predominant among them is that owed to nurses. How could a health agency possibly function without nurses? Their contributions are many and well known. And then there are the invaluable multiplier effects as well as unique functions of the social case worker and the health educator. And finally, how could any of those mentioned know what the problems were and how best to attack them without the combined efforts of the vital statistician and the laboratory staff? It is to a consideration of these crucial supportive professions and disciplines that the chapters in this part are addressed.

> *America's two greatest contributions*
> *to public health were the Panama Canal*
> *and the public health nurse.*
>
> WILLIAM H. WELCH

CHAPTER 36

# Public health nursing services

## HISTORICAL DEVELOPMENT

Among the various professional persons engaged in public health work, one group, that of public health nurses, merits particular mention. Aside from the fact that a large proportion of public health funds and positions is devoted to them, nurses are of special significance in that, considered as a group, they probably have closer personal contact with greater numbers of the public than does the rest of the professional staff of the health department. To many citizens the public health nurse represents the health department. It is she who reduces the work of the organization to its lowest common denominator—direct service to the individual in his home. As a matter of fact, many health departments owe their start to communities' becoming convinced of the value of the services rendered by one or two visiting nurses. One review[1] of the subject has stated it in this way:

It is precisely in the field of the application of knowledge that the public health nurse has found her great opportunity and her greatest usefulness. In the nationwide campaigns for the early detection of cancer and mental disorders, for the elimination of venereal disease, for the training of new mothers and the teaching of the principles of hygiene to young and old; in short, in all measures for the prevention of disease and the raising of health standards, no agency is more valuable than the public health nurse.

The public health nursing movement owes its inception to William Rathbone of Liverpool, who in 1859 was impressed by the care and comfort given by a nurse to his fatally ill wife. Already a philanthropist, he promoted the establishment of a visiting nurse service for the sick poor of his city. It is somewhat surprising to find that despite the enormous existing demand for therapeutic nursing of the sick, the first nurse, Mary Robinson, was directed not only to give direct care to her patients but to instruct them and their families in the care of the sick, the maintenance of clean, tidy homes, and other matters that contribute to healthful living. As the previously mentioned review[1] stated:

. . . This went far beyond mere nursing, and the work of the visiting nurse was thus bound up with and made part of a general health movement—the nurse herself becoming perforce a social worker as well as a nurse. And the highly constructive educational work all this involved put new life and vitality into the age-old charity of visiting the sick poor, gave it enormously increased importance, and brought about its later amazing development.

So that qualified nurses would be available for the work, Rathbone enlisted the assistance of Florence Nightingale and established a training school in affiliation with the Royal Infirmary of Liverpool. Interestingly, Miss Nightingale from the beginning referred to the graduates who engaged in home visiting as "health nurses."

Early in 1873 Bellvue Hospital in New York City opened the first school of nursing in the United States. It was patterned after Miss Nightingale's principles. One of its first graduates, Frances Root, went out to work with poor patients in their homes and thus pioneered community nursing.[2] In 1877 in the United States, as in England, the first visiting nurses were employed by a voluntary agency, the Women's Branch of the New York City Mission.

The idea soon spread to other communities. Meanwhile official health organizations were being established, and it was only natural that eventually they recognized the unique contribution that nurses could make to their programs. At first, resort was made to the visiting nurses of the voluntary agencies. Thus the nurses of the New York City Mission carried out the orders of the school medical inspectors, visited the pupils' homes, instructed the mothers in general health and infant care, and took sick children to the dispensary.[3]

The first visiting nursing associations per se were established in Buffalo in 1885 and in Boston and Philadelphia in 1886. Originally those of Buffalo and Philadelphia were named District Nursing Societies and that of Boston was referred to as the Boston Instructive District Nursing Association. Eventually all their names were changed to Visiting Nurse Associations. They depended on lay contributions for their support, and small service charges where indicated. At the beginning not only were they administratively under the direction of lay boards but the actual work of the nurses themselves was supervised by lay persons. Within a short time, however, the Philadelphia organization led the way by providing for a supervising nurse. It is interesting that each of these three early voluntary field nursing organizations is still active and influential in its respective community, and in Buffalo, until recently, the organization provided almost all of the public health nursing services for the official health department. The Philadelphia Visiting Nurse Society, as will be described subsequently, joined with the public health nursing staff of the health department in 1959.

With the expanding concept of public health it was inevitable that nurses be employed directly by official health departments. The first city to do so was Los Angeles in 1898. The initial purpose was to provide visiting nursing care to the sick poor rather than to engage in educational or health promotional activities. The first official public health nurse, although paid with tax funds and responsible to the health officer, was assigned to the Los Angeles Settlement Association. As more nurses were added, however, there was established in 1913 a bureau of municipal nursing in the health department. The first state to legally approve the employment of public health nurses by local boards of health was Alabama in 1907.

In earlier days of public health work it was easier to focus public attention on special individual problems and to obtain public and private funds for their solution than it was to gain support for a broad general program. As a result, most public health nursing programs were originally organized on a specialized basis; nurses were employed specifically as tuberculosis nurses, school nurses, maternal and child health nurses, communicable disease nurses, and, later, industrial nurses. This trend was given further strength by the activities of the National Tuberculosis Association, by the passage of the Sheppard-Towner Act, and by the growing interest of school officials in the health of the schoolchild. On the other hand, the demonstration of the value of county health units sponsored by the Public Health Service and the Rockefeller Foundation and of the Town and Country Nursing Service sponsored in many parts of the nation by the American National Red Cross indicated distinct advantages to the generalization of visiting nursing activities.

Over several years therefore one of the outstanding controversies in public health nursing administration centered around the question of specialization as opposed to generalization of nursing services. It was argued, on the one hand, particularly by clinicians, that a nurse specially trained for tuberculosis work, for example, was equipped to render much more adequate care and service to the tuberculous patient than was a generalized nurse. Similarly, school administrators, wishing complete administrative control over the nurses working with schoolchildren, usually argued strongly for specialized school nurses. On the other hand, those favoring the generalization of nursing services had several strong arguments to put forth. One was that it was people and families who were served rather than diseases or physical situations. Furthermore, it was pointed out that seldom does only one problem exist in a family and that a specialized nurse was likely to close her eyes to all but one problem. A practical objection to specialized nursing was the frequency with which a family with several health problems would be overwhelmed by the successive visits of a series of specialized nurses, where a single, well-trained generalized public health nurse could cope with all situations that might arise. Eventually a consensus developed in favor of generalized public health nursing programs with only a few exceptions, for example, industrial nursing and full-time specialized clinic activities.

## THE SUPPLY OF NURSES

Nursing represents one of the greatest professional shortage areas in the health field. In 1970 there were about 850,000 registered professional nurses in the United States. One problem is, however, that only about 530,000 are in active nursing practice and about one fourth of these are working only part time. By 1970 the shortage of nurses in the nation was placed at 150,000.[4] But there is still another part of the problem. Not only is the population growing but so is its expectancy for health services, including nursing. Furthermore, with the widespread coverage by health service insurance plans, Medicare, and similar programs, new sources of funds for such services have become available. By virtue of intensified recruitment, the provision of training stipends, and other devices, the number of nursing graduates significantly increased from about 34,000 in 1966 to 52,000 in 1967. In 1962, however, the Surgeon General's Consultant Group on Nursing actually called for 80,000 new admissions to nursing schools by 1966. Furthermore, projections into the next half decade indicate that no significant increase is probable.[5] The situation is compounded by almost 1,000 vacancies on the faculties of nursing schools.

Although the nursing shortage affects hospitals the most severely, other health service fields, including public health nursing, also suffer. Among the standards that have been developed throughout the years have been some dealing with the number of nurses needed to fulfill satisfactorily the needs of the average community. It is generally recommended that there be at least 1 public health nurse for each 5,000 people and that, if bedside nursing services are included, the population base should be reduced to 2,500. Taken as a whole, the nation is still far below these minimal standards, despite the great increase in the number of public health nurses. The figures available indicate a growth in the number of nurses employed in all types of public health work, except industry, from 130 in 1901 to 48,742 full-time and 1,750 part-time in 1968. Until the early 1920s the majority of field nurses were employed by voluntary agencies. Since that time, the distribution has changed considerably, and the latest increase in total employment is largely due to a gain in the number of nurses employed by local boards of education, where over the years the rise has been both constant and substantial. In contrast a steady and continuing decline is seen in the number of nurses employed both by health departments and visiting nursing societies in relation to population. Table 36-1 presents the numbers of public health nurses employed in 1968 in different types of agencies exclusive of industry.[6]

Indicative of the shortage that exists throughout the entire field of public health nursing is a comparison of those employed in local official agencies in 1964 with the minimum suggested

**Table 36-1.** Nurses employed for public health work, by agencies, United States, Puerto Rico, the Virgin Islands, and Guam, January 1968*

| Type of agency | Number of agencies | Registered nurses | | | Licensed practical nurses | | |
|---|---|---|---|---|---|---|---|
| | | Total | Full time | Part time | Total | Full time | Part time |
| National agency | 9 | 518 | 513 | 5 | | | |
| University agency | 191 | 618 | 567 | 51 | | | |
| State agency | 111 | 1,490 | 1,424 | 66 | 10 | 10 | |
| Local agency | 9,684 | 46,116 | 41,255 | 4,861 | 1,740 | 1,637 | 103 |
| Official | 2,622 | 19,070 | 17,183 | 1,887 | 723 | 689 | 34 |
| Nonofficial | 765 | 5,625 | 4,605 | 1,020 | 610 | 563 | 47 |
| Combination | 100 | 2,461 | 2,269 | 192 | 150 | 142 | 8 |
| Hospital-based | 127 | 315 | 230 | 85 | 50 | 40 | 10 |
| Board of Education | 6,070 | 18,645 | 16,968 | 1,677 | 207 | 203 | 4 |
| Total agencies | 9,995 | 48,742 | 43,759 | 4,987 | 1,750 | 1,647 | 103 |

*From U. S. Public Health Service: Nurses in public health, PHS pub. no. 785 (revised), Washington, D. C., 1969.

in Emerson's report, *Local Health Units for the Nation*.[7] Table 36-1 shows that in 1968 there were public health nurses employed full time in local health departments. This is little more than two-thirds the number (26,390) recommended by Emerson in his report. It should be noted, furthermore, that this is despite the fact that at the time of Emerson's recommendations there were only 48 states with a population of 131,669,300, as compared to the present 50 states with about 200 million inhabitants. At the present time the national average is 1 nurse for every 12,800 people. Few states, most of them in New England and along the northeastern seaboard, plus several western states, have a sufficient number of nurses to meet the standards of the American Public Health Association.

It should be noted further that only about a third of the staff nurses working in public health nursing have received 1 year or more of academic training in public health nursing, although at supervisory level and above a majority have had 1 or more academic years of public health training. To further illustrate the nursing personnel shortage 1 out of every 20 budgeted positions for public health nurses in state and local health departments is currently vacant. Actually this figure is low, since several states and large cities do not report and their nursing vacancies therefore are not included in the count. It is estimated that about 20,000 additional public health nurses are needed in the United States to meet minimum desirable standards. It is also estimated that by 1975 a total of 50,000 public health nurses will be needed. This is based on the proportion of 1 nurse per 5,000 population for local areas, the current ratio of administrative and supervisory personnel, the current number of nurses in state agencies, and an additional 1,500 nurses to assist in programs for the home care of the sick. Overall it is estimated that by 1975 the nation will need about 1 million registered nurses and over 500,000 licensed practical nurses.[4]

Meanwhile some significant steps have been taken during recent years to extend the effectiveness of public health nursing staffs by the training and use of a variety of auxiliary personnel.[8] Thus the increase in the number of practical nurses employed has been extraordinary—from 137,000 in 1950 to 250,000 in 1964. In the same interval the number of approved training programs tripled to about 900, with current graduates numbering about 35,000

each year. A similar increase has occurred in the on-the-job training and employment of other types of individuals who take some of the burden off fully qualified nurses. Thus between 500,000 and 750,000 nursing aides, orderlies, and attendants were employed in the nation's hospitals by 1970. In the community and in the home the public health nurse is receiving similar assistance.[9] Between 1950 and 1963 the number of home health aids and homemakers multiplied phenomenally, from 500 to 3,900. "In view of the health insurance provisions of Social Security [Medicare], it is expected that this category of supportive and personal care services into the home of the individual will expand even more in the decades ahead and their services will become increasingly integrated into the personal health care team."[5] Estimates of the number of individuals employed in the several categories mentioned at the beginning of 1966 were as follows[10]:

| | |
|---|---|
| Professional nurses | 621,000 |
| Practical nurses | 282,000 |
| Aides, orderlies, attendants | 500,000 |
| Home health aides, homemakers | 6,000 |

In addition, much of the burden of epidemiologic case finding and follow-up is being taken off the shoulders of the public health nurse by disease control investigators.

## FIELD NURSING AGENCIES

In the evolution of community health programs the contribution of nurses has been increasingly recognized on all levels.

### National level

On the federal level several programs of the Public Health Service conduct activities in public health nursing. They operate essentially by providing grants-in-aid and consultation service to the states and through them to local health departments and by participating in the development of proper standards and qualifications. For a period of years the Office of Indian Affairs provided direct nursing service to its wards by means of public health field nurses stationed on the various reservations. In 1953 this activity was transferred to the Public Health Service and has been significantly expanded. Among other activities it promotes nursing as a career among young Amerindians. In general, the work is the same as that performed by public health nurses employed in local health departments. Three nonofficial agencies that are active on the national level are the National

League for Nursing, the American Nurses' Association, and the Town and Country Nursing Service of the American National Red Cross.

**State level**

By 1937 all of the states employed public health nurses in their state health organizations. The manner of their placement in the organization varies. The majority of state health departments have separate bureaus or divisions of public health nursing, although a few place it under maternal and child health, preventive medicine, or local health administration. Individual nurses may be assigned to functional units of the department by the nursing unit and in a few instances are employed directly by the specialized service. The functions and responsibilities of nurses in state health departments depend on the legislative basis of the department. In the majority of instances they act as advisors to local health departments, boards of education, voluntary health agencies, and other state agencies. In a few state health departments that have been given broader responsibilities and powers the nurses may actually supervise and administer certain direct services, local as well as state, and may have some inspectional powers such as are related to midwives, nurseries, baby boarding homes, nursing or convalescent homes, and hospitals. The latter function is becoming more important in relation to the Medicare portion of the 1965 and 1972 Amendments to the Social Security legislation. Other important activities of state health department nurses include demonstrations of particular services or of total public health nursing programs and the conducting of in-service training courses.

All state health departments are active in the promotion of home public health nursing services for prenatal and postnatal patients, infants, and preschool children. In order to do so they function either through the direct assignment of state nurses to local areas, through emergency loan of state nurses to specially selected local communities, or through subsidy of local nursing programs. In recent years a number of state health departments, often in conjunction with philanthropic foundations, have experimented with the provision of nursing service for home deliveries.

**Local level**

Generally speaking, field nurses today may be placed into two general categories—those employed by official health agencies primarily to carry out preventive and promotive health functions, and those engaged almost always by voluntary agencies primarily to render home nursing care to the sick. Despite some differences of opinion regarding terminology, it is convenient for our purposes to refer to the first group as *public health nurses* and to the second group as *visiting nurses*. It should be pointed out, however, that neither of these terms can be interpreted strictly. The functional differences between the two groups are becoming increasingly obscured. Both visiting nurses and public health nurses visit homes and perform what are considered public health functions. Furthermore, there are many indications of a trend toward the inclusion of bedside nursing care of the sick in the functions of the publicly or officially employed field nurse. In other words the distinction between the two groups of nurses, if indeed a real distinction exists, depends merely on the manner of their employment and compensation—in one case by government, in the other case by a private yet publicly supported agency.

On the local level nurses are employed by several different agencies. Outstanding, of course, is the official local health department, the nurses of which render direct personal service to individuals and families. In addition, many local boards of education employ special school nurses. Of a quasi-official nature is the nursing program of the American National Red Cross, which began in Ohio in 1912 and has since spread to many parts of the country, particularly in rural areas. From the beginning its policy has been to promote and assist in the establishment of local public health nursing programs and of full-time local health departments to which it eventually turns over its work. The American National Red Cross also played an important role in the promotion of public health nursing units in state health departments.

The majority of public health nurses employed in a nonofficial capacity are found in the many local visiting or voluntary nursing associations. These organizations are primarily concerned with bedside care of the sick. It should not be assumed, however, that their function is limited to this, since the typical home visit includes much public health education and promotion as well as bedside nursing services. An important consideration in this respect is the fact that increasingly nurses of visiting nursing associations and of official health departments receive similar training and frequently interchange positions.

Two other groups that until recently provided visiting nursing services should be mentioned. Some of the larger insurance companies, particularly Metropolitan Life and John Hancock, for many years offered home nursing service to persons holding certain types of policies. The manner in which this was done varied, depending on the size of communities, the number of policyholders, and the existence of other qualified nursing agencies agencies in the community. In some areas nurses were employed directly by the insurance companies, whereas in others the service was purchased on a cost per visit or on a contract basis from local private nursing agencies. These programs were phased out some years ago on the basis of the services' having become readily available from other sources.

Another source of nursing service that has played an important role in some parts of the country is the large private occupational medical and health programs, many of which employ not only industrial clinic nurses but also nurses whose function it is to attend sick employees and sometimes members of their families in their homes. With the broadening scope of occupational health and safety and the interests of labor unions in health services, such programs often include health protection and promotion activities provided by industrial clinic and home visiting nurses.

Before leaving the subject of public health nursing agencies, reference should be made to the National Organization for Public Health Nursing. Although it did not render direct service to the public, it played a dominant role in the advancement of this field. The NOPHN was organized in 1912 as the national professional society for those engaged or interested in this work and became recognized as the spokesman for the profession. No other single agency contributed so much to the improvement of educational and service standards and to the promotion of the public acceptance of and respect for the work of the public health nurse. By 1952, however, concern developed about the growing number of nursing agencies and the need for coordination. As a result, in that year the NOPHN joined the National League of Nursing Education and the Association of Collegiate Schools of Nursing to form the National League for Nursing. At the same time the bylaws of the American Nurses' Association were changed to provide for cooperation with the new National League for Nursing. Mean-while the National Association of Colored Graduate Nurses also went out of existence, and its functions were integrated into the other organizations. As a result there are now only three national nursing organizations: the American Nurses' Association, the National League for Nursing, and the American Association of Industrial Nurses.[11]

## FUNCTIONS AND RESPONSIBILITIES

The following statement is accepted as the definition of public health nursing.

Public health nursing is a field of specialization within both professional nursing and the broad area of organized public health practice. It utilizes the philosophy, content, and methods of public health and the knowledges and skills of professional nursing. It is responsible for the provision of nursing service on a family centered basis for individuals and groups, at home, at work, at school, and in public health centers. Public health nursing interweaves its services with those of other health and allied workers and participates in the planning and implementation of community health programs.*

The statement of functions and qualifications for public health nurses, first prepared in 1931 by the Subcommittee on Functions of the National Organization for Public Health Nursing, has undergone several revisions. The most recent statements of functions and qualifications were prepared by a committee of the Public Health Nurses Section of the American Nurses' Association in 1964.[12] They represent the combined thinking of practitioners of public health nursing from every state and territory of the United States. These statements are grouped by classification and include functions, standards, and qualifications for public health nurses in staff positions; administrative, supervisory, and consultative positions are listed separately.

The following are the functions of public health nurses in staff positions employed by departments of health, boards of education, and voluntary agencies:

### ASSESSING

#### Function I
**Identifies present and potential needs and resources related to the health of individuals, families, and the community**
   A. Uncovers health needs and problems through observation, interviews, analysis of records, and use of vital data

*Statement presented and adopted at the National League for Nursing Biennial Convention, May 1959.

B. Observes, explores, and evaluates the patient's physical and emotional condition, reaction to drugs or treatments

C. Considers age, sex, culture, economic status, or geographic location that may influence the incidence or prevalence of health problems

D. Recognizes attitudes that influence individual and community health

E. Estimates the ability and readiness of individuals and families to recognize and meet their own health needs

F. Identifies the availability and utilization of community resources

G. Evaluates the urgency and complexity of the need in determining priority of action

### Function II
**Shares in identifying present and potential needs and resources related to the agency's program and the nurse's job responsibilities**

A. Appraises community health and social needs and resources for interpretation to administrative and planning groups

B. Appraises the adequacy of public health nursing services in her district in relation to the community needs and the agency program

C. Determines through her contacts with patients, families, members of related disciplines, and others, the extent of their knowledge of the agency's program

D. Estimates the effectiveness of intra- and extra-agency communications

E. Participates in the exploration and identification of her own needs in relation to the job

## PLANNING

### Function I
**Plans for comprehensive nursing service to individuals and families in their homes**

A. Interprets nursing and other services of the agency to patients and families as a part of planning

B. Plans with the individual, family, physician, and other concerned members of the health team for care which is appropriate

C. Plans with other individuals and agencies for continuity of patient care

### Function II
**Participates in planning for public health nursing service in special settings such as schools, places of employment, nursing homes and similar institutions, hospitals, clinics, and health conferences**

A. Helps develop and arrange for public health nursing services in special settings

B. Develops plans for group teaching to meet the special needs of various groups

### Function III
**Contributes to planning for the development and operation of the public health agency**

A. Contributes to the development of philosophy, purposes, policies, and procedures of the public health nursing services in the agency

B. Participates in planning nursing aspects of new and ongoing programs

C. Contributes to the preparation and revision of the nursing budget

D. Participates in planning the administrative procedures of the nursing office

E. Participates in planning continuing education programs for agency personnel

### Function IV
**Participates in planning with other agencies for community health programs**

A. Advises or participates in community group planning related to nursing and health

B. Plans with professional organizations and civic groups for the improvement and advancement of the practice of nursing and public health

## IMPLEMENTING

### Function I
**Helps provide comprehensive nursing service to individuals and families in their homes**

A. Gives skilled care to patients requiring part-time professional nursing service and teaches and supervises the family and other members of the nursing team

B. Interprets extent and limitations of available nursing service

C. Gives preventive and therapeutic treatment under medical or dental direction, and teaches positive health measures

D. Utilizes her understanding of behavior patterns in giving nursing service

E. Initiates nursing measures to prevent complications and to minimize disabilities

F. Helps the individual and family to develop attitudes that permit them to make optimum use of available resources and health facilities

G. Helps the family accept and assume its responsibility for providing and arranging care, and guides it toward self-help

H. Helps the patient and family understand implications of the diagnosis and recommended treatment consistent with their readiness and with the knowledge of the physician

I. Helps individuals and families to utilize their capabilities and make the best possible adjustment to their limitations

J. Helps individuals and families understand patterns of growth and development, and encourages attitudes and actions that will promote optimum health for each individual

K. Aids in effecting changes in the environment or in the organization of activities for the elimination or modification of health hazards

L. Communicates with other professional workers regarding the individual and family, and refers pertinent information to the appropriate agency

M. Participates in conferences with other disciplines to coordinate services and plan joint action

N. Assists the physician and dentist with examinations and treatments when nursing skills are required

O. Obtains laboratory specimens, performs diagnostic tests when indicated, and interprets the significance of the results to individuals and families when authorized

P. Participates in recruiting, training, and supervising volunteer workers

Q. Maintains necessary records and reports

**Function II**

**Provides public health nursing service in special settings**

A. Gives direct or consultative nursing services in such settings as schools, clinics, hospitals, or places of employment

B. Provides nursing service, on a demonstration or temporary basis, to convalescent and nursing homes and similar institutions

C. Carries out inspections of institutions when delegated by the licensing authority for the purpose of making nursing recommendations

D. Participates in the teaching of selected individuals and groups

**Function III**

**Participates in the development and operation of the public health agency**

A. Keeps the agency informed about changes in the community and in nursing practice which may have an effect on the program

B. Assists with orientation and guidance of new staff members, volunteers, citizen committes, and boards

C. Participates in the public information and promotion activities of the agency

**Function IV**

**Participates in community health programs**

A. Teaches basic principles of healthful living in relation to changing needs of individuals in all age groups

B. Provides for or encourages others in the community to provide for group instruction related to health

C. Represents the agency in her professional organizations and community groups when so designated

D. Interprets to the community the need for and meaning of health laws and regulations, and reports violations to the appropriate authority

E. Participates in community health surveys and epidemiologic studies, and other organized health programs

F. Interprets health and welfare needs to appropriate community groups

**EVALUATING**

**Function I**

**Appraises performance**

A. Evaluates the effectiveness of her nursing service to individuals and families

B. Evaluates the effectiveness of her service in health programs in special settings

C. Contributes to the evaluation of workers for whom she shares supervisory responsibility

D. Uses available help to study and evaluate her own job performance and plan for continuing professional growth

**STUDYING AND RESEARCHING**

**Function I**

**Engages in surveys, studies, and research**

A. Identifies problem areas related to her functions in assessing, planning, implementing, and evaluating

B. Participates in defining problems for study

C. Participates in the conduct of surveys, studies, and research related to her clinical and functional responsibilities

**Function II**

**Applies pertinent research findings**

## QUALIFICATIONS OF PUBLIC HEALTH NURSES

The recommended qualifications for public health nurses in staff positions include:

**A. Licensure**

Holds a license to practice professional nursing in the state in which employed.

**B. Education**

Completion of a baccalaureate degree program approved by the National League for Nursing for public health nursing preparation or post-baccalaureate study which includes content approved by the National League for Nursing for public health nursing preparation. (It is essential that there be continued self-improvement through supervision, sharing in evaluation, utilization of educational opportunities such as staff education, workshops, institutes, self-directed reading, continuation of formal education, and active participation in professional and related organizations.)

**C. Characteristics**

Abilities that contribute to the practice of public health nursing develop with experience and maturity. However, even at a beginner's level, each of the following qualities is required to some degree:

Willingness and ability to

1. Act with integrity

2. Understand and accept people with individual and cultural differences

3. Understand individual behavior

4. See and evaluate self in relation to others

5. Accept the public health nurse's role and interpret this role to others

6. Work with others toward a common goal

7. Adapt to the realities of a situation while adhering to fundamental principles

8. Gain satisfaction from helping others to help themselves

9. Use help from available sources
10. Maintain receptive and cooperative attitude toward change
11. Communicate effectively
12. Accept responsibility in professional and community activities
13. Observe desirable health practices

Qualifications for nurses in supervisory, administrative, and consultative positions require a master's degree with a major in administration, supervision, consultation, or in a special field, or a master's degree in public health from a school approved by the American Public Health Association.

## ADMINISTRATIVE RELATIONSHIPS

An important administrative consideration influencing the value and efficiency of public health nursing programs is the nature of the relationships that exist among the various nursing and social agencies in the community, the public, and the members of other healing professions. The demand for public health nursing services is so great that if all available personnel in an area were employed in a single ideally efficient agency, it would still be inadequate. This being true, it is important and necessary that agencies engaged in this work cooperate fully to correlate and coordinate their respective programs as much as possible for the maximum efficiency.

### Relationships within the health department

The professional relationships of public health nurses take place in two areas: (1) within the health department itself and (2) in contacts with other agencies and individuals in the community. Within the health department the relationship between the public health nursing staff and the administrative health officer is of paramount importance. All too often adequate and satisfactory relationships and understanding between the nursing staff and the health officer are falsely assumed to exist. It is not unknown for health officers merely to support the nursing program quantitatively according to standards such as 1 nurse per 5,000 population, but, once obtaining nursing personnel, to neglect to participate in the planning and administration of the public health nursing program and activities.

Apparently some health officers, thinking that they know nothing about nursing problems, follow the path of least resistance by allowing the nursing division to proceed almost as if it were an independent agency. Inevitably this policy leads to difficulty both within and outside of the department. The health officer by virtue of his position is ultimately responsible for all phases of the health program of the department and, to a considerable extent, of the community as a whole. With respect to the nursing aspects of the program the health officer should carefully select a well-qualified director or supervisor, provide her with adequate administrative support, and see that general policies and interagency relationships are cleared at the top of the organization by him rather than perhaps haphazardly and inadequately lower down by his staff nurses and the staff workers of other agencies. He should maintain constant interest in the nursing program and endeavor to learn enough about it to assist the nurses to see how their activities really fit into the total community health picture. It is significant that within the past few years several of the schools of public health have established courses in public health nursing supervision and administration specifically for medical health officers.

With reference to public health nursing programs within a health department, Ross[13] stated, "No division of nursing can rise above the level of performance set by its health officer and no division of nursing will get far without his active and understanding support. The quality of the public health nursing program in official agencies country-wide is, in the last analysis, in the hands of health officers; if it is to become grade A only they can decide." In contrast with the foregoing are the occasional situations in which members of a nursing staff circumvent their nursing supervisor or director and approach the health officer with their problems and complaints. This practice should never be condoned for obvious administrative reasons. If permitted to come about and continue, it can result only in disastrous damage to the morale of the organization. Again it is up to the health officer and his nursing director to see that organizational channels are understood and followed by the staff nurses.

The public health nurse and the staff working in environmental health may on the surface seem unrelated. However, they are part of the same organization and should work in a helpful as well as cordial relationship. In the course of her daily field visits the alert public health nurse is certain to become aware of many insanitary situations. Often they have a direct or indirect bearing on her own professional interests and activities. A policy of prompt and effective intraagency referral should be developed to handle such situations. The same applies conversely to the engineer and sanitarian.

## Relationships with other nursing agencies

One of the most important extra-agency relationships of public health nurses is with the staffs of other agencies that render nursing services in the community. In view of the necessity of maintaining desirable interagency relationships and of the considerable scarcity of nursing personnel at the present time, it is important that public health nursing functions be carefully analyzed to make the most efficient use of the time of those employed. One writer[14] has stated: "The discriminating review of our nursing functions which was forced upon us as a war expediency helped us to set up standards of priority in our home visiting programs which should continue to be of assistance to us in our present and future planning. However, this review also exposed the fact that the qualities of ready adaptability which have made public health nurses such a valuable adjunct to public health staffs have also resulted in wasteful use of our nurses' professional skills. We found that many of the time-consuming duties our nurses had carried did not require highly technical skill. However, they absorbed so much of the time of our well-prepared nurses that the teaching and other skills they had acquired were not utilized to the best advantage." The considerable expansion of this point of view has since been forced by the many dynamic changes that have been occurring in public health in general during recent years and the increased regard of health services as a continuum.[15]

Among the sound recommendations that have recently been made and increasingly followed are those for the elimination of public health nurses in strictly routine clinical activities that can be carried out under their supervision by auxiliaries; the increased use of nurses without public health training, practical nurses, nurse aides, community service assistants, neighborhood health workers, and lay volunteers for certain activities; and the elimination insofar as possible of strictly clerical activities of public health nurses by the employment of an adequate office staff and the constant scrutiny of record requirements. By such means the strictly public health nursing activities of many agencies may be increased considerably.

## Consolidation of nursing services

There is little if any justification for more than two field nursing groups in any given community: (1) the public health nurses working as employees of the official health department and (2) the staff of the nonofficial visiting nursing association. Accordingly, the trend has been to explore ways of effectively and equitably merging even these two groups. Regardless of the number involved, the correlation and coordination of the work of all agencies providing nursing services in a community are obviously necessary and desirable in order best to serve the needs and interests of the public. Since there is no one answer to how this may be accomplished, each community must work out a solution best suited to its particular needs and backgrounds. The number and variety of possible arrangements in a given community may be somewhat as follows. If there are several voluntary or nonofficial agencies such as a visiting nursing association, cancer societies, tuberculosis societies, and occupational health organizations that render nursing services in the community, they may (1) remain completely independent of each other in an inefficient uncoordinated manner, (2) retain their individual identities but coordinate their programs by means of a central nursing advisory committee in which each agency participates, or (3) combine their programs to form a single community public health nursing agency. The voluntary agencies singly or united may limit their activities to bedside care, leaving most or all educational, promotional, and legal control measures to the nurses of the official health department. On the other hand, the health department may delegate some or even all of its public health nursing responsibilities to the voluntary nursing agency. In the few communities where this procedure is followed, it is usually attributable to two influences, that is, the existence of a long-established, well-supported, and accepted visiting nursing association, and a weak official health department or one of relatively recent origin and tenuous support.

The completely satisfactory consolidation of community nursing services is as yet relatively rare, usually strongly resisted, and in some situations premature. One of the most successful solutions developed up to the present time was effected in Seattle, Wash. The official and voluntary nursing agencies agreed on a cooperative, completely generalized public health nursing program that includes all preventive, promotive, educational, and bedside services but retains the board of directors of the voluntary nursing agency as an advisory committee that controls its own contribution to the total cost of the program by means of an annual contract with the official health department. Where carefully prepared for and put into effect, this plan has worked well and has brought about an increased efficiency and economy, and both groups of nurses have found more professional job appeal and stimulation from it.

In 1959 Philadelphia proceeded to merge its several field nursing services in still a different manner that appears to be successful and acceptable to all concerned.[16] There were three groups involved: (1) the nursing staff of the department of public health, (2) the nursing staff of the long-established and highly reputed Visiting Nurse Society of Philadelphia, and (3) the nursing staff of a smaller voluntary nursing agency restricted to one section of the city. After careful study and planning by representatives of all three agencies plus several additional unaffiliated citizens and consultants, it was decided that no one agency should absorb the others. Instead a completely new and distinct agency was established—the Community Nursing Services of Philadelphia. Each of the three existing agencies formally agreed to place at the disposal of the new organization all of its personnel and noncapital material resources. Each contributed a proportionate share of funds to employ an outstanding public health nursing administrator, her secretary, and part-time financial and legal assistance. These are literally the only direct employees of the new organization.

It was agreed that the sum of the nature and level of services of the respective cooperating agencies at the time of the merger would serve as the base line of activities, any addition to or subtraction from which would require concurrence by the Board of Directors of the new Community Nursing Services organization. This consists of individuals equally designated by the city government and the directors of the Visiting Nurse Society (which still continues its separate existence in order to own property, to accept gifts and contributions, and to receive monetary support from the United Fund). The Commissioner of Health is an ex officio member of the Community Nursing Services' Board of Directors, and the Director of the department's Community Health Services routinely meets with the board as a consultant and advisor.

As a first step a group of particularly well-suited and experienced nurses from all three agencies worked together in one district of the city for 1 year to find potential operational trouble spots, develop new policies, records, and the like. Meanwhile an extensive indoctrination and retraining program was begun on a phased basis with the remainder of the personnel. As each new group was ready to begin a merged operation in some additional district of the city, some of those who had already been working in the trial area were transferred to help get them started. The top administrative and consultative staff is housed in the Community Health Services headquarters building, and in all cases the Community Nursing Services' field nursing staffs are housed in district health centers with the respective multidisciplinary staff of the general health program.

Meanwhile a medical advisory committee was established and began to function in connection with the many technical problems that continually arise in a nursing program. In addition, to maintain a balanced and up-to-date activity a program committee was established to review any suggested program changes of major import, to study community needs, and to make recommendations to the Board of Directors regarding any indicated policy and program changes. By agreement the Director of Community Health Services is an ex officio member of the medical advisory committee and is chairman of the program committee. This assures a constant channel to and from the general health program of the community. To date, the organization and its program have been functioning well and smoothly, and there is reason to believe that the community is obtaining more and better service per nurse and per dollar expended. Probably the greatest virtue of this approach is that no one organization can feel that it was absorbed or swallowed by any other organization or group. To the contrary, the very structure connotes and requires cooperative action.

With reference to the joining or merger of nursing services, in 1946 The Association of State and Territorial Health Officers adopted as a general guide a resolution that included the following recommendations:

The community should adopt one of three patterns of organization that will provide the type of coordinated public health service most feasible under local conditions and that will best fit into the general plan advocated by the state department of health in each state. The organization patterns are:

1. All public health nursing service, including care

of the sick at home, administered and supported by the health department. This is the most satisfactory pattern for rural communities.

2. Preventive services carried by the health department, with one voluntary agency working in close coordination with the health department, carrying responsibility for bedside nursing and some special fields. At present this type of organization is the most usual one in large cities.

3. A combination service jointly administered and jointly financed by official and voluntary agencies with all field service rendered by a single group of public health nurses. Such a combination of services is especially desirable in smaller cities because it provides more and better service for each dollar expended.

### Medical relationships

The nurse in public health work has traditionally served at the right hand of the physician. Therefore the relationship of the public health nurse with physicians practicing in her community has become of great importance. In most of her daily work the public health nurse repeatedly comes in contact with people who either are or should be under the care of a physician. She must always realize that private physicians as a group constitute the most powerful and most important weapon against ill health. Accordingly the public health nurse, working in the field with families and individuals, must assume as one of her primary functions the interpretation of medical service in the community. She must act as a sort of implementor, seeking out those who need the care of physicians, helping them to obtain it, and assisting them in putting the advice of their physician into effect.

It is advantageous to a health department and particularly to its nursing staff that there be a medical advisory committee with whom to discuss, clear, and implement matters of medical policy. The members of the committee should be appointed by the local medical society. Frequently the public health committee of the medical society serves the purpose adequately. A committee of this nature is particularly helpful in planning new projects or programs in which the public health nursing staff may be engaged. Another valuable service of the medical advisory committee is the formulation of written policies for the nurses of the health department. It is obviously of mutual benefit for the director of nurses and the health officer to meet with the medical advisory committee.

On entering a home, the public health nurse whenever possible, should relate her visit to the wishes of the family physician. To do this successfully the astute public health nurse should acquaint herself with the wishes and policies of each physician in her area and constantly keep him apprised concerning the status of his patients. This she may do by means of personal interviews, telephone conversations, or written reports. Some agencies have a policy that the first contact with a physician must be through an interview or at least by phone. These policies are basic to good relationships and are appreciated by medical practitioners.

It is important that public health nurses observe professional ethics the same as they do in the hospital situation. In the typical community everyone who receives nursing care, particularly of a bedside nature, should be under medical supervision. Permission and instructions should be obtained from the attending physician beforehand to make the nursing services of greatest value, to maintain desirable patient-physician relationships, and to develop a feeling of professional partnership between the public health nurse and the private physician. Diagnoses and treatments must never be criticized or contradicted. If the nurse believes that she possesses information that might alter the medical management of the case, she should discuss it in a cordial, respectful manner with the medical attendant, but never with the patient or his family.

The selection of a physician should be the prerogative of the patient to be served. Frequently the nurse, and for that matter other health department employees, is asked to name an acceptable medical attendant. If possible, no single physician should ever be suggested. The person making the request should be given the names and addresses of several capable and creditable practitioners, preferably from a list agreed on by the local medical society. The complaint is sometimes heard that public health nurses take patients away from private physicians by referring them to health department and other free clinics. Unfortunately this claim occasionally may have been justified. The amount of the services for which private physicians are uncompensated is fairly common knowledge. Many prefer to maintain contact with their patients through poor times as well as good. This being true, in the interests of a good professional relationship it is important that no such referral ever be made except after the signed release of the patient by his physician.

### Community nursing councils

Somewhat similar in nature and purpose to the medical advisory committee that has been previously recommended is a community nursing council. This advisory group should assist in studying, planning, improving, and coordinating all of the nursing activities in the community. Its membership is usually fairly large, including representatives from all official and nonofficial agencies that render nursing services, from organized professional groups such as medicine, dentistry, nursing, and social work, and from the public at large.

At the present time a great many communities have a council of social agencies, often in close affiliation with a community chest or fund. The council plays a most important role in the development of joint analyses, planning, and implementation by all of the many social agencies that exist in the typical community. It usually functions by means of several standing and ad hoc committees with representatives of various interested and pertinent agencies. The health committee, which is almost universally one of the standing committees, often has a subcommittee on public health nursing. Occasionally this subcommittee serves effectively in the absence of a community nursing council.

## PUBLIC HEALTH NURSING AND SOCIAL WORK

The association of the official health nursing program with the other social agencies in the community emphasizes the fact that in a certain sense the public health nurse is essentially a highly specialized type of social worker. Her approach to individual and family problems, however, must of necessity be from a somewhat different basic point of view from that of the usual professional social case worker. Nevertheless, because of the complex nature of all social problems, of which illness and its prevention are one, mutual understanding and cooperation between the two groups is of great importance. As a team, they can be invaluable. The more they know about each other's special training and abilities the better will be their individual and joint performance. The role of social services in public health is considered in Chapter 37. For her part the public health nurse should first be familiar with each of the social agencies in her community and second should know what each does, where its interests and contributions cut across, supplement, or complement those of the public health nursing program. She should have available for ready reference a directory or file indicating the interests, resources, location, and leadership of each one.

Usually the social welfare programs consist of six basic community services: child welfare services, family services, medical social services, psychiatric social work, public assistance, and recreation. Occasionally most or all of these are found in a single agency. However, the usual pattern is for several official and nonofficial agencies to be involved. Some of the types of programs in which they are variously concerned with administering are those dealing with aid to dependent children, the care of neglected and delinquent children, child guidance, mental health clinics, old-age assistance, unemployment insurance, aid to the blind, vocational rehabilitation, and retirement.

One of the important practical reasons for familiarity with the social agencies of a community is for purposes of referral. A case of tuberculosis, for example, may appear to be primarily the concern of the health department through its public health nurse. However, problems of hospitalization and its costs, family support in the absence of the breadwinner, the placement of dependent children, and rehabilitation, to mention a few, will usually arise. The public health nurse cannot solve all of these singlehandedly. She must therefore refer certain aspects of the total family problem, which has been cryastallized by the appearance of tuberculosis, to other appropriate community resources.

Of great value to the nurse in such instances is the existence of a social service exchange. This is a clearinghouse wherein are registered identifying data regarding cases on the registers of the various community agencies. Its purpose is to enable all community agencies to serve the needs of the distressed individual or family more satisfactorily. The following types of patients or families should usually be registered by public health nurses: (1) those with pressing or complex social problems, (2) those to be referred to social agencies or other health agencies, (3) those having long-time health problems such as tuberculosis, (4) those receiving free services for which a charge is usually made, and (5) readmissions that were previously registered with the exchange. These patients or families are cleared again as a means of obtaining new data about them.

## ADMINISTRATIVE AIDS IN PUBLIC HEALTH NURSING

As in other professional areas, public health nursing has found it practical to apply certain well-proved administrative aids.

### Supervision

Unquestionably the most valuable administrative aid is the supervision provided at each level within a public health nursing agency. Supervision is necessary for the properly balanced development of the nursing service to public health programs and for the maintenance of its standards. Total responsibility for such supervision rests on the nurse administrator and, depending on the size of the agency, assistants and one or more supervisors. At the staff level supervision ensures the quality and quantity of the service through both administrative and educational processes. With a ratio of 1 supervisor to every 6 to 8 staff nurses it should be possible for the supervisor to offer sufficient guidance and counsel to the field or staff nurses to maintain the standard of the service offered and individually develop each staff nurse to the maximum of her ability to serve the patient and his family. The nursing supervisor is in fact also a liaison person who serves as a two-way link between the staff nurses and the administrative officers of the agency. The supervisor interprets policies and methods of application and may also transmit the impressions of the staff, together with suggestions for additions or changes in policies, to the administration centers of the agency. In this way it is possible for the field staff to play an important role in the formation or modification of policies and program.

### Standard procedures

In any situation where several persons perform similar work toward a common purpose, it is desirable that they each follow the same procedures with regard to certain aspects of their work. To avoid misunderstanding and confusion it is helpful, even in the smaller agencies, to have available a manual that sets forth clearly the policies of the agency and details of technical procedure. This should include statements of the exact responsibilities and authority of the personnel, standing orders used by the agency, and descriptions of techniques that are considered safe, effective, and ethically acceptable. Although each agency will find it necessary to develop its own manual, attention is directed to the *Manual of Public Health Nursing*, which has been prepared and is periodically revised by the National League for Nursing (formerly the NOPHN). Many state health departments have also prepared excellent nursing manuals for use by local health departments. There also should be a record manual in which the purpose and proper use of each record used by the public health nursing staff is explained and illustrated. It must be remembered that, valuable as these administrative manuals are, they quickly become useless unless continually kept up to date.

### Clerical staff

Although much of the recording, particularly that relating to details of field visits, must of necessity be done by the nurses themselves, there is much clerical work that is most efficiently carried on by an office clerical staff. Despite this, it is by no means uncommon to find the professional nurses of many organizations devoting large proportions of their worktime to details of record keeping and analysis in the office. This is particularly unfortunate in the face of significant shortage in nursing personnel. The false reasoning appears to be prevalent that, as long as nurses must be employed in the public health nursing program, they might as well do all or most of the clerical work involved. It should always be realized that the records are also a necessary part of the program and that proper personnel for their handling is wholly justified. Furthermore, it is well to remember that the use of the relatively expensive time of a professionally trained public health nurse for office work, which may more efficiently and effectively be turned over to lesser trained employees in lower salary scales, is poor administration.

### REFERENCES

1. Department of Philanthropic Information, Central Hanover Bank and Trust Co.: The public health nurse, New York, 1938, reprinted by the National Organization for Public Health Nursing.
2. Birth of nursing at Bellevue, Md. **17:**68, April 1973.
3. Waters, Y.: Visiting nursing in the United States, New York, 1909, Charities Publication Committee.
4. The need for nurses, New York, 1971, National League for Nursing.
5. National Commission on Community Health Services: Health manpower, Washington, D. C., 1967, Public Affairs Press.
6. U. S. Public Health Service: Nurses in public health, PHS pub. no. 785 (revised), Washington, D. C., 1969.

7. Emerson, H.: Local health units for the nation, New York, 1945, Commonwealth Fund.

8. Freeman, R., and Holmes, E.: Administration of public health services, Philadelphia, 1960, W. B. Saunders Co.

9. Ryder, C. F., Stitt, P. G., and Elkin, W. F.: Home health services—past, present, future, Amer. J. Public Health **59:**1720, Sept. 1969.

10. U. S. Public Health Service: Health resources statistics, PHS pub. no. 1509, Washington, D. C., 1965.

11. New structure of nursing organizations, Public Health Rep. **67:**1258, Dec. 1952.

12. Functions and qualifications in the practice of public health nursing, New York, 1964, Public Health Nurses Section, American Nurses' Association.

13. Ross, G.: Is the health officer fulfilling his responsibility in relation to the nursing program? Amer. J. Public Health **29:**305, April 1939.

14. Johnson, M. L.: Public health nursing administration in the changing order, Public Health Nurs. **39:**333, July 1947.

15. Freeman, R.: The expanding role of nursing, some implications, Int. Nurs. Rev. **19:**351, April 1972.

16. Wilson, D., Andrews, M., and Hall, M.: Community nursing services of Philadelphia, Nurs. Outlook **9:**612, Oct. 1961.

CHAPTER 37

# Social services

## HEALTH AS A SOCIAL PHENOMENON

One of the most interesting aspects of the medical and public health movements has been the progressive growth of the use of sociologic methods to explain and better understand the etiology and epidemiology of disease. In the early history of public health, for example, during the Middle Ages, disease was considered to be punishment for sins; thus it was more of an individual, internally oriented explanation rather than one that involved interpersonal or intergroup relationships to any significant extent. This interpretation was later considered to be inadequate for explaining the presence of disease, and people began to accept the theory of communicability of many diseases. Doctrines relating to these initial propositions evolved into more public concern, leading to a preventive concept of disease, involving social processes. Efforts were made to deal with the sanitary problems of the towns, quarantine was used widely, hospitals were developed, and medical care was provided. The era of microbiology offered a great stimulus to public interest in health problems, but it led to a temporary setback in the understanding of the importance of the environment because of its unitary causation theory, in which emphasis was placed on a specific cause and specific treatment for each specific ailment.

Increased urbanization, industrialization, and specialization revived an awareness of the significance of social factors in relation to disease. Health problems that developed as a result of the crowded industrial civilization led to the appreciation of social effects and aspects of disease and to the necessity of new means of disease prevention that required community effort. Special attention was given to the health problems of the poor and of the working classes. Malnutrition was rampant, infant and maternal mortality was high, housing was pitiful, and other general health conditions were unsatisfactory. Toward the end of the nineteenth and during the early twentieth century, various governmental and voluntary organizations were established to provide needed community services and to educate the public. Child welfare programs expanded, school services for children evolved, public health nursing was established, and other important health programs were developed. The need was firmly established to incorporate the study of social processes in considering diseases, both mental and physical, now recognized as of multiple causation. In present society the need is especially great because of the shift in importance from infectious to chronic illness. The high social and economic costs of these conditions have brought about greater concern for the welfare of patients and their families; the need for more and better facilities for medical care, including such things as home care, nursing homes, and rehabilitation centers; and a demand for more effective health education of youth and adults as well. All this is possible only through a total, organized community effort.

The future of the application of sociology to public health appears promising, Indications are that it will help medical and public health personnel to understand better the relationship of social processes to the etiology and epidemiology of disease and to develop more effective action to cope with the exigencies that arise. It was indicated that all public health problems involve economics, education, cultural attitudes, and many other factors. In the normal conduct of their activities public health workers must involve themselves to an increasing degree with the solution of these other aspects of the problems with which they deal. Public health nurses have been particularly active and successful in this regard. However, the recognition and adequate handling of such problems and the dealing with certain types of individuals and agencies often require special training and skills that the traditional health worker has only partially acquired in his training and experience. Only relatively recently have public health agencies, especially official health departments, realized the great potential value of social workers to the public health program. Some specific examples will be referred to subsequently.

Public health and social workers should understand and relate to each other with relative ease and to mutual advantage, since both groups are concerned with overlapping aspects of the multifaceted problems of individuals and families. To be successful both professions must be family and society oriented rather than merely individual oriented. Social case work, public health nursing, and in fact public health activities in general attempt to assist the individual or group in the understanding of its problems, to rationalize, and to explain. Far more can be accomplished by all concerned if they work as members of a team.

On the basis of experience with a children's center in a housing project, Robinson[1] has suggested that critical attention be given to the effectiveness of intensive medical, nursing, and social work as a unit in obtaining maximum return on the deployment of scarce personnel, facilities, and especially in multiproblem communities. As Goodrich[2] says, "The future effectiveness of social service in comprehensive medical care depends largely on the concerted efforts of allied medical fields such as physicians, nurses, social service personnel, public health officials, and personnel in other health agencies developing and successfully implementing the problem of communication." The importance of this has been described by Ebie[3] in relation to solving the sociomental

problems of families in Edinburgh, Scotland, where the facility is actually a multidisciplinary social case work center with social workers backed by psychiatrists, psychologists, marriage counselors, and others as necessary. The nature of their case load is illustrated by a sample of 134 individuals—94 requested material help (money, food, clothing, or housing), 10 needed psychologic help, 4 required a combination of material and psychologic help, and 18 required other kinds of help. Two individuals were referred because of child neglect. It is interesting that in 32 instances temporary relief of some type was sought for a period when the mother was to be in the hospital.

Health legislation enacted during recent years in the United States, especially that relating to regional medical programs, the Medicare, Medicaid, and comprehensive child health components of the Social Security law, and the comprehensive health planning acts, has forced public health workers to take a much broader viewpoint than in the past, including a greater realization of the importance of social casework in the achievement of health goals. Barnett[4] has stated the case clearly in a paper prepared for the Third National Conference on Public Health Training:

If health is perceived to include more than medical or biologic entities, and is a by-product of social systems, then social work is intimately related to public health. Family planning, alcoholism, suicide and drug addiction are public health and social problems. The major social problems of today—juvenile delinquency, racial discrimination and violence, poverty, crime, child neglect, marital incompatibility and divorce, deterioration of the inner city and expanding suburbia relate to health and to welfare. These are social and health problems. These situations are crucial. In planning it is recognized that health and social problems are interrelated and have interwoven etiologies. Thus far, social problem intervention has been carried out through one social system and health problem intervention through another. There has not been consensus on social-health issues, problems, and decisions either by the people in need, the professional service groups, or the decision makers. Medicine, education, and social work are concerned with the individual, the family, and the community. They all have a concern for prevention, early casefinding and early mobilization of high quality care provided through a network of specialized services. The hitherto sharp lines of demarcation between institutional care and home care, physical disability and mental disability, health and welfare needs, are blurring. There is a general movement toward a more holistic interpretation and operational definition of the principles of primary, secondary, and tertiary prevention.

## DEVELOPMENT OF THE FIELD

Social work in relation to health and medical programs had its beginnings early in the twentieth century when Richard Cabot and Ida Cannon introduced the concept at the Massachusetts General Hospital. They based their action on the philosophy that the patient's understanding and cooperation were needed to overcome illness, over and above anything the physician and the hospital might do. Furthermore, they recognized that there were many other factors involved in recovery, among them the family economy, the living conditions in the home and neighborhood, social relationships, and the like. They recognized also that there were usually available in the community numerous resources that might be tapped for the best ultimate solution of all aspects of the case, provided the physician had time to seek them out or if he had someone to do it for him and the patient.

The success and spread of these ideas in medical and hospital practice are well known. Social work and its involvement in health and medical programs has progressed considerably as a profession since it was presented to hospitals as an economy measure to preclude giving free care to people who might be able to pay. From this it passed to a concern for assisting individuals with the social and economic problems that contributed to or arose out of their medical problems.[5] Today, as indicated by Silver and Stiber[6] and by Wittman,[7] the emphasis is more on prevention, and the social worker's role in the health team is to seek out potential sources of disaster that lie within the personality of individuals or family relationships, and attempt to modify the situation favorably. As they suggest, this may involve working with a child in a family rather than directly with his disturbed mother or with a husband rather than with his sick wife. In other words, the emphasis now is often on strengthening the supporting factors as much as on helping to treat the individual who is ill. Under such circumstances, as Rice[8] warns, the social worker is confronted with a difficult decision as to the most effective balance between the nature and extent of services to give to persons who already have problems and need immediate help as against those who are in situations or groups that may make them vulnerable to potentially harmful societal stresses. In the latter role the emphasis must be on analysis, anticipation, and neutralization or at least diversion of the undesirable social forces. Among the areas, especially in young families, where Rice sees social workers to be useful are the following:

1. Experience of families in crises, such as the birth of a congenitally handicapped child, acquired handicapping conditions due to trauma or disease, the birth of a premature baby, a patient newly diagnosed as having tuberculosis or cancer, a death, or a miscarriage. These all are crises in families to which individuals will react intensely. Knowing this and working with them at the time of crisis, or preferably in advance of an anticipated crisis, will help to lessen the impact on the individual and family.

2. Early years of marriage and pregnancies at an early age.

3. Separation of the child from the family or separation of the parent from the child. Hospitalization of a parent often results in unfortunate experiences for the child.

4. Assumption of a new responsibility, such as becoming a spouse, a parent, or meeting the difficulties of widowhood.

5. Pressures on both mothers and children because mothers are working.

6. Siblings of sick, disabled, or handicapped children.

7. Supportive services to adolescents who are trying to make their adjustments to adult life.

8. Children who leave school early, to become often unemployed in the labor market, or marry young, or who frequently are added to the group of our juvenile delinquents in a community.

To take a long step back in time it is interesting to note that a Sociological Section was established in the American Public Health Association as early as 1910. At that time John M. Glenn,[9] General Director of the Russell Sage Foundation, stated that "the purpose of the section is to increase the social workers' knowledge of health problems and their interest in them, to bring social worker and health officer into closer touch with each other with a view to securing closer and larger cooperation between them; to bring to both a clearer recognition of the fundamental relation between social and health problems; and thus to develop the potential power of both to win and hold the interest and support of the public." Mr. Glenn went on to point out that already "Many social workers have recognized the value of the American Public Health Association and felt that acquaintance and close alliance with its members was essential to the success of their work. . . . Health officer and social worker has each his field to cultivate; but each will do his own work more thoroughly and effectively if he knows more about what the other knows and is aiming at. . . . Close alliance, with mutual confidence, between health officer and social worker is inevitably necessary to victory in the war against disease and its promoters."

Rosen[10] describes regretfully the subsequent struggle of the Sociological Section to find a meaningful place and role in the organization. Despite active support and participation by several of the leading medical figures in the association, it finally faded away by 1923. As Rosen indicates, considering the period, it was a product of unusually progressive thinking, whose day had not yet come. In the time since, numerous social workers have become active members of the professional public health society but have done so by joining a variety of specialized sections. Perhaps in terms of ultimate effect this process of unintended infiltration of other disciplines will produce the greatest result. Meanwhile, for several years a Conference of Social Workers in the American Public Health Association has met in conjunction with the annual meeting of the association.

## PRESENT STATUS

By 1972 there were 80 graduate schools of social work in the United States accredited by the Council on Social Work Education. Three others are working toward accreditation. These schools enroll more than 15,000 full-time students, of whom about 14,500 are in the master's program, with the rest in post-master's degree programs. They graduate about 6,000 individuals each year. About 800 colleges and universities offer undergraduate social work education. Three fourths are accredited and graduate about 1,800 baccalaureates each year. An estimated 137,000 social workers were employed in the nation in 1970; only 25,500, however, worked in health and related programs, 16,800 worked in psychiatric, and 8,700 worked in medical settings.[11] After the adoption of their services by hospitals, numerous voluntary health agencies began to employ social workers, and more recently, because of the increasing emphasis on the social and community aspects of health as well as the trend to integrate preventive and promotive health activities with therapeutic medical care and rehabilitation, increasing numbers of official health agencies have been adding social workers to their staffs.

Despite this, the valuable adjunct of social work is still utilized only to a fraction of its potential by health agencies. Currently only one quarter of all hospitals in the United States have social services available in the hospital to the patients who need them.[12] In 1950 there were only slightly more than 400 positions for qualified social workers in health agencies in the United States, exclusive of positions in hospitals, clinics, and other medical care institutions. Most positions were on the staffs of official state and local health departments and of agencies concerned with crippled children or vocational rehabilitation services. Others were on the staffs of voluntary health agencies on national, state, and local levels. During the following decade from 1950 to 1960, only a 3% increase occurred in employment of medical and psychiatric social workers by governmental noninstitutional health agencies and only a 1% increase by voluntary health agencies. A study[13] of 131 state and local health departments in 1961 showed a social work vacancy rate of 15.8% in contrast with an overall vacancy rate of 7.7%. Social work had the highest percentage of vacancies of any category in the health field. Ironically, despite the overall shortage of qualified personnel in this field, another study revealed that of all social workers with 2 years of training and a master's degree, 47% reported field instruction in either medical or psychiatric social work.[14] Between 1960 and 1970 the number who sought field instruction in a health setting increased significantly. At present, health programs rank fourth in the 10 possible fields of social work practice among students and graduates.[11] It appears therefore that far more of the inadequate number of social workers wish to work in the health field than can find satisfactory employment in it.

The social and health legislative advances of recent years, as well as legislation to increase and improve social work education, are certain to bring about a great acceleration in the employment of social workers in the health field. This will be necessary in view of the increased emphasis on comprehensiveness and continuity of care on a family and neighborhood basis, mental health programs, the health needs of the socioeconomically disadvantaged, aged dependants, and addictive diseases. When a national health insurance program is enacted, there will be an especially great need for more social caseworkers in the health field. It is difficult if indeed possible to estimate the number of social workers ultimately needed in health programs in view of the extremely labile and transitional nature of the current situation.[12] This difficulty lends weight to Wittman's[15] comment, "There is an urgent need to capitalize on the current upsurge of interest in expansion of health services. . . . There will be high value in the achievement of more precise definitions of practice in public health social work and medical social work. An immediate task for public health social work is the exploration of the potential contributions of group work training and preparation in community organization in the health services. There should be more experimentation with combinations of practice methods which would seem to lend themselves in a better way to improved and extended health services."

## ROLE OF THE SOCIAL WORKER IN PUBLIC HEALTH

The range of the social worker's activities in a health agency is necessarily determined by the size, scope, and changing purposes and priorities of the agency, the vision and understanding of its administration, and the availability of social work personnel. One basic question must be answered with respect to their function in a health department: What is the extent of direct service through personal contact with individuals in need of assistance, in contrast with working essentially through other members of the staff, especially the public health nursing staff? An ancillary factor here is the extent to which other members of the staff have been prepared to understand and accept the potential professional contribution of the social worker and are willing to accept her as a specialized consultant. In most instances in which social workers have been brought into programs of local health departments, many individual and family contacts were initially anticipated and emphasized. Repeatedly, however, it has been found that the most efficient and fruitful use of the limited number of social workers and of their time is as staff consultants, fellow program planners, and as liaisons with the many other pertinent community agencies. Despite the limited number of social workers active in public health agencies, a substantial literature is developing to describe the wide areas in which social workers are already contributing significantly. Among the many examples that could be mentioned are in child health clinics,[16] family planning programs,[17] mental

health,[18,19] epilepsy, diabetes, and arthritis,[20] heart disease,[21] geriatrics,[22] prepaid medical care plans,[23] health maintenance clinics,[24] and ghetto health programs.[25] The last reference, incidentally, includes several examples that illustrate "a new role for Social Service students and staff: to reach clients on a different level at which some of their basic needs and problems beyond the immediate health problems might be addressed; to engage them in meaningful change in their own life situation—which should be ego developing and reinforcing in order to counteract the years of deprivation and apathy."

## SOCIAL WORK FUNCTIONS IN PUBLIC HEALTH

The increased need for and employment of social workers in public health programs led to the establishment in the Committee on Professional Education of the American Public Health Association of a subcommittee on Educational Qualifications of Social Workers in Public Health Programs. This subcommittee, in collaboration with the American Association of Medical Social Workers, not only developed a series of sound qualifications for the different levels of social work in health agencies but also produced the following excellent statement of social work functions in health and medical programs[26]:

1. **Social work consultation services.** Consultation is a major responsibility of social workers in public health. It is often available on any aspect of the health department's program. More commonly it is related to the social problems of an individual or family, to problems met by other agencies, to social needs within the community, to coordination of the services of the health department with other community services, to agency administration, and to program and policy development within the department. Depending on the situation, the social worker may provide consultation service alone or as a member of an interprofessional team, as in evaluation of particular aspects of a community or institutional program.

2. **Program planning, implementation, and policy formulation.** Social workers in public health usually have responsibility for participating in program planning and policy development in the agency. On the basis of their professional equipment and the cumulative evidence from day-to-day activity, they are generally in a position to know how policies affect individuals or groups, or what standards and programs need to be strengthened, modified, or developed.

Social workers participate, with other personnel,

**Table 37-1.** Social components in health department programs: a guide developed by the social service staff, California State Department of Public Health*

| I | II |
|---|---|
| Analyzing the social needs of people in the community and the resources available as they affect the total public health program. | Planning programs with consideration of social factors in health department services and how people are affected by the ways in which the services are given. |
| *Program determination* | |
| Who are the people mainly served by the health department? From what economic, national, and racial groups do they come? To what health problems do these factors contribute? | Determining through evaluation by health department personnel what problems, such as resistance to care, exist in tuberculosis, crippled children's services, and maternal and child health and determining whether solutions should be found within the health department and/or in cooperation with other agencies. |
| *Economic factors* | |
| Where can families and individuals served by the health department turn in times of financial stress? What are the prevailing community attitudes toward giving and receiving help? What are legislative and administrative policies and how are they interpreted? | Ascertaining how interpretations of special needs in relation to health should be done if economic deprivation or transiency is a major community problem and stringent policies are in effect. |
| *Psychosocial aspects* | |
| What facilities (casework services, foster homes, day care, vocational rehabilitation, psychiatric, housekeeping, etc.) are available and how adequately are these provided? Are there gaps or duplications? | Considering, over and above financial assistance, what services people want, what seem needed, and what cooperation and leadership the health department can give in using or developing services having a bearing on the maintenance of health. |
| *Community participation* | |
| What are the working agreements and relationships between the health, social, and education agencies in the community? | Deciding with which agencies there is need to work on a continuing basis concerning referral procedures and cooperative services to people. |

*From Social components in health department programs, editorial, Amer. J. Public Health **45:**97, Jan. 1955.

| *III* | *IV* |
|---|---|
| Maintaining a public health program that recognizes and deals directly or indirectly with concomitant social problems. | Investigating through research psychosocial and economic factors related to the maintenance or breakdown of health and to the use of health facilities by such projects as: |
| Carrying out policies and procedures in health department programs which consider basic needs of children and adults as well as individual and group differences, including staff and community education around these concepts. | Studying the use of health department facilities by various groups such as migrant, national, and ethnic. |
| Referring patients to agencies for financial assistance and having a continuing relationship with these agencies, bringing regularly to their attention case situations where restrictions aggravate public health problems, and encouraging appropriate referrals from these agencies. | Studying the incidence of a specific disease in relation to socioeconomic status. |
| Helping individuals and groups served by the health department to use existing services, within or outside the health department, which best meet their health, social, and emotional problems. | Studying normal and premature births in relation to marital stability, planned or unplanned pregnancy, fear of childbirth, reasons for delayed or no prenatal care, etc. |
| Bringing to the attention of the community the need for modification and extension of services and programs and reaching an understanding with agencies as to types of referrals and exchange of information that will be mutually helpful. | Studying cases to determine if there is a need for a proposed resource or if existing facilities are meeting current needs. |

in the development of joint projects; in the stimulation of activity on problems which fall within the jurisdiction of the health agency; and in the determination of program priorities. As a member of an interprofessional staff, social workers have the added responsibility of conferring with and advising health officers and program chiefs and supervisors in other professional areas on appropriate matters, or help in determining the most satisfactory solutions to social problems.

In most health agencies, administrative and supervisory responsibilities for the social work services are assigned to one person, who is often designated chief social worker, director of social work, or chief social work program consultant.

In some instances, primarily in mental health agencies, social workers carry out the major administrative responsibility for development of the total program of the agency.

3. **Social work services to individuals and families, social case work.** Social case work in public health involves social study and evaluation leading to services for individuals or families who are having difficulty in social functioning, primarily as it affects their health and their ability to use health services. The problems may be those "which impinge upon the family unit or individual from the social or physical environment" or those "which the individual brings into being, in whole or in part, by modes of behavior and interaction between himself and other persons and situations." Individuals or families needing social case work may be brought to the attention of the social case worker by the members of the health team, by other agencies, by the individual or family, or they may belong to a group already identified, needing social case work on the basis of diagnosis or the type of situation. Persons within selected categories may be routinely referred for the purpose of identifying social factors which affect the individual's health problems or his use of needed health and medical services. The social worker initiates case work services in instances where resolution of social and emotional problems helps to prevent problems or facilitates care. Collaboration with other professional staff is an essential part of the case work process.

Social case work service may be provided temporarily for the purposes of demonstration, in order to develop methods of effective referrals to appropriate agencies, or to facilitate more comprehensive study and treatment by the health agency.

Opportunity for direct case work services is most often provided in local agencies, less frequently in state programs, and least often in programs at the national level.

4. **Social work services to groups.** Increased use of the group process in resolving social problems is a definite trend in social work in public health. The social worker in public health may act as leader of groups of patients or family members, or as a consultant or resource person to groups or to their leaders. This group process may be used by social workers with patients in a single diagnostic category, with relatives of patients who have the same health problem, or with other groups where there is a health need.

Social group workers, especially trained in social work methods, have been used more frequently in hospitals and mental health programs than in other public health programs, although the opportunities in all are apparent.

5. **Social work services to the community.** All members of the public health team contribute to the provision of community services. In public health, the social worker places a major emphasis on this activity, in which he applies his social work knowledge of individuals, groups, and communities and of community process, his understanding of social welfare as a social institution, and his knowledge of social work organization to the task of community planning.

The social worker in public health is in a strategic position to identify, evaluate, and document social problems relating to health needs, to discover ways of preventing them, and to plan new services or to strengthen those already in existence. He serves also as an interpreter of social resources to other team members and of health services to social agencies. He thus assists in improving collaboration and in coordination of programs for health and social welfare, and in modifying or developing services to meet new needs.

Social workers especially trained in the social work method of community organization have been used more often in voluntary health programs than in public health departments.

6. **Research, studies, and surveys.** Research is carried on by social workers, both independently and in collaboration with other professions in public health, mental health, and medical care programs.

7. **Educational responsibilities.** The social worker is responsible for the supervision of social work students assigned to the agency for field instruction. He also participates in the preparation of students from other professions with respect to promoting an understanding of the social and health needs of individuals, groups, and communities, and ways of preventing and meeting these needs. He contributes to and benefits from the educational program of the health agency by participation in programs of staff education within the agency and in the community.

With the purpose of pulling these various roles and functions together into a meaningful guide, the social service staff of the California State Department of Health developed a useful summary of social components in health department programs,[27] which is presented in Table 37-1. It indicates basic social work functions in relation to program planning, economics, psychosocial factors, and community participation.

Wittman[15] in trying to fit social work into the public health context, advised that "The social work profession is only one of several concerned with means for the prevention and treatment of disease and disability in this country. It should make every effort to take its place beside the others in a concerted attack on the problems of ill health." As stimulating evidence of its intent and ability to do just that, Corwin,[28] in an excellent discussion of new dimensions of social work practice in health, takes the initiative by stating that "Any referral may be in the form of a request for consultation or for direct service. Subsequently a decision can be reached with the other staff members as to future management. In addition, some conditions are so fraught with social implications that, by their very nature, some type of social work intervention to alleviate distress, limit disability, and assist in rehabilitation seems indicated." Then she suggests and discusses the following circumstances as outstanding examples in the second category:

1. Out-of-wedlock pregnant women and other pregnant women who for one reason or another require social work service
2. Battered children and children in need of care and protection
3. Families in which there is a diagnosis of mental illness in the mother
4. Multiproblem families
5. Individuals who resist medical care, especially if children are involved
6. Children who are mentally retarded or have other handicapping conditions

Earlier the importance of interprofessional communications and cooperation was discussed. It has been suggested[29] that interactions among agencies or professions in these regards are affected by three factors: (1) the nature of the functions they perform, which in turn determine the elements they need; (2) their access to elements from outside the system of health and welfare agencies or conversely, their relative dependence on the local system of other health and welfare agencies; and (3) the degree to which domain consensus exists within the system of health and welfare agencies. If these points are valid, as they probably are, it is suspected that the social worker in the health agency is possibly the best fitted to satisfy them in their most favorable sense.

## REFERENCES

1. Robinson, D.: Effectiveness of medical and social supervision in a multiproblem population, Amer. J. Public Health **58:**252, Feb. 1968.
2. Goodrich, C. H.: Social work in medical and health services, New Jersey Public Health News, p. 8, Jan. 1966.
3. Ebie, J. C.: A multidisciplinary social casework center with a staff psychiatrist, HSMHA Health Rep. **86:**863, Oct. 1971.
4. Barnett, E. M.: Social work training needs. Background paper prepared for Third National Conference on Public Health Training, Washington, D. C., Aug. 1967, U. S. Department of Health, Education, and Welfare.
5. Goldstine, D, editor: Readings in the theory and practice of medical social work, Chicago, 1954, University of Chicago Press.
6. Silver, G., and Stiber, C.: The social worker and the physician, J. Med. Educ. **32:**324, May 1957.
7. Wittman, M.: Preventive social work—a goal for practice and education, Social Work **6:**19, Jan. 1961.
8. Rice, E. P.: Concepts of prevention as applied to the practice of social work, Amer. J. Public Health **52:**266, Feb. 1962.
9. Glenn, J. M.: Sociological section; Report of the section committee, Amer. J. Public Health **3:**645, Nov. 1913.
10. Rosen, G.: The sociological section of the American Public Health Association, 1910-1922, Amer. J. Public Health **61:**2515, Dec. 1971.
11. U. S. Department of Health, Education, and Welfare: Health resources statistics, DHEW pub. no. (HSM) 73-1509, Rockville, Md., 1973.
12. Closing the gap in social work manpower. Task Force report on social work education and manpower, Washington, D. C., 1965, U. S. Department of Health, Education, and Welfare.
13. Hill, E. L., and Kramer, L. M.: Training for service and leadership in the health professions, Department of Health, Education, and Welfare Indicators, Aug. 1964.
14. Salaries and working conditions of social welfare manpower in 1960, New York, 1961, National Social Welfare Assembly, Inc.
15. Wittman, M.: Social work manpower in the health services, Amer. J. Public Health **55:**393, March 1965.
16. Corwin, R. A., et al.: Social work in a child health clinic, Amer. J. Public Health **55:**821, June 1965.
17. Mednick, M. F.: The social worker's responsibility in family planning, In Gorman, J. F., editor: The social worker and family planning, PHS pub. no. 2166, Rockville, Md., 1970, U. S. Department of Health, Education, and Welfare.
18. National Institute of Mental Health: The social worker's role in mental health, PHS pub. no. 351, Rockville, Md., 1954.
19. McCaffrey, I., Cumming, E., and Rudolph, C.: Mental disorders in socially defined populations, Amer. J. Public Health **53:**1025, July 1963.
20. Rander, M. A.: Expanding role of the social worker in the health field, Amer. J. Public Health **62:**1102, Aug. 1972.
21. Peay, R. E.: What social services offer to patients

who undergo cardiac surgery, Public Health Rep. **78:**1045, Dec. 1963.

22. Goldman, F.: Social service in homes for the aged, Public Health Rep. **76:**625, July 1961.

23. Alt, E. S.: Social work consultation in a prepayment medical care plan, Amer. J. Public Health **49:**350, March 1959.

24. Stoeckle, J. D., Sittler, R., and Davidson, G. E.: Social work in a medical clinic: the nature and course of referrals to the social worker, Amer. J. Public Health **56:**1570, Sept. 1966.

25. Russell, M. V.: Social work in a black community hospital: its implications for the profession, Amer. J. Public Health **60:**704, April 1970.

26. Educational qualifications of social workers in public health programs, Amer. J. Public Health **52:**317, Feb. 1962.

27. Social components in health department programs, editorial, Amer. J. Public Health **45:**97, Jan. 1955.

28. Corwin, R.: Some new dimensions of social work practice in a health setting, Amer. J. Public Health **60:**860, May 1970.

29. Levine, S., White, P. E., and Paul, B. D.: Community interorganizational problems in providing medical care and social services, Amer. J. Public Health **53:**1183, Aug. 1963.

*If you are planning for a year ahead, sow rice;*
*for ten years, plant trees;*
*for a hundred years, educate people.*

CHINESE PROVERB

## CHAPTER 38

# Health education*

### ACTION REQUIRES UNDERSTANDING

That remarkable universal man of American history, Thomas Jefferson, once observed, "Health is no more than learning." In considering the important subject of health education the following statement is pertinent:

The time has gone by when people can be dragooned into cleanliness, or be made virtuous by police regulations, and hence it is that the most thoughtful among practical reformers of the present day base their hopes of sanitary progress on the education of the masses as the real groundwork of national health. The people must be taught that good conduct, personal cleanliness, and the avoidance of all excesses, are the first principles of health, hand-in-hand in the rearing and guidance of youth. . . . They must be interested systematically in the general results of sanitary progress, and become more intimately acquainted with the social and material causes by which it is impeded.[2]

This quotation from the first report of the Maryland State Board of Health, dated 1875, emphasized that the public's health is dependent on the public's convictions about health.

Health education in some form has always been an important activity of public health personnel. It was not until the second quarter of the century, however, that it became formally recognized as a specialty and as a major function in public health. The transition has been gradual. In the earlier eras of public health that focused on the sanitation of the environment and the control of communicable disease,

---

*For a useful bibliographic guide, see Roberts and associates.[1]

public health activity was interpreted to consist of doing things *to* and *for* people, with heavy reliance on legislative and police power. With the development of the newer interpretation of public health as the summation of personal health, there developed an appreciation of the need to do things *with* people and to get people to accept an increasing responsibility for their own health. This change in point of view was summarized by Governor Franklin Roosevelt in the foreword to "The Report on Public Health in New York State by the State Health Commission of 1931." He compared the report with that of 1913 as depicting the transition of the public health movement from the single problem of attaining mass health to the double task of maintaining mass health and controlling preventable disease in the individual. He stated:

This is a more difficult task than that of establishing wholesale preventive measures in which the people themselves are not required to take an initiative. It involves the fullest use of public health education, so that citizens may understand and cooperate with activities necessary for their own welfare. Important as are the laws which the Commission has recommended, of far greater importance is intelligent action on the part of the individual and of the community.

### DEVELOPMENT OF HEALTH EDUCATION

Chapter 16 presented a discussion of the development and role of the voluntary health movement in the United States. It was indicated that one of their earliest and continuing activities has been an attempt to improve the knowledge about, hence action against, their respective disease interests on the part of the

**669**

general public. Because of these early activities, priority in the field of health education may rightfully be assigned to the voluntary health agencies and especially to the antituberculosis societies. These set the pattern that was followed for about a third of a century—conscious involvement of large numbers of citizens as small contributors and/or as neighborhood volunteer workers, and the development of "impact" visual aids that depicted graphically and dramatically the medical and social consequences of the particular disease in question. Exhibits, leaflets, pamphlets, newspaper articles, health talks, lantern slides, children's parades, plays in school, and many other imaginative techniques were used. As time passed, motion pictures, popular magazines, radio, and television were added.

In 1914 the New York City Health Department established the first bureau of health education in an official agency, followed promptly in the same year by a similar unit in the New York State Health Department. Over the years these two agencies have employed significant numbers of workers in various aspects of the field and have done outstanding work, especially in the use of mass media for popular and professional health education. Soon after the New York units were established the Detroit Department of Health formed a separate organizational division of health education that pioneered in the development of neighborhood health groups, clubs, and guilds that intimately and effectively involved the targets of the health educational efforts, especially the socioeconomically disadvantaged, consisting for the most part of immigrants from Central Europe and both white and black transmigrants from the southern United States. Progress was by no means rapid; by 1929 health publications were being issued by only 52 city and 35 state health departments, and only a few had full-time directors of health education.

In the meantime, however, the field had received its specialty name, *health education*, at a conference called in 1919 by the Child Health Organization of America, which also offered the first fellowship in health education the following year. It is interesting to note that this organization was formed by a pediatrician, L. Emmett Holt, and a nurse, Sally Lucas Jean, both of whom were convinced that emphasis on child health promotion through education and nutrition would accomplish much more than dogged, never-ending diagnosis and treatment of existing ills.[3] By 1922 there were sufficient numbers of people working in the field to merit the establishment of a separate specialty section in the American Public Health Association.

However, retrogression set in, and at the time that the United States became involved in World War II a mere 13 state and local health departments reported employment of health educators (44 persons in all). Wartime needs spurred action, and special curricula were established in several of the accredited schools of public health. The rapidity of response was indicated by the fact that by 1947 over 300 persons, all of whom had completed graduate courses in recognized Schools of Public Health, were employed as health educators in official and voluntary health agencies. Concurrent was an important change in attitude on the part of health officers and other more traditional health workers from one of skepticism and suspicion to welcome and professional acceptance. This trend continued, and in 1951 two organizations, the Society of Public Health Educators and the International Union for Health Education of the Public, were formed.

As time passed, the philosophy, objectives, and methods of health education underwent significant change. This has been summarized by Rosen[4] as follows:

It has been recognized that it is not enough simply to present information; what counts is whether and how this knowledge is applied. Furthermore, it has been realized that the community is an organized structure, and that in health education, as in other health work, a coordinated program is needed that will touch each segment of the community in accordance with its nature and its needs. Finally, it is accepted in principle that when the members of a community have a chance to learn about their health problems and how they might deal with them, they will do so, but this was obscured during the early decades of the century by an excessive emphasis on tools and techniques.

## NEEDS IN HEALTH EDUCATION

It is paradoxical that despite extensive advances in literacy and education as well as vastly improved methods of communication, there still exists a great gap between existing medical and health protective knowledge and the public's acceptance and use of it. Professional journals are replete with reports of surveys of schoolchildren, college students, and the adult public that present discouraging and embarrassing evidence of failure in this field.

Many parents still do not obtain immunization for their children, and many drivers still invite injury and death by drinking and driving and by not using seat belts. The use of cigarettes and patent medicines is still widespread. One of the handicaps of public health work, of course, is the usual absence of pain and urgency (except when an epidemic occurs). Indeed, this is becoming even more true as the public health profession progresses from attacks on communicable diseases to an attempted control of chronic illnesses. There is little difficulty in motivating to prompt action an individual with a high fever from typhoid or a severe abdominal pain from acute appendicitis. To bring about a change in dietary or behavioral habits or to secure health maintenance examinations against possible future difficulty is something else. Results are less dramatic or rapid; cause and effect are less readily apparent.

The clearly evident inadequacy and ineffectiveness of health education up to the present obviously calls for considerable evaluation and experimentation. Steps in this direction are already under way by the Society of Public Health Educators and the Public Health Education Section and the School Health Section of the American Public Health Association. The American School Health Association is similarly concerned, and it is hoped that this will become true of the National Education Association. Skillfully developed and properly used, health education can become a powerful force in social improvement and change. Its ultimate goal, of course, should be to encourage and assist the public in taking individual and group actions to protect and improve its own health.

Several reasons have been put forward to explain the inadequacies of health education at the present time. A practical starting point is consideration of Swinehart's[5] observation that "Information presented through the channels commonly used by public health and voluntary associations is fairly easy for most potential audiences to avoid, since these audiences are not 'captive.' Even if they are exposed to communication, there is no guarantee that this will lead to learning and action." So in the field of health education public health workers begin the game with two psychologic strikes against them.

In more detail a committee of the New York Academy of Medicine presented the following points to consider[6]:

1. It is easier to sell symptomatic relief of illness or the promise of a cure than it is to sell health and prevention of disease.

2. Education is a catchall—a ready solution and means of disposition but one that is all too seldom put into action. Whenever there is a problem in a community, someone is sure to say, "The answer is education." And usually, that is where the problem rests.

3. Health education does not have high prestige. In the schools it is treated as a subordinate subject or as an additional chore to be passed out to a teacher whose main interest is not too remotely related. It is frequently made the responsibility of an athletic coach or physical training teacher.

4. In general, the people charged with health education programs lack special training and are not qualified.

5. Departments of education and health do not work together in programming, planning curricula, and raising standards of teaching health in the schools.

6. There is a lack of overall organization in the field of health education with a unified program and a single-minded objective. An effective and dynamic program of health education must include: intercommunication of ideas, selection of priorities, formulation of program, and assignment of responsibility. As matters stand now, there is a great deal of shifting of responsibility from school to home to church to community organization.

Beyond this it is self-evident that health education has been regarded too much in the past as private preserve by the professionals in public health, medicine, and education; to be perfectly honest they have tended to be stuffy, overly didactic, and lacking in understanding of what really worries the average and less educated components of the population. This was forcefully brought out by an official of one of the most successful public relations and advertising companies in America in an address to a public health conference that he entitled "Public Health is no Private Preserve (or things I never knew 'till now, no thanks to you)." This unusually well-educated man stated, "I was asked by your chairman to talk about selling public health. I, like most people, know very little about public health. I have no ready answers for your problems. I'm not even sure I understand the problems themselves. But I do know this: You are not communicating—you are not getting through to people. . . . I am amazed at the amount of effort, time, and money needed to safeguard my health and that of my family . . . yet the average citizen has no awareness of your efforts and actually impedes your work through ignorance."[7] The same concerns have also been voiced from within public health itself. Lifson[8] warns, "Health education is one of the subjects which sometimes has come under attack as a 'frill.'" Hoff[9] emphasizes the preconceived and rigid attitudes and interpretations of public health workers as a major obstacle.

Concern over the foregoing reached a national focus in 1971, when a presidential Committee on Health Education was established to study the nature of the problem and what might be done toward improvement. After a 14-month nationwide study the committee concluded that health education in America was "a neglected, underfinanced, unhealthily fragmented activity," and "School health programs for 60 million American children are in disarray, and are scheduled for rainy days when children have nothing else to do." The committee director, Victor Weingarten, president of the Institute of Public Affairs pointed out that of the $75 billion spent on "health" in the United States during 1971, about 92% was spent after illness occurred and only 0.5% was spent on health education. And most of that, he complained, went into "packaged information" that is irrelevant and ineffective.[10]

Three conclusions appear obvious: (1) personal and community health education are fundamental to any public health advancement; (2) significant improvements are necessary in the field of personal and community health education; and (3) the major fault and challenge rests with the schools, health agencies, and the health professions, and far better joint planning and coordination of their efforts are necessary before the current inadequate record is improved.

## SCOPE OF HEALTH EDUCATION

The content and methodology of health education is peculiarly difficult to define. Many have tried, but it can be fairly said that all attempts seem to have something lacking or unstated. One problem is the variety of interpretations of intent and purpose of the field. Necessarily related to this are the different ways in which health educators are used by health officers and others to whom health educators report and on whom they must depend for guidance and support. Still another problem is the variety of knowledge and techniques a competent health educator must have in his armamentarium—pedagogy, public health, public relations, journalism, social science, and visual aids, to mention only some.

One of the best known and still most applicable definitions of health education is one of the earliest. In 1926 Wood[11] described health education as the "sum of experiences which favorably influence habits, attitudes, and knowledge relating to individual, community, and racial health." The term *health education,* or what might better be regarded as the selling of sound health understanding and behavior,* usually gives consideration to at least five phases or types of activities: analysis, sensitization, publicity, education, and motivation. They are in no sense mutually exclusive but tend to be sequential, overlap generously, and be dependent on each other. The first, *analysis,* is of course fundamental. It involves a study of the problems of an area or a group, the factors that generated the problems and tend to maintain them, and the characteristics of the individuals or groups that may contribute to or hinder the application of sound knowledge or techniques toward the solution of the problems.

The next phase is *sensitization.* Here the intent or expected result is not an addition to health knowledge per se or an evident change in the health habits of a person or a community; rather, it is a process by which the individual and the community are made aware of the existence of certain things: a health department, a disease, a service. Sensitizing procedures such as slogans, spot announcements on radio or television, billboards, and the like are not expected to give the public more knowledge about a subject or to make them do something they otherwise might not do. The best examples are found in commercial advertising, where a manufacturer merely attempts to make potential customers aware of the existence of his product in competition with those of other manufacturers. He may accomplish this by bombarding the public's eyes and ears, and in some recent instances even the olfactory sense, with simple reminders of his product. The techniques used are manifold and include everything from repetitive spot radio announcements urging one to eat "Oaties," to sky writing, huge billboards, and even the perfuming of newspaper advertisements. In doing this the manufacturer and his advertising agent do not expect the public to rush to the nearest

---

*The reader is referred to a charming essay, "The Pebble in the Bell," which deals with the application of advertising to health.[12]

store to purchase his product. What he does hope for is that when those who comprise the public are in a situation that requires them to make an immediate decision, "Shall I buy or not?" or "Shall I buy this brand or that?" they will choose the product the name of which is now familiar as a result of an almost subconscious sensitizing process. Therefore when a health department by any of the audiovisual methods asks, "Is your baby protected against diphtheria?" or states, "Diphtheria kills children," it is merely sensitizing the listeners or readers so that they will be receptive to subsequent more detailed information.

On thing is certain—people cannot be sensitized by the term *health education*. The term is not well understood by professionals, much less by laymen. The concept must be made meaningful by relating it to readily recognized problems and services that are already known to be practical and useful to the individual or the community.[13]

The third phase of health education is *publicity*. This is closely related to the foregoing and, like it, is of considerable importance in the public relations program of the organization. In one sense, publicity might be considered an elaboration of sensitizing procedures, presenting more details about the items mentioned in the simple concise statements or exhortations. Examples of activities that might be included in this category are press releases that relate to the program of the health department, announcements of clinics available for various purposes, and statements about the seriousness of certain conditions in the community.

The fourth phase of health education is *education* in the more literal sense. In the final analysis this is really accomplished only in a rather intimate manner and involves personal contact between the one who imparts the information and those who receive it. It must be realized that education in health or in anything else is never something given by one person to another. The mere act of presenting information and knowledge accomplishes nothing. To use an extreme example, a gibbon might be exposed to the constant expostulations of the world's greatest philosophers, but it is doubtful that he would learn anything, simply because of inability to absorb and interpret the sounds he hears. For a large segment of the human race the word inability may well be changed to unwillingness. In other words learning takes place only through the efforts of the learner. To impart

information to increase the knowledge of others or to change concepts, personal discussions carried out in terms familiar to the listener and related to his personality and circumstances are required. Derryberry[14] has described a demonstration of the truth of this in the experience of the United States Government in selling war bonds: "The most extensive use possible was made of all known information media, including news articles, billboards, radio, exhibits, pamphlets, motion pictures, etc., in an effort to induce people to buy bonds, not only for financing the war but also for curbing inflation. When final tabulation was made, it was found that over 80% of individual purchases were made on personal solicitation, which shows the need for intimate and personal contact in order to induce overt action in a large proportion of the population."

A similar experience was observed in Detroit some years ago in connection with a program to control tuberculosis. Unusual publicity facilities were placed at the disposal of the health department. For weeks, generous front-page space and occasionally even headlines were made freely available for the purpose. News stories were written by one of the country's outstanding popular writers. Free radio time was provided for the presentation of excellent dramas, professionally prepared, produced, and enacted. The city was exposed to a profusion of posters, streetcar advertisements, pamphlets, and similar material. A significant special appropriation made possible the employment of a large number of additional public health nurses to engage primarily in home visits for the promotion of examinations for tuberculosis. After all this had gone on for a while a study was conducted of those who responded to determine which approach prompted them to go to their physician or to a clinic for an examination. Despite the almost ideal publicity methods, it was found that the visits of the public health nurses and the back-fence discussions between neighbors accounted for most of the positive responses. More recently Gordon[15] made the same observation in a comparative study of various communications media in health projects in Baltimore.

The fifth or final phase of health education is concerned with *motivation*. The mere transmission of information or knowledge, even if it is accepted, is not enough, since in itself it does not necessarily imply action or a change in habit or conduct. Among those who die each year from preventable diseases are many who have been exposed to much publicity relating to them and have even acquired considerable knowledge about them. Only a fraction of the parents of children who needlessly acquire and even die from communicable disease are either ignorant of the availability of protective measures or opposed to them. In other words the acquisition of knowledge in itself is not an accomplishment; it is the extent to which that knowledge is translated into action that makes the difference. A note of caution is indicated with reference to motivation. It must be used cautiously or it might "backfire." An example was an intensive drug education program in a junior high school which apparently so stimulated curiosity that there resulted a sharp increase in the use of drugs.[16]

Various aspects of motivation are discussed in Chapter 5. It is well recognized that to motivate people to use health knowledge it must be presented to them in a manner comprehensible and acceptable to them. It should take into consideration their basic emotional needs and wants, their cultural attitudes, beliefs, and prejudices, their fears, ambitions, jealousies, determinations, pride, malice, or any combination of these.[17] Rosenstock and colleagues[18] have summarized the problem well: "It is known that human behavior is determined more by one's belief about reality than by reality itself, and that people vary markedly in their interpretations of reality." As a consequence, it has been pointed out that effective health education can be achieved only by linking what is taught to the endogenous motivation of the individual or group addressed. Kost[19] points to the success of the advertising industry, which long ago found that one cannot reach everyone with the same message, so it selects specific audiences and talks in their terms to their interests. In the health field he says that if public health workers have a message for a certain group, they should write and promote the message for that group. If it is a low socioeconomic group with a low level of education, they should couch the message in terms different from those for a middle class, suburban population. The trouble, he adds, is that "those who would be heard also must be willing to listen. In public health, we haven't been listening enough. Only by listening can you find out what is important to the people you are trying to reach." Whitehorn,[20] in seeking a working concept of human nature, has listed a basic set of motiva-

tional emotional needs and satisfactions that may be useful: (1) the desire for affection, (2) the desire for emotional security and trust, and (3) the desire for personal significance. He believes that since these sources of motivation are endogenous or arise from within, education efforts based on them are more likely to strike a responsive chord and bring forth understanding and action.

In an interesting study of commercial advertising as a health education technique, inquiry was made with regard to the use of patent medicines. Of those interviewed, 60% said they used products of this nature before calling a physician. Although the majority recognized that the claims for the products were not substantiated, the investigation indicated that the patent medicines resorted to most frequently were those for which the advertising played on emotions (especially fear), vanity, and desire for personal gain and those which promised or implied unequivocal cure and relief. It is because of the foregoing considerations that the health educator is often referred to as a "catalyst," one of whose chief functions is the provision of learning situations, preferably based on an understanding and adroit use of community organization.

On the other hand, health educators and others in the health field should not be too ready to condemn the various "nonprofessionals" who provide question-and-answer columns in newspapers, in magazines, or on radio or television. Neither should the public be criticized for contacting them. The mere fact that they do gives reason for professional introspection, and their advice and counsel is not necessarily bad. As Hemming[21] has pointed out in relation to the "Agony Aunties" in the British press, they apparently provide some commodities, such as reassurance and courage, that we "professionals" so often ignore.

## PERSONNEL IN HEALTH EDUCATION

Everyone involved in or concerned with health in any way is a health educator. A long list of such persons could be developed. The most important, however, are all of the members of the health department staff, private practitioners of medicine, dentistry, and nursing, teachers, the personnel of many voluntary and community organizations, and last but not least, parents. These are the people who in effect are on the "firing line" of health education. It is they who in their daily person-to-person contacts are responsible for the actual transmission of knowledge relating to health. In addition, as has been indicated in the section on the development of health education, in recent years there has developed a specialized worker, the health educator, who is trained to act as a combined stimulator, catalyst, correlator, co-ordinator, implementor, extender, and resource person for all of the potential abilities and activities of the entire staff of the health agency.[22] Beginning in 1943, training programs were set up in several of the schools of public health to provide training for this new type of personnel. Graduates of these curricula have been found increasingly useful by official and voluntary health agencies on all levels and in school health programs. Both the present actual and the potential demand for this new professional group is great, and it would appear that within a remarkably short period of time they have carved a definite niche for themselves in the health programs of the communities and states of the nation.

## FUNCTIONS IN HEALTH EDUCATION

As in all other phases of the public health program, the functions in health education vary in the different levels of government. In its 1957 *Report on Educational Qualifications and Functions of Health Educators*[23] the Committee on Professional Education of the American Public Health Association listed the functions of the health educator on the community level in the following categories:

A. Program planning and evaluation
  1. Study, survey, and research in assessing health education needs and possibilities
  2. Analysis of present knowledge, interests, beliefs, and practices of the people in terms of aids or barriers to the educational process
B. Organization and promotion of health education activities
  1. Development of groups for health action
  2. Assistance in establishing and maintaining close cooperative working relationships between those agencies and groups of citizens which contribute to the health education of the public; in this the public health educator often serves as a liaison person among public, civic, professional, official, and voluntary organizations
  3. Assistance in planning preservice education for public health, school, or other personnel
  4. Stimulation, organization, or guidance of in-service education for employed personnel in health departments, schools, or other agencies
  5. Provision of technical assistance and service as a resource person in the development and guidance of health education programs in schools, parent-teacher associations, clubs, adult education services, extension services, study groups, and libraries
  6. Assistance in interpreting the value of health activities to the community in the development of community interest and support
  7. Leadership in the use of various educational teaching or group work procedures as applied to public health activities
C. Extension of health education through communication
  1. Development, preparation, and use of mass media of communication
  2. Establishment of health library facilities
  3. Organization of a speaker's bureau, conferences, and meetings
  4. Organization and operation of an information service

Functions in health education on the state level, by virtue of removal from the immediate scene of action, are similar in purpose and design to those of many other activities of a state health department. Derryberry[14] suggested the following functions and activities in which a division of health education in a state health department might engage, depending on the size of the state, its resources, the extent of its coverage with local health units, and the presence or absence of trained health educators in local areas:

  1. Planning, developing, and administering a statewide program in public health education
  2. Encouraging and promoting the development of programs in local health departments, utilizing trained personnel who are capable of working in all phases of the public health program and are also sufficiently competent in education to work with the schools

3. Recruiting personnel and arranging for their training and assignment
4. Assisting the medical, nursing, and sanitation personnel in their educational work by providing them with an educational mechanism and advice on effective techniques of education in various local situations
5. Consulting with local health departments and local health educators on all matters pertaining to health education
6. Maintaining relations with the press and the public, preparing articles and approving special stories and speeches by department personnel
7. Preparing or securing public health education material and distributing it through useful channels
8. Correlating the educational endeavors of the divisions or bureaus in the state health department
9. Coordinating the activities of all agencies in the state interested in health education
10. Developing and maintaining a continuing in-service program of training for public health personnel
11. Evaluating continually the materials and methods being used both in the state and in the local departments

Health education on the federal level has been a particular interest of the Public Health Service. Necessarily its attention is focused on the national approach to problems and situations and the encouragement of the state, and through them, local health agencies in activities in this field. Coffey[24] presented the following particular responsibilities of the Public Health Service in health education:

1. To focus attention on health problems of national scope as they arise
2. To give consultation service and assistance in program planning and execution and in the preparation of materials when such assistance is requested
3. To stimulate the training of personnel and hold high the standards for their training and accomplishment
4. To serve as a clearinghouse for new ideas, methods, and materials
5. To summarize new developments in science and show its applicability to the subject matter of health education
6. To prepare high quality materials that have national application
7. To conduct an information service for the many inquiries received

8. To conduct research on methods and materials of health education and evaluate programs with the purpose of making all our efforts more effective

It has been observed[25] that in more recent years public health educators are more involved in programs that require joint planning and action with other people and agencies as well as in community organization and interpersonal communication as a whole. Fewer health educators are devoting their own time and energy to school health activities and mass media.

It is not the purpose of this book to discuss the many and various techniques in health education. Attention is called, however, to Chapter 14, which deals with public relations, much of which has a direct bearing on the subject of the moment. A few additional words are indicated to emphasize several general considerations. The term *community organization* is one of the most commonly encountered at the present time, especially in connection with health education programs. Its exact meaning often appears elusive to many. Perhaps the simplest manner of restating it would be to say, "Find out everything you can about your community, its inhabitants, interests, prejudices, facilities, subdivisions, and the like, and proceed to work through them." The first prerequisite to a sound health education program, and therefore a sound public health program, is a thoroughgoing community survey, diagnosis, or analysis. Every organized group and every influential person or agency must be noted with their particular interests and potentialities. They must be approached insofar as they represent segments of the population. The method of approach must be carefully considered.

One of the easiest mistakes that may be made is to speak a language foreign to that of one's listeners. Too many long, technical, and complicated words and phrases may be used. Public health workers have been taken severely to task in this respect.[26] One editorial statement is especially worthy of repetition and should be heeded by everyone who works in this field: "The use of jargon becomes a bad habit with public health workers. They come to depend upon it to confuse and mystify the public and to help create a favorable impression of their work. . . . But perhaps the main reason that public health workers use jargon is that it makes them feel important. It impresses the public and it adds to their own feeling of well-being to hear the long and musical words rolling from their lips. After all, it takes a pretty smart fellow to be able just to make the sounds, to say nothing of knowing what they mean and less of knowing how to translate them into appropriate and effective action."[27]

## SCHOOL AND HEALTH DEPARTMENT RELATIONS

The school represents a most important learning situation for a large and significant group of the population. What is learned by a child tends to have a deep and lasting influence on his happiness, opinions, and behavior throughout his life. The child is reached and influenced primarily through two channels, his parents and his teachers. Unfortunately the influence of some parents, chiefly because of limitations in their childhood, is not always of the best. As a result, the importance of the teacher in the development of desirable health knowledge and practices is doubly magnified and serves to emphasize the importance of teacher training in health and the maintenance of the personal well-being of those in this important relationship to children.

It has been pointed out[28] that the schools contain all of tomorrow's "public" and affect most of today's. However, the national School Health Education Study of the late 1960s, like the subsequent President's Committee on Health Education, concluded that in most communities the next generation will be little better equipped to separate the basic facts concerning health and disease from the vast amount of misinformation that troubles the present generation. These considerations prompted the School Health Section of the American Public Health Association in 1967 to reaffirm that not only is school health education a logical adjunct of a comprehensive community health program but one of high priority.

A certain amount of misunderstanding and self-defeating competition sometimes develops between public health agencies and departments of education from their mutual interest in the development of health knowledge and instruction of children. It is strongly believed that no real cause for conflict exists. In some areas both the health department and the school department reach for the school health education program with attitudes of equal proprietorship. The fact is that it belongs to both of them or, more correctly, that both belong to it. Each organization has its place and its function. The

personnel of health departments must always remember that teaching is a professional specialty in itself and that in the final analysis it is the classroom teacher who does the teaching of the children. On the other hand, school personnel should bear in mind that the school health program and its educational component are merely parts of the larger total community health program. This does not necessarily imply a right for the official health department to usurp the activities of the schools in this field any more than this overall responsibility and concern entitles the health department to take over the private practice of medicine or the management of food industries. The need is obvious. What is indicated is the coordination, in friendly, professional, and cooperative terms, of the contributions and abilities of those interested in health education, whether employed in a health agency, a school system, or elsewhere. The important fact to consider at this point in time is that the job that needs to be done is great, that neither group alone can accomplish it, and that neither group has been very successful so far. The conclusion is clear—greater resources, much better joint planning, and truly coordinated action.

Many communities employ a person referred to as a school health coordinator. Usually this person is on the staff of the school system, occasionally on the staff of health departments and sometimes employed jointly. There is an increasing tendency to require that they obtain training in a school of public health. Such professional persons in company with the health educator of the health department may accomplish wonders in the improvement of the program. Similar trends are observable on the state and federal levels, where joint planning committees and interagency consultations are frequent.

## ORGANIZATION OF ACTIVITIES FOR HEALTH EDUCATION

Within public health departments the organization of activities for health education poses problems similar to those arising in relation to public health statistics. Although each functional unit of the agency should be engaged in health education to some degree, there are certain overall aspects of the field that must be treated in a more central manner. The questions arise therefore concerning whether the work should be completely centralized in one health education unit and whether such a unit should be a line or a staff agency. Every possible variation may be observed both in state and local health departments. Centralized health education units are organized sometimes as a separate line unit and sometimes as a staff agency in close proximity to the health officer. Not infrequently, on the other hand, all activities for health education are completely decentralized and dispersed throughout the various parts of the organization. Beyond these are numerous illogical arrangements, usually arising from expediency, wherein health education is placed in a division of vital statistics, of maternal and child health, or of communicable disease control. This has little to recommend it, since it usually results in provincialization of the service.

Certain general conclusions may be drawn. It would seem manifestly impossible to centralize completely the activities for health education. Even if this could be accomplished, the rest of the health department would lose the major part of its effectiveness. Therefore the functional units, augmented and supported by a central unit of health education staffed by specialists in that field should be encouraged to engage freely in these activities. These persons, among other ways, should function as consultants and advisors to the line divisions of the agency. It would probably be best, in most circumstances, for the central health education unit to be a staff unit closely associated with the administrator, with whom overall community planning and programming may be effected.

Much of what has been presented in this chapter may appear derogatory to those directly involved in health education. If so, it has not been intended as such. There is no question of the fundamental, even critical importance of this field. The problem is the essential nature of human nature. Health educators are confronted by a group of formidable obstacles,—so formidable that it is unrealistic to expect ready success. But obstacles are also challenges, and without challenges there can develop no grounds for some measures of satisfaction. When the Society of Public Health Educators met in 1971, it issued a statement that in its expanded horizon should give additional insight and courage to all in its profession:

Health education's effect on the quality of life can be broadened through political and social interventions as well as through the educational process, through interaction with consumers of all backgrounds—including labor and political office holders—and through a deeper understanding and sensitivity to the determinants of the quality of life.

In commenting on this, Dallas[29] noted three common threads that health educators would do well to bear in mind:

1. Quality of life implies choice—knowledge of all the available options, freedom to choose any option, and an understanding of the effects once a choice has been made.

2. Quality of life implies increased individual responsibility for health.

3. Quality of life implies the development of new skills and roles for health educators as well as the full use of existing strategies.

## REFERENCES

1. Roberts, B. J., Grossman, J., and Griffith, W.: The public health educator's bookshelf, Amer. J. Public Health **53:**531, April 1963.
2. Report of the Maryland State Board of Health, 1875. (Courtesy Clemens W. Gaines, Executive Office, 1965.)
3. Rosen, G.: A history of public health, New York, 1958, MD Publications.
4. Rosen, G.: Evolving trends in health education, Canad. J. Public Health **52:**499, Dec. 1961.
5. Swinehart, J. W.: Voluntary exposure to health communications, Amer. J. Public Health **58:**1265, July 1968.
6. Health education: its present status; Report by the Committee on Public Health, New York Academy of Medicine, Bull. N. Y. Acad. Med. **41:**1172, Nov. 1965.
7. Anderson, R. E.: Public health is no private preserve (or things I never knew 'till now, no thanks to you), Mich. Health, May-June, 1965.
8. Lifson, S. S.: What's wrong with health education in the schools? Nat. Tuberc. Ass. Bull. p. 12, Dec. 1965.
9. Hoff, W.: Why health programs are not reaching the unresponsive in our communities, Public Health Rep. **81:**654, July 1966.
10. U. S. Department of Health, Education, and Welfare: Report of the President's Committee on Health Education, Washington, D. C., 1973, Government Printing Office.
11. Wood, T. D.: In fourth yearbook of the Department of Superintendent of the National Education Association, Washington, D. C., 1926, National Education Association.
12. Marti-Ibanez, F.: The pebble in the bell, MD **15:** 13, July 1971.
13. Conant, R. K., DeLuca A. J., and Levin, L. S.: Health education—a bridge to the community, Amer. J. Public Health **62:**1239 Sept. 1972.
14. Derryberry, M.: The role of health education in a public health program, Public Health Rep. **62:** 1633, Nov. 1947.

15. Gorden, J.: Evaluation of communications media in two health projects in Baltimore, Public Health Rep. **82:**651, July 1967.
16. Amer. Med. News, Dec. 11, 1972.
17. Bauer, W. W.: What is health education? Amer. J. Public Health **37:**641, June 1947.
18. Rosenstock, I. M., Derryberry, M., and Carriger, B. K.: Why people fail to seek poliomyelitis vaccination, Public Health Rep. **74:**98, Feb. 1959.
19. Kost, K.: A communicator talks back, Environ. News Digest, Nov.-Dec. 1970.
20. Whitehorn, J. C.: Motivating pattern of the normal individual. In Psychological dynamics of health education, New York, 1951, Columbia University Press.
21. Hemming, J.: Agony Aunties and their contribution to health education, Roy. Soc. Health J. **5:**246, May 1972.
22. Education for healthier living, currents in public health, Ross Laboratories, vol. 2, no. 7, July-Aug. 1962.

23. Committee on Professional Education: Educational qualifications and functions of health educators, Amer. J. Public Health **47:**114, Jan. 1957.
24. Coffey, E. R.: Planning for health education in war and post-war periods—the national program, Public Health Rep. **59:**904, July 1944.
25. Bowman, R. A., Bowman, V. A., and Roccella, E. J.: Comparison of duties and responsibilities of public health educators, 1957 and 1969, HSMHA Health Rep. **86:**551, June 1971.
26. Bross, I.: Prisoners of jargon, Amer. J. Public Health **54:**918, June 1964.
27. Editorial: By his tongue shall ye know him, Amer. J. Public Health **38:**264, Feb. 1948.
28. Editorial: School health education; a public health concern Amer. J. Public Health **57:**2061, Dec. 1967.
29. Dallas, J. L.: Health education: enabler for a higher quality of life, Health Services Rep. **87:**910, Dec. 1972.

CHAPTER 39

# Vital statistics

## THE IMPORTANCE OF DATA

Vital statistics, the bookkeeping of public health, is an essential activity of every public health agency on every level of government. Not only is it a legal responsibility of health agencies but it also provides the foundation on which all other parts of the public health program are constructed. It is impossible to imagine a sound program of maternal and child health, communicable disease control, environmental health, or even laboratory services in the absence of this invaluable adjunct. Its influence, if properly used, permeates every part of the organization. At one point it determines what visits should be made by staff nurses or sanitarians; at another it assists in deciding matters of policy for the top administrator.[1]

When satisfactorily organized and conducted, the vital statistics office may serve literally as the brain center, continually giving answers to "What is the score?" and "What next?" Its constituent parts taken in toto present the composite life history of a community, state, or nation. It is the storehouse of indispensable information that reflects the strengths and foibles, successes and failures, joys and sorrows of the group. It is the key that opens the door to a competent, sound, and efficient community health administration. The applications of statistics in public health have been summarized to include (1) population estimation and prediction, (2) surveys of population characteristics, health needs, and problems, (3) analysis of health trends, (4) epidemiologic research, (5) treatment and program evalua-

tion, (6) program planning, (7) budget preparation and justification, (8) operational and administrative decision making, and (9) health education.[2]

It is difficult, if not impossible, for a public health worker to be either successful or satisfied without an intelligent and sympathetic appreciation of the vital data of the area he serves. Unfortunately too many regard this activity as a chore or necessary evil to be delegated to a few inadequately trained clerks working in an out-of-the-way office. It should be realized that although the real material of statistics may appear to be scraps of paper containing crooked little integers, each represents a human interest story that with its fellows leads to a critically important end product—a philosophic plan for the alleviation of human misery and the attainment of health for all.

## ORIGINS OF VITAL STATISTICS

The compilation of vital statistics is of ancient origin. Enumerations of people were carried out long before the birth of Christ, notably in China, Egypt, Persia, Greece, and Rome, primarily for purposes of taxation and to determine the military manpower. Data relating to births, deaths, and marriages were recorded in elementary form in the old church registers of England. The oldest known copy of these so-called "Bills of Mortality" can be seen in the British Museum and is dated November 1532. These bills were compiled by parish priests and clerks for more than a century before John Graunt in 1662 published his book *Natural*

**680**

*and Political Observations Mentioned in a Following Index and Made Upon the Bills of Mortality.* Vital statistics in the modern sense can be considered to have originated from the publication of this book.

The late eighteenth century saw the beginning of the modern national census. Priority is somewhat open to question. The outstanding claims are Canada, 1666; Sweden, 1749; and England and the United States, 1790. Regardless of the earliest claim, it may be stated that the United States Census had a significant influence on the spread of the idea throughout the rest of the world. The institution of a national census in the United States has, with good reason, been called a political accident, since the provision for the decennial enumeration arose from the conflict between the small and large states. The former demanded equal representation in the national legislature, whereas the latter considered that their larger populations justified more power.

The compromise solution was to establish a bicameral legislature consisting of the Senate, in which states were equally represented, and the House of Representatives, with representation in proportion to population. This compromise solution made necessary some provision for the periodic inventory of the population. As a result, the following was included in the Constitution: "Representatives shall be apportioned among the several States according to their respective numbers, counting the whole number of persons in each State, excluding Indians not taxed. The actual enumeration shall be made within three years after the first meeting of the Congress of the United States, and within every subsequent term of ten years, in such manner as they shall by law direct."*

It should be noted that all which was required was a simple count. From this basic purpose and requirement there has developed a national census of great complexity and detail that provides data of value far beyond what was envisioned by the framers of the Constitution. Similarly the value and use of vital data in general now extends far beyond what was initially visualized. Few parts of the nation's social, political, economic, and industrial systems could possibly operate without it.[3]

It is significant that the collection and analysis of vital statistics or more specifically

*Article I, Section 2, Paragraph 3, modified by the Fourteenth Amendment.

public health statistics has always been considered one of the basic functions in public health. With substantial reason it may be stated that all of the other functions depend essentially on the adequate fulfillment of this primary function for their success. Statistics have come to be regarded as an indispensable administrative tool for the proper planning, performance, and evaluation of any modern business or public program. Certainly it is inconceivable that intelligent or meaningful public health programs could be planned, implemented, monitored, and evaluated without a reasonably solid vital data base. It is fundamental to all aspects of public health.[4]

## SOURCES OF PUBLIC HEALTH STATISTICS

Woolsey and Lawrence,[5] regarding health statistics broadly, list five basic types of data necessary to a sound attack on health problems of a community: (1) counts of people, (2) measures of their health, (3) health services received, (4) health resources of manpower and facilities, and (5) the state of the environment. Would that all statisticians shared this breadth of viewpoint!

The most fundamental information on which activities in public health must be predicated is a knowledge of the quantitative and qualitative characteristics of the population to be served. This implies some form of a count or estimate of the people within a jurisdiction. On the surface it would appear that the decennial census, to which reference has been made, would supply whatever data are necessary. This was the case in the more stable or immobile societies that preceded the era of paved highways, rapid transportation, and industrialization. Reasonably adequate intercensal populations could be estimated by means of rather simple arithmetic or geometric projections. The situation was changed drastically, however, as a result of World War II. In 1940 an extremely detailed census had been carried out. However, within little more than a year the nation became engaged in an international conflict of great magnitude that required the enlistment and draft of several millions of citizens. In addition, new and old industries underwent spectacular expansion, necessitating the movement of additional millions of persons to serve them. Many communities within a short space of time found their populations doubled or trebled, whereas others were noticeably depleted. It soon became evident that neither the 1940 census data, which by this time had been released, nor any estimates based on them could serve much useful purpose.

Many attempts were made to find suitable substitutes in the form of school attendance records, work records, or food ration card applications. Of the group, the latter was probably the most useful during the World War II years. Social Security registration provided some additional measure of the population, with the handicaps, however, of not including children and certain groups of the employable and not giving an indication of population movement. It was hoped that the confused situation would be temporary, but soon statisticians, economists, and public health workers were convinced that the national mode of life had been so deeply affected as to require some new form of population determination and analysis. During the same period of time, a new business and social study technique, the sample survey or poll, came on the scene and began to serve a valuable purpose in the health and other fields.[6] These surveys and the National Health Survey, which was subsequently developed, came to play an extremely important role, especially during intercensal years and to obtain answers to special questions.

Next in importance to the population base are data obtained from administrative registration and reporting procedures. Responsibility for this function in the United States rests with the respective states. The most significant of these activities relate to the vital events of birth, death, and morbidity. Again, so that these data may be of value in the planning of public health programs, there must be some assurance of their qualitative and quantitative dependability. This need led to the establishment of birth and death registration areas by the Bureau of the Census. The death registration area was organized in 1900 and included the states of Connecticut, Indiana, Maine, Massachusetts, Michigan, New Hampshire, New Jersey, New York, Rhode Island, Vermont, and the District of Columbia. At that time these areas contained about 40% of the total population of the United States. The birth registration area was established in 1915 and included originally Connecticut, Maine, Massachusetts, Michigan, Minnesota, New Hampshire, New York, Pennsylvania, Rhode Island, Vermont, and the District of Columbia, accounting for 31% of the total population. By 1933 all states had become members of both the birth and the death regis-

tration areas. Membership is based on two criteria: satisfactory state registration laws and at least 90% completeness in reporting.

## ACCURACY OF VITAL DATA

Certain limitations are found in relation to the value of birth and death reports. The most obvious is the fact that as yet some of these events may be unrecorded. This has become relatively unimportant in recent years. An analysis in 1950 by the Bureau of the Census indicated that after 35 years of birth registration 97.8% completeness had been achieved, although it was then estimated that each year in the United States about 50,000 babies were born who were not registered. Much of this discrepancy, however, was remedied by late registration when individuals enter school, the Armed Forces, or apply for a Social Security number in the process of employment. Other problems are related to the inadequate reporting of stillbirths and babies born out of wedlock. These problems have been essentially eliminated by almost all deliveries occurring in hospitals and by changed attitudes toward illegitimacy.

Nevertheless, the assurance of prompt and adequate reporting of both live and stillbirths requires constant vigilance on the part of registrars and directors of vital statistical offices. Many different approaches have been used, and it would appear that no one alone is satisfactory. Education of the public, of attendants at birth, and of hospitals must be conducted constantly. In addition to this is the use of many types of checks. Hospital records, baptismal records, and, of much less value, newspaper announcements have been used for this purpose. Probably the most common and accurate check of completeness of birth reporting is that of deaths of infants under 1 year of age. When corrected for residence, this group constitutes a more or less representative sample of the infants born in an area. Other groups that have been used are entering school children in states that require a birth certificate for school attendance, and children attending well-baby or child health clinics. In many states hospitals prepare a birth certificate at the time the prospective mother enters the hospital, complete except for the date of birth, sex, and name of the child. These can be readily added after birth at the time the physician signs the certificate. In addition to producing highly satisfactory results, this procedure has added value in that the certificates are usually typed and therefore are more legible than they otherwise might be.

The problem of reporting illegitimate births has been approached in three different ways by the various states. One is to make mandatory provision for the attendant at birth to file the birth certificate of an illegitimate child directly with the state office of vital statistics rather than to have it pass through the hands of the local registrar. Some believe that this weakens the local registration system and is therefore undesirable. Another approach is the provision that the certificate of an illegitimate child not differ from that of a legitimate child—once the child in question has been adopted or legitimized. An objection to this is the necessity of preparing new certificates. A third and least desirable method is to delete the item of legitimacy entirely. This has been successfully promoted in a few states by welfare agencies and certain other groups. The objection, of course, is that this precludes knowledge concerning the extent of illegitimacy and of the many social and health problems relating to it. It may also give rise to several legal complications.

Two compromises should be mentioned that offer perhaps the best solutions up to the present. Many states have removed the item of legitimacy from the certificate proper and have placed it on a supplementary portion. Perhaps more satisfactory is the policy of a few states of including the item on the certificate but eliminating it on certified copies of the certificate, usually by the general use of an abbreviated copy of the certificate.

One other phase of birth reporting that causes difficulty is delayed registration of births. This problem came to a head during the first half of the 1940s, when a birth certificate, as evidence of citizenship, was required for employment in the large numbers of war industries. Two problems arose. What evidence should be required to support the application for delayed registration of a birth? Should this evidence be reviewed by the registrar or by the courts? The manual on Uniform Procedures for Delayed Registration prepared jointly by the American Association of Registration Executives and the National Center for Health Statistics seems to provide the answers as to the nature of acceptable evidence. Since routine court evaluation is unwieldy, particularly by virtue of the numbers of applications involved, most states now have the evidence reviewed by the state registrar, with recourse to the courts in case of a rejection. This seems to be a satisfactory and advisable pattern.

Because of burial requirements, deaths are reported to a greater degree of completeness than are births. The value of death certificates is impaired, however, not only by some inadequate reporting but also by the subjective nature of much of the data requested on the form. It is still not rare for the cause of a death to be misstated deliberately to circumvent potential social stigma. This occurs not only in relation to suicides and syphilis but also in some degree to tuberculosis, cancer, and some hereditary ailments. Incorrect diagnoses present a constant problem to the vital statistician. Numerous studies have been made regarding the degree of accuracy of the physician's statement of cause of death. The figure varies considerably by time and place. The magnitude of this error is subject to steady reduction by virtue of improved medical education and the development and use of new laboratory and clinical diagnostic techniques. Beyond this the most that can be hoped for at present is that each jurisdiction for its own purposes attempt some estimate of this source of error by means of checking with autopsy reports and by consultations. Even the most conscientious physician is faced with the difficult problem of deciding the primary cause of death as against contributing causes. This problem has been partially solved by the publication and wide adoption of the World Health Organization's International Classification of Diseases, Injuries, and Causes of Death,[7] which presents primary and secondary causal preferences for all possible combinations of diseases.

## REPORTING PROCEDURES

Almost all states and territories place responsibility for vital records management in their state health department, and in the majority of instances the state health officer is designated by law as the state registrar of vital statistics. In all instances actual collection is accomplished through local registrars who receive reports directly from attending physicians, midwives, undertakers, and others. The routing of reports of births and deaths is subject to much variation. In some states certificates are either filed with the county health officers, who transmit them to the state health departments, or are routed by the local registrars through the county health departments. More commonly, local registrars send the certificates directly to their state health departments. In one state the local registrars also send copies to the county health departments for their use. In about one half of the states the two procedures just described are combined. Certificates are forwarded by local registrars directly to the state health departments, except that in counties or districts with full-time local health departments certificates are sent to them for transmission to the state office.

In almost all states, birth and death certificates are forwarded to the state health department once a month. Whatever routing procedure is followed, four basic principles should be adhered to:

1. Certificates should be made promptly by medical or other attendants.

2. There should be a system of routine checking by registrars of all certificates for correctness and completeness.

3. Certificates should be forwarded to the state agency at intervals of not longer than 1 month.

4. Pertinent data on certificates should be made readily and promptly available to local health departments, preferably by means of their acting as intermediaries in the transmission of certificates from local registrars to the state department. If this is not provided for, much of the value of the reporting is lost.

Morbidity reporting presents an extremely difficult problem. Information relating to the incidence of disease in a community is obviously necessary for a public health program of any logical design. On these data depend whatever steps the organization may take in many of its other activities. The incidence of various types of disease points to the extent of hospital, laboratory, and home nursing facilities needed. The prevalence of enteric diseases gives an index of the adequacy of the environmental sanitation and the food and milk control programs. Information concerning disease is one of the most potent items in the armamentarium of the health educator. With increased interest in problems of older citizens, data depicting their illnesses are fundamental to the crystallization of a program for their benefit.

Completeness of morbidity reporting is subject to great variation, depending on the state laws and local regulations, the presence or absence and adequacy or inadequacy of local health departments, the types and severity of diseases common in the area, the professional and social attitudes of the physicians practicing

in the area, and the customs and economy of the people.

There is considerable variation among the states both in the total number of diseases reportable and in the specific diseases included. Table 21-5 (p. 402) lists the diseases usually considered reportable. Reports of occupational diseases are required in addition in many states. All states require the reporting of conjunctivitis, diphtheria, measles, meningitis, poliomyelitis, scarlet fever, smallpox, syphilis, typhoid fever, tuberculosis, undulant fever, and whooping cough. Similar variation is noted with respect to morbidity reporting methods. Only two requirements are uniform in all the states. First, every state requires that cases of notifiable disease be reported by the attending physician or in the absence of a physician by householder, head of the family, or person in charge of the patient. Second, the reports are to be made to the local health authority. Of the 50 states, 46 use report cards. Seventeen states use the same card for all diseases, 13 states have a special card for tuberculosis, and 29 states have a special card for cases of venereal diseases. Format varies from no regular form (4 states), to single (27 states) and multiple (9 states) case penalty cards, stamped cards (2 states), cards requiring postage (3 states), and forms other than a postcard (4 states).

The usual practice is to route morbidity reports through the local health department to the state health department. Some states require only that copies of daily, weekly, or monthly summaries be sent to the state health department. A few states follow the unreasonable practice of requiring physicians to send reports both to the local and to the state health departments.

## PRACTICAL CONSIDERATIONS

Certain factors must be considered in regard to morbidity reports. Fundamental is the need to prepare and educate those in the community from whom reports are expected to be obtained. The most important of these are private physicians, hospitals, and schools. Two other sources worthy of mention are the dental profession and industry. Too often there is an inclination to require reports of too many diseases and in too much detail, whether or not any practical use can be made of the information. Generally when this is done, physicians and other reporting agencies eventually question the practicality of the request and the use made of it. If they decide that the information is merely received and filed away, they soon become careless in their reporting. In all fairness they can hardly be blamed if no one takes the trouble to explain the purpose of the items requested.

An additional important factor is the amount of work involved in making the report. Busy practitioners are loath to spend much time in writing out details of cases for official agencies. The problem of "red tape" is very real. The average physician practicing in an American community today finds it necessary to have readily available an increasing number of different official and semiofficial report forms that must be filled out for births, deaths, communicable diseases, premarital examinations, medical care, acts of violence, workmen's compensation, veteran's benefits, and insurance examinations, to mention only a few. By now, as Wilson[8] puts it, the components of the health care system groan under the load of information requested and forms required by an ever-increasing number of programs, agencies, and organizations. The least that can be done is to standardize and simplify some of these forms and procedures insofar as possible.

In the case of morbidity reporting, requirements and methods should be reduced to the barest essentials. Thus an increasing number of official health agencies accept reports of cases of communicable diseases in the form of telephone calls or preaddressed postcards, requiring only the diagnosis and the name, age, and address of the person affected. It is significant that the patient's name, address, and age and the name of the disease are the only items common to the morbidity report forms of all of the states. From there on it is the responsibility of the public health personnel to obtain what further details appear necessary for the adequate public health management of the case.

West,[9] in an analysis of the completeness of morbidity reporting, found that whereas physicians were the most important and in some areas almost the only source, in other areas hospitals, schools, visiting nurse associations, industrial plants, health department clinics, staff members, and householders were also valuable reporting sources. Within given areas she found that some diseases, particularly scarlet fever, were reported almost entirely by physicians, whereas other sources were more important for certain other diseases, notably tuberculosis. As a result, she suggested the use of certain indices for the estimation of the level of reporting of various diseases. In the areas studied it was found that for the childhood diseases—chickenpox, diphtheria, German measles, measles, mumps, scarlet fever, and whooping cough—the level of reporting of cases included in the school records furnished useful information as to the completeness of reporting.

For meningococcal meningitis, pneumonia, and poliomyelitis the completeness of reporting of cases in general hospitals provides a useful index. For diseases for which there is available no one source representative of the population at risk, an index representing an upper limit to the completeness of reporting can be obtained by combining the available data in the form:

$$\frac{\text{All reported cases}}{\substack{\text{All reported cases} + \text{Unreported cases from} \\ \text{all relevant sources}}}$$

In the case of rheumatic fever, for instance, no single source was found to be satisfactory. Here an upper limit based on data from hospital, school, and death records provides an index. For tuberculosis an upper limit based on the reporting of cases found in hospital, sanatorium, death certificate, and health department data provides the most useful index.

It is concluded that it is impossible to devise any final or universally applicable index, since such shifting factors as the occurrence of an epidemic or a change in the population will temporarily alter the level of reporting of particular diseases. However, West[9] states, "The need of the local health officer is not for refined figures which could be developed from protracted study, but for approximate figures which will assist him in interpreting and evaluating the morbidity program of his own department and in planning the better utilization of reporting sources."

## MORBIDITY SURVEYS

Since 1925 there have been many proposals for the establishment of a morbidity reporting area similar to the birth and death registration areas. It has been increasingly suggested that public health agencies obtain morbidity data for administrative planning by means of special detailed studies and sample surveys rather than to depend on routine reports that are subject to so many limitations.[10] This approach to the problem has already been put into effect in several instances, notable among which are the Hagerstown studies and more recently the United States National Health Survey.[11] The use that has already been made of the continuing outflow of data collected in these two instances has more than justified their cost, and it points to the need for further application and development of these techniques.

Langmuir[12] has stated the following viewpoint:

The morbidity survey is a particularly useful epidemiological tool in that data on both the sick and the well are obtained concurrently. The problems arising from underreporting of cases, from arbitrary classifications of causes of death, and from unknown shifts of population between census years are largely eliminated. . . . Its unique advantage lies in the detailed information that can be collected about the population. Frequency rates, specific for a wide variety of social and environmental factors, can be determined. Such comparisons are not obtainable by matching routine morbidity reports and death certificates with census figures.

He further points out the interrelationships between the simple survey and the special study:

The simple morbidity survey has one inherent limitation—only general data can be obtained. The questions asked by the interviewers must be simple and understandable to the informants. Few specific diseases can be adequately counted by this method. Special studies are necessary to collect such definitive epidemiological information.

## NATIONAL VITAL DATA

To obtain vital data for the nation as a whole, states routinely transmit the information they obtain to the National Center for Health Statistics in the Public Health Service for collation, analysis, and publication. Numerous useful documents are prepared and made available. Among them are the annual *Vital Statistics of the United States*[13] and the *Morbidity and Mortality Weekly Report,*[14] which present data for the nation as a whole and for each state, including comparisons with the year before and indications of trends. In addition, the weekly report includes descriptions of unusual or particularly important epidemiologic occurrences. The National Center in its turn submits its data and analyses to the World Health Organization for inclusion in the development of the worldwide picture[15,16] and for epidemiologic intelligence purposes.

The confusion and complexity that characterize the present situation with reference to health data have led to the current development of a Cooperative Federal-State-Local Health Statistics System.[17] In time it is hoped that it will encompass the different data collection components—ambulatory and long-term care, health facility, health manpower inventories, health care expenditures, household interview and other survey data, to name a few of the information sources necessary to provide continuing statistical evidence covering the health of the entire population and the entire health industry. A critical challenge in its achievement is the development of record linkages and methods of central recording, processing, storing, analyzing, retrieving, and feedback of information at all levels of the system.[18,19] The importance of doing this has been well described by Acheson[20]:

Today time acts on a different scale. The predominant diseases creep upon us over years or decades, the onset may be insidious and the course prolonged. What matters are the habits of a lifetime. . . . No single record made in one place or at one time can describe the evolution of such diseases. Whether it is required to study the etiology, evaluate the treatment or estimate the prognosis of these conditions, it will be necessary to accumulate information about people over long periods of time. Nevertheless, our [England's] system of public health intelligence remains, in principle, unchanged since 1837. It is organized in terms of events rather than in terms of the persons experiencing those events.

## ADMINISTRATIVE USES OF VITAL STATISTICS

The collection and analysis of public health statistics are at best costly and difficult tasks. The only real justification for performing it is the administrative use to which the resulting information may be put. Reports of vital and of related events, such as the services rendered by the personnel of a health department, constitute important legal records. Their personal value arises in connection with proof of citizenship, the right to attend school, to vote, to marry, to enter the Armed Services, and to draw benefits of many types. Records of births and deaths are of particular significance in the establishment of inheritance rights and in the prevention of capital crime. Not infrequently health department service records play an important role in litigation relating to property use and condemnation.

Of particular importance, however, are the uses to which statistical data may be put in the administration and management of the public health program. For statistical data to be of real value in the public health program, efforts far beyond the strict legal responsibilities imposed upon public health agencies are required. Too often the minimal acts of registration and reporting have been conducted as the sole activity in this field. Registration may be relegated to an untrained clerk who routinely accepts, transcribes, and files the documents after a most cursory examination. This procedure can make statistics nothing but "dead" in the most literal sense. When, on the other hand, all the statistics available to a health department are correlated, they become of fourfold value in that they make possible (1) the definition of the problem, (2) the development of a logical program for its control, (3) the planning of records and procedures for the administration and analysis of the program as it progresses, and (4) the evaluation of the results of the program.

Trauger[21] makes this point emphatically, saying that the ultimate test of any reporting system is "How many important questions does it answer and how well?" If the ultimate test of the system is its power to answer questions, he says that the number of questions is not a valid test. "What is important is whether the system provides (a) solid information rather than merely a basis for estimates of guesses, (b) a basis for perceiving the development or change of trends soon enough to permit administrative reaction, and (c) output sufficiently selective to answer the most important questions without overwhelming the potential user or the person who compiles the report." With specific reference to disease reports Kraus[2] also urges the deemphasis of the "fishing expedition" or "shotgun" approach to epidemiologic investigation. Rather, he recommends the development of specific hypotheses regarding causative and preventive factors through consideration of clinical knowledge and thorough analysis of geographic or spatial distribution of cases and variation in incidence or mortality rates with age, sex, and time. This is in part a recognition that although statistical information can assist in reaching executive conclusions and making executive decisions, much more than statistics must be considered in these conclusions and decisions.

An example may serve to illustrate these points. The crude number of deaths occurring in a community is of relatively little value. It must be fixed to some standard, the most convenient and useful being a unit of population. This involves an appreciation of the adequacy of reporting and the availability of a dependable population count or estimate. The death rate may then be found to be 9.5 per 1,000 inhabitants. A series of questions now arise: Is this high or low? Comparison must be made with the rates of other communities of a similar nature or adjusted for the differences. If it is decided that the single figure is relatively low, is that true of all groups in the community? Age is one basis for grouping. Calculation of age-specific death rates may show a much higher than average mortality under the age of 1 year. Further breakdown may localize the problem in the neonatal period, involving particularly infants born prematurely. What can be done to alleviate the situation? Perhaps an analysis of certain other factors may point the way. Correlation of birth and infant death certificates may point to premature infants born at home or in a particular hospital as accounting for a majority of the deaths. The health department may then strive for the installation of special facilities, incubators, and specially trained nurses in the hospital in question. To include those few who might have been born at home it is imperative that birth certificates be sent to the local health department within 24 hours after birth, in which case they should be routinely screened for prematures. A somewhat better solution would be the arrangement of a discussion of prematurity with the local medical society and the adoption of a policy of telephoning the health department immediately on delivery of a premature infant in the home. In either of these ways it becomes possible for the health department to detail a public health nurse to the care of the infant within the first few crucial days of life.

Perhaps analysis of the statistical data relating to births and infants deaths indicated a higher incidence of prematurity and premature death among certain racial or nationality groups. It then becomes the task of the public health staff to study the habits and customs of these groups in an attempt to discover causal relationships. If such relationships are discovered, a difficult but fascinating task is laid before the health education and public health nursing staffs.

Fig. 39-1 presents another example, this time of the use of the birth certificate in the diphtheria prevention program of one city. It should be noted that the birth certificates represent the key to the approach and also that for public relations reasons a constant running check is made against reports of infant deaths.

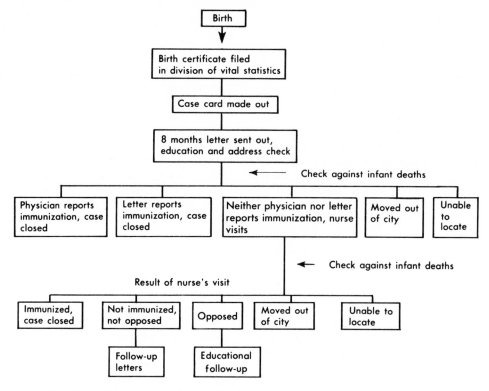

**Fig. 39-1.** Diagrammatic sketch of diphtheria prevention program, Detroit, Mich.

## PRESENTATION OF VITAL DATA

Of increasing importance in the planning and operation of modern public health programs is the use of fractionated data and of certain graphic devices. There is nothing particularly new or difficult about the breakdown of crude or general data into its component parts. The possible number and types of such breakdowns are practically infinite, and the public health worker must decide which are going to be most useful. With all statistical analyses much depends on the form in which the material is arranged for study and presentation. A mass of figures is generally incomprehensible. It is desirable therefore to depict the data in some manner that makes it possible to grasp the total picture and all of the details. One of the most common methods is the simple spot or pin map, which gives an instant overall answer to the question of where the problem is located. An example is presented in Fig. 39-2, which shows for a large city the residences of persons who died from tuberculosis known to the health department as of a certain date. Since the information is based on a constantly moving point in time, this should preferably be in the form of a pin map. This would make possible the shifting of pins as cases are added or dropped and would also allow for the use of different-colored pins to indicate the present status of each case as to severity and hospitalization.

By itself a spot map of a disease or other single item is limited in that it does not indicate the extent to which the group is affected. One general approach to this problem is to distribute the data on the basis of various personal characteristics such as age, race, sex, or economic status. Fig. 39-3 illustrates one method of doing this. The city to which the figure relates has a low tuberculosis death rate. But note how this analysis and presentation point specifically to tuberculosis as an important cause of death in one particular age group. A few of the many other facts it brings to the surface are that cancer and heart disease are important even as early as the young adult years, that the greatest risk of death is during the first year of life particularly because of prematurity, and that accidents are of great significance throughout childhood and young adulthood. Naturally information of this sort will largely determine the nature of the public health program of the area.

**Fig. 39-2.** Spot map. Distribution of reported deaths from tuberculosis, Philadelphia, 1957.

An effective and easily comprehended method of relating specific problems to other factors and to the group is by means of transparent overlay maps. This is particularly useful if there is available for use as a base a map such as Fig. 39-4, which shows the distribution of the population of the area. Thus if spot maps such as Fig. 39-2 are of the same size and are made on transparent material, they may be superimposed on the population map or on each other for visual correlation. (It must be recognized that the purpose of these figures is to illustrate techniques and not to present presently applicable statistical data.)

The procedures described are obviously cumbersome, time consuming, and also easily subject to human error. Techniques have been developed in recent years to achieve the same visual and analytic ends by means of computer mapping printouts.[22]

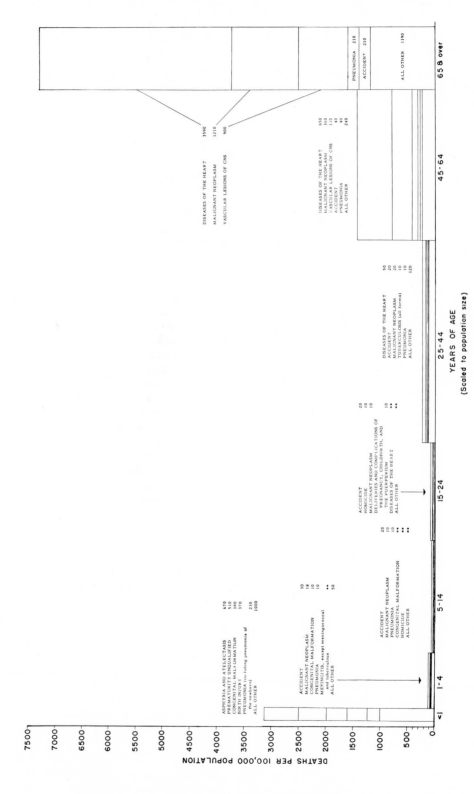

**Fig. 39-3.** Five principal causes of death by age group per 100,000 estimated population, Philadelphia, 1957.

**Fig. 39-4.** Distribution of total population, Philadelphia, 1955.

In recent years public health administrators have come to realize that the health programs of large cities are best administered through decentralized neighborhood health centers. These centers are usually decentralized administrative units of the central health department and are often planned to serve populations of about 200,000. Merely to determine the best locations of the health centers it is necessary to have detailed information concerning the various subdivisions of the jurisdiction. It is strange that although data have long been available for small villages and towns, this has not been generally true of the neighborhood units of large cities until the 1940 census. Too often programs have been based on data limited to the incidence of cases and deaths and have totally ignored the composition of the matrix among whom the cases and deaths were occurring. To be of more than limited use and significance these vital statistics must be related to the places people live, the way they live, the kinds of work they do, and the problems they face. Because of this, the Bureau of the Census for several decades has broken down and made available much of the enormous fund of information it gathers on the basis of census tracts.

A census tract is a small area with definite and permanent boundaries, including a population of between 3,000 and 6,000. It is usually fairly homogeneous with respect to race, nativity, economic status, and general living conditions. This has made it worthwhile for public health administrators in turn to tabulate the vital statistical data of their jurisdictions on the basis of smaller administrative areas. The correlation of these two sources of information has two great advantages: (1) Health statistics compiled on a census tract basis serve to show the geographic distribution of health problems, and (2) health statistics compiled on a census tract basis may be related to other social and economic factors also available by census tracts. As Dunn[23] has stated, the ability to spot births, deaths, communicable disease cases, nurses' visits, and other pertinent data on a tract map shows the health administrator where his business is. Classes for mothers should be organized in areas where births are most frequent. There should be special effort and specific preventive measures in areas where stillbirths and infant deaths predominate. Well-baby clinics should be located in the areas where the babies live. Venereal disease and tuberculosis clinics should be located in the areas where venereal disease and tuberculosis cases are concentrated. Similarly public health education programs on venereal disease and tuberculosis should be stressed in these areas. Special preventive measures should be taken in areas where certain other communicable diseases occur. Accident prevention programs should be stressed in areas where most accidents occur and where persons who are involved in accidents reside. Outpatient hospital clinics should be located in areas where the people who use them reside. Nurses' areas should be designed according to the distribution of demand for nurses' services. Housing inspections and inspections of food establishments are presumably made on a citywide basis. It is a good idea to design inspectors' areas by census tracts and to keep inspection records on this basis. Problem areas may be easily spotted, and special attention can be given these areas.

It is not practical, of course, to establish a health center or clinic in each census tract. Furthermore, because of the small numbers of births, deaths, and cases of disease occurring in each tract, any rates computed in this relatively small population base are of doubtful significance. In using the information therefore the health officer usually finds it desirable to recombine the census tract data in a manner most convenient and best suited to his needs. The usual practice is to form health or sanitary districts, the boundaries of which coincide with those of several census tracts. It is then possible to compute statistically significant rates and ratios that may be presented in one or several ways, as has been done in Fig. 39-5.

A particularly valuable and illustrative method of presentation of fractionated data for administrative purposes is in the form of what has been called the epidemiologic master chart. This type of chart makes possible the presentation at one time of the most complex yet comprehensible pictures of the total public health situation. An example is shown in Fig. 39-6, which presents a detailed and interrelated analysis of a great many important factors bearing on the public health program of the city of Philadelphia. It presents vital data in a form that makes it possible to compare the health districts of the city with one another and to gain a composite view of a large number of factors within each district. The total width of the bars represents 100% of the population of Philadelphia. The width of the 10 subdivisions in each bar indicates the percentage of the total population residing in each district. The numerical percentage is indicated for each district, at the top of the first bar. The height of the two bars for race and age groups represents 100% of the population that resides in each district, the subdivisions indicating the percentage of persons in each age and race group. In the remaining bars are shown rates of birth, death, infant deaths, and deaths from important causes, with the scale placed at the left of each bar. On the right, opposite the title of each bar, is noted the rate for the city as a whole, this being shown further by a horizontal line drawn across each bar.

## RATES AND RATIOS

Although it is in no sense the purpose of this chapter to discuss statistical methodology, there are several computations that public health workers have found particularly useful in judging their programs and in gauging their problems. The simplest of these is the crude death rate. This commonly used rate is merely the number of deaths occurring within a certain

City Wide
P = 2,190,000
BR = 23.2
DR = 11.4
IMR = 31.6
MMR = 1.3
DEI = 47.1

P = 208,000
BR = 17.9
DR = 6.8
IMR = 20.6
MMR = 1.0
DEI = 22.6

10

9
P = 261,000
BR = 20.4
DR = 11.6
IMR = 26.3
MMR = 0.8
DEI = 32.2

8
P = 269,000
BR = 18.0
DR = 11.6
IMR = 22.1
MMR = ***
DEI = 28.2

7
P = 267,000
BR = 20.7
DR = 10.3
IMR = 19.5
MMR = 0.7
DEI = 25.5

5
P = 216,000
BR = 27.1
DR = 11.0
IMR = 44.9
MMR = 3.2
DEI = 93.5

6
P = 208,000
BR = 22.9
DR = 12.4
IMR = 44.3
MMR = 1.4
DEI = 69.2

4
P = 201,000
BR = 22.7
DR = 12.7
IMR = 39.4
MMR = 2.5
DEI = 61.7

P = 227,000
BR = 21.0
DR = 12.2
IMR = 26.5
MMR = 1.3
DEI = 38.3

1
P = 119,000
BR = 18.9
DR = 16.4
IMR = 50.8
MMR = ***
DEI = 73.1

P = 214,000
BR = 22.0
DR = 10.2
IMR = 28.7
MMR = 2.3
DEI = 48.6

3

2

PHILADELPHIA PUBLIC HEALTH SERVICE AREAS

SCALE IN MILES

**Fig. 39-5.** Estimated population, birthrate, death rate, infant mortality rate, maternal mortality rate, and death from diseases of early infancy by health district, Philadelphia, 1957. *P*, Population; *BR*, birthrate; *DR*, death rate; *IMR*, infant mortality rate; *MMR*, maternal mortality rate; *DEI*, diseases of early infancy.

time period, usually 1 year, relative to a convenient unit of population, usually 1,000 persons. Thus a community of 23,460 persons that experiences 220 deaths during a year has a crude death rate of $\dfrac{220 \times 1,000}{23,460} = 9.4$ deaths per 1,000 population. This figure has obvious limitations, all of which arise from the many factors its innate crudeness may conceal. It is easily possible, for example, for a community to have a low crude death rate and yet experience serious mortality from certain particular diseases. Similarly one community may have a lower death rate than another merely by virtue of a greater proportion of young adults in its population. Despite these handicaps, how-

*Text continued on p. 698.*

**Fig. 39-6.** Epidemiologic master chart, Philadelphia, 1957.

**Fig. 39-6, cont'd.** Epidemiologic master chart, Philadelphia, 1957.

*Continued.*

**Fig. 39-6, cont'd.** Epidemiologic master chart, Philadelphia, 1957.

**Fig. 39-6, cont'd.** Epidemiologic master chart, Philadelphia, 1957.

ever, the crude death rate is still the single most commonly used basis for comparison by time and place.

Less commonly used is the vital index or birth-death ratio. This is obtained by dividing the number of births by the number of deaths occurring during a year and multiplying by 100 as a base. If this ratio exceeds 100, the population is growing; it is less than 100, the population is decreasing because of biologic factors alone. One limitation of the figure is that a prolific community may have a vital index of more than 100 in the face of unhealthy conditions and many deaths, whereas the index of another and perhaps healthier community may be low merely because of small families or an older average age of the population.

An interesting although not commonly used, rate is the discratic index. It presents the relationship between the infant mortality rate and the mean age at death. It is considered a good measure of the state of well-being of a community, since it takes into consideration both the tendency of death during the sensitive first year of life in relation to the total number born and the average length of life of the total dynamic population, which is necessarily influenced by all sanitary measures and preventable causes of death along each phase of life. The population under 1 year of age is subject to all of the conditions that tend to raise or lower the infant mortality. If the mean age at death is low, it indicates that diseases are destroying life in the younger age groups of childhood and early adulthood where preventive medicine and public health measures offer the greatest benefits up to the present time. The discratic index has been defined by de Shelley-Hernandez[24] as "the reflection of the sanitary condition of the community as seen through the observed relation between the mean age at death of the inhabitants and the force of infant mortality. It is obtained by dividing for a given year the coefficient in terms of 1,000 live births of the infant deaths, by the mean age at death or average duration of life of the inhabitants of the same community." For the practical application of this interesting and useful index de Shelley-Hernandez suggested the following standards:

| Discratic index | Sanitary and health conditions |
|---|---|
| 1 | Very good |
| 2 | Good |
| 3 | Almost good |

| Discratic index | Sanitary and health conditions |
|---|---|
| 4 | Almost bad |
| 5 | Bad |
| 6 | Very bad |

Another type of statistical index of fundamental importance to health officers is the endemic index. This may be developed in several ways. If one wishes to compare the current frequency of a disease with some standard for the community in the recent past, the experience for several years might be averaged to obtain a mean. If for the previous 5 years the experience of each calendar week is averaged, there results a 5-year moving mean. If a disease demonstrates cyclicity, as does measles, an endemic and epidemic moving mean may be calculated and graphed for comparison with the current experience and for estimating to a certain limited degree the probable anticipated incidence. Similarly an endemic median and a 3-, 5-, or 7-year moving median may be obtained. Fig. 21-4 presents several charts of this type.

An increasingly important use of vital statistics is in connection with the allocation of federal funds to state health departments and of state funds to local health departments. Various aspects of this subject have been discussed in Chapter 8. It will suffice here to call attention to the bases on which grants-in-aid may be made. Just as population serves as the basic factor in the computation of incidence and death rates, population or per capita data form the most significant single factor in the allocation of public health funds. Beyond this various fiscal formulas include provisions for supplemental grants beyond the per capita grants based on special problems. The existence of these is determined by morbidity data, prevalence rates, facilities available or needed, mortality, natality, and rate of population increase.

Statistical data are of further administrative importance in the sense that they provide a measure of the degree of compliance of local health departments with established standards and a means for the evaluation and comparison of the programs of health departments.

Elsewhere it has been stated that every progressive health department has a responsibility to accept research as one of its functions. The word *research* almost automatically makes one think of statistics. They are mutually interdependent. Unfortunately, too few official health departments on either the state or local level engage in special statistical research projects. The potentialities here are great. To conduct such investigations obviously requires highly trained statistical personnel. When they are available and engaged by the health department, a problem arises as to their relationship with the rest of the personnel of the vital statistics unit. This logically draws attention to the question of the organization of statistical services in public health agencies.

## ORGANIZATION OF STATISTICAL ACTIVITIES

In rural counties and small communities the local health officer is usually designated as the registrar of vital statistics. Ordinarily he in turn delegates this responsibility to some member of his office staff who, although seldom specifically trained, in some instances is referred to as a statistical clerk. This person acts as a sort of combination record clerk and clearinghouse for the reports that come to the health department. Certificates of birth and death are received, checked, transcribed, indexed, and filed. His analytic activities are usually confined to the compilation of simple tabulations for the annual report. He also receives the reports of cases of morbidity that are transmitted to the health officer or whatever person is responsible for their control. In connection with this he often maintains files and registers of active and closed cases. In most instances he has no responsibility for the service and activity records of the health department personnel who usually take care of their own. Where systems such as the family or household folder are used, however, he is often put in charge. The general picture therefore is one of simplicity and almost informality, brought about by the combination of small staff, proximity to problems, and lack of statistically trained personnel and of funds to employ them.

When the public health departments of large cities and states are considered, one would expect to find a more or less uniform plan of statistical organization, since the needs and problems are essentially similar in such situations. Interestingly enough this is not the case. From the viewpoint of organizational principles the statistical activities of these larger units are of two types: functional or line (in the sense of the routine collection, preservation, and transcription of vital statistical documents) and staff (in the sense of the activities related to studies, research, consultation, fiscal and program control). Herein lies the origin of most of the organizational problems and variations.

Analysis indicates five basic patterns of organization of state health department statistical services: (1) no central statistical organization, (2) a division of vital statistics with some central statistical services, (3) a division of vital statistics with an independent central tabulating unit, (4) a central statistical division with an independent division of vital records, and (5) a central statistical division covering all registration and statistical activities.

In the states in the first category the collection, preservation, and tabulation of the routine vital records is a function of a separate line division or bureau of vital statistics. Beyond this each major subdivision of the health department is individually responsible for all of its own record keeping, reporting, and statistical functions.

In the second category are state health departments in which certain limited statistical services to other divisions are rendered by the line division or bureau of vital statistics. In most instances this resulted from attempts at economy and efficiency by pooling all mechanical tabulating equipment and specialized statistical personnel. The usual pattern is for the functional divisions to collect and edit data and to plan tabulations. The vital statistics division then processes and tabulates the data, after which the completed information is returned to the program divisions for analysis and use.

The state health departments in the third category have what amounts to an adaptation of the foregoing in that they maintain a division of vital statistics and a central tabulating unit, which, however, are not combined. The typical pattern is a line division of vital statistics and a central tabulating unit as a staff agency in the division of administration. Some state health departments have established independent units for statistical services in addition to line divisions responsible for vital records. As in the third category, the central statistical service is organized as a staff agency responsible to the director of health. The difference, however, lies in the purpose of the central statistical unit. In this instance it has no routine administrative or operating responsibilities. Rather, it exists to provide staff services and technical assistance to all parts of the department and to local health departments in the state. It serves essentially for the purpose of "thinking the program through" and for planning, analysis, and interpretation. Needless to say, this necessitates highly qualified leadership and a well-trained staff.

The states in the fifth category, an increasing number, have centralized all statistical services in one unit. The pattern that is usually followed is to form subdivisions or sections that deal with vital records, tabulation, analysis and reports, and consultation service.

Administrators appear to be divided into two groups with regard to centralization of statistical services. One group strongly believes that except for routine activities, such as vital records and tabulating, all statistical functions should be left in the various functional divisions. The primary reason given reflects fear that centralization of statistical records and activities might detract from their adequacy and usefulness. The majority of administrators, however, believe that some form of centralized statistical unit is necessary in large public health organizations to ensure efficiency, correlation of data and activities, and more profitable use of statistical personnel. It is probably desirable that so much variation exists. Among other things variation indicates ingenuity and experimentation, two characteristics that continue to be greatly needed in this and many other fields of public health.

This brings up a final important point—the ever-present need for interdisciplinary communications, which leads to improved understanding and effectiveness. The case was well stated by two prominent statisticians in the following terms[5]:

Statisticians must learn to talk to the planners, and they to us. It is our impression that right now we are not speaking the same language. In particular, we are frustrated because they have not yet been able to articulate their needs for data in terms we can understand, and they are frustrated because of our long lag-times, and seeming lack of appreciation for the kinds of statistical detail needed for input to the planning process. Yet planners are obviously looking to health statistics offices to serve their needs, and one of our functions is to provide hard data for this purpose. Somehow, we must all learn better communication.

## REFERENCES

1. Mattison, B. F.: The administrative value of statistics to a local health officer, Public Health Rep. **67:**747, Aug. 1952.
2. Kraus, A. S.: Efficient utilization of statistical activities in public health, Amer. J. Public Health **53:**1075, July 1963.
3. Aune, H. V.: The importance of vital records in today's society, Public Health Rep. **74:**1029, Nov. 1959.
4. Schweitzer, M. D., et al.: Information systems in public health, Public Health Rep. **83:**343, May 1968.
5. Woolsey, T. D., and Lawrence, P. S.: Moving ahead in health statistics, Amer. J. Public Health **59:**1820, Oct. 1969.
6. Sirken, M. G., Pifer, J. W., and Brown, M. L.: Survey procedures for supplementing mortality statistics, Amer. J. Public Health **50:**1753, Nov. 1960.
7. International classification of diseases, injuries, and causes of death, Geneva, 1957, World Health Organization.
8. Wilson, V. E.: In Highlights of the Fourteenth National Conference on Records and Statistics, Health Services Rep. **87:**709, Oct. 1972.
9. West, M. D.: Morbidity reporting in local areas, Public Health Rep. **63:**329, March 12, 1948; and **63:**1187, Sept. 10, 1948.
10. Morbidity surveys—a symposium, Amer. J. Public Health **39:**737, June 1949.
11. Linder, F. E.: The national health survey, Science **127:**1275, May 30, 1958.
12. Langmuir, A. D.: The contribution of the survey method to epidemiology, Amer. J. Public Health **39:**747, June 1949.
13. Vital Statistics of the United States, Washington, D. C., (issued annually), Government Printing Office.
14. Morbidity and Mortality Weekly Report, Washington, D. C., (issued weekly), Government Printing Office.
15. Epidemiological and Vital Statistics Report, Geneva (issued monthly), World Health Organization.
16. Annual Epidemiological and Vital Statistics, Geneva (issued annually), World Health Organization.
17. U. S. Public Health Service: The Cooperative-Federal-State-Local Health Statistics System, pub. no. (HSM) 72-1209, Rockville, Md., 1972.
18. White, K. L.: Improved medical care statistics and the health services system, Public Health Rep. **82:**847, Oct. 1967.
19. Gertzog, J.: The changing concept of medical records, Public Health Rep. **85:**673, Aug. 1970.
20. Acheson, E. D.: Medical record linkage, London, 1967, Oxford University Press.
21. Trauger, D. A.: What is a good statistical report, Health Services Rep. **87:**693, Oct. 1972.
22. Lewis, R., and Chadzynski, L.: Evolutionary changes in the environment, population, and health affairs in Detroit, 1968-1971, Amer. J. Public Health **64:**557, June 1974.
23. Dunn, H. L.: Health and social statistics for the city, Amer. J. Public Health **37:**740, June 1947.
24. de Shelley-Hernandez, R.: Statistics applied to biological science, Caracas, Venezuela, 1939, El Comercio, Ministerio de Hacienda.

*The origin of all science is
in the desire to know causes.*

WILLIAM HAZLITT

CHAPTER 40

# Laboratory services

## DEVELOPMENT OF PUBLIC HEALTH LABORATORIES

Because of the need for scientific guidance in an era rife with epidemic disease, early recognition was given to the importance of laboratory procedures in public health programs. It is not surprising therefore that most of the older public health laboratories owed their inception to some catastrophe such as an epidemic and that, generally speaking, they were developed in congested cities and towns before they became common on the state level. For example, the first municipal laboratory in the United States was established in 1892 when New York City suffered a severe outbreak of cholera. At about the same time the first state laboratory was established in Michigan, followed by Rhode Island in 1894. Other state laboratories, however, were slow to develop. This relatively early resort to laboratory procedures by health departments was perhaps more fortunate than is ordinarily realized. In a sense it established a philosophy or point of view and encouraged a constantly inquiring attitude. Without it many public health programs up to recent times would have been based on sheer guesswork. The benefits that accrued from this relationship between laboratory and program were stated by William H. Welch[1] in the following terms:

The development of laboratories connected with boards of health is one which is peculiarly American. The appreciation of the need of such laboratories, of what can be accomplished by them and of the benefits which the general public derive from them, has been greater in this country than else-

where. We have led in this particular direction. . . . The foundation of such laboratories has had a very important stimulating influence upon boards of health, both local and state. It has introduced a scientific spirit into the work; it has brought into connection with executive officers the younger men who are full of enthusiasm with reference to studies along these lines, and I think that we may say that the general tone of boards of health has been elevated and stimulated by the foundation of laboratories of this character.

## FUNCTIONS OF PUBLIC HEALTH LABORATORIES

Schaeffer[2] has identified an unfortunate and contradictory phenomenon in laboratory science: "During an era of advancement in the biological and chemical sciences, research laboratories have flourished beyond expectation, but the service laboratories have not kept pace. This has occurred though physicians and health officers require more and greater varieties of services from clinical and public health laboratories." He explains that antiobiotics have almost eliminated many infections, thereby leading to a false sense of security and largely eliminating the diagnostic microbiologic laboratory. In this respect he observes that "medical microbiology is almost a lost art, and few medical bacteriologists are being trained to replace the rapidly dwindling handful of old ones." This is to be regretted and feared in view of the shrinking world, increased travel, and the concomitant risk of reintroduction of various communicable diseases.

On the other hand, although it is true that

701

public health laboratories until recently have been primarily concerned with problems of sanitation and epidemiology, the scope of their potential role has been greatly broadened by the very changes that have been occurring in society and public health in general. This is implied by the *American Journal of Public Health* in an editorial consideration of "Research and the Public Health"[3]:

As the problems of communicable disease have declined in urgency and scope in the United States, the community health program has been broadened to include, wherever feasible, other elements and situations that may adversely affect physical, social, and psychological well-being. The widening horizons of public health have in recent years come to focus on control of new aspects of the physical environment, chronic disease, and medical care. With our changing and expanding industrial technology have come environmental alterations of increasing complexity. The once dominant problems of bacterially contaminated air, water, and food have now been replaced in considerable degree by chemical pollution. The other major problem area concerns chronic disease and medical care or, more broadly, the area of personal health services.

Within the health department the laboratory continues to serve as a guide and tool for each of the other activities. It furnishes the clue to the types and extensiveness of communicable and increasingly of noncommunicable disease problems. It not only indicates the effectiveness of the sanitation program but even provides the basis of design of engineering structures in that field. It is of great importance in certain phases of the maternal and infant health programs. In the final analysis it may be said that, aside from research, by itself laboratory service is of little value and that of necessity it must be used as an adjunct or in relation to other programs and activities. Beyond serving the component parts of the health department, although individual medical management is primarily the concern of the private practitioner, the modern public health laboratories have found it worth while to assist him by ensuring, inasmuch as possible, the availability of essential aids to diagnosis, prevention, and treatment. Increasingly, however, because of improved technology, increased demands for medical care, and the extended application of prepaid health insurance and Social Security provisions, the medical profession has turned to private laboratories for such services.[4] This has given rise to an additional problem in that now there are an estimated 100,000 people working in

12,000 to 14,000 clinical laboratories in the United States.[5] Studies by the National Center for Disease Control indicate erroneous results in more than 25% of their tests.[6] Obviously there is a great need for standards, inspection, and supervision.

At the present time the activities of at least the larger public health laboratories fall into the following six categories:

1. Provision of facilities for physicians, hospitals, and health workers for the diagnosis, prevention, and management of disease
2. Establishment and maintenance of standards through chemical and bacteriologic examination of food, milk, water, streams, air, pharmaceuticals, narcotics, liquors, and other substances
3. Supervision, especially by state laboratories, of the practices, procedures, personnel, and products of local and private laboratories
4. Manufacture and/or distribution of sera, toxins, antitoxins, vaccines, and other biologic materials for diagnosis, prevention, and therapy; some state laboratories also determine standards of quality and potency of such substances
5. Training of technologists
6. Research

The following discussion is limited essentially to the larger laboratories located in major cities and particularly in state health departments, which because of the populations they serve, are in a position or find it necessary to engage in a wide variety of activities. In a sense the laboratories of smaller communities that have limited facilities and resources may be considered subsidiaries or local outposts of the more extensive laboratories of larger governmental units.

All states assume responsibility for providing laboratory services at least for the diagnosis and control of communicable diseases. Ordinarily the spectrum of diseases for which such services are available is broad. Because of the number of specimens and state legislation pertaining to it, serologic tests for syphilis account for a significant proportion of the examinations performed by state public health laboratories. An additional reason is the inability of most laboratories in smaller jurisdictions to perform the tests and their tendency to transfer the responsibility to the larger state unit.

Because of the magnitude of the work and the customary responsibility of the state for supervision, most state health department laboratories carry on routine bacteriologic and chemical analyses of public supplies of drinking water. Private water supplies are usually tested on special request by private citizens as well as physicians and public health workers. Frequently a fee is charged for this service. A charge for testing private water supplies is more common than for any other type of public health laboratory service; in fact it is rare for any other charges to be made. In several instances state universities also make analyses of drinking water, either independently or cooperatively with the health department.

Interestingly facilities and procedures for the testing of food, milk, and drugs are much more varied than those relating to disease diagnosis and water examination. This is largely the result of different allocations of responsibility by the states for surveillance over food, milk, and drugs. Although state health department laboratories are most commonly charged with this responsibility, in 24 states, two or more agencies are involved. Most frequently the other agency is the department of agriculture, and in three instances it has exclusive jurisdiction over all aspects of milk and food laboratory control. In addition, in about a dozen instances independent state laboratories or laboratory departments, state chemists, agricultural experiment stations, livestock sanitary boards, state university laboratories, or boards of pharmacy analyze milk, foods, and drugs from standpoints of significance to public health.

Altogether 30 states have established facilities for the laboratory study and control of industrial dusts, gases, fumes, and other toxic substances to which workers may be exposed. In 25 states the work is done by the public health laboratory; in 3 states the department of labor performs this function alone; and in the other 2 states the departments of health and labor share responsibility.

At the present time, one of the major functions of many state health department laboratories is the distribution of biologics, pharmaceuticals, and other materials for diagnosis, prevention, and therapy to local health departments and through them to hospitals and private physicians. About one half of the state laboratories manufacture at least a few of the materials they distribute. The most common are typhoid fever vaccine and silver nitrate solution for the prevention of ophthalmia neonatorum. Several states prepare rabies vaccine, diphtheria

toxoid, and toxin for Schick tests. Other products occasionally manufactured in state laboratories include smallpox vaccine, diphtheria antitoxin, scarlet fever antitoxin, tuberculin, pneumonia serum, antimeningitis serum, and convalescent sera for measles, scarlet fever, and several other diseases. A few manufacture multiple antigens, particularly diphtheria-tetanus-pertussis combined antigens. In the past, several southern states have distributed antimalarial and anthelmintic drugs. Generally, however, because of cost and other factors, health agencies are purchasing biologic materials from the large pharmaceutical companies for whom production costs are less due to mass production methods and in which quality control measures are more easily applied.

Technical procedures, methods of transporting specimens, and reports of findings have been well standardized. Much of the credit for this is due the American Public Health Association, and particularly its laboratory section. This section is composed of several committees, among which are those relating to diagnostic procedures and reagents, examination of water and sewage, examination of dairy products, analysis of frozen desserts, examination of shellfish, biology of laboratory animals, and biologic products. Each committee studies procedures and recommends those most practical for use by public health laboratories. Among its many contributions has been the issuance over many years of a series of manuals of standard laboratory methods and procedures.

In the field of chronic diseases progressive public health laboratories have added significantly to their technical armamentarium and provided an ever-lengthening list of test procedures. The Clinitron, Auto Analyzers, and similar equipment have made possible rapid, inexpensive, and broad-ranging test results. These devices have contributed greatly to the feasibility of mass screening and diagnostic programs against many chronic noncommunicable illnesses. With reference to the scope of procedures many public health laboratories have long since performed blood grouping, blood sugar, and blood cholesterol tests. Some already do certain other tests related to heart disease.[7] The Papanicolaou test is now commonly performed, as are tests for gastric acid in relation to asymptomatic cancer of the stomach, several tests for rheumatoid arthritis, and fluorescent antibody procedures as applied to rheumatic fever and other conditions.[8,9] A few laboratories are already exploring the use of a variety of tests related to schizophrenia.[10] Increasingly public health laboratories have become involved in the diagnosis of genetic conditions such as phenylketonuria,[11] sickle-cell anemia,[12] erythroblastosis (Rh disease),[13] galactosemia,[14] glycine deficiency, maple syrup urine disease, histidinuria, Wilson's disease, and other causes of mental retardation.[15] It is also reasonable to anticipate public health laboratory programs including analyses of amniotic fluid for early indications of congenital malformations.

The potential role of the public health laboratory in environmental health has already gone far beyond the simple tests of water, milk, and food.[16] The greatly increased hazards of air pollution and ionizing radiation have presented the laboratory with significant new challenges and opportunities. Its contribution to air pollution control programs includes standard setting, support of air monitoring systems, development of methods for analysis and epidemiologic applications, research on the chemical and physical nature of air pollutants, and the relating of air pollution research results to other health programs.[17] Similarly the public health laboratory can be of assistance in radiologic control programs.[18]

The development of standard methods and the great increase in various legally required serologic tests have served to place responsibility on state health department laboratories for the supervision and control of techniques used by local public and private laboratories. The origin of this role dates back about a half century, when the Sanitary Code of the City of New York made the health department responsible for the supervision of clinical laboratories. Soon afterward, in 1925, the code was amended again to establish qualifications of laboratory directors, to provide for examination of technical personnel, and to allow for inspection of laboratory premises. The laboratory of the health department was given the responsibility for enforcement.[2]

The supervisory function of the public health laboratory is carried out by means of inspections, analyses in the state laboratory of duplicate test specimens from the local laboratory, licensing of local laboratories, and setting qualifications for and approval of locally employed laboratory personnel. With reference to public health laboratory personnel themselves the American Public Health Association itself

has for several years issued statements of qualifications.[19] At present one third of the states specifically require that laboratories performing serologic tests for syphilis be approved and periodically checked by the state laboratory. Nine states extend this supervision to include all types of diagnostic tests of public health significance. Increasingly, even in states with no provisions for regulation, approval by state laboratories is being sought voluntarily by private laboratories as a mark of recognition. Unfortunately, however, in too many states there is neither licensing nor listing of the local private laboratories. In fact, a person totally untrained in laboratory science can often operate a clinical laboratory. As a result, large numbers of clinical laboratories operate without adequate or with only token supervision.[2]

Unfortunately the action by New York City, now a half century ago, did not prompt similar action elsewhere. The states that should have provided leadership did not. Thus by 1966 when the Medicare program began, only 6 states provided any type of laboratory licensure. It was hoped that the Medicare program would rapidly stimulate other states, but the extent to which this occurred has been limited. Meanwhile, in 1967 the Clinical Laboratory Improvement Act (P.L. 90-174) was passed. It provided for federal licensure of clinical laboratories engaged in interstate commerce.[20] This law appears to be having more effect than Medicare on the development of local and state regulations. One important advantage is that whereas Medicare regulations emphasize personnel qualifications, the Clinical Laboratory Improvement Act emphasizes accuracy of performance through proficiency testing and internal quality control. Hopefully, as a result of the combination of these measures, most clinical laboratories in the United States will operate under comparable high standards. The pursuit and surveillance of this should be regarded as a high priority public health function.[6]

**FUNCTIONAL CHANGE**

In view of the current rapid changes occurring in society, public health, and the delivery of personal health services in the United States, some fundamental functional changes are indicated for public health laboratories. Up to the present they have operated for the most part as service facilities, accepting and inviting a wide variety of specimens on which, in the name of protection of the public's health, they gratuitously performed and reported the results of various tests. Conscientiously over the years they added to the list of services available, often severely stretching their resources. Increasingly, however, it has become evident that this is not their most influential potential role.

As Evans[21] puts it, "The massive volume of routine work has hobbled the proper and efficient development of public health laboratories . . . just as traditional and unimaginative public health duties have burdened the epidemiologist." He continues pertinently, "The economic and social pressures now evolving point us in new directions: reference work, quality control, extension training, and surveillance. Proper utilization of this opportunity," he opines, "may yield important advances for public health." Among his thoughtful recommendations are the following: (1) a closer working relationship between the public health epidemiologist and the laboratory (it is worth nothing that this once existed and now apparently must be rediscovered and reinstituted); (2) the epidemiologic orientation of the laboratory director and his staff; (3) the greater development of the application of computer systems for the processing of laboratory data; (4) the more extensive development and use of sera reference banks; and (5) a change in emphasis from the provision of direct and routine services to specialized studies, reference work, test evaluations, demonstration programs, and assistance in quality control to community laboratories. He predicts that the social and economic changes which will result from the various national health service programs and the greater development and use of automated laboratory procedures "create a new lease on life for the public health laboratory."

Evans' views and predictions merit careful consideration. They are in line to a great extent with the policy statement for the improvement of laboratory services by the Committee on Evaluations and Standards of the American Public Health Association, issued October 25, 1967.[22] It states that to meet the serious need for improvement of laboratory services concerned with the maintenance of the health of man, the following steps are recommended:

1. State legislation requiring *licensure* of laboratories concerned with health, such as clinical, public health, agricultural, industrial and commercial health related laboratories, other than those of individual physicians performing tests for their own patients. Licensing should be the responsibility of the State Health Departments and should be on as uniform a basis as possible throughout the Country.

2. *Certification* of professional laboratory personnel, through the utilization of suitable current certification programs, and coordination of efforts of all competent organizations concerned with certification.

3. Improved *training* of laboratory personnel by
   a. Accreditation of schools for the training of such professional laboratory personnel as microbiologists, laboratory technologists, laboratory technicians and clinical chemists.
   b. Continuing education of all professional and technical personnel.
   c. Educational programs, including fellowships to upgrade personnel.

4. Improvement of laboratory services by means of quality control programs including inspections and submission of unknown samples, preferably conducted by State Health Departments. *Proficiency testing* should be a condition of continued licensure.
   Mechanisms for periodic review of state health laboratories should be expanded.

5. Increased *consultation* services by selected laboratories, such as State Health Departments, the National Center for Communicable Disease Control, the National Center for Urban and Industrial Health and other appropriate agencies.

6. Provision of adequately trained *supervisory personnel*.

*Additional problems requiring attention*

1. Recent but well-known research techniques should be adapted to current routine laboratory services.

2. Research should develop new laboratory procedures which will make evaluation of the environment and detection of disease agents more sensitive, accurate and rapid.

3. Better methods for sample collection should be developed, including considerations of time as well as space, especially in fields such as air, water and food.

*Definitions*

For the purposes of this policy statement, the following definitions apply:

*Accreditation*—approval of courses, training or education by nationally recognized organizations.

*Certification*—approval of the education and training of individuals by appropriate professional organizations, boards or state agencies.

*Licensure*—authorization to conduct business issued by official governmental agencies to approved individuals or laboratories.

*Registration*—listing of those individuals who are certified or those institutions which are accredited. (This differs from the Center for Disease Control's definition which does not imply approval, only a listing of the location of facilities and the character of program and services.)

## RESEARCH

No public health agency can remain progressive and effective without constantly seeking ways of improving its work, services, and methods. Although research is needed and possible in all phases of public health, one place where particularly fruitful investigations may be carried out is in the laboratory. An opportunity exists here both for pure laboratory research and for investigations carried on in conjunction with other functional divisions of the health department or other community or even national agencies. Thus the majority of large laboratories engage in special research projects in addition to their routine activities.

Among the general areas of investigation worthy of mention are studies on the diagnosis and reporting of disease and disease patterns, descriptive epidemiology, surveillance methodology, retrospective, current, and prospective studies on the incidence and prevalence of disease, and the relationship between the occurrence of disease and factors in the environment. Far from being set apart, the laboratory should consider itself and should be very much in the middle of all that goes on in the public health program. Its opportunities are unique. Evans[21] states it cogently noting that the contributions of the public health laboratory are possible by virtue of the large volume of materials submitted, the geographic distribution of the sources, and the availability of correlative clinical and epidemiologic data from public health departments or hospital records. He also emphasizes the special relationship between the epidemiologist and the public health laboratorian, indicating that by working closely together they have a tremendous opportunity for important and fruitful investigation.

Attention is called to the possibilities of developing immunologic and biochemical profiles of populations based on the study of sera obtained from samples of blood submitted for syphilis testing, from blood donors, and from various other sources.[23] Occasionally special local funds are appropriated for particular research projects, and special personnel are assigned or employed full time to carry them out. Increasingly, however, federal and private research funds have been placed at the disposal of the large, well-equipped, and well-staffed public health labora-

tories. Frequently investigations are designed to improve currently used techniques or to compare them with new procedures. Much also has been done by public health laboratories in the development, testing, and production of new products and techniques. In addition, an increasing amount of pure research is being done. Of particular note are investigations concerned with diagnostic tests for cancer, diabetes, and fluorescent antibody techniques as well as with various aspects of immunization against influenza, rabies, pneumonia, diphtheria, pertussis, brucellosis, poliomyelitis, staphylococcic and streptococcic infections, and histoplasmosis.

## LABORATORY ORGANIZATION

Despite the fact that the public health laboratory is essentially auxiliary to the program units of the public health organization, one seldom finds it located organizationally in the manner theoretically recommended for auxiliary agencies. The practical reasons for this are the technical nature of the laboratory's activities and its frequently large size. With reference to size, in several states, notably Michigan, New York, California, and Massachusetts, the laboratory itself is of about the same magnitude in budget, physical size, and number of employees as the rest of the health department. The pattern therefore has been for the laboratories of state and large city health departments to be major functional line units in the organization. Among the states only a few exceptions are found to this rule. In two states more than one bureau has laboratory functions; in one state the laboratory is in the bureau of local health services. In another it is an entirely independent agency.

The general lack of attention to the development of local laboratory facilities, because of their highly technical nature and cost, has tended to make the public health laboratory highly centralized. Yet, having centralized all but the simplest procedures in the state health department laboratory, there is now a tendency toward decentralization. This usually takes the form of branch or regional counterparts of the state laboratory rather than an actual return to dependence on small local laboratories.

More than half of the state health departments maintain branch laboratories at strategic points throughout their areas. Usually such branch laboratories serve as localized points for the distribution of biologics and specimen equipment received from the central state laboratory and for the collection of specimens to be transmitted to the central laboratory. In addition, certain analyses that are within the competency of the local laboratory are performed there, whereas more difficult or complex procedures are sent to the central laboratory for reasons of competency or efficiency.

Several states make additional use of their supervisory authority by designating certain local public health and even private laboratories as branches or local agents. This procedure has much merit in that it encourages those laboratories to maintain their standards and stimulates others to improve theirs. A few states emphasize the development and use of local public health laboratories by subsidizing laboratories in local health departments. The subsidy may take the form of funds, personnel, or equipment.

In some places the development of a joint hospital-health department laboratory has been found advantageous, since the additional financial resources allow the utilization of better qualified personnel. Some small cities with more than one hospital have found it effective to have a single director administer the health department laboratories and the several hospital laboratories. This arrangement makes possible a well-integrated laboratory service and enables the community to obtain a director of higher caliber.

A similar problem that has occasionally arisen is concerned with the extent to which laboratory services should be centralized or decentralized within the structure of the health department itself. In the past it was not rare to find that several divisions within a health department had developed their own separate specialized laboratory service. Thus the division of communicable disease control might operate its own small laboratory in addition to the main laboratory, as might perhaps a special venereal disease or tuberculosis division, the sanitary engineering division, the food and milk division, and so on. The organization chart of State B (Fig. 10-4) provides an illustration. There are many objections to this. It involves the problem of vertical in contrast to horizontal organization and administration. The inefficiency resulting from duplication of materials, equipment, and personnel is obvious. It is difficult enough to find competent laboratory directors without multiplying the problem and usually settling for persons with less than adequate qualifications and ability. Often the directors of the various

units involved, such as engineering, have attempted personally to supervise the work of their laboratories. However, the proper direction of a laboratory is a specialized full-time responsibility, and an engineer rarely makes a good laboratory director. Furthermore, a multiplicity of smaller unit laboratories tends to divide the total work of the organization into tight little compartments, no one of which is aware of the others or how they might act to mutual benefit.

Three different arrangements therefore are possible: The first and by far the most desirable is the organization of a single central division or bureau of laboratory services, which functions as a major unit of the health department and provides all laboratory services to all programs of the department. The second and least desirable is the operation of a series of smaller, specialized laboratories within each of several functional units of the department. The third approach, which is a compromise and is sometimes necessary in deference to convenience, tradition, or personality, is maintenance of certain small departmental facilities for the performance of certain relatively simple procedures, in addition to a large central laboratory.

In Chapter 10, which dealt with the organizational aspects of public health, decentralization of programs and services, especially in larger cities, was discussed. In places where programs are decentralized by means of health districts with district health centers, it is frequently useful to provide a limited amount of space and personnel for the immediate on-the-spot performance of certain simple but important laboratory tests. The decision depends, of course, on the nature of the programs being carried out in the district. Especially as public health agencies become more involved in programs of chronic noncommunicable disease and adult health maintenance, the provision of basic laboratory facilities in health centers will become more practical and necessary.

During recent years several states have experimented with the use of mobile laboratories as a substitute for or in addition to branch laboratories. Some have expressed doubt as to the usefulness of these laboratories, and a few have discontinued them. It is possible that dissatisfaction might be attributed to failure to appreciate their essential purpose and therefore to use them improperly or inefficiently. They should always be considered an adjunct to rather than a substitute for the central and branch laboratories. In this respect they should be under the technical and preferably under the administrative supervision of the central laboratory. Their effective function requires good working relationships among the staffs of the mobile laboratory, of the central laboratory, and of the local health department or local governmental officials. It is desirable that they be kept flexible rather than geared for only one particular function or activity. In this way the mobile laboratory can be a multipurpose resource. In an age of good roads and rapid transit the mobile laboratory could possibly occupy a significant place in the overall public health program, particularly in certain areas and for specialized time-limited efforts. This is most likely to be true of emergencies, field epidemiologic investigations, stream pollution studies and control, resort sanitation, occupational health activities, and some aspects of food and milk control.

The distribution of biologic products and the collection and transmission of biologic specimens require careful planning and timing on the part of the health department laboratory personnel. Arrangements must be made for temporary storage and for prompt pick-up. Delivery and pick-up services for materials going to and from the state laboratory must be coordinated with the time schedules of public carriers such as railroad, air, and bus lines. Containers for specimens and for their safe shipment must be designed and distributed. Furthermore, provision must be made for 24-hour availability of certain products, particularly antitoxins and antisera, for use in emergencies. In small communities, reliance is usually placed on the cooperation and concern of the local health officer or pharmacist.

In large cities it has been possible for health departments to make highly satisfactory arrangements for the provision of collection and distribution stations throughout their areas. Some are located in fire or police stations, and others are in pharmacies where refrigerators are placed at the disposal of the health department. All large city health departments provide for their own messenger service for the collection of specimens and for the daily replenishment of supplies at the distribution stations. It is worth while to include report forms with the supplies made available, and many communities require that identifying data concerning cases be provided at the time biologic materials are obtained from distribution stations.

**REFERENCES**

1. Welch, W. H.: Relations of laboratories to public health. (Lecture.)
2. Schaeffer, M.: Health department's role in improving operations of clinical laboratories, Public Health Rep. **81:**71, Jan. 1966.
3. Editorial: Research and the public health, Amer. J. Public Health **57:**1259, Aug. 1967.
4. Freeborn, D. K., et al.: Determinants of medical care utilization: physicians' use of laboratory services, Amer. J. Public Health **62:**846, June 1972.
5. Conference on manpower for the medical laboratory, National Commission for Careers in Medical Technology and the National Center for Disease Control, College Park, Md., Oct. 11-13, 1967.
6. Brooke, M. M.: Quality clinical laboratory services for the American people, Pub. Health Rep. **85:** 155, Feb. 1970.
7. Berliner, R. W., and Stewart, W. H.: The public health laboratory in the community control of heart diseases, Amer. J. Public Health **47:**719, June 1957.
8. Chapman, A. L.: The chronic disease laboratory in public health, Public Health Rep. **73:**1070, Dec. 1958.
9. Peeples, W. J., Spielman, D. W., and Moody, M. D.: Field application of fluorescent antibody technic for identification of Group A streptococcus, Public Health Rep. **76:**651, July 1961.
10. Bachbinder, L., and Ferguson, A.: Does the public health laboratory have a role in mental health? Amer. J. Public Health **58:**573, April 1958.
11. Guthrie, R., and Susi, A.: A simple phenylalanine method for detecting phenylketonuria in large populations of newborn infants, Pediatrics **32:** 338, Sept. 1963.
12. Lin-Fu, J. S.: Sickle cell anemia: review of the literature, pub. no. (HSM) 71-5104, Rockville, Md., 1965, U. S. Department of Health, Education and Welfare.
13. Umansky, I., et al.: A state program for prevention of sensitization to Rh factor, HSMHA Health Rep. **86:**212, March 1971.
14. Help from the biochemist, World Health, Aug.-Sept. 1966.
15. David, W. D.: The developing role of laboratories in chronic disease programs, Amer. J. Public Health **78:**13, Jan. 1963.
16. Hardy, A. V.: The public health laboratory—looking to the future, Amer. J. Public Health **50:**927, July 1960.
17. Helwig, H. L., and Maga, J. A.: The role of the public health laboratory in air pollution programs, Amer. J. Public Health **50:**933, July 1960.
18. Gilcreas, F. W., and Morgan, G. B.: The role of the public health laboratory in radiological science, Amer. J. Public Health **50:**619, May 1960.
19. Educational qualifications of public health labora-

tory workers, Amer. J. Public Health **57:**523, March 1967.

20. Center for Disease Control: Licensure of clinical laboratories and personnel, Atlanta, 1966, U. S. Department of Health, Education, and Welfare.

21. Evans, A. S.: Epidemiology and the public health laboratory, Amer. J. Public Health **57:**1041, June 1967.

22. American Public Health Association: Policy statement for improvement of laboratory services, Oct. 25, 1967, The Association.

23. Paul, J. R.: Clinical epidemiology, Chicago, 1966, University of Chicago Press.

# PART TWELVE

# The future of public health

The role of the prognosticator at any time and under all circumstances is fraught with difficulties and dangers. Change is known to be inevitable in a biologic complex such as that in which we humans play a dominant role. The nature and extent of the change, however, present different questions. It is here that one challenges credulity, stubs one's intellectual toes, and risks one's reputation. Nevertheless, prognostication is justified and serves a useful purpose. When based on considered analysis and judgment of things past and present, it forms the best possible and in fact the only reasonable basis for determining sound planning and action for the future.

CHAPTER 41

# The past as prologue

## QUO VADIMUS

During recent years public health workers in the United States have experienced increasing introspection and have raised several provocative questions: What is the future of our profession? Have we served our essential purpose and should we begin to phase out? Is public health at crossroads? Have our training and our programs kept up with the times, or have we become passé? Are we sufficiently dynamic, or have we become static? What are the next steps in public health? Questions such as these increasingly have been the keynotes or themes of local, state, and national professional meetings and discussions. Events of the past several years have made increasingly critical the need to find adequate answers to these and related questions.

What is the background against which public health workers should judge themselves and determine the future course of public health? At this point it is insufficient merely to look over one's shoulder at the events of the past 5, 10, or 25 years. Rather, it is necessary to turn full-face about and view the entire past of the human species to obtain a proper perspective.

## A LOOK AT THE PAST

This planet was formed about 3 billion years ago. Based on the discoveries of Louis Leakey in the Olduvai Gorge of Tanzania, it was only about 1 to 2 million years ago that the first creature who might be called man appeared. He was distinguished by his ability to grasp with an opposing thumb and by his development of the power of conceptual thought and means of transmitting the results of his thinking, information, and knowledge to others. Although he possessed these remarkable innovations, man nevertheless progressed extremely slowly and tortuously. For all except a tiny part of his history the conditions of his existence have been decidedly primitive, and, indeed, in major parts of the world today they remain so. This primitive existence consisted of obtaining food, avoiding death from the elements, wild beasts, and other men, reproducing, and attempting to establish an understanding of and relationship with some superhuman force or being. For most of the period man obtained food merely as a predator living off the fruits of the land as they occurred naturally. This, of course, had its limitations.

Eventually, after some hundreds of thousands of years, man made and applied several truly fundamental discoveries, that is, the control of fire, the domestication of animals, and the development of planned agriculture. These three great advances led to further discoveries and made possible all subsequent development of the species. However, they all took time. Thus countless generations passed before man progressed beyond the digging stick, before he smelted metal and made useful tools therefrom, and before he developed even simple methods of food preservation. Only recently and only in certain areas did man reach the point at which he could produce not only enough food for himself and his family but also a surplus with which to support the now specialized fabricators of his tools and clothing. The latter began to concentrate in convenient places, usually determined by proximity to natural means of transport or to natural strongholds. Thus the first urban centers came into being, and with them came new problems, including many of a public health nature. These urban centers with their attendant developing cultures probably first appeared about 3500 B.C. in the Tigris and Euphrates valleys of Mesopotamia and in the Nile valley of Egypt. Similar unique centers developed subsequently in Crete, in the Indus valley, along the lower Yellow River of China, in Central America, and on the coast and Andean highlands of what are now Peru and Bolivia.

The urban centers became increasingly important for several reasons, that is, as trading places, as headquarters for those who governed and the military who supported them, as convenient and desirable living locations for those who in one way or another had gained control over large areas of land and all they contained, as the focal points for the religions that developed, as repositories of acquired knowledge, and eventually as centers of learning and research. Gradually some of these urban civilizations grew, reached their zeniths, then faded due to conquest, plague, or famine. Others grew, spread, and continued their influence in adapted forms in other parts of the world. Remarkable throughout most of this period, however, was the slowness of improvement and the small number of people involved.

At the time the Roman Empire reached its peak in the second century A.D., Italy had a population of only about 14 million, almost 10% of whom resided in Rome. By the time of the Norman Conquest in A.D. 1066 there were only about 1 million people in the British Isles. As recently as the beginning of the eighteenth century the population of the British Isles had grown only to about 7 million persons, almost 10% of whom inhabited the city of London. From about this point on in history, however, great discoveries and events began to occur at an accelerating rate: the discovery, exploration, and colonization of new lands; the use of coal; the discovery of steam power and its application to transportation and industry; advances in medical and related sciences; the belated planting and nurturing of the seeds of social consciousness and democratic self-government. These and other types of revolutions led to a sudden spurt in the size and distribution of the human race, in effect, to a human explosion. As previously pointed out, to appreciate the recency and magnitude of this human explosion it should be realized that whereas during the tremendous period before A.D. 1650 the world population grew to only 450 million, in the mere 300 years since there has been a sevenfold increase to more than 3.6 billion.

Even from this sketchy résumé of man's background it is clear that public health is still a new concept, that man has been exposed to its benefits for only a tiny fraction of his total time span, and that of necessity up to the present the new public health profession has been addressing itself essentially to a vast accumulated backlog of problems and needs and, incidentally, with signal success.

If the eventual goal is the ultimate possible length and quality of human life, considering all of man's past, present, and future, it may be contended that public health through time must consist of three phases, that is, cleanup, repair, and building. It is clear that the public health profession has been devoting its attention so far to the first and to some extent the second of these, and it is hoped that the continuation of this period will be of limited duration. It is the construction phase, the positive building and maintenance of good health, that must endure through the long period of man's future as the goal. This is the goal that henceforth should occupy a major share of the attention and effort of society in general and of public health workers in particular. In other words the public health profession has merely begun, and the best is yet to come.

## OUR EXPLODING ERA

Irvine[1] has observed, "The public health is necessarily a reflection of the times, our culture, our social system, and level of knowledge." To understand the proper place and role of the public health profession in the present and future and to understand the environment in which it must work, let us again examine the world at large. Man is living in the midst of what is undoubtedly the most revolutionary period of his history. Historically it had its origin in the remarkable period of the late eighteenth century, which saw, among other things, the French and American Revolutions and the Industrial Revolution. In a sense this period might be considered to represent the lighting of the fuse, and the present full force of its consequences to represent a series of intimately interrelated explosions, that is, demographic, economic, social and political, cultural, and scientific and technologic. All of these revolutions or explosions bear great significance to the direction that public health must take in the future.

**The demographic revolution**

Because of its complexity and the number of variables involved, an adequate explanation of the current demographic revolution is not easy. Some of the many factors were discussed briefly elsewhere in this book. With specific reference to the United States several recent phenomena of consequence may be noted. The country has never experienced such an increase in marriages, such a reduction in the average age of marriage and parenthood, and such an absolute and relative increase in births as during the 1940s and 1950s. These had a considerable positive effect on the population but were followed during the 1960s by significant changes in social and sexual mores and a decline of the rate of births to about a maintenance level. One effect has been that the prediction of 5 million births by 1970 was actually only 3.7 million. What the long- or even short-term results will be are unknown. The fact is that despite a lowered birthrate, the sheer number of people is increasing. The millions of babies born during the late 1940s and early 1950s became fecund during the 1960s and, human attitudes and events being transient, could well give rise to a spurt of births during the late 1970s.

Added to this is the effect of greater longevity due to the successful application of public health measures, improved nutrition, and similar beneficial factors. At the turn of the century of every 1,000 infants born alive, approximately 200 died within their first year. Now fewer than 18 infants succumb. Notestein[2] emphasized this by pointing out that a white female born in the United States in 1957 had a better chance of living to age 60 years than she had of surviving to her fifth birthday in 1900. The benefits have not been restricted to children. In 1900 more than 25% of children born in the United States faced the prospect of becoming orphans by the time they reached 18 years of age. This grim figure, fraught with so many social implications, has now been reduced to about 5%.

The unforeseen dramatic extension of the length of life is well illustrated by the many correct predictions of the imaginative Jules Verne. In most things time proved him to be amazingly accurate. However, in 1890, when the average length of life was 37 years, he optimistically predicted that 1,000 years later, by the year 2890, the average life-span would reach 58 years! Actually, life expectancy at birth has increased from 47.3 years in 1900 to over 70 years at the present time, with a high of almost 75 years for white females. Undoubtedly this trend will continue for some time, and it is entirely conceivable that by 1980 the average age expectancy of life at birth might be 80 years. As a result, it is reasonably certain that the population will increase 10% to 12% per decade during the next two to three decades. This will bring about a total population in 1980 of about 250 million people.

One result of the foregoing is that whereas in 1900 only 13 million persons, or 18% of the total population, were in the age group over 45 years of age, now the corresponding figures are about 67 million and about 33%. Furthermore, it is estimated that by 1975 almost 50% of the labor force in the United States will be over 40 years of age. Similar shifts are occurring at the other end of the scale. Thus it is estimated that within a decade, whereas 10% of the population of the United States will be over 65 years of age, about 50% will be under 25 years of age. In brief, then, the current population boom is characterized by considerable increases at both ends of the life-span. Incidentally, these are the periods of life that ordinarily demand the greatest amount of medical and public health attention.

**The economic revolution**

There are many characteristics of the current economic revolution that do and will affect the nature of public health problems and programs. There is a distinct and rapid trend toward economic equality among people. In the United States, for example, this is evidenced by continued broadening of the Social Security coverage, the development of the concept of the guaranteed annual wage not only for industrial workers but even for everyone, the increased purchase of insurance and retirement policies, and the ever-widening corporate ownership. As a result, the standard of living has reached very high levels, with a strong trend to equalization among all groups and classes of the population.

**The social and political revolution**

The effects of the rapidly expanding economy are closely linked with the recent striking social and political changes. It is interesting that in introducing a colloquium on *Governing Urban*

*Society,* James E. Webb,[3] former Administrator of the National Aeronautics and Space Administration, predicted the following:

There is a strong possibility that this century will be noted neither for its technology nor for its science. For today there is a growing conviction among people and among nations that it may now be possible to eliminate human suffering and human misery—that it may now be possible to build a world society which offers human dignity and the opportunity for self realization to all. Despite the enormity of such an undertaking, it is significant that the question is no longer whether such a goal *should* be met; nor is the question now whether such a goal *can* be met. The questions perplexing us today are those of *how* the goal can be achieved and *how long* will be required. . . . Perhaps this alone is enough to distinguish the twentieth century far more profoundly than could achievements in science and technology.

As applied specifically to the United States at this time, one can point to the overriding concerns for an all-out drive to eliminate all remaining pockets of poverty, the provision of equal opportunity, and the guarantee of complete civil rights to everyone.

Increased labor has not been the price of the rapid improvements in the standard of living. Quite the contrary, the annual days of work required, if anything, are becoming fewer, and work itself is becoming physically easier. With the increasing use of electronics and automation and the beginning availability of atomic power, even greater changes may be expected. These changes apply to farming as well as to industry, as evidenced by the fact that whereas 50 years ago the United States required 13 million farmers for a population of 106 million, now only 7 million farmers are needed for a population of 200 million. It is anticipated by the Secretary of Agriculture that in the year 2000, with a population of over 300 million, only about 2 million farmers will be necessary.[4]

A work week of as few as 3 or 4 days is not impossible to anticipate. The implications of more time for cultural and recreational pursuits, on the one hand, and of additional behavioral and mental health problems, on the other hand, should not be overlooked. Expanded use of automation will mean less tedium, less job fatigue, and fewer opportunities for industrial accidents and illness. It should be noted that the number of women in the labor force has increased to about 30% of the total. Significant also is the change in the types of women's occupations, from domestic, farm, and semiskilled labor to clerical, semiskilled, skilled,

and professional activities. Possible consequences may be an increase in the number of women involved in industrial and vehicular accidents and in the number who have physical and mental disabilities attributable to chronic tensions.

Of great social significance is the strong trend toward urbanization and metropolitanization. In the past 50 years the urban population has increased from one half to about three fourths of the total population of the United States, with only 15% now left on farms. Even so, the 15% living on farms produce surpluses of many food products. The last two decades have seen the appearance around every city of large numbers of relatively self-sufficient suburban developments of moderately to highly priced homes or apartment dwellings, usually centered around self-contained decentralized shopping and recreational centers. It would appear that these are destined to become the social, economic, and political units of the future and should represent important points of impact for public health education and the programs it promotes.

The combination of expressways, industrial decentralization, suburbanization, and metropolitanization has led to the appearance of two new phenomena: the town that appears almost overnight around a single decentralized industrial park, and the so-called "strip city," which results from the coalescence of several cities or metropolises and their merged suburbia. A dramatic example is the strip that extends almost unbroken from north of Boston to Richmond, Va. A number of others are in various stages of formation in other parts of the country. These phenomena bring with them many new and challenging problems in public health, sanitary engineering, and the provision of medical and hospital care. Prominent among these problems is the "central rot" of the older cities and the concentration in them of socially and economically underprivileged groups—the elderly, the chronically ill, the undereducated, the poor, and the various emergent groups. In addition are the needs for urban redevelopment, problems of stream and air pollution, the development of suburban slums, and the search for an adequate source of revenue to finance local services.

One other characteristic of the present social change is the remarkable mobility of the American and European. With work car pools, frequent changes in employment, business

716 THE FUTURE OF PUBLIC HEALTH

trips, and vacations, a viewer from the higher atmosphere would obtain an impression of Brownian movement. The extent of the movement may be realized by the fact that about one fifth of the population of the United States changes residence each year. The shallow social roots that result have far-reaching implications with regard to family stability and cohesiveness, the patient-physician relationship, and the epidemiologic factors of susceptible-immune ratios and exposure. In addition to the millions of travelers within the country, more than 1 million United States citizens travel abroad each year, and millions more cross the borders into Mexico and Cánada. In the process of visiting all parts of the world, United States tourists spent approximately $2 billion each year. The injection of this amount of money into other national economies must have some ultimate beneficial effect on their standards of living, including health services, but also with the risk of inflation.

## The cultural revolution

John W. Gardner,[5] former Secretary of Health, Education, and Welfare, in opening The White House Conference on Health in 1965, observed, "Health frees the individual to live up to his potential." Hints of the significant cultural changes to come are many. Already there is ever-increasing attention given to education, both quantitatively and qualitatively. This is as true for adults as it is for children. But it must be meaningful education. There is more time for leisure, social interests, family activities, and intelligent consideration of current social and political issues, including those related to personal and community health, and the needs for and possible methods of providing adequate medical and hospital care for all. The combination of rising labor costs and of more free time has brought about a considerable interest in hobbies and do-it-yourself activities; these activities are good for mental health, on the one hand, but risky in terms of increased chances for home accidents, on the other hand. With the lowered age at marriage, parents may really be young with their children, and the trend toward disintegration of family ties may stop and be reversed. These factors cannot help but contribute to improved family relationships and improved mental health. Furthermore, with a change for the better in the status of women, younger mothers with better education, more leisure, and a somewhat more sophisticated outlook will, of course, have an effect on the birthrate, family size, child health, maternal health, and insistence on adequate medical and institutional care. This is part of the phenomenon to which several have called attention: the shift from the era of the dominant father to the era of the dominant mother, and especially of the dominant child.

## The scientific and technologic revolution

In the crucible in which the scientific and technologic revolution is occurring, many wonders that bid well for the future may be found. The British scientist Bronowski[6] foresees three outstanding scientific changes that will dominate the next 50 years: (1) change in the source and use of energy, that is, nuclear fission, (2) change in the control of energy, that is, automation, and (3) results of the biologic revolution. The amazing advances in the medical and surgical fields are common popular knowledge and undoubtedly will become increasingly popular news items. One thing is clear—people want to know about anything that will make them well and keep them that way.

New techniques, instruments, drugs, and antibiotics are appearing with a dizzy rapidity that makes it literally impossible to remain adequately informed. There appears to be no limit in this field, and the future is certain to bring forth products more remarkable than those already developed. It has been estimated that the rate of major medical developments has been about one per century before 1900, about one per decade between 1900 and 1940, and one or more per year since 1940. New pharmaceuticals are being developed, tested, and mass-produced on a calculated investigative production-line basis. This is reflected in a survey which disclosed that 90% of the prescriptions now written in the United States are for medications and prophylactic products that did not even exist 10 years ago. Oral agents for immunization against several infections are now being tried with apparently good results, and the ultimate development of a universal antigen is not beyond the realm of possibility. Significant pharmaceutical cracks have been made in the walls of certain cardiovascular diseases. Viable, infectious, and reproducing DNA has been synthesized. Organ transplants, even of the human heart, have been achieved, only to be followed by synthetic substitutes.

During the past two decades, the death rate from stroke among American males aged 45 through 64 years dropped from 128 to 87 per 100,000, whereas the death rate from hypertension in the same group declined from 93 to 40 per 100,000. The amount of decline was even greater among females. Because of the dramatic pharmaceutical and surgical advances, numerous scientists are already sufficiently optimistic to anticipate the relegation of deaths from heart disease to a secondary role by the end of the twentieth century. Similar great advances are being made with reference to several metabolic diseases, especially arthritis, and certain mental illnesses. Another advance of considerable significance is the recent appearance of an effective and safe oral contraceptive based on progestational steroids. As an additional example, it is probable that eventually a chemical or hormonal means of significantly delaying menopause will be developed. Meanwhile there are already in wide use oral hormonal substances that minimize menopausal distress. The social, moral, medical, economic, and demographic effects of such discoveries are far reaching.

An area of important technical advance is in the construction industry. New materials and methods of construction of dwellings are being tried on large scales. It may be expected that out of these efforts will come more satisfactory and more sanitary low-cost and medium-cost housing, which will help to eradicate one of the contributing causes of physical and mental ill health and juvenile and adult delinquency. At the same time it may be anticipated that increased activities in the fields of community planning and traffic engineering will result in fewer vehicular accidents.

Of all technical advances, those relating to the use of nuclear energy of course overwhelm everything else. All health workers are increasingly aware of and concerned about the problems it will bring as well as its blessings. On the one hand, public health workers view hopefully its application to the treatment of malignancies, to portable x-ray equipment, to food preservation, to sewage treatment, and many other things. On the other hand, public health workers must view with concern the problems of civil defense, disposal of radioactive industrial wastes, and the like. The potentials of the peaceful application of nuclear energy are so great, however, as to contraindicate anything but a hopeful, optimistic viewpoint of the future.

General David Sarnoff, speaking as Chairman of the Board of the Radio Corporation of America, made the challenging comment: "Our atomic age is like a knife; in the hands of a surgeon it can save a life; in the hands of an assassin it can take one. But to blame the knife is ridiculous."

## COURSE OF ACTION

In the light of man's past history and of all of these momentous current events, what must be the course of action in the field of public health? Reference was made previously to the three phases—cleanup, repair, and building—that public health must consist of through time. It would seem logical that their counterparts during this present period of public health history should be (1) consolidation of past successes, (2) remediation of the backlog of disabilities, and (3) a truly vigorous, carefully planned attack on both new problems and unsolved old problems.

### Consolidation of past successes

Consolidation of past successes really consists of unfinished business. There is a tremendous amount yet to be accomplished in the areas for which the public health profession now has adequate tools and knowledge for rather complete success. Consider the area of health statistics. The gathering and processing of relevant data form an essential part of the approach whereby the problems that confront public health workers are studied, understood, and attacked. Excellent and current data are available on the circumstances surrounding births and deaths in the United States. But the public health profession still falls far short of the more important goal of satisfactory morbidity data, that is, the incidence and distribution through time and space of illness, the types of illnesses, susceptibility to illness, and many other analyses. There is a serious need, particularly at this time, to extend the use of proved procedures such as sampling techniques and the full collation of available data. The National Health Survey has provided much leadership in this field. Beyond this, public health agencies, the medical profession, hospitals and clinics, insurance companies, business and industry, and various social agencies must soon work out a much more adequate means of standardizing and pooling their respective data concerning illness. Similarly more extensive use must be made of longitudinal studies of health and disease. In addition there are certain customary categories such as cardiovascular disease and cancer that should be broken down to pinpoint and expedite future attack on their components. What is greatly needed, of course, is a comprehensive community, state, and national epidemiologic intelligence and surveillance system that would constantly keep score and point up the problems as they are developing.

There is still a vast amount of unfinished business in the control of diseases against which the public health profession already has effective tools. It is entirely reasonable to visualize that during the next 20 to 25 years tuberculosis, the venereal diseases, poliomyelitis, brucellosis, meningococcic meningitis, tetanus, rabies, trichinosis, and several other diseases might for all practical purposes be eradicated in this country and even in the world. Tuberculosis and syphilis still account for about 4,500 deaths per year in the United States. Certainly these deaths are needless in view of the expanding economy, existing knowledge, the increased availability of hospital beds, isoniazids, PAS, and the everbroadening spectrum of antibiotics.

Eradication is admittedly a strong word; but 30 years ago how many people would have believed that by now deaths from typhoid fever, small pox, malaria, typhus fever, diphtheria, scarlet fever, pertussis, measles, and several other previously important diseases would no longer occur to any practical extent in the United States? Yet today these triumphs are realities. On the international level the nations of the world are working with the World Health Organization toward the goal of worldwide eradication of smallpox and malaria. In fact, the complete demise of smallpox is expected by 1976.

There are still many other diseases that, although not yet eradicable, can be depressed to a fraction of their present level. Among these are pneumonia, influenza, dysenteries, diabetes, appendicitis, and many maternal and infant deaths. Not including the approximately 57,000 infant deaths, these conditions alone result in the loss of almost 100,000 lives each year. A nonfatal but important pathologic condition that can be expected to decrease substantially is dental caries.

In the area of environmental health much remains to be done, not merely with old problems but especially with the burgeoning manmade environmental hazards. As pointed out elsewhere, there are still many small communities with populations totaling 2 to 3 million that have no public water systems. A large proportion of existing systems need improve-

ment or expansion. With reference to sewerage systems the situation is as bad or worse. Sprawling suburbs are compounding both of these problems. There is a great need to discover and develop more adequate solutions to the environmental health problems of these areas. The political scientist will probably contribute to this as significantly as the sanitation scientist.

Disease outbreaks traceable to food, milk, or water, although fewer each year, still occur to a significant extent. Workers in the field of environmental health still have before them the application or provision of customary sanitary services and safeguards to the great number of new suburban communities, the extension of occupational health and safety to the large number of smaller plants, and the challenge of the rapid economic and industrial development of the South and West.

A great social challenge still facing public health workers and others is the complete equalization of opportunities for health among the races. Thus the infant mortality for white babies in 1970 was 17.4 per 1,000 live births, in comparison with 31.4 per 1,000 live births of black babies. With reference to life expectancy at birth, in 1970 for white males it was 67.5 years, in contrast to 60.1 years for nonwhite males. For females the comparison is 74.9 years for white females to 67.5 years for nonwhite females. Obviously these discrepancies can no longer be tolerated in an affluent civilized society. The relationship of poverty to illness, disability, and malnutrition is now accepted. With greater equalization of educational and employment opportunities, wealth, foods, and goods, and the ever-rising standard of living, the differences in health potential should become much less. To accomplish this, however, the development of a more effective working interrelationship among agencies in related fields will be necessary as well as the development of new and more effective methods of providing comprehensive health services on a neighborhood basis.

For several years investigators have discussed and promoted the concept of complete coverage of the nation with adequate local health services. Yet many significant areas remain unserved or are served by too few professional workers. More is involved than the mere quantitative filling-in of a geographic jigsaw puzzle. Quality of personnel and comprehensiveness of programs are involved too, with adequate backup by suitable hospital, convalescent, and rehabilitative services. In addition, there is the necessity of further practical administrative decentralization of local health services to serve more adequately the multiplying and growing neighborhood and suburban housing developments, possibly through their shopping centers, and with appropriate participation by those who are to be served.

Perhaps the most important area for consolidation, and one that affects most of the others, is assurance of the availability of adequate medical and hospital services for all of the population. The development of this has been extremely difficult because of many complex economic problems and traditional political and professional philosophies. Actually, much progress has been made in recent years, especially by means of voluntary group medical and hospital insurance, now augmented by Titles V, XVIII, and XIX of the Social Security Amendments of 1965 and 1972. Each recent year has seemed to be one of final fulfillment, but the nation still waits while political adversaries, special interests, and even some professionals maneuver for advantage. Meanwhile arrangements for handling emergencies are almost chaotic. In all of this it is hoped that the public health profession will play a significant role as a catalyzer, a coordinator, and possibly as an administrative agent for all interested parties. Whereas the basic problem at the moment is to provide a way to lighten the burden caused by catastrophic illness or injury, it must also be considered in the light of the eventual development of an all-inclusive medical, hospital, nursing, and social service with strong if not major emphasis on positive health promotion, early diagnosis, and prevention of disease.

To meet the foregoing needs certain personnel problems must be solved. The public health profession must develop more successful methods of recruitment into all of the health fields. A more aggressive and carefully planned approach to high school and college students must be pursued. But before attempting to interest students in the field of public health, the profession must define its future goals and must be sure of what it is trying to accomplish and in what it is trying to interest them. Needless to emphasize, more equitable salaries and benefits must be secured for public health workers, competitive with those in the private sector. Beyond this, however, is the necessity to work out some equitable means of transfer of accumulated benefits, such as retirement and pension rights, from one location to another when public health workers change their locus of employment. One of the greatest personnel needs is a national career service of which public health workers could all be members, regardless of the location or agency of their work. Public health work by its very nature is often an itinerant profession that requires frequent change of employment and residence. The obvious economic disadvantages of this should be eliminated. This is common in education and in private enterprise—why not in public health?

Over a relatively short interval of history there has been a development of numerous splendid training centers related to the health sciences: schools of medicine, nursing, engineering, and public health. They have developed high standards and practical methods of teaching and have contributed greatly to the world's knowledge through their research. Nevertheless it would seem imperative that their goals, curricula, and facilities be reviewed particularly carefully and continuously at this time in relation to the revolutionary changes that are occurring with such rapidity and are shaping the future. It is probable that a rather considerable retooling job is needed in all quarters. Certainly the time has come for health workers in all fields to have a much better background than heretofore in sociology, social pathology, behavioral science, community analysis and dynamics, and political science. Medical schools and schools of public health must place more stress on subjects such as the medical and health problems that arise from exposure to fissionable material, accident prevention, mental health, chronic disease control, physical medicine and rehabilitation, and especially geriatrics and preventive and promotive medicine. The health department of tomorrow will obviously have to include geriatricians, as yesterday it included the services of pediatricians.

A final personnel problem is the inability to supply and pay for a qualified staff of sufficient size to meet the needs and demands of the citizenry. This is especially true on the local level. As a result, the public health profession must be willing to explore possible satisfactory compromises that will provide more efficient service to more people. The potentials of joint employment with other health agencies and with agencies in related fields should be explored further. The public health agency must experiment with the use of auxiliary personnel such as physician-assistants, nurse-associates, nonmedical administrators, epidemiologic field investigators, nurses' aides, and neighborhood health workers recruited from the neighborhoods in which they serve. More satisfactory and effective relationships and division of responsibilities must be worked out between sanitary engineers and sanitarians and between public health nurses, social workers, and health educators. It may be useful to consider blends of public health nurses, social workers, health educators, and other personnel. Possibly it may be worth while to develop some entirely new categories of personnel that will more adequately meet the new challenges that are on the horizon.

### Remediation of the backlog of disabilities

What sometimes has been referred to as the fourth phase of medicine forms the second part of public health's present and future concern—the remediation of the great backlog of disabilities to the point where the certain amount of inevitable current disabilities may be handled with relative ease and economic efficiency. Two aspects of this are important to realize at this time, that is, the size of the backlog and its economic significance. With regard to extent it has been estimated that there has accumulated in the United States at the present about 2.5 million persons with orthopedic impairments, about the same number with unremedied hearing defects, and about 250,000 blind individuals. Furthermore, about 250,000 disabilities due to accidents, illness, or congenital defects are added each year.

Experience has established the fact that a great many of all types of handicapped persons are capable of making real and significant social and economic contributions if given an opportunity to readjust to the demands of working and living situations. In every community there are disabled persons in need of assistance, but how many public health agencies have really addressed themselves to this challenge? The public health agency obviously cannot be expected to do the whole job, but it can serve as the catalyzer in the first instance for the establishment of a sound program, as a rallying point for all public and private agencies involved. Beyond that it may provide certain specific activities in the field of physical and mental rehabilitation. It may also make known to the public and to special groups the needs,

methods, and opportunities for prevention and rehabilitation of disabilities. It is impossible, of course, to predict, but the incidence of disabilities may not necessarily continue at its present level. Progress in control of tuberculosis, immunization against poliomyelitis, prevention of a few of the congenital malformations, potential advances in the prevention of accidents or better management of their consequences, and prevention of cardiovascular diseases and mental illness may result in a smaller annual addition to the number of disabilities.

### Attack on new and unsolved old problems

There are so many new areas left for aggressive pioneering attack that it is difficult to know where to begin. All of these are problems to which various persons, groups, or agencies have addressed themselves to some extent. It must be admitted, however, that in many respects public health efforts have been partial, poorly planned, and uncoordinated. Of one thing the public health profession can be sure—the abatement and if possible the control of the so-called chronic noncommunicable diseases will be one of its major concerns for a long time into the future. With regard to these conditions the importance of early diagnosis of predisposition or actual illness has logically been stressed. In this connection periodic physical or so-called health examinations have been discussed and promoted for many years. Yet it must be admitted that the reception of the idea both by the public and unfortunately by many of the medical profession has been disappointingly poor. There are several reasons for this, each representing a challenge. There is the matter of economics. The physician is entitled to a fee for his professional service, but many people are either insufficiently sophisticated to seek out or economically unable to afford medical attention in the absence of a frank illness or disability.

A serious deterrent is general medical disinterest in the periodic physical examination. One has only to canvass several conscientious enlightened citizens who have sought to obtain this sort of medical service to learn of their all too common disillusionment. Too often the physician is so preoccupied and overloaded with patients who have frank ills and injuries that he essentially pats the apparently well patient on the back, tells him he appears healthy, and sends him on his way. In addition, as mentioned previously, the fact that health insurance plans still pay only for care of illness or injury but not for preventive or health promotive services acts as a powerful economic and psychologic deterrent. There are also the factors of misguided modesty or fear, which delay many people from seeking periodic physical examinations until the development of definite signs or symptoms drives them to it. All of these deterrents represent real challenges for the medical profession, medical educators, medical economists, public health administrators, public health educators, and behavioral scientists.

Let us pass on to some of the chronic noncommunicable diseases that are now of such high incidence and consider briefly some of the prospects for the future. The total picture, although at the moment somewhat overwhelming, is not necessarily entirely dark. Recognition must be given to the remarkable advances that have been made in only recent years in the better understanding of the physical chemistry and physicopathology of many of these diseases and to the progress in the fields of biochemistry, pharmacology, and chemical and industrial antibiotic production. Consider cardiovascular disease, the current captain of the causes of death. It accounts for 50% of the total death toll in the United States. Actually it is a complex of different conditions, that is, congenital heart disease, rheumatic heart disease, arteriosclerotic heart disease, hypertensive heart disease, cardiac syphilis, thyroid heart disease, and various other organic and functional cardiac conditions. Some of these are potentially eradicable, whereas the incidence and seriousness of others may be reduced.

Eradication of heart disease from rheumatic fever, syphilis, and thyroid dysfunction is well within the realm of possibility. Some reduction in congenital heart disease may be expected from the assurance of rubella and other viral infections in women before marriage and pregnancy. Discovery of the significance of familial tendency, obesity, and personality also have done much to point to ways of prevention or abatement of hypertension. More recently the discovery of the dramatic effects of tranquilizers, and other drugs on hypertension, with few adverse effects, opens a whole new vista for optimism. Recent advances provide a possible means of prevention of atherosclerosis. There are indications that this condition may be delayed or its effects kept to a minimum by lipotropic factors such as choline and inositol, which reduce high blood cholesterol levels. It may be possible to prevent or control the disease by a diet low in cholesterol.

The practical potentials in this field are illustrated by recent analyses, which indicate that during the decade that ended in 1965 death rates from heart disease declined by 5%; from hypertension, 46%; from stroke, 20%; and from rheumatic heart disease, 33%. Although coronary heart disease death rates rose 11%, they have since fallen by 2%. The recently accentuated national focus on cancer and hypertension should accelerate the decline in incidence of these current major killers.

In all of these and related situations there are many possible points of action for public health agencies, that is, administrative organization, promotion, and possibly management of positive health maintenance by means of periodic health examinations; use of chest x-ray examinations for screening of certain cardiac defects and tuberculosis; generalized and individualized nutrition education, especially with regard to obesity; adequate provision of protective factors, and in some instances low-cholesterol diets; activities in the field of mental health especially as it relates to personality factors; and general health education. Two important and encouraging points should be borne in mind with regard to cardiovascular diseases: (1) the inevitable beneficial effect of the recent considerable and widespread improvement in the standard of living, including nutrition; and (2) the fact that sulfonamides, penicillin, and the host of other antibiotics have been used for only about 35 years. There is reason to expect that mankind has not yet even begun to reap some of the long-term delayed-action benefits of these and other factors and that their effects will show up partly in future lowered incidence of some of the cardiovascular diseases.

Cancer represents perhaps the most difficult disease problem for the present and for the future. There seems to be no question of a real increase. Some reasons for encouragement do exist, however. Detection at earlier stages of cancerous lesions not readily accessible is becoming more common through the wider use of radioactive tracers and the Papanicolaou technique of cytologic examination. The health officer might well devote attention to the physical and economic availability of these procedures to all who might benefit from them. Considerable progress is being made also in treatment with radioactive isotopes, improved deep x-ray equipment, and improved surgical techniques. The large sums of money now going into research on the causes, prevention, and treatment of cancer also give reason for a substantial degree of optimism.

Meanwhile public health personnel may participate further not only through increased general public education but also by extending control over certain environmental factors, urging and arranging for periodic physical and laboratory examinations and encouraging continued and extended good obstetric and gynecologic practice. Most specifically, all health workers have a great responsibility to work toward the reduction and elimination of cigarette smoking, which has been shown so conclusively to be involved in cancer of the lung and larynx as well as emphysema and coronary heart disease.

About 275,000 people who suffer from mental disorders now occupy about one half of the hospital beds in the United States. There is some question whether there is a real or an apparent increase in mental disorders. The public is much more aware of the problem than ever before and is now willing to discuss it in other than hushed terms. As a result, many more people are seeking treatment than previously. Also more conditions are being recognized as mental aberrations. The shortages of hospital beds, psychiatrists, and psychiatric social workers and the inadequate psychiatric training among public health personnel are serious problems. On the other hand, in addition to improved fever and shock therapy the door to a new approach has been opened by the discovery of some remarkably effective drugs such as tranquilizers. With pharmacologic limitation of some of the changes usually associated with the climacteric a decrease in involutional melancholia and senile psychosis should be expected.

On the other hand, the American society is becoming ever more stressful. Aggression, suicide, addictions, alcoholism, and other forms of escape or "compensation" are increasingly indulged in. Usually they are ignored or condemned by the public and the professions alike. Here is a significant field related to sociology, psychiatry, mental health, and community education that public health workers with few exceptions have completely ignored. Local health departments, in addition to public education, should provide or arrange for around-the-clock guidance services for despondent individuals, somewhat similar to the activities of Alcoholics Anonymous. Such a program should use the collaborative help of religious, medical,

and other groups in the community. Related to this is the potential contribution that public health workers might make to the solution of the problem of juvenile delinquency and other manifestations of the disease-delinquency-dependency syndrome that have been presented.

Finally, to touch briefly on a completely different area, environmental health requires vigorous action. Consider the relatively meager and ineffective manner in which public health workers individually and collectively have addressed themselves to the public health aspects of the control of water and air pollution, the disposal of radioactive wastes, the prevention of home accidents, and the improvement of housing and neighborhoods. Some may complain that "lead action and responsibility" in these fields have been removed from public health in many jurisdictions. That may be true organizationally, but the field of public health can never remove itself from concern about the effects of these hazards on human health. These are "musts" and will continue to be so into the future.

## CONCLUSION

Challenges? No end of them. Shortly before his death the great inventor and industrialist Charles F. Kettering said, "The achievements of the past 50 years will be dwarfed by the things to come if we just keep our minds open and willingly contribute each day an honest day's work." This is well complemented by a statement by General David Sarnoff, "We may be a privileged generation who, by taming our fears, our hungers, our terrible weapons, are asked to pay the price of the transition to a golden hour."

As participants in one of the most successful and significant endeavors in history, each public health worker must keep his mind open and contribute a share of thoughtful imagination to the solution of the fascinating challenges of the future, and in so doing remember that intelligent mankind is still very young and that the future will last a long, long time.

## REFERENCES

1. Irvine, E. D.: Public health: what of the future? Roy. Soc. Health J. **2:**106, 1962.
2. Notestein, F. W.: As the nation grows younger, The Atlantic **200:**131, Oct. 1957.
3. Webb, J. E.: Governing urban society: new scientific approaches, Philadelphia, 1967, American Academy of Political and Social Science.
4. Freeman, O. L.: Agriculture/2000, Address pre-

sented to the National Science Teacher's Association, Detroit, March 20, 1967 (mimeographed).

5. Gardner, J. W.: A great move forward. Address presented at the White House Conference on Health, Washington, D. C., Nov. 3, 1965 (mimeographed).

6. Bronowski, J.: The shape of the future, Roy. Soc. Health J. **3:**127, 1962.

# Index